INSTRUCTOR'S GUIDE
to Accompany

Second Edition

PHARMACOTHERAPY
Casebook

a patient-focused approach

INSTRUCTOR'S GUIDE
to Accompany

Second Edition

PHARMACOTHERAPY
Casebook

a patient-focused approach

Edited by
Terry L. Schwinghammer, PharmD, FCCP, FASHP, BCPS
Associate Professor, Department of Pharmaceutical Sciences
School of Pharmacy, University of Pittsburgh
Pittsburgh, Pennsylvania

with

Joseph T. DiPiro, PharmD, FCCP
Panoz Professor, College of Pharmacy, Head, Department of Clinical
and Administrative Sciences
University of Georgia College of Pharmacy
Clinical Professor of Surgery, Medical College of Georgia
Augusta, Georgia

Robert L. Talbert, PharmD, FCCP, BCPS
Professor and Division Head, College of Pharmacy
University of Texas at Austin
Professor, Departments of Medicine and Pharmacology
University of Texas Health Science Center at San Antonio
San Antonio, Texas

Gary C. Yee, PharmD, FCCP
Professor and Chair, Department of Pharmacy Practice,
College of Pharmacy,
University of Nebraska Medical Center
Omaha, Nebraska

Gary R. Matzke, PharmD, FCP, FCCP
Professor of Pharmaceutical Sciences and Medicine
Schools of Pharmacy and Medicine
Center for Clinical Pharmacology,
University of Pittsburgh
Pittsburgh, Pennsylvania

Barbara G. Wells, PharmD, FASHP, FCCP, BCPP
Professor and Dean, Idaho State University College of Pharmacy
Pocatello, Idaho

L. Michael Posey, RPh
President
Pharmacy Editorial and News Services
Athens, Georgia

APPLETON & LANGE
Stamford, Connecticut

Notice: The authors and the publisher of this volume have taken care to make certain that the doses of drugs and schedules of treatment are correct and compatible with the standards generally accepted at the time of publication. Nevertheless, as new information becomes available, changes in treatment and in the use of drugs become necessary. The reader is advised to carefully consult the instruction and information material included in the package insert of each drug or therapeutic agent before administration. This advice is especially important when using, administering, or recommending new or infrequently used drugs. The authors and publisher disclaim all responsibility for any liability, loss, injury, or damage incurred as a consequence, directly or indirectly, of the use and application of any of the contents of this volume.

Copyright © 2000 by Appleton & Lange
Copyright © 1997 by Appleton & Lange

All rights reserved. This book, or any parts thereof, may not be used or reproduced in any manner without written permission. For information, address Appleton & Lange, Four Stamford Plaza, PO Box 120041, Stamford, Connecticut 06912-0041.

www.appletonlange.com

99 00 01 02 / 10 9 8 7 6 5 4 3 2 1

Executive Editor: Cheryl L. Mehalik
Development Editor: Kathleen McCullough
Senior Production Editor: Jeanmarie Roche
Art Manager: Eve Siegel
Production Service: Rainbow Graphics, LLC
Designer: Mary Skudlarek

PRINTED IN THE UNITED STATES OF AMERICA

Contributors

Marie A. Abate, PharmD, Professor and Associate Chair of Clinical Pharmacy; Director of the West Virginia Drug Information Center, West Virginia University School of Pharmacy, Morgantown, West Virginia

Cesar Alaniz, PharmD, Clinical Assistant Professor, University of Michigan College of Pharmacy; Clinical Pharmacist, University of Michigan Hospitals, Ann Arbor, Michigan

Peter L. Anderson, PharmD, Fellow in Antiviral Pharmacology, Department of Clinical Pharmacology, College of Pharmacy, University of Minnesota, Minneapolis, Minnesota

Edward P. Armstrong, PharmD, BCPS, FASHP, Associate Professor, Department of Pharmacy Practice and Science, University of Arizona College of Pharmacy, Tucson, Arizona

Tana R. Bagby, PharmD, Adjunct Assistant Clinical Professor, Department of Pharmacy Practice, University of Georgia College of Pharmacy, Athens, Georgia

Laura A. Bartels, PharmD, Assistant Professor of Pharmacy, Department of Pharmacy Practice, Albany College of Pharmacy, Union University, Albany, New York

Leslie L. Barton, MD, Professor of Pediatrics and Pediatric Infectious Diseases; Director, Pediatric Residency Program, Department of Pediatrics, University of Arizona School of Medicine, Tucson, Arizona

Susan D. Bear, BS, PharmD, Clinical Specialist, Department of Pharmacy, University Hospital, Charlotte, North Carolina

Karen Beauchamp, BPharm, RPh, Pharmacy Practice Resident, Southwest Washington Medical Center, Vancouver, Washington

Amy J. Becker, PharmD, Hematology-Oncology Clinical Pharmacy Specialist, University of Iowa Hospitals & Clinics, Iowa City, Iowa

Reina Bendayan, PharmD, Assistant Professor, Faculty of Pharmacy, University of Toronto, Toronto, Ontario, Canada

William H. Benefield, Jr., PharmD, BCPP, FASCP, Clinical Assistant Professor of Pharmacy, University of Texas at Austin; Clinical Assistant Professor of Pharmacology, University of Texas Health Sciences Center at San Antonio; Clinical Pharmacologist, San Antonio State School, San Antonio, Texas

Brian K. Bond, PharmD, was Doctor of Pharmacy Candidate, West Virginia University School of Pharmacy, Morgantown, West Virginia at the time of this writing

Karim A. Calis, PharmD, MPH, BCPS, BCNSP, FASHP, Coordinator, Drug Information Service and Endocrinology Clinical Pharmacy Specialist, Warren G. Magnuson Clinical Center, National Institutes of Health, Bethesda, Maryland; Associate Clinical Professor, Medical College of Virginia, Virginia Commonwealth University, Richmond, Virginia; Clinical Associate Professor, University of Maryland, Baltimore, Maryland

Bruce R. Canaday, PharmD, BCPS, FASHP, FAPhA, Clinical Professor, University of North Carolina Schools of Pharmacy and Medicine; Pharmacotherapy Director, Coastal Area Health Education Center, Wilmington, North Carolina

Bruce C. Carlstedt, PhD, Professor, Department of Pharmacy Practice, Purdue University School of Pharmacy and Pharmacal Sciences, West Lafayette, Indiana

Daniel T. Casto, PharmD, FCCP, was Associate Professor, College of Pharmacy, University of Texas at Austin and Department of Pediatrics and Pharmacology, University of Texas Health Science Center, San Antonio, Texas at the time of this writing

Marie A. Chisholm, PharmD, Assistant Professor, Department of Pharmacy Practice, University of Georgia College of Pharmacy, Athens, Georgia

Susan Chuck, PharmD, Infectious Diseases Fellow, Department of Pharmacy Practice, University of Illinois at Chicago College of Pharmacy, Chicago, Illinois

Lawrence J. Cohen, PharmD, BCPP, FASHP, FCCP, Professor of Pharmacy, Psychiatry, and Behavioral Sciences, University of Oklahoma Health Sciences Center, Oklahoma City, Oklahoma

Julie A. Cold, PharmD, BCPP, Assistant Professor, Department of Pharmacy Practice, Mercer University Southern School of Pharmacy, Atlanta, Georgia

James D. Coyle, PharmD, Assistant Professor, Department of Pharmacy Practice and Administration, Ohio State University College of Pharmacy, Columbus, Ohio

Brian L. Crabtree, PharmD, BCPP, Associate Professor of Clinical Pharmacy Practice, Department of Clinical Pharmacy Practice, University of Mississippi School of Pharmacy, Jackson, Mississippi

Simon Cronin, PharmD, MS, Clinical Assistant Professor, University of Michigan School of Pharmacy, Ann Arbor, Michigan

Contributors

Terri G. Davidson, PharmD, Chief Executive Officer, Clinical Pharmacy Associates, Inc.; Senior Medical Writer, Cortex Communications, Inc., Tucker, Georgia

Andrea Eggert, PharmD, BCPP, Was Clinical Assistant Professor of Pharmacy, Department of Pharmacy Practice and Administration, University of Texas at Austin at the time of this writing

Victor A. Elsberry, PharmD, BCNSP, Assistant Professor, Department of Pharmacy Practice and Science, University of Arizona College of Pharmacy, Tucson, Arizona

Brian L. Erstad, PharmD, FASHP, FCCM, Associate Professor, Department of Pharmacy Practice and Science, University of Arizona College of Pharmacy, Tucson, Arizona

Charles W. Fetrow, PharmD, Clinical Pharmacist, Department of Pharmacy Services, St. Francis Medical Center, Pittsburgh, Pennsylvania

John O. Fleming, MD, Associate Professor, Department of Neurology, University of Wisconsin, Madison, Wisconsin

Courtney V. Fletcher, PharmD, Professor, Department of Clinical Pharmacology, College of Pharmacy, University of Minnesota, Minneapolis, Minnesota

Rex W. Force, PharmD, BCPS, Assistant Professor, Departments of Pharmacy Practice and Family Medicine, Idaho State University, Pocatello, Idaho

Carla B. Frye, PharmD, BCPS, Associate Professor, Department of Pharmacy Practice, Butler University College of Pharmacy and Health Sciences, Indianapolis, Indiana

Ashesh J. Gandhi, PharmD, Clinical Cardiology Specialist, Department of Pharmacy, Allegheny University Hospitals—Hahnemann, Philadelphia, Pennsylvania

Marie E. Gardner, PharmD, Clinical Associate Professor, Department of Pharmacy Practice and Science, University of Arizona College of Pharmacy, Tucson, Arizona

Barry E. Gidal, PharmD, Associate Professor, School of Pharmacy and Department of Neurology, University of Wisconsin, Madison, Wisconsin

Patrick P. Gleason, PharmD, BCPS, Assistant Professor, Department of Pharmaceutical Sciences; Assistant Professor of Medicine, Department of General Internal Medicine, University of Pittsburgh Schools of Pharmacy and Medicine, Pittsburgh, Pennsylvania

Barry R. Goldspiel, PharmD, FASHP, Oncology Clinical Pharmacy Specialist, Pharmacy Department, National Institutes of Health Clinical Center, Bethesda, Maryland

Jean-Venable (Kelly) R. Goode, PharmD, BCPS, Assistant Professor, Department of Pharmacy, Virginia Commonwealth University School of Pharmacy, Richmond, Virginia

Elizabeth S. Gray, PharmD, Assistant Professor, Department of Pharmacy, Virginia Commonwealth University School of Pharmacy, Richmond, Virginia

Paige Robbins Gross, RPh, Staff Pharmacist, University of Pittsburgh Medical Center, Pittsburgh, Pennsylvania

Amy J. Guenette, PharmD, BCPS, Clinical Coordinator, Department of Pharmacy, Wausau Hospital, Wausau, Wisconsin

Wayne P. Gulliver, MD, FRCPC, Associate Professor of Medicine (Dermatology), Faculty of Medicine, Memorial University of Newfoundland, St. John's, Newfoundland, Canada

John G. Gums, PharmD, Professor, Department of Pharmacy Practice, Community Health and Family Medicine, University of Florida College of Pharmacy, Gainesville, Florida

R. Donald Harvey III, PharmD, BCPS, Hematology/Oncology Resident, University of North Carolina at Chapel Hill, Chapel Hill, North Carolina

Amy M. Heck, PharmD, Specialized Resident in Drug Information and Pharmacotherapy, Warren G. Magnuson Clinical Center, National Institutes of Health, Bethesda, Maryland

Richard N. Herrier, PharmD, Assistant Professor, Department of Pharmacy Practice and Science, University of Arizona College of Pharmacy, Tucson, Arizona

Mary M. Hess, PharmD, Assistant Professor, Department of Pharmacy and Therapeutics, University of Pittsburgh School of Pharmacy; Critical Care Specialist, Department of Pharmacy, University of Pittsburgh Medical Center, Pittsburgh, Pennsylvania

Kimberly Heying, PharmD, Oncology Pharmacy Resident, Department of Pharmacy Services, University Hospital, Cincinnati, Ohio

Catherine A. Heyneman, PharmD, MS, Assistant Professor, Department of Pharmacy Practice, Idaho State University College of Pharmacy, Pocatello, Idaho

Mark T. Holdsworth, PharmD, BCPS, Associate Professor, University of New Mexico School of Pharmacy, Albuquerque, New Mexico

Jon D. Horton, PharmD, Clinical Pharmacist, Department of Pharmacy, York Health System, York, Pennsylvania

Denise L. Howrie, PharmD, Associate Professor of Pharmacy and Pediatrics, Schools of Pharmacy and Medicine, University of Pittsburgh; Clinical Coordinator, Pharmacy Services, Children's Hospital of Pittsburgh, Pittsburgh, Pennsylvania

Jonathan P. Hubbard, DO, Resident Physician, Department of Family Medicine, Idaho State University, Pocatello, Idaho

Timothy J. Ives, PharmD, MPH, FCCP, BCPS, Associate Professor, Department of Family Medicine, University of North Carolina, Chapel Hill, North Carolina

Linda A. Jaber, PharmD, Associate Professor, Department of Pharmacy Practice, Wayne State University College of Pharmacy, Detroit, Michigan

Mark W. Jackson, MD, FACG, Private Practice in Gastroenterology, Knoxville, Tennessee

Scott Jacober, DO, CDE, Associate Professor of Medicine, Department of Internal Medicine, Division of Endocrinology, Metabolism and Hypertension, Wayne State University School of Medicine, Detroit, Michigan

Michael W. Jann, PharmD, FCP, FCCP, Professor of Pharmacy Practice, Mercer University Southern School of Pharmacy, Atlanta, Georgia

Douglas D. Janson, PharmD, BCNSP, Clinical Pharmacy Specialist in Nutrition Support, University of Pittsburgh Medical Center; Assistant Professor, Department of Pharmacy and Therapeutics, University of Pittsburgh School of Pharmacy, Pittsburgh, Pennsylvania

Donna M. Jermain, PharmD, BCPP, Assistant Professor, Department of Medicine and Psychiatry, Texas A&M University Health Sciences Center; Coordinator of Pharmacy Research and Education, Department of Pharmacy, Scott & White Memorial Hospital, Temple, Texas

Kjel A. Johnson, PharmD, BCPS, Clinical Specialist, Health America of Pennsylvania, Inc.; Assistant Professor, Department of Pharmaceutical Sciences, University of Pittsburgh School of Pharmacy, Pittsburgh, Pennsylvania

Steven V. Johnson, PharmD, BCPS, Clinical Instructor, University of Minnesota College of Pharmacy, Minneapolis; Clinical Pharmacy Specialist/Manager, Regions Hospital, St. Paul, Minnesota

Melanie S. Joy, PharmD, Clinical Instructor and Research Coordinator, School of Medicine, Division of Nephrology and Hypertension, University of North Carolina, Chapel Hill, North Carolina

Barbara L. Kaltenbach, PharmD, Pharmacy Practice Resident, Department of Pharmacy, University of Iowa Hospitals and Clinics, Iowa City, Iowa

Daniel T. Kennedy, PharmD, BCPS, Assistant Professor, Department of Pharmacy, Virginia Commonwealth University School of Pharmacy, Richmond, Virginia

Tien T. Kiat-Winarko, PharmD, BSc, Assistant Professor of Clinical Pharmacy, University of Southern California School of Pharmacy; Director of Pharmacy, USC Pharmacy at the Doheny Eye Institute, Los Angeles, California

Aaron D. Killian, PharmD, BCPS, Assistant Professor, Department of Pharmacy Practice, School of Pharmacy, Texas Tech University Health Sciences Center at Amarillo, Amarillo, Texas

Krista M. King, PharmD, BCOP, Clinical Pharmacy Specialist in Lymphoma, Division of Pharmacy, University of Texas MD Anderson Cancer Center, Houston, Texas

Cynthia K. Kirkwood, PharmD, Assistant Professor, Department of Pharmacy, Virginia Commonwealth University School of Pharmacy, Richmond, Virginia

Daren L. Knoell, PharmD, Assistant Professor, Department of Pharmacy Practice and Administration, Ohio State University College of Pharmacy, Columbus, Ohio

Cynthia P. Koh-Knox, PharmD, Pharmacy Practice Resident, Clarian Health Partners—Methodist Hospital, Indianapolis, Indiana

Robert J. Kuhn, PharmD, Professor and Vice Chair of Ambulatory Services, Division of Pharmacy Practice and Science, University of Kentucky College of Pharmacy, Lexington, Kentucky

Lyle K. Laird, PharmD, BCPP, Assistant Professor, Department of Pharmacy Practice, University of Colorado School of Pharmacy, Denver, Colorado

Nancy P. Lam, PharmD, BCPS, Assistant Professor, Colleges of Pharmacy and Medicine, and Pharmacotherapist, Digestive and Liver Diseases, University of Illinois at Chicago, Chicago, Illinois

Rebecca M. Law, PharmD, Associate Professor, School of Pharmacy, Memorial University of Newfoundland, St. John's, Newfoundland, Canada

Cara Lawless-Liday, PharmD, Assistant Professor, Department of Pharmacy Practice and Administrative Sciences, College of Pharmacy, Idaho State University, Pocatello, Idaho

W. Greg Leader, PharmD, Assistant Professor, Department of Clinical Pharmacy, West Virginia University School of Pharmacy, Morgantown, West Virginia

Mary Lee, PharmD, BCPS, FCCP, Associate Dean and Professor, Department of Pharmacy Practice, Chicago College of Pharmacy, Downer's Grove, Illinois

Christine A. Lesch, PharmD, Infectious Diseases Research Fellow, Department of Pharmacy Practice, University of Illinois at Chicago College of Pharmacy, Chicago, Illinois

James S. Lewis II, PharmD, Pharmacy Practice Resident, Department of Pharmacy, Southwest Washington Medical Center, Vancouver, Washington

Celeste C. Lindley, PharmD, MS, FASHP, FCCP, BCPS, Associate Professor, School of Pharmacy, University of North Carolina at Chapel Hill, Chapel Hill, North Carolina

Sherry Luedtke, PharmD, Assistant Professor, Department of Pharmacy Practice, Texas Tech University Health Sciences Center School of Pharmacy, Amarillo, Texas

Mark S. Luer, PharmD, Assistant Professor, Department of Pharmacy Practice, College of Pharmacy, University of Arkansas for Medical Sciences, Little Rock, Arkansas

Steven J. Martin, PharmD, BCPS, Assistant Professor, Department of Pharmacy Practice, University of Toledo College of Pharmacy, Toledo, Ohio

Barbara J. Mason, PharmD, Professor of Pharmacy, Department of Pharmacy Practice, Idaho State University College of Pharmacy; Ambulatory Care Clinical Pharmacist, Veterans Affairs Medical Center, Boise, Idaho

Rae Ann Maxwell, RPh, PhD, Director of Pharmacy, Western Psychiatric Institute and Clinic; Director of the Investigational Drug Service, University of Pittsburgh Medical Center; Assistant Professor, Department of Pharmacy and Therapeutics, University of Pittsburgh School of Pharmacy, Pittsburgh, Pennsylvania

James W. McAuley, RPh, PhD, Assistant Professor, Departments of Pharmacy Practice and Neurology, Ohio State University, Columbus, Ohio

Alex K. McDonald, PharmD, Specialty Resident in Drug Information, University of North Carolina and Glaxo-Wellcome Inc., Chapel Hill, North Carolina

Elaine McGhee, MD, Clinical Assistant Professor, Department of Pediatrics, University of Pittsburgh School of Medicine, Pittsburgh, Pennsylvania

William McGhee, PharmD, Clinical Pharmacist, Children's Hospital of Pittsburgh; Assistant Professor, Department of Pharmacy and Therapeutics, University of Pittsburgh School of Pharmacy, Pittsburgh, Pennsylvania

Margaret E. McGuinness, PharmD, Assistant Professor of Pharmacy Practice, Oregon State University College of Pharmacy; Clinical Pharmacist—Internal Medicine and Oncology, Portland Veterans Affairs Medical Center, Portland, Oregon

Renee-Claude Mercier, PharmD, Assistant Professor of Pharmacy, University of New Mexico College of Pharmacy, Albuquerque, New Mexico

Joette M. Meyer, PharmD, was Clinical Assistant Professor, Department of Pharmacy Practice, University of Illinois at Chicago College of Pharmacy, Chicago, Illinois at the time of this writing

Laura Boehnke Michaud, PharmD, Clinical Pharmacy Specialist—Breast Oncology, Division of Pharmacy, University of Texas MD Anderson Cancer Center, Houston, Texas

W. Alexander Morton, PharmD, BCPP, Professor of Pharmacy Practice, College of Pharmacy; Associate Professor of Psychiatry and Behavioral Sciences, Department of Psychiatry and Behavioral Sciences, Medical University of South Carolina, Charleston, South Carolina

Laura Mulloy, DO, Acting Chief of Nephrology and Associate Professor of Medicine, Department of Medicine, Medical College of Georgia, Augusta, Georgia

Pamela J. Murray, MD, MPH, Associate Professor of Pediatrics and Obstetrics, Gynecology and Reproductive Sciences, University of Pittsburgh School of Medicine, Pittsburgh, Pennsylvania

James J. Nawarskas, PharmD, Assistant Professor of Pharmacy, University of New Mexico College of Pharmacy, Albuquerque, New Mexico

B. Nhi Nguyen, PharmD, Cardiology Fellow, Department of Clinical Pharmacy, University of Tennessee College of Pharmacy, Memphis, Tennessee

Dannielle C. O'Donnell, PharmD, BCPS, Assistant Professor, University of Texas at Austin College of Pharmacy, Austin, Texas

Michael A. Oszko, PharmD, BCPS, Associate Professor, Department of Pharmacy Practice, University of Kansas School of Pharmacy, Kansas City, Kansas

Linda M. Page, PharmD, Clinical Research Associate, Ventures-Drug Delivery Business, Medtronic Neurological, Minneapolis, Minnesota

Robert B. Parker, PharmD, Associate Professor, Department of Clinical Pharmacy, University of Tennessee College of Pharmacy, Memphis, Tennessee

Beth Bryles Phillips, PharmD, Clinical Pharmacist in Ambulatory Care, Department of Pharmaceutical Care, University of Iowa Hospitals & Clinics, Iowa City, Iowa

Bradley G. Phillips, PharmD, Assistant Professor, Division of Clinical and Administrative Pharmacy, University of Iowa College of Pharmacy, Iowa City, Iowa

Page H. Pigg, PharmD, Pharmacist Account Manager, First Health Services Corporation, Glen Allen, Virginia

Charles D. Ponte, PharmD, BCPS, CDE, FAPhA, FASHP, FCCP, Professor, Department of Clinical Pharmacy and Family Medicine, Schools of Pharmacy and Medicine, Robert C. Byrd Health Sciences Center, West Virginia University, Morgantown, West Virginia

Tara L. Posey, PharmD, Ambulatory Care Clinician, University of Pittsburgh Medical Center; Assistant Professor, Department of Pharmacy and Therapeutics, University of Pittsburgh School of Pharmacy, Pittsburgh, Pennsylvania

Jane M. Pruemer, PharmD, FASHP, Oncology Clinical Pharmacy Specialist, Department of Pharmacy Services, University Hospital, Cincinnati, Ohio

Thomas W. Redford, PharmD, Assistant Professor, Division of Clinical and Administrative Pharmacy, University of Iowa College of Pharmacy, Iowa City, Iowa

Richard S. Rhodes, PharmD, Associate Professor, Department of Pharmacy Practice, Idaho State University College of Pharmacy, Pocatello, Idaho

Denise H. Rhoney, PharmD, Assistant Professor, Department of Pharmacy Practice, Wayne State University College of Pharmacy and Allied Health Professions, Detroit, Michigan

Ted L. Rice, MS, BCPS, Pharmacy Specialist—Trauma, University of Pittsburgh Medical Center; Associate Professor, Department of Pharmacy and Therapeutics, University of Pittsburgh School of Pharmacy, Pittsburgh, Pennsylvania

Milissa A. Rock, RPh, CDE, Community Practice Resident and Clinical Instructor of Pharmacy, Department of Pharmacy, Virginia Commonwealth University School of Pharmacy, Richmond, Virginia

Keith A. Rodvold, PharmD, FCCP, BCPS, Professor of Pharmacy Practice and Associate Professor of Medicine in Pharmacy, Departments of Pharmacy Practice and Infectious Diseases, University of Illinois at Chicago, Chicago, Illinois

Carol J. Rollins, MS, RD, PharmD, BCNSP, Coordinator, Nutrition Support Team and Clinical Pharmacist for Home Infusion Therapy, Arizona Health Sciences Center, Tucson, Arizona

Meredith L. Rose, PharmD, Assistant Professor, Department of Pharmacy and Therapeutics, University of Pittsburgh School of Pharmacy; Clinical Specialist, University of Pittsburgh Medical Center, Pittsburgh, Pennsylvania

Daniel Sageser, PharmD, Oncology Clinical Specialist and Hospice Pharmacy Team Leader, Southwest Washington Medical Center, Vancouver, Washington

Nannette A. Sageser, PharmD, Clinical Pharmacist and Director of the Anticoagulation Service, Southeast Washington Medical Center, Vancouver, Washington

Beata Saletnik, PharmD, Adjunct Clinical Faculty, Idaho State University College of Pharmacy; Veterans Affairs Medical Center, Boise, Idaho

Kristine E. Santus, PharmD, Ambulatory Care Resident, Department of Pharmacy, University of Pittsburgh Medical Center; Clinical Instructor, Department of Pharmacy and Therapeutics, University of Pittsburgh School of Pharmacy, Pittsburgh, Pennsylvania

Jennifer L. Schoelles, PharmD, Pediatric Specialty Resident, University of Kentucky Children's Hospital, Lexington, Kentucky

Rowena N. Schwartz, PharmD, Associate Professor, Department of Pharmacy and Therapeutics, University of Pittsburgh School of Pharmacy; Coordinator of Pharmacy Programs, University of Pittsburgh Cancer Institute, Pittsburgh, Pennsylvania

Terry L. Schwinghammer, PharmD, FCCP, FASHP, BCPS, Associate Professor, Department of Pharmaceutical Sciences, University of Pittsburgh School of Pharmacy, Pittsburgh, Pennsylvania

Mollie Ashe Scott, PharmD, BCPS, Assistant Professor, Department of Pharmacy Practice, Campbell University School of Pharmacy, Buies Creek, North Carolina; Clinical Specialist in Family Medicine, Duke University, Durham, North Carolina

Amy L. Seybert, PharmD, Assistant Professor, Department of Pharmacy and Therapeutics, University of Pittsburgh School of Pharmacy; Clinical Specialist, University of Pittsburgh Medical Center, Pittsburgh, Pennsylvania

Susan Shaffer, PharmD, Specialty Resident in Drug Information, University of North Carolina School of Pharmacy and Glaxo-Wellcome Inc., Chapel Hill, North Carolina

Penny S. Shelton, PharmD, BCPP, FASCP, Assistant Professor, Department of Pharmacy Practice, Campbell University School of Pharmacy, Buies Creek, North Carolina; Clinical Specialist in Geriatrics, Dorothea Dix Hospital, Raleigh, North Carolina

Susan J. Skledar, RPh, MPH, Clinical Instructor, Department of Pharmacy and Therapeutics, University of Pittsburgh School of Pharmacy, Pittsburgh, Pennsylvania

Jill Slimick-Ponzetto, PharmD, BCPS, Clinical Pharmacist, Department of Pharmacy, Veterans Affairs Medical Center; Instructor, Department of Pharmacy and Therapeutics, University of Pittsburgh School of Pharmacy, Pittsburgh, Pennsylvania

Ralph E. Small, PharmD, FCCP, FASHP, FAPhA, Professor of Pharmacy and Medicine, School of Pharmacy, Medical College of Virginia, Virginia Commonwealth University, Richmond, Virginia

Catherine A. Smith, PharmD, Hematology/Oncology Pharmacy Resident, Department of Pharmaceutical Services, Emory University Hospital, Atlanta, Georgia

Jerry D. Smith, PharmD, Manager of Pharmacy Services, Simkin, Inc., and Clinical Assistant Professor, Department of Community Health and Family Medicine, College of Medicine, University of Florida, Gainesville, Florida

Judith A. Smith, PharmD, Oncology Pharmacy Practice Resident, Pharmacy Department, National Institutes of Health Clinical Center, Bethesda, Maryland

Renata Smith, PharmD, Infectious Disease Specialty Resident, Department of Pharmacy Practice, University of Illinois at Chicago College of Pharmacy, Chicago, Illinois

Denise R. Sokos, PharmD, Specialty Pharmacy Resident in Adult Internal Medicine, West Virginia University Hospitals, Morgantown, West Virginia

Christine L. Solberg, PharmD, BCPS, CSPI, Research Associate, Department of Surgery, Regions Hospital, St. Paul, Minnesota

Alka Z. Somani, PharmD, Clinical Pharmacist in Ambulatory Care/Transplantation, Department of Pharmacy, University of Pittsburgh

Medical Center; Assistant Professor, Department of Pharmacy and Therapeutics, University of Pittsburgh School of Pharmacy, Pittsburgh, Pennsylvania

Suellyn J. Sorensen, PharmD, BCPS, Assistant Professor of Pharmacy Practice, Department of Pharmacy Practice, Butler University College of Pharmacy and Health Sciences; Clinical Pharmacist in Infectious Diseases, Clarian Health Partners, Indianapolis, Indiana

William J. Spruill, PharmD, Associate Professor, Department of Clinical and Administrative Sciences, University of Georgia College of Pharmacy, Athens, Georgia

Mary K. Stamatakis, PharmD, Assistant Professor, Department of Clinical Pharmacy, West Virginia University School of Pharmacy, Morgantown, West Virginia

Virginia L. Stauffer, PharmD, BCPS, Clinical Pharmacist, Department of Geriatric Medicine, Methodist Medical Group, Indianapolis, Indiana

Jennifer Stoffel, PharmD, BCPS, Assistant Professor, Department of Pharmacy and Therapeutics, University of Pittsburgh School of Pharmacy; Transplant Clinical Pharmacist, University of Pittsburgh Medical Center, Pittsburgh, Pennsylvania

Jennifer A. Torma, PharmD, Clinical Assistant Professor, Rutgers University College of Pharmacy and Oncology Pharmacy Specialist, Hackensack University Medical Center, Hackensack, New Jersey. At the time of this writing, she was Oncology Specialty Pharmacy Resident, University of Pittsburgh Medical Center, Pittsburgh, Pennsylvania

Sharon M. Tramonte, PharmD, Clinical Assistant Professor, Department of Pharmacy and Pharmacology, University of Texas Health Sciences Center at Austin; Clinical Pharmacologist, Department of Pharmacology, San Antonio State School, San Antonio, Texas

James A. Trovato, PharmD, Assistant Professor, Department of Pharmacy Practice and Science, School of Pharmacy, and Greenebaum Cancer Center, University of Maryland, Baltimore, Maryland

Tate N. Trujillo, PharmD, Critical Care Resident, Cardiopulmonary Care Center, Clarian Health Partners, Indiana University Hospital, Indianapolis, Indiana

Gretchen M. Tush, PharmD, BCPS, Assistant Professor, Department of Pharmacy, Virginia Commonwealth University School of Pharmacy, Richmond, Virginia

J. Edwin Underwood, Jr., PharmD, Associate Professor, Samford University McWhorter School of Pharmacy, Birmingham; Clinical Pharmacist, Lloyd Noland Hospital and Ambulatory Center, Fairfield, Alabama

Chad M. VanDenBerg, PharmD, Clinical Neuroscience Fellow, Department of Pharmacy Practice, Mercer University of Southern School of Pharmacy, Atlanta, Georgia

William E. Wade, PharmD, FASHP, FCCP, Associate Professor, Department of Clinical and Administrative Sciences, University of Georgia College of Pharmacy, Athens, Georgia

Mary Louise Wagner, MS, PharmD, Associate Professor, Department of Pharmacy Practice, Rutgers University College of Pharmacy, Piscataway, New Jersey

Donna S. Wall, PharmD, BCPS, Clinical Pharmacist, Cardiopulmonary Care Center, Clarian Health Partners, Indiana University Hospital, Indianapolis, Indiana

Carla Wallace, PharmD, BCPS, Assistant Professor, Department of Pharmacy Practice, St. Louis College of Pharmacy, St. Louis, Missouri

Amy L. Whitaker, PharmD, Community Pharmacy Practice Resident, Virginia Commonwealth University School of Pharmacy, Richmond, Virginia

Dennis M. Williams, PharmD, FASHP, FCCP, BCPS, Assistant Professor, Department of Pharmacy Practice, University of North Carolina School of Pharmacy, Chapel Hill, North Carolina

Susan R. Winkler, PharmD, BCPS, Clinical Assistant Professor, Department of Pharmacy Practice, University of Illinois at Chicago College of Pharmacy, Chicago, Illinois

Maria Yaramus, PharmD, PharmD Candidate, Duquesne University Mylan School of Pharmacy, Pittsburgh, Pennsylvania

Peggy C. Yarborough, MS, CDE, FAPP, FASHP, NAPP, Associate Professor, Campbell University School of Pharmacy, Buies Creek, North Carolina; Director of Pharmacotherapy—Wilson, Area L Area Health Education Center, Rocky Mount, North Carolina

Winnie M. Yu, PharmD, BCPS, Assistant Professor, Department of Pharmacy and Therapeutics, University of Pittsburgh School of Pharmacy; Clinical Specialist, University of Pittsburgh Medical Center, Pittsburgh, Pennsylvania

Nancy S. Yunker, PharmD, Assistant Professor, Department of Pharmacy, Virginia Commonwealth University School of Pharmacy, Richmond, Virginia

Margaret B. Zak, PharmD, Assistant Professor, Department of Pharmacy and Therapeutics, University of Pittsburgh School of Pharmacy; Clinical Specialist in Infectious Disease, Department of Pharmacy, University of Pittsburgh Medical Center, Pittsburgh, Pennsylvania

William C. Zamboni, PharmD, Assistant Professor, Department of Pharmacy Practice and Science, School of Pharmacy; Department of Developmental Therapeutics, Greenebaum Cancer Center, University of Maryland, Baltimore, Maryland

Basil J. Zitelli, MD, FAAP, Professor of Pediatrics, Department of Pediatrics, Children's Hospital of Pittsburgh, Pittsburgh, Pennsylvania

Contents

Preface xvii

Acknowledgments xix

PART ONE
Principles of Patient-focused Therapy
Terry L. Schwinghammer, PharmD, FCCP, FASHP, BCPS, Section Editor

Chapter	1	Introduction: How to Use This Casebook 1
		Terry L. Schwinghammer, PharmD, FCCP, FASHP, BCPS
Chapter	2	Active Learning Strategies 7
		Elizabeth S. Gray, PharmD, Gretchen M. Tush, PharmD, BCPS, Cynthia K. Kirkwood, PharmD
Chapter	3	Case Studies in Patient Communication 11
		Marie E. Gardner, PharmD, Richard N. Herrier, PharmD
Chapter	4	Documentation of Pharmacist Interventions 16
		Timothy J. Ives, PharmD, MPH, FCCP, BCPS
		Bruce R. Canaday, PharmD, BCPS, FASHP, FAPhA
		Peggy C. Yarborough, MS, CDE, FAPP, FASHP, NAPP

PART TWO
Disorders of Organ Systems

SECTION 1
Cardiovascular Disorders 21
Robert L. Talbert, PharmD, FCCP, BCPS, Section Editor

Chapter	1	Cardiopulmonary Resuscitation 21
		Tate N. Trujillo, PharmD, Donna S. Wall, PharmD, BCPS
Chapter	2	Hypertension 23
		J. Edwin Underwood, Jr., PharmD
Chapter	3	Hypertensive Urgency 27
		James J. Nawarskas, PharmD
Chapter	4	Heart Failure 30
		Jon D. Horton, PharmD
Chapter	5	Ischemic Heart Disease 32
		Amy J. Guenette, PharmD, BCPS
Chapter	6	Acute Myocardial Infarction 36
		B. Nhi Nguyen, PharmD, Robert B. Parker, PharmD
Chapter	7	Ventricular Tachycardia 40
		Ashesh J. Gandhi, PharmD

Chapter	8	Atrial Fibrillation 42
		Bradley G. Phillips, PharmD
Chapter	9	Hypertrophic Cardiomyopathy 45
		Laura A. Bartels, PharmD
Chapter	10	Deep Vein Thrombosis 47
		Nannette A. Sageser, PharmD
Chapter	11	Pulmonary Embolism 49
		Amy L. Seybert, PharmD, Ted L. Rice, MS, BCPS
Chapter	12	Chronic Anticoagulation 52
		Beth Bryles Phillips, PharmD
Chapter	13	Ischemic Stroke 55
		Susan R. Winkler, PharmD, BCPS, Mark S. Luer, PharmD
Chapter	14	Hyperlipidemia: Primary Prevention 58
		Laura A. Bartels, PharmD
Chapter	15	Hyperlipidemia: Secondary Prevention 61
		Kjel A. Johnson, PharmD, BCPS
Chapter	16	Peripheral Vascular Disease 64
		Susan D. Bear, BS, PharmD
Chapter	17	Hypovolemic Shock 67
		Brian L. Erstad, PharmD, FASHP, FCCM

SECTION 2
Respiratory Disorders 70
Robert L. Talbert, PharmD, FCCP, BCPS, Section Editor

Chapter	18	Acute Asthma 70
		Daniel T. Kennedy, PharmD, BCPS
		Ralph E. Small, PharmD, FCCP, FASHP, FAPhA
Chapter	19	Chronic Asthma 73
		Dennis M. Williams, PharmD, FASHP, FCCP, BCPS
Chapter	20	Chronic Obstructive Lung Disease 77
		Daren L. Knoell, PharmD
Chapter	21	Respiratory Distress Syndrome 80
		Jennifer L. Schoelles, PharmD, Robert J. Kuhn, PharmD
Chapter	22	Cystic Fibrosis 83
		Robert J. Kuhn, PharmD

SECTION 3
Gastrointestinal Disorders 86
Joseph T. DiPiro, PharmD, FCCP, Section Editor

Chapter	23	Gastroesophageal Reflux Disease 86
		Meredith L. Rose, PharmD

xii Contents

Chapter	Title	Page
Chapter 24	Peptic Ulcer Disease	90
	Marie A. Chisholm, PharmD, Mark W. Jackson, MD, FACG	
Chapter 25	Stress Ulcer Prophylaxis/Upper GI Hemorrhage	92
	Steven V. Johnson, PharmD, BCPS	
	Christine L. Solberg, PharmD, BCPS, CSPI	
Chapter 26	Ulcerative Colitis	95
	Nancy S. Yunker, PharmD	
	Ralph E. Small, PharmD, FCCP, FASHP, FAPhA	
Chapter 27	Nausea and Vomiting	99
	Amy J. Becker, PharmD	
Chapter 28	Diarrhea	102
	Marie A. Abate, PharmD	
	Charles D. Ponte, BS, PharmD, BCPS, CDE, FAPhA, FASHP, FCCP	
Chapter 29	Pediatric Gastroenteritis	105
	William McGhee, PharmD, Basil J. Zitelli, MD, FAAP	
Chapter 30	Constipation	108
	Barbara L. Kaltenbach, PharmD	
	Beth Bryles Phillips, PharmD	
Chapter 31	Cirrhotic Ascites	111
	Joette M. Meyer, PharmD	
Chapter 32	Esophageal Varices	115
	Cesar Alaniz, PharmD	
Chapter 33	Hepatic Encephalopathy	117
	Nancy P. Lam, PharmD, BCPS	
Chapter 34	Acute Pancreatitis	119
	Charles W. Fetrow, PharmD, Maria Yaramus, PharmD	
Chapter 35	Viral Hepatitis	122
	Nancy P. Lam, PharmD, BCPS	

SECTION 4
Renal and Genitourinary Tract Disorders 126
Gary R. Matzke, PharmD, FCP, FCCP, Section Editor

Chapter	Title	Page
Chapter 36	Drug-induced Acute Renal Failure	126
	Mary K. Stamatakis, PharmD	
Chapter 37	Progression of Chronic Renal Disease	130
	Reina Bendayan, PharmD, Winnie M. Yu, PharmD, BCPS	
Chapter 38	End-stage Renal Disease	134
	James D. Coyle, PharmD	
Chapter 39	Renal Transplantation	139
	Marie A. Chisholm, PharmD, Tana R. Bagby, PharmD	
	Laura Mulloy, DO	
Chapter 40	Chronic Glomerulonephritis	141
	Melanie S. Joy, PharmD	
Chapter 41	Syndrome of Inappropriate Antidiuretic Hormone Release	145
	Rex W. Force, PharmD, BCPS, Jonathan D. Hubbard, DO	
Chapter 42	Hypokalemia and Hypomagnesemia	147
	Denise R. Sokos, PharmD, W. Greg Leader, PharmD	
Chapter 43	Hyperkalemia, Hyperphosphatemia, and Hypocalcemia	152
	Brian K. Bond, PharmD, Mary K. Stamatakis, PharmD	
Chapter 44	Hypercalcemia	156
	James S. Lewis II, PharmD, Daniel Sageser, PharmD	
Chapter 45	Metabolic Acidosis	158
	Melanie S. Joy, PharmD	
Chapter 46	Metabolic Alkalosis	161
	Jennifer Stoffel, PharmD, BCPS	
Chapter 47	Benign Prostatic Hyperplasia	164
	Catherine A. Heyneman, PharmD, MS	
	Richard S. Rhodes, PharmD	
Chapter 48	Neurogenic Bladder and Urinary Incontinence	167
	Mary Lee, PharmD, BCPS, FCCP	
Chapter 49	Erectile Dysfunction	170
	Cara Lawless-Liday, PharmD, Rex W. Force, PharmD, BCPS	

SECTION 5
Neurologic Disorders 175
Barbara G. Wells, PharmD, FASHP, FCCP, BCPP, Section Editor

Chapter	Title	Page
Chapter 50	Multiple Sclerosis	175
	Barry E. Gidal, PharmD, John O. Fleming, MD	
Chapter 51	Complex Partial Seizures	178
	James W. McAuley, RPh, PhD	
Chapter 52	Status Epilepticus	180
	Sharon M. Tramonte, PharmD	
Chapter 53	Acute Management of the Head Injury Patient	183
	Denise H. Rhoney, PharmD, Mark S. Luer, PharmD	
Chapter 54	Parkinson's Disease	187
	Mary Louise Wagner, MS, PharmD	
Chapter 55	Pain Management	191
	Karen Beauchamp, BPharm, RPh, Daniel Sageser, PharmD	
Chapter 56	Headache Disorders	194
	Mark S. Luer, PharmD, Susan R. Winkler, PharmD, BCPS	

SECTION 6
Psychiatric Disorders 198
Barbara G. Wells, PharmD, FASHP, FCCP, BCPP, Section Editor

Chapter	Title	Page
Chapter 57	Attention-deficit Hyperactivity Disorder	198
	William H. Benefield, Jr., PharmD, BCPP, FASCP	
	Donna M. Jermain, PharmD, BCPP	
Chapter 58	Anorexia Nervosa	200
	Rae Ann Maxwell, RPh, PhD	

Chapter	59	Alzheimer's Disease 208
		Cynthia P. Koh-Knox, PharmD
		Virginia L. Stauffer, PharmD, BCPS
Chapter	60	Alcohol Withdrawal 205
		Jill Slimick-Ponzetto, PharmD, BCPS
Chapter	61	Nicotine Addiction 207
		Julie A. Cold, PharmD, BCPP
Chapter	62	Schizophrenia..211
		William H. Benefield, Jr., PharmD, BCPP, FASCP
		Lawrence J. Cohen, PharmD, BCPP, FASHP, FCCP
Chapter	63	Major Depression 214
		Brian L. Crabtree, PharmD, BCPP
Chapter	64	Bipolar Disorder 216
		Andrea Eggert, PharmD, BCPP
		William H. Benefield, Jr., PharmD, BCPP, FASCP
Chapter	65	Generalized Anxiety Disorder.............................220
		Michael W. Jann, PharmD, FCP, FCCP
		Chad M. VanDenBerg, PharmD
Chapter	66	Panic Disorder 222
		W. Alexander Morton, PharmD, BCPP
Chapter	67	Obsessive-Compulsive Disorder 225
		Lyle K. Laird, PharmD, BCPP
Chapter	68	Insomnia 228
		Penny S. Shelton, PharmD, BCPP, FASCP
		Mollie Ashe Scott, PharmD, BCPS

SECTION 7
Endocrinologic Disorders 232
Robert L. Talbert, PharmD, FCCP, BCPS, Section Editor

Chapter	69	Type 1 Diabetes Mellitus 232
		Scott Jacober, DO, CDE, Linda A. Jaber, PharmD
Chapter	70	Type 2 Diabetes Mellitus 234
		Milissa A. Rock, RPh, CDE
		Jean-Venable (Kelly) R. Goode, PharmD, BCPS
Chapter	71	Hyperthyroidism: Graves' Disease 238
		Kristine E. Santus, PharmD, Tara L. Posey, PharmD
Chapter	72	Hypothyroidism 241
		Tara L. Posey, PharmD
Chapter	73	Cushing's Syndrome.....................................243
		Jerry D. Smith, PharmD, John G. Gums, PharmD
Chapter	74	Addison's Disease 246
		Cynthia P. Koh-Knox, PharmD, Bruce C. Carlstedt, PhD
Chapter	75	Hyperprolactinemia 248
		Amy M. Heck, PharmD
		Karim A. Calis, PharmD, MPH, BCPS, BCNSP, FASHP

SECTION 8
Gynecologic Disorders 252
Barbara G. Wells, PharmD, FASHP, FCCP, BCPP, Section Editor

Chapter	76	Contraception...252
		Carla B. Frye, PharmD, BCPS
Chapter	77	Premenstrual Dysphoric Disorder 256
		Donna M. Jermain, PharmD, BCPP
Chapter	78	Hormone Replacement Therapy 258
		Alka Z. Somani, PharmD

SECTION 9
Immunologic Disorders..261
Gary C. Yee, PharmD, FCCP, Section Editor

Chapter	79	Systemic Lupus Erythematosus............................261
		Thomas W. Redford, PharmD
		Ralph E. Small, PharmD, FCCP, FASHP, FAPhA

SECTION 10
Bone and Joint Disorders....................................264
L. Michael Posey, RPh, Section Editor

Chapter	80	Osteoporosis 264
		Carla B. Frye, PharmD, BCPS
Chapter	81	Rheumatoid Arthritis.....................................267
		Ralph E. Small, PharmD, FCCP, FASHP, FAPhA
		Thomas W. Redford, PharmD, Amy L. Whitaker, PharmD
Chapter	82	Osteoarthritis..271
		Michael A. Oszko, PharmD, BCPS
Chapter	83	Gout and Hyperuricemia 274
		Page H. Pigg, PharmD
		Ralph E. Small, PharmD, FCCP, FASHP, FAPhA

SECTION 11
Eyes, Ears, Nose, and Throat Disorders..................277
L. Michael Posey, RPh, Section Editor

Chapter	84	Glaucoma..277
		Tien T. Kiat-Winarko, PharmD, BSc
Chapter	85	Allergic Rhinitis 280
		W. Greg Leader, PharmD

SECTION 12
Dermatologic Disorders 285
L. Michael Posey, RPh, Section Editor

Chapter	86	Acne Vulgaris..285
		Rebecca M. Law, PharmD,
		Wayne P. Gulliver, MD, FRCPC
Chapter	87	Psoriasis...288
		Rebecca M. Law, PharmD

SECTION 13
Hematologic Disorders 292
Gary C. Yee, PharmD, FCCP, Section Editor

Chapter 88   Iron Deficiency Anemia 292
        William E. Wade, PharmD, FASHP, FCCP
        William J. Spruill, PharmD

Chapter 89   Vitamin B_{12} Deficiency 294
        Barbara J. Mason, PharmD, Beata Saletnik, PharmD

Chapter 90   Folic Acid Deficiency 297
        Beata Saletnik, PharmD, Barbara J. Mason, PharmD

Chapter 91   Sickle Cell Anemia 299
        R. Donald Harvey III, PharmD, BCPS
        Celeste C. Lindley, PharmD, MS, FASHP, FCCP, BCPS

PART THREE
Diseases of Infectious Origin
Joseph T. DiPiro, PharmD, FCCP, Section Editor

Chapter 92   Using Laboratory Tests in Infectious Diseases 303
        Steven J. Martin, PharmD, BCPS

Chapter 93   Bacterial Meningitis 305
        Sherry Luedtke, PharmD

Chapter 94   Community-acquired Pneumonia 308
        Patrick P. Gleason, PharmD, BCPS

Chapter 95   Otitis Media 311
        Carla Wallace, PharmD, BCPS

Chapter 96   Streptococcal Pharyngitis 314
        Denise L. Howrie, PharmD, Elaine McGhee, MD

Chapter 97   Rhinosinusitis 317
        Aaron D. Killian, PharmD, BCPS

Chapter 98   Pressure Sores 321
        Richard S. Rhodes, PharmD
        Catherine A. Heyneman, PharmD, MS

Chapter 99   Diabetic Foot Infection 324
        Renee-Claude Mercier, PharmD

Chapter 100   Infective Endocarditis 328
        Renata Smith, PharmD
        Keith A. Rodvold, PharmD, FCCP, BCPS

Chapter 101   Pulmonary Tuberculosis 331
        Susan Shaffer, PharmD
        Dennis M. Williams, PharmD, FASHP, FCCP, BCPS

Chapter 102   *Clostridium difficile*-associated Diarrhea 334
        Margaret B. Zak, PharmD

Chapter 103   Intra-abdominal Infection 337
        Renee-Claude Mercier, PharmD

Chapter 104   Pelvic Inflammatory Disease and Other Sexually Transmitted Diseases 339
        Denise L. Howrie, PharmD
        Pamela J. Murray, MD, MPH

Chapter 105   Lower Urinary Tract Infection 342
        Christine A. Lesch, PharmD
        Keith A. Rodvold, PharmD, FCCP, BCPS

Chapter 106   Acute Pyelonephritis 345
        Margaret E. McGuinness, PharmD

Chapter 107   Syphilis 348
        Alex K. McDonald, PharmD
        Dennis M. Williams, PharmD, FASHP, FCCP, BCPS

Chapter 108   Genital Herpes and Chlamydial Infections 350
        Suellyn J. Sorensen, PharmD, BCPS

Chapter 109   Osteomyelitis 354
        Edward P. Armstrong, PharmD, BCPS, FASHP
        Victor A. Elsberry, PharmD, BCNSP, Leslie L. Barton, MD

Chapter 110   Gram-negative Sepsis 355
        Mary M. Hess, PharmD

Chapter 111   Systemic Fungal Infection 358
        Aaron D. Killian, PharmD, BCPS

Chapter 112   Dermatophytosis 361
        Winnie M. Yu, PharmD, BCPS

Chapter 113   Bacterial Vaginosis 364
        Charles D. Ponte, PharmD, BCPS, CDE, FAPhA, FASHP, FCCP

Chapter 114   Antimicrobial Prophylaxis for Surgery 367
        Susan J. Skledar, RPh, MPH, Paige Robbins Gross, RPh

Chapter 115   Pediatric Immunization 370
        Daniel T. Casto, PharmD, FCCP

Chapter 116   Cytomegalovirus (CMV) Retinitis 372
        Winnie M. Yu, PharmD, BCPS

Chapter 117   Treatment of HIV Infection 375
        Susan Chuck, PharmD
        Keith A. Rodvold, PharmD, FCCP, BCPS

Chapter 118   HIV Infection and PCP Pneumonia 380
        Linda M. Page, PharmD, Peter L. Anderson, PharmD
        Courtney V. Fletcher, PharmD

PART FOUR
Oncologic Disorders
Gary C. Yee, PharmD, FCCP, Section Editor

Chapter 119   Breast Cancer 385
        Laura Boehnke Michaud, PharmD

Chapter 120   Non-small Cell Lung Cancer 388
        Kimberly Heying, PharmD, Jane M. Pruemer, PharmD, FASHP

Chapter 121	Colon Cancer 391	

Daniel Sageser, PharmD

Chapter 122	Prostate Cancer 392	

Judith A. Smith, PharmD, Barry R. Goldspiel, PharmD, FASHP

Chapter 123	Malignant Lymphoma......................................396	

Krista M. King, PharmD, BCOP

Chapter 124	Ovarian Cancer 400	

William C. Zamboni, PharmD, James A. Trovato, PharmD

Chapter 125	Acute Lymphocytic Leukemia 403	

Mark T. Holdsworth, PharmD, BCPS

Chapter 126	Chronic Myelogenous Leukemia......................407	

Terri G. Davidson, PharmD, Catherine A. Smith, PharmD

Chapter 127	Melanoma 411	

Jennifer A. Torma, PharmD, Rowena N. Schwartz, PharmD

Chapter 128	Bone Marrow Transplantation 415	

Simon Cronin, PharmD, MS

PART FIVE
Nutrition and Nutritional Disorders
Gary R. Matzke, PharmD, FCP, FCCP, Section Editor

Chapter 129	Parenteral Nutrition 419	

Douglas D. Janson, PharmD, BCNSP

Chapter 130	Adult Enteral Nutrition 423	

Carol J. Rollins, MS, RD, PharmD, BCNSP

Chapter 131	Obesity...427	

Dannielle C. O'Donnell, PharmD, BCPS

Note: Additional cases with questions and suggested answers may be found on the Internet at www.pharmacy.pitt.edu/ce/pharmacotherapy.

Preface

This guide is designed to help instructors use the book, *Pharmacotherapy Casebook: A Patient-focused Approach,* efficiently. In this volume, case authors have provided suggested answers to the questions posed in the casebook itself. Because the casebook complements the textbook *Pharmacotherapy: A Pathophysiologic Approach,* 4th edition, case authors sometimes refer the reader to specific sections of the corresponding textbook chapter for more detailed explanations. After reading the relevant textbook chapter, studying the case materials, and considering the answers provided herein, instructors should be capable of guiding student discussions about individual cases. Because the students themselves will be considering therapeutic alternatives and making decisions about the case, instructors facilitating the discussions do not necessarily have to be content experts in the disease state specialty at hand.

The instructor should use the information in this *Instructor's Guide* as a reference source to focus and direct student discussions but not to provide lectures. The instructor should develop clearly defined objectives for the case, conduct the session so that students employ analytical and decision-making skills, and maximize participation of the students. Directed questions may be asked to focus the discussion and keep it on track, but the instructor should not dominate the conversation. Judicious use of a blackboard to highlight important points and summarize major issues can help to keep the discussion focused.

The answers provided in this manual should not necessarily be considered to be the single "right" answer. Just as in real-life clinical situations, there is often more than one acceptable plan or "right" answer. Students should be expected to arrive at their own answers and therapeutic plan, either individually or in small groups, and be able to defend their decisions orally or in written form. Experienced discussion leaders quickly learn that thoughtful students often arrive at decisions that are perfectly appropriate (and even novel) but that may have been overlooked by the instructor.

As with any tertiary reference source, the material contained herein may become obsolete or incomplete as new drugs are approved or practice standards change. Also, clinicians may disagree about any component of a therapeutic plan. Differences of opinion should be aired openly and the advantages and disadvantages of each plan be given careful consideration in discussions with students.

It is imperative that instructors unfamiliar with the *Pharmacotherapy Casebook* read the introductory chapters contained therein. Chapter 1 describes the structure and format of the cases, including the directed patient-focused approach that is applied to each case. Chapter 2 describes the philosophy of active learning strategies and how these techniques can be used to enhance the education of students. Chapter 3 describes an efficient approach to patient counseling, and Chapter 4 outlines two processes (SOAP and FARM notes) for documenting and communicating pharmaceutical care plans to other health care providers. The information contained in the latter two chapters should be applied to each of the individual scenarios described in the patient casebook. Students should be given the opportunity to practice their verbal counseling skills through simulated counseling sessions or by other means. They should also be required to compose a written communication note to other health professionals outlining their pharmacotherapeutic plan. Several independent self-study assignments are also included with each case that are designed for students to complete outside of class.

This *Instructor's Guide* is provided in limited distribution to instructors only and is not intended for use by students. Access by students would greatly diminish the usefulness of the casebook as a tool for learning and practicing the skills required to solve the drug-related problems of patients. Your ability to preserve the integrity of the manual will ensure that the casebook will retain its usefulness for students in subsequent years.

Readers of the first edition will note improvements in this second edition of the *Instructor's Guide*. Most importantly, the answers to case questions are more thorough and complete. The appearance of the guide has also been improved. A concise bullet-point format is employed, and drug names are printed in italics when they first appear in the Alternative Treatments section. The editors and case authors hope that you find both the casebook and instructor's guide to be valuable tools for developing the clinical problem-solving skills of your students. I invite your comments and suggestions for improving future editions of this educational product. Please also contact me if you have ideas for cases or are interested in serving as a case author in the future. My e-mail address is schwing+@pitt.edu.

I would like to thank the 165 case and chapter authors from 84 schools of pharmacy, hospitals, and other institutions who contributed their scholarly efforts to this casebook. My sincere appreciation is also extended to the other Section Editors of this casebook whose careful review and critique of the cases also contributed to the quality of the final product. I am also grateful for the secretarial assistance of Ms. Diane Kenna at the University of Pittsburgh School of Pharmacy.

I am indebted to the following colleagues for their assistance in obtaining and interpreting illustrations to assist in the learning process: Lydia C. Contis, MD, Division of Hematopathology, William Pasculle, MD, Department of Microbiology, and Orlando F. Gabriele, MD, Department of Radiology, University of Pittsburgh Medical Center (UPMC); Terence W. Starz, MD, Department of Medicine, University of Pittsburgh School of Medicine; Philip J. Nerti, RPh, Health Center Pharmacy Central, Pittsburgh; and Jason Lazar, MD, Winthrop University Hospital, Long Island, New York. The expert photography of Donald Koch and Lisa Dehainaut of the Creative Services/Medical Photography Department at UPMC is also gratefully acknowledged.

I would like to thank Cheryl L. Mehalik, Editor-in-Chief/Health Related Professions, Jeanmarie Roche, Senior Productions Editor, Robin Lazrus, Acquisitions Editor, and Jessica Hirshon, Associate Editor/Health Related Professions, at Appleton & Lange. Their cooperation, advice, and commitment were instrumental in bringing this publication from concept to reality. The meticulous production service provided by Bennie Sauls and the staff at Rainbow Graphics, LLC, are also appreciated.

My greatest debt of gratitude is owed to my wife, Donna, and children, Amanda and Steven, who shared in large measure in the production of this work by virtue of their sacrifice of hundreds of weekend and evening hours with me. Their understanding, support, and encouragement were vital to the successful completion of this book.

Terry L. Schwinghammer, PharmD, FASHP, FCCP, BCPS

PART ONE

Principles of Patient-focused Therapy

Terry L. Schwinghammer, PharmD, FCCP, FASHP, BCPS, Section Editor

CHAPTER 1

Introduction: How to Use This Casebook

Terry L. Schwinghammer, PharmD, FCCP, FASHP, BCPS

WHY DO CASE STUDIES ENHANCE LEARNING IN THE CURRICULUM?

The main goals of the case method are to develop the skills of self-learning, critical thinking, and decision making. When case studies are used in the formal curricula of the health care professions or for independent study by health care professionals, the focus of attention should be on learning the *process* of solving drug-related problems, rather than simply finding the scientific answers to the problems themselves. Students do learn scientific facts during the resolution of case study problems, but they usually learn more of them from their own independent study and from discussions with their peers than they do from the instructor. Information recall is reinforced by working on subsequent cases with similar problems. Traditional programs in the health care professions that rely heavily on the lecture format tend to concentrate on scientific content and the rote memorization of facts rather than the development of higher-order thinking skills.

Case studies provide the personal history of an individual patient and information about one or more health problems that must be solved. The learner's job is to work through the facts of the case, analyze the available data, gather more information, develop hypotheses, consider possible solutions, arrive at the optimal solution, and consider the consequences of his or her decisions.[1] The role of the teacher is to serve as coach and facilitator rather than as the source of "the answer." In fact, in many cases there is more than one acceptable answer to a given question. Because instructors do not need to possess the correct answer, they need not be experts in the field being discussed. Rather, the students become teachers and learn from each other through thoughtful discussion of the case.

FORMAT OF THE CASEBOOK

Background Reading

The patient cases in this casebook are intended to be used as the focal point for independent self-learning by individual students and for in-class problem-solving discussions by student groups and their instructors. If meaningful learning and discussion are to occur, students must come to discussion sessions prepared to discuss the case material rationally, propose reasonable solutions, and defend their pharmacotherapeutic plans. This requires a strong commitment to independent self-study prior to the session. The cases in this book were prepared to correspond with the scientific information contained in the fourth edition of *Pharmacotherapy: A Pathophysiologic Approach*.[2] For this reason, thorough familiarity with the corresponding textbook chapter is recommended as the primary method of student preparation. Other primary and tertiary literature should also be consulted as necessary to supplement the textbook readings. For some of the cases in this second edition of the casebook, there is no corresponding textbook chapter. It therefore becomes mandatory that students explore other reference materials for the necessary background information before completing the answers to these cases.

The cases selected for inclusion in the casebook represent common dis-

2 Principles of Patient-focused Therapy

eases likely to be encountered by general pharmacy practitioners. As a result, not all of the *Pharmacotherapy* textbook chapters have an associated patient case in the casebook. On the other hand, some of the textbook chapters have several corresponding cases in the casebook.

Levels of Case Complexity

In this second edition, each case is identified at the top of the first page as being one of three levels of complexity. Instructors may use this classification system to select cases for discussion that correspond to the experience level of the student learners. These levels are defined as follows:

Level I. An uncomplicated case; only the single textbook chapter is required to complete the case questions. Little prior knowledge of the disease state or clinical experience is needed.

Level II. An intermediate-level case; several textbook chapters or other reference sources may be required to complete the case. Prior clinical experience may be helpful in resolving all of the issues presented.

Level III. A complicated case; multiple textbook chapters and substantial clinical experience are required to solve all of the patient's drug-related problems.

Developing Ability Outcomes

At the beginning of each case, four to five ability outcomes are included for student reflection. The focus of these outcomes is on achieving competency in the clinical arena, not simply on learning isolated scientific facts. These items indicate some of the functions that the student should be expected to be able to perform in the clinical setting as a result of studying the case, preparing a pharmacotherapeutic plan, and defending his or her recommendations.

The ability outcomes provided are meant to serve as a starting point to stimulate student thinking, but they are not meant to be all inclusive. In fact, students should also generate their own personal ability outcomes and learning objectives for each case. By so doing, students take greater control of their own learning, which serves to improve personal motivation and the desire to learn.

PATIENT PRESENTATION

The format and organization of cases reflect those usually seen in actual clinical settings. The patient's medical history and physical examination findings are provided in the following standard outline format.

Chief Complaint

The chief complaint is a brief statement of the reason why the patient consulted the physician, *stated in the patient's own words*. In order to convey the patient's symptoms accurately, no medical terms or diagnoses are used.

HPI

History of present illness is a more complete description of the patient's symptom(s). General features usually included in the HPI are:

- Date of onset
- Precise location
- Nature of onset, severity, and duration
- Presence of exacerbations and remissions
- Effect of any treatment given
- Relationship to other symptoms, bodily functions, or activities (e.g., activity, meals)
- Degree of interference with daily activities

PMH

The past medical history includes serious illnesses, surgical procedures, and injuries the patient has experienced previously. Minor complaints (e.g., influenza, colds) are generally omitted.

FH

The family history includes the age and health of parents, siblings, and children. For deceased relatives, the age and cause of death are recorded. In particular, heritable diseases and those with a hereditary tendency are noted (e.g., diabetes mellitus, cardiovascular disease, malignancy, rheumatoid arthritis, obesity).

SH

The social history includes not only the social characteristics of the patient, but also the environmental factors and behaviors that may contribute to the development of disease. Items usually included are the patient's marital status, number of children, educational background, occupation, physical activity, hobbies, dietary habits, and use of tobacco, alcohol, or other drugs.

Meds

The medication history should include an accurate record of the patient's current prescription and non-prescription medication use. Because pharmacists possess extensive knowledge of the thousands of prescription and non-prescription products available, they can perform a valuable service to the health care team by obtaining a complete medication history that includes the names, doses, schedules, and duration of therapy for all medications, including herbal therapies and non-traditional remedies.

All

Allergies to drugs, food, pets, and environmental factors (e.g., grass, dust, pollen) are recorded. An accurate description of the reaction that occurred should also be included. Care should be taken to distinguish adverse drug effects ("upset stomach") from true allergy ("hives").

ROS

In the review of systems, the examiner questions the patient about the presence of symptoms related to each body system. In many cases, only the pertinent positive and negative findings are recorded. In a complete ROS, body systems are generally listed starting from the head and working toward the feet and may include the skin, head, eyes, ears, nose, mouth and throat, neck, cardiovascular, respiratory, gastrointestinal, genitourinary, endocrine, musculoskeletal, and neuropsychiatric systems. The purpose of the ROS is to evaluate the status of each body system and to prevent the omission of pertinent information. Information that was included in the HPI is not repeated in the ROS.

PE

The exact procedures performed during the physical examination vary depending upon the chief complaint and the patient's medical history. A suitable physical assessment textbook should be consulted for the specific procedures that may be conducted for each body system. The general sections for the PE are outlined as follows:

Gen (general appearance)
VS (vital signs)—blood pressure, pulse, respiratory rate, temperature; weight and height are usually included in this casebook, although they are not technically considered to be vital signs)
Skin (integumentary)
HEENT (head, eyes, ears, nose, and throat)
Lungs/Thorax (pulmonary)
Cor or CV (cardiovascular)
Abd (abdomen)
Genit/Rect (genitalia/rectal)
MS/Ext (musculoskeletal and extremities)
Neuro (neurologic)

Labs

The results of laboratory tests are included with almost all cases, and reference ranges for most tests are included in **Appendix A.** Occasionally, another reference text will be needed to identify the usual reference range. It should be noted that reference values differ among laboratories, so the values given in Appendix A should be considered as a general guide only. Institution-specific reference ranges should be used in actual clinical settings.

All of the cases include some physical examination and laboratory findings that are within normal limits. For example, a description of the cardiovascular examination may include a statement that the point of maximal impulse is at the fifth intercostal space; laboratory evaluation may include a serum sodium of 140 mEq/L. The presentation of actual findings (rather than simple statements that the heart examination and the serum sodium were normal) reflects what will be seen in actual clinical practice. More importantly, listing both normal and abnormal findings requires students to carefully assess the complete database and identify the pertinent positive and negative findings for themselves. A valuable portion of the learning process is lost if students are only provided with findings that are abnormal and are known to be associated with the disease being discussed.

The patients described in this casebook have been given fictitious names in order to humanize the situations and encourage students to remember that they will one day be caring for patients, not treating disease states. However, in the actual clinical setting, patient confidentiality is of utmost importance, and patient names should not be used during group discussions in patient care areas unless absolutely necessary. In order to develop student sensitivity to this issue, instructors may wish to avoid using these fictitious patient names during class discussions. In this casebook, patient names are given only in the initial presentation; they are not used in subsequent questions or other portions of the case.

The issues of race, ethnicity, and gender also deserve thoughtful consideration. The traditional format for case presentations usually begins with a description of the patient's age, race, and gender, as in: "The patient is a 65-year-old white male. . . ." Single-word racial labels such as "black" or "white" are actually of limited value in many cases and may actually be misleading in some instances.[3] For this reason, racial descriptors have been excluded from the opening line of each presentation. When ethnicity is pertinent to the case, this information is presented in the social history or physical examination. Finally, patients in this casebook are referred to as men or women, rather than males or females, to promote sensitivity to human dignity.

The patient cases in this casebook include medical abbreviations and drug brand names, just as medical records do in actual practice. Although these customs are sometimes the source of clinical problems, the intent of their inclusion is to make the cases as realistic as possible. A list of abbreviations used in the casebook is included in **Appendix B.** This list is limited to commonly accepted abbreviations; thousands more exist, which makes it difficult for the novice practitioner to efficiently assess patient databases. Most institutions have an approved list of accepted abbreviations; these lists should be consulted in practice to facilitate one's understanding and to avoid using abbreviations in the medical record that are not on the official approved list.

The casebook also contains some photographs of commercial drug products. These illustrations are provided as examples only and are not intended to imply endorsement of those particular products.

Pharmaceutical Care and Drug-related Problems

Modern drug therapy has played a crucial role in improving the health of people by enhancing the quality of life and extending life expectancy. The advent of biotechnology has led to the introduction of unique compounds for the prevention and treatment of disease that were unheard of a decade ago. Each year the Food and Drug Administration approves approximately two dozen new drug products that contain active substances that have never before been marketed in the United States. Although the cost of new therapeutic agents has received intense scrutiny in recent years, drug therapy actually accounts for a relatively small proportion of overall health care expenditures. Appropriate drug therapy is cost effective and may actually serve to reduce total expenditures by decreasing the need for surgery, preventing hospital admissions, and shortening hospital stays.

Improper use of prescription medications is a frequent and serious problem and has been estimated to cause approximately 200,000 deaths, 9 million hospitalizations, and expenditures of $76 billion annually in direct patient care costs. A societal need for better use of medications clearly exists. Widespread implementation of pharmaceutical care has the potential to positively impact this situation by the design, implementation, and monitoring of rational therapeutic plans to produce defined outcomes that improve the quality of patients' lives.[4]

The new mission of the pharmacy profession is to render pharmaceutical care. Schools of pharmacy are implementing new instructional strategies to prepare future pharmacists to provide pharmaceutical care. New entry-level PharmD programs have an increased emphasis on patient-focused care, as evidenced by more experiential training, especially in ambulatory care. Many programs are structured to promote self-directed learning, develop problem-solving and communication skills, and instill the desire for lifelong learning.

In its broadest sense, pharmaceutical care involves the identification, resolution, and prevention of potential drug-related problems. A drug-related problem is an event or circumstance involving drug therapy that actually or potentially interferes with the patient's ability to achieve an optimal medical outcome. Eight major types of drug-related problems have been identified that may potentially lead to an undesirable event that has physiologic, psychological, social, or economic ramifications.[5] These problems include:

1. *Untreated indications.* The patient needs drug therapy for a specific indication but is not receiving it.

2. *Improper drug selection.* The drug currently prescribed is either ineffective or toxic.
3. *Subtherapeutic dosage.* Too little of the correct drug has been prescribed.
4. *Failure to receive drugs.* The patient is not taking or receiving the drug prescribed.
5. *Overdosage.* Too much of the correct drug is being given.
6. *Adverse drug reactions.* The patient has a medical condition resulting from an adverse drug reaction.
7. *Drug interactions.* A medical problem has resulted from a drug–drug, drug–food, or drug–laboratory interaction.
8. *Drug use without indication.* The patient is taking a drug for which there is no valid medical indication.

Because this casebook is intended to be used in conjunction with the *Pharmacotherapy* textbook, one of its purposes is to serve as a tool for learning about the pharmacotherapy of disease states. For this reason, the primary problem to be identified and addressed for most of the patients in the casebook is the need for drug treatment of a specific medical indication (problem #1). Other actual or potential drug-related problems may coexist during the initial presentation or may develop during the clinical course of the disease.

Patient-focused Approach to Case Problems

In this casebook, each patient presentation is followed by a set of patient-focused questions that remain essentially the same for each case. These questions are applied consistently from case to case to demonstrate that a systematic patient care process can be successfully applied regardless of the underlying disease state(s). The questions are designed to enable students to identify and resolve problems related to pharmacotherapy. They help students recognize what they know and what they do not know, thereby guiding them in determining what information must be learned to satisfactorily resolve the patient's problems.[6] A description of each of the steps involved in solving drug-related problems is included in the following paragraphs.

1. Identification of real or potential drug-related problems

The first step in the patient-focused approach is to collect pertinent patient information, interpret it properly, and determine whether drug-related problems exist. Some authors prefer to divide this process into two or more separate steps because of the difficulty that inexperienced students may have performing these complex tasks simultaneously.[4,7] This step is analogous to documenting the subjective and objective patient findings in the SOAP format. It is important to differentiate the process of identifying the patient's drug-related problems from making a disease-related medical diagnosis. In fact, the medical diagnosis is known for the majority of patients seen by pharmacists. However, pharmacists must be capable of assessing the patient's database to determine whether drug-related problems exist that warrant a change in drug therapy. In the case of pre-existing chronic diseases such as asthma or rheumatoid arthritis, one must be able to assess information that may indicate a change in severity of the disease. This process involves reviewing the patient's symptoms, the signs of disease present on physical examination, and the results of laboratory and other diagnostic tests. Some of the cases require the student to develop complete patient problem lists. Potential sources for this information in actual practice include the patient or his or her advocate, the patient's physician or other health care professionals, and the patient's medical chart or other records.

After the drug-related problems are identified, the clinician should determine which of them are amenable to pharmacotherapy. Alternatively, one must also consider whether any of the problems could have been caused by drug therapy. In some cases (both in the casebook as well as in real life), not all of the information needed to make these decisions will be available. In that situation, providing precise recommendations for obtaining additional information needed to satisfactorily assess the patient's problems can be a valuable contribution to the patient's care.

2. Determination of the desired therapeutic outcome

After pertinent patient-specific information has been gathered and the patient's drug-related problems have been identified, the next step is to define the specific goals of pharmacotherapy. The primary therapeutic outcomes include:

- Cure of disease (e.g., bacterial infection)
- Reduction or elimination of symptoms (e.g., pain from cancer)
- Arresting or slowing of the progression of disease (e.g., rheumatoid arthritis)
- Preventing a disease or symptom (e.g., cardiovascular disease)

Other important outcomes of pharmacotherapy include:

- Not complicating or aggravating other existing disease states
- Avoiding or minimizing adverse effects of treatment
- Providing cost-effective therapy
- Maintaining the patient's quality of life

Sources of information for this step may include the patient or his or her advocate, the patient's physician or other health care professionals, medical records, and the *Pharmacotherapy* textbook or other literature references.

3. Determination of therapeutic alternatives

Once the intended outcome has been defined, attention can be directed toward identifying the kinds of treatments that might be beneficial in achieving that outcome. The clinician should ensure that all feasible pharmacotherapeutic alternatives available for achieving the predefined therapeutic outcome(s) are considered before choosing a single therapeutic regimen. Non-drug therapies (e.g., diet, exercise, psychotherapy) that might be useful should be included in the list of therapeutic alternatives when appropriate. Useful sources of information on therapeutic alternatives include the *Pharmacotherapy* textbook and other references, as well as the clinical experience of the health care provider and other involved health care professionals.

4. Design of an optimal individualized pharmacotherapeutic plan

The purpose of this step is to determine the drug, dosage form, dose, schedule, and duration of therapy that are best suited for a given patient. Individual patient characteristics should be taken into consideration when weighing the risks and benefits of each available therapeutic alternative. For example, an asthma patient who requires new drug therapy for hypertension might better tolerate treatment with a thiazide diuretic rather than a β-blocker. On the other hand, a hypertensive patient with gout may be better served by use of a β-blocker rather than a thiazide diuretic.

The reason for avoiding specific drugs should be stated in the therapeutic plan. Potential reasons for drug avoidance include drug allergy, drug–drug or drug–disease interactions, patient age, renal or hepatic impairment, adverse effects, poor compliance, and high treatment cost.

The specific dose selected may depend upon the indication for the drug. For example, the dose of aspirin used to treat rheumatoid arthritis is much higher than that used to prevent myocardial infarction. The likelihood of compliance with the regimen and patient tolerance come into play in the selection of dosage forms. The economic, psychosocial, and ethical factors that are applicable to the patient should also be given due consideration in design of the pharmacotherapeutic regimen. An alternative plan should also be in place that would be appropriate if the initial therapy fails or cannot be used.

5. Identification of parameters to evaluate the outcome

One must identify the clinical and laboratory parameters necessary to assess the therapy for achievement of the desired therapeutic outcome and for detection and prevention of adverse effects. The outcome parameters selected should be specific, measurable, achievable, directly related to the therapeutic goals, and have a defined end point. As a means of remembering these points, the acronym SMART has been used (*S*pecific, *M*easurable, *A*chievable, *R*elated, and *T*ime bound). If the goal was to cure a bacterial pneumonia, one should outline the subjective and objective clinical parameters (e.g., relief of chest discomfort, cough, and fever), laboratory tests (e.g., normalization of white blood cell count and differential), and other procedures (e.g., resolution of infiltrate on chest x-ray) that provide sufficient evidence of bacterial eradication and clinical cure of the disease. The intervals at which data should be collected are dependent upon the outcome parameters selected and should be established prospectively. It should be noted that expensive or invasive procedures may not be repeated after the initial diagnosis is made.

Adverse effect parameters must also be well defined and measurable. For example, it is insufficient to state that one will monitor for potential drug-induced "blood dyscrasias." Rather, one should identify the likely specific hematologic abnormality (e.g., anemia, leukopenia, or thrombocytopenia) and outline a prospective schedule for obtaining the appropriate parameters (e.g., obtain monthly hemoglobin/hematocrit, white blood cell count, or platelet count, respectively).

Monitoring for adverse events should be directed toward preventing or identifying serious adverse effects that have a reasonable likelihood of occurrence. For example, it is not cost effective to obtain periodic liver function tests in all patients taking a drug that causes mild hepatic abnormalities only rarely, such as omeprazole. On the other hand, serious patient harm may be averted by outlining a specific screening schedule for drugs associated more frequently with hepatic abnormalities, such as methotrexate for rheumatoid arthritis or troglitazone for diabetes mellitus.

6. Provision of patient counseling

The concept of pharmaceutical care is based on the existence of a covenantal relationship between the patient and the provider of care. Patients are our partners in health care, and our efforts may be for naught without their informed participation in the process. For chronic diseases such as diabetes mellitus, hypertension, and asthma, patients may have a greater role in managing their diseases than do health care professionals. Self-care is becoming more widespread as increasing numbers of prescription medications receive over-the-counter status. For these reasons, patients must be provided with sufficient information to enhance compliance, ensure successful therapy, and minimize adverse effects. Chapter 3 describes patient interview techniques that can be used efficiently to determine the patient's level of knowledge. Additional information can then be provided as necessary to fill in knowledge gaps. In the questions posed with individual cases, students will be asked to provide the kind of information that should be given to the patient who has limited knowledge of his or her disease. Under the Omnibus Budget Reconciliation Act (OBRA) of 1990, for patients who accept the offer of counseling, pharmacists should consider including the following items:

- Name and description of the medication (which may include the indication)
- Dosage, dosage form, route of administration, and duration of therapy
- Special directions or procedures for preparation, administration, and use
- Common and severe adverse effects, interactions, and contraindications (with the action required should they occur)
- Techniques for self-monitoring
- Proper storage
- Prescription refill information
- Action to be taken in the event of missed doses

Instructors may wish to have simulated patient interviewing sessions for new and refill prescriptions during the case discussions to practice medication counseling skills. Factual information should be provided as concisely as possible to enhance memory retention. An excellent source for information on individual drugs is the *USP-DI Volume II: Advice for the Patient*.[8]

7. Communication and implementation of the pharmacotherapeutic plan

The most well-conceived plan is worthless if it languishes without implementation because of inadequate communication with prescribers or other health care providers. Permanent, written documentation of significant recommendations in the medical record is important to ensure accurate communication among practitioners. Oral communication alone can be misinterpreted or transferred inaccurately to others. This is especially true because there are many drugs that sound alike when spoken but that have different therapeutic uses.

The SOAP format (*S*ubjective, *O*bjective, *A*ssessment, *P*lan) has been used by clinicians for many years to assess patient problems and communicate findings and plans in the medical record. However, writing SOAP notes may not be the optimal process for learning to solve drug-related problems, because several important steps taken by experienced clinicians are not always apparent and may be overlooked. For example, the precise therapeutic outcome desired is often unstated in SOAP notes, leaving others to presume what the desired treatment goals are. Health care professionals using the SOAP format also commonly move directly from an assessment of the patient (diagnosis) to outlining a diagnostic or therapeutic plan, without necessarily conveying whether careful consideration has been given to all available feasible diagnostic or therapeutic alternatives. The plan itself as outlined in SOAP notes may also give short shrift to the monitoring parameters that are required to ensure successful therapy and to detect and prevent adverse drug effects. Finally, there is often little suggestion provided as to the treatment information that should be conveyed to the most important individual involved: the patient. If SOAP notes are used for documenting drug-related problems, consideration should be given to including each of these components.

In Chapter 4 of this casebook, the FARM note is presented as a useful method of consistently documenting therapeutic recommendations and implementing plans.[9] This method can be used by students as an alternative to the SOAP note to practice communicating pharmacotherapeutic plans to other members of the health care team. Although preparation of written communication notes is not included in written form with each set of case questions, instructors are encouraged to include the composition of a SOAP or FARM note as one of the requirements for successfully completing each case study assignment.

Clinical Course

The process of pharmaceutical care entails an assessment of the patient's progress in order to ensure achievement of the desired therapeutic outcomes. A description of the patient's clinical course is included with many of the cases in this book to reflect this process. Some cases follow the progression of the patient's disease over months to years and include both inpatient and outpatient treatment. Follow-up questions directed toward ongoing evaluation and problem solving are included after presentation of the clinical course.

Self-study Assignments

Each case concludes with several study assignments related to the patient case or the disease state that may be used as independent study projects for students to complete outside class. These assignments generally require students to obtain additional information that is not contained in the corresponding *Pharmacotherapy* textbook chapter.

References

Selected literature references that are specific to the case at hand are included with most cases. These references may be useful to students for answering the questions posed. The *Pharmacotherapy* textbook contains a more comprehensive list of references pertinent to each disease state.

DEVELOPING ANSWERS TO CASE QUESTIONS

The use of case studies for independent learning and in-class discussion may be unfamiliar to many students. For this reason, it may initially be difficult for students to devise complete answers to the case questions. **Appendix C** contains the answers to three cases in order to demonstrate how case responses might be prepared and presented. Additional cases with questions and suggested answers may be found on the Internet at www.pharmacy.pitt.edu/ce/pharmacotherapy. The recommended answers provided in the appendix and on the Website were contributed by the authors of the cases, but they should not necessarily be considered the sole "right" answer. Thoughtful students who have prepared well for the discussion sessions may arrive at additional or alternative answers that are also appropriate.

With diligent self-study, practice, and the guidance of instructors, students will gradually acquire the knowledge, skills, and self-confidence to develop and implement pharmaceutical care plans for their own future patients. The goal of the casebook is to help students progress along this path of lifelong learning.

References

1. Herreid CF. Case studies in science: A novel method of science education. J College Sci Teaching 1994;23:221–229.
2. DiPiro JT, Talbert RL, Yee GC, et al., eds. Pharmacotherapy: A Pathophysiologic Approach, 4th ed. Stamford, CT, Appleton & Lange, 1999.
3. Caldwell SH, Popenoe R. Perceptions and misperceptions of skin color. Ann Intern Med 1995;122:614–617.
4. Hepler CD, Strand LM. Opportunities and responsibilities in pharmaceutical care. Am J Hosp Pharm 1990;47:533–543.
5. Strand LM, Morley PC, Cipolle RJ, et al. Drug-related problems: Their structure and function. Drug Intell Clin Pharm 1990;24:1093–1097.
6. Delafuente JC, Munyer TO, Angaran DM, Doering PL. A problem-solving active-learning course in pharmacotherapy. Am J Pharm Educ 1994;58:61–64.
7. Winslade N. Large-group problem-based learning: A revision from traditional to pharmaceutical care-based therapeutics. Am J Pharm Educ 1994;58:64–73.
8. Micromedex, Inc. USP-DI volume II: Advice for the Patient, 19h ed. Englewood, CO, 1999.
9. Canaday BR, Yarborough PC. Documenting pharmaceutical care: Creating a standard. Ann Pharmacother 1994;28:1292–1296.

CHAPTER 2
Active Learning Strategies

Elizabeth S. Gray, PharmD
Gretchen M. Tush, PharmD, BCPS
Cynthia K. Kirkwood, PharmD

INTRODUCTION

Everyone is faced with situations daily that require use of problem-solving skills. For example, trying to find the quickest route to a gas station in a major city, or determining the most effective method to train your dog not to bark at the neighbors. In the hospital, you may need to identify the etiology of nausea and vomiting in a patient on your internal medicine service. In order to solve problems, we call upon our previous experiences with similar situations, observe, investigate, ask appropriate questions, and finally come to a conclusion or resolution.

Students who graduate from pharmacy school will have the opportunity to pursue many different career paths. They must be prepared to take direct responsibility for patient outcomes by practicing pharmaceutical care. Pharmacists will need to use their skills in communications, problem solving, independent learning, drug information retrieval, and knowledge of disease state management.[1,2] In order to prepare students to practice in this manner, pharmacy educators are moving away from traditional methods of teaching and are using active learning strategies in the classroom. In therapeutics courses, students are given actual written patient cases as the basis for learning. Students may be asked to identify the significant findings, develop a drug-related problem list, create an assessment statement, consider all feasible therapeutic alternatives, make therapeutic recommendations, develop a monitoring plan, formulate a written communication note for other health care providers, and decide how they would educate the patient about new drug therapies. This process actively engages students in problem solving because it requires them to integrate knowledge gained in other areas of the curriculum with specific patient information. As a result, students learn skills that they will use on a daily basis in their future practice sites.

TRADITIONAL TEACHING

In pre-pharmacy course work, and even in some pharmacy school courses, most students are taught using traditional methods. The student comes to class, and the teacher lectures on a predetermined subject that does not require student preparation. Students are passive recipients of information and are usually tested by written examinations that employ a multiple-choice or short answer format. With this method, students are tested primarily on their ability to recall isolated facts and do not learn to apply their knowledge to situations that they will ultimately encounter in pharmacy practice. They are rewarded only by receiving an exam or course grade that may or may not reflect their actual ability to use knowledge to improve patient care. In order to teach students to be lifelong learners, it is essential to stimulate them to be inquisitive and actively involved with the learning that takes place in the classroom. This requires that teachers move away from more comfortable teaching methods and learn new techniques that will help students "learn to learn."

ACTIVE LEARNING STRATEGIES

During the last 15 years, active learning has been defined in many ways, and various methods are described in the educational literature. Simply put, active learning means involving students in the learning process.[3] In classes with active learning formats, students are involved in much more than listening. The transmission of information is de-emphasized and replaced with the development of skills. Most proponents agree that active learning allows students to become engaged in the learning process while developing cognitive skills. Learning is reinforced when students actually apply their knowledge to new situations.[4] In order for active learning to be successful, it requires willing students, innovative teachers, and administrative support within the school.[5] Control of learning must be shifted from the teacher to the students; this provides an opportunity for students to become active participants in their own learning. Although it sounds frightening at first, students *can* take control of their own learning. Knowledge of career and life goals can help students make decisions about how to spend their educational time. Warren[6] identifies several traits that prepare students for future careers:

- Analytical thinking
- Polite assertiveness
- Tolerance
- Communication skills
- Understanding of one's own physical well-being
- The ability to continue to teach oneself after graduation

After going through the active learning process, most students realize that knowledge is easily acquired, but developing critical thinking skills aids in lifelong learning.[5]

Teachers implement active learning exercises into classes in a variety of ways. Some of the active learning strategies give students the opportunity to pause and recall information, cooperate and collaborate in groups, solve problems, and generate questions.[7] More advanced methods include use of simulation, role-playing, debates, peer teaching, problem-based learning, and case studies.[8] Tests and quizzes evaluate student comprehension of material. Each of these strategies allows students to demonstrate their skills.

Didactic lectures can be enhanced by several active learning strategies. The "pause procedure" is designed to enhance student retention and comprehension of material.[9] It involves 15- to 20-minute mini-lectures with 2- to 3-minute pauses for students to rework their notes, discuss the material with their peers for clarification, and develop questions.[10] This strategy can be incorporated into a 50-minute lecture up to three times. Students are able to assess their understanding of the material and formulate opinions. The pause procedure is a useful method for classes that require retention of factual information.[8] With the "think-pair-share" exercise, students are asked to write down the answer to a question and turn to a classmate to compare answers. This method provides immediate feedback to students.[11]

Another active learning technique for classroom sessions is to involve the students in short writing assignments. Writing helps students identify knowledge deficits, clarify understanding of the material, and organize thoughts in a logical manner. Students can be asked to write questions related to the reading assignment and submit them for discussion at the next class session. Alternatively, students can formulate questions and answers before class, and then discuss them in small groups. The "shared paragraph exercise" requires students to write a paragraph at the end of class summarizing the major concepts that were presented. The paragraph is then shared with a partner to clarify the material and receive feedback.[8] Discussions of any misconceptions can be conducted in class or one-on-one with the teacher. Sample test questions may also be used to assess student comprehension of the presentation and facilitate class discussion.

Tests and quizzes are effective tools to help students review the class presentations or reading assignments. Quizzes can be administered several times during class and may or may not be graded. Quizzes given at the beginning of class help stimulate students to review information they did not know and listen for clarification during lecture. Quizzes at the end of the class session allow students to use their problem-solving skills by applying what they have just learned to a patient case or problem.

Problem-solving skills can be developed during a class period by applying knowledge of disease state management to a patient case. Application reinforces the previously learned material and helps students understand the importance of the topic in a real-life situation. Problem-based learning (PBL) is a teaching method in which a problem is used as the stimulus for developing critical thinking and problem-solving skills for acquiring new knowledge. The process of PBL starts with the student identifying the problem in a case. The student spends time either alone or in a group exploring and analyzing the problem and identifying learning resources needed to solve the problem. After acquiring the knowledge, the student applies it to solve the problem.[12] Small or large groups can be established for case discussions to help students develop communication skills, respect for other students' opinions, satisfaction for contributing to the discussion, and the ability to give and accept criticism.[12]

Cooperative or collaborative learning strategies involve students in the generation of knowledge.[8] Students are randomly assigned to groups of 4 to 6 at the beginning of the school term. Several times during the term, each group is given a patient case and a group leader is selected. Each student in the group volunteers to work on a certain portion of the case. The case is discussed in class and each member receives the same grade. After students have finished working in their small groups or during large group sessions, the teacher serves as a facilitator of the discussion rather than as a lecturer. The students actively participate in the identification and resolution of the problem. The integration of this technique helps with development of skills in decision making, conflict management, and communication.[7] Group discussions help students develop concepts from the material presented, clarify ideas, and develop new strategies for clinical problem solving. These skills are essential for lifelong learning and will be used by the students throughout their careers.

CASE STUDIES

Case studies are used by a number of pharmacy schools to teach disease state management.[1,13,14] Case studies are a written description of a real-life problem or situation. Only the facts are provided, usually in chronological sequence similar to what would be encountered in a patient care setting. Many times, as in real life, the information given is incomplete or important details are not available. When working through a case, the student must distinguish between relevant and irrelevant facts and become accustomed to the fact that there is no single "correct" answer. The use of cases actively involves the student in the analysis of facts and details of the case, selection of a solution to the problem, and defense of his or her solution through discussion of the case.[15]

Students enrolled in such courses find that the case study method requires a large amount of preparation time outside of class. In class, active participation is essential for the maximum learning benefit to be achieved. Because of the various backgrounds of the students in class, students learn different perspectives when dealing with patient problems. Some general steps proposed by McDade[15] for students when preparing for class include:

- Skim the text quickly to establish the broad issues of the case and the types of information presented for analysis.
- Reread the case very carefully, underlining key facts as you go.
- Note on scratch paper the key issues and problems. Next, go through the case again and sort out the relevant considerations and decisions for each problem.

- Prioritize problems and alternatives.
- Develop a set of recommendations to address the problems.
- Evaluate your decisions.

EXPECTATIONS OF STUDENTS AND TEACHERS

Active learning provides students with an opportunity to take a dynamic role in the learning process. The students are expected to participate in class discussions and be creative in formulating their own opinions. This method also requires that students listen and be respectful of the thoughts and opinions of their classmates. Assigned readings and homework must be completed before class in order to use class time efficiently for questions that are not answered in other reference material. In order to prepare answers or appropriate therapeutic recommendations, students may have to look beyond the reference materials provided by the teacher; they may have to perform literature searches and use the library to retrieve additional information. It is important for students to justify their recommendations. The active learning strategies outlined previously allow students to comprehend the material presented, participate in peer discussions, and formulate opinions as in real-life situations.

In order to implement active learning strategies in the classroom, teachers must overcome the anxiety that change often creates. Experimenting with active learning methods such as the pause technique and slowly implementing a change in the classroom may work best. Using any of the active learning strategies requires teachers to encourage as much classroom discussion as possible instead of lecturing. Use of a wireless microphone is helpful in encouraging student participation in large classrooms. Teachers should make an effort to learn the names of all students so they can more easily interact with them. In addition, teachers should have a preconceived plan for how the class discussion will go and stick to it. Hutchings recommends envisioning what the chalkboard should look like at the end of the session before beginning.[16]

MAXIMIZING ACTIVE LEARNING OPPORTUNITIES: ADVICE TO STUDENTS

Taking initiative is the key to deriving the benefits of active learning. It is crucial to recognize the three largest squelchers of initiative: laziness, fear of change, and force of habit.[17] You will find that time management is important. Be sure to schedule adequate time for studying, prepare for class by reading ahead, use transition times wisely, identify the times of day that you are most productive, and focus on the results rather than the time to complete an activity.[6]

In active learning, you are expected to talk about what you are learning, write about it, relate it to past experiences, and apply it to your daily life. In a sense, you repeatedly manipulate the information until it becomes a part of you. Some techniques to use when studying are to compare, contrast, and summarize similarities and differences between disease states and pharmacotherapy. In class, take advantage of every opportunity to present your own work. Attempt to relate personal experiences or outside events to topics discussed in class, and always be an active participant in class or group discussions.[18]

When reading assignments, summarize the information and take notes. These will be your notes to study for the course exams and to review for the pharmacy state board examination. While taking notes in class, leave a wide margin on the left to write down questions that you generate later when reviewing the notes.[11] Alternatively, make lists of questions from class or readings to discuss with your colleagues or faculty or try to answer them on your own. When time allows, seek out recent information on subjects that interest you. In class, always try to determine the "big picture."[18]

Some other methods for maximizing active learning are to review corrected assignments and exams for information that you do not understand and seek clarification from faculty. Complete assignments promptly and minimize short-term memorization. Attend class regularly and ask questions when you do not understand something. Give others a chance to contribute and try not to embarrass other students.[18]

In active learning, much of what you learn you will learn on your own. You will probably find that you read more, but you will gain understanding from reading. At the same time, you are developing a critical lifelong learning skill. Your reading will become more "depth processing" in which you focus on:

- The intent of the article
- Actively integrating what you read with previous parts of the text
- Trying to use your own ability to make a logical construction
- Thinking about the functional role of the different parts of an argument

In writing, consider summarizing the major points of each class. Writing about a topic develops critical thinking, communication, and organization skills. In classes that involve active learning, you may write for "think-pair-share" exercises, quizzes, summary paragraphs, and other activities. Stopping to write allows you to reflect on the information you have just heard and reinforces learning. Discussions may occur in large or small groups. Discussing material helps you to apply your knowledge, verbalize the medical and pharmacologic terminology, engage in active listening, think critically, be a leader or a follower, and develop interpersonal skills. When working in groups, all members should participate in problem solving. Teaching others is an excellent way to learn the subject matter.[6]

HOW TO USE THE CASEBOOK

This casebook has been prepared to assist in the development of each student's understanding of a disease and its management as well as problem-solving skills. It is important for students to realize that learning and understanding the material will be guided through problem solving. Students are encouraged to solve each of the problems individually or with others in a study group before discussion of the problem and topic in class. Being prepared for class is essential!

As problems are solved, the student begins to understand that each problem may not have a single solution or answer. The student will begin to appreciate the variety and complexity of diseases that are encountered in different patient populations. In some cases, more detailed information from the patient will play a pivotal role in drug therapy selection and monitoring. In others, most of the diagnoses may be resolved through use of laboratory analysis or specific medical tests. Some cases may require a much more in-depth assessment of the patient's disease state and treatment rendered so far. Other cases may involve initiation of both nonpharmacologic and pharmacologic therapy, ranging from single to multiple drug regimens.

Regardless of disease and/or treatment complexity, students must rely on knowledge previously learned in the areas of anatomy, biochemistry, microbiology, immunology, physiology, pathophysiology, medicinal chemistry, pharmacology, pharmacokinetics, and physical assessment. As a consequence, it will be necessary for the student to review previous notes, handouts, or textbooks. Students can use MEDLINE searches for primary literature, drug reference books, the Internet, and faculty experts as information sources. These resources and the textbook *Pharmacotherapy: A Pathophysiologic Approach* will be essential in supporting each student's ability to solve the problems successfully. Understanding the usefulness and limitations of these resources will be beneficial in the future. Likewise, discussions in study groups and class should lead to a further understanding of disease states and treatment strategies.

SUMMARY

The use of case studies and other active learning strategies will enhance the development of essential skills necessary to practice in any setting, including community pharmacy, health-system pharmacy, long-term care, home care, managed care, and the pharmaceutical industry. The role of the pharmacist will change dramatically in the next century; thus, it is important for students to acquire knowledge and develop the lifetime skills required for continued learning. Teachers who incorporate active learning strategies into the classroom are facilitating the development of lifelong learners who will be able to adapt to any changes that may occur in the profession of pharmacy.

References

1. Winslade N. Large-group problem-based learning: A revision from traditional to pharmaceutical care-based therapeutics. Am J Pharm Educ 1994;58:64–73.
2. Kane MD, Briceland LL, Hamilton RA. Solving problems. US Pharmacist 1995;20:55–74.
3. Tanenbaum BG, Cross DS, Tilson ER, et al. How to make active learning work for you. Radiol Technol 1998;69:374–376.
4. Moffett BS, Hill KB. The transition to active learning: A lived experience. Nurs Educator 1997;22:44–47.
5. Rangachari PK. Active learning: In context. Adv Physiol Educ 1995;13:S75–S80.
6. Warren G. Carpe Diem: A Student Guide to Active Learning. Landover, MD, University Press of America, 1996.
7. Bonwell CC, Eison JA. Active Learning: Creating Excitement in the Classroom. ASHE-ERIC Higher Education Report no. 1. Washington, DC, George Washington University, School of Education and Human Development, 1991.
8. Shakarian DC. Beyond lecture: Active learning strategies that work. JOPERD May–June 1995, 21–24.
9. Ruhl KL, Hughs CA, Schloss PJ. Using the pause procedure to enhance lecture recall. Teacher Educ Spec Educ 1987;10:14–18.
10. Rowe MB. Pausing principles and their effects on reasoning in science. In: Brawer FB, ed. Teaching the Sciences. New Directions for Community Colleges, no. 31. San Francisco, Jossey-Bass, 1980.
11. Elliot DD. Promoting critical thinking in the classroom. Nurs Educator 1996;21:49–52.
12. Walton HJ, Matthews MB. Essentials of problem-based learning. Med Educ 1989;23:542–558.
13. Hartzema AG. Teaching therapeutic reasoning through the case-study approach: Adding the probabilistic dimension. Am J Pharm Educ 1994;58:436–440.
14. Delafuente JC, Munyer TO, Angaran DM, et al. A problem-solving active-learning course in pharmacotherapy. Am J Pharm Educ 1994;58:61–64.
15. McDade SA. An Introduction to the Case Study Method: Preparation, Analysis, and Participation. New York, Teachers College Press, 1988.
16. Hutchings P. Using Cases to Improve College Teaching. Washington, DC, American Association of Higher Education, 1993.
17. Robbins A. Awaken the Giant Within. New York, Simon & Schuster, 1991.
18. Chickering AW, Gamson ZF, Barsi LM. Seven Principles for Good Practice in Undergraduate Education. Racine, WI, The Johnson Foundation, 1989.

CHAPTER 3

Case Studies in Patient Communication

Marie E. Gardner, PharmD
Richard N. Herrier, PharmD

PATIENT CASES

This guide contains the suggested answers to each question posed in the casebook. These facilitator's answers are meant as guides to direct discussions with the students about how to best approach each situation.

Case No. 1: Sally M. Johnson

> 1. Before talking with the patient, what concerns do you have about counseling this patient? What else would you like to know about your patient?

A review of Sally's profile indicates that she is a middle-aged woman who has been recently diagnosed with breast cancer. *Of greatest concern is her emotional state* at the moment of the counseling, but keep in mind that this is an issue to be evaluated every time you see this patient. It is not known whether she has family. What will her support system be to help her deal with having cancer? Does she have children? Is she wondering about her responsibilities as a mother, wife, or caregiver, and who will take over if she dies? It would be helpful to have this information. How should one address this? The pharmacist must evaluate the patient as the consultation proceeds. Sally may be very open and use "talk" therapy to discuss all sorts of issues. The pharmacist needs the skills of good listening, reflective responding, and perhaps limit-setting. Avoid saying, "I know how you feel" unless you have had her experience, or she may not be open to discussing her problems. As the consultation unfolds, look for opportunities to address her concerns. For example, she may say, "What's going to happen to all those people who depend on me?" An appropriate response might be, "It sounds as if you are worried about who will take care of your family if something happens." This reflecting response shows the patient that you have some sense of her thoughts and concerns. You need not say more than this. Listen for her next comment, and continue using reflecting responses when "feelings" issues arise.

This patient is no doubt in one of the stages of death described by Kübler-Ross. These stages include shock and illness denial, anger, bargaining, depression, and acceptance. Patients may move through these stages at various speeds, may experience only some of them, or may get "stuck" in one stage. Sally may be in denial; if so, her affect may be happy or unconcerned. She may be angry, and this anger may be displaced on you, as when patients complain of the high cost of medication or having to wait too long for their prescriptions to be filled. She may appear depressed and unwilling to take the medication or inattentive during the consultation. Watch the patient's body language and eye contact as you counsel her. A tired body posture and poor eye contact may suggest that she is depressed and/or overwhelmed by the news of her cancer. Use "repeating back" when you think she is not listening. For example, the *final verification* is a useful strategy.

It would be helpful to know what type of cancer she has, what was done during the surgery, what her prognosis is, and whether tamoxifen is being given as prevention or treatment. Is she undergoing other chemotherapy, and might we expect other medications to be taken (e.g., antiemetics or analgesics)?

> 2. How are you going to begin the consultation?

First, protect the patient's privacy and dignity. Second, use the *Prime Question* technique since it is a new prescription. With respect to process issues in

Sally's case, the counseling should be conducted in as private an area as possible. Pay attention to any nonverbal signs that indicate distress or disinterest. If such signs appear, ask the patient if there is a better time to discuss the medication. It may be helpful to ask the patient outright, "How do you feel about taking this medication?" Sometimes the direct approach is most revealing. Patients have the right to refuse treatment. Since the pharmacist is often not equipped with the entire clinical history of the patient, it is best to refer the patient back to the physician or call the physician yourself if the patient indicates she will not comply.

The facilitator may wish to discuss with the group what to do if the patient refuses counseling up front. The patient may be too overwhelmed to sit through the consultation or may decide there is no hope and the medication is not worth taking, and thus may not want the counseling.

3. Listed below are three different responses by the patient to the first *Prime Question*. For each statement, consider what each statement reveals about what the patient knows or feels, and state what should happen next in the consultation.

*Patient Response A: *"He gave it to me after my surgery."*

The patient seems "closed" and doesn't want to talk about cancer. The fact that she said "surgery" without attaching other descriptors may indicate that she is embarrassed about it or is in a stage of illness denial. It is possible that the patient is unaware of her diagnosis. Alternatively, she may be uncomfortable physically and wants to end the conversation quickly. Observing the patient's non-verbal signs may be helpful, but keep in mind that in such a case there can be many and mixed emotions. Her answer does not indicate whether she knows what the medication is for. One option is to proceed with additional questioning such as, "What is it supposed to do for you?" Another option is to proceed with the counseling and see whether the patient reveals the diagnosis. This option may be preferred, because dealing with factual information is an acceptable way to handle sensitive issues.

An appropriate response would be to proceed to *Prime Question* #2 and assess the patient's verbal and non-verbal responses throughout the rest of the consultation.

Patient Response B: *"I just had surgery for breast cancer."*

The patient has already voiced the word "cancer," indicating that she is aware of her diagnosis. It would be ideal to find out what the patient knows about tamoxifen's use, but this answer will suffice, given time constraints. The appropriate response is to proceed to the second *Prime Question*. Depending on the patient's tone of voice and expression, an empathic response may be needed. An example is, "It sounds as if you've been through a lot."

Patient Response C: *"I know what it's for."*

This kind of response may indicate several things. It may be that the patient has full understanding of what the medication is for, that the patient is in a hurry and doesn't want to talk about it, or that the patient is unwilling to discuss it for some reason. It is probably best to reserve judgment and move to the second *Prime Question*. Keep monitoring the patient's verbal and non-verbal expressions, and look for opportunities to ask pointed questions.

4. Listed below are three different responses to the second *Prime Question*. Consider what each tells you, and state what you would do next in the consultation.

Patient Response A: *"I'm going to take it twice a day."*

The patient's response indicates that she already knows the correct dosage. You can move to *Prime Question* #3.

Patient Response B: *"It's on the label, isn't it?"*

The patient is either in a hurry or is in denial and is closed to talking about her clinical situation. The patient's non-verbal behavior would be key in interpreting the difference. In either situation, the patient presents a barrier to learning about the medication. If you want to press on with the consultation, first use a reflecting response such as "I can see that you have a lot on your mind, but this will just take a minute." The best solution is to find a mutually convenient time to discuss the medication. Ask the patient when it would be good to call her and discuss it. Heavy-handed tactics to convince the patient of the importance of knowing about the medication will be fruitless.

Patient Response C: *"I don't remember. He didn't tell me."*

The patient's body language may again indicate that she is not in a receptive mood. Poor eye contact, fidgeting, or a slumped body posture may indicate a depressed or anxious state. The appropriate response is to review the dosage instructions and proceed to *Prime Question* #3.

5. Listed below are three different responses to the third *Prime Question*. Consider what each tells you, and state what you would do next in the consultation.

Patient Response A: *"I hope it will keep my cancer in check."*

The patient is optimistic and expects a good response. The response says nothing about her knowledge of adverse effects. Provide positive feedback (e.g., "I hope so, too"). Ask "What side effects did the doctor tell you about?" and provide necessary missing information. Then close the consultation with the *final verification*.

Patient Response B: *"The doctor says things look good, but I thought I heard something about uterine cancer?"*

The patient seems optimistic and was listening to the doctor, but she is concerned about deleterious effects. She may be worried that the situation is worse than the doctor said. She may be in denial if she focuses concern on a side effect that has not yet happened to avoid dealing with the problem she already has. Depending on your assessment of the situation, appropriate responses include providing information on side effects orally and with written supplements. An empathic response may be warranted. For instance, "I can see that this (uterine cancer risk) concerns you. Let's talk about that." Referral to her physician would be appropriate.

Patient Response C: *"Nothing. I'm not sure anything is going to help me now."*

---

*Patient statements A, B, and C do not necessarily correspond throughout the consultation.

Pharmacists are often uncomfortable with this type of response. It triggers personal emotional reactions to the situation. You may be tempted to agree with the patient, but you know that is not the appropriate response. Avoid giving false reassurance. Statements such as "I'm sure things will work out" or "Medicines can do wonders these days" completely undermine the bond of trust between you and the patient. The patient's statement also conveys a suggestion that she will be non-compliant. Avoid trying to talk her into taking the medication.

The best *first* response is an empathic response. It must be carefully stated, since the patient is voicing despair over her condition. Acceptable examples include "It sounds as if you don't think the medication will help" or "I can see this is very difficult for you." Use of *minimal facilitators* (brief remarks to keep the conversation going) is good, as is silence and appropriate touching. Minimal facilitators include "I see," "Oh, my," and similar remarks commonly used.

Offer help at the patient's request and do not force the consultation. The opportunity to ask the patient "How do you feel about taking this medication?" may present itself. Despite the fact that the patient says "nothing can help," she is at the pharmacy, with some need. Facilitators may wish to discuss from their own experience what it means when a patient presents to the pharmacist for a medication they appear not to want to take. Confrontational strategies (e.g., "If you don't want the medicine, why are you here?") sound accusatory and create more barriers to patient–pharmacist interaction. Another option is to ask, "All right, so you don't want to take the medication. How do you think I can help?" The objective is to have the patient specify what he or she wants from you without consuming your time or having to retread ground already covered. Once the patient's specific request is identified, it is usually easy to determine whether you can meet it, or whether the patient needs referral to another party.

In cases where the patient is willing to try the medication and the *Prime Questions* have been addressed, close the consultation with the *final verification* and an offer to help.

Case No. 2: Thomas Gordon

> 1. What concerns do you have based on review of the patient's medication profile? What else would you like to know about your patient? Before talking with the patient, what concerns do you have about counseling this patient? What are the goals of the consultation?

This middle-aged patient has diabetes and an infection. The two main goals of the consultation are to verify understanding of proper use of the new medication and explore issues related to his diabetes, including potential non-compliance with therapy.

Consultation skills needed for this case include profile review, use of the *Prime Question* technique for new prescriptions, recognizing "pink flags" during counseling, and probing a new symptom with the *Key Symptom Questions*. Also, either a *reflecting response* or a *supportive compliance probe* will be needed to address the lateness of the tolazamide (*assume that he does not get the medication elsewhere*).

An important concern is possible poor compliance as manifested by late refills on the glipizide. This is objective evidence that must be verified during the consultation. One reason for his non-compliance could be that he is asymptomatic. His profile indicates that he is otherwise healthy. The fact that he is a busy person may mean that he "can't be bothered" with taking medication or can't fit it into his schedule. Therefore, both functional and attitudinal barriers to compliance may exist and might need to be explored during the consultation.

Specific points of information one would want to know include whether he is under treatment for diabetes at present (since he may be getting his medication elsewhere), how he monitors his clinical condition, and what he perceives to be the risks and benefits of treatment.

> 2. How are you going to begin the consultation?

Begin the consultation with the *Prime Questions* addressing the cephalexin prescription. Reserve discussion of the antidiabetic medication until the new prescription has been reviewed. During the consultation, listen carefully to the patient's answers for any mention of his diabetes, as that would be an appropriate moment to discuss the glipizide use.

> 3. Listed below are Tom's responses to the *Prime Questions*. Consider what each response reveals about what the patient knows or feels, and state how you would address any concerns you detect.

Pharmacist: "What did the doctor tell you the medication was for?"
Tom: "He said he was giving me an antibiotic for this infection on my arm. It started as just a scratch, but it's gotten really bad."
Pharmacist: "How did the doctor tell you to take the medicine?"
Tom: "I don't know. He said it was on the label. I know I'm supposed to take it all."
Pharmacist: "What did the doctor tell you to expect?"
Tom: "I guess it will kill the infection and make the cut heal."

Tom's answer to *Prime Question* #1 indicates that he knows the purpose of the medication. His non-verbal language may indicate worry about the infection. If it does, use reflecting responses. If Tom's comment about the scratch doesn't seem to concern him, then proceed to *Prime Question* #2.

Tom's answer to the second *Prime Question* suggests that the physician didn't explain all the instructions for taking the medication, or that Tom was preoccupied when instructed. Therefore, the first goal is to "fill in the blanks" with the needed information for proper medication-taking behavior. Include additional open ended questions such as "What does four times a day mean to you?" or "How will you fit this into your busy schedule?"

The fact that he knows to take it all may mean that he has learned this from past experience or from the doctor's advice. The words "supposed to" often represent subtle suggestions about a patient's intent. Statements such as "My doctor says I'm supposed to . . ." or "I'm supposed to take it three times a day" herald uncertainty or ambivalence in the patient's view. Since patients want to please and *not* to be scolded for not following instructions, they may use such words to indicate what is supposed to be happening versus what is reality. Often, we ignore these "pink flags" or subtle clues to a potential problem and simply agree with the patient. Recognizing "pink flags" and using reflecting responses in follow-up help reveal the truth in a non-threatening manner. Contrast Tom's response, "I know *I'm supposed to* take it all" with "I'm going to take it all." His remark indicates that he knows the right thing to do, but will he do it? Is he concerned about how to remember to take it? Is he thinking he recovered in the past with fewer days of therapy? Is he thinking it's not a serious infection, and he doesn't need all the medication? Since you do not know the basis for the patient's hesitation, ask. Do this by using a reflecting response such as "It sounds as though you're unsure about that." The word "unsure" reflects the ambivalence within the patient. The patient must make the next move. *Don't presume;* let the patient tell you his concern. The next statement usually reveals a more specific barrier such as the questions listed above, which you can then address.

Regarding the third *Prime Question*, the patient says "*I guess* it will kill the infection . . ." Again, the "pink flag" reflects some uncertainty, perhaps about the efficacy of the medication, perhaps about the condition itself. When patients use these words often during the consultation, it may reflect attitudinal issues. Patients may be in denial about their illness, disagree with the doctor about what they have, or be ambivalent about treatment. Since patients may not be consciously aware of these internal inconsistencies, their hesitations and concerns appear in disguise. Caution must be exercised in applying reflecting responses to not "polly parrot" everything the patient says. Because the patient understood the purpose of the medication, he should expect the infection to clear and the cut to heal. A reflecting response is not really needed here. If you think the patient is concerned that the antibiotic is not going to work, you might ask directly, "Are you concerned that the antibiotic won't be effective?" If the patient agrees, a simple "What makes you think/say that?" could be asked next. If you choose not to probe into this last concern or are finished addressing it, then proceed to the *final verification*.

Two opportunities exist for addressing the potential non-compliance with glipizide. His answer to the second *Prime Question* might suggest that he did not anticipate that the scratch would become infected. During consultation, pay attention to the patient's body language while he says this. Does he look worried? Is he curious about why it is worse than expected? If so, a helpful response would be a reflecting response used to probe for more information on what the patient knows. For example, "It seems as though you weren't expecting that." The patient may agree. One option in the consultation is to discuss *at that moment* the relationship between glucose control in diabetes and infections. Avoid critical statements that "point the finger," such as "You got this infection because your diabetes is not in control." Although perhaps true, this communication strategy will put the patient in a defensive posture, creating a barrier to trust and openness. A *universal statement* which makes inferences to the patient can be used, such as "Patients with diabetes are at risk for infections like this." If the patient seems interested, more discussion is in order. Providing such information may help the patient realize the benefits of complying with both therapies. What happens if the consultation about the antibiotic proceeded without an opportunity to mention the diabetes? In that case, after the *final verification* for cephalexin, use a *supportive compliance probe* to open the discussion of the glipizide. "Mr. Gordon, I noticed while reviewing your profile that you are about two months late in getting your glipizide refilled."

> 4. Listed next is Tom's answer to your inquiry about the glipizide. Consider what the statement reveals, and state how you would address his concerns. "Yeah, well, I'm really busy with my business and it's hard to remember to take it."

The patient is raising a functional or practical barrier to complying with the regimen. However, this is a once-a-day medication that should be more easily incorporated into a daily habit. Therefore, one might wonder whether the "forgetfulness" is really an excuse. In any case, since the goal is helping the patient find a way to remember taking the medication, it is appropriate to ask the patient, "What daily activity would remind you to take your medicine?" Partnering with the patient and helping him choose the system are more likely to be associated with change on the patient's part.

Case No. 3: William Hodges

> 1. Review the patient's profile. What concerns do you have based on your review of the patient profile? What are the goals of the consultation?

The patient's profile does not contain any evidence of compliance problems by pill count, except that he did not obtain refills for digoxin and nifedipine before he went on vacation in May. If no problems are detected during counseling, the pharmacist could gently probe using a *supportive compliance probe* or a *universal statement* after the consultation was completed.

Supportive compliance probe: "I noticed that you didn't pick up a vacation supply of your digoxin or nifedipine in May."
Universal statement: "Many of our customers have trouble remembering to take their medication. What kind of problems have you encountered?"

> 2. How are you going to begin the consultation?

Begin by introducing yourself and identifying the patient: "I'm _____, your pharmacist, and you are _____? I just want to take a moment to make sure nothing has changed since your last visit." Then begin the *Show-and-Tell* technique, going through all three questions on digoxin, then repeating the procedure with captopril.

> 3. Listed below are Bill's responses to *Show-and-Tell* questions. What do you notice?

Two potential compliance problems are detected during the consultation. One, the patient is taking the digoxin only once daily rather than the alternating schedule the doctor thinks he is on. Two, the patient provided the pharmacist with two clues to problems with captopril. A very subtle "pink flag" when he hesitated about how he takes captopril and a more obvious "pink flag" when he asked about potential side effects.

> 4. How should you respond to Bill's last question?

The most appropriate response to Bill's question about side effects is, "Why do you ask?" Hopefully, the patient will explain the problem in more detail. If the patient is still hesitant, a reflecting response such as "You seem concerned about side effects" should prompt a revelation about their concerns. In this case, the first question yields the following response: "Well, I felt real funny the first few days I took it."

> 5. Bill tells you that captopril made him feel funny when he first started taking it. What should be your next response, and what technique should you now use?

With a symptom or chief complaint from the patient, the student should shift gears and begin interviewing using the *Key Symptom Questions*. The initial response should be "What do you mean by feeling funny?" The pharmacist can then begin clarifying the problem using the focused open-ended questions.

6. What clinical assessment do you make from these responses?

The patient is describing what appears to be orthostatic hypotension, possibly due to a sudden fall in blood pressure in a volume-depleted patient (seen with ACE inhibitors) or just a hypotensive response from a high dose.

7. Before taking action to correct the problem, what should you do now in the consultation?

Before any further action, the student should summarize what the patient has told him to verify the accuracy of his determination. "So you began to feel dizzy the next day. The dizziness was worse when you stood up suddenly, occurred every time, and you almost passed out on several occasions. You tried getting up slowly which helped, but you ended up stopping the medication which made the problem stop. You then restarted about two weeks ago at one tablet twice a day and increased it to one tablet three times a day without the problem, and you are planning to slowly increase it. Since you have been taking it, you have been feeling much better with less breathlessness and increased ability to do daily activities."

8. What about the problem with his digoxin?

This could have been dealt with at the time of discovery or postponed until just before the end of the consultation. The disadvantage of bringing it up immediately is that it interferes with the efficient flow of the consultation. The disadvantage to waiting in this case, where another problem is discovered, is that you may forget about this one while working on the other one.

A *supportive compliance probe* can be used to begin the dialogue about the digoxin. "I noticed that you said you take the digoxin once a day. It appears that the doctor thinks you are taking an extra pill on Tuesday, Thursday, and Sunday." Patients who are unaware may respond with surprise. Those who have had trouble remembering can tell you when they changed. They may tell you that the doctor knows and said it was all right.

9. You need to call Dr. Ames. How would you phrase your comments to Dr. Ames regarding the two problems you detected?

"Dr. Ames, this is _____, the pharmacist at _____. Your patient, William Hodges, stopped by for his prescriptions today, and while counseling him I discovered two things that you may not be aware of. As you know, he is doing much better, but he told me that he is only taking his digoxin 0.125 mg once a day. He said he just couldn't get the hang of remembering those extra doses on Tuesday, Thursday, and Sunday."

"In addition, he developed dizziness about 24 hours after starting captopril. It occurred mostly when he got up from a sitting or standing position. He says he almost passed out several times. He tried getting up slowly with minimal success, so he stopped taking the captopril for 24 hours and then restarted it at 25 mg twice daily. After about 2 weeks without dizziness, he increased it to 25 mg TID and is doing fine on that dose. He is planning to continue to slowly increase the dose towards what you prescribed. I was concerned and decided to call."

This approach mimics how doctors in training or in practice communicate patient information with each other. Using this format will improve receptivity by the provider, especially those who are unfamiliar with your expertise and interest. It also prevents wasted time, because many times the physician will try to ascertain a symptom-specific patient history by questioning you. Finally, do not make a recommendation to the physician yet. Let the physician digest what you have said. He or she may tell you what he or she wants to do or may ask for your suggestions. In either case, in the physician's eyes, he or she remains in charge of the care of the patient; you are not challenging this control or usurping the physician's prerogative.

10. What would you recommend to Dr. Ames?

Because the patient is improved and doing well after implementing his own plan (digoxin 0.125 mg QD and upward titration of captopril), this seems to be a reasonable approach for the present. Close follow-up monitoring will be required.

CHAPTER 4

Documentation of Pharmacist Interventions

Timothy J. Ives, PharmD, MPH, FCCP, BCPS
Bruce R. Canaday, BCPS, PharmD, FASHP, FAPhA
Peggy C. Yarborough, MS, CDE, FAPP, FASHP, NAPP

INTRODUCTION

If there is no documentation, then it didn't happen! This philosophy is the standard in all health care settings as physicians, nurses, respiratory therapists, physical therapists, social workers, and other health care providers generate and maintain detailed notes regarding the patient's situation and their efforts to achieve the best possible outcomes for the patient. Documentation chronologically outlines the care the patient received and serves as a form of communication among health care providers, so that each practitioner involved knows what evaluation has occurred, what the plan for the patient's treatment is, and who will provide it. Furthermore, third-party payers require reasonable documentation from practitioners that assures that the services provided are consistent with the insurance coverage.[1] General principles for documentation include:

- A complete and legible record.
- Documentation for each encounter with a rationale for the encounter, physical findings, prior test results, assessment, clinical impression (or diagnosis) and plan for care.
- Identified health risk factors.
- The patient's progress, response to and changes in treatment, and revision of the original diagnosis/assessment.

Much of this documentation is derived from a systematic patient care process of evaluation that is standardized within each discipline. For example, physicians are taught to perform a history and physical examination based upon a standardized review of body systems and to document their results using a universally accepted, standardized, systematic process.

Several evaluation/documentation systems have been suggested for health care professionals. Over 30 years ago, the use of a Problem-oriented Medical Record was proposed,[2] and most physicians, nurse practitioners, physician associates, and other health care practitioners have been taught to write progress notes using the *S*ubjective, *O*bjective, *A*ssessment, *P*lan (SOAP) format. Variations of this standard exist,[3] but the underlying process is the same. For example, institutional consultant notes often use an abbreviated version of the SOAP format. This abbreviated version usually includes Findings (i.e., subjective and objective information), Assessment (or Impression), and Diagnosis (or Recommendations). Historically, pharmacy has not had a corresponding standard approach to the evaluation and documentation of the patient's pharmacotherapy that is applicable to all types of pharmacy practice settings. Thus, pharmacy has not been as active as other disciplines in documenting its contributions to patient care.

IMPORTANCE OF DOCUMENTATION

Pharmaceutical care uses a process through which a pharmacist cooperates with a patient and other health care professionals in designing, implementing, and monitoring a therapeutic plan that will produce specific therapeutic outcomes for the patient.[4] This process involves three major functions:

1. Identifying potential and actual drug-related problems
2. Resolving actual drug-related problems
3. Preventing potential drug-related problems

These functions aid in the provision of patient care through the identification of medication-related problems, development of a pharmacotherapeutic plan to address the problems, and the ultimate resolution or prevention of those problems.

As described in Chapter 1, a systematic approach is used in this casebook to identify and resolve the medication-related problems of patients. These steps are summarized as follows:

1. Identification of real or potential medication-related problems
2. Determination of the desired therapeutic outcome
3. Determination of therapeutic alternatives
4. Design of an optimal pharmacotherapeutic plan for the patient
5. Identification of parameters to evaluate the outcome
6. Provision of patient counseling
7. Communication and implementation of the pharmacotherapeutic plan

The final step is crucial; the tenets of pharmaceutical care suggest that pharmacists should document, at the very least, the actual or potential medication-related problems identified, as well as the associated interventions that they desire to implement or have implemented. The pharmacist must adequately communicate his or her recommendations and actions to non-pharmacy health care practitioners (e.g., physicians, nurses), the patient or caregiver (e.g., parents), or other pharmacists. The goal is to provide a clear, concise record of the actual/potential problem, the thought process that led the pharmacist to select an intervention, and the intervention itself. Additionally, the ability to receive remuneration for services provided necessitates an acceptable documentation strategy.

TRADITIONAL DOCUMENTATION FORMAT: SOAP NOTES

In the SOAP note format, the subjective (S) and objective (O) data are recorded and then assessed (A) to formulate a plan (P). Subjective data include patient symptoms, things that may be observed about the patient, or information obtained about the patient. Subjective information is by nature descriptive and generally cannot be confirmed by diagnostic tests or procedures. Much of the subjective information is obtained by speaking with the patient while obtaining the medical history, as described in Chapter 1 (chief complaint, history of present illness, past medical history, family history, social history, medications, allergies, and review of systems). Important subjective information may also be obtained by direct interview with the patient after the initial medical history has been performed (e.g., a description of an adverse drug effect, rating of pain severity using standard scales).

A primary source of objective information (O) is the physical examination. Other relevant objective information includes laboratory values, serum drug concentrations (along with the target therapeutic range for each level), and the results of other diagnostic tests (e.g., ECG, x-rays, culture and sensitivity tests). Risk factors that may predispose the patient to a particular problem should also be considered for inclusion. The communication note should include only the pertinent positive and negative findings. Pertinent negative findings are signs and symptoms of the disease or problem that are not present in the particular patient being evaluated.

The assessment (A) section outlines what the practitioner thinks the patient's problem is, based upon the subjective and objective information acquired. This assessment often takes the form of a diagnosis or differential diagnosis. This portion of the SOAP note should include all of the reasons for the clinician's assessment. This helps other health care providers reading the note to understand how the clinician arrived at his or her particular assessment of the problem.

The plan (P) may include ordering additional diagnostic tests or initiating, revising, or discontinuing treatment. If the plan includes changes in pharmacotherapy, the rationale for the specific changes recommended should be described. The drug, dose, dosage form, schedule, route of administration, and duration of therapy should be included. The plan should be directed toward achieving a specific, measurable, goal or end point, which should be clearly stated in the note. The plan should also outline the efficacy and toxicity parameters that will be used to determine whether the desired therapeutic outcome is being achieved and to detect or prevent drug-related adverse events. Ideally, information about the therapy that should be communicated to the patient should also be included in the plan. The plan should be reviewed and referred to in the note as often as necessary.

AN ALTERNATIVE APPROACH TO DOCUMENTING DRUG-RELATED PROBLEMS AND PLANS

There is a pharmacist equivalent of a physician's progress note in a systematized approach for the construction and maintenance of a record reflecting the pharmacist's contributions to care.[5] This process includes provisions for the identification and assessment of actual or potential medication-related problems, description of a therapeutic plan, and appropriate follow-up monitoring of the problems. Although there is no current uniform documentation system for the profession of pharmacy, students are encouraged to try this system as they learn to document patient interventions and compare its effectiveness with the SOAP format. In this system, problems that have been identified are addressed systematically in a pharmacist's note under the headings *Findings, Assessment, Resolution,* and *Monitoring.* The sections of the pharmacist's note can be easily recalled with the mnemonic "FARM."

Identification of Drug-related Problems

The first step in the construction of a FARM note is to clearly state the nature of the drug-related problem(s). Each problem in the FARM note should be addressed separately and assigned a sequential number. Understanding the types of problems that may occur facilitates identification of pharmacotherapy problems. Eight types of medication-related problems have been identified (see Chapter 1).[6] These problems include:

1. Untreated indications
2. Improper drug selection
3. Subtherapeutic dosage
4. Failure to receive drugs
5. Overdosage

6. Adverse drug events
7. Drug interactions
8. Drug use without indication

Use of a classification system such as this for the various types of medication-related problems offers at least two advantages. First, it presents a framework, applicable in any practice setting, to assure that the pharmacist has considered each possible type of problem. Second, categorization allows optimal data analysis and retrieval capabilities. Thus, problems as well as the interventions to resolve them can be stored in a standardized format in a computer. When later analysis of this information is needed, such as determining how much money was saved through an intervention, how outcomes were improved by the pharmacist, or how many problems of a certain type have occurred, the problems and interventions can be reviewed by groups rather than individually.

Documentation of Findings

Each statement of a drug-related problem should be followed by documentation of the pertinent findings (F) indicating that the problem may (potential) or does (actual) exist. Information included in this section should include a summary of the pertinent information obtained after collection and thorough assessment of the available patient information. Demographic data that may be reported include a patient identifier (name, initials, or medical record number), age, race (if pertinent), and gender. As noted earlier under the section on SOAP notes, medical information included in the note should include both subjective and objective findings that indicate a drug-related problem.

Assessment of Problems

The assessment (A) section of the FARM note includes the pharmacist's evaluation of the current situation (i.e., the nature, extent, type, and clinical significance of the problem). This part of the note should delineate the thought process that led to the conclusion that a problem did or did not exist and that an active intervention either was or was not necessary. If additional information is required to satisfactorily assess the problem and make recommendations, this data should be stated along with its source (e.g., the patient, pharmacist, physician). The severity or urgency of the problem should be indicated by stating whether the interventions that follow should be made immediately or within one day, one week, one month, or longer. The desired therapeutic outcome should be stated. This may include both short-term goals (e.g., lower blood pressure to < 140/90 mm Hg in a patient with primary hypertension) and long-term goals (e.g., prevent cardiovascular complications in that patient).

Problem Resolution

The resolution (R) section should reflect the actions proposed (or already performed) to resolve the drug-related problem based upon the preceding analysis. The note should convey that, after consideration of all appropriate therapeutic options, the option(s) considered to be the most beneficial was either carried out or suggested to someone else (e.g., the physician, patient, or caregiver). Recommendations may include non-pharmacologic therapy, such as dietary modification or assistive devices (e.g., canes, walkers); the rationale for this method of treatment should be described. If pharmacotherapy is recommended, a specific drug, dose, route, schedule, and duration of therapy should be specified. It is not sufficient to simply provide a list of choices for the prescriber. Importantly, the rationale for selecting the particular regimen(s) should be stated. It is reasonable to include alternative regimens that would be satisfactory if the patient is unable to complete treatment with the initial regimen because of adverse effects, allergy, cost, or other reasons. If patient counseling is recommended, the information that will be included in the counseling session should be included. Conversely, if certain types of information will be withheld from the patient, the reasons for doing so should be stated. If no action is recommended or was taken, that should be documented as well. In this situation, the note serves as a record of the pharmacist's involvement in the patient's care. The pharmacist then has documentation that patient care activities were performed.

Monitoring for Outcomes

It is not enough, however, to only provide a clear, concise record of the nature of a problem, the assessment that led to the conclusion that a problem exists, and the selection of a plan for resolution of the problem. In the spirit of pharmaceutical care, the patient must not be abandoned after an intervention has been made. A plan for follow-up monitoring (M) of the patient must be documented and adequately implemented. This process is likely to include questioning the patient, gathering laboratory data, and performing the ongoing physical assessments necessary to determine the effect of the plan that was implemented to assure that it results in an optimal outcome for the patient.

Monitoring parameters to assess efficacy generally include improvement in or resolution of the signs, symptoms, and laboratory abnormalities that were initially assessed. The monitoring parameters used to detect or prevent adverse reactions are determined by the most common and most serious events known to be associated with the therapeutic intervention. Potential adverse reactions should be precisely described along with the method of monitoring. For example, rather than stating "monitor for GI complaints," the recommendation may be to "question the patient about the presence of dyspepsia, diarrhea, or constipation." The frequency, duration, and target end point for each monitoring parameter should be identified. The points at which changes in the plan may be warranted should be included. For example, in the case of a patient with dyslipidemia, one may recommend to "obtain fasting HDL, LDL, total cholesterol, and triglycerides after 3 months of treatment. If the goal LDL of < 100 mg/dL is not achieved with good compliance at 3 months, increase simvastatin to 40 mg po once daily. If goal LDL is achieved, maintain simvastatin 20 mg po once daily and repeat fasting lipoprotein profile annually."

SUMMARY

A SOAP or FARM progress note constructed in the manner described identifies each drug-related problem and states the pharmacist's *F*indings observed, an *A*ssessment of the findings, the actual or proposed *R*esolution of the problem based upon the analysis, and the parameters and timing of follow-up *M*onitoring. Either form of note should provide a clear, concise record of process, activity, and projected follow-up. When written for each medication-related problem, these notes should provide data in a standardized, logical system. In particular, FARM notes provide a convenient format for progress notes for all pharmacists, applicable to any practice setting.

SAMPLE CASE PRESENTATION

The following case presentation illustrates how such a system can be used in practice. Franklin Jones is a 9-year-old Caucasian male seen on rounds Monday morning, who was admitted the previous evening with a painful right ear and fever ($T_{max} = 102°F$). He has a 6-year history of asthma. At home, he uses Theo-Dur 300 mg twice daily and albuterol 2 puffs TID. The admitting physician noted no wheezing. A theophylline level on admission was 19 µg/mL. His white blood cell count was $16.0 \times 10^3/mm^3$ with 12% bands and no eosinophils. The physician's working diagnosis is otitis media. Upon admission Sunday night, orders were written for acetaminophen 325 mg po Q 6 H PRN temp >101°F and ciprofloxacin 500 mg po BID.

Construction of a SOAP Note

S: Pt complains of right ear pain.
O: Inflamed right TM, fever ($T_{max} = 102°F$). He has a 6-year history of asthma, well controlled on Theo-Dur 300 mg po BID and albuterol MDI 2 puffs TID. Chest clear to A & P. Theophylline level on admission (i.e., random) was 19 µg/mL. Admission WBC = 16,000 with a left shift. He was started last night on acetaminophen 325 mg po Q 6 H PRN temp > 101°F and ciprofloxacin 500 mg po BID.
A: Right otitis media, with inappropriate antibiotic selection.
P: D/C ciprofloxacin, and start co-trimoxazole 1 tablet po BID × 10 days. Reassess clinical condition on a daily basis. Follow temps every shift. Follow improvement in pain, changes in TMs. Monitor fever every shift, and obtain daily WBC count. Obtain a theophylline level if toxicity is suspected. Educate the patient to take each dose with a full glass of water and to complete the entire course of therapy.

Construction of a FARM Note

F: Franklin Jones is a 9 yo WM presenting with a right otitis media and fever ($T_{max} = 102°F$). He has a 6-year history of asthma, well controlled on Theo-Dur 300 mg po BID and inhaled albuterol 2 puffs TID. His chest was clear to A & P. Theophylline level on admission was 19 µg/mL. WBC on admission was 16,000 with a left shift. He was begun last night on acetaminophen 325 mg po Q 6 H PRN temp > 101°F and ciprofloxacin 500 mg po BID.

Problem # 1: *Chronic Asthma*
A: Controlled on current medication.
R: Continue current condition daily.
M: Monitor clinical condition daily. Obtain theophylline level if exacerbation occurs.

Problem # 2: *Right Otitis Media*
A: Ciprofloxacin presents a problem for several reasons:
1. The broad spectrum may lead to superinfection.
2. It is not indicated in children due to risk of arthropathy and osteochondrosis.
3. Ciprofloxacin may elevate serum theophylline levels, resulting in toxicity.

R: Discontinue ciprofloxacin. Begin sulfamethoxazole/trimethoprim 1 double-strength tablet po BID × 10 days.
M: Monitor clinical improvement in pain, TMs. Follow fever and WBC count daily.

Problem # 3: *Fever*
A: Fever is controlled on current medication.
R: Continue acetaminophen.
M: Monitor temperature every shift.

References

1. Documentation Guidelines for Evaluation and Management Services. Washington, DC, Health Care Finance Administration, August 1997.
2. Weed LL. Medical records that guide and teach. N Engl J Med 1968;278:593–600, 652–657.
3. Larimore WL, Jordan EV. SOAP to SNOCAMP: Improving the medical record format. J Fam Pract 1995;41:393–398.
4. Hepler CD, Strand LM. Opportunities and responsibilities in pharmaceutical care. Am J Hosp Pharm 1990;47:533–543.
5. Canaday BR, Yarborough PC. Documenting pharmaceutical care: Creating a standard. Ann Pharmacother 1994;28:1292–1296.
6. Strand LM, Morley PC, Cipolle RJ, et al. Drug-related problems: Their structure and function. Ann Pharmacother 1990;24:1093–1097.

PART TWO

Disorders of Organ Systems

SECTION 1

Cardiovascular Disorders

Robert L. Talbert, PharmD, FCCP, BCPS, Section Editor

1 CARDIOPULMONARY RESUSCITATION

▶ A Near-death Experience (Level II)

Tate N. Trujillo, PharmD
Donna S. Wall, PharmD, BCPS

Three days after coronary artery bypass grafting, ventricular fibrillation occurs in a 62-year-old woman with coronary artery disease and multiple other medical problems. Resuscitation efforts are initiated, and the patient eventually converts to normal sinus rhythm with premature ventricular contractions. Students are asked to use the treatment algorithm for CPR based on the ACLS Guidelines to evaluate the drug therapy that was administered during the arrest. An appropriate pharmacotherapeutic plan is then needed to maintain the patient's stability on a long-term basis. Monitoring for efficacy and adverse effects is an important part of the pharmaceutical care plan, especially in light of the patient's end-stage renal disease and other medical problems.

▶ Questions

Problem Identification

1. a. *What actual and potential drug-related problems does this patient have just prior to the development of ventricular fibrillation?*

Actual Problems

- Patient requires DVT prophylaxis but is not receiving it (i.e., SQ unfractionated or LMW heparin).
- ESRD: metabolic complications are inadequately managed with Nephrocaps (hyperphosphatemia) and PhosLo (hypocalcemia); patient has metabolic acidosis (CO_2 20 mEq/L) and is not receiving alkali therapy; hypermagnesemia may require dialytic control.
- Anemia due to ESRD with no treatment given.
- Inadequate control of HTN on present regimen of diltiazem, furosemide, and clonidine.

Potential Problems

- Close monitoring is needed to maintain cardiovascular stability (i.e., nitrates, vasopressors, vasodilators may be needed).
- Caution is required to ensure adequate dosage adjustment for all medications in ESRD.
- Needs appropriate diet for ESRD, HTN, hyperlipidemia, and healing post-surgical procedure; serum albumin is low (2.5 g/dL), which may indicate poor long-term nutrition.
- Type 2 DM presently treated with sliding scale insulin and unknown long-term control.
- Hyperlipidemia treated with atorvastatin; control unknown.
- CAD, S/P CABG: patient appears to be receiving adequate pain control (but no data are given) and antibiotic prophylaxis.

1. b. *Discuss the possible causes for the development of ventricular fibrillation.*

Ventricular fibrillation (VF) is an electrical anarchy of the ventricle resulting in no cardiac output and cardiovascular collapse. Causes need to be identified very quickly to prevent death. Possible causes of VF in this patient include:

- Electrolyte imbalance: She is an ESRD patient and 36 hours S/P CABG. Either of these may result in abnormal potassium or magnesium serum levels, increasing cardiac irritability.
- Metabolic imbalance: In ESRD, a high BUN could produce acidemia. She also has a history of DM. A high blood glucose resulting from a relative or absolute lack of insulin may produce diabetic ketoacidosis.
- History of CAD and acute MI: Although she is immediately S/P CABG, there could be another area in which the plaque became unstabilized. Surgery has its own risk factors for AMI, such as hypoxemia, thrombosis of a new graft, or spasm of a graft or vessel. Other causes of an AMI in this patient may be hypoglycemia, hemorrhage, or an anaphylactic or hypersensitivity reaction.
- Hypotension: The patient could be experiencing a pulmonary embolism, hemorrhage, sepsis, or a low intravascular volume leading to altered tissue perfusion.

Desired Outcome

2. What are the short-term goals of pharmacotherapy for this patient?

- Return to and maintain NSR
- Assure oxygenation
- Prevent additional adverse outcome (i.e., stroke, anoxic injury)

Therapeutic Alternatives

3. a. What non-pharmacologic maneuvers should be undertaken immediately in a patient with ventricular fibrillation?

- The first interventions that must be undertaken may be remembered by the mnemonic "ABCD"[1]:
  ✓ *Airway.* Open the airway.
  ✓ *Breathing.* Provide positive-pressure ventilation.
  ✓ *Circulation.* Give chest compression.
  ✓ *Defibrillation.* Three escalating wattage shocks.
- After those interventions, the second "ABCD" includes the following measures[1]:
  ✓ *Airway.* Endotracheal intubation.
  ✓ *Breathing.* Continue to provide positive-pressure ventilations.
  ✓ *Circulation.* Obtain IV access to administer fluids and medications, continue CPR.
  ✓ *Differential diagnosis.* Identify possible causes for the arrest.

b. What pharmacotherapeutic agents are available for the acute therapy of this patient's condition?

- *Epinephrine* is the drug of choice for cardiac arrest if VF is still present after implementation of the ABCDs including defibrillation with three direct current countershocks. Its primary effect is peripheral vasoconstriction that leads to increased cerebral and cardiac perfusion. Epinephrine's α-adrenergic effects make VF more susceptible to direct current countershock. The standard dose is 1 mg (10 mL of a 1:10,000 solution) given by IV push every 3 to 5 minutes. Although higher doses may increase the initial resuscitation success rate, their use is controversial because they do not improve survival to discharge or neurologic outcome. Higher doses (0.1 mg/kg) are not specifically recommended but are acceptable and may be beneficial.[1]
- *Lidocaine* is considered the next treatment option. It suppresses VF by decreasing the automaticity of cardiac tissue and may terminate reentry arrhythmias by affecting the conduction in those pathways. It is given as a 1.0 to 1.5 mg/kg IV bolus that may be repeated in 3 to 5 minutes.[1]
- *Bretylium* is the next agent to use after defibrillation, epinephrine, and lidocaine. Bretylium has multiple mechanisms of action. First, it releases norepinephrine from adrenergic nerve endings followed by an inhibition of norepinephrine release from peripheral adrenergic terminals. It also increases the VF threshold in both normal and infarcted myocardium. It simultaneously increases the duration of the action potential, which in effect increases the refractory period of the ventricular muscles and Purkinje fibers. Bretylium is administered as a 5 mg/kg IV push and may be repeated once at the same dose.[1]
- *Magnesium sulfate* is considered the agent of choice in patients with torsades de pointes and hypomagnesemia. Magnesium is essential for the function of sodium–potassium ATPase pumps and can act as a physiologic calcium channel blocker and neuromuscular block. One to two grams of magnesium sulfate is usually sufficient when treating hypomagnesemia, but doses as high as 5 to 10 g may be needed when treating torsades de pointes.[1]
- *Procainamide* is the last agent to be considered for treatment of VF. It suppresses ventricular ectopy by reducing the automaticity of all pacemakers in the cardiac tissue. It also slows intraventricular conduction. Caution must be taken when using procainamide due to its hypotensive and negative inotropic effects, and it is contraindicated in torsades. Procainamide is used in refractory VF by continuous IV infusion of 30 mg/min until the arrhythmia is suppressed, hypotension occurs, the QRS widens 50% above baseline, or a total dose of 17 mg/kg has been infused.[1]
- *Calcium chloride* is indicated in this patient since she is hypocalcemic even after a correction for a low albumin (corrected calcium 7.9 mg/dL). Calcium is the primary ion responsible for interaction between actin and myosin, and it increases the force of myocardial contractions. It can be given as a slow IV push at a dose 2 to 4 mg/kg of a 10% calcium chloride solution.[1]
- *Sodium bicarbonate* may be used in patients with known preexisting hyperkalemia. Alkalinization of the blood will cause potassium to move intracellularly. Sodium bicarbonate is also used to treat metabolic acidosis in cardiac arrest when a life-sustaining heart rhythm does not occur within 15 to 20 minutes.[1]

Optimal Plan

4. a. A pharmacist was not available to participate in this resuscitation effort. Assess the appropriateness of the treatment used to obtain a cardiac conversion in this patient.

- *Treatment of torsades de pointes.* There was no mention of the use of magnesium sulfate once the patient developed torsades. Magnesium sulfate 1 to 2 g IV over 1 to 2 minutes followed by the same amount over 1 hour is considered treatment of choice, although a 4- to 6-g total dose may be needed to break this arrhythmia.[2] Antiarrhythmics that prolong repolarization (quinidine, procainamide) are contraindicated because they may

worsen torsades. Epinephrine and atropine will have no real effect on the torsades rhythm, but they might be beneficial in overdrive pacing of the ventricular rate. Lidocaine will not convert a patient in torsades but will do no harm to the patient.
- *Medication administration and timing.* According to the current ACLS guidelines,[1] medications should be administered followed by a defibrillation before another medication is administered. From the documented patient record, it looks as if epinephrine, atropine, and lidocaine were all administered at the same time, not following the drug-shock-drug-shock method.

b. *Upon conversion to normal sinus rhythm, what is your pharmacotherapeutic plan to maintain the patient's stability?*

The patient's problem began with multifocal PVCs. She is now in NSR with occasional PVCs. Treatment should now be focused toward minimizing the arrhythmia and its cause.
- *Lidocaine infusion* is the first antiarrhythmic to use for the treatment of VF. Lidocaine boluses totaling 150 mg were administered during the code, and the patient converted to NSR. It is recommended to start a lidocaine infusion at a rate of 2 to 4 mg/min since the patient converted after the lidocaine IV bolus. Serum concentrations should be followed to keep the patient within an effective suppressive range of 1.5 to 6 μg/mL. The need for additional bolus doses of lidocaine should be guided by clinical response or plasma lidocaine concentrations. Lidocaine is hepatically metabolized; therefore, there is no need to adjust the dose due to her renal impairment. Patients with heart failure are prone to increased serum lidocaine concentrations because of decreased blood flow to the liver.
- *Bretylium* is considered second-line therapy after lidocaine because of a greater potential for adverse hemodynamic effects.[2] It should be considered in patients with refractory malignant ventricular arrhythmias. The dose for refractory or recurrent ventricular tachycardia (which differs from that used for VF) is a bolus of 500 mg diluted in 50 mL to be run over 10 minutes. Alternatively, a continuous infusion may be run at a rate of 2 mg/min.
- *Amiodarone* given IV can be effective in patients with refractory polymorphic ventricular tachycardia. Its efficacy appears to be similar to bretylium, and it may be better tolerated hemodynamically. In an emergency situation, an initial IV loading dose of 150 mg is given at a rate of 15 mg/min. It is followed by an infusion of 1 mg/min for 6 hours and then a maintenance infusion of 0.5 mg/min. Supplemental IV boluses of 150 mg may be given if arrhythmias occur during the infusion. The acute antiarrhythmic effect of the drug is not seen if the bolus is omitted.
- *Magnesium supplementation* may reduce the incidence of postinfarction ventricular arrhythmias. As stated previously, magnesium is a treatment of choice in patients with torsades de pointes. However, this patient's ESRD complicates the therapy. Serum magnesium levels need to be evaluated and supplementation supplied if low.
- *Procainamide* is a second-line therapy for patients with ventricular arrhythmias. Due to the patient's ESRD, its use is not recommended.

Outcome Evaluation

5. *How should the patient be monitored to assess drug efficacy and to prevent and detect adverse effects? Describe how the therapy should be adjusted if adverse events occur.*

Assessment of Drug Efficacy

- Monitor ECG (HR and rhythm) continuously due to the patient's recent history of ventricular fibrillation.
- Obtain electrolytes (Na, K, Cl, CO_2, BUN, SCr, Glucose, Mg every 6 to 8 hours; check Ca and PO_4 once daily.
- Assess acid–base balance (blood gases) after ventilator changes and every 6 hours after ventilator stabilization.
- Adjust antiarrhythmic doses appropriately given the patient's ESRD (see question 4b.).
- Check vital signs every hour.
- Check CBC with differential every 12 hours.
- Monitor pulse oximetry continuously with a goal O_2 sat >96%.

Evaluation of Adverse Drug Effects

- *Lidocaine.* Assess for neurologic changes (i.e., drowsiness, disorientation, muscle twitching); check vital signs and serum concentrations daily to prevent myocardial and circulatory depression.
- *Bretylium.* Check vital signs for postural hypertension, hypertension, or tachycardia.
- *Amiodarone.* Perform baseline liver function and thyroid function tests, a chest radiograph, and ophthalmologic examination prior to prolonged treatment with amiodarone. Hepatic enzymes should then be monitored periodically to detect elevations that may lead to clinical hepatitis. Amiodarone can also affect thyroid function and ophthalmologic performance. Interstitial pneumonitis and pulmonary fibrosis may occur and may be severe. Repeat chest x-ray and thyroid function tests periodically (e.g., every 3 to 6 months).
- *Magnesium.* Assess for flushing, sweating, mild bradycardia, and hypotension that may occur from too rapid administration.

References

1. Cummins RO, ed. Advanced Cardiac Life Support. American Heart Association, 1997.
2. Lopez LM, Scheife RT, eds. Acute management of ventricular arrhythmias: Focus on new developments. Pharmacotherapy 1997;17(2 Pt 2):56S–88S.

2 HYPERTENSION

▶ No More Time for Complacency (Level I)

J. Edwin Underwood, Jr., PharmD

A 61-year-old man with hypertension, chronic sinus drainage, and symptoms of benign prostatic hyperplasia (BPH) presents to his new primary care physician for a follow-up evaluation. Physical examination reveals inadequately controlled hypertension (150/98 mm Hg) on hydrochlorothiazide/triamterene with evidence of ophthalmic and cardiac target organ damage. The patient is also taking several medications that may interfere

24 Hypertension

with his blood pressure control. He is also hyperglycemic (FBG 172 mg/dL), which may be partially attributable to the thiazide diuretic. Patient education on life-style modifications is the first intervention that should be undertaken. A change in drug therapy is also warranted, but the usual first-line medications, diuretics and β-blockers, may not be optimal for this patient. An antihypertensive that would also treat his BPH (i.e., an α_1-antagonist) is a reasonable choice for this patient. The case points out the need to treat each patient as an individual and that first-line drug therapies are not always the best choice.

▶ Questions

Problem Identification

1. a. Create a list of this patient's drug-related problems.

- Hypertension inadequately treated with present regimen and possibly aggravated by current medication use.
    - ✓ Sudafed (pseudoephedrine) and Aleve (naproxen) both may increase BP through different mechanisms. It would be better to use a local decongestant such as normal saline spray as needed and use acetaminophen for elbow pain, reserving the OTC NSAID use for acetaminophen failure.
    - ✓ Flunisolide (Nasalide), a fluorinated corticosteroid, should achieve a local anti-inflammatory effect and should not contribute to his elevated BP. Theoretically, it may raise BP if he is using it too frequently. Systemic corticosteroids can increase BP primarily due to increased volume.
    - ✓ It appears that Dyazide (hydrochlorothiazide 25 mg/triamterene 50 mg) is probably not the best antihypertensive for this patient. Despite the proven benefit of thiazide diuretics in preventing morbidity and mortality associated with HTN, it is not achieving the desired BP goal even though the patient confirms compliance. It may also be contributing to his elevated fasting blood sugar, even though he is on a low dose. Furthermore, the cause of his glucose intolerance may be multifactorial, and thiazide therapy may make his blood glucose and dyslipidemia more difficult to manage. Given his life-style, FH, obesity, abnormal FBS, and lipid profile, he may be hyperinsulinemic. Nevertheless, a thiazide diuretic (even at a low dose of 25 mg per day) appears to be a poor choice in this patient with no room to increase the dose to control BP.
    - ✓ His current life-style (sedentary life-style, overweight, excessive salt and alcohol) are likely hindering BP control and the effectiveness of the Dyazide as well.
- The patient reports increasing urinary hesitancy over the past 6 months, straining to urinate, and frequent nocturia without dysuria; his prostate is enlarged on physical exam. Further evaluation may be needed to determine whether he has benign prostatic hyperplasia, which may respond to drug treatment. If desired, a symptom score can be assigned using the American Urological Association's questionnaire to further clarify watchful waiting versus drug treatment.[1] Hence, this may be an opportunity to use one drug to both decrease BP and improve urine flow. Because the patient is less than 70 years old and has a life expectancy greater than 10 years, a PSA level should also be determined.
- He complains of occasional tendinitis and left elbow pain that he self-treats with OTC naproxen. As stated earlier, naproxen should be replaced with a trial of acetaminophen.
- The patient has a history of chronic sinus drainage that has been treated with multiple antibiotics. The exact etiology of this problem is not stated; presumably the flunisolide is helping to reduce the severity of this problem.

b. Outline the steps for obtaining a proper blood pressure measurement. Please demonstrate if a cuff is available (see Figure 2–1).

- Mercury sphygmomanometers are the most accurate measurement devices but are not practical for home use due to their high cost. Aneroid sphygmomanometers and electronic devices, if validated, can be accurate and serve well for home use. Finger monitors are inaccurate and should be avoided. Refer to Chapter 10 of the textbook for the steps involved in proper BP measurement.

c. This patient has established disease and has already been diagnosed with hypertension. What evidence supports that his BP has been poorly controlled?

- This patient has early evidence of target organ damage (TOD) based on his funduscopic examination and echocardiogram. His BP remains elevated despite medication compliance. Since there is evidence of mild TOD, the patient is not adhering to appropriate life-style measures, and his medication has not been adjusted for 8 years, one may assume that this patient probably has been diagnosed and treated as "hypertensive," yet little has been done to manage his disease appropriately. Emphasize to students that proper follow-up is necessary to ensure a good outcome for their patients.

d. What pathophysiologic mechanisms might explain the etiology of the elevated BP in this patient?

- Several life-style habits (sedentary life-style, overweight, excessive salt and alcohol) are likely contributing to his elevated BP.
- The patient should be asked to quantify his alcohol intake, asked if he ever binge drinks, and fully assess this habit to determine if alcohol is significantly contributing to his elevated BP.
- His OTC medication use should be quantified. If he is using naproxen and pseudoephedrine on a chronic basis, they may be contributing to increased BP.
- If he is hyperinsulinemic, this may indirectly increase BP.
- In addition, he has a strong family history for HTN as well as cardiovascular disease.
- The underlying cause of essential (primary) HTN is typically multifactorial. Factors contributing to his elevated BP may be related to a presumed hyperinsulinemia and obesity. However, it is not as important to identify the cause of essential HTN as it would

be for secondary HTN. The latter is usually correctable (usually surgically) and the former requires life-style modifications often in combination with drug therapy. Refer to the textbook for well-accepted and theoretical etiologies of essential and secondary HTN.

e. Based on the most recent guidelines from JNC VI, classify this patient's hypertension.

With an average BP of 150/98 mm Hg, evidence of early TOD, and other cardiovascular risk factors and the likelihood of NIDDM, this patient best fits into Stage 1, Risk Group C, according to JNC VI.[2]

Desired Outcome

2. List the goals of antihypertensive therapy for this patient, including the desired BP range.

- The general goal when treating HTN is to prevent or reduce morbidity resulting from uncontrolled high BP—retinal damage leading to blindness, renal dysfunction, stroke, CHF, and acute MI—and mortality with the least intrusive means possible.
- The measurable objective is to maintain a SBP <140 mm Hg and DBP <90 mm Hg and improve other modifiable risk factors of coronary artery disease when present.

Therapeutic Alternatives

3. a. What non-pharmacologic therapies are necessary for this patient to obtain and maintain adequate BP reduction?

- Life-style modifications should always be employed first and continued if drug therapy is warranted. As previously mentioned, he has several modifiable risk factors that directly influence BP.
  ✓ Decreasing intake of alcohol and salt (quantified below) will serve to directly decrease BP.
  ✓ An appropriate increase in physical activity will reduce cardiovascular risks and help achieve weight reduction.
  ✓ Reducing overall caloric intake and dietary fat and cholesterol will help achieve weight reduction, lipid normality, and better glucose tolerance, thereby reducing his BP and cardiovascular risks.
  ✓ He no longer smokes, but remind students that tobacco may acutely raise BP and that smoking is a significant risk factor for cardiovascular disease.

b. What reasonable pharmacotherapeutic options are available for controlling this patient's BP?

- If the patient is having significant adverse effects and/or not responding to the current medication, the most reasonable option is to discontinue the current therapy and substitute a drug from a different class.
- If the patient is tolerating the current medication but has not achieved full response, it may be reasonable to add a low dose of a drug from a different class with a different mechanism of action (usually a thiazide or β-blocker if not chosen initially).
- It may be reasonable to increase the dose of the initial drug toward its maximum using discretion not to increase the frequency of adverse effects.
- If a patient has a coexisting disease state (e.g., angina, cardiac dysrhythmias), an attempt should be made to select drug therapy that will treat both conditions and certainly NOT hinder treatment or exacerbate the other disease state.[2] For example, propranolol would be a poor choice for a patient with severe asthma and HTN. Alternatively, diltiazem or verapamil may be a reasonable choice for a patient with angina or atrial fibrillation existing with HTN.
- The option chosen should be patient specific and should take into account current disease states, predilection to disease exacerbation, and likely adverse effects, especially if these may lead to noncompliance.
- If drug therapy has been used in the past, any history of intolerance to an antihypertensive medication should be documented, and that drug should be avoided.
- This patient has not responded fully to the current regimen despite compliance. Furthermore, for reasons previously discussed, increasing his current Dyazide dose is not the most reasonable option. Once appropriate diet, life-style changes, and pharmacotherapy have been implemented to control his obesity, hyperglycemia, and dyslipidemia, it may be reasonable to reintroduce a low-dose thiazide if necessary.
- Similarly, adding a second agent while continuing the Dyazide may achieve BP control but will hinder the appropriate management of his glucose intolerance and dyslipidemia. Therefore, it is the author's opinion that the current therapy should be discontinued and a drug from a different class selected. This selection should take into account his current health status and concomitant disease states.

Optimal Plan

4. a. Outline an appropriate regimen of specific life-style modifications for this patient.

- *Reduce body weight.* This patient is about 14 kg (30 lb) over his ideal body weight and has a BMI of 27, which is associated with increased BP. Obesity is also a risk factor for other diseases such as diabetes, dyslipidemia, and coronary artery disease.[2]
- *Reduce dietary fat and cholesterol.* Reduction of these substances will not directly affect BP but will help with weight reduction, enhance dyslipidemia therapy, and reduce his risks for coronary artery disease.
- *Moderate dietary sodium intake and increase dietary potassium.* Excessive sodium intake can increase BP and blunt the effectiveness of some antihypertensive medications. Encourage the use of salt substitutes instead. However, these should be used with caution and appropriate monitoring if the pharmacotherapy includes an ACE inhibitor or potassium-sparing diuretic. The patient and his wife (since she does the food preparation) need to be educated not to use more than 6 grams of sodium chloride (table salt) per day (2.4 g sodium) and to read food labels to select foods low in sodium. Consultation with a registered dietician would be ideal for this patient and his wife.
- *Implement an appropriate exercise program.* Some type of regular aerobic exercise (moderately intense physical activity) will be necessary. This may be achieved with 30 to 45 minutes of brisk walking most days of the week.[2] Because this patient has early ev-

idence of hypertensive cardiomyopathy despite his normal ECG, this patient should probably have a cardiac stress test before beginning a moderate exercise program. A cardiac rehabilitation exercise program may be helpful.
- *Moderate alcohol intake.* The patient should be counseled that excessive intake may result in elevated BP, medication failure, stroke, brain abnormalities, increased heart size, osteoporosis, and liver disease. However, moderate alcohol consumption (daily ingestion of 1 ounce ethanol, 2 ounces of 100 proof whiskey, 2 cans of beer, or 2 glasses of wine) may produce beneficial effects on his dyslipidemia. The patient needs to understand that anything over these amounts is potentially harmful.
- *Continue to avoid tobacco.* Smoking is another risk factor for cardiovascular disease.

b. *Outline a specific and appropriate pharmacotherapy regimen for this patient, including drug, dosage form, dose, and schedule.*

- There are several appropriate options for this patient. Use of an α_1-receptor antagonist is reasonable due to the presence of a mildly enlarged prostate and clinical symptoms of BPH. Because of its potential detrimental effects, discontinue the Dyazide and initiate doxazosin (Cardura) 2 mg po QD. Doxazosin is an α_1-blocker that works peripherally to decrease BP and has a beneficial effect on enhancing urine flow. The α_1-receptor antagonists also have favorable effects on lipids and glucose tolerance, at least early in therapy. These beneficial effects may not be sustained long term but can be an advantage at this time. Furthermore, doxazosin will not alter resting heart rate and should indirectly improve cardiac output by reducing afterload. Doxazosin may be less expensive than terazosin and generally causes less orthostasis than prazosin.
- Another option is to discontinue the Dyazide and initiate doxazosin 2 mg po QD plus a low dose of an ACE inhibitor (e.g., enalapril 2.5 to 5 mg po QD-BID). The patient's UA did not indicate proteinuria, and further work-up will be necessary to determine if he is a true type 2 diabetic. However, a low-dose ACE inhibitor would potentially help lower BP, prevent microalbuminuria, and improve cardiac output by decreasing afterload without adversely affecting any coexisting conditions.
- Doxazosin 2 mg po QD combined with a low dose of the dihydropyridine CCB nicardipine should effectively decrease BP and may delay or prevent proteinuria as well.[3]
- Enalapril and nicardipine were selected because they have been extensively studied in diabetics for the treatment and prevention of diabetic nephropathy. Although other dihydropyridine CCBs have not been shown to have these effects, other ACE inhibitors have been found to produce similar beneficial renal effects in diabetics.[3]
- Since β-blocker therapy could worsen this patient's dyslipidemia, decrease insulin secretion, and further decrease his resting heart rate, it may not be the best option for this patient at this time.
- Despite the proven ability of β-blockers and thiazide diuretics to decrease morbidity and mortality associated with HTN, these agents should be avoided in light of this patient's response to initial therapy with Dyazide and his current medical problems. In addition, neither of these agents will effectively manage the patient's BPH symptoms, and he would require additional drug therapy for this. Stress to students that β-blockers and thiazide diuretics are not necessarily contraindicated in patients with dyslipidemia or diabetes. For example, if our patient had a PMH of acute MI, the benefit of β-blocker therapy would probably outweigh the risk of this therapy, and more aggressive management of his dyslipidemia would be in order.

Outcome Evaluation

5. *Based on your recommendations, what parameters should be monitored after initiating these changes and throughout the treatment course?*

- Monitor accomplishment of life-style modifications including dietary adjustments. Because of the close interrelationship of these with HTN and cardiovascular risks, life-style modifications should be reinforced as necessary throughout the course.
- BP should be rechecked in 1 to 2 months to assess efficacy of both life-style adjustments and pharmacotherapy.
- Improvement of BPH symptoms should also be assessed.
- The patient should be monitored for significant adverse effects of drug therapy. If an α_1-receptor antagonist was chosen this would include, but not be limited to, significant hypotension (especially with the first dose), cognitive dysfunction, and impotence. Peripheral edema may also be a problem due to reflex increase in renin secretion with subsequent sodium and water retention unless an ACE inhibitor was also chosen. Refer to the textbook for commonly encountered adverse effects of the particular antihypertensive chosen.

Patient Counseling

6. *Based on your recommendations, provide appropriate counseling to this patient.*

Alpha$_1$-receptor antagonist (e.g., doxazosin)

- This medication is sometimes associated with a large decrease in BP with the first dose and with future dosage increases, if those become necessary. Therefore, take the first dose at bedtime or, if taken during the day, avoid driving and tasks requiring agility and balance. This effect will most likely occur 2 to 6 hours after the first dose, but you should use caution during the first 24 hours of therapy. This side effect does not usually occur with subsequent doses of the medication.
- This medication should also benefit your bladder or prostate problem by improving the flow of urine and decreasing your night time urination frequency.
- This medicine may help increase your good cholesterol and decrease the bad cholesterol and help improve your blood sugar. However, these beneficial effects will likely diminish in the future. At that time, your other medications and diet will help improve these conditions.
- Call your physician or me if you experience any adverse effects such as memory problems, swelling in your feet or ankles, or trouble obtaining an erection. Not everyone experiences these side effects but it is important to report them so that another more tolerable medication can be prescribed for you if they occur.
- I encourage you to let me check your sitting and standing BP with each refill or between refills if you would like.

- Because some of the medications you have used in the past may cause elevated blood pressure, follow your Nasalide directions closely and do not exceed the recommended dose. It may be best to minimize use of pseudoephedrine and use acetaminophen (Tylenol) instead of Aleve.

▶ Follow-up Questions

1. *What advice and counseling should you give the patient at this point in his therapy?*

   - The patient should be complimented on his hard work in achieving the goals set forth to decrease his BP and cardiovascular risks. He should be reminded that these need to continue in order to live a longer healthier life.

2. *Suppose the patient now complains of intolerable adverse effects due to the current antihypertensive drug therapy. Outline an appropriate change to his current therapy.*

   This answer is based on the selection of an α_1-receptor antagonist. Refer to the textbook for a list of commonly encountered adverse effects if another antihypertensive was chosen.

   - If the patient is experiencing impotence or peripheral edema, discontinue the doxazosin and initiate an ACE inhibitor such as benazepril 10 mg po QD.
   - If he is experiencing intolerable orthostatic effects, discontinue the doxazosin and initiate a calcium channel blocker such as nicardipine or amlodipine. These CCBs should not decrease resting heart rate and may prevent proteinuria.

3. *Suppose the patient is tolerating the current drug therapy but has not achieved the desired BP control (average BP = 142/92 mm Hg). Outline an appropriate change to his current therapy.*

   - Appropriate options would include increasing the dose of initial drug(s) or adding a second agent from a different class if the patient received only one drug initially.
   - Because of their proven benefits in large randomized controlled trials, JNC VI recommends that a diuretic or β-blocker should usually be added at this point.[2] However, as stated earlier, these agents may not be the best choices for this particular patient. It would not be unreasonable to add a very low dose of a thiazide diuretic (e.g., hydrochlorothiazide 6.25 mg po QD) now that his FBS and lipid profile are improved. The risk versus benefit should be weighed and discussed with the patient and an appropriate choice made.
   - Other logical choices include increasing doxazosin to 4 mg po QD or adding a low dose of an ACE inhibitor (e.g., enalapril 2.5 mg to 5 mg po QD-BID), CCB (if not chosen initially), or adding a low-dose thiazide diuretic as described above. Beta-blockers without the property of intrinsic sympathomimetic activity (ISA) are best avoided in this patient because he has a low resting heart rate (56 bpm).

References

1. Barry MJ, Fowler FJ, O'Leary MP, et al. The American Urological Association symptom index for benign prostatic hyperplasia. The Measurement Committee of the American Urological Association. J Urol 1992;148:1549–1557.
2. Joint National Committee on Prevention, Detection, Evaluation, and Treatment of High Blood Pressure. Sixth report. Arch Intern Med 1997;157:2413–2446.
3. Baba T, Ishizaki T. Recent advances in pharmacological management of hypertension in diabetic patients with nephropathy. Effects of antihypertensive drugs on kidney function and insulin sensitivity. Drugs 1992;43:464–489.

3 HYPERTENSIVE URGENCY

▶ My Doctor Made Me Do It   (Level I)

James J. Nawarskas, PharmD

Discontinuation of antihypertensive medications several months prior leads to the development of hypertensive urgency (BP 230/127 mm Hg) in a 72-year-old man undergoing pre-operative assessment for an unrelated condition. The patient has no symptoms or evidence of target organ damage. In determining optimal therapy for this patient, students must choose between the parenteral and oral routes, determine whether hospitalization is necessary, select an appropriate medication regimen, outline monitoring parameters with defined end points, and provide patient counseling about chronic outpatient antihypertensive therapy.

▶ Questions

Problem Identification

1. a. *Create a list of the patient's drug-related problems.*

   - Hypertensive urgency requiring drug treatment due to discontinuation of antihypertensive therapy.
   - Possible misinterpretation of the physician's directions regarding antihypertensive treatment or possible discontinuation of antihypertensive treatment, presumably warranted, by his physician without proper follow-up.

   b. *What classifies this patient's situation as a hypertensive urgency?*

   - This patient has a severely elevated BP (diastolic BP ≥ 115 mm Hg), without severe symptoms or evidence of severe, progressive target organ dysfunction.[1] Target organ damage (TOD) typically involves the eyes, heart, kidneys, and CNS and may manifest as visual disturbances, chest pain, palpitations, hematuria, proteinuria, elevated serum creatinine and BUN concentrations, and various CNS disturbances.

   c. *How does this situation differ from a hypertensive emergency?*

   - A hypertensive emergency is a condition in which BP is elevated with concomitant acute and progressing TOD.[2] A hypertensive emergency requires immediate BP reduction to prevent or limit TOD.³ A diastolic BP >120 mm Hg in the presence of TOD typically constitutes a hypertensive emergency.

d. *How does this patient's underlying pancreatitis affect the severity of his hypertension?*

- Chronic pancreatitis does not fall under the classification of acute, progressive target organ dysfunction and therefore does not fulfill the criteria for a hypertensive emergency in this patient. Refer to textbook Chapter 10 for examples of hypertensive emergencies.

e. *What other signs and symptoms are present that may be related to this patient's hypertension?*

- Signs and symptoms of HTN are frequently not readily apparent, especially in the earlier stages of the disease. This patient, a 25-year veteran of HTN, reports no symptoms, but left ventricular hypertrophy and a systolic ejection murmur with a prominent S_2 are signs of a chronically elevated BP.

Desired Outcome

2. a. *What are the goals of pharmacotherapy for this patient's hypertension?*

- The ultimate goal of therapy is to prevent TOD. This is most easily achieved through BP reduction. The degree and quickness of BP reduction depend on the patient. Whereas persistent HTN increases the risk of TOD, too much or too rapid reduction in BP may precipitate renal, cerebral, or coronary ischemia due to a sudden drop in perfusion pressure.³ Patients with strong risk factors for atherosclerotic vascular disease or a history of coronary or cerebral vascular disease should therefore be approached very cautiously.¹ While this patient does not specifically fall into this category, he is elderly, which limits his ability to tolerate relative hypotension.¹
- A reduction of diastolic BP to between 100 and 110 mm Hg over 6 to 24 hours is a reasonable approach to reduce BP while attempting to avoid relative hypotension.

b. *If this patient had a hypertensive emergency, how would the goals of treatment differ?*

- Due to the increased risk of TOD in a hypertensive emergency, treatment tends to be more aggressive. The desired degree of BP reduction may be similar to, but is usually desired faster than, that seen in a hypertensive urgency.
- JNC VI guidelines specify a reduction in mean arterial BP of not more than 25% within minutes to 2 hours, then towards 160/100 mm Hg within 2 to 6 hours.³

Therapeutic Alternatives

3. a. *What non-drug therapies might be useful for this patient?*

- A short period of supine rest in a dark, quiet room may reduce BP to an acceptable level. A 15% to 20% decrease in diastolic BP has been seen after 30 to 120 minutes of quiet rest in patients with very severe hypertension.¹ However, since this patient's hypertensive urgency seems related to his discontinuation of antihypertensive therapy, pharmacologic therapy seems inevitable.

b. *What feasible pharmacotherapeutic alternatives are available for the treatment of this patient's hypertension?*

- *Parenteral versus oral therapy.* The first determination that should be made is whether this patient should receive IV or oral medications. Parenteral antihypertensives are typically reserved for true hypertensive emergencies. Their use in hypertensive urgencies tends to be considered only in patients who require the tightly regulated and easily reversible BP reduction not possible with oral agents. Examples of such patients include older patients with cardiovascular risk factors or patients with known vascular disease.¹ Although this patient is elderly and has cardiovascular risk factors [LVH, (+) FH, male gender and age >60], the chronicity of the BP elevation is an important consideration in this (and every) patient. This patient most likely has had an elevated BP ever since discontinuing his antihypertensive regimen about 2 months ago. Since the body's homeostatic mechanisms seem to be compensating for his HTN (evidenced by lack of symptoms), it is therefore questionable whether or not rapid BP reduction with IV medications is really necessary.⁴

- *Choice of drug.* While most clinicians would forego parenteral therapy in this patient, one could argue in favor of this, considering the patient's age and underlying cardiovascular risks. Nitroprusside sodium is perhaps the most commonly used parenteral agent for acute BP reduction due to its efficacy and ease of titration. Other IV medications that effectively lower BP in hypertensive crises include labetalol, nitroglycerin, diazoxide, trimethaphan camsylate, hydralazine, nicardipine, phentolamine, and enalaprilat. Due to its rapid onset and offset of action, esmolol is gaining popularity for this indication. Compared with nitroprusside, fenoldopam has demonstrated comparable BP lowering while eliminating the risks of thiocyanate toxicity. IV medications, while providing tight, predictable BP lowering, are expensive to administer and require close monitoring, usually resulting in hospitalization.

- For these reasons, oral agents are most frequently used. The drugs most commonly used are captopril, labetalol, and clonidine. Prazosin, losartan, minoxidil, and nimodipine have also been used effectively. Sublingual nifedipine has been widely used for this purpose but has recently fallen into disfavor because of its unpredictable response and reports of serious adverse effects. The JNC VI guidelines now classify sublingual nifedipine as unacceptable for use in reducing BP in hypertensive emergencies.³

c. *The attending physician requests that the medical resident write prescriptions for Procardia XL 120 mg po QD and Zestril 40 mg po QD (the patient's previous antihypertensive regimen) and discharge the patient from the urgent care center. The resident does not feel comfortable with this and proceeds to phone the patient's cardiologist, who wants the patient admitted. What do you think is the most appropriate course of action for this patient?*

- Cogent arguments may be made for both courses of action. Since the patient is asymptomatic, is likely to be experiencing a chronic (versus acute) episode of HTN, and the etiology of this hyperten-

sive urgency is most likely due to the discontinuation of Procardia and Zestril, which controlled his BP well in the past, gradual BP reduction with appropriate maintenance therapy may be effective.
- On the other hand, the patient is elderly with underlying pancreatitis as well as cardiovascular risk factors, which may necessitate more intense monitoring in a hospital setting.
- A reasonable hybrid of these choices would be to place the patient in an observation unit, administer appropriate therapy, and monitor the patient for several hours for response. This is a practice commonly employed with hypertensive urgencies since it avoids a hospital admission while providing appropriate monitoring in a controlled setting.

Optimal Plan

4. What drug, dosage form, schedule, and duration of therapy are best for this patient?

- Based on the previous answer, oral therapy would be most appropriate for this patient. As mentioned earlier, the most commonly used oral agents for the treatment of hypertensive urgencies are captopril, clonidine, and labetalol, although JNC VI guidelines mention that any drug with a relatively fast onset of action may be used. Examples of these include loop diuretics, β-blockers, ACE inhibitors, α_2-agonists, or calcium antagonists.[3] An exception to this is sublingual nifedipine, for reasons mentioned earlier. Since reinstitution of maintenance therapy will ultimately be required in this patient, a drug that will facilitate this should be selected. Since this patient has had success in the past with nifedipine and lisinopril and will likely go back on that regimen, either a calcium antagonist or an ACE inhibitor would be best to achieve this. Due to its experience in treating hypertensive urgencies, captopril is usually considered the ACE inhibitor of choice for this indication.
- Another consideration is the patient's heart rate. Because he already has borderline tachycardia, it would be preferable to give a drug that does not promote reflex tachycardia.[4] Clonidine and labetalol tend to decrease heart rate while captopril may rarely (1% of patients) increase heart rate. However, captopril has a quick onset of action (≤ 30 minutes) as opposed to the longer onsets of action of clonidine and labetalol (2 hours). Since captopril typically does not increase heart rate, acts quickly, and this patient has had success with ACE inhibitors in the past, captopril may be the preferred agent, although labetalol and clonidine are also reasonable choices.
- Captopril is typically given as 25 mg po, but in this elderly patient 12.5 mg may be more appropriate, repeated in 1 to 2 hours if necessary.
- Clonidine is given as 0.1 to 0.2 mg po (0.1 mg in elderly patients), repeated every 1 to 2 hours as necessary to a maximum of 0.8 mg.
- Labetalol is administered as 200 to 400 mg po (200 mg with liver dysfunction or in elderly patients), repeated every 2 to 3 hours as necessary.

Outcome Evaluation

5. What clinical and laboratory parameters are necessary to evaluate your therapy for reducing this patient's blood pressure and monitoring for adverse events?

- Regardless of the drug chosen, BP and heart rate are the primary clinical end points. While there are no specific guidelines for the extent and speed of BP lowering, a reduction in diastolic BP to 100 to 110 mm Hg is a reasonable end point to be achieved within 6 to 24 hours after initiating pharmacologic therapy.
- BP and heart rate should be obtained every 15 to 30 minutes after drug administration until the desired response is achieved.
- The patient should also be instructed to report any feelings of dizziness, lightheadedness, or headache, which are common side effects of each of these drugs.

Patient Counseling

6. The patient received the treatment and monitoring regimen you recommended and is now ready to be discharged on Procardia XL 60 mg po QD and Zestril 20 mg po QD. What information will you provide to the patient to enhance compliance, ensure successful therapy, and minimize adverse effects?

- Procardia XL (generic name nifedipine) is a drug that prevents calcium from getting into your blood vessels and increasing blood pressure. Zestril (generic name lisinopril) is a drug called an ACE inhibitor that interferes with an enzyme (called ACE) which leads to an increase in blood pressure. Both drugs are used to lower blood pressure.
- Procardia XL and Zestril are both taken as a tablet once a day. The dose of Procardia XL is 60 mg and the dose of Zestril is 20 mg. You will take both drugs indefinitely until your clinician determines this is no longer necessary. Your clinician will determine this by measuring your blood pressure at each office visit. You should also monitor your blood pressure and pulse frequently at home while taking these drugs.
- Remain seated for about an hour after you take the first few doses of each drug since they may cause dizziness. Common side effects of Procardia XL include dizziness, flushing, and headache, which should eventually go away after a few days once your body gets adjusted to the medicine. Fluid retention may also occur with Procardia XL. When you have a bowel movement, the outer coating of the Procardia XL tablet may be visible in your stool, which is normal.
- Zestril may cause dizziness, headache, or upset stomach that usually goes away after a few days of taking the drug. Zestril may also cause a dry, hacking cough and taste disturbances. Contact your clinician immediately if you experience a rash, swelling of the hands, feet, or tongue; difficulty breathing; or yellowing of the skin or eyes.
- If you forget to take a dose, take it as soon as you remember. If it is almost time to take your next dose when you remember, skip the missed dose and go back to your regular schedule. Do not take two doses at once.
- These drugs should be stored at room temperature in a tightly closed container, away from heat and light.

References

1. Thach AM, Schultz PJ. Nonemergent hypertension. New perspectives for the emergency medicine physician. Emerg Med Clin North Am 1995;13:1009–1035.
2. Abdelwahab W, Frishman W, Landau A. Management of hypertensive urgencies and emergencies. J Clin Pharmacol 1995;35:747–762.

3. Joint National Committee on Prevention, Detection, Evaluation, and Treatment of High Blood Pressure. Sixth report. Arch Intern Med 1997;157:2413–2446.
4. Gales MA. Oral antihypertensives for hypertensive urgencies. Ann Pharmacother 1994;28:352–358.

4 HEART FAILURE

▶ The Pump Organist   (Level III)

Jon D. Horton, PharmD

A 65-year-old man with multiple medical problems is hospitalized because of weight gain, pitting peripheral edema, progressive dyspnea on exertion, orthopnea, and tachycardia; a chest x-ray shows evidence of heart failure, and an ECG indicates atrial fibrillation. Patient management requires initiation of diuretic therapy and optimization of the patient's current ACE inhibitor and digoxin therapy. Beta-adrenergic blocker therapy with carvedilol is subsequently initiated for control of the ventricular response, to reduce exacerbations of heart failure, and to improve survivability. Appropriate patient education on the potential benefits and adverse effects of this complex medical regimen is an important aspect of the case.

▶ Questions

Problem Identification

1. a. *Create a list of this patient's drug-related problems.*

   Drug-related Problems Requiring Attention at This Time

   - Symptomatic heart failure requiring drugs and other treatment
   - Atrial fibrillation with inadequate rate control on digoxin
   - Hypertension inadequately treated with a low dose of lisinopril
   - Hypercholesterolemia in a patient S/P CVA, with LDL above target level of 100 mg/dL on low pravastatin dose

   Chronic, Stable Drug-related Problems Requiring No Intervention at This Time

   - Type 2 diabetes well controlled on metformin and glyburide
   - Cerebrovascular disease treated with warfarin

   b. *What signs and symptoms indicate the presence and severity of the patient's heart failure?*

   - *Signs.* Peripheral edema, jugular venous distension, hepatojugular reflux, displaced point of maximal impulse, crackles 2/3 of the way up the lung fields, diminished peripheral pulses, pulmonary effusion, pulmonary edema, S_3 gallop, cardiomegaly on CXR.
   - *Symptoms.* Dyspnea on exertion, dyspnea at rest, paroxysmal nocturnal dyspnea, nocturia, orthopnea, 10-kg weight gain, exercise intolerance, tachypnea.
   - Refer to textbook Table 11–5 for other signs and symptoms of CHF.

   c. *What functional classification and hemodynamic subset is this patient upon presentation?*

   - New York Heart Association (NYHA) Functional Class III
   - Hemodynamic subset Class II (pulmonary congestion)
   - See textbook Chapter 11 for a discussion of the hemodynamic subsets of acute heart failure

   d. *Could any of this patient's problems have been caused by drug therapy?*

   - A more thorough history could be elicited to assess the use of OTC analgesics (i.e., NSAIDs) for his recent headaches. Atrial fibrillation could be exacerbated by inadequate magnesium and potassium intake (especially considering digoxin use).
   - See textbook Table 11–4 for drugs that may precipitate heart failure.

Desired Outcome

2. a. *What are the goals for the pharmacologic management of heart failure in this patient?*

   - Improve or resolve the patient's symptoms
   - Improve his exercise tolerance
   - Reduce the potential for mortality
   - Avoid iatrogenic complications and maximize his quality of life

   b. *Considering his other medical problems, what other treatment goals should be established?*

   - Establish blood pressure control (goal BP ≤135/85 because of his diabetes)
   - Establish rate control of atrial fibrillation
   - Maintain glycemic control to prevent further end organ damage (ideally, HbA_{1c} <7%)
   - Maintain therapeutic INR (2.0 to 3.0)
   - Achieve an LDL-cholesterol level of ≤100 mg/dL to reduce cardiovascular and cerebrovascular events

Therapeutic Alternatives

3. *What medications are indicated in the long-term management of this patient's heart failure?*

   - ACE inhibitors have been shown to improve mortality and morbidity associated with heart failure.
   - Diuretics reduce patient morbidity by significantly improving the patient's symptoms.

- Digoxin does not reduce mortality associated with heart failure but does improve patient symptoms. Clinical studies have shown that patients who have been withdrawn from digoxin have a significantly higher incidence of exacerbations and hospitalizations.
- Beta-blockers (i.e., **metoprolol** and **carvedilol**) appear to be beneficial in the management of chronic heart failure.[1] They should not be used in the acute setting unless the potential benefits of rate control outweigh the risks of initiation in the acute setting.

Optimal Plan

4. What drugs, doses, schedules, and duration are best suited for the management of this patient?

- Intravenous diuretics (e.g., IV furosemide 40 to 80 mg) should be the initial intervention to maintain adequate urine output and resolve pulmonary congestion and its associated symptoms. Doses can be doubled every 30 to 60 minutes until an adequate response has been achieved. After resolution of pulmonary congestion, the patient should be switched to chronic oral therapy, titrating to slowly reestablish baseline weight and resolution of peripheral edema.
- An ACE inhibitor should be titrated to maximal tolerated doses without symptoms of hypotension or signs of hypoperfusion (e.g., increased serum creatinine or reduced urine output). The results of the ongoing ATLAS trial (a study evaluating the utility of maximal ACE inhibitor doses in heart failure) will provide some guidance for what doses are most appropriate (high versus low), but at present there is little data to support low-dose ACE inhibitors.[2]
- An IV "mini-loading" dose of digoxin should be administered to provide a serum drug concentration of 1.8 to 2.5 ng/mL to maximize rate control. The oral dosing regimen should then be re-instituted at a slightly increased dose to maintain this serum concentration.
- IV potassium chloride and magnesium sulfate should be administered to establish a serum potassium ≥4.0 mEq/L and a serum magnesium of 1.7 to 2.2 mEq/dL. Chronic oral supplementation should be considered pending patient needs.

Outcome Evaluation

5. What clinical and laboratory parameters are needed to evaluate the therapy for achievement of the desired therapeutic outcome and to detect and prevent adverse events?

Efficacy Parameters

- Fluid intake and urine output should be monitored daily during the acute initial stages of diuresis.
- The patient should be assessed for improvement in his exercise tolerance.
- Body weight should be evaluated daily initially to assess the efficacy of diuresis; the long-term goal is to return his body weight to his baseline level.
- The patient's quality of life can be assessed using standard scales.

Toxicity Parameters

- Symptoms of hypovolemia (e.g., lightheadedness).
- Signs of hypovolemia (e.g., hypotension, tachycardia); vital signs should be measured frequently during the initial stages of diuresis.
- Renal function tests (BUN, serum creatinine) should be assessed daily initially to monitor for pre-renal azotemia resulting from overdiuresis.
- Serum electrolytes, especially sodium and potassium, should be monitored daily initially and then periodically thereafter.
- Serum digoxin concentrations, fasting lipid profiles, glucose, and HbA_{1c} should be monitored periodically.

Patient Counseling

6. What patient information should be provided to the patient about the medications used to treat his heart failure?

- *General information.* It is important for you to take each medication daily exactly as prescribed. Contact your doctor if you notice any sudden changes in your weight, exercise tolerance, shortness of breath, urine output, and overall sense of well-being. It is advisable to weigh yourself several times a week. Check with your doctor or pharmacist before starting any new medications, including non-prescription remedies. Be sure to keep all follow-up appointments with your doctor.
- *Lisinopril* is in a class of drugs called ACE inhibitors. They are used to control blood pressure and reduce the workload of the heart. This medication can be taken by mouth once daily. If you forget to take a dose, take it as soon as you remember. If it is almost time for your next dose, skip the missed dose and go back to your regular schedule. This medicine may cause dizziness, lightheadedness, or fainting, especially during hot weather. Notify your doctor if you notice difficulty breathing; reduced urine output; swelling of the face, lips, or tongue; a dry, persistent cough; or skin rash or itching.
- *Digoxin* is used to slow the heart and increase the strength of contractions. It should be taken once a day on an empty stomach (1 hour before or 2 hours after meals). If a dose is missed and you remember within 12 hours of when you normally take your dose, then go ahead and take the dose at that time. If it is closer to the time of your next dose, then only take the next dose. Notify your doctor if you experience nausea and/or vomiting; visual color changes; loss of appetite; slow irregular heart rate; fast heart rate; and dizziness or drowsiness. I will teach you how to take your radial pulse so you can better monitor the effects of digoxin on heart rate.
- *Furosemide* is a diuretic that is used to help control blood pressure and maintain appropriate fluid balance in patients with heart failure. You will notice an increase in the amount of urine or in your frequency of urination, so take the daily dose in the morning rather than at bedtime. If you miss a dose, take it as soon as you remember, unless it is almost time for your next dose. This medicine sometimes causes dizziness and lightheadedness, especially when getting up from the lying or sitting position. Contact your doctor if you experience dry mouth and/or increased thirst associated with decreased urine output, skin rash, tingling or loss of hearing, irregular heartbeat, fever or chills associated with sore throat, nausea and vomiting, or mood changes.

▶ Follow-up Questions

1. What medications could be used to provide better rate control, and which of these alternatives would be most appropriate considering the patient's heart failure?

- The dosage of digoxin can be increased to determine if rate control is improved at higher serum drug concentrations. Care must be taken to avoid potential toxicity, and adequate serum electrolyte concentrations must be maintained.
- Verapamil or diltiazem would provide good rate control but have been shown to increase morbidity and mortality associated with heart failure. Caution would need to be exercised because of the potential drug interaction with digoxin.
- Beta-blockade with metoprolol or carvedilol could provide rate control but caution must be exercised to avoid exacerbating heart failure in the short term. The concomitant administration of carvedilol and vasodilators should be avoided.
- Amiodarone could be potentially beneficial in this situation,[3] but caution is needed because of its long-term adverse effects (which should be minimized at appropriate doses) and the potential drug interactions with warfarin (which may require a 50% to 75% reduction in dose) and digoxin (which may require a 50% reduction in dose).

2. *Outline a therapeutic plan for employing a β-blocking agent in this patient.*

- Initiate metoprolol 6.25 mg or carvedilol 3.125 mg po BID in patients who are medically stable. Patients should probably be monitored for several hours after initiation of therapy to avoid potential complications. Titration should be carried out every 2 to 4 weeks or at longer intervals as tolerated by patients.
- Dosage goals for metoprolol have not been established, but typically should be between 75 and 100 mg/day. Carvedilol should be titrated to 25 mg po BID for patients weighing less than 85 kg and to 50 mg po BID for those weighing more than 85 kg.

3. *The patient was started on carvedilol at an approriate starting dose. What information should be provided to the patient about common adverse effects? Describe how they should be managed if they occur.*

- This medication may cause dizziness and lightheadedness (symptoms of vasodilation). If these effects occur, take this medication with food. Avoid taking your lisinopril at the same time as the carvedilol. If these measures do not resolve the dizziness or lightheadedness, the clinician should consider decreasing the dose of the diuretic, vasodilator, or ACE inhibitor (e.g., lisinopril 15 mg po QD). If symptoms still persist, consideration should be given to reducing the dose of carvedilol.
- This medication may cause leg swelling, weight gain, or shortness of breath, which may indicate worsening heart failure. If you notice a 5-pound weight gain after two consecutive weighings, take an extra 40 mg of furosemide, an extra 400 mg of magnesium oxide, and an extra 40 mEq of potassium chloride. The clinician should consider potential sources of exacerbation (i.e., diet and/or medication non-compliance). If the patient does not note improvement in the next 12 hours or if he experiences any worsening symptoms, he should call the clinic to be evaluated. The clinician should subsequently consider increasing the dose of the diuretic. If symptoms continue, the dosage of carvedilol may need to be reduced. If bradycardia or prolonged AV conduction occurs, the carvedilol dosage should be reduced.

4. *What information should you convey to the patient about his current perspective on the usefulness of carvedilol?*

- The patient should be made aware that early in dosage titration, patients often complain of worsening feelings, and that this is to be expected. He should also be made aware that this medication provides long-term improvements in terms of reduced exacerbations of heart failure and improved survivability.

References

1. Packer M, Bristow MR, Cohn JN, et al. The effect of carvedilol on morbidity and mortality in patients with chronic heart failure. N Engl J Med 1996;334: 1349–1355.
2. Vagelos R, Nojedly M, Willson K, et al. Comparison of low versus high dose enalapril therapy for patients with severe congestive heart failure (CHF). J Am Coll Cardiol 1991:275A. Abstract.
3. Hammill SC, Packer DL. Amiodarone in congestive heart failure: Unraveling the GESICA and CHF-STAT differences. Heart 1996;75:6–7. Editorial.

5　ISCHEMIC HEART DISEASE

▶ Neither Hale Nor Hearty　　　　(Level II)

Amy J. Guenette, PharmD, BCPS

A 65-year-old man with known coronary artery disease, s/p MI and CABG, asthma, and hypertension returns for follow-up with continued complaints of exertional angina despite isosorbide mononitrate and a recent increase in his nifedipine XL dose. His concurrent asthma and reduced left ventricular ejection fraction must be considered when selecting additional antianginal medication. Two months after modification of his antianginal regimen, the patient requires angioplasty with consideration of concomitant abciximab therapy because of unstable angina and a high-grade lesion at the site of his previous bypass graft. In addition to the selection and monitoring of the patient's anginal therapy, the case provides the opportunity to discuss the evolving role of glycoprotein IIb/IIIa receptor antagonists as adjunctive therapy in coronary angioplasty.

▶ Questions

Problem Identification

1. a. *What drug-related problems appear to be present in this patient?*

- Poorly controlled angina on dual drug therapy (inadequate treatment).
- Mildly symptomatic asthma on subtherapeutic dosage of inhaled steroid and inappropriately scheduled doses of albuterol (rather than PRN).

- Renal insufficiency with hyperkalemia—possibly due to ACE inhibitor and triamterene (in Dyazide) therapy.
- Microcytic, hypochromic anemia (presently untreated)—may be amenable to drug treatment.

b. *Could any of these problems potentially be caused or exacerbated by his current therapy? Would any additional information be helpful to you in making this judgment?*

- Renal insufficiency may potentially be secondary to Mavik (trandolapril) therapy. However, this is difficult to assess without pre-ACE inhibitor laboratory data. Knowing this information would allow an assessment of the potential contributory effect of trandolapril to the present renal insufficiency.
- Certainly, the present hyperkalemia could be exacerbated, if not caused, by ACE inhibitor (plus the triamterene in Dyazide) therapy.

c. *What information presented in this case supports the diagnosis of ischemic heart disease and provides insight into the severity of this disease?*

- The patient carries a diagnosis of IHD by history, and indeed has had an acute MI followed by CABG surgery seven years ago. He underwent a cath one month prior to this visit, which showed CAD progression but no interventional targets. He describes his chest pain as typical for his angina. It possesses commonly described qualities for classical angina pain (i.e., substernal, crushing). The symptoms appear with limited and predictable levels of physical exertion.
- Although his angina symptoms possess some properties of unstable angina (history implies symptoms have accelerated in frequency and intensity in the relatively recent past, and he was probably classified as having unstable angina at the time of his cath), he would likely be considered at present to be exhibiting stable angina because of the predictable nature of the symptoms provoked by known exertional triggers. He has also shown some response to an increase in therapy.
- LVEF is decreased on cath to 45%, which is a likely result of long-standing ischemic disease and his MI.

Desired Outcome

2. *What are the goals of pharmacotherapy for IHD in this case?*

- Reduction in symptoms of chest pain
- Improvement in exercise tolerance
- Prevention of second MI (with ASA)

Therapeutic Alternatives

3. a. *Does this patient possess any modifiable risk factors for IHD? If so, would addressing them improve his condition?*

- There are a number of modifiable risk factors for IHD that are discussed in greater detail in the textbook chapter. Briefly, they include obesity, HTN, smoking, hyperlipidemia, Type A personality, sedentary life-style, and treatment with certain drugs (including thiazides and most β-blockers, which exhibit adverse effects on lipid profiles). Unfortunately this patient does not seem to possess many modifiable factors.
- He does have a diagnosis of HTN, which appears to be controlled on his present regimen. Modification of HTN as a risk factor appears most beneficial for primary prevention of IHD, although control of BP is important for maintaining a favorable myocardial oxygen demand profile in the presence of known CAD. His body weight appears to be near ideal. He is also a nonsmoker. He is forcibly sedentary at the present time due to angina symptoms. The degree to which this can be modified will depend on his response to therapy.
- His lipid profile is very good at present—within the ranges recommended by NCEP II for secondary prevention (i.e., LDL ≤100 mg/dL). He should be encouraged to continue helpful life-style modifications. It is unknown whether he exhibits Type A personality traits.

b. *What pharmacotherapeutic options are available for treating this patient's IHD? Discuss the items in each class with respect to their relative utility in his care.*

- *Nitrates* are useful as antianginals because of their ability to dilate coronary and systemic vessels, leading to reductions in preload and afterload. The alternatives in this class differ significantly from each other only in their onset and duration of activity. Products with rapid onset and short duration are most useful in terminating acute attacks or preventing anticipated acute attacks due to exertion. Agents with longer durations of action must be used for long-term prophylaxis. Regardless of the product used, all nitrates can produce tolerance. Generally, a 10- to 12-hour nitrate-free interval is recommended to avoid the development of tolerance in long-term prophylaxis regimens. Oral nitroglycerin (NTG) products are generally not used for prophylaxis. NTG patches allow for once-daily application, whereas NTG paste is typically applied 3 to 4 times daily. Oral isosorbide dinitrate (ISDN) products are typically given 3 to 4 times daily when used prophylactically. Isosorbide mononitrate (ISMN) is available in two types of formulations: (1) a tablet that must be taken orally in two divided doses 7 hours apart (Monoket, Ismo), and (2) an extended-release tablet that may be taken once daily (Imdur). All of these long-term prophylactic regimens are effective, but they differ with respect to cost and convenience. This patient is presently receiving Imdur 60 mg daily. This product has the advantage of a nitrate-poor interval built into its once-daily extended-release formulation. There is no evidence that he is not tolerating the agent well, and its once-daily dosing is good for compliance. There is also room to increase the dosage of this drug to 120 mg daily. As long as the patient can afford this product (which is somewhat more expensive than some of the other options in this class) it may continue to be a viable option for him.
- *Calcium channel antagonists* (CCAs) are useful in treating angina because of their ability to dilate systemic arterioles and coronary arteries, thus reducing afterload and coronary vascular resistance. Some agents, namely verapamil and diltiazem, also have the potential to reduce myocardial oxygen demand by reducing myocardial contractility. In the normal heart, reflex sympathetic stimulation effectively tempers reductions in contractility. In individuals unable to mount or respond to such

stimulation, negative inotropic effects may become apparent. The other major class of CCAs, the dihydropyridines, are noted for clinically exerting very little negative inotropic effect due to induction of a reflex sympathetic response brought about by their marked systemic vasodilatory capacity. The sympathetic response induced by dihydropyridines can also lead to tachycardia. There are relatively few contraindications to the use of CCAs. Two of the most notable examples are the requirements for extra caution in the presence of heart failure or conduction disease (as verapamil and diltiazem can be strong negative inotropes and can slow conduction through the AV node). This patient has a relatively high heart rate for an angina patient (88 bpm). Recall that heart rate is a determinant of myocardial oxygen demand. Nifedipine therapy may be contributing to this elevated heart rate, or at least will not be helpful in reducing it. An agent that does not produce sympathetic activation and that has the propensity to produce a negative chronotropic effect (such as verapamil or diltiazem) may be desirable in his case. This patient is known to have a reduced EF but does not presently seem to be exhibiting signs or symptoms of heart failure. However, selection of verapamil or diltiazem as his CCA therapy would require observing him carefully for development of symptomatic heart failure. His case presentation also does not mention any conduction system abnormalities. Should one of these drugs be chosen, effects on the conduction system must be evaluated and considered. Many once-daily and sustained-release CCAs are available to enhance compliance.

- *Beta-blockers* are useful as antianginals because of their ability to reduce myocardial oxygen demand. The reduction in demand is brought about by reductions in heart rate, contractility, and blood pressure. Beta-blockers have a good track record in ischemic disorders, including when used in patients who have suffered a previous MI. Beta-blockers are available as both cardioselective and non-selective agents. Cardioselective blockers are relatively specific for the β_1-receptor, although this specificity is lost at higher doses. Non-selective agents antagonize both β_1 and β_2 receptors throughout the dose range. Due to their pharmacologic properties, β-blockers may be contraindicated (either relatively or absolutely) in a variety of conditions including CHF, obstructive airway disease, diabetes mellitus, and peripheral vascular disease. No specific β-blocker appears to possess superior antianginal efficacy. This patient has asthma that appears to be at least somewhat symptomatic at present. The history indicates that his cardiologist has elected not to use a β-blocker because of the asthma. Use of an agent with β_1-selectivity may potentially be feasible in this patient. However, more information is required before such a decision could be made. It would be helpful to have a more complete assessment of the severity of his asthma (i.e., PFTs, history of oral steroid use, hospitalizations, ICU admissions, or intubation). Receptor selectivity is a relative phenomenon that is lost at higher doses, and the risk of using even selective β-blocker doses in highly reactive patients could be substantial. It would also be prudent to learn if the patient has ever had a trial of β-blockade, and whether he was able to tolerate its addition to his regimen. The simple fact that a β-blocker is not part of his regimen at this time with his history of long-standing disease and MI tends to raise the suspicion that his asthma may be too severe to tolerate therapy. However, not enough information is provided to adequately consider this issue. As with diltiazem and verapamil, the presence of pre-existing conduction system disease or significant LV dysfunction must be considered if a β-blocker is to be used.

- Aspirin has antiplatelet effects that have been shown to reduce primary and secondary risk of MI. Thus, aspirin therapy is an important part of his IHD regimen.

Optimal Plan

4. *Given the patient information provided, construct a complete pharmacotherapeutic plan for optimizing his IHD management.*

- It is unclear from the information provided what details concerning asthma were important in the cardiologist's decision to avoid β-blockers. The reasons may be substantial, since this patient has a long-standing history of IHD and has had an AMI. In the absence of a significant clinical contraindication, he would stand to benefit from a β-blocker. One could make a reasonable argument for addressing with the cardiologist the issue of proceeding with a cautious trial of a β_1-selective agent. When given at low doses (bearing in mind the dose relation of receptor selectivity), a β_1-selective agent can often be tolerated in the presence of mild airway disease. Given the good track record of β-blockers as therapeutic agents in IHD, a considered evaluation should be conducted before the idea of their use is summarily dismissed due to the presence of a relative contraindication. If the cardiologist agrees to a trial, β_1-selective agents and initial regimens include the following:

  ✓ Metoprolol XL 50 mg po QD (range 50 to 450 mg/day, cardioselective to 100 mg)
  ✓ Atenolol 25 mg po QD (range 25 to 200 mg/day, cardioselective to 100 mg)
  ✓ Betaxolol 10 mg po QD (range, 10 to 40 mg/day)
  ✓ Bisoprolol 5 mg po QD (range 5 to 10 mg/day)

  If such an approach is chosen by the student, suggest maintaining ASA, Imdur, and Procardia XL therapies at present dosages during addition of the β-blocker. If the patient can tolerate β-blocker therapy, then attempt discontinuation of CCA therapy and consider an increase in the doses of the long-acting nitrate and β-blocker as needed and as tolerated.

- Operating on the assumption that such a significant contraindication exists as evidenced by the cardiologist's choice to avoid β-blockade, first preference would be for the following regimen:

  ✓ Diltiazem CD 240 mg po QD (range 120 to 480 mg/day)
  OR
  ✓ Verapamil SR 120 mg po BID (range 240 to 480 mg/day)
  ✓ Verapamil given as CoveraHS 240 mg po QD at bedtime may be used if once-daily dosing is necessary for compliance

  These drugs are less likely to cause heart rate increases than is nifedipine and will provide a good substitute for it. They may even produce a reduction in heart rate, which would have a beneficial effect on myocardial oxygen demand. Although he has a mildly reduced LVEF at 45% and verapamil and diltiazem can be potent negative inotropes, many patients with this level of LV dysfunction can be treated with these agents without development of CHF symptoms. It is possible a student may choose Tarka (verapamil SR/trandolapril) to treat this patient since he is already receiving trandolapril. However, for reasons discussed later in the case, it may be desirable to avoid ACE inhibitor therapy in this patient's plan of care.

- Isosorbide mononitrate may be continued. Although many long-acting nitrates would be acceptable, the patient is already receiving this drug and is apparently tolerating it satisfactorily. It also has the advantage of providing an "effortless" nitrate-free interval built into its formulation to prevent tolerance. As long as cost factors are not a major consideration, it should be continued. Increasing the dose to 120 mg po QD (the maximum daily dose) from his present dose of 60 mg po QD may improve his antianginal response.
- A rapid-onset nitrate for acute use (e.g., sublingual NTG 0.4 mg tablets given PRN) should be added to the regimen. The patient should be instructed to place one tablet under the tongue as needed for chest pain; he may repeat this for a total of three doses 5 minutes apart. Sublingual aerosol NTG 400 µg/spray given in the same dosing regimen is also a feasible choice. The patient may also be instructed to use one dose just before activities known to provoke an anginal attack. This is likely to be especially useful for him because of the predictability of his anginal events.
- Enteric coated ASA 325 mg po QD should be continued for secondary prevention of MI.

Outcome Evaluation

5. *When the patient returns to the clinic in 2 weeks for his follow-up visit, how will you evaluate the response to his new antianginal regimen for efficacy and adverse effects?*

    - *Efficacy.* Ask him about the number and severity of anginal attacks and the provocative factors for attacks. Is the character and duration of attacks similar to before? What distance can he walk before experiencing symptoms? Does sublingual NTG relieve the pain? How many SL NTGs have been used per day or per week? Have any attacks occurred at rest?
    - *Adverse effects.* Obtain an ECG to observe for AV block. Assess blood pressure for control and for hypotension. Check heart rate for bradycardia. Ask the patient about symptoms of dizziness, lightheadedness, headache, and facial flushing. Check for signs and symptoms of CHF (edema, pulmonary congestion, rales, JVD, orthopnea, PND) with diltiazem, verapamil, or β-blockers and worsening of asthma symptoms in relation to β-blockers (if selected). Assess for constipation with CCAs.

Patient Counseling

6. *What information will you communicate to the patient about his antianginal regimen to help him experience the greatest benefit and fewest adverse effects?*

    - *General information.* Keep all medicines in original containers to avoid confusing them, and keep them out of reach of children. Do not stop any of your medicines abruptly without talking to your physician. Your doctor may need to stop some of them gradually. Keep track of the number of chest pain episodes you experience on the new medicine. Keep track of how many NTG tablets you use.
    - *Cardizem CD.* This medication is prescribed to prevent episodes of chest pain; it will not relieve an attack that has already begun. It is replacing the Procardia XL you were taking. Do not take both of these medications. It is important to take this medicine every day as prescribed by your doctor. You will be taking one 240-mg capsule every day. Swallow the intact capsule; do not break it open. Report dizziness, leg swelling, or shortness of breath to your doctor. If you are able to check your blood pressure at home, please do so and bring the readings with you to your next doctor's visit. Call the doctor if the top number is less than 100. If you miss a dose, take the missed dose as soon as possible unless your next dose is due soon (about 8 hours or less). Do not double doses.
    - *Imdur (isosorbide mononitrate extended-release tablets).* This medicine is for prevention of chest pain attacks as well. You will be taking one 120-mg tablet once daily. Take it each day as directed by your doctor. Do not break, crush, or chew it before swallowing. If you miss a dose, take it as soon as possible; if it is within 6 hours of your next dose, skip the missed dose and return to your regular schedule. This medicine can cause dizziness or lightheadedness, especially when getting up from a lying or sitting position. It may also cause headache, rapid pulse, and flushing of the face and neck.
    - *Nitroglycerin sublingual tablets.* This medicine should be used at the start of an attack to relieve chest pain. You may also use this medicine by taking it just before doing something that you think will cause chest pain. Dissolve one tablet under the tongue; do not swallow it. If necessary, additional tablets can be taken every 5 minutes for a total of 3 tablets. If the pain persists, you should notify your doctor or call 911 immediately. You should not try to drive to the hospital. These tablets should be kept in their original container with the cap tightly closed. They should be stored away from excessive heat and moisture. Taking them out of the original container causes them to break down faster. These tablets should be replaced every 6 months after the original container has been opened. This medicine has similar side effects to Imdur. They may be more obvious or severe because this medicine acts much more quickly than Imdur.
    - *Enteric-coated aspirin.* Aspirin has been prescribed to help prevent another heart attack. You should take it once daily with food as directed by your doctor. You should report stomach pain, black stools, or any easy bleeding or bruising. If you miss a dose, take it as soon as you remember, but not if your next dose is due soon. Do not double doses.
    - If the student has chosen an alternative regimen which includes a β-blocker, the following information specific to β-blocker therapy should be conveyed.

    Toprol XL (metoprolol extended-release tablet). This medicine is intended to prevent episodes of chest pain; it will not work on an attack that has already started. One 50-mg tablet should be taken by mouth every day as directed. This medicine may cause dizziness, lightheadedness, or drowsiness. Contact your doctor if any of these occur. If you can check your blood pressure and pulse at home, please do so and bring the results with you to your next appointment. Call your doctor if your top blood pressure number is less than 100 or if your pulse is 50 or less. If you miss a dose, take it as soon as possible, but not if it is within 8 hours of when your next dose is due. Do not double doses.

▶ Follow-up Questions

1. *What role does abciximab play in the setting of PTCA?*

    - Abciximab (ReoPro) was approved by the FDA in 1994 for use as an adjunct in patients undergoing PTCA who are considered at high risk for abrupt reocclusion of the affected vessel. The EPIC trial[1] showed that patients who received abciximab in a bolus and continuous infusion regimen in combination with standard heparin and aspirin therapy experienced a significant decrease in rates of death, nonfatal MI, and need for other acute revascularization efforts. However, abciximab therapy was associated with a twofold greater risk of serious bleeding complications.

- A follow-up study called EPILOG[2] examined use of abciximab in a broader population of angioplasty recipients. Similar reductions in end points were noted with abciximab therapy as in the EPIC trial. Bleeding complications were reduced in this study with the use of weight-adjusted heparin and abciximab infusion dosing.

- A third evaluation, CAPTURE,[3] examined abciximab use in refractory unstable angina patients for whom a percutaneous coronary intervention (PCI) was planned within 24 hours. This evaluation employed a different administration method for abciximab but yielded results of reduction in cardiac endpoints consistent with the results of EPIC and EPILOG.

- The indications for this product were expanded in 1997 to include a broad indication for patients undergoing PCI or patients with unstable angina not responding to conventional medical therapy when PCI is planned within 24 hours. This drug product is expensive, with an average cost per patient of $1500.

2. What is this patient's risk/benefit assessment for abciximab therapy?

- In the setting of unstable angina, he is at high risk for abrupt closure of the affected vessel. Under different circumstances, he might be considered to be poised to benefit from abciximab treatment. However, his age puts him on the cusp of a group (>65 years of age) who may be at greater risk for major hemorrhage. Furthermore, his recent history of CVA (within the preceding two years) is a contraindication to abciximab therapy. Therefore, this patient would not be a likely candidate for abciximab use.

3. Given the information provided, what changes, if any, would you make in the therapy for his other drug-related problems?

- Although there is evidence for ACE inhibitor benefit in the presence of LV dysfunction, trandolapril should be discontinued due to renal insufficiency and hyperkalemia. This will also help prevent hypotension that may otherwise result from adding a β-blocker or increasing the CCA dose in the antianginal regimen. If hyperkalemia persists, discontinuation of triamterene should be considered.

- The current regimen of inhaled corticosteroids is inadequate at the present bedtime dose. The dose and frequency of inhalations should be increased or a longer acting agent should be chosen. Also, a longer acting β-agonist (e.g., salmeterol) may be favorable in this patient because of his nocturnal symptoms (coughing paroxysms). In addition to these measures, a short-acting β-agonist such as albuterol may be placed on board for quick symptom relief. However, it should be employed on a PRN rather than a scheduled basis.

- The patient is anemic. Based on his heme (+) rectal exam and his microcytic, hypochromic RBC indices, he may be suffering from iron deficiency anemia. Iron/TIBC studies should be considered. Although his heme (+) stool may be a consequence of ASA therapy, investigation of the source of his GI blood loss should be pursued, especially in light of his recent weight loss and poor appetite. Addressing anemia is important in this patient to improve myocardial oxygen supply by improving oxygen-carrying capacity of the blood.

References

1. EPIC investigators. Use of a monoclonal antibody directed against the platelet glycoprotein IIb/IIIa receptor in high-risk coronary angioplasty. N Engl J Med 1994;330:956–961.
2. EPILOG investigators. Platelet glycoprotein IIb/IIIa receptor blockade and low-dose heparin during percutaneous coronary revascularization. N Engl J Med 1997;336:1689–1696.
3. CAPTURE investigators. Randomised placebo-controlled trial of abciximab before and during coronary intervention in refractory unstable angina: The CAPTURE study. Lancet 1997;349:1429–1435.

6 ACUTE MYOCARDIAL INFARCTION

▶ **Not Just for Men Alone** (Level II)

B. Nhi Nguyen, PharmD
Robert B. Parker, PharmD

Severe, substernal chest pain that radiates to the neck and arms, shortness of breath, and diaphoresis occur in a 66-year-old woman who is about to undergo an intravenous pyelogram. An ECG shows changes consistent with an acute anterior wall MI. The patient has a known history of coronary artery disease, hypertension, type 2 diabetes mellitus, and hyperlipidemia. Acute management is directed toward agents that reduce oxygen demand (morphine, nitroglycerin, β-blockers, and ACE inhibitors) and those that increase oxygen supply (thrombolytics, aspirin, and heparin). Students are asked to select specific dosage regimens for each of these agents and develop appropriate monitoring plans. When thrombolytic therapy is unsuccessful, the patient undergoes rescue PTCA with placement of a coronary artery stent. The patient is ultimately discharged on a complex regimen of medications that necessitates extensive patient education efforts.

▶ **Questions**

Problem Identification

1. a. What findings in this patient's case history are consistent with acute myocardial infarction?

- Crushing, substernal (squeezing) chest pain radiating to the neck and both arms that has lasted for at least 20 minutes. SL NTG provided incomplete relief.
- Nonspecific findings of SOB and diaphoresis are also commonly found in acute MI.
- ECG showing ST segment elevation (minimum of 2 to 3 mm re-

quired for MI diagnosis) in leads V2 to V6 is consistent with anterior MI.
- Cardiac isoenzymes are normal at this point since they were drawn so early in the presentation. Expect the CPK and CK-MB to rise beginning 3 to 12 hours after the onset of symptoms, peak within 18 to 24 hours, and become undetectable after 48 hours.
- Expect troponin I to rise 3 to 12 hours after the onset of symptoms, peak within 24 hours (sooner if given a thrombolytic), and return to the normal range in 5 to 10 days.

b. *What risk factors for the development of coronary artery disease are present in this patient?*

- Female ≥55 years of age (postmenopausal status)
- Positive family history of premature MI (father died of MI before the age of 55)
- Hypertension
- Dyslipidemia (elevated LDL cholesterol and borderline low HDL cholesterol)
- Diabetes mellitus

Note: A hysterectomy alone in premenopausal women does not increase the risk for ischemic heart disease if the ovaries are still intact and producing estrogen. However, the deprivation of estrogen after natural or surgical (oophorectomy) menopause places a woman at risk for ischemic heart disease.

Desired Outcome

2. *What are the goals of pharmacotherapy in this patient?*

- Minimize infarct size and salvage viable myocardium, since the size of the infarction is the main determinant of prognosis. Therapies to achieve these goals will be directed toward decreasing myocardial oxygen demand and increasing myocardial oxygen supply.
- Relieve patient symptoms (e.g., chest pain)
- Prevent or minimize complications
- Decrease mortality

Therapeutic Alternatives

3. a. *What feasible pharmacotherapeutic alternatives are available to treat this patient?*

General Measures
- Admission to a coronary care unit with continuous monitoring of vital signs and ECG
- Oxygen by nasal prongs or mask
- Stool softeners

Drugs That Decrease Oxygen Demand
- *Analgesics.* Pain and anxiety may increase heart rate and blood pressure resulting in increased oxygen demand. Morphine is also an arterial and venous vasodilator resulting in decreases in afterload and preload, respectively.
- *Nitroglycerin* decreases oxygen demand by reducing preload (may also reduce afterload at higher doses). Venodilation results in less infarct expansion. NTG also increases myocardial oxygen supply by coronary vasodilation.
- *Beta-blockers* decrease oxygen demand by slowing heart rate and decreasing blood pressure and myocardial contractility. They are particularly useful in patients with tachycardia and hypertension.
- *ACE inhibitors* limit post-infarction left ventricular dilatation and hypertrophy.

Drugs That Increase Oxygen Supply
- *Thrombolytics.* Thrombolytics improve oxygen supply by dissolving the thrombus that is responsible for precipitating acute MI and restoring blood flow to the ischemic myocardium. This in turn leads to reduction in infarct size and lower morbidity and mortality.
- *Aspirin.* Inhibition of platelet aggregation by aspirin prevents rethrombosis and reinfarction in patients receiving thrombolytic therapy.
- *Heparin.* The antithrombotic effect of heparin prevents rethrombosis and reocclusion of the coronary artery.

b. *What non-pharmacologic alternative therapies might be used in this patient?*

- Primary percutaneous transluminal coronary angioplasty (PTCA) can be considered as an alternative to thrombolytic therapy. Current guidelines recommend primary PTCA as an alternative to thrombolytic therapy only if performed in a timely fashion by individuals skilled in the procedure (more than 75 procedures per year) and supported by experienced personnel in high-volume centers (more than 200 PTCA procedures per year).[1]
- If thrombolytic therapy fails to restore antegrade coronary flow (10% to 15% of patients), then rescue PTCA or emergency coronary artery bypass grafting (CABG) may be attempted.

Optimal Plan

4. *Based on the history and presentation, what drug therapy is indicated in this patient?*

Drugs That Decrease Oxygen Demand
- Morphine given IV is the drug of choice in most patients and should be administered in doses of 2 to 5 mg every 5 to 15 minutes as needed for pain.
- Nitroglycerin is usually given as a continuous IV infusion in acute MI beginning at 5 to 10 μg/min, and titrated upward based on chest pain, blood pressure, and heart rate. The goal is to relieve chest pain.
- Beta blockers such as metoprolol 5 mg IV every 5 minutes × 3 doses followed by 50 mg po every 6 hours for 48 hours, then 100 mg po every 12 hours. Other β-blockers are also effective, including both non-selective and cardioselective drugs. Agents with intrinsic sympathomimetic activity (ISA) should be avoided. See Tables 13–3 to 13–5 in the textbook for indications, contraindications, and doses of β-blockers.
- ACE inhibitors such as captopril 6.25 mg po, followed 2 hours later by 12.5 mg po, followed 10 to 12 hours later by 25 mg po, then 50 mg po BID for 28 days. Lisinopril is another reasonable alternative (5 mg po titrated to 10 mg po QD for 6 weeks).

Drugs That Increase Oxygen Supply
- A thrombolytic is indicated in this case. Many patients eligible for thrombolytic therapy never receive it. The time from symptom onset to initiation of therapy is extremely important. Unless contraindicated, thrombolytics should be given to patients who present with an acute MI within 12 hours of the onset of chest pain and have ST elevations in two contiguous leads on ECG or a new left bundle branch

block.² The sooner treatment is started, the greater the myocardial salvage and improvement in survival (i.e., time is muscle). Alteplase (TPA) is the thrombolytic of choice in this patient who presents within 2 hours of symptom onset, has an anterior MI, and is less than 75 years old (see textbook Figure 13–5 for an algorithm on the use of TPA versus streptokinase). The dosage regimen is 100 mg IV over 1.5 hours given as a 15-mg bolus followed by 50 mg over 30 minutes and then 35 mg over 1 hour.

- The first dose of aspirin (160 to 325 mg) should be chewed and swallowed as soon as the clinical impression of an acute MI is entertained. Therapy can then be continued at 160 to 325 mg per day. Even if the patient takes an aspirin daily, an additional tablet should be given in the ED.
- IV heparin should be administered for at least 48 hours adjusted to maintain an aPTT 1.5 to 2.0 times control in patients who receive alteplase or reteplase. Similarly, those who receive streptokinase or anistreplase and are at high risk for systemic emboli (large or anterior MI, atrial fibrillation, previous emboli, or known LV thrombus) should receive IV heparin.
- Patients not treated with a thrombolytic agent should receive subcutaneous heparin 7500 units twice daily or IV heparin, as just described, for those at high risk for systemic emboli.

Outcome Evaluation

5. How should the recommended therapy be monitored for efficacy and adverse effects?

- For analgesics, pain relief is the desired therapeutic end point. Continue therapy until pain relief is achieved or systolic blood pressure is <100 mm Hg. Adverse effects include hypotension, respiratory depression, and bradycardia.
- Nitroglycerin's efficacy is assessed by heart rate and blood pressure reduction, relief of chest pain, and resolution of ECG abnormalities (e.g., ST segment elevation returns to baseline). Adverse effects include hypotension, bradycardia, tachycardia, and headache.
- Efficacy parameters for β-blockers include heart rate and blood pressure reduction, and resolution of chest pain. Refer to the algorithm in Table 13–3 in the textbook describing early use of β-blockers. Adverse effects include bradycardia, AV block, hypotension, and heart failure. See Table 13–4 in the textbook for absolute and relative contraindications to β-blocker therapy.
- Efficacy of ACE inhibitors is judged by ejection fraction and reduction in clinical signs of heart failure. Adverse effects include hypotension, angioedema, hyperkalemia, hyponatremia, and renal dysfunction.
- Thrombolytic efficacy is assessed by normalization of ST segment elevation, relief of chest pain, reperfusion arrhythmias, and early peak of CK enzymes. See Table 13–6 in the textbook for absolute and relative contraindications to thrombolytic therapy. The most serious adverse effect is bleeding, including intracerebral hemorrhage. Refer to the algorithm in Figure 13–3 for management of thrombolytic associated bleeding.
- Aspirin's efficacy can be monitored by signs and symptoms of recurrent ischemia. Adverse effects include bleeding, GI complaints (abdominal pain, heartburn, nausea), and allergic reactions. GI effects may be minimized by using enteric-coated aspirin chronically, but non-enteric coated aspirin should be used for the first dose.
- The efficacy of heparin is assessed by observing for signs and symptoms of recurrent ischemia. The aPTT should be maintained between 1.5 and 2.0 times control. The half-life of heparin is 1.0 to 1.5 hours, so an aPTT should be obtained no sooner than 4 to 6 hours after the heparin infusion is started or after any dosage changes. The most common adverse effects in this setting include bleeding (monitor hemoglobin and hematocrit) and thrombocytopenia.

Patient Counseling

6. a. What discharge medications would be most appropriate for this patient?

- Aspirin reduces risk of vascular death, nonfatal reinfarction, nonfatal stroke, and the combined end point of nonfatal MI and sudden death. Typical doses range from 81 to 325 mg po QD. However, some centers administer aspirin twice daily for the first 4 to 6 weeks after stent placement based on the results of a randomized, controlled trial.[3] After this period, patients are switched to once-daily aspirin.
- Beta blockers reduce post-MI mortality. Metoprolol, propranolol, and timolol are FDA-approved for this indication and are reasonable choices; other β-blockers without ISA could also be used. Drugs with ISA have not been shown to decrease post-MI mortality.
- ACE inhibitors have been shown to reduce mortality when initiated within 24 hours of the onset of chest pain and are given for 4 to 6 weeks post MI regardless of the EF. Recommended doses include captopril 50 mg po BID for 4 weeks or lisinopril 10 mg po QD for 6 weeks. Chronic, long-term ACE inhibitor therapy is indicated for post-MI patients with an ejection fraction < 40%. When started at least 3 days post-MI, ACE inhibitors reduce mortality, slow the progression of CHF, and decrease reinfarction rates in these patients.[4]
- An HMG-CoA reductase inhibitor would be a better choice than gemfibrozil for this patient's dyslipidemia. Any reductase inhibitor would probably be a reasonable choice. However, in patients with clinical evidence of coronary heart disease, only fluvastatin, pravastatin, and lovastatin are FDA-approved to slow the progression of coronary atherosclerosis, and only pravastatin and simvastatin are FDA-approved to reduce the risk of acute coronary events (at the time of this writing). The gemfibrozil should be discontinued and replaced with a reductase inhibitor such as pravastatin 20 mg po Q HS with the goal of achieving an LDL of ≤100 mg/dL in this patient. Hepatic transaminases (AST, ALT) should be checked at baseline, 6 and 12 weeks after starting therapy, and then periodically thereafter.
- Warfarin prevents mural thrombus development and stroke in patients with an anterior MI. The dose should be titrated to an INR of 2.0 to 3.0 and continued for 3 months. (*Note:* patients usually receive ticlopidine, or in some cases clopidogrel, for 4 to 6 weeks after coronary artery stent placement. Since the combined use of warfarin and one of these agents would increase her risk for bleeding, warfarin alone is acceptable in this situation. However, her warfarin dose should be titrated to an INR of 3.5 to 4.5 for the first 6 weeks of therapy to prevent thrombosis of the coronary stent.[3] After this 6-week period, the warfarin dose should be decreased to maintain an INR of 2.0 to 3.0.)

- Estrogen replacement therapy for cardiovascular protection is controversial because of the breast cancer risk associated with its use. Observational studies suggest that in women with cardiovascular disease, the benefits of estrogen replacement outweigh the risks. Nevertheless, this decision is highly individualized. Given the severe cardiac history in this patient and lack of evidence of breast cancer, conjugated equine estrogen 0.625 mg po QD would be a reasonable choice. Note that fewer data are available on the estrogen patches, and although they seem to be better tolerated, the lipoprotein benefits are less than those received with oral estrogen. If this patient still had an intact uterus, then progestin must be given with estrogen for protection from endometrial cancer.
- Glyburide should be continued for ongoing control of her type 2 diabetes mellitus.
- Sublingual NTG should be prescribed for the patient to take PRN for treatment of acute ischemic episodes.

b. *What patient counseling information should you provide to this patient?*

Risk Factor Modification
Weight loss
Step 2 American Heart Association diet (see textbook for details)
Control of blood sugar
Exercise program

Drug Therapy
- *Aspirin.* Take this medication once daily as prescribed. Take this with food to avoid stomach upset. Consult your pharmacist or physician before taking any over-the-counter medications, as many of them contain aspirin. Be aware of signs/symptoms of bleeding including easy bruising; nosebleeds; bleeding gums; pink, red, or brown urine; red or black tarry stools; vomiting of blood; coughing up blood; severe headache.
- *Metoprolol.* Take this medication twice daily. Do not suddenly stop taking this medication. If you miss a dose, take it as soon as possible. If you do not remember to take the missed dose and your next regularly scheduled dose is less than 4 hours away, skip the missed dose and take only the next scheduled dose. This medication may cause dizziness, lightheadedness, fatigue, cold hands or feet, slow heart beat, confusion, and nightmares. Contact your doctor if any of these are severe. This may also cause drowsiness. Use caution when driving or performing other tasks requiring alertness until you become familiar with the medication's effects. Notify you doctor immediately if you experience shortness of breath (either on exertion or when lying down), feet/ankle swelling, or chest pain.
- *Captopril.* Take this medication on an empty stomach twice daily for 4 weeks, then stop. Notify your doctor immediately if you notice any trouble breathing, or swelling of any part of the head or neck. You may develop a rash or a dry, persistent cough while taking this medicine. Contact your doctor if these are severe or troublesome. These side effects will go away when you stop the medicine.
- *Pravastatin.* Take this every night at bedtime. Notify your doctor immediately if you notice any muscle weakness or aches.
- *Warfarin.* Take this medication once daily at the same time each day; it can be taken with or without food. Avoid extreme changes in eating habits. Avoid vitamins containing vitamin K. Examples include Geritol Extend, Family Tabs with Iron, and ABC Plus. Avoid alcohol while taking this medication. Do not start or stop taking any other medication unless you consult with your doctor or pharmacist; this includes any over-the-counter medications. Do not stop taking this medication or change the dose unless directed by your doctor. If you miss a dose, take it as soon as possible. If you do not remember the missed dose until the next day, do not take the missed dose; only take the scheduled dose for that day. Be aware of signs/symptoms of bleeding, as described above for aspirin. If your toes develop a purple discoloration, call your doctor. Keep all follow-up appointments with your doctor.
- *Glyburide.* Take this medication twice daily. Be sure to eat after taking this medication.
- *Sublingual NTG.* Take only as needed for chest pain. Do not swallow the tablets. Place one tablet under the tongue at the first sign of chest pain. If the pain is not relieved in 5 minutes, place another tablet under the tongue. If the pain is not relieved in 5 minutes, place a third tablet under the tongue. If the pain continues, call 911 immediately. Do not attempt to drive to the hospital or your doctor's office. Sit down before taking this medication. This may cause a tingling sensation under the tongue, headache, dizziness, lightheadedness, and flushing. Store these tablets in their original brown glass container and keep the container closed tightly after each use.

▶ **Follow-up Question**

1. *The patient returns to the cardiology clinic in 6 weeks for a follow-up visit. She reports feeling fine. What do you recommend at this time?*

- Check an INR. Since 6 weeks has passed since placement of the coronary stent, you can now decrease her warfarin dose to achieve a goal INR of 2.0 to 3.0 (rather than 3.5 to 4.5). She should be kept on warfarin for a total of 3 months from the date of her anterior MI.
- Check a fasting lipid profile now. Sufficient time has passed such that the acute phase of her MI would not interfere with her cholesterol readings. LFTs are recommended at 6 and 12 weeks after initiation or elevation in dose of HMG-CoA reductase inhibitors.

References

1. Ryan TJ, Bauman WB, Kennedy JW, et al. ACC/AHA guidelines for percutaneous transluminal coronary angioplasty: A report of the American College of Cardiology/American Heart Association Task Force on Assessment of Diagnostic and Therapeutic Cardiovascular Procedures (Committee on Percutaneous Transluminal Coronary Angioplasty). J Am Coll Cardiol 1993;22:2033–2054.
2. Ryan TJ, Anderson JL, Antman EM, et al. ACC/AHA guidelines for the management of patients with acute myocardial infarction: A report of the American College of Cardiology/American Heart Association Task Force on Practice Guidelines (Committee on Management of Acute Myocardial Infarction). J Am Coll Cardiol 1996;28:1328–1428.
3. Schömig A, Neumann FJ, Kastrati A, et al. A randomized comparison of antiplatelet and anticoagulant therapy after the placement of coronary-artery stents. N Engl J Med 1996;334:1084–1089.
4. Pfeffer MA, Braunwald E, Moye LA, et al. Effect of captopril on mortality and

morbidity in patients with left ventricular dysfunction after myocardial infarction. Results of the Survival and Ventricular Enlargement (SAVE) trial. N Engl J Med 1992;327:669–677.

7 VENTRICULAR TACHYCARDIA

▶ Hello, 911 Operator?   (Level III)

Ashesh J. Gandhi, PharmD

A 41-year-old man with a history of hypertension dials 911 after experiencing two episodes of crushing chest pain that radiates down his left arm. After paramedics arrive, he requires defibrillation when ventricular tachycardia (VT) degenerates into ventricular fibrillation (VF). The patient is subsequently found to have an anterior wall MI and undergoes PTCA with stent placement. During his hospitalization, he develops sustained asymptomatic VT and multiple episodes of asymptomatic non-sustained VT. Students are asked to weigh the therapeutic alternatives for treatment of acute-onset VT and select the optimal drug and regimen for this patient. With appropriate antiarrhythmic therapy, the patient experiences no further episodes of VT and is discharged. Because of his stent placement, he is discharged on multiple medications, which requires conscientious patient education to prevent bleeding and other complications.

▶ **Questions**

Problem Identification

1. a. *What are the possible causes of sudden cardiac death and VT in this patient? What information presented in the case suggests these causes?*

   Possible Risk Factors
   - Structural heart disease (e.g., coronary artery disease, cardiomyopathies, valvular disease, or lesions of molecular structure including congenital long QT syndrome)
   - Reperfusion arrhythmias
   - Systemic factors (e.g., hypoxemia, acidosis, electrolyte imbalance)
   - Toxic cardiac effects (e.g., dose-dependent proarrhythmia, idiosyncratic proarrhythmia)

   Patient Risk Factors
   - In this particular patient, sudden cardiac death or primary VF occurred most likely due to myocardial ischemia. An external event such as physical exertion may have triggered the activation of the sympathetic nervous system, which led to an increase in the heart rate, blood pressure, platelet aggregation, and blood viscosity while inhibiting the native fibrinolytic system. These changes may have led to coronary plaque rupture and subsequent platelet aggregation that eventually leads to unstable angina and MI. The ischemic area in the myocardium then serves as a substrate for reentrant and potentially fatal arrhythmias to occur.
   - Recurrence of VT occurred as a result of reperfusion to the area of the myocardium that was not being supplied with blood. Reperfusion (with thrombolytics or interventional procedures such as angioplasty) appears to induce electrical instability by mechanisms such as reentrant and triggered activity. Hypertrophied hearts (generally due to chronic, uncontrolled hypertension) appear to be more prone to generating reperfusion-induced arrhythmias.

   b. *How are VT and NSVT characterized on the ECG?*
   - VT appears on the ECG with the occurrence of 3 or more consecutive premature ventricular complexes whose QRS duration is >120 msec. The R–R interval can be regular or sometimes may vary. Depending on the type of VT, the rates range from 70 to 250 bpm. The QRS complexes can be unchanging (uniform, monomorphic) or can vary randomly (multiform, polymorphic). VT is a sustained rhythm lasting for more than 30 seconds and if rapid enough, can lead to hemodynamic collapse, thereby requiring emergent resuscitation. In this case, the QRS complex is 140 msec in duration, the rate is 105 bpm, and the R–R interval is regular. The QRS complexes are monomorphic in nature and the rhythm lasted for more than 30 seconds.
   - Nonsustained VT (NSVT) has the same ECG criteria as VT except that the rhythm does not last for 30 seconds and terminates spontaneously.

Desired Outcome

2. *What are the goals of treatment for acute-onset VT?*
   - Rapid assessment of the patient's signs and symptoms and diagnosis of VT
   - Restoration of sinus rhythm quickly to prevent degeneration of VT to VF
   - Correction of precipitating factors to prevent recurrence of VT

Therapeutic Alternatives

3. a. *What non-drug therapies may be useful for treating acute VT in this patient?*
   - If severe symptoms are present with hemodynamic collapse, defibrillation should be instituted immediately to restore sinus rhythm. If the patient is hemodynamically stable, a transvenous pacing wire can be inserted and VT terminated by overdrive pacing.

   b. *What pharmacotherapeutic alternatives are available for the treatment of acute-onset VT?*

The following antiarrhythmic agents are recommended to be administered in order based on the most recent ACLS guidelines[1] after defibrillation and epinephrine administration.

- *Lidocaine* is the drug of choice in the setting of acute MI when treatment is indicated for VT or VF. Lidocaine is recommended as the first antiarrhythmic agent to be used in cardiac arrest patients with persistent VT/VF despite defibrillation and epinephrine. It is also indicated to prevent recurrence, to control non-sustained ventricular tachycardia requiring therapy, and to treat wide complex tachycardia of uncertain type.
- *Bretylium* is indicated for the treatment of resistant VF and hemodynamically unstable/pulseless VT. According to the current ACLS guidelines, it is only recommended after defibrillation, epinephrine, and lidocaine have failed to convert VF (or pulseless VT), or after VF has recurred despite epinephrine and lidocaine.
- *Procainamide* is listed as potential therapy in the ACLS guidelines for VF and pulseless VT refractory to defibrillation and epinephrine, but only after lidocaine, bretylium, and magnesium have failed. Procainamide may be used as potential therapy in patients with hemodynamically stable VT, but only after lidocaine has been tried.
- *Beta-blockers (metoprolol, atenolol, and propranolol)* have been shown to reduce the incidence of VF in patients with acute MI and have also been shown to reduce mortality that is arrhythmia related. In the pre-thrombolytic era, β-blockers initiated soon after MI reduced mortality by as much as 20% in the subsequent 2 to 3 years.[2] Beta-blockers are also particularly useful in the setting of recent MI with recurrent VT/VF that is unresponsive to standard antiarrhythmic therapy.
- *Amiodarone* given IV is presently only indicated for the treatment and prophylaxis of frequently recurring VF and hemodynamically destabilizing VT. It is suggested that the acute termination of VT seen after amiodarone administration is more as a result of β-blockade rather than a class I, III, or IV effect.
- *Magnesium* is recommended in the ACLS guidelines as potential therapy in patients with VF and pulseless VT refractory to defibrillation and epinephrine after lidocaine and bretylium have been administered. It is also recommended in patients with documented magnesium deficits, especially those receiving diuretics before onset of infarction and for episodes of torsade de pointes.

Optimal Plan

4. *What drug, dosage form, schedule, and duration of therapy are best for this patient for the treatment of acute-onset VT?*

- This patient suffered from VT, s/p MI with a heart rate of 105 bpm while maintaining his blood pressure. Lidocaine is generally considered the drug of choice in this situation. It acts preferentially on the ischemic myocardium, has a rapid onset and high degree of effectiveness, and is easily administered.
- Lidocaine is given in an initial IV bolus of 1.0 to 1.5 mg/kg (75 to 100 mg); additional boluses of 0.5 to 0.75 mg/kg can be given every 5 to 10 minutes if needed up to a maximum dose of 3 mg/kg. An infusion of lidocaine is then started at a rate of 1 to 4 mg/min and reduced after 24 hours to 1 to 2 mg/min. The dose of lidocaine should be decreased by 50% in the setting of heart failure, hepatic congestion, liver disease, cimetidine administration, or β-blockade.
- Lidocaine may be continued for 24 to 48 hours or until the patient is stable and then discontinued. There is no need for long-term antiarrhythmic therapy once the precipitating factor (i.e., ischemia) has been corrected. However, the patient must be closely observed in the telemetry unit for additional recurrences of arrhythmia.

Outcome Evaluation

5. *What monitoring parameters are necessary to evaluate the therapy for achievement of the desired therapeutic outcome and to prevent toxicity?*

Efficacy Parameters

- Serum lidocaine concentration; the therapeutic range is 1.4 to 5.0 μg/mL.
- Suppression of VT.
- Widening of QRS complex.

Toxicity Parameters

- CNS adverse reactions such as drowsiness, numbness, speech disturbances, dizziness, and blurred vision may occur, especially in patients over 60 years of age.
- Sino-atrial arrest is a possibility, especially during co-administration of other drugs that potentially depress nodal function.
- Bradyarrhythmias.
- Toxic effects such as seizures are usually associated with lidocaine concentrations exceeding 9.0 μg/mL.

Patient Counseling

6. *What information should be provided to the patient to enhance patient understanding and compliance upon discharge?*

- *Warfarin.* This medication is to be taken once a day. It is a blood thinner that prevents a clot from forming in the stent placed in your heart vessel. This medication is to be taken for a period of 4 weeks, at which point your doctor will determine whether you need to continue it or not. Watch for any abnormal signs of bleeding including nosebleeds, abnormal bruising, blood in the stools or urine, unusually heavy bleeding from cuts, bleeding gums, and coughing up blood. If any of these occur, contact your doctor immediately. Also, do not drink alcohol with this medication and do not alter your diet in eating green leafy vegetables. If you have a headache or pain, do not use aspirin but use Tylenol instead. You will need to go to the clinic periodically to check how thin your blood is and whether your warfarin dose needs to be adjusted. This test is called the INR. If you go to another doctor or dentist, you must tell them that you are on warfarin. If you decide to take an over-the-counter medicine or you get another prescription, ask your pharmacist if it is okay to take this medication with warfarin.
- *Enteric-coated aspirin.* This medication is to be taken once daily and must be taken whole and not crushed. This medicine is used to prevent another heart attack from occurring and also to thin your blood so that a clot does not form in your stent. Do not use more of this medication if you have a headache or pain; use Tylenol instead. This medication is to be taken every day as long as you live.
- *Ticlopidine.* Take one tablet twice a day for 1 month. This medica-

tion is also used to prevent a clot from forming in the stent. It affects blood clotting similar to aspirin, and you must watch for any abnormal signs of bleeding. Report to the doctor at once if you experience any sign of infection such as fever, chills, or sore throat. Also report any sores, ulcers, or white spots in the mouth immediately. Tell all doctors, dentists, and pharmacists that you are taking this medication.

- *Metoprolol.* Take one tablet every 12 hours. This medication is used to prevent another heart attack or chest pain and also to prevent any abnormal heartbeats from occurring. It will also slow down your heart rate and decrease your blood pressure. You may feel easily fatigued when you try to exercise or do any strenuous activity. Do not take any over-the-counter cough or cold medicines without first talking to your pharmacist or doctor. Some of these cough medicines may increase your blood pressure. Also, report any of the following side effects to your doctor: decreased sexual ability, dizziness or light-headedness, trouble sleeping, fast or slow heartbeats, and unusual tiredness or weakness.
- *Quinapril.* Take this medication once daily. You were taking this medication for your high blood pressure before you came into the hospital. You may experience dizziness or light-headedness. Check with your doctor if any of the following occur: dry cough, fever and chills, sudden trouble in breathing or swallowing, or itching of the skin.
- For all these medications, if you miss a dose, take it as soon as possible. However, if it is almost time for your next dose, skip the missed dose and go back to your regular dosing. Do not double the doses. Also, keep the medications out of the reach of children; store medications away from heat and direct light; do not store in damp places such as the bathroom since moisture may make the medicine ineffective; do not take or keep outdated medicine.

▶ Follow-up Question

1. *Create a list of the patient's drug-related problems.*

- The patient may have been receiving the wrong drug for outpatient treatment of his hypertension before his MI. Prior to admission and before suffering from an MI, the patient had a medical history of hypertension only. Unless there are compelling indications for the use of an ACE inhibitor (e.g., presence of comorbid disease states such as CHF, diabetes [type 1 with proteinuria] or MI [based on the JNC VI guidelines]), the initial therapy of choice for hypertension is a diuretic or β-blocker. These are the only classes of drugs that have been shown to decrease mortality in patients with hypertension.[3] ACE inhibitors are indicated for most patients post-MI unless contraindications exist.
- The dose of metoprolol post-MI was too low. In two major trials (MIAMI and TIMI-II), the dose of metoprolol used was 15 mg IV in three divided doses in patients with an evolving MI. In the MIAMI trial,[4] the oral dose used after the IV dose was 50 mg Q 6 H for 48 hours, then 100 mg BID thereafter. In the TIMI-II trial,[5] the oral dose was 50 mg BID for one day and then 100 mg BID thereafter. This dosing led to a significant decrease in mortality, subsequent reinfarction, and recurrent ischemia. The dose of metoprolol in this case should have been increased to 100 mg po BID, especially since the patient did not have any bradyarrhythmias or hypotension and because he did have multiple episodes of NSVT.
- The target INR for warfarin dosing was set too low. In patients who are at high risk for subacute thrombosis after stent placement, the combination of aspirin (indefinitely), ticlopidine (1 month duration), and warfarin/low-molecular-weight heparin (1 month duration) is recommended. Low-intensity warfarin should be used to maintain a target INR of 2.0–2.5 and not 1.8–2.0 as in this case.[6] Also, there is no need to overlap low-molecular-weight heparin with warfarin until the INR is therapeutic.

References

1. Hazinski MF, Cummins RO, eds. 1997 Handbook of Emergency Cardiac Care for Healthcare Providers. Dallas, American Heart Association, 1996.
2. Yusuf S, Peto R, Lewis J, et al. β-blockade during and after myocardial infarction: An overview of the randomized trials. Prog Cardiovasc Dis 1985;27:335–371.
3. Joint National Committee on Prevention, Detection, Evaluation, and Treatment of High Blood Pressure. Sixth report. Arch Intern Med 1997;157:2413–2445.
4. MIAMI Trial Research Group. Metoprolol in acute myocardial infarction. Am J Cardiol 1985;56:1G–57G.
5. TIMI Study Group. Comparison of invasive and conservative strategies after treatment with intravenous tissue plasminogen activator in acute myocardial infarction: Results of the thrombolysis in myocardial infarction (TIMI) phase II trial. N Engl J Med 1989;320:618–627.
6. Dalen JE, Hirsh J, eds. Fourth ACCP Consensus Conference on Antithrombotic Therapy. Antithrombotic therapy in patients undergoing coronary angioplasty. Chest 1995;108(4 suppl):486S–501S.
7. Moss AJ, Hall WJ, Cannom DS, et al. Improved survival with an implanted defibrillator in patients with coronary disease at high risk for ventricular arrhythmia. Multicenter Automatic Defibrillator Implantation Trial Investigators. N Engl J Med 1996;335:1933–1940.
8. American College of Cardiology/American Heart Association Task Force on Practice Guidelines (committee on management of acute myocardial infarction). ACC/AHA guidelines for the management of patients with acute myocardial infarction. J Am Coll Cardiol 1996;28:1328–1428.

8 ATRIAL FIBRILLATION

▶ If It's Not Love, Head for the ER (Level II)

Bradley G. Phillips, PharmD

The onset of heart palpitations and dizziness cause a 63-year-old man to seek medical attention at the Emergency Department. He has a history of hypertension (uncontrolled due to noncompliance), COPD, and benign prostatic hyperplasia. Issues that students must address in the case include achieving and maintaining control of ventricular response rate, restoring normal sinus rhythm, and preventing thromboembolic events. Because this patient has several comorbid disease states that may have contributed to the development of atrial fibrillation, students should be expected to discuss how treatment for this patient differs from that for a patient with lone atrial fibrillation.

▶ Questions

Problem Identification

1. a. List and prioritize the patient's drug-related problems.

- Symptomatic atrial fibrillation requiring acute drug therapy to control ventricular response.
- COPD with wheezing despite therapy with albuterol and ipratropium.
- Hypertension reportedly uncontrolled by single antihypertensive therapy (terazosin).
- Alpha blockers are not generally recommended as single-agent therapy for HTN.
- Documented noncompliance with terazosin therapy, contributing to poor BP control.
- BPH appears to be a chronic, stable drug-related problem controlled with terazosin therapy, as the patient reports no difficulty with urination.

b. Does this patient have "lone" atrial fibrillation?

- No; the diagnosis of lone atrial fibrillation is made when there is no identifiable cause for the arrhythmia. This patient's HTN is the most likely cause of his new onset atrial fibrillation. He has a history of medication noncompliance and has evidence of retinal and renal damage, supporting the contention that his HTN is poorly controlled.
- Furthermore, COPD may also contribute to atrial fibrillation. As Mr. Jacobson has suffered from both HTN and COPD for the last 15 years, it is likely that both diseases are associated with his atrial fibrillation.
- Other common causes of atrial fibrillation (not present in this patient) include myocardial ischemia or infarction, valvular disorders, and congestive or obstructive cardiomyopathy.

c. Considering his presenting signs and symptoms, how would you characterize the severity of this patient's atrial fibrillation? State the rationale for your answer.

- This patient has mildly symptomatic atrial fibrillation. Despite his arrhythmia, he is able to ambulate and can maintain a BP that is only causing mild symptoms (i.e., dizziness). He may become more symptomatic upon physical exertion because of increased adrenergic tone. For example, he first noticed palpitations and became dizzier while he was pushing his lawn mower. Atrial fibrillation in patients like this who have preserved left ventricular function tends to be less symptomatic because the heart relies less on the atria's contribution (atrial kick) to cardiac output.
- Patients with syncope are classified as having severely symptomatic atrial fibrillation. In these patients, electrical cardioversion is employed without delay to restore normal sinus rhythm and hemodynamics.

Desired Outcome

2. What are the acute goals for pharmacotherapy in this case?

The goals of therapy for this patient are[1]:

- *Control ventricular response rate.* In atrial fibrillation, the atria can beat up to 600 bpm. However, fewer impulses are conducted to the ventricles through the AV node, causing the ventricles to beat between 120 and 180 bpm. In general, a target ventricular response rate is <100 bpm. Alternatively, attaining a ventricular response rate that relieves the symptoms associated with the arrhythmia would also be appropriate. For this patient, a ventricular response rate of <100 bpm or a rate that relieved his dizziness and palpitations would be optimal.
- *Restore normal sinus rhythm.* Following ventricular rate control, cardioversion of atrial fibrillation to normal sinus rhythm may be performed electrically (by direct current cardioversion) or chemically. Chemical cardioversion is preferred over electrical cardioversion in those patients without severely symptomatic atrial fibrillation.
- *Prevent thromboembolic events.* As a result of atrial fibrillation, concerted atrial contraction is absent. For this reason, there is a risk for thrombus formation and subsequent thromboembolic events. Although it is not known how long it takes thrombi to form in the atria, it is recommended that patients with atrial fibrillation of more than 48 hours in duration receive anticoagulation therapy for 3 weeks prior to cardioversion. This patient presented to the ED within 4 hours of noticing palpitations and experiencing dizziness and therefore is less likely to have a thrombus in his atria. However, it is clinically difficult to determine the exact time his atrial fibrillation started. For example, he may have had asymptomatic atrial fibrillation for several days that only became symptomatic during physical exertion (pushing his lawn mower). In cases where the duration of atrial fibrillation is unknown, a transesophageal echocardiogram can help determine if a thrombus is present and guide subsequent therapy.[2] Patients who present to the hospital in atrial fibrillation are routinely started on heparin to keep the aPTT 1.5 to 2.0 times control. Heparin therapy will be continued in those patients who present within 48 hours from the onset of their atrial fibrillation until cardioversion. Patients who have had atrial fibrillation for more than 48 hours or who have a thrombus on echocardiogram will be started on warfarin therapy for 3 weeks until they are cardioverted.

Therapeutic Alternatives

3. Describe the benefits and risks of drugs that can be used to achieve and maintain ventricular rate control in patients with atrial fibrillation.

- *Intravenous digoxin, calcium channel antagonists, and β-blockers* may be used to achieve and maintain ventricular rate control in patients with atrial fibrillation. The selection of the best agent depends on the severity of atrial fibrillation, the presence of underlying diseases, and the clinician's experience in using specific agents. Characteristics of an ideal drug would include an agent with (1) rapid onset of action, (2) low potential for toxicity, (3) dose easily adjusted to maintain tight ventricular rate control or to lessen potential drug-induced side effects (e.g., hypotension), and (4) cost effectiveness.
- *Digoxin* has traditionally been the mainstay for ventricular rate control in patients with atrial fibrillation. However, with the advent of more rapid acting agents (see below), digoxin has fallen out of favor. Ventricular rate control is achieved slowly, usually over a 24- to 48-

hour period, after repeated IV doses.³ Other disadvantages include the need to monitor digoxin levels and the potential for digoxin toxicity. In patients with pre-existing congestive heart failure, digoxin may be the preferred agent to achieve and maintain ventricular rate control because it lacks negative inotropic activity.

- *Beta-blockers (metoprolol or esmolol)* can be given as an IV bolus to achieve acute ventricular rate control and then as an IV infusion to maintain rate control. Each drug can be titrated quickly to control ventricular response and to avoid possible side effects (e.g., hypotension). The disadvantages associated with β-blocker therapy include exacerbation of underlying diseases such as diabetes mellitus, COPD, and congestive heart failure. Since this patient has COPD, β-blocker therapy for acute ventricular rate control should be avoided.
- *Calcium channel antagonists (diltiazem or verapamil)* can be given in IV bolus doses to achieve acute ventricular rate control. Each drug can also be administered as a continuous IV infusion and titrated to control ventricular response and avoid possible side effects (e.g., hypotension). The disadvantages associated with these agents include hypotension and worsening of systolic function in patients with pre-existing congestive heart failure. Diltiazem and verapamil are equally effective in achieving and maintaining ventricular response, but verapamil is associated more frequently with hypotension.⁴

Optimal Plan

4. Which agent and dosage regimen would you recommend to achieve and maintain control of this patient's ventricular response rate?

- IV diltiazem or verapamil therapy is the best choice for ventricular rate control in this patient. These drugs are equally effective, but verapamil is more commonly associated with hypotension.
- Diltiazem 20 mg (0.25 mg/kg) may be given as an IV bolus over 2 minutes. If the patient tolerates the initial dose but does not achieve ventricular rate control, a second bolus dose of 25 mg (0.35 mg/kg) may be given 15 to 30 minutes later. If the patient responds, an IV infusion can be started at 10 mg/hr, which can be titrated to response and tolerability; the maximum recommended infusion rate for diltiazem is 15 mg/hr.
- Verapamil 5 mg (0.075 mg/kg) may be given as an IV bolus over 2 minutes. If the patient tolerates the initial dose but does not achieve ventricular rate control, a second bolus dose of 5 to 10 mg (0.075 to 0.15 mg/kg) may be given in a similar fashion 15 to 30 minutes later if no response is achieved. If the patient responds, an IV infusion can be started at 5 mg/hr and titrated to response and tolerability; the usual maximum infusion rate is 10 mg/hr.
- Beta-blocker therapy should be avoided because the patient has COPD. Digoxin may be considered, but due to its delayed onset of action it would be more appropriate as an alternate therapy.

Outcome Evaluation

5. How would you monitor and adjust the IV infusion to control his ventricular response rate?

- A positive response to therapy is generally defined as a >10% reduction from baseline ventricular rate with resolution of symptoms or achieving a ventricular response rate of <100 bpm.
- This patient was actually given a single 20-mg IV bolus dose of diltiazem over 2 minutes. After 15 minutes his ventricular rate decreased from a baseline value of 131 bpm to 95 bpm (see Casebook Figure 8–1). This is a 27% reduction from baseline with a rate of <100 bpm. He stated that he felt better and did not notice the fluttering in his chest, and his BP remained stable. Diltiazem was therefore well tolerated and effective in achieving ventricular rate control. A continuous diltiazem infusion at 10 mg/hr was started to maintain his ventricular response.
- The goal now is to maintain control of the patient's ventricular response rate (rate <100 bpm) with a continuous infusion. Diltiazem can be infused at an initial rate of 10 mg/hr and can be titrated to a recommended maximum of 15 mg/hr. Diltiazem or verapamil infusion can be increased at 60-minute intervals by 2 to 3 mg/hr if needed to maintain his ventricular response rate <100 bpm. At 10-minute intervals and just prior to increasing the infusion rate, his rhythm, ventricular response rate, and BP should be monitored. If his systolic BP falls below 90 mm Hg or if he has symptomatic hypotension, the infusion should be held and then restarted at a lower dose once his BP stabilizes.

▶ Follow-up Questions

1. Is it possible that the drug therapy you recommended to control the ventricular response rate will also convert his atrial fibrillation to normal sinus rhythm?

- No; diltiazem, and other agents such as verapamil, β-blockers, or digoxin, will not convert the arrhythmia to normal sinus rhythm. However, he may spontaneously convert to sinus rhythm irrespective of his diltiazem therapy. This would also apply if verapamil, digoxin, or β-blocker therapy was administered. Approximately 25% of patients who present with atrial fibrillation will spontaneously convert to normal sinus rhythm. Conversion to normal sinus rhythm without antiarrhythmic therapy (e.g., quinidine) is attributable to spontaneous cardioversion.

2. If the cardiology team decides to chemically cardiovert the patient, why is it important to first control his ventricular rate?

- Antiarrhythmic therapy (e.g., quinidine) can cause a paradoxical increase in ventricular response in patients with atrial fibrillation. The number of atrial-generated impulses that the AV node is able to conduct to the ventricular conduction system depends, in part, on the refractoriness of the AV node and the cycle length between impulses. As the time between atrial impulses decreases (i.e., faster atrial rates) the more refractory the AV node becomes, leading to a decrease in the number of atrial impulses (although still rapid) that are conducted through the AV node to the ventricular conduction system.
- Antiarrhythmics like quinidine produce a slowing of atrial conduction, thereby decreasing the number of impulses that are presented to the AV node. Thus, because quinidine slows the atrial rate (i.e., increases cycle time between impulses), the AV node is less refractory and is now able to conduct a larger number of impulses. This causes a paradoxical increase in ventricular response and most likely hemodynamic instability.
- It is imperative that agents that slow conduction through or increase refractoriness of the AV node be administered before chemical cardioversion is initiated. An exception to this rule is patients with atrial

fibrillation who present with a low ventricular response, usually indicating pre-existing SA or AV nodal disease (sick sinus syndrome).[1]

3. *Assuming that the patient is successfully cardioverted, should the therapy you prescribed to control his ventricular response be prescribed long term?*

- Chronic diltiazem (or verapamil) therapy would not be needed if he had lone atrial fibrillation or if his atrial fibrillation was secondary to a reversible underlying cause. However, since there is a good chance (because of long-standing HTN and COPD) that he may have paroxysmal atrial fibrillation, longer-term therapy will help avoid hemodynamic instability if he reverts back into atrial fibrillation. Diltiazem or verapamil will not prevent the recurrence of atrial fibrillation but will help protect him from becoming symptomatic (i.e., decrease ventricular responsiveness) if atrial fibrillation recurs.

References

1. Prystowsky EN, Benson W, Fuster V, et al. Management of patients with atrial fibrillation. A statement for healthcare professionals from the Subcommittee on Electrocardiography and Electrophysiology, American Heart Association. Circulation 1996;93:1262–1277.
2. Seto TB, Taira DA, Tsevat J, et al. Cost-effectiveness of transesophageal echocardiographic-guided cardioversion: A decision analytic model for patients admitted to the hospital with atrial fibrillation. J Am Coll Cardiol 1997;29:122–130.
3. Roberts SA, Diaz C, Nolan PE, et al. Effectiveness and costs of digoxin treatment for atrial fibrillation and flutter. Am J Cardiol 1993;72:567–573.
4. Phillips BG, Gandhi AJ, Sanoski CA, et al. Comparison of intravenous diltiazem and verapamil for the acute treatment of atrial fibrillation and atrial flutter. Pharmacotherapy 1997;17:1238–1245.

9 HYPERTROPHIC CARDIOMYOPATHY

▶ Having a Big Heart Is Not Always a Good Thing (Level I)

Laura A. Bartels, PharmD

A 17 yo male is referred to a cardiologist after experiencing fatigue, shortness of breath, orthopnea, chest pressure, palpitations, and lightheadedness. A complete cardiac evaluation confirms the diagnosis of hypertrophic caridomyopathy (HCM). The goals of treatment are to reduce the patient's symptoms, improve exercise tolerance, and slow the progression of the disease. Non-selective β-blockers, calcium channel antagonists (especially verapamil), and antiarrhythmics such as disopyramide and amiodarone have been shown to be beneficial in this condition. Students are asked to select the appropriate drug for this patient and titrate the dosage regimen to achieve the maximum tolerated dose. Monitoring parameters include not only blood pressure and pulse, but also assessment of the degree of symptom relief. It is important that patient counseling efforts include the potential benefits of the medication in retarding disease progression so that compliance will be maximized.

▶ Questions

Problem Identification

1. *What signs and symptoms indicate the presence or severity of the patient's HCM?*

- This patient has experienced fatigue, orthopnea, dyspnea, lightheadedness, and palpitations prior to his doctor's visit.
- The echocardiographic findings confirm the diagnosis of HCM. Findings consistent with HCM include a low normal end-diastolic dimension, septal wall thickness of 16 mm, and septal-to-posterior wall thickness ratio of 1.5:1 (refer to textbook Chapter 15 for more detailed information).

Desired Outcome

2. *What are the goals of pharmacotherapy in this case?*

- The severity of HCM correlates with the severity of the patient's symptoms. Since there is no known cure or ways to prevent HCM, methods to minimize the consequences of the disease should be sought. Therefore, the goals of treatment should be to reduce symptoms, improve exercise tolerance, and retard disease progression to improve the patient's prognosis.
- Of major concern is the incidence of sudden cardiac death (SCD), especially in younger patients (10 to 35 years of age). Occasionally, the first manifestation of the disease is SCD. Risk factors for SCD in patients with HCM include (1) presentation at a younger age, (2) marked left ventricular hypertrophy, (3) family history of SCD, and (4) the presence of non-sustained ventricular tachycardia on ambulatory ECGs.[1] One long-term study showed that 68% of patients with HCM died of SCD.[2] Factors associated with SCD included age <30 years old and left ventricular end-diastolic pressures >20 mm Hg.
- Other concerns include a variety of other rhythm abnormalities such as supraventricular and ventricular tachycardias, bradyarrhythmias, aberrant atrioventricular nodal pathways, complete heart block, and a prolonged QT interval.[3,4]

Therapeutic Alternatives

3. a. *What non-drug therapies might be useful for this patient?*

- It is recommended that young patients refrain from competitive athletics even in the absence of symptoms (refer to the section on Natural History/Prognosis in textbook Chapter 15).

b. *What feasible pharmacotherapeutic alternatives are available for the treatment of HCM?*

- Agents that decrease cardiac contractility, improve diastolic dysfunction, and suppress arrhythmias have been used with some success. The three primary therapies that have been used include β-blockade, calcium channel antagonists (especially verapamil), and disopyramide.

- *Propranolol* in high doses (320 mg/day or more) is the most widely used agent and frequently reduces symptoms. The nonselective β-blockers such as propranolol have been shown to retard the progression of HCM as well as alleviate symptoms. Propranolol and verapamil increase exercise tolerance to the same extent. Cardioselective β-blockers are less desirable than nonselective drugs because they affect the outflow tract to a lesser extent. Therefore, they should be reserved for patients with COPD. Beta-blockers with intrinsic sympathomimetic activity (ISA) may not reduce the resting heart rate sufficiently and should be avoided in patients with HCM.[3]
- *Verapamil* (in doses of about 360 mg/day) may be beneficial in patients with asthma or other contraindications to the use of β-blockers. Verapamil is a very logical therapy to relieve the diastolic relaxation problems found in hypertrophic cardiomyopathy.[3,5] Contraindications to the use of verapamil in patients with HCM include a pulmonary capillary wedge pressure >20 mm Hg, a history of nocturnal dyspnea or orthopnea, sick sinus syndrome or atrioventricular nodal disease in the absence of a permanent pacemaker, and low systolic blood pressure.[6] Verapamil has been reported to have occasional dangerous or even lethal side effects, most likely due to the fact that its afterload reducing effect is more vigorous than its negative inotropic effect, so that outflow tract obstruction is precipitated. For this reason, nifedipine is also contraindicated in patients with resting obstruction.
- *Disopyramide* 150 mg po QID has demonstrated to be hemodynamically better than propranolol 40 mg po QID or placebo in a small group of patients, in that the subaortic pressure gradient was virtually abolished by disopyramide versus propranolol.[7] However, the use of propranolol alleviates other symptoms the patient experiences. Disopyramide is also a less desirable agent because its side effects include blurred vision, dry mouth, and urinary retention.
- *Amiodarone* has also been used for the management of HCM. It has negative inotropic, chronotropic, and coronary vasodilating properties. Amiodarone may also relieve symptoms and prolong exercise duration in some patients.[3] Unfortunately, SCD may still occur.

Optimal Plan

4. *What drug, dosage form, dose, and schedule, and duration of therapy are the best for this patient?*

- Start propranolol 40 mg po QID for one week and monitor heart rate to ensure that it does not drop below 60 bpm. Most patients respond to a maximum of 80 mg po QID or 320 mg po QD of a sustained-release preparation. The maximum tolerated dose of a β-blocker should be used in all patients with HCM. Any other non-selective β-blocker could also be used in equivalent doses (refer to the section on Treatment in textbook Chapter 15).
- This patient has relative contraindications to verapamil therapy because he has experienced orthopnea and has a family history of SCD.
- Disopyramide is a less desirable agent for the long-term therapy of HCM due to its side-effect profile.
- Amiodarone has a long half-life, which makes management of complications difficult should they occur.

Outcome Evaluation

5. *What clinical and laboratory parameters are necessary to evaluate the therapy for achievement of the desired therapeutic outcome and to detect or prevent adverse effects?*

- Daily recording of the patient's blood pressure and pulse should be done to monitor for hypotension and bradycardia. Because the patient is young, he should refrain from athletic activity to maintain his heart rate between 60 bpm and 130 bpm. Any variation beyond these boundaries should be recorded in a journal. Symptoms of decompensation (SOB, fatigue, lightheadedness, inability to conduct daily activities, orthopnea, and palpitations) should also be recorded in the journal, which can be reviewed by his doctor at regularly scheduled follow-up visits.
- The patient should also be asked whether he is obtaining relief of his symptoms of shortness of breath, orthopnea, palpitations, lightheadedness, and chest pain. His activity level at the time of symptoms should also be assessed (e.g., climbing a flight of stairs versus resting in a chair).
- He should be asked about the presence of side effects of propranolol at high doses, such as fatigue, impotence, depression, nightmares, insomnia, lethargy, and, rarely, psychotic changes.

Patient Counseling

6. *What information should be provided to the patient to enhance compliance, ensure successful therapy, and minimize adverse effects?*

- Your doctor has prescribed propranolol for your heart condition called "hypertrophic cardiomyopathy." This is why your heart muscle is thicker than in most other young men your age. This medication will slow your heart rate, which will allow your heart to rest better and slow the progression of your condition.
- Take one 40-mg tablet four times a day for the next week. Your doctor may decide to increase the dose at that time if you are tolerating the medicine well. It is important that you do not stop this medication on your own without first checking with your doctor.
- When you take this medication, swallow the tablet whole with a glass of water. Try not to miss any doses, because this medication needs to be taken on a regular basis to improve your condition. If you do forget to take a dose, take it as soon as you remember. However, if it is within 4 hours of your next dose, skip the missed dose and go back to your regular dosing schedule. Do not double doses.
- Store this medication out of the reach of children, and away from heat and direct light. Do not store this medication in the bathroom, near the kitchen sink, or in other damp places. Heat and/or moisture may cause this medication to break down. Do not keep outdated medication any longer than needed and discard any unused portion out of the reach of children.
- It is important that your doctor check your progress at regularly scheduled visits. This is to make sure that this medication is working for you and to allow the dosage to be changed if needed. Your doctor may want you to carry a medical identification card stating that you are taking this medication. Make sure that you have enough medication on hand to last you through this week before you see your doctor again for your next prescription.

- Make sure that you discuss with your doctor the safe amount of exercise for your condition.
- Do not take other medications unless they have been discussed with your doctor. This includes over-the-counter medications for colds, cough, sinus problems, and appetite control.
- This medication may cause you to feel tired at first. In time, you may build a tolerance to this effect once a steady dose is maintained. Notify your doctor as soon as possible if any of the following effects occur: breathing difficulty or wheezing, cold hands and feet, confusion or dizziness, irregular heartbeat, mental depression, vivid dreams or nightmares, skin rash, a slow heart beat (<50 beats per minute), or swelling of ankles, feet, or lower legs.
- To monitor your therapy it is a good idea to take your pulse and blood pressure and record them in a daily log. Also record any activity you recently finished or are currently doing when you took the measurements. It is ideal to have your heart rate be above 60 beats per minute while awake and go no higher than 130 beats per minute during the amount of physical exercise allowed by your doctor. Call your doctor right away if your heart rate or blood pressure is out of the ordinary.
- If you have any questions, concerns, or desire further information about this medication or your medical condition, please ask your doctor, nurse, or me.

▶ Follow-up Question

1. *Are any adjustments in his medication dosage warranted at this time?*

    - The patient has been taking propranolol 40 mg QID for 1 week and monitoring his heart rate to go no less than 60 bpm while awake. At this point, an increase in dosage should be made to achieve the maximum tolerated dose of the β-blocker to slow the progression of his disease. As stated above, most patients respond to 80 mg po QID of a prompt-release product or 320 mg po QD of a sustained-release preparation.
    - One common method is to give 80 mg po QID for 1 week before switching to a sustained release preparation (320 mg once daily). Should complications arise during this second week, it will be easier to titrate the dose to patient needs if the shorter-acting preparation is being used. Once the maximum tolerated dose is established, the patient may be switched to a sustained-release preparation.

References

1. Maron BJ, Roberts WC. Hypertrophic cardiomyopathy. In: Schlant RC, Alexander RW, eds. Hurst's The Heart, 8th ed. New York, McGraw-Hill, 1994: 1621–1635.
2. Koga Y, Ogata M, Kihara K, et al. Sudden death in hypertrophic and dilated cardiomyopathy. Jpn Circ J 1989;53:1546–1556.
3. Maron BJ, Bonow RO, Cannon RO III, et al. Hypertrophic cardiomyopathy. Interrelations of clinical manifestations, pathophysiology, and therapy. N Engl J Med 1987;316:780–789, 844–852.
4. Martin AB, Garson A, Perry JC. Prolonged QT interval in hypertrophic and dilated cardiomyopathy in children. Am Heart J 1994;127:64–70.
5. Hopf R, Kaltenbach M. Management of hypertrophic cardiomyopathy. Annu Rev Med 1990;41:75–83.
6. Rosing DR, Idanpaan-Heikkila U, Maron BJ, et al. Use of calcium channel blocking drugs in hypertrophic cardiomyopathy. Am J Cardiol 1985;55:185B–195B.
7. Pollick C. Disopyramide in hypertrophic cardiomyopathy. II. Noninvasive assessment after oral administration. Am J Cardiol 1988;62:1252–1255.

10 DEEP VEIN THROMBOSIS

▶ From San Diego to Portland (Level I)

Nannette A. Sageser, PharmD

An 83-year-old man with a history of deep vein thrombosis (DVT) and postphlebitic syndrome develops left lower leg swelling, aching, and warmth after completing a long trip by automobile. Diagnostic tests indicate the presence of a left lower extremity DVT with no evidence of pulmonary embolism. Based on pre-determined criteria, this patient is a good candidate for home-based treatment of DVT with subcutaneous low-molecular-weight heparin (LMWH) and oral warfarin. Students are asked to evaluate the LMWH and warfarin regimen the patient received and recommend suitable changes in therapy. Initiation of appropriate monitoring parameters and patient education on warfarin use and side effects are important aspects of this case.

▶ Questions

Problem Identification

1. a. *Create a list of the patient's drug-related problems.*

    - Left lower extremity DVT requiring anticoagulation management.
    - Chronic stable problems requiring no intervention at this time include hypothyroidism controlled with levothyroxine (TSH within normal range) and benign prostatic hypertrophy (BPH) treated with terazosin (although the patient has complaints of nocturia and recent history of reduced frequency of urination, which may require attention if they become more troublesome or severe).

    b. *What risk factors for DVT are present in this patient?*

    - Prior history of DVT with postphlebitic syndrome (venous obstruction from any cause)
    - History of colon cancer (hypercoagulable state due to multiple factors)
    - Long car trip (immobility leading to venous stasis)
    - Elderly patient (venous stasis due to poor venous return/circulation)

    c. *What subjective and objective evidence is suggestive of a lower extremity DVT?*

    Subjective Evidence
    - Calf about "double" the normal size

- Aching/pain in the LLE
- LLE feels warm to the touch
- Sock feels tight on the left lower leg

Objective Evidence
- Left calf is 6 cm larger in circumference than right calf, left ankle swelling
- (+) Homan's sign with palpable cord
- (+) Doppler ultrasound

Desired Outcome

2. What are the immediate and long-term therapeutic goals for this patient?

- The immediate goal is to minimize extension of the DVT and prevent embolization with appropriate anticoagulation using heparin and warfarin.
- The primary long-term goal is to prevent future embolic events by using warfarin chronically or indefinitely, since this is his second episode.
- Maximize warfarin therapy while minimizing any adverse outcomes or side effects related to anticoagulation management.

Therapeutic Alternatives

3. a. What are the therapeutic alternatives for the initial anticoagulation management of this patient?

- *Unfractionated IV heparin therapy and oral warfarin.* The patient could be admitted to the hospital and started on standard IV heparin. To minimize the recurrence of venous thromboembolism, it is desirable to reach a therapeutic aPTT within the first 24 hours after starting heparin therapy. Several nomograms have been published to aid in reaching this goal. Hull and associates suggest an initial heparin loading dose of 5000 to 10,000 units followed by a maintenance infusion of 1300 units/hr.[1] Using a widely accepted weight-based nomogram,[2] one would use a loading dose of 6400 units (80 units/kg) followed by a continuous heparin infusion of 1400 units/hr (18 units/kg/hr) in this patient. Once the aPTT is within the therapeutic range (1.5 to 2.5 × control), start warfarin 5 mg po QD and titrate to achieve an INR of 2.0 to 3.0. Once the INR is therapeutic for 24 hours (or 2 consecutive levels), discontinue the heparin infusion. The patient could then be discharged to home on a maintenance dose of warfarin for follow-up with his PCP or the anticoagulation service.
- *LMWH therapy and warfarin.* Certain criteria must be met in order for a patient to be considered a good candidate for home-based treatment of DVT. Patients must be willing to participate in their own care, including self-injection of medication and daily follow-up for warfarin dosing adjustments. Exclusion criteria for home-based treatment of DVT may include: suspected PE, high risk of bleeding (malignant HTN, PUD, recent surgery, known bleeding disorder, fall risk, or thrombocytopenia), pregnancy, inability to follow-up for daily PT/INR monitoring, and financial constraints. The two pharmacologic options available at the time of this writing include enoxaparin 1 mg/kg SQ twice daily, or dalteparin 200 units/kg SQ once daily.[3]

  LMWH should be started immediately after diagnosis of DVT and should be administered for a minimum of 5 days. Warfarin therapy should be initiated on the same day as the LMWH or the day after. Obtain daily PT/INRs, and titrate warfarin to achieve an INR of 2.0 to 3.0. Once the INR is therapeutic for 24 hours (or 2 consecutive levels), discontinue the LMWH. The patient is then maintained on warfarin alone.
- *Thrombolytic therapy.* This is not a good choice for this patient; thrombolytics are usually reserved for selected patients with extensive proximal vein thrombosis or life-threatening pulmonary embolism. Thrombolytic therapy has not been shown to be more effective than anticoagulant therapy in the management of DVT. Routine use of thrombolytic therapy is not recommended because of the increased risk of hemorrhage and the higher cost of therapy.

b. What alternatives are available if this patient were to have a history of heparin-induced thrombocytopenia (HIT)?

- There is >90% immune cross-reactivity between standard heparin and LMWH. In contrast, cross-reactivity is much less common (approximately 10%) with danaparoid sodium. If available, the physician could use danaparoid SQ instead of heparin or LMWH with less risk of developing HIT syndrome.

Optimal Plan

4. Do you agree with the above plan made by the patient's PCP? If not, what would you recommend at this point in therapy?

- The physician recommended a 40% increase in the total weekly dose of warfarin (from 25 to 35 mg/week), which could lead to a supratherapeutic INR. A practical dosing adjustment is achieved by calculating the total milligrams per week and using approximately 10% of that number to make an increase or decrease in total weekly dose.[4] Because the patient's INR is 1.85, a total weekly dose increase of about 10% would be reasonable. For example, his new dose of warfarin could be 5 mg po on Monday, Wednesday, Friday, and Saturday, and 2.5 mg po on Tuesday, Thursday, and Sunday (27.5 mg/week). Preference for which days to use half-tablets is left up to the clinician managing the warfarin. Using a dosing regimen that utilizes single-strength tablets (e.g., 5 mg) minimizes the opportunity for dosing errors. A great deal of flexibility can be achieved by using half-tablets and whole tablets and basing dosing instructions accordingly. If the tablet strength of warfarin was changed with each dosage adjustment, the patient may become confused because of the various strengths of warfarin tablets he or she has on hand (and all the different colors).
- An alternative to this dosing could be 4 mg po QD (28 mg/week,) since this would still be approximately a 10% increase in total weekly dose. Also, when a dosage adjustment is made, follow-up in 4 weeks is insufficient. The patient should have a repeat PT/INR in 10 to 14 days.
- NOTE: This patient was placed on the Coumadin brand of warfarin, but generic warfarin also could have been used. In general, it is best to maintain a patient on the product that was used initially. Avoid switching back and forth between brand and generic products to minimize PT/INR fluctuations.

Outcome Evaluation

5. What clinical and laboratory monitoring parameters should be as-

sessed to ensure the efficacy and safety of chronic warfarin therapy in this patient?

Clinical Parameters

- Assess leg for swelling, pain, redness, or increased warmth to touch (suggesting recurrent DVT) at each anticoagulation clinic visit. The patient should also assess these parameters at home and call or go to the ED if necessary.
- Assess the patient for coughing, SOB, chest pain, or blood-tinged sputum (suggesting progression of DVT to PE). Assess these parameters by thoroughly questioning the patient at each anticoagulation clinic visit. Patient home assessment is also needed; he should be directed to call or go to the ED if these symptoms develop.
- Excessive bruising, bloody nose or gums, or blood in urine or stool may indicate overanticoagulation. Assess for these findings at each anticoagulation clinic visit visually and through extensive patient questioning. Patient home assessment is needed, and he should be instructed to call or go to the ED if these symptoms appear.
- Severe headache, weakness, numbness or tingling of extremities, or visual disturbances may also indicate overanticoagulation. These complications should be assessed at each anticoagulation clinic visit by questioning the patient.

Laboratory Parameters

- Check PT/INR every 4 to 6 weeks (if stable); more frequent testing should be done after each dosage adjustment until the INR is again stable. The exact timing of retesting depends on how far the patient is from the therapeutic range.
- Obtain U/A, stool guaiac, and CBC with platelets every 6 months to assess for internal bleeding.

Patient Counseling

6. *What information should be provided to the patient to enhance compliance and minimize adverse effects of warfarin therapy?*

- Warfarin decreases the clotting ability of the blood and therefore decreases the chance of developing harmful clots in the blood vessels. It is sometimes called a blood thinner, but it does not actually thin the blood. Warfarin does not dissolve clots, but it can prevent the clots from becoming larger and causing more serious problems.
- Many different medications can affect the way warfarin works in your body. It is very important to tell your health care provider if you are taking any other prescription, non-prescription, or herbal products. Also inform them of any dosage changes that occur with your current medications. Inform your provider if you become sick and have an elevated temperature, diarrhea, or vomiting.
- Take the warfarin only as directed. Take your dose of warfarin at the same time each day, and take it at a time that is easy for you to remember to help with compliance. Your doctor or pharmacist will check your protime on a regular basis and may need to make adjustments in the amount of warfarin you take each day. It is very important to keep your protime appointments.
- If you miss a dose of warfarin, take it as soon as possible. If you do not remember until the next day, do not take the missed dose and do not double the next one (this may cause bleeding). Instead, go back to your regular dosing schedule and tell your provider about the missed dose of warfarin.
- While you are taking warfarin, it is important to avoid sports or activities that may cause you to be injured. Be careful to avoid cutting yourself.
- The warfarin can be affected by the amount of vitamin K in your diet. Eat a normal, well-balanced diet, and check with your provider before starting any new vitamins, nutritional supplements, or fad diets. It is important to be consistent in the amount of vitamin K that you take in each day through the foods that you eat. You do not have to avoid these foods; just use them in moderation. Some common foods that contain higher levels of vitamin K include broccoli, spinach, cabbage, kale, brussel sprouts, and liver. Your health care provider can give you a complete list of foods and their vitamin K content.
- Alcohol can also affect how the warfarin works in your body. Avoid binge drinking or drinking more than 1 to 2 drinks at a given time. Notify your provider if the amount of alcohol you consume changes substantially.
- Call your doctor immediately if any of the following side effects occur: unexplained bruising, bleeding from the nose, blood in the urine, bloody or black stools, coughing up blood, severe headache, unusual tiredness, or weakness.

References

1. Hull RD, Raskob GE, Rosenbloom D, et al. Optimal therapeutic level of heparin therapy in patients with venous thrombosis. Arch Intern Med 1992;152:1589–1595.
2. Raschke RA, Reilly BM, Guidry JR, et al. The weight-based heparin dosing nomogram compared with a "standard care" nomogram: A randomized controlled trial. Ann Intern Med 1993;119:874–881.
3. Chaffee BJ. Low-molecular-weight heparins for treatment of deep vein thrombosis. Am J Health-Syst Pharm 1997;54:1995–1999.
4. Oertel LB. Managing maintenance therapy. In: Ansell JE, Oertel LB, Wittkowsky AK, eds. Managing Oral Anticoagulation Therapy: Clinical and Operational Guidelines. Gaithersburg, MD, Aspen, 1997:4B-3:1–3:4.

11 PULMONARY EMBOLISM

▶ **The Clot Thickens** (Level I)

Amy L. Seybert, PharmD
Ted L. Rice, MS, BCPS

A 22-year-old woman taking oral contraceptives presents to the Emergency Department with pleuritic chest pain, shortness of breath, and cough of 11 days' duration. Physical examination and initial diagnostic studies are inconclusive for thromboembolic disease, but the decision is made to initiate empiric treatment for pulmonary embolism until further confirmatory studies are completed. Students are asked to select the appropriate therapy and design an optimal dosing regimen for this situation. When a pulmonary angiogram indicates the presence of a pulmonary embolism (PE), students must decide on the most appropriate therapy to minimize the duration of hospitalization and initiate therapy for outpatient management of PE. The case gives students the opportunity to respond to actual changes in therapy that were made based on coagulation tests and to consider use of a new outpatient treatment approach employing low-molecular-weight heparin and warfarin.

Pulmonary Embolism

▶ Questions

Problem Identification

1. a. *What risk factors for the development of a pulmonary embolus are present in this patient?*

   - The primary risk factor for thromboembolism in this patient is current estrogen use (an oral contraceptive agent).[1] Estrogens have been shown to increase clotting factors and induce hypercoagulability in a dose-dependent fashion. There also appears to be an increased risk of venous thrombosis associated with the progestin component of oral contraceptives.[2]
   - Other risk factors for PE (for which there is no evidence in this patient) include:
     ✓ Immobility (i.e., as part of Virchow's triad)
     ✓ Obesity, cigarette smoking, and hypertension have been identified as risk factors for the development of pulmonary embolism in women[3]
     ✓ Lupus anticoagulant
     ✓ Deficiencies of endogenous anticoagulant factors

   b. *What subjective and objective evidence is suggestive of a pulmonary embolus in this patient? (see Figure 11–1).*

   - Subjective: Chest pain (acute onset), shortness of breath when talking, cough.
   - Objective: Hemoptysis, tachycardia, tachypnea.
   - Note that the Homan's sign was negative in this patient. A positive sign is discomfort in the calf on forced dorsiflexion of the foot, which may indicate thrombosis in the calf veins. However, this is a non-specific and insensitive test that lacks diagnostic accuracy (refer to the section on Clinical Presentation in Chapter 17 of the textbook).

Desired Outcome

2. *What are the goals of therapy for this patient?*

   - Prevent mortality and reduce morbidity from the acute event
   - Prevent the recurrence of thromboembolic events
   - Minimize the potential for adverse drug reactions
   - Minimize the cost of therapy and length of hospital stay
   - Provide an alternative method of birth control without risk for thromboembolic events

Therapeutic Alternatives

3. a. *What non-pharmacologic therapeutic alternatives are available for the acute treatment of pulmonary embolism?*

   - Surgical pulmonary embolectomy is uncommon and is indicated in emergency situations where massive pulmonary embolism compromises cardiopulmonary function. Embolectomy is not indicated in this case because the patient is not demonstrating cardiopulmonary instability.
   - Surgical interruption of the inferior vena cava by ligation has been largely supplanted by percutaneous placement of a transvenous filter or umbrella. Insertion of such a device may be indicated when anticoagulation is ineffective or unsafe in a particular patient. In some situations, concomitant therapy with an intracaval device and anticoagulants is used.

   b. *What pharmacotherapeutic alternatives are available for the acute treatment of pulmonary embolism?*

   - The traditional method of treating acute PE is initial anticoagulation with IV unfractionated heparin followed by long-term anticoagulation with oral warfarin. One standard method is to give an IV heparin bolus of 5000 units followed by a continuous IV infusion starting at 1000 units/hr. Subcutaneous heparin injection of 15,000 to 17,500 units twice daily has also been used. More recently, weight-adjusted dosing has been shown to be more effective than administration of the same dosage to all patients. In one method, an IV bolus dose of 80 units/kg is followed by a continuous infusion of 18 units/kg/hr.[4] When compared to standard care (5000 unit bolus followed by 1000 units/hr), this weight-based dosing regimen resulted in a shorter time to achieve a therapeutic aPTT. Recurrent venous thromboembolism also occurred less frequently in patients who received weight-based dosing.
   - Warfarin can be started within the first day of heparin therapy. It is essential that the heparin dosing regimen achieves a therapeutic aPTT rapidly and that the period of overlap of heparin and warfarin is sufficient to allow the full antithrombotic effects of warfarin to be expressed (i.e., 4 to 5 days).
   - An even more recent method of anticoagulation in patients at low risk of recurrent PE consists of initial dosing with low-molecular-weight heparin (LMWH) with concomitant warfarin started at 5 mg/day for long-term anticoagulation.[5] Subcutaneous administration is more convenient than IV administration and may permit self-administration by the patient on an outpatient basis, thereby reducing the length of hospitalization. For these reasons, this method is an attractive alternative to continuous IV unfractionated heparin. However, only limited data are available at the time of this writing and this treatment strategy has not yet become a universally accepted standard of care.
   - Thrombolytic therapy with the fibrinolytic enzymes streptokinase, urokinase, or alteplase (tissue plasminogen activator, TPA) accelerates the rate of emboli dissolution.[6] However, thrombolytic therapy is associated with an increased risk of bleeding, is more expensive than heparin, and most patients do well with anticoagulant therapy. For these reasons, only about 10% of PE cases are treated with thrombolysis in the United States. Thrombolytic therapy is primarily indicated in patients with a massive/submassive pulmonary embolism and associated hemodynamic compromise.

Optimal Plan

4. a. *Design a pharmacotherapeutic plan for the empiric treatment of pulmonary embolism in this patient.*

   - This patient has no absolute contraindications to anticoagulant therapy and should receive heparin. An IV heparin infusion should be administered using weight-based doses such as the Raschke method.[4] Using that regimen, this patient should receive an initial bolus of 5000 units (80 units/kg) followed by a continuous infusion of 1100 units/kg/hr (18 units/kg/hr). Note that calculated doses should be rounded to achieve numbers that are easily administered and adjusted by the clinical staff with less potential for error.

b. *Based on the new information, what additions or changes need to be made to the current therapy?*

- The V/Q scan demonstrated defects in the left lower lobe that do not indicate a massive pulmonary embolus. The patient is also stable hemodynamically. Therefore, surgical pulmonary embolectomy is not indicated.
- The patient has no contraindication to anticoagulation and does not appear to have a history of recurrent PEs while on adequate anticoagulation; therefore, placement of an IVC filter is not indicated.
- Finally, the patient is not a candidate for thrombolytic therapy because she is not hemodynamically compromised.
- The patient should therefore be continued on the initial regimen of continuous IV heparin.
- Oral anticoagulation with warfarin should be started (initial dosage range 5 to 10 mg/day × 3 days and adjust based on INR), overlapped with heparin (which the patient was started on in the ED) until the INR is in the therapeutic range for 1 to 5 days. Warfarin should be continued for at least 3 months. Warfarin therapy should be initiated promptly (i.e., day 1 or 2) once the decision for long-term anticoagulation is made to reduce the patient's length of hospitalization.
- Because erythromycin inhibits the hepatic cytochrome P450 system and the metabolism of warfarin, erythromycin should be changed to an antimicrobial agent that does not affect warfarin pharmacokinetics, such as azithromycin, levofloxacin, or ofloxacin.

Outcome Evaluation

5. a. *What monitoring parameters should be used to assess efficacy and toxicity of anticoagulation?*

- Heparin therapy is usually monitored by the aPTT, and warfarin therapy is usually monitored by the PT and INR.
- Obtain a baseline assessment of aPTT, PT/INR, and CBC with platelet count.
- An aPTT should be obtained no sooner than 6 hours after heparin therapy initiation or after any heparin dose adjustment; because the half-life of heparin is about 90 minutes, it takes about 6 hours for the maximum effect of dosage initiation or dosage change to be seen. The target aPTT is 1.5 to 2.5 times the baseline value. Check the aPTT at least once daily during heparin therapy to maintain the aPTT in the therapeutic range.
- Beginning on the second day of warfarin therapy, check the PT and INR daily until stable. Dosage adjustments should be based on the INR; the target range is 2.0 to 3.0.
- Obtain hemoglobin, hematocrit, and platelet count every 3 days to identify occult bleeding and thrombocytopenia associated with heparin therapy.
- Monitor daily for visual signs of obvious bleeding, such as hematomas, epistaxis, and hematemesis. Diagnostic tests for occult bleeding can be performed, such as identification of guaiac-positive stools and the presence of hematuria identified by urine dipstick test in addition to visual evidence.

b. *What is your assessment of the appropriateness of these interventions?*

- The aPTT value on day one of hospitalization, 6 hours after heparin was started, was less than desired. The rate increase of 400 units/hour (or about 6 units/kg/hour) was excessive and this became apparent with the 6-hour post rate increase aPTT of 90 sec. The Raschke weight-based heparin nomogram recommends re-bolusing with 80 units/kg (or 5000 units) and increasing the rate by 4 units/kg/hour (to 1400 units/hour). The heparin dose was appropriately decreased and maintained throughout the remainder of the hospitalization.
- The warfarin loading regimen of 5 mg/day on the first 3 days of therapy, or a non-aggressive dosing approach, was appropriate since urgent anticoagulation was not necessary. If rapid anticoagulation is required, warfarin could be initiated as an initial dose of 10 mg/day for two days, with the INR checked and the dose adjusted accordingly. An initial warfarin dose of 10 mg offers no clear advantage over a 5 mg initial dose and carries a greater risk of excessive anticoagulation. An INR within the desired range of 2.0 to 3.0 was obtained on day 5 of hospitalization; therefore, since the patient was stable and had no further complications, she could be discharged to home.
- Warfarin inhibits vitamin K-dependent coagulation factors, such as protein C. After warfarin initiation in some patients, there can be a decline in circulating levels of protein C. This can result in a transient hypercoagulable state leading to thrombosis of the microvasculature and necrosis of the surrounding skin. This complication has been associated with protein C deficiency and protein S deficiency (less commonly), but can occur in nondeficient patients. The most common sites for warfarin-induced skin necrosis are the breast, thigh, and buttocks. It is proposed that warfarin and heparin therapy should be overlapped because of the delayed onset of warfarin's effect and the potential for hypercoagulabilty following initiation of warfarin. Therefore, it could be argued that this patient's heparin was discontinued too soon and should have been continued until the INR was within the therapeutic range for at least 2 days.

Patient Counseling

6. *What medication counseling about warfarin should this patient receive at the time of hospital discharge?*

- Warfarin is being prescribed for you to minimize the risk of developing future blood clots. Do not stop taking this medication unless your doctor tells you to do so. To avoid missing a dose, take warfarin at the same time each day. Record each dose on a calendar when you take it. Remember to follow-up with your doctor for the necessary blood work (INR, PT) to check your response to this medication and make any dosage adjustments if necessary.
- You may wish to carry a card or wear a medical bracelet indicating that you are receiving warfarin. Be sure to inform all medical personnel that you are taking warfarin.
- Although side effects of warfarin are not common, they can occur.

Some side effects include signs of bleeding, including nosebleeds, black stools, bleeding gums, red/brown urine, easy bruising, excessive menstrual bleeding, weakness, or dizziness. Contact your doctor immediately if any of these signs or symptoms occur. It may be necessary to adjust the warfarin dose or administer an antidote.
- Do not increase or decrease your normal consumption of foods containing vitamin K, such as green leafy vegetables, broccoli, and cauliflower. An increase in your intake of vitamin K may reduce the effects of warfarin.
- Do not take or discontinue other medications (prescription or nonprescription) without approval from your doctor. If you need a pain reliever, acetaminophen is the agent of choice. A recent report suggests that total weekly acetaminophen intake should be less than 9 g (18 extra-strength tables) per week to avoid the risk of overanticoagulation.[7]
- Avoid alcoholic beverages while taking warfarin.
- Do not use this medication if you are pregnant. Warfarin can cross the placenta and cause abnormalities to the unborn child. If you think that you could be pregnant, contact your physician immediately.
- Avoid activities associated with high risk of injury.
- Store warfarin in the container it came in and out of the reach of children. Store it at room temperature and away from light.

References

1. Price H. Deaths from venous thromboembolism associated with combined oral contraceptives. Lancet 1997;350:450.
2. Rosing J, Tans G, Nicolaes GA, et al. Oral contraceptives and venous thrombosis: Different sensitivities to activated protein C in women using second- and third-generation oral contraceptives. Br J Haematol 1997;97:233–238.
3. Goldhaber SZ, Grodstein F, Stampfer MJ, et al. A prospective study of risk factors for pulmonary embolism in women. JAMA 1997;277:642–645.
4. Raschke RA, Reilly BM, Guidry JR, et al. The weight-based heparin dosing nomogram compared with a "standard care" nomogram. A randomized controlled trial. Ann Intern Med 1993;119:874–881.
5. Simonneau G, Sors H, Charbonnier B, et al. A comparison of low-molecular-weight heparin with unfractionated heparin for acute pulmonary embolism. N Engl J Med 1997;337:663–669.
6. Goldhaber SZ. Contemporary pulmonary embolism thrombolysis. Chest 1995;107(1 suppl):45S–51S.
7. Hylek EM, Heiman H, Skates SJ, et al. Acetaminophen and other risk factors for excessive warfarin anticoagulation. JAMA 1998;279:657–662.

12 CHRONIC ANTICOAGULATION

▶ A Delicate Balance   (Level II)

Beth Bryles Phillips, PharmD

A 59-year-old man with GERD and recurrent thromboembolism presents for follow-up evaluation of his chronic warfarin therapy. He reports having an episode of epistaxis, and his INR increased from 2.7 to 3.5 over the last month. He stated that he has been taking vitamin E 1000 IU daily for about 4 weeks to prevent a heart attack. He is also experiencing GERD symptoms that will require pharmacologic intervention. Students are asked to consider all possible reasons for the patient's over-anticoagulation and to recommend alternatives to reduce the INR to the target range. Institution of effective therapy for GERD during concomitant warfarin therapy also needs to be addressed. Once interventions are made, an appropriate monitoring plan must be devised, and education about warfarin use should be reviewed with the patient.

▶ Questions

Problem Identification

1. a. *Identify this patient's drug-related problems.*

    - Supratherapeutic INR at the present time
    - Potential drug interaction between vitamin E and warfarin
    - Suboptimal treatment of GERD symptoms

   b. *Do any signs or symptoms indicate that this patient is over-anticoagulated?*

    - *Symptoms*. The patient reports one episode of epistaxis.
    - *Signs*. The present INR is 3.5, which is above the desired range of 2.0 to 3.0.[1]

   c. *What questions would you ask this patient to assess his current warfarin therapy?*

    - Have you started any new medications recently, including prescription, OTC, and alternative therapies? It is especially important to ask patients about OTC medications (particularly OTC NSAIDs) and alternative therapies, because patients will often forget to mention these agents because they have not been prescribed. However, they can have a substantial impact on warfarin therapy.
    - Have you stopped taking any medications recently?
    - What dose of warfarin are you taking? (Verify dose and color of tablet.)
    - Have you had any recent changes in your diet? (i.e., alteration in consumption of vitamin K-containing foods, alcohol intake)
    - Have you missed any doses?
    - Have you taken any extra doses recently?
    - Have you had any episodes of bleeding, unexplained bruises, or bruises that do not seem to heal?

Desired Outcome

2. *What are the goals of oral anticoagulant therapy in this patient?*

    - Minimize risk of recurrent DVTs and PEs in this patient

- Minimize adverse effects (i.e., bleeding) associated with warfarin therapy
- Maintain the INR between 2.0 and 3.0 to ensure adequate anticoagulation with a minimum of adverse effects

Therapeutic Alternatives

3. a. What medications other than warfarin could be used to prevent recurrent thromboembolism in this patient?

- Although not as popular as warfarin, dose-adjusted subcutaneous (SQ) heparin may be used to prevent recurrent TBE. Dose-adjusted SQ heparin is usually reserved for patients who are unable to take warfarin (e.g., pregnant women). In addition to being more difficult to administer than warfarin, this delivery method is associated with the risk of heparin-induced osteoporosis (risk increases with dose and duration of therapy). For these reasons, patients and clinicians generally prefer warfarin therapy. Because this patient has no contraindication to warfarin therapy, dose-adjusted SQ heparin was not considered for him.
- Another option is to use a low-molecular-weight heparin (LMWH) product (e.g., enoxaparin, dalteparin). A potential advantage of these agents is the reduced need for laboratory monitoring. A predictable dose–response relationship eliminates the need for laboratory monitoring in most patients. Disadvantages include cost (price per dose is much higher than warfarin) and route of administration (injectable versus oral). Because this patient requires chronic anticoagulant therapy and has done well on warfarin, LMWH therapy was not considered in his case.

b. Because the patient is experiencing symptoms of GERD, the physician would like to prescribe a medication to relieve his symptoms. He would like to initiate therapy with an H_2-receptor antagonist (H2RA), but he thinks there are drug interactions with these agents and warfarin. Instead, he is considering a proton pump inhibitor (PPI) because his understanding is that these agents do not interact with warfarin. He asks you if this is correct and if you could recommend an appropriate agent. What would you recommend?

- There are agents in both the H2RA and PPI classes that can interact with warfarin. In the H2RA class, a significant interaction exists between cimetidine and warfarin. However, the other agents appear to be safer to use with warfarin. Although not as pronounced as cimetidine, the PPI omeprazole has been reported to interact with warfarin.[2] When considering this class of agents, lansoprazole is a safer choice in a patient who has been stabilized on a particular warfarin dose. Both cimetidine and omeprazole can increase patient response to warfarin by reducing the clearance of R-warfarin through inhibition of the hepatic cytochrome P450 enzyme known as CYP 3A4.[3] This patient has tried some life-style modifications (avoiding food known to aggravate GERD, elevating the head of his bed, eating small meals, wearing loose-fitting clothing, and avoiding alcohol), but smoking cessation and weight loss should also be attempted. Since the patient has failed OTC antacids and his symptoms do not seem to be severe, prescription H2RAs are also a reasonable consideration. Alternatives include famotidine 20 mg po BID, nizatidine 150 mg po BID, and ranitidine 150 mg po BID (refer to textbook Chapter 30 for more detailed information).

Optimal Plan

4. Based on today's laboratory result, what is your recommendation for this patient's warfarin therapy?

- Given the patient's stable warfarin dose of 5 mg for at least the previous 6 months, one must consider other possible explanations for the elevated INR. Other factors known to raise INR values were ruled out by patient history (alcohol use, weight loss, history of disease states known to affect warfarin therapy, taking an incorrect dose, recent change in diet, and initiation of other medications known to interact with warfarin).
- One possible reason is an interaction between warfarin and the vitamin E he started 4 weeks ago. The medical literature contains conflicting results on this interaction. Several older studies reported that vitamin E can augment the anticoagulant effect of warfarin.[4–6] However, a more recent randomized, double-blind study found that vitamin E in daily doses up to 1200 IU had no effect on the INR.[7] Unfortunately, it is not uncommon to find contradictory reports of drug–drug interactions in the medical literature. Because no other factors were found to account for the increased INR in this patient, and because the vitamin E was not prescribed by a physician for a defined medical condition, it is appropriate to recommend discontinuing the vitamin E and monitoring the patient's INR closely. The current warfarin dose of 5 mg po QD should be maintained, and a follow-up PT/INR should be scheduled in about two weeks.

Outcome Evaluation

5. How will you monitor this patient's warfarin therapy?

- The INR should be maintained between the range of 2.0 to 3.0. Patients with supratherapeutic INRs are at an increased risk of bleeding. It is important to note that although the patient's *risk* of bleeding is increased, it does not mean that the patient *will* bleed. Patients may develop a bleeding episode with therapeutic INRs and may have no evidence of bleeding with very high INRs (e.g., >5.0). The patient in this case did happen to experience a minor bleeding episode with a slightly elevated INR. Patients with a subtherapeutic INR are at an increased risk of developing a TBE.
- Because many factors can alter a patient's response to warfarin therapy, the INR should be monitored on a routine basis. Upon initiation of therapy, it is wise to monitor the INR frequently until the patient has been stabilized on an individualized warfarin dose. Once the patient has been stabilized (i.e., documented stable therapeutic INRs on the same dose), the INR may be followed on a monthly basis. As stated above, this patient should have an INR checked in about 2 weeks to assess the effect of medication changes made.
- Patients should be educated on common sites of bleeding and instructed to notify their physician or pharmacist if any signs or symptoms of bleeding occur. Common sites include bleeding from the nose and gums (often after brushing teeth), and blood in the stool or urine (it is usually more difficult to detect blood in the urine, but the urine becomes a rusty color). In addition, patients should be told to watch for unexplained bruises and bruises that do not seem to heal.

At each appointment, patients should be asked if they have noticed any symptoms of bleeding.
- Symptoms of a recurrent DVT include unilateral pain, tenderness, swelling, and discoloration in a lower extremity. Symptoms of a PE include dyspnea, pleuritic chest pain, cough, tachypnea, and tachycardia. Patients with these symptoms should be referred for a medical evaluation.

Patient Counseling

6. *What information should this patient know about his warfarin therapy?*

- *Warfarin* is an oral anticoagulant, which means it decreases the body's ability to make clots. It is also sometimes called a blood thinner. Although warfarin does not actually "thin" the blood, it does help prevent new clots from forming.
- *Laboratory monitoring.* This drug requires close monitoring of blood clotting by periodic laboratory monitoring of blood tests. The prothrombin time (PT) measures how long it takes your blood to form a clot. To standardize the PT test between laboratories, another test called the international normalized ratio or INR is also reported. The goal is to keep your INR between 2.0 and 3.0. If the INR is above 3.0, you are at an increased risk of bleeding. If the INR is below 2.0, you are at an increased risk of developing another clot.
- *Warfarin dose.* Because we want your blood tests to stay within a certain range, your warfarin dose will probably be changed in response to those results. It is important to know exactly what warfarin dose you are taking at all times. It is a good idea to keep a medication list in your wallet. As your warfarin dose changes, the color of your tablet(s) may also change. Each strength of warfarin is a different color. It is important to remember the color of tablet you are taking at any given time.
- *Compliance.* It is very important that you take your warfarin dose every day. Even if you miss one dose, your blood tests will show a difference. If you do forget to take a dose one day, you should not take an extra dose the next day to "catch up." In the event that you happen to forget a dose, it is important to notify your physician or pharmacist because it will show up in your blood tests. A good way to organize your warfarin is to use a medication box. This is a good way to know that you have taken your dose every day, and it will also show you if you have missed a dose.
- *Administration time.* It is important that you take your warfarin dose at the same time every day, preferably in the afternoon or evening.
- *Drug–drug interactions.* Many medications can interact with warfarin and cause you to be at an increased risk of bleeding or for developing a clot. It is important that you notify all of your health care providers that you are taking warfarin. This includes doctors, pharmacists, nurses, and dentists. Both prescription and non-prescription medications can interact with warfarin. It is important that you not take any over-the-counter products containing aspirin unless specifically instructed by your doctor. In addition, you should not take ibuprofen (e.g., Motrin IB, Advil), naproxen (Aleve), or ketoprofen (Orudis KT) without your doctor's knowledge. If you have a headache or need a pain reliever, acetaminophen (Tylenol) is a safer option, but you should even limit how much of this you use. You should check with your pharmacist before taking any non-prescription medications, herbal medications, dietary supplements, vitamins, or other alternative therapies, because they may also interact with warfarin.
- *Drug–food interactions.* Certain foods can alter your response to warfarin therapy. These foods contain vitamin K and include dark green leafy vegetables, certain meats, oils, mayonnaise, and nutrition products. It is important that keep your intake of these foods consistent. You should not drastically change your intake of these foods from week to week. Alcohol can also alter your response to warfarin. You should consult your doctor before drinking alcohol while taking warfarin. It is preferable to avoid alcohol altogether if you can.
- *Side effects.* Call your doctor immediately if you experience any abdominal pain or swelling, back pain, coughing up blood, or vomiting of blood (this may look like coffee grounds), as these symptoms might indicate internal bleeding from warfarin. You should also tell your doctor if you notice a blue or purple color and pain in the toes.
- *Medical Alert bracelet.* It is a good idea to get a Medical Alert bracelet for anticoagulants. This will notify health care providers that you are taking warfarin in the event that you are unable to tell them yourself.
- *Proper storage.* Your warfarin should be kept in a cool (room temperature), dry place that is out of the reach of children. Refrigerators and bathroom cabinets are not good places to keep medicines due to the humidity.
- *Pregnancy.* Women of child-bearing age must take precautions not to become pregnant while receiving this medication, because warfarin may cause harm to the unborn child. For this reason, never share your medication with any other person.

▶ Follow-up Question

1. *Based on this information, what are your recommendations for his warfarin therapy?*

- Since the INR is now within the therapeutic range and has been stable in the past on this warfarin dose, it is reasonable to recommend continuing warfarin 5 mg po QD.

References

1. Hirsh J, Dalen JE, Deykin D, et al. Oral anticoagulants: Mechanism of action, clinical effectiveness, and optimal therapeutic range. Chest 1995;108(4 suppl):231S–246S.
2. Unge P, Svedberg E, Nordgren A, et al. A study of the interaction of omeprazole and warfarin in anticoagulated patients. Br J Clin Pharmacol 1992;34;509–512.
3. Gibaldi M. Stereoselective and isozyme-selective drug interactions. Chirality 1993;5:407–413.
4. Corrigan JJ, Ulfers LL. Effect of vitamin E on prothrombin levels in warfarin-induced vitamin K deficiency. Am J Clin Nutr 1981;34:1701–1705.
5. Schrogie JJ. Coagulopathy and fat-soluble vitamins. JAMA 1975;232:19.
6. Corrigan JJ. The effect of vitamin E on warfarin-induced vitamin K deficiency. Ann NY Acad Sci 1982;393:361–368.
7. Kim JM, White RH. Effect of vitamin E on the anticoagulant response to warfarin. Am J Cardiol 1996;77:545–546.

13 ISCHEMIC STROKE

▶ Brain Attack (Level II)

Susan R. Winkler, PharmD, BCPS
Mark S. Luer, PharmD

A 67-year-old man with hypertension, dyslipidemia, and a seizure disorder is brought to the Emergency Department after experiencing an acute ischemic stroke. Initial treatment goals are directed toward reducing secondary brain damage by reestablishing and maintaining adequate perfusion to ischemic areas of the brain. In considering therapeutic alternatives, students must determine that this patient meets inclusion criteria for treatment with the thrombolytic agent alteplase. An appropriate dosage regimen and monitoring plan for alteplase must then be implemented. The primary long-term goal is to prevent recurrent stroke by pharmacotherapeutic means and modification of patient risk factors. Reasonable therapeutic alternatives include aspirin, warfarin, ticlopidine, and clopidogrel. Students should be expected to select an appropriate drug and regimen and be able to provide the rationale for their choice of agent.

▶ Questions

Problem Identification

1. a. *Create a list of the patient's drug-related problems.*

   - Acute ischemic stroke in the left hemisphere requiring drug or other therapy
   - Hypertension, currently untreated with pharmacotherapy
   - Hypercholesterolemia, inadequately treated with present dose and schedule of lovastatin
   - Cigarette smoking with probable nicotine dependence
   - The seizure disorder is a chronic, stable problem that is currently controlled with therapeutic concentrations of phenytoin.

   b. *What risk factors for acute ischemic stroke are present in this patient?*

   - Hypertension
   - Hypercholesterolemia
   - Cigarette smoking
   - Increased hematocrit
   - Age (>55 years old)
   - Race (African American)
   - Gender (male)

   c. *What signs and symptoms indicate the presence of an acute ischemic stroke?*

   - Motor deficit in both the right upper and lower extremities
   - Confusion
   - Abrupt onset of symptoms
   - Previous symptoms 2 weeks prior to this event

Desired Outcome

2. *What are the initial and long-term goals of pharmacotherapy in this case?*

   Initial Goals
   - Reduce secondary brain damage by reestablishing and maintaining adequate perfusion to marginally ischemic areas of the brain
   - Protect these areas from the effects of ischemia (i.e., neuroprotection)

   Long-term Goals
   - Prevention of a recurrent stroke through reduction and modification of risk factors

Therapeutic Alternatives

3. a. *What non-drug therapies might be useful for this patient?*

   - *Carotid endarterectomy.* It is unknown at this time if this procedure is of value when performed emergently in acute stroke.[1] It appears that patients with mild to moderate neurologic deficits, crescendo TIAs, or stroke-in-evolution can be operated on safely early after the onset of symptoms. Patients with more severe neurologic deficits should only be considered for carotid endarterectomy when the procedure can be performed within the first few hours after the onset of symptoms. It is not indicated for patients with permanent deficits from a moderate to severe completed stroke.
   - *Middle cerebral artery embolectomy.* This procedure remains controversial in the acute treatment of stroke. Patients who may benefit from this procedure are those who have good collateral circulation and can be operated on within the first few hours after the onset of symptoms.

   b. *What feasible pharmacotherapeutic alternatives are available for the treatment of acute ischemic stroke?*

   - *Heparin* given IV is commonly used in acute stroke therapy; however, no adequately designed trials have been done to establish efficacy and safety. The literature suggests that IV heparin should not be used on a routine basis in patients with TIAs and not at all in those with completed stroke, due to the risk of intracranial hemorrhage and lack of proven benefit. IV heparin is commonly used in patients with progressing stroke, severe stenosis of large intracranial or extracranial arteries, and in cardioembolic stroke. Early heparin therapy is generally avoided in large strokes or in patients with uncontrolled hypertension due to the risk of intracranial hemorrhage.
   - *Low-molecular-weight (LMW) heparins* are undergoing clinical trials for acute stroke treatment.
   - *Alteplase (rt-PA)*, an IV thrombolytic, was approved for acute stroke treatment in June 1996 based on the results of the National Institute of Neurological Disorders and Stroke (NINDS) rt-PA

Stroke Trial.[2] Based on several assessment scales, patients treated with rt-PA were 30% more likely to have minimal or no disability at 3 months compared with patients given placebo. Intracerebral hemorrhage within 36 hours after stroke onset occurred in 6.4% of those given rt-PA versus 0.6% in those given placebo (p<0.001). There was no significant difference in mortality between the two groups at 3 months. Thus, in carefully selected patients, alteplase appears to be effective in limiting the infarct size and protecting brain tissue from ischemia and cell death by restoring blood flow. Treatment must be given within 3 hours of the onset of symptoms, and a CT scan must be done prior to alteplase therapy to rule out an intracranial hemorrhage. A dose of 0.9 mg/kg (maximum 90 mg) is recommended; the first 10% is given as an IV bolus and the remainder is infused over one hour.

- *Streptokinase* is not indicated for use in acute stroke, as all of the large randomized trials evaluating it were stopped early due to a high incidence of hemorrhage in the streptokinase-treated patients.
- *Intra-arterial thrombolytics* cannot be recommended until more data are available.
- *Aspirin*. Patients who received aspirin within 48 hours of the onset of acute stroke were less likely to suffer early recurrent stroke. Early aspirin can be recommended in patients with acute stroke who do not receive alteplase.
- *Pentoxifylline* may be effective in the first 1 to 4 days after the onset of symptoms, but it is ineffective after that time.
- *Ancrod*. Several small trials have been done showing a trend toward improved outcomes with this investigational drug. However, due to the small number of patients enrolled, further studies are needed. Previous studies also used a 6-hour treatment window, which may partially explain the lack of success.
- *Gangliosides (e.g., GM1)* provide a neuroprotective effect against glutamate and other excitatory amino acids and provide a neurotrophic effect for maturation and repair of neuronal tissue. Early data suggest that GM1 may provide a beneficial effect early after symptom onset. Further clinical studies of these investigational agents are needed.
- *NMDA receptor inhibitors, inhibitors of lipid peroxidation, free radical scavengers,* and *lazaroids* have shown promise, but further clinical studies are needed.
- *Naloxone* and *hemodilution* have been used, but further clinical studies are required.
- *Calcium channel blockers, beta blockers, epoprostenol,* and *LMW Dextran* have not been shown to be effective in acute ischemic stroke.

Optimal Plan

4. What initial therapy would you recommend for this patient?

Emergent Supportive Interventions

- Optimize blood pressure; however, hypertension should not be treated initially in acute stroke patients as this may cause decreased blood flow in areas of ischemia. The cautious use of antihypertensive medications may be necessary in patients who are candidates for thrombolytic therapy, those with a severely elevated BP (systolic >220 mm Hg or MAP >130 mm Hg), and those with other medical disorders. In this patient, no treatment is necessary at this time for the elevated BP. If treatment were required, 10 to 20 mg labetalol IVP over 1 to 2 minutes could be given. This dose may be repeated or doubled every 20 minutes to a maximum dose of 150 mg. Avoid using sublingual calcium channel blockers, as these may lower BP too rapidly.
- Optimize oxygenation if required. Measure the oxygen saturation using pulse oximetry and supplement if necessary.
- Correct the blood glucose if required, as both hyperglycemia and hypoglycemia may worsen brain ischemia. If the patient is hypoglycemic, bolus with 50% dextrose immediately. A blood glucose >300 mg/dL should be lowered using insulin.
- If the patient is febrile, treat with acetaminophen, as fever may also worsen brain ischemia.
- Heparin 5000 units subcutaneously Q 12 H should be given for DVT prophylaxis in patients who are not candidates for IV alteplase or IV heparin. In patients receiving IV alteplase, the administration of heparin should be delayed 24 hours to avoid bleeding complications.

Thrombolytic Therapy (Alteplase)

This patient is a candidate for IV alteplase as he meets all of the inclusion criteria and none of the exclusion criteria used in the NINDS study.[2]

- Inclusion criteria:
  - ✓ 18 years of age or older
  - ✓ Clinical diagnosis of ischemic stroke causing a measurable neurologic deficit
  - ✓ Time of symptom onset well established to be less than 180 minutes before treatment would begin
- Exclusion criteria:
  - ✓ Evidence of intracranial hemorrhage on pretreatment head CT
  - ✓ Only minor or rapidly improving stroke symptoms
  - ✓ Clinical presentation suggestive of subarachnoid hemorrhage even with a normal head CT
  - ✓ Active internal bleeding
  - ✓ Known bleeding diathesis, including but not limited to (1) platelet count <100 × 10^3/mm^3; (2) heparin within 48 hours with an elevated aPTT; or (3) current oral anticoagulant use (e.g., warfarin) or recent use with an elevated PT (>15 seconds) or INR
  - ✓ Intracranial surgery, serious head trauma, or previous stroke within 3 months
  - ✓ History of gastrointestinal or urinary tract hemorrhage within 21 days
  - ✓ Major surgery or serious trauma within 14 days
  - ✓ Recent arterial puncture at a noncompressible site
  - ✓ Lumbar puncture within 7 days
  - ✓ History of intracranial hemorrhage
  - ✓ Known arteriovenous malformation or aneurysm
  - ✓ Witnessed seizure at the same time as the onset of stroke symptoms occurred
  - ✓ Recent acute myocardial infarction
  - ✓ SBP >185 mm Hg or DBP >110 mm Hg at the time of treatment, or patient requires aggressive treatment to reduce blood pressure to within these limits
- For this patient, 58 mg total should be given, with the first 6 mg given as an IV bolus and the remaining 52 mg infused over 1 hour.

- Antiplatelet agents, anticoagulants, and invasive procedures such as the insertion of a central line or the placement of a nasogastric tube should be avoided for 24 hours after the infusion of alteplase to prevent bleeding complications. Bladder catheterization should also be avoided for 30 minutes post-infusion.

Aspirin and IV Heparin Therapy

Aspirin should be administered if this patient was *not* a candidate for IV alteplase, as there was no evidence of hemorrhage on the CT scan. The patient should then be evaluated for IV heparin.

Outcome Evaluation

5. *What clinical and laboratory parameters are necessary to evaluate the chosen therapy for achievement of the desired effect and to detect or prevent adverse effects?*

Efficacy With IV Alteplase

- The primary measures of efficacy are the elimination of existing neurologic deficits and the long-term improvement in neurologic status and functioning based on neurologic examinations and other outcome measures.
- In the NINDS trial, neurologic function was assessed 24 hours after the administration of alteplase using the National Institutes of Health stroke scale (NIHSS). This scale quantifies neurologic deficits in patients who have had a stroke.
- At 3 months, four outcome measures were used: the Barthel Index, modified Rankin scale, Glasgow outcome scale, and the NIHSS. The Barthel Index is a measure of the ability to perform activities of daily living; the modified Rankin scale is a simplified overall assessment of functioning, and the Glasgow outcome scale is a global assessment of functioning.

Adverse Effects of IV Alteplase

- The primary adverse effects are bleeding, including intracerebral hemorrhage and serious systemic bleeding. Mental status changes and a severe headache may indicate an intracerebral hemorrhage. Signs of bleeding include easy bruising; hematemesis; guaiac-positive stools; black, tarry stools; hematoma formation; hematuria; bleeding gums; and nosebleeds.
- Blood pressure should be monitored every 15 minutes × 2 hours, then every 30 minutes × 6 hours, then every 60 minutes × 16 hours. Blood pressure should be maintained below 185/110 mm Hg to prevent complications.

Efficacy With Heparin

- An improvement in neurologic function has not been established in clinical trials; however, heparin may prevent early recurrent stroke in patients with cardioembolic stroke and may prevent stroke progression in patients with severe stenosis.
- IV and SC heparin will significantly decrease the risk of developing DVT post-stroke.

Adverse Effects With Heparin

- The major complications of heparin include evolution of the ischemic stroke into a hemorrhagic stroke, bleeding, and thrombocytopenia. The occurrence of a severe headache and mental status changes may indicate an intracerebral hemorrhage.
- Signs of bleeding include those described above for alteplase. The hemoglobin, hematocrit, and platelet count should be obtained at least every 3 days to detect bleeding and thrombocytopenia.

▶ **Follow-up Questions**

1. *What non-drug therapies might be useful for preventing recurrent stroke in this patient?*

- A major goal in the long-term treatment of ischemic stroke involves the prevention of a recurrent stroke through the reduction of risk factors. These factors include hypertension, cardiac disease, atrial fibrillation, diabetes mellitus, cigarette smoking, alcohol abuse, and hyperlipidemia.
- Encourage the patient to enroll in a smoking cessation program.
- Instituting a diet low in saturated fats and sodium would be beneficial for hyperlipidemia and hypertension.
- Increase physical activity, when appropriate, as it impacts risk factors for cardiovascular disease, promotes weight loss, lowers blood pressure, and positively affects blood cholesterol.
- Carotid endarterectomy may be beneficial for preventing stroke in patients with symptomatic carotid stenosis 70% or greater. Trials are ongoing to evaluate if carotid endarterectomy is beneficial for patients with moderate stenosis (30% to 69%). It is not beneficial for carotid stenosis less than 30%.
- Cerebral angioplasty is typically restricted to patients who are refractory to medical therapy and are not surgical candidates.

2. *What feasible pharmacotherapeutic alternatives are available for the secondary prevention of acute ischemic stroke?*

- *Aspirin* will decrease the risk of recurrent stroke by approximately 25% in patients with both small and large vessel disease. It is considered to be the first line preventative agent for ischemic stroke.
- *Warfarin* has not been adequately studied in noncardioembolic stroke, but it is often recommended in patients after antiplatelet agents fail. One small retrospective study suggests that warfarin is better than aspirin.[3]
- *Ticlopidine* has been shown to be slightly more beneficial in stroke prevention than aspirin in both men and women. The usual recommended dosage is 250 mg po BID. Ticlopidine is very costly, and side effects include bone marrow suppression, rash, diarrhea, and an increased cholesterol level. Neutropenia is seen in approximately 2% of patients. Monitoring of the CBC is required every 2 weeks for the first 3 months of therapy. Ticlopidine is a reasonable alternative in patients who cannot tolerate or who have failed aspirin therapy.
- *Clopidogrel* has been shown to be slightly more effective than aspirin with a relative-risk reduction of 7.3% greater than that provided by ASA.[4] The usual dose is 75 mg po QD. Clopidogrel has a significantly lower incidence of diarrhea and neutropenia than ticlopidine, and laboratory monitoring is not required.
- *Low-dose aspirin and ticlopidine combination therapy* has been shown to inhibit all three pathways for platelet aggregation and may provide a benefit. Clinical testing must be performed to determine the role of combination therapy in the secondary prevention of acute ischemic stroke.
- *Dipyridamole* has no role in stroke prevention. There is one study

suggesting that the combination of dipyridamole and aspirin is better than placebo.
- Sulfinpyrazone has no role in stroke prevention.

3. *What drug, dosage form, dose, schedule, and duration of therapy would you recommend for the secondary prevention of acute ischemic stroke in this patient?*

- Aspirin has been shown to decrease the risk of subsequent stroke by approximately 25% in both men and women with TIA or stroke. A wide range of doses has been used; however, enteric-coated aspirin 325 mg po QD is the most widely used regimen.

4. *How should the therapy you recommended be monitored?*

- The efficacy endpoint with aspirin therapy is prevention of a recurrent ischemic stroke.
- Adverse effects include GI intolerance, GI bleeding, and hypersensitivity reactions.

5. *In addition to the management of the ischemic stroke, what other therapeutic interventions should be undertaken for this patient?*

- Monitor the blood pressure regularly to determine if an antihypertensive agent is needed. Patients often have an elevated blood pressure post-stroke, however, and may not need long-term drug therapy.
- Measure the fasting lipid profile to determine if an increase in the lovastatin dose is needed. Lovastatin should be given with the evening meal rather than at bedtime to obtain optimal absorption. A change to a more potent reductase inhibitor (e.g., simvastatin, atorvastatin) may ultimately be required if the patient's LDL-cholesterol is high. The maximum lovastatin dose of 80 mg is being approached, and the patient's goal LDL level is ≤100 mg/dL because of the presence of atherosclerotic disease.
- Continue phenytoin 300 mg po Q HS. Obtain an EEG to evaluate the need for anticonvulsant therapy, as this patient has been seizure free for 2 years.
- Recommend that the patient attend a smoking cessation program. Nicotine replacement therapy may be considered, but bupropion should be avoided in this patient due to the history of seizures.

Patient Counseling

6. *What information should be provided to the patient about the secondary preventive therapy you recommended?*

- It is important to take one 325-mg coated aspirin every day as prescribed. This will help to prevent another stroke.

- Signs of bleeding from the intestinal or urinary tract include black stools and pinkish urine. Report these to your doctor if they occur.
- Limit the amount of fat in your diet. Take the lovastatin as directed to lower your cholesterol level and decrease your risk of stroke.
- Limit the amount of sodium in your diet. Try to avoid canned foods and processed foods. Avoid the salt shaker when cooking.
- You will need to monitor your blood pressure regularly to determine if a medicine is needed to lower your blood pressure. Decreasing your blood pressure is important because it will help to prevent another stroke.
- Another important life-style change you can make is to stop smoking.

References

1. Camarata PJ, Heros RC, Latchaw RE. "Brain attack": The rationale for treating stroke as a medical emergency. Neurosurgery 1994;34:144–158.
2. National Institute of Neurological Disorders and Stroke rt-PA Stroke Study Group. Tissue plasminogen activator for acute ischemic stroke. N Engl J Med 1995;333:1581–1587.
3. Chimowitz WI, Kokinos J, Strong J, et al. The warfarin–aspirin symptomatic intracranial disease study. Neurology 1995;45:1488–1493.
4. CAPRIE Steering Committee. A randomised, blinded, trial of clopidogrel versus aspirin in patients at risk of ischaemic events (CAPRIE). Lancet 1996;348:1329–1339.

14 HYPERLIPIDEMIA: PRIMARY PREVENTION

▶ **What, Me Worry?** (Level I)

Laura A. Bartels, PharmD

A 55-year-old man with hypertension, a high LDL-cholesterol (208 mg/dL), and several other risk factors for coronary heart disease (CHD) returns for a follow-up evaluation. He has been nonadherent with the dietary, exercise, and smoking cessation programs that have been recommended in the past. In addition to these non-drug interventions, pharmacotherapy is required in order to achieve the 34% reduction in LDL that is recommended for this patient. Although other drug classes may be considered, an HMG-CoA reductase inhibitor is the most likely single drug to achieve this magnitude of reduction. The case requires students to consider the differences among agents in this class and to select an optimal regimen and monitoring plan for this patient.

▶ Questions

Problem Identification

1. a. *Create a drug-related problem list for this patient.*

- Newly diagnosed hyperlipidemia, presently inadequately treated with failed dietary interventions.

- Hypertension, presently uncontrolled on present drug regimen.
- Potential adverse effects of HCTZ on the patient's lipid profile. HCTZ may cause an increase in TC by 10%, LDL by 11%, and triglycerides by 11%.[1] Diuretics have the ability to impair glucose metabolism, which may then contribute to the cause of hyperlipidemia. Although this may be a contributing factor to dyslipidemia, it is unlikely to be the only factor in this patient.
- Alcohol consumption should be limited to one ounce per day in

patients with hyperlipidemia. Levels of VLDL and triglycerides may accumulate with chronic alcohol consumption. Alcohol usually has no effect on LDL-C. One ounce of alcohol per day may have a beneficial effect on HDL levels, and a high HDL is a negative risk factor for CHD.
- The patient's obesity and cigarette smoking may be detrimental to his health; these may be considered to be drug-related problems if pharmacotherapy is implemented to help control them.

b. *What signs, symptoms, and laboratory values indicate the presence and severity of hyperlipidemia in this patient?*

- Hyperlipidemia is an asymptomatic disease in the majority of patients. Patients may not realize that they have elevated cholesterol levels until an outpatient screening is conducted, as in this patient's case. This patient's lipid concentrations vary from the desirable levels of total cholesterol <200 mg/dL, LDL <130 mg/dL, and HDL ≥35 mg/dL. His triglyceride levels are classified as normal (<200 mg/dL).[2] In addition to his dyslipidemia, he has multiple other risk factors for CHD, which places him at high risk for cardiovascular events in the future if treatment is not initiated.

c. *In addition to an elevated LDL-cholesterol, what other risk factors does this patient have for the development of coronary heart disease (CHD)?*

- Low HDL-C (<35 mg/dL)
- Hypertension (BP ≥140/90 or taking antihypertensive drugs)
- Male gender and age ≥45 years old
- Family history of premature CHD (definite MI or sudden death in his father before age 55)
- Current cigarette smoking
- The only major risk factor *not* present in this patient is diabetes mellitus

d. *What additional information is needed to satisfactorily assess this patient?*

- Critical evaluation of his diet
- Determination of his exercise level
- Assessment of the patient's efforts to stop smoking (e.g., past enrollment in a smoking cessation program)
- Assessment of the patient's motivation to improve his lipid levels and overall health

Desired Outcome

2. *What is the desired therapeutic outcome for this patient?*

- The goals of treatment are to reduce total and LDL cholesterol in order to prevent the development of CHD. This includes preventing formation of new atherosclerotic plaques in coronary arteries, stopping progression of established lesions, and causing existing lesions to regress.
- Clinical trials have shown that such interventions will reduce new CHD events and CHD mortality in primary prevention (patients without known CHD).[2]
- This patient has more than two risk factors for CHD, but he has no evidence of CHD or other clinical atherosclerotic disease. Therefore, his goal LDL-C level is <130 mg/dL, a reduction of approximately 34% from the present level (refer to textbook Chapter 19).

Therapeutic Alternatives

3. a. *What non-drug therapies might be useful in the initial management of this individual?*

- Dietary education should be provided; with dietary modification this patient's LDL-C level may be reduced by 5% to 15% depending upon his compliance.
- Information on smoking cessation should be provided to the patient, and an appropriate exercise program should be encouraged.

b. *What feasible pharmacologic alternatives are available?*

- Lipid-lowering drugs may be required when dietary and risk factor management fails, when cardiovascular drugs are not implicated in causing dyslipidemia, and when there are no underlying diseases. The major types of lipid-lowering drugs are bile acid sequestrants, nicotinic acid, the fibrates, and the HMG-CoA reductase inhibitors. These drugs act in different ways to produce beneficial effects on lipids (see the section on Drug Therapy in textbook Chapter 19).
- *Bile acid sequestrants (cholestyramine, colestipol)* bind bile acids in the intestine and interrupt their enterohepatic recirculation. This causes a compensatory increase in hepatic LDL-receptors so that blood LDL-C is more rapidly removed and total cholesterol falls. Sequestrants are usually given as powders that must be mixed with liquid or sprinkled on food and given in divided doses two or three times daily. The most common side effects are related to the GI tract, including constipation, heartburn, and flatulence; steatorrhea occurs rarely. Many patients may need encouragement from their physician or pharmacist to continue therapy in the face of these side effects. The majority of patients cannot manage more than a low dose, which may be useful when used with other lipid-lowering agents. Sequestrants may also interfere with the absorption of digoxin, warfarin, thyroxine, and thiazides; these medications should be taken 1 hour before or 4 hours after the sequestrant.
- *Nicotinic acid (or niacin)* is the cheapest compound and can be purchased over-the-counter. Since it is a non-prescription product, some third-party payers may not reimburse the patient for the cost. Nicotinic acid has numerous side effects but most can be minimized by cautiously increasing the dose. Common side effects that are often dose limiting include prostaglandin-mediated symptoms such as flushing, dizziness, and palpitations. Impaired glucose tolerance, increased serum uric acid concentrations, hepatic dysfunction, and rashes may also occur. A history of gout, peptic ulcer, or diabetes is a relative contraindication to the use of this medication.
- The *fibrates (gemfibrozil, fenofibrate,* and the investigational drug *bezafibrate*), may be preferred in conditions in which high blood triglycerides are the primary abnormality. These drugs carry the risk of a myositis-like syndrome, especially in patients with renal impairment or during co-therapy with a reductase inhibitor. Other side effects include abdominal discomfort, muscle pains, decreased libido, and cholesterol gallstones. The effects of warfarin may also be potentiated. Bezafibrate may be a useful agent for diabetics because (unlike gemfibrozil) it tends to reduce plasma glucose levels.[3]

- *HMG-CoA reductase inhibitors* (or statins) include *lovastatin, simvastatin, pravastatin, fluvastatin, atorvastatin,* and *cerivastatin.* These agents can produce the largest reductions in total and HDL-cholesterol, have relatively few side effects, and can be dosed once daily. They can reduce LDL-C by 20% to 40% or more, which is comparable to the reductions that have been shown to reduce major CHD events.[4] The most common side effects are headache and GI complaints such as flatulence, diarrhea, constipation, and nausea. Potentially serious but rare effects are myositis and liver damage. Myositis with rhabdomyolysis and the associated risk of acute renal failure are more likely to occur during co-therapy with fibrates, nicotinic acid, or cyclosporine. Hepatic enzymes should be monitored periodically in patients receiving these drugs (see below). Based on dose-equivalence ratios in clinical trials, simvastatin was determined to be twice as potent as lovastatin, and lovastatin and pravastatin are equally potent.[5] Fluvastatin has been suggested to have a dose-equivalence ratio similar to lovastatin (1:1).[5] Direct comparisons of cerivastatin with other statins are needed to determine its dose-equivalence ratio. Atorvastatin was shown to be more effective than simvastatin in reducing LDL-C and TG in a 1-year, blinded, randomized study.[6] In this study, atorvastatin 10 to 20 mg QD reduced LDL-C by 37% and TG by 23% versus 30% and 15%, respectively, for simvastatin 10 to 20 mg QD ($P < 0.05$).

Optimal Plan

4. *What drug, dosage form, dose, schedule, and duration of therapy are best for this patient?*

- This patient requires a 34% reduction in LDL-C, which is beyond the means of dietary modification within the next 6 months. According to his history, this patient has tried dietary modification unsuccessfully over the past 10 years to lower his blood pressure. This patient therefore requires potent pharmacologic treatment for his LDL-C. An HMG-CoA reductase inhibitor would be the most likely class of drug to help him achieve his target LDL of <130 mg/dL. Initial once-daily oral doses of the reductase inhibitors are atorvastatin 10 mg, lovastatin 20 mg, pravastatin 20 mg, simvastatin 10 mg, fluvastatin 20 mg, and cerivastatin 0.2 mg.
- Since some medications are more beneficial when dosed in the evening, timing needs to be taken into consideration to achieve an optimal effect. Pravastatin, simvastatin, and fluvastatin should be taken once daily at bedtime and cerivastatin may be taken without regard to meals in the evening. Because intestinal absorption of lovastatin is increased by about 50% when it is given with food,[5] it should be taken once daily with the evening meal. Atorvastatin may be taken any time of the day; this may be due to its long elimination half-life of 14 hrs. Since this patient currently takes the majority of his medications in the morning it may be advisable to continue emphasizing this pattern of medication administration, which would make atorvastatin a good choice for him. It also appears to be the most potent reductase inhibitor.
- Bile acid sequestrants, fibrates, and approved doses of fluvastatin cannot achieve the 34% reduction in LDL-C that is needed. Niacin has a highly variable response and many adverse drug reactions, making it a less optimal choice.
- In addition to pharmacotherapy, the patient should be strongly encouraged to adhere to a diet and lose weight to improve his overall health.

Outcome Evaluation

5. *What clinical and laboratory parameters are necessary to evaluate the therapy for achievement of the desired therapeutic outcome and to detect or prevent adverse effects?*

- LDL-C, HDL-C, and triglycerides should be monitored and evaluated at baseline and at 3 months after the initiation of dietary therapy and drug therapy. Annual evaluations may be made thereafter.
- Hepatic enzymes (AST, ALT) should also be monitored at baseline (before starting treatment) and periodically thereafter in patients receiving reductase inhibitors. For most drugs, AST/ALT should be obtained at 6 and 12 weeks into therapy or after dosage increases, and then periodically (e.g., semiannually), thereafter. Revised labeling for pravastatin indicates that testing is needed only at 12 weeks after initiation of therapy or dosage escalation. Labeling for simvastatin has been revised to recommend testing at the start of therapy and then periodically (e.g., semiannually) for the first year of therapy.

Patient Counseling

6. *What information should be provided to the patient to enhance compliance, ensure successful therapy, and minimize adverse effects?*

General Information

- LDL-cholesterol is the "bad" cholesterol. It is important to lower the level of this cholesterol because it increases your chances for having heart disease, chest pain, or a heart attack.
- Your LDL-cholesterol level was high at 198, and your goal is 130, so you need to reduce it by approximately 34%. If you stick to your diet and take your medication once a day, you may be able to reach this goal without having to take any other medication for your LDL-cholesterol.
- Being on a good diet is very important and with your family history, I recommend that you see a dietitian for a complete dietary consultation. Smoking cessation and an exercise program would be highly beneficial for you as well.

Atorvastatin

- This medication is called Lipitor (or atorvastatin). You are to take one 10-mg tablet every day to help lower your LDL-cholesterol.
- You may take it with your other medications once a day. If you forget to take a dose, you may take it later on that day. However, if you do not remember to take the dose until the next day, skip that dose and go back to your regular schedule. Do not double the dosing of this medication without the permission of your doctor.
- This drug sometimes causes a slight headache, constipation, diarrhea, and gas. In rare instances it may cause muscle aches and pains; notify your doctor if these effects occur.
- Please keep this medication out of the reach of children and store it in a dry place at normal room temperature.

Follow-up Question

1. *What is your assessment of the effectiveness of the interventions? Is any other type of pharmacologic intervention required at this time?*

   - Atorvastatin 10 mg/day and dietary compliance produced a reduction in LDL-C of approximately 29%. The patient tolerated the medication well. Hepatic enzyme tests should be repeated at this 6-month interval. If they are normal, atorvastatin may be increased to 20 mg/day to achieve further lowering of LDL-C. In addition, positive feedback and strong encouragement should be given to the patient to continue his compliance with the dietary and medication regimens. This would also be a good time to start a graded exercise regimen and consider a smoking cessation program.

References

1. Pollare T, Lithell H, Berne C. A comparison of the effects of hydrochlorothiazide and captopril on glucose and lipid metabolism in patients with hypertension. N Engl J Med 1989;321:868–873.
2. National Cholesterol Education Program. Second report of the National Cholesterol Education Program (NCEP) Expert Panel on detection, evaluation, and treatment of high blood cholesterol in adults (Adult Treatment Panel II). Circulation 1994;89:1329–1445.
3. Pazzucconi F, Mannucci L, Mussoni L, et al. Bezafibrate lowers plasma lipids, fibrinogen and platelet aggregability in hypertriglyceridemia. Eur J Clin Pharmacol 1992;43:219–223.
4. Holme I. Cholesterol reduction and its impact on coronary artery disease and total mortality. Am J Cardiol 1995;76:10C–17C.
5. Lennernas H, Fager G. Pharmacodynamics and pharmacokinetics of the HMG-CoA reductase inhibitors. Similarities and differences. Clin Pharmacokinet 1997;32:403–425.
6. Dart A, Jerums G, Nicholson G, et al. A multicenter, double-blind, one-year study comparing safety and efficacy of atorvastatin versus simvastatin in patients with hypercholesterolemia. Am J Cardiol 1997;80:39–44.

15 HYPERLIPIDEMIA: SECONDARY PREVENTION

▶ **The Mushroom Hunter**   (Level I)

Kjel A. Johnson, PharmD, BCPS

A 53-year-old man with chronic stable angina pectoris and s/p myocardial infarction presents to a pharmacy-managed clinic because of dyslipidemia that has been difficult to control on the maximum recommended dose of gemfibrozil. The current LDL-cholesterol is 140 mg/dL, so the patient requires a 29% reduction to achieve his target LDL of ≤100 mg/dL. Adherence to dietary therapy and an appropriate exercise program are important treatment measures, but alternative drug therapy will be required to attain the desired reduction in LDL. The reductase inhibitors pravastatin and simvastatin are the only lipid-lowering agents thus far to have shown a reduction in total mortality in secondary prevention. When the patient returns 6 weeks after new treatment is initiated, the LDL is still elevated above the desired level. Students are asked to make recommendations for further treatment based on this information. The case also offers the opportunity to discuss appropriate combination therapy should the patient not respond optimally to maximum doses of a single agent.

Questions

Problem Identification

1. *a. Create a list of the patient's drug-related problems.*

   - The patient has back and hip pain, which may or may not be amenable to drug therapy, depending on its cause. The clinician must determine if the patient's pain is anginal or musculoskeletal in nature. The PE and ECG do not suggest pain of cardiac origin, since the pain waxes and wanes with movement and no ST-segment changes were seen in any ECG leads. Further probing as to possible causes of this non-cardiac pain is needed. If the pain is found to be musculoskeletal due to his recent fall, NSAIDs are first-line agents, and short-term treatment with an OTC NSAID such as ibuprofen 400 mg po Q 6 H PRN or naproxen sodium 220 mg Q 8–12 H PRN may be recommended.
   - The patient's dyslipidemia is inadequately controlled with the present drug regimen. This patient requires more aggressive cholesterol reduction to reach his goal LDL-C level (≤100 mg/dL for patients with existing CAD). This target is not achievable with gemfibrozil, as he currently is receiving the maximum recommended daily dose. Furthermore, only HMG-CoA reductase inhibitors have shown reproducible reductions in total and cardiovascular mortality.
   - The patient's other chronic, stable medical problems that appear to be adequately treated with present therapy include S/P MI, chronic stable angina pectoris, HTN, and ulcerative colitis.

   b. What signs, symptoms, or laboratory tests indicate presence or severity of this individual's hyperlipidemia?

   - As expected, the patient reports no symptoms of dyslipidemia. However, all fractions of his cholesterol profile do not meet the goals established by the National Cholesterol Education Program (NCEP).[1] LDL-C should be ≤100 mg/dL and HDL-C should be ≥35 mg/dL. The higher the HDL, the lower the patient's risk of another cardiovascular event. The NCEP classifies triglycerides (TG) as normal (<200 mg/dL), borderline-high (200 to 400 mg/dL), high (400 to 1000 mg/dL), and very high (>1000 mg/dL). The relationship between CHD and TG levels is complicated and may be due to the association with low HDL and particularly atherogenic forms of LDL.

c. *What additional information is needed to satisfactorily assess this patient's dyslipidemia?*

- Determination of the patient's compliance with both non-pharmacologic and pharmacologic therapy is essential. Medication compliance and adherence to a low-cholesterol diet can be assessed by medication refill history and the short dietary questionnaire,[1] respectively. Many clinicians consider patients compliant with their medication if 8 of the past 10 refills were received on time.

Desired Outcome

2. *What is the desired therapeutic outcome for this patient?*

- The overall goal in treating patients with dyslipidemia in the face of a history of MI or angina is to prevent a second event, such as sudden cardiac death, fatal MI, non-fatal MI, or stroke.
- It is well known that elevations in LDL-C and low levels of HDL-C correlate with increases in risk of these CHD events. Therefore, surrogate markers for predicting event risk include HDL and LDL, and the goal LDL-C goal in patients who are being treated for secondary prevention is ≤100 mg/dL (see textbook Chapter 19 for tables on classification and treatment decisions).
- In addition, this patient's HDL-C should be increased to further reduce risk of CHD events. HDL should be elevated to the highest obtainable level.
- Most clinicians prefer to have TG levels <250 mg/dL, although the guidelines for TG are currently poorly defined. In addition, it is not known if elevated TG is an independent risk factor for CHD.
- The goal for treatment of the patient's pain is to have the patient assessed medically for a specific diagnosis. The pain may be musculoskeletal in nature, in which case treatment with analgesics would be appropriate.

Therapeutic Alternatives

3. a. *What non-drug therapies may be used in the management of this patient's dyslipidemia?*

- The combination of aggressive diet therapy with pharmacologic modification of cholesterol results in an additive effect on LDL cholesterol. Although dietary therapy is important, it must be remembered that it leads to only a 5% to 15% reduction in total cholesterol, depending upon the patient's level of motivation and compliance. This patient reports a modest adherence to his diet, but it certainly can be improved. This should be stressed as an important part of his treatment, and he should be taught the difference between saturated and unsaturated fats, as well as how to read food labels. However, it is unlikely that dietary intervention alone will reduce the patient's LDL to goal, since a 29% reduction in LDL is required. Most clinicians proceed directly to drug therapy in secondary prevention patients who are unlikely to achieve LDL-C goal (those who have an LDL-C >120 mg/dL at baseline), although diet is always stressed.
- Regular exercise, such as 20 minutes of walking thrice weekly, can increase HDL-C and may reduce LDL-C.
- The inclusion of one or two servings of alcohol daily has been shown to increase HDL; however, the exact reduction in cardiovascular events resulting from this increase in HDL (predominantly the HDL_3 fraction) is unknown. It is known that alcohol itself will reduce risk for CAD likely through a blood thinning effect. The benefits of alcohol must always be weighed against the potential risks of abuse. In patients treated for secondary prevention, the risks of alcohol use are often accepted.

b. *What feasible pharmacologic alternatives are available for the treatment of this individual's dyslipidemia?*

A large number of dyslipidemic agents are available (refer to the table on drug therapy in textbook Chapter 19 for a detailed list).

- *Bile acid sequestrants colestipol and cholestyramine* have not been studied in secondary prevention, may lead to an exacerbation of hypertriglyceridemia, will likely not achieve the LDL-C goal in this patient, and are difficult regimens to adhere to.
- *Niacin*, while very effective at decreasing LDL-C, increasing HDL-C, and decreasing triglycerides, has also not been studied in secondary prevention and is difficult for patients to adhere to.
- *HMG-CoA reductase inhibitors (atorvastatin, cerivastatin, fluvastatin, lovastatin, pravastatin, simvastatin)* include the only drugs that have been shown to reduce total mortality in primary *and* secondary prevention. For this reason, they are now considered the drugs of choice in the management of patients with dyslipidemia
  - ✓ *Simvastatin* was shown to reduce LDL-C by 35% in patients given the drug for secondary prevention in the 4S study.[2] The result after 4 years was a 30% reduction in total mortality risk, a 42% reduction in risk of cardiovascular mortality, and a 44% reduction in risk of suffering a secondary event.
  - ✓ *Pravastatin* reduced CHD risk in patients treated for secondary prevention who had either mild or moderate elevations in LDL-C post-infarction. The CARE Study[3] demonstrated a 24% reduction in major coronary events, and the LIPID Study[4] reduced all-cause mortality by 23%. Both studies compared pravastatin to placebo after an infarction.

Therefore, simvastatin and pravastatin are the only reductase inhibitors FDA approved for the reduction of coronary events in patients with CAD. All others in this class are capable of reducing the patient's LDL-C to NCEP goal but have not been studied in secondary prevention. In addition, only lovastatin, pravastatin, and simvastatin have long-term (more than 5 years) safety data. Recently, simvastatin and atorvastatin were approved for mixed dyslipidemia (elevations in LDL-C and TG). The reductions in TG are dose related and depend on baseline TG concentration; reductions of up to 30% may be achieved with each agent. Because simvastatin has been shown to save lives, decrease events in patients with CAD, and is approved for mixed dyslipidemia, it may be the best choice for this patient.

Optimal Plan

4. *What drug doses, schedules, and duration of therapy are best suited for management of this patient's dyslipidemia?*

- A reductase inhibitor dosage that is capable of decreasing his LDL-C to ≤100 mg/dL should be instituted. The once-daily doses of each drug that would be required are atorvastatin 10 mg, cerivastatin 0.3 mg, fluvastatin 40 mg, lovastatin 40 mg, pravastatin 40 mg, or simvastatin 20 mg. As stated above, only pravastatin and simvastatin

have been shown to decrease mortality/morbidity in patients treated for secondary prevention. Patients in the 4S trial were initiated with simvastatin 20 mg once daily, and patients in both pravastatin trials received 40 mg once daily.
- If goal LDL-C is not reached on the initial dosage chosen, simvastatin may be increased to 40 mg and then 80 mg once daily. It is expected that each doubling of the daily dose of any reductase inhibitor leads to an additional 6 mg/dL reduction in LDL-C over the starting dose.[5] Therefore reductions in LDL-C of near 50% can be obtained with this agent.

Outcome Evaluation

5. *What parameters should be assessed to determine the effectiveness and adverse effects of the therapy you recommended?*

- A full lipid panel should be evaluated 6 weeks after any changes in the patient's antihyperlipidemic regimen. LDL-C should be lowered to ≤100 mg/dL, and HDL-C should be increased as much as possible. All reductase inhibitors increase HDL to the same extent (approximately 8 mg/dL). Once at goal, a total lipid panel should be evaluated every 6 months.
- Liver function tests (AST and ALT) may occasionally be elevated with reductase inhibitor use. The elevation is often transient and most patients can continue therapy. Most reductase inhibitors require hepatic enzymes to be measured at 6 and 12 weeks after initiating therapy or after a dosage increase, and then periodically (semiannually) thereafter. The FDA has granted pravastatin and simvastatin a more relaxed hepatic enzyme evaluation regimen; the tests should be evaluated prior to initiation of treatment and at 3 and 12 months with these agents. Annual evaluations are performed for the duration of drug therapy.
- Muscular pain should be evaluated after initiating therapy or after a dosage increase. Approximately 5% of patients will complain of GI disturbances, but this incidence does not differ from that seen with placebo.

Patient Counseling

6. *What information should be provided to the patient about his new therapy?*

Simvastatin
- This medication is called simvastatin (Zocor), and it has been shown to save lives and reduce the chance of another heart attack in patients such as you who have had a heart attack. In fact, it reduces your chance of dying in the next 5 years by 30%. In these studies, 20 mg of simvastatin was taken once daily, and that is the dose prescribed for you.
- Take this medication in the evening, because most of your cholesterol production occurs late in the day. Many patients take this medication with dinner to help them remember to take it.
- This medication is called a "reductase inhibitor" or "statin," and like all of the medications in this class, it is generally well tolerated. Occasionally, muscle pain occurs, but the chance of this happening is only slightly greater than not taking the medication at all. If you do get muscle aches with usual exertion or if the aches persist for more than 3 days, call your physician or me.
- It is imperative that you take this medication daily. If you forget to take the medication, and it is later in the evening than normal, still take your dose. If it is almost time for your next dose, skip the missed dose and go back to your regular schedule. We will increase your dose until your LDL cholesterol (the bad type) is less than 100.

▶ **Follow-up Questions**

1. *Based on this new information, what interventions, if any, should be made at this time?*

- Increase the dose of the reductase inhibitors until the maximum recommended dose is reached or the NCEP goal is met (e.g., increase simvastatin from 20 to 40 mg once daily). A repeat fasting lipid profile should be obtained in another 6 weeks. The patient's liver function tests remain within normal limits, indicating that it is safe to continue therapy. Because of the dosage increase, it would be prudent to repeat these tests when the next lipid panel is obtained.

2. *If the patient's goal lipid levels cannot ultimately be obtained with the maximum dose of the initial agent chosen, what therapeutic options are available?*

- Approximately 15% of patients will require combination therapy. Bile acid sequestrants have been shown to reduce coronary events, but not total mortality, in patients treated for primary prevention. However, because treatment with one of these drugs may result in increases in triglycerides of up to 40%, these medications may not be good medications to add to this particular patient's regimen.
- Niacin and fibric acid derivatives, when used with reductase inhibitors, increase the risk of myopathy. However, the risk of this adverse event with combination therapy remains relatively low. Historically, clinicians have instituted niacin at 100 mg po TID, and then titrated the dose upward until at least 1 g daily is taken. Compliance with this regimen has been poor,[5] so many clinicians now start with niacin 250 mg po Q HS for 1 week, and increase in 250-mg increments until a dose of 1 g Q HS is reached. This can result in reductions in LDL-C and TG and increases in HDL-C. Therefore, the most appropriate combination therapy for this patient is probably niacin therapy.

References

1. National Cholesterol Educational Program. Second report of the expert panel on detection, evaluation, and treatment of high blood cholesterol in adults (adult treatment panel II). Circulation 1994;89:1333–1445.
2. Scandinavian Simvastatin Survival Study Group. Randomised trial of cholesterol lowering in 4444 patients with coronary heart disease: The Scandinavian Simvastatin Survival Study (4S). Lancet 1994;344:1383–1389.
3. Sacks FM, Pfeffer MA, Moye LA, et al. The effect of pravastatin on coronary events after myocardial infarction in patients with average cholesterol levels. Cholesterol and Recurrent Events Trial investigators. N Engl J Med 1996;335:1001–1009.
4. Tonkin A, et al. Long-term intervention with pravastatin in ischemic disease (LIPID Study). American Heart Association Meeting, November 1997, Orlando.
5. Jones P, Kafonek S, Laurora I, et al. Comparative dose efficacy study of atorvastatin versus simvastatin, pravastatin, lovastatin, and fluvastatin in patients with hypercholesterolemia (the CURVES study). Am J Cardiol 1998;81:582–587.

16 PERIPHERAL VASCULAR DISEASE

▶ The Colors of the Flag   (Level II)

Susan D. Bear, BS, PharmD

A 67-year-old woman with systemic sclerosis and other medical problems presents with signs and symptoms of Raynaud's phenomenon. Several of her present medications could be contributing to her recent complaints. A number of non-drug therapies are useful for preventing and treating the painful symptoms associated with Raynaud's phenomenon. Peripheral vasodilators are the most effective therapeutic agents, and the dihydropyridine calcium channel blocker nifedipine has been shown to be effective in several clinical trials. This particular agent may also be beneficial for treating this patient's concurrent hypertension. Topical nitroglycerin ointment could be added if adequate symptomatic relief is not obtained from oral nifedipine therapy.

▶ Questions

Problem Identification

1. a. *Create a list of this patient's drug-related problems.*

   - Untreated Raynaud's phenomenon
   - Untreated renal insufficiency
   - Non-optimal drug therapy selection for hypertension (β-blockers may worsen Raynaud's)
   - Unmonitored ibuprofen (Advil) usage (ibuprofen may worsen Raynaud's)
   - Untreated anemia with heme (+) stool
   - Untreated GERD, with gastritis, erosive esophagitis, and esophageal hypomotility
   - Untreated malabsorption syndrome
   - No regimen for control of painful joint symptoms

   b. *What signs, symptoms, and laboratory values indicate the presence of Raynaud's phenomenon?*

   - Raynaud's phenomenon or syndrome is characterized initially by digital arterial vasospasm resulting in fingertip whiteness (pallor). Digital blood flow is greatly reduced during the initial attack. As vasoconstriction abates, digital vessels are partially filled with blood. Cyanosis is evident when this blood deoxygenates. As the episode resolves (e.g., because of digital warming) and blood flow returns to the digits, erythema and rubor replace cyanosis. Numbness, tingling, throbbing, and pain accompany digital blood flow return. These episodes classically occur in response to cold exposure or emotional stress.
   - Primary Raynaud's disease is not associated with another disorder. When it is secondary to another disease or cause, it is termed Raynaud's phenomenon or syndrome. Raynaud's phenomenon is often associated with connective tissue disease. It is the initial manifestation of disease in 70% of patients with systemic sclerosis.[1] Raynaud's phenomenon may be present for many years prior to the clinical presentation of connective tissue disease.
   - During the course of illness, the patient describes the following symptoms consistent with Raynaud's disease:
     ✓ Ulceration of fingertips
     ✓ Numbness, tingling, and burning of fingers when exposed to cold
     ✓ Blanching and pallor of fingers followed by cyanosis when exposed to cold
     ✓ Rubor and pain of fingers upon warming
   - No laboratory measurement serves as a diagnostic standard for Raynaud's disease. Changes in skin surface temperature, alterations in rewarming time, thermographic changes, and laser Doppler flowmetry are all used in clinical research but are of little value in clinical practice. Thorough clinical assessment and subjective patient information are still the best diagnostic tools.
   - A review of the patient's laboratory results identifies elevated ESR, positive ANA, and elevated RA. These values along with a diagnosis of systemic sclerosis identify her Raynaud's as secondary rather than primary. Patients with primary Raynaud's disease usually require only conservative therapy. Digital ischemia and loss of digital tissue are rare. Patients with secondary disease have a far graver prognosis and usually require pharmacotherapeutic intervention.

   c. *Could any of the patient's peripheral vascular symptoms have been caused by drug therapy?*

   - The patient's ibuprofen usage has been significant over the last 2 weeks. Advil usage could exacerbate Raynaud's phenomenon through inhibition of prostaglandin synthesis.
   - Propranolol (Inderal LA) is not a drug of choice for this patient's hypertension. Beta-adrenergic blocking agents may worsen symptoms of Raynaud's phenomenon. These agents block vasodilating mechanisms in the digits and may also enhance the vasoconstriction produced by endogenous norepinephrine.

Desired Outcome

2. *What are the goals of therapy for this patient's Raynaud's phenomenon?*

   - Decrease the frequency of Raynaud's attacks
   - Minimize the duration and severity of symptoms associated with Raynaud's attacks
   - Promote healing of existing digital ulcerations and minimize future recurrences
   - Prevent digital ischemia and associated tissue loss
   - Minimize disease-related limitations of daily living activities
   - Educate the patient about emotional, occupational, and environmental attack triggers

- Adjust the pharmacotherapeutic regimen to eliminate agents that may trigger Raynaud's attacks
- Educate the patient about avoidance of non-prescription drugs that may exacerbate Raynaud's symptoms

Therapeutic Alternatives

3. a. What non-drug therapies could be useful for the treatment of the patient's painful symptoms associated with exacerbation of Raynaud's phenomenon?

- Non-drug measures are not usually curative in secondary Raynaud's but are an essential part of a comprehensive treatment plan. She should be instructed to:
    - ✓ Avoid cold exposure when possible
    - ✓ Minimize exposure to air conditioning
    - ✓ Dress warmly (including gloves or mittens and socks) if exposure to cold is unavoidable
    - ✓ Protect the face and trunk from cold (exposure of other body parts may induce reflex vasoconstriction)
    - ✓ Use electric hand and foot warmers if cold exposure is unavoidable (proper instruction is essential)
    - ✓ Avoid external sources of stress and exhaustion that may trigger activation of the sympathetic nervous system
    - ✓ Avoid long periods of standing that could produce lower extremity vasoconstriction
    - ✓ Avoid tobacco, which can cause cutaneous vasoconstriction
    - ✓ Use insulated containers for cold foods and beverages
    - ✓ Recognize and terminate attacks by returning to warmth and placing the hands in warm water or using an electric hair dryer to warm the digits and induce vasodilation
    - ✓ Practice biofeedback techniques to minimize the stress and the emotional component, as well as techniques to voluntarily raise body temperature to minimize frequency, duration, and severity of attacks
    - ✓ Practice good hand hygiene to minimize ulcer formation and avoid infection
    - ✓ Use finger cages to protect ulcerated digits and improve healing
    - ✓ Consult her pharmacist or physician prior to selecting any over-the-counter medications

b. What pharmacotherapeutic alternatives are available for the treatment of Raynaud's disease?

- Therapy is directed toward smooth muscle relaxation, relief of vasospasm, and increasing resting blood flow to digits with resolution of ischemia. It is believed that a combination of many defects involving hormones, structural abnormalities, circulating mediators, neural signals, and alterations in alpha adrenoreceptor sensitivity all contribute to symptoms. Based on the pathophysiology, vasodilators, platelet inhibitors, serotonin antagonists, and fibrinolytics have been used with varying degrees of success.
- *Dihydropyridine calcium channel antagonists* are first-line therapy for Raynaud's syndrome. These agents derive therapeutic benefit through vascular smooth muscle relaxation and peripheral vasodilation. They may also be helpful because of antiplatelet effects. In addition to being more potent vasodilators, dihydropyridines are less likely than other calcium channel blockers to suppress cardiac contractility and slow cardiac conduction.
    - ✓ *Nifedipine* has been studied the most extensively in placebo-controlled, randomized trials. Patients receiving nifedipine 10 to 20 mg po TID experienced a significant and sustained decrease in the number of Raynaud's attacks. However, the intensity of attacks did not differ from placebo.[1] Headache, dizziness, ankle edema, palpitations, and pruritus were the most common side effects reported. Clinical observation suggests that the extended-release product may be better tolerated and allow a more convenient dosage interval to be used.[2] Current studies with controlled-release dosage forms are not double blind and placebo controlled. Ankle edema is the most frequently reported adverse event associated with the extended-release dosage form.
    - ✓ *Felodipine, isradipine,* and *amlodipine* have proven useful in small studies and may be considered therapeutic alternatives for patients who do not tolerate the adverse effects of nifedi-pine. Nicardipine was beneficial in one trial but no better than placebo in another study.[1]
- *Diltiazem* (a non-dihydropyridine calcium channel blocker) has been found to be useful in short-term studies. Its side effect profile was similar to nifedipine but not as severe. Diltiazem is a less potent vasodilator, and therefore has decreased effectiveness when compared to agents in the dihydropyridine class.
- *Verapamil* (another non-dihydropyridine calcium channel blocker) has not been shown to be effective in relieving symptoms of Raynaud's phenomenon.
- *Topical nitroglycerin paste* applied locally along the course of the digital artery has been reported anecdotally to improve symptoms of ischemia by improving capillary blood flow.[1] Adverse effects include headache and hypotension. Nitrate tolerance is a theoretical limitation to successful long-term therapy. Controlled clinical trials to document efficacy have not been performed.
- *Methyldopa*, a sympatholytic agent, was shown in early studies to reduce the frequency and severity of Raynaud's attacks. Doses of 1 to 2 g/day were used. Results also showed prevention of cold-induced pain, increased digital blood flow, and decreased time to digital warming. These results were only evident in primary Raynaud's disease and not secondary Raynaud's phenomenon, as seen in this patient.[1] Clinical studies do not indicate that this patient would obtain significant symptom resolution.
- *Aspirin* and *dipyridamole* have not been shown to decrease frequency or severity of symptoms.[1]
- *Pentoxifylline* 400 mg po TID has been reported to have beneficial effects, but the evidence comes from small open studies that evaluated subjective measures of symptom improvement.[2]
- *ACE inhibitors* have been studied less extensively than calcium channel blockers. This drug class inhibits the breakdown of bradykinin, resulting in vasodilation.
    - ✓ *Captopril* has been shown to improve cutaneous blood flow, but patients experienced no subjective improvement in severity or number of attacks.[1] In theory, these agents should be beneficial, but to date no controlled studies support the use of

ACE inhibitors as first-line therapy for Raynaud's phenomenon.
- *Prostaglandins* are potent vasodilators, platelet aggregation inhibitors, and have biologic functions that may improve vascular reactivity. Prostacyclin and alprostadil are available in the United States for IV use only. The role of oral prostaglandin analogs has yet to be defined; they may ultimately be indicated as second-line therapy in patients who are refractory to other agents.
  - ✓ *Iloprost* is a chemically stable oral prostacyclin analog not available in the United States. Several double-blind, placebo-controlled trials have shown clinical benefit in the treatment of Raynaud's exacerbation. In a comparative trial of iloprost versus nifedipine, both medications reduced the number, duration and severity of attacks, but nifedipine was associated with more frequent adverse effects.[3]
  - ✓ *Misoprostol* did not show positive reversal of cold-induced vasospasm in one small study of patients with primary disease.
- *Prazosin*, a postsynaptic α-blocking agent, decreased the number of attacks in one double-blind crossover study. These effects were not seen in patients with systemic sclerosis. Its side effect profile was unacceptable and included headache, dizziness, syncope, and rash.[1] The available scientific evidence does not support the use of prazosin as first-line therapy for this patient with a diagnosis of systemic sclerosis.
- *Stanozolol* normalizes the impaired fibrinolytic system seen in secondary Raynaud's phenomenon. This was evaluated by laboratory measurement, but patients did not experience objective or subjective improvement in symptoms. Undesirable anabolic steroid side effects also render this agent of little value for this patient.
- *Ketanserin*, a serotonin receptor antagonist with slight α-adrenergic antagonist activity, has shown promise in clinical trials. Although it is not available in the United States at the time of this writing, it is presently being evaluated in large multicenter studies.
- Other agents in clinical trials include thromboxane synthetase inhibitors, thromboxane receptor antagonists, tissue plasminogen activator, calcitonin gene-related peptide, and endothelin receptor antagonists.[1-4]

Optimal Plan

4. a. What drug, dose, and schedule would be most appropriate for treating this patient's Raynaud's phenomenon?

- Nifedipine has been proven to be the most efficacious agent as first-line therapy. The dosage strategy includes initiation of low doses with gradual titration. After dose titration with the prompt-release form, transition to the long-acting product will minimize adverse effects and allow for the ease of once-daily administration. Therapy should be initiated at 10 mg twice daily. The dose should be advanced after 7 to 10 days to 10 mg po TID. The dose can further be titrated to 20 mg BID and then to 20 mg TID if necessary.[2] Dose changes should be made slowly (e.g., every 7 to 10 days) based on clinical response. The lowest effective dose should be used. When the target dose is achieved, the patient can be changed to the once-daily product in the equipotent dose. In clinical practice, many practitioners initiate therapy with a once-daily sustained-release nifedipine product (i.e., 30 mg po QD). This does not allow such precise flexibility of dose titration but may improve patient compliance during therapy initiation.
- Amlodipine, felodipine, isradipine, or nisoldipine could be used if the patient fails a trial of nifedipine due to intolerance. These agents are administered once daily at the beginning of therapy. Because they produce therapeutic effects by the same mechanism of action, it is unlikely that they would be effective if the patient fails to respond to nifedipine. They may provide a more favorable adverse event profile for patients who achieve symptom improvement with nifedipine but cannot tolerate its side effects.
- Topical nitroglycerin ointment could be selected as initial therapy. However, headache is a common side effect that may render this therapy undesirable. Topical nitroglycerin has been shown to improve healing of digital ulceration, which is present in this patient.[1] To avoid the adverse effects associated with polypharmacy, nitroglycerin could be added if maximum symptomatic relief is not obtained from oral nifedipine therapy.
- The efficacy of aspirin, dipyridamole, pentoxifylline, and ACE inhibitors has not been substantiated by clinical trials and would not be used as first-line therapy for this patient. ACE inhibitor therapy could be evaluated as second-line therapy because it may also benefit her concomitant hypertension, renal insufficiency, systemic sclerosis, and NIDDM.
- The therapeutic benefit of prazosin has not been convincingly demonstrated. Clinical trials do not show symptom improvement in patients with systemic sclerosis.

4. b. In addition to initiating the new therapy that you suggested for control of the patient's peripheral vascular symptoms, what other adjustments would you make to her current drug regimen?

- She should be instructed to avoid ibuprofen, aspirin, and all other NSAIDs, as they can worsen peripheral vascular symptoms. Acetaminophen can be used for minor pain relief.
- Propranolol should be discontinued because β-blockers have the potential to worsen Raynaud's symptoms. Nifedipine could be used successfully to treat the patient's hypertension.
- Discontinuation of hydrochlorothiazide should be considered. Thiazide diuretics can elevate serum lipids and elevate glucose.

Outcome Evaluation

5. What clinical and laboratory parameters are needed to evaluate the patient's therapy for achievement of therapeutic goals and avoidance of adverse events?

- Therapeutic goals include decreasing the frequency of Raynaud's exacerbations with associated decrease in pain, numbness, tingling, and digital ulceration.
- Success of symptom resolution may be obtained from the patient diary.
- Nifedipine monitoring should include heart rate and blood pressure. A BP of <130/85 mm Hg is optimal for minimizing end-organ damage in patients with diabetes mellitus.
- The patient should also be monitored for signs and symptoms of bradycardia, ankle edema, and CHF.

Patient Counseling

6. *What information should be provided to the patient to enhance compliance, ensure successful therapy, and minimize adverse events?*

General Information

- Continue to practice all of the other strategies that we talked about such as avoiding cold, wearing gloves, and using insulated drinking glasses.
- It would be helpful to keep a diary or notebook. Write down when you have pain and what you were doing at the time. We can then review the diary and see how well the drug is working for you.

Nifedipine Capsules

- This new drug is called nifedipine. It will help reduce the pain and tingling in your fingers.
- This drug will also help to lower your blood pressure. We will have you stop taking the hydrochlorothiazide and taper the Inderal LA. It will be slowly stopped over the next week.
- Take this medication every day. It will not work if you only take it when you have pain in your fingers.
- Take this medication once in the morning and once at bedtime. Do not take more than two capsules per day.
- Swallow the capsule whole, and do not chew or bite the capsule.
- You can take this medication with or without food. If it bothers your stomach, try taking it with food.
- This drug sometimes causes dizziness. Get up slowly from sitting or lying down until you see how the drug affects you. Be careful when driving or using any machinery if the drug makes you drowsy.
- If you miss a dose, take it as soon as you remember. However, if it is close to the time for your next dose when you remember, skip the missed dose and go back to your regular schedule.
- Call your doctor if you have difficulty breathing or notice swelling, severe dizziness, or irregular heartbeat.
- Do not suddenly stop taking the drug without your physician's knowledge. Call your doctor if side effects become troublesome or severe.
- Store this medication safely away from children.
- Make sure that you get your refills on time. Do not let yourself run out of medication.
- Ask your pharmacist or physician to help you select any medications for cough, cold, pain, or indigestion. Using the wrong product could make your Raynaud's symptoms worse.

References

1. Bolster MB, Maricq HR, Leff R. Office evaluation and treatment of Raynaud's phenomenon. Cleve Clin J Med 1995;62:51–61.
2. Belch JJ, Ho M. Pharmacotherapy of Raynaud's phenomenon. Drugs 1996;52:682–695.
3. Ferro CJ, Webb DJ. The clinical potential of endothelin receptor antagonists in cardiovascular medicine. Drugs 1996;51:12–27.
4. Wigley FM, Flavahan NA. Raynaud's phenomenon. Rheum Dis Clin North Am 1996;22:765–781.

17 HYPOVOLEMIC SHOCK

▶ **A Glass Half Full** (Level II)

Brian L. Erstad, PharmD, FASHP, FCCM

A 47-year-old man who had a liver transplant 6 months ago is hospitalized because of nausea, anorexia, diarrhea, fatigue, and decreased oral intake. One of his immunosuppressant medications, tacrolimus, is temporarily withheld because of renal impairment. The patient has clinical signs of hypotension and dehydration that indicate the early stages of hypovolemic shock. When considering alternatives for intravascular volume repletion, students must weigh the benefits and limitations of crystalloids versus colloids. The potential need for adjunctive therapies such as inotropic agents and vasopressors should also be considered. Dosage adjustment of concomitant medications in the face of renal impairment may be necessary. Monitoring parameters should be directed toward achieving successful fluid resuscitation while minimizing the likelihood of fluid overload.

▶ Questions

Problem Identification

1. a. *Create a list of the patient's drug-related problems.*

- This patient is in early stages of shock (hypotension, dehydration) with hyponatremia; this will require treatment with fluids and electrolytes.
- Possible adjustment and/or discontinuation of medications that may be either contributing to renal dysfunction (tacrolimus, acyclovir) or have elimination altered by it (acyclovir, famotidine, fluconazole, mycophenolate).
- Possible medication non-compliance resulting from nausea and diarrhea.
- Possible ongoing rejection as noted by recent biopsy; this may require adjustment of immunosuppressant dosing.

b. *What information (signs, symptoms, laboratory values) indicates the presence or severity of hypovolemic shock?*

- The presence of the early stages of shock is determined from inadequate oral intake of fluids and diarrhea, decreased blood pressure, skin pallor, weak pulse, third-spaced fluid (ascites, edema), pre-renal azotemia (BUN:SCr ratio 22:1) leading to decreased urine output and renal failure. The renal failure is evidenced by the elevated BUN and creatinine, decreased urine output, and by the increased serum phosphorus concentration, since it accumulates in the presence of renal dysfunction.

Desired Outcome

2. What are the goals of pharmacotherapy in this case?

- Prevent progression of shock to a potentially life-threatening situation
- Reverse organ dysfunction (e.g., renal dysfunction) related to shock
- Eliminate the patient's symptoms of dehydration and shock
- Slow or arrest the toxicity of medications that may have contributed to renal dysfunction by appropriate resuscitation with particular emphasis on plasma volume expansion, and withholding nephrotoxic medications (as is being done for tacrolimus)
- Adjust medications with elimination affected by renal dysfunction to prevent medication toxicity

Therapeutic Alternatives

3. a. What non-drug therapies might be useful for this patient?

- *Subacutely.* Possible need for withdrawal of ascitic fluid given the patient's increase in weight and ascitic fluid volume (e.g., positive fluid wave) with decreasing breath sounds probably secondary to fluid impinging on lungs.
- *Chronically.* Dietary compliance. In the post-transplant patient calorie requirements are approximately 15% to 20% above basal energy expenditure with <30% of calories obtained from saturated fat. Protein requirements typically average 1 g/kg/day. Sodium is preferably restricted to 2 to 3 g/day.

b. What feasible pharmacotherapeutic alternatives are available for treatment of shock?

- The treatment of shock is usually initiated with crystalloid infusion with near-isotonic, salt-containing fluids such as *lactated Ringer's* or *normal saline solution*.[1] These fluids fill the extracellular space (all 1000 mL of 1000 mL infused), which is more important than intracellular filling in symptomatic patients with obvious intravascular depletion.
- Dextrose solutions for patients with intravascular depletion are not appropriate since only a small amount of the solution is retained in the extracellular space (e.g., one-third of amount infused for 5% dextrose in water).
- Colloid therapy such as 5% *albumin* or 6% *hetastarch* solutions should be considered if at least two liters of crystalloid solution has been administered without an adequate response in monitoring parameters. While these solutions initially are restricted to the intravascular space, substantial leakage to the interstitial space begins to occur within hours even in patients without altered capillary permeability. A recent review of randomized trials of colloids versus crystalloids found that colloid use was associated with an increased absolute mortality risk of 4%, or four extra deaths for every 100 patients resuscitated.[2] The authors concluded that these data do not support the continued use of colloids for volume replacement in critically ill patients.
- There is no advantage to using *plasma protein fraction* instead of 5% albumin, since plasma expansion is similar with the two products and adverse effects related to plasma protein fraction (e.g., vasomotor reactions) may be greater. Theoretically, administration of 25% albumin would cause fluid to shift from the interstitial to the intravascular space, which might decrease the amount of third-space fluids. However, the albumin will eventually leak across the capillary membrane into the interstitial space and pull fluid with it.
- Colloid therapy should also be considered if the patient develops dyspnea, rales, or radiographic evidence of substantial interstitial fluid accumulation, assuming such findings are consistent with interstitial fluid accumulation due to crystalloid administration despite inadequate responses in monitoring parameters (e.g., blood pressure, urine output). If such problems develop, oxygen therapy, titrated by arterial blood gas determinations and/or oximetric recordings, will also be indicated.
- Inotropic agents such as *dobutamine* are considered (with or without right heart catheter monitoring) if there is an inadequate response to plasma expanders as determined by vital signs, hemodynamic indices, urine output, and physical examination.
- Vasopressors (e.g., *norepinephrine, phenylephrine,* high-dose *dopamine*) are used as a last resort and only when other therapies for shock have produced an inadequate response.

Optimal Plan

4. What drug, dosage form, dose, schedule, and duration of therapy are best for this patient?

- Plasma expansion using either crystalloid or colloid (much more expensive) therapy is necessary for preventing the progression of shock. Begin by infusing 15 mL/kg of crystalloid solution (such as 0.9% sodium chloride or lactated Ringer's) over approximately 2 hours. Administration of additional fluids is based on physical examination findings, heart rate, blood pressure (arterial if not rapidly responding to fluid resuscitation), and urine output (catheterize if not rapidly responding to fluid resuscitation).
- Since the patient does not have a history of renal failure, it is possible that the renal dysfunction will reverse relatively quickly with adequate fluid resuscitation. Therefore, rather than immediately adjusting all doses of renally eliminated medications, it may be more appropriate to temporarily hold the doses of the medications for the first 24 hours to see if renal function improves quickly. If not, the famotidine would be the only medication that would need to be decreased during the first week, since the other medications are already being given in relatively low (some would argue too low) doses. In renal failure, the appropriate famotidine dose is 10 mg every 24 hours.

Outcome Evaluation

5. What clinical and laboratory parameters are necessary to evaluate the therapy for achievement of the desired therapeutic outcome and to detect or prevent adverse events?

- Physical examination findings (e.g., skin turgor), heart rate, blood pressure (preferably arterial), urine output (by bladder catheterization), mental status, and possibly PAOP measurements if there is prolonged or complicated resuscitation. Initially, these parameters should be monitored every 10 to 15 minutes and then with decreas-

ing frequency as compensation for fluid losses is achieved. In general, an adult patient will require 35 to 40 mL/kg/hr of fluids to maintain euvolemia, so even larger amounts are required for patients with hypovolemia.
- As successful resuscitation occurs, one would expect the skin to have normal mobility and turgor. The heart rate and blood pressure recordings should return to normal pretreatment values. Urine output in healthy adults should be at least 0.5 mL/kg/hr (assuming the patient is catheterized). Other signs and symptoms related to volume depletion (e.g., fatigue, dry oral mucosa, weakness) should abate with successful resuscitation.
- Laboratory parameters (renal function tests, calcium, phosphorus, and magnesium) should be monitored daily until stable. Fluid intake and output should be monitored at least every nursing shift until stable, and then decreased to daily. Daily weights should be obtained.
- The most likely adverse effects of crystalloid and colloid therapies are fluid overload due to interstitial space expansion (usually seen as increasing ascitic fluid accumulation and leg edema as in this patient) and pulmonary edema as noted by auscultation and/or radiographic evidence. Development of CHF is a concern in patients with poor LV function.
- For monitoring tacrolimus therapy, an admission blood tacrolimus concentration should be obtained. Once the drug is restarted, tacrolimus can be monitored with additional blood levels and concentrations of other laboratory parameters. The total bilirubin, AST/ALT, and GGT concentrations can be used to assess possible rejection. The serum creatinine and/or creatinine clearance measurements will indicate renal function status. Electrolytes and blood glucose should be obtained, as tacrolimus can cause hyperkalemia, hypomagnesemia, and hyperglycemia. All labs should be obtained at least daily until the patient is stable. Clinical signs and symptoms of toxicity (hypertension, tremor, headache, diarrhea, nausea) or organ rejection (liver function tests mentioned and/or biopsy) should also be evaluated regularly.
- All medications that are renally eliminated will need to be adjusted as renal function improves or worsens (as noted by serum creatinine concentrations and urine output).

Patient Counseling

6. What information should be provided to the patient to enhance compliance, ensure successful therapy, and minimize adverse effects?

- After transplantation, it is essential that you maintain appropriate fluid and food intake. When you do not drink enough liquids your body cannot work properly and it may be harmful to many organs including your new liver. When you ingest too many fluids, especially those containing large amounts of sodium, you may worsen the fluid accumulation in your gut and legs that can make you uncomfortable. We will have a dietitian see you regarding a healthy diet now that you have had your transplant.
- If you have problems such as nausea or fatigue in the future, contact your physician or me for helpful advice, which may prevent you from having to be hospitalized.
- Finally, it is very important that you take your medications exactly as ordered. If you feel you are having a problem related to a medication, contact your physician or me for further instructions. Do not take any other medication, even over-the-counter products such as aspirin or antacids, without consulting one of us first.

▶ Follow-up Question

1. Why might this patient have changes in urine output, heart rate, and other parameters that are consistent with volume depletion even though he has edema on physical examination and his admission weight was indicative of volume overload?

- Although the patient has increased total body water, much of it has been distributed to third spaces and is not readily accessible to the vasculature. Therefore, he is intravascularly volume depleted, even though he has excess interstitial fluid resulting in edema.

References

1. Vermeulen LC Jr, Ratko TA, Erstad BL, et al. A paradigm for consensus. The University Hospital Consortium guidelines for the use of albumin, nonprotein colloid, and crystalloid solutions. Arch Intern Med 1995;155:373–379.
2. Schierhout G, Roberts I. Fluid resuscitation with colloid or crystalloid solutions in critically ill patients: A systematic review of randomised trials. BMJ 1998;316:961–964.

SECTION 2

Respiratory Disorders

Robert L. Talbert, PharmD, FCCP, BCPS, Section Editor

18 ACUTE ASTHMA

▶ **Living With Restricted Spaces**   (Level I)

Daniel T. Kennedy, PharmD, BCPS
Ralph E. Small, PharmD, FCCP, FASHP, FAPhA

A 20-year-old man with a history of asthma, GERD, and depression presents to the ED with an acute asthmatic attack thought to have been precipitated by exposure to paint fumes. He is presently on a prednisone taper following a recent exacerbation. The patient has a number of drug-related problems that students are asked to identify. Initiation of oxygen therapy and specific regimens of inhaled β_2-agonists and corticosteroids are required for acute treatment. Students are also asked to create a pharmacotherapeutic plan for this patient upon discharge. The case provides the opportunity for students to practice educating patients on inhalation technique for metered-dose inhalers and use of peak flow meters.

▶ **Questions**

Problem Identification

1. a. *Create a list of the patient's drug related problems.*

   - Acute asthma attack secondary to paint fumes requiring appropriate pharmacologic treatment.
   - Improper drug selection; the anticholinergic agent ipratropium bromide (Atrovent) has not been shown to be effective for chronic asthma.
   - Improper dosing interval; triamcinolone acetonide (Azmacort) is presently given QID when BID dosing is effective in most patients.
   - Inadequate treatment of heartburn/GERD (patient complains of recent heartburn), which may be a trigger for this patient's worsening asthma control.
   - Patient has not been monitoring peak flows as an outpatient, which may result in inability to detect pulmonary decompensation.
   - Hypokalemia potentially due to albuterol nebulizations and/or corticosteroid use.

   b. *What information (signs, symptoms, laboratory values) indicates the severity of the acute asthma attack?*

   - History of intubations × 5
   - Currently on prednisone taper for recent exacerbation
   - Patient reports "breathing fine" earlier in the day
   - Increased pulse and respiratory rate
   - Sinus tachycardia on ECG
   - Bilateral decreased breath sounds, tight air movement, high-pitched wheezes bilaterally
   - pco_2 42 mm Hg; respiratory drive is typically increased in acute asthma, so a pco_2 >40 mm Hg may indicate severe airflow obstruction and increased risk of respiratory failure
   - Difficulty speaking
   - Labored breathing, using accessory muscles
   - Pneumomediastinum on L heart border most likely due to barotrauma of acute asthma attack

- Peak flow 150 L/min (31% of baseline)
- Hypokalemia (3.2 mEq/L) potentially secondary to albuterol nebulizations and/or corticosteroid use

Note: A theophylline level of 6.3 mg/L is adequate according to National Asthma Education and Prevention Program Expert Panel Report 2 guidelines, which state that a therapeutic range of 5 to 15 mg/L has equal efficacy and less adverse drug reactions than a range of 10 to 20 mg/L.[1]

Desired Outcome

2. *What are the goals of pharmacotherapy in this case?*

   Short-term Goals
   - Rapid reversal of airway obstruction (response to therapy above 70% of baseline PEF or FEV_1)
   - Decrease pco_2 and maintain $po_2 \geq 80\%$ and O_2 sat $\geq 90\%$
   - Response sustained at least 60 minutes from last treatment
   - Relieve the patient's symptoms/physical distress
   - Normal physical examination
   - Correct hypokalemia

   Long-term Goals
   - Reduce the rate of recurrent asthma symptoms
   - Prevent ED visits, hospitalization, and intubation through patient education and proper pharmacotherapy

Therapeutic Alternatives

3. a. *What non-drug therapies might be useful for this patient?*
   - Oxygen is recommended for most patients experiencing an acute asthma exacerbation.[1] Administer supplemental oxygen by nasal cannulae or mask to achieve an O_2 sat $\geq 90\%$. Those with heart disease or who are pregnant should achieve an O_2 sat $\geq 95\%$. Oxygen saturation should be continuously monitored to gauge efficacy of bronchodilator therapy. Intubation must also be seriously considered in patients with a $pco_2 \geq 42$ mm Hg or any other indications that respiratory failure is imminent. The exact time to intubate is based on clinical expertise and knowledge. Once the decision has been made to intubate, the procedure should not be delayed because respiratory failure can advance quickly and is difficult to reverse.[1]

   b. *What feasible pharmacotherapeutic alternatives are available for the treatment of acute asthma?*
   - *Inhaled short-acting β_2-agonists* are the treatment of choice for an acute asthma attack. Nebulized albuterol (5 mg/mL) at a dose of 2.5 to 5 mg every 20 minutes for 3 doses, then 2.5 to 10 mg every 1 to 4 hours as needed, or 10 to 15 mg/hr continuously may be used. Albuterol via MDI can also be used at a dose of 4 to 8 puffs every 20 minutes up to 4 hours, then every 1 to 4 hours as needed. Use of a nebulizer often is a simpler method of administration and results in a quicker onset of action in the acute asthma case. However, recent data support the use of an MDI over nebulization of β_2-agonists in those patients who are able to demonstrate adequate inhaler technique during status asthmaticus.[2,3]
   - *Systemic corticosteroids* have an onset of action of 6 to 12 hours to resolve airway obstruction and prevent acute asthma relapses. *Oral prednisone, prednisolone,* or *IV methylprednisolone* may be used in 3 to 4 divided daily doses for the first 48 hours, then QD–BID until PEF reaches 70% of predicted or personal best (refer to Pharmacologic Management in textbook Chapter 24). It is important to note that oral administration of prednisone has been shown to be as effective as IV administration of methylprednisolone and is less invasive.[4]
   - *Systemic sympathomimetics (SQ epinephrine or terbutaline)* have no proven advantage over inhaled short-acting β_2-agonists and should be reserved for patients who are unable to adequately move air.
   - *Anticholinergics (e.g., ipratropium bromide or Atrovent)* should not be used as a first-line therapy but may be used in combination with β_2-agonist therapy for the treatment of acute asthma.
   - *Methylxanthines (e.g., IV aminophylline)* are not generally recommended because they provide little benefit over optimal inhaled short-acting β_2-agonist therapy for acute asthma.[5] For patients taking a theophylline preparation on an outpatient basis who present with acute asthma, a serum theophylline concentration is indicated to rule out potential toxicity.

   c. *What psychosocial considerations are applicable to this patient?*
   - For an asthmatic prison inmate, issues such as availability of medications for PRN use are major considerations for the health care professional. Also, trigger control (e.g., mold, humidity, paint fumes) cannot be easily modified in the prison setting.

Optimal Plan

4. a. *What drug, dosage form, dose, schedule, and duration of therapy are best for this patient?*
   - Continue oxygen supplementation (e.g., 4 to 6 L).
   - Nebulized albuterol (5 mg/mL) at a dose of 2.5 to 5 mg every 20 minutes for 3 doses, then 2.5 to 10 mg every 1 to 4 hours as needed, or 10 to 15 mg/hr continuously may be used. Initially, continuous nebs may be indicated because of the pco_2 level and this patient's unwillingness to be intubated.
   - Methylprednisolone 125 mg IV Q 6 H for 24 to 48 hours. Methylprednisolone IV or prednisone po can be dosed at 1 to 2 mg/kg Q 6 H for 24 to 48 hours, or until severe symptoms diminish, then reduce to 1 to 2 mg/kg Q 12 H. Refer to the medication dosage table in textbook Chapter 24 for further recommendations.
   - Supplement potassium via IV replacement fluids (up to 10 mEq/hr diluted) or orally (10 to 25 mEq po QD).
   - IV magnesium sulfate would be considered only if the patient does not respond or worsens with the above standard therapy.

   b. *What pharmacotherapy would you recommend for this patient upon discharge?*
   - Continue albuterol MDI 2 puffs BID PRN. Long-acting β_2-agonists (e.g., salmeterol) should be withheld at this time because the patient has not been optimized on inhaled corticosteroid therapy.
   - Make available albuterol via nebulization (5 mg) to be used PRN for wheezing or SOB.
   - Continue Azmacort (triamcinolone acetonide) since this is what

the patient had been receiving previously, but increase the dose to 8 puffs BID. Other inhaled corticosteroids may also be considered, such as Flovent (fluticasone propionate) 220 μg/puff, 2 puffs BID. Cost, likely patient adherence, and formulary issues are important factors in selecting the optimal agent for a particular patient.
- Continue Theo-Dur 200 mg po BID for the time being. If the patient can gain control of the disease with the increased Azmacort dosage, attempt to discontinue theophylline in 1 to 2 months.
- Begin a prednisone taper, such as prednisone 20 mg po BID × 7 days, then 20 mg po QD × 3 days, then 10 mg po QD × 3 days, then discontinue. Other tapering schedules may also be appropriate. A taper is necessary because the patient has been on corticosteroid therapy for longer than 2 weeks.
- Discontinue Atrovent because the effectiveness of anticholinergics in the long-term management of asthma has not been demonstrated.[6]
- Consider increasing omeprazole to 20 mg po BID for added heartburn/GERD coverage.
- Continue doxepin for depression at the dose used upon admission.
- Question the continuation of guaifenesin, as it has no proven benefit in asthma. Ask the patient if he feels the guaifenesin benefits his symptoms in any way before stopping it.
- Peak flow monitoring must be initiated in this patient while in prison. Peak flow monitoring will help guide further pharmacologic decisions.
- Consider the addition of leukotriene modifiers and/or salmeterol in the future if asthma symptoms are not controlled with maximal doses of the inhaled corticosteroid.

Outcome Evaluation

5. a. *What are the long-term goals of asthma therapy for this patient?*

- Prevent chronic and troublesome symptoms
- Maintain near "normal" pulmonary function
- Maintain normal activity levels, including exercise and other physical activity
- Prevent recurrent exacerbations of asthma and eliminate ED visits and/or hospitalizations
- Provide optimal pharmacotherapy with minimal adverse effects
- Meet patient's expectations of and satisfaction with asthma care

b. *What will you monitor to assess the efficacy of asthma pharmacotherapy in this patient?*

- Improvement in PEF, wheezing, and breathing
- Number of β_2-agonist canisters used/month
- Frequency of use of PRN albuterol nebulizations
- Need for oral prednisone in the future
- Patient adherence with the drug regimen
- Number of ED visits/hospitalizations

c. *What will you monitor to assess the side effects of drug therapy?*

- *Albuterol:* Nervousness, anxiety, skeletal muscle tremor, headache, hypokalemia, cardiac arrhythmias, palpitations
- *Triamcinolone (Azmacort):* Cough, dysphonia, oral thrush (candidiasis)
- *Theophylline (Theo-Dur):* Insomnia, gastric upset, aggravation of ulcer or reflux, nausea and vomiting, tachyarrhythmias, CNS stimulation, headache, tremors

d. *What laboratory tests or other objective measures are necessary to monitor therapy?*

- Evaluation of PEF/FEV_1 every 1/2 to 1 hour initially in ED
- Evaluation of peak flow readings monthly after discharge
- Theophylline level every 3 months after discharge
- Potassium level every 3 to 6 months after discharge

Patient Counseling

6. *Describe the information that should be provided to this patient regarding inhaler technique, the differences between quick-relief and long-term-control medications, and the use of a peak flow meter (see Figures 18–2 and 18–3).*

Inhaler Technique

- Some of the medications you take for asthma are inhaled into the lungs. It is important that I check your inhaler technique often to make sure that the medications give you the best control of your asthma. I will be happy to observe and assess your inhalation technique. Follow these steps when using your inhaler:
  ✓ Remove the cap and hold the inhaler upright.
  ✓ Shake the canister well for 3 to 4 seconds.
  ✓ Tilt your head back slightly and breathe out slowly.
  ✓ Position the inhaler using the open-mouth, closed-mouth, or spacer/holding chamber technique (students will have to choose the appropriate technique for an individual patient).
  ✓ Press down on the inhaler to release medication as you start to breathe in slowly.
  ✓ Breathe in slowly for 3 to 5 seconds.
  ✓ Hold your breath for 10 seconds to allow the medicine to reach deeply into your lungs.
  ✓ Exhale slowly.
  ✓ Wait 1 to 2 minutes before inhaling the next puff to give the medicine some time to work. Then repeat the above steps.

Differences Between Quick-relief and Long-term-control Medications

- Your quick-relief medication is your albuterol inhaler. This is a short-acting bronchodilator that relaxes the muscles around your airways. You should use this medication to relieve the wheezing and shortness of breath during an asthma attack. Use this medication only if you need it to help with the symptoms of an acute attack. This medication should work quickly to open your airways and make you breathe easier. If this medication doesn't help your symptoms during an asthma attack, or if your breathing gets worse, contact your doctor or pharmacist immediately for further assistance.
- Your long-term-control medications are the Azmacort inhaler and Theo-Dur tablets. These medications prevent asthma symptoms from occurring by decreasing the swelling that can close your airways. These medications need to be taken every day in regularly spaced doses to be effective in controlling asthma symptoms. They will not relieve an asthma attack that has already started. The Azmacort inhaler has a built-in spacer-mouthpiece that makes the inhaler easier to use and may allow more medicine to reach your lungs. Rinsing

your mouth with water after each use of the Azmacort may help prevent dryness of the mouth and oral thrush. Contact your doctor or pharmacist if any of these symptoms occur.

Use of a Peak Flow Meter
- A peak flow meter is a device used to determine your asthma control by measuring how well air moves out of your lungs. Peak flow meters are used to check your asthma the way that blood pressure cuffs are used to check high blood pressure. Your personal best peak flow number is the highest peak flow number you can achieve over a 2 to 3 week period. Your treatment plan will be based on your own personal best peak flow number. To find out what your personal best peak flow number is, take peak flow readings at least twice a day for 2 to 3 weeks. The steps for using a peak flow meter are as follows:
  ✓ Attach the mouthpiece to the peak flow meter (if one is needed).
  ✓ Make sure the indicator is at the bottom of the scale.
  ✓ Hold the peak flow meter so that your fingers do not block the opening or the indicator on the scale.
  ✓ Take a deep breath (inhale and exhale).
  ✓ Take another deep breath, filling your lungs completely, and place your mouth firmly around the mouthpiece. Do not put your tongue inside the hole.
  ✓ Blow out as hard and fast as you can in a single blow.
  ✓ Repeat these steps two more times. Record the highest of the three readings along with the date and time in your asthma diary.
- Once you know your personal best peak flow number, your doctor or pharmacist will set up an action plan. In the action plan, the peak flow numbers are placed into zones that are set up like a traffic light. You only need to measure your peak flow once a day, the first thing in the morning before you take your asthma medications. Record the result in your asthma diary. The action plan will tell you what to do when your peak flow changes.
- Note the presence of the green, yellow, and red zones:
  ✓ The green (top) zone indicates that your breathing is within 80% to 100% of your personal best peak flow reading. No asthma symptoms are present. Take your asthma medicines as usual.
  ✓ The yellow (middle) zone indicates 50% to 80% of your personal best and signals caution. An acute asthma attack may be present, and a temporary increase in your albuterol use or the addition of oral prednisone may be indicated.
  ✓ The red (bottom) zone indicates that your breathing is below 50% of your personal best and signals a medical alert. Use your inhaled or nebulized albuterol immediately. Call your doctor or dial 911 if peak flow results stay in the yellow or red zone.

▶ **Follow-up Question**

1. *What other actions could be taken to control the factors contributing to this patient's asthma severity?*

- Avoid exposure to allergens to which he is sensitive (e.g., paint fumes)
- Identify other allergen exposures
- Avoid the use of β-blockers and/or sulfite-containing and other foods to which he is sensitive
- Determine if the patient has a history of sensitivity to aspirin or NSAIDs, and if so, avoid these medications
- Monitor efficacy of GERD treatment
- Administer annual influenza vaccine

References

1. National Asthma Education and Prevention Program. Expert Panel Report 2: Guidelines for the Diagnosis and Management of Asthma. Bethesda, National Institutes of Health, 1997. www.nhlbi.nih.gov/nhlbi/nhlbi.
2. Idris AH, McDermott MF, Raucci JC, et al. Emergency department treatment of severe asthma. Metered-dose inhaler plus holding chamber is equivalent in effectiveness to nebulizer. Chest 1993;103:665–672.
3. Mandelberg A, Chen E, Noviski N, et al. Nebulized wet aerosol treatment in emergency department—Is it essential? Comparison with large spacer device for metered-dose inhaler. Chest 1997;112:1501–1505.
4. Ratto D, Alfaro C, Sipsey J, et al. Are intravenous corticosteroids required in status asthmaticus? JAMA 1988;260:527–529.
5. Murphy DG, McDermott MF, Rydman RJ, et al. Aminophylline in the treatment of acute asthma when beta-2-adrenergics and steroids are provided. Arch Intern Med 1993;153:1784–1788.
6. Kerstjens HA, Brand PL, Hughes MD, et al. A comparison of bronchodilator therapy with or without inhaled corticosteroid therapy for obstructive airways disease. N Engl J Med 1992;327:1413–1419.

19 CHRONIC ASTHMA

▶ A Tale of Cats, Colds, Compliance, and
  Corticosteroids   (Level I)

Dennis M. Williams, PharmD, FASHP, FCCP, BCPS

A 20-year-old woman college student with a history of persistent asthma and perennial allergic rhinitis presents to the student health service with complaints of increased shortness of breath, wheezing, poor exercise tolerance, and nasal stuffiness. She is admitted for 2 days and improves substantially after receiving oxygen, bronchodilators and corticosteroids. Students are asked to consider the possible factors that may have precipitated this acute exacerbation of asthma. A number of nonpharmacologic therapies should be considered in an attempt to prevent future episodes, reduce interactions with the health care system, and improve the patient's quality of life. Changes in her pharmacotherapeutic regimen may also be required. Feasible first-line alternatives include increasing the inhaled steroid dose or adding cromolyn or nedocromil sodium, theophylline, or a leukotriene antagonist. Home peak flow monitoring will allow the patient to assess her own disease control and take appropriate measures during impending exacerbations.

Chronic Asthma

▶ Questions

Problem Identification

1. a. *Create a list of the patient's drug-related problems.*

    - Poorly controlled moderate persistent asthma with an acute exacerbation currently treated with inhaled Azmacort (triamcinolone acetonide), Serevent (salmeterol), PRN Proventil HFA (albuterol that does not contain chlorofluorocarbons as the propellant), and an oral prednisone taper.
    - Uncontrolled perennial allergic rhinitis (on a corticosteroid nasal spray but with boggy nasal mucosa and nasal smear containing numerous eosinophils).
    - Heartburn (possible gastroesophageal reflux disease; currently untreated).
    - Family planning may be an issue, as the patient is taking oral contraceptives.

    b. *What information indicates the presence of uncontrolled chronic asthma and an acute asthma exacerbation?*

    - Signs of poorly controlled asthma in this case include the frequent symptoms that the patient reports, nighttime awakenings, and chest tightness.
    - She has had numerous ED visits and hospitalizations.
    - This acute exacerbation is classified as moderate to severe based on her signs and symptoms, including shortness of breath, wheezing, decreased exercise tolerance, decreased pulse oximetry, decreased peak flow (<50% of personal best), tachypnea, tachycardia, and the use of suprasternal accessory muscles to breathe.[1]

    c. *Could any of the patient's problems have been caused by drug therapy?*

    Not directly, but several factors should be addressed in her management:
    - She may be continually exposed to asthma triggers, and strategies to avoid or minimize these should be addressed (see question 3a, below).
    - Additional reasons for her noncompliance should be sought. She has stated some potential problems and concerns already, but she may be experiencing side effects or have fears about the safety of her therapies that should be addressed. Improved compliance may be achieved by modifying her regimen to make it more convenient or seeking alternative therapies.
    - Her technique in using the inhalation devices should be assessed. A limiting factor in getting optimal benefit from therapy is often related to poor inhalation technique. Her inhalation technique should be observed periodically and corrected if needed. If she has difficulty, alternative or ancillary devices should be considered (e.g., dry powder inhalers, holding chambers).
    - She has indicated a problem with her nebulizer. Nebulizer performance can vary; her present equipment should be checked and replaced if needed, since the patient perceives that this is a problem. A general method of determining if there is a problem is to observe the performance of the equipment when administering a dose of medication. Within a few seconds of turning the equipment on, a steady stream of aerosol gas should be noted from the mouthpiece. Also, the time required to administer the dose of medication provides a general estimate of the efficiency of output. In this patient, her previous nebulizer treatment was complete within 6 to 8 minutes, and with the current nebulizer the time required has been 12 to 15 minutes. The clinician should determine whether there has been a change in brands and attempt to provide her with the same nebulizer type previously used.
    - Poorly controlled upper airway allergies and GERD can aggravate asthma. It is important to assess the adequacy of treatment for her allergic rhinitis and to determine if her symptoms of heartburn are attributable to GERD. If so, appropriate nonpharmacologic or pharmacologic therapy can be instituted.[1]

Desired Outcome

2. *What are the goals of pharmacotherapy in this case?*

    - Preventing chronic symptoms of asthma (e.g., coughing or breathlessness at night, in the early morning, or after exertion)
    - Maintain near normal lung function
    - Maintain normal activity levels (including exercise and other physical activity)
    - Prevent recurrent exacerbations and minimize the need for hospitalization or ED visits
    - Provide optimal pharmacotherapy with minimal or no adverse effects
    - Meet patient's and families' expectation of and satisfaction with asthma treatment and care
    - Improve the patient's quality of life
    - In addition to the above goals, the patient should be asked if she has any personal goals that she would like to achieve

Therapeutic Alternatives

3. a. *What non-drug therapies might be useful for this patient?*

    - In addition to pharmacotherapy, the other components of asthma management include avoidance of asthma triggers, patient education, and objective monitoring through the use of a peak flow meter.
    - She has a history of allergies to salicylates and cats. She should be counseled about the risk of taking aspirin-containing products or other NSAIDs. She can be advised to check with her physician or pharmacist before taking any OTC products since many of them contain an NSAID for fever or pain. She should also include this allergy when providing medical information to any health care professional. The issue of her boyfriend and the cat should be discussed. If it is not possible to remove the pet from the environment or for her to not be exposed, the contact should be minimized as much as possible, and pretreatment with an inhaled β-agonist might provide some benefit.
    - Another common asthma trigger is the house dust mite. Since she has perennial allergies and asthma, she may have house dust mite sensitivity. She can be questioned about potential exposure to verify this. Simple measures to reduce exposure to house dust mite antigen include the use of mattress and pillow covers and weekly washing of bedding in hot water. Removal of carpet from the bedroom and the use of dehumidifiers can also be considered.

Allergy skin testing is recommended to identify specific allergies for some patients so that targeted strategies can be used.
- She should be educated about the triggers of asthma and the disease process. The role of each medication should be reviewed, and her inhalation technique must be assessed. She should receive an action plan whereby her medication is adjusted based on changes in her peak flow rates.
- In addition to the strategies described, certain conditions are known to worsen asthma control. These include upper airway allergies, sinusitis, and GERD. She is confirmed to have upper airway allergies, and interventions for those have been discussed. She can be questioned about the presence of symptoms for the other two conditions, and appropriate drug and non-drug therapies can be recommended if they are identified.

b. *What feasible pharmacotherapeutic alternatives are available for treatment of this patient's chronic asthma?*

- *Cromolyn or nedocromil sodium.* These nonsteroidal anti-inflammatory therapies are safe and useful alternatives to inhaled corticosteroids but are less effective for moderate to severe persistent asthma. Based on her history of moderate persistent asthma, they would not likely be effective. Some clinicians would add them to inhaled corticosteroids in order to reduce the steroid dose; however, this increases cost and reduces convenience of the regimen.
- *Theophylline.* Long-acting dosage forms prevent or control bronchospasm and are particularly useful for patients with nocturnal symptoms. Theophylline may be less effective than salmeterol and more difficult to use due to pharmacokinetic variability and drug interactions. Therefore, salmeterol enjoys more frequent use.
- *Leukotriene modifiers.* These newer oral agents block the effects of leukotrienes, which are potent inflammatory mediators in asthma. Data from clinical trials suggest that they are effective for mild to moderate forms of asthma. The expert panel asthma guidelines recommend them as an alternative to inhaled corticosteroids, cromolyn, or nedocromil for patients with mild persistent asthma. The only therapy that is known to alter the course of asthma is the inhaled corticosteroids, so they are preferred first-line treatment.[2] Newer studies have been designed to compare them to inhaled steroids or to evaluate their utility in reducing doses of inhaled steroids. Although they show promise, additional clinical experience is needed to determine their role in persistent asthma.[3] There are now three products available in the United States:
  - ✓ *Zileuton* (a 5-lipoxygenase enzyme inhibitor) has several limitations, including a QID dosing schedule and the potential for hepatotoxicity. Drug interactions with theophylline and warfarin have also been reported.
  - ✓ *Zafirlukast* (a leukotriene receptor antagonist) is dosed twice daily, and it also may interact with warfarin. Cases of Churg–Strauss syndrome have occurred in patients receiving zafirlukast while tapering oral corticosteroids, although direct causality has not been proven. This syndrome is characterized by flu-like symptoms and pulmonary infiltrates with eosinophilia.
  - ✓ *Montelukast* (a leukotriene receptor antagonist) may offer the most promise of the available agents; it is dosed once a day and currently has no known drug interactions. It also is indicated for patients 6 years of age and older, whereas the others are labeled only for ages 12 and older. For this patient, these agents might be considered as a future alternative if she is unable to be adequately controlled with her current therapy or if there is a strong preference for an oral therapy instead of inhaled medication.[3]
- Another alternative in this case is to increase the inhaled corticosteroid dose. This is an effective method of gaining better control of inflammation. However, other interventions (e.g., education, allergen avoidance) should be instituted first. The use of salmeterol with inhaled corticosteroids provides better symptom relief and peak flow rates than increased doses of inhaled corticosteroids.[4]

Optimal Plan

4. a. *Outline an optimal plan of treatment for this patient's chronic asthma.*

- She will be completing a short course of oral corticosteroids (prednisone 60 mg daily tapered over 10 days) for this resolving exacerbation. Tapering of the steroid dose is commonly employed in situations like this; however, there is no evidence that this is necessary. Although she has evidence of poor control for an extended period, her previous medication regimen may be adequate. Nevertheless, several areas can be addressed. Upper respiratory viral infections are the most common cause of acute asthma exacerbations and that may be the trigger in this case. Also, her uncontrolled allergic rhinitis may aggravate asthma control.
- The role of each medication should be reviewed and clarified (quick relief vs. long-term control therapy). In her regimen, the inhaled corticosteroid and the salmeterol prevent or control inflammation and bronchospasm. The albuterol is her quick relief agent and can be administered either via an MDI (2 to 4 puffs as needed) or nebulizer (2.5 mg in normal saline) based on the severity of her symptoms or convenience.
- Her technique in using the various inhalation devices should be evaluated and corrected if necessary.
- Allergic rhinitis and GERD (if the diagnosis is established) are two common conditions that can aggravate asthma and should be controlled. Similarly, exposure to cigarette smoke and cats should be avoided. She has evidence of an allergic component to her disease as indicated by a nasal and peripheral eosinophilia.
- Her inhaled corticosteroid regimen can be switched to a BID regimen without any loss of efficacy. She should be treated with 8 to 12 puffs per day of triamcinolone.
- Her salmeterol is a long-term control therapy used as 2 inhalations twice daily. This patient should not increase the use of salmeterol and should not use it as rescue therapy.
- Although a comprehensive assessment of her nebulizer performance is not warranted, its performance in producing an aerosol stream and the time required for a treatment can be observed. If the patient perceives this nebulizer to be part of the problem, replacement should be considered. It would be appropriate to provide her with the same brand previously used.

- A self-management plan and action plan should be reviewed and modified based on symptoms or peak flow values. She should receive specific instructions about when to seek help.

b. *What alternatives would be appropriate if the initial therapy fails?*

- If reestablishment of her chronic regimen fails to control her asthma, she can intensify her triamcinolone daily dose or switch to a more potent inhaled steroid (fluticasone or budesonide), which would allow fewer daily inhalations.
- Theophylline or leukotriene modifiers could be added to her regimen. Theophylline use for moderate persistent asthma should be dose-titrated to a serum concentration of 5 to 15 μg/mL. The usual doses of the oral leukotriene modifiers are zileuton 600 mg QID, zafirlukast 20 mg BID, and montelukast 10 mg daily.
- Oral corticosteroids (e.g., prednisone) in low doses could be added to her regimen. This represents a last resort when the patient is not adequately controlled on other therapies. Starting doses of 60 mg daily should be titrated down to the lowest dose that controls symptoms and administered on an alternate day basis if possible.
- Other medications that are employed in severe cases in order to reduce the use of systemic corticosteroid therapy include troleandomycin, cyclosporine, methotrexate, gold, intravenous immunoglobulin, dapsone, and hydroxychloroquine. These therapies should be used with caution and only under the supervision of an asthma care specialist.
- She may benefit from an electronic peak flow meter device that would allow her to be followed more closely by her physician. With these devices, data can be transmitted to the patient's clinician so that appropriate interventions can be made.

Outcome Evaluation

5. a. *What clinical and laboratory parameters are necessary to evaluate the therapy for achievement of the desired therapeutic effect and to detect or prevent adverse effects?*

- Peak flow monitoring will provide the most useful data for this patient. Her control can be assessed, impending exacerbations can be detected, and step-down in therapy can be attempted based on well-controlled asthma.
- A peak flow-based action plan should help her to better control her asthma, avoid ED visits and hospitalizations, and feel more in control of her condition. With a written plan, she can make adjustments in her medications based on symptoms or a change in peak flow rates. Typical strategies include rescue doses of short-acting β-agonists and short-term scheduled use during exacerbations, increased (doubling) doses of inhaled steroids for short-term periods, and a short course of oral corticosteroids (prednisone). The frequency of use and implementation of an action plan should be monitored by a physician or pharmacist to determine if changes in the chronic treatment regimen are needed.[1]
- The eosinophilia seen on her peripheral smear suggests uncontrolled exposure to allergens. This should resolve with avoidance and treatment with corticosteroids. Similarly, amelioration of her nasal eosinophilia will indicate better control of asthma and allergic rhinitis.
- The major side effects of concern are related to the inhaled corticosteroid therapy. The primary effects are oral candidiasis, dysphonia, and reflex coughing. She should use a holding chamber to reduce oropharyngeal deposition of drug and rinse her mouth with water after use. The short-term use of the oral corticosteroids should not result in any significant problems.

Patient Counseling

6. *What information should be provided to enhance compliance, ensure successful therapy, and minimize adverse effects?*

General Information

- In addition to general education about asthma, the role of various medications, and proper inhaler technique, the goals of therapy should be reviewed with this patient, and she can identify her own goals and expectations.
- She can be reassured about the safety of all her therapies, including the use of corticosteroids with holding chambers.
- Her medications should be scheduled in the most convenient manner for her life-style. Twice daily regimens are easily achieved with her medication.
- She should understand and be comfortable with her action plan based on a change in symptoms or peak flow rates, and know when to seek help.
- She can pre-treat herself with albuterol before a planned event known to cause her asthma symptoms.
- For patients on long-term inhaled steroids, some clinicians recommend calcium and vitamin D supplementation.
- It is important not to miss any doses. If a dose is missed, it should be taken as soon as remembered; if it is almost time for next dose, skip the missed dose and return to regular schedule. Do not take double doses.
- To keep track of the amount of medication in your inhalers, calculate the number of doses in each canister divided by the number of puffs per day you are using. This will tell you when to request a refill. For your rescue therapy, estimate the number of times you have used it over a certain period of time and this will give you an idea of the amount remaining.

Oral Corticosteroids (Prednisone)

- You are receiving a short course of oral prednisone in order to control the inflammation in your lungs. With prolonged use, this medication can cause serious side effects; however, you will only receive it for a week or so. With this short-term use, you may notice an increase in your appetite, weight gain, and fluid retention. These problems should disappear when you complete the therapy.

Inhaled Corticosteroids (e.g., Triamcinolone)

- To control your asthma, you will receive therapy with an inhaled steroid. This is to allow these medications to be used safely. This medication is part of the long-term control therapy for your asthma. You should use it twice a day every day even if you have no symptoms.
- Your inhalation technique is very important to get the benefit from the medication, so the pharmacist will check it periodically. Your

medication has a spacer device to reduce drug deposition in the back of your throat that can cause sore throat, hoarseness, or cough. You should also rinse your mouth with water after use and spit the water out in the sink.

Serevent (Salmeterol)
- This is a long acting medicine to relax your breathing tubes and allow you to breathe easier. It also should be used on a regular basis twice daily whether or not you have any symptoms of asthma. You can use this at the same time as your Azmacort inhaler.
- In some people, this medication causes nervousness and a hand tremor when first used, but this usually improves over the next week.
- This medication should only be used as prescribed. Do not increase the dose above 2 puffs twice a day, and do not use this medication during an acute asthma attack.

Proventil HFA (Albuterol)
- This medication is your rescue therapy for asthma. It works in just a few minutes to relax your breathing when you have asthma symptoms (coughing, wheezing, and shortness of breath). You should always carry this medication with you in case you need it. It is usually not used on a regular (scheduled) basis, but rather when you have symptoms of asthma.
- When first used, this medication may cause nervousness and a hand tremor. Patients develop a tolerance to this over a week or so and don't usually have problems after that.

References

1. Clinical Practice Guidelines. Expert Panel Report 2: Guidelines for the Diagnosis and Management of Asthma. NIH pub. no. 97-4051. April 1997. Also available on the Internet at http://www.nhlbi.nih.gov/nhlbi/lung/asthma/prof/asthgdln.htm.
2. Haahtela T, Jarvinen M, Kava T, et al. Effects of reducing or discontinuing inhaled budesonide in patients with mild asthma. N Engl J Med 1994;331: 700–705.
3. Gross NJ. Leukotriene modifiers: What place in asthma management? J Resp Dis 1998;19:245–261.
4. Greening AP, Ind P, Northfield M, et al. Added salmeterol versus higher-dose corticosteroid in asthma patients with symptoms on existing inhaled corticosteroid. Lancet 1994;344:219–224.

20 CHRONIC OBSTRUCTIVE LUNG DISEASE

▶ **Waiting to Exhale** (Level II)

Daren L. Knoell, PharmD

A 64-year-old man with a history of cirrhosis, hypertension, COLD, and asthma presents to the ED with complaints of increasing shortness of breath, cough, and sputum production. He is treated with oxygen, bronchodilators, corticosteroids, and empiric antibiotic therapy and then admitted to the hospital where similar treatment is continued. Students are asked to design an optimal pharmacotherapeutic regimen for the patient upon discharge from the hospital. The patient has several drug-related problems that need to be addressed for proper drug therapy management. The case provides the opportunity for students to learn and practice the proper technique for using metered-dose inhalers.

▶ **Questions**

Problem Identification

1. a. *Create a list of this patient's drug-related problems prior to treatment in the ED.*

   - Acute exacerbation of COLD/asthma requiring intensive pharmacologic therapy and oxygen.
   - Possible respiratory tract infection concomitant with COLD exacerbation; empiric antimicrobial therapy is warranted until infection can be ruled out.
   - Inadequate doses of Atrovent (ipratropium bromide) and albuterol to control the patient's COLD chronically.
   - Wrong drug for treatment of hypertension (nadolol); in general, all β-blockers (even those with $β_1$-receptor selectivity) should be avoided if possible in patients with asthma.
   - Atrovent, an anticholinergic agent, can cause blurred vision if inadvertently sprayed into the eyes; this may be occurring due to his poor inhalation technique.
   - Hypokalemia (possibly from furosemide or albuterol use), requiring potassium replacement therapy.
   - Alcoholic cirrhosis with ascites, inadequately treated with a small daily dose of furosemide.

   b. *What signs, symptoms, and laboratory data provide evidence that this patient is experiencing a COLD exacerbation? Based on the evidence, is his presentation more consistent with emphysema or chronic bronchitis?*

   Signs
   - Increased heart rate and respiratory rate
   - Inspiratory and expiratory wheezes
   - Decreased breath sounds
   - Thin, elderly male

   Symptoms
   - Three day history of SOB, cough, increased sputum production in a cigarette smoker with known COLD

   Laboratory Data
   - Abnormal ABG on admission (respiratory acidosis)
   - Abnormal CXR (flattened diaphragm)
   - Abnormal PFTs with decreased DL_{CO}

   The patient's presentation is more consistent with emphysema (e.g., thin patient with tachypnea, diminished breath sounds, flattened diaphragm on CXR). However, he is also having an acute asthma exacerbation, which can mimic chronic bronchitis. The patient lacks some findings of chronic bronchitis (e.g., right-sided heart failure, increased hematocrit, and digital clubbing). Although clubbing can also occur in end-stage emphysema when the heart becomes involved, it occurs more commonly and usually earlier in chronic bronchitis due to right-sided heart failure.

c. *What additional information do you need to satisfactorily assess the adequacy of COLD treatment in this patient before he presented to the ED?*

- Medication history, with emphasis on COLD and asthma medications
- History of corticosteroid use if any (systemic and inhaled)
- History of ED visits and hospitalizations over the past 2 years
- Observation and assessment of the patient's MDI technique
- History of occupational/environmental exposure to inhaled irritants (e.g., insulation)
- Knowledge of living arrangements, physical activity, and limitations
- Recent exposure to others with colds, influenza, or pneumonia
- Nutritional status

Desired Outcome

2. *What are the desired goals for the treatment of this patient's COLD?*

- Acute improvement of COLD and stabilization for long-term management
- Treatment and prevention of acute exacerbations
- Reduction of the rate of progression of the disease
- Improvement of physical and psychological well-being so that daily activities can be resumed or maintained
- Reduction in hospitalization, morbidity, and mortality
- Improvement/stabilization of ABG and PFT
- Smoking cessation to prevent further cardiopulmonary damage

Therapeutic Alternatives

3. a. *What non-drug therapies would be useful to improve this patient's COLD symptoms?*

- Enrollment in a smoking cessation program that may include psychological counseling as well as pharmacologic support with nicotine patches, gum, or other drug therapy
- Counseling to cease alcohol consumption
- Enrollment in a pulmonary rehabilitation program if possible; components would include:
    ✓ Assessment of nutrition and caloric intake
    ✓ An exercise program to improve mechanics of breathing
    ✓ Psychological counseling regarding the disease and smoking
    ✓ Potential for peak flow monitoring since the patient has an asthmatic component to his obstructive disease

b. *What feasible pharmacotherapeutic alternatives are available for the treatment of COLD in this patient, particularly those that can be continued as an outpatient?*

- The patient needs optimization of his current regimen before changing to alternative therapy. However, there are many options from which to choose if additional therapy is needed.[1]
- Continue Atrovent, but increase the dose frequency to QID.
- Continue albuterol (or another β_1-selective agonist), but increase the dose frequency to QID.[2]
- Replace use of the two single drugs above with Combivent (ipratropium/albuterol) if necessary to improve compliance.
- Consider use of the long-acting β-agonist Serevent (salmeterol).
- Consider use of inhaled corticosteroids, particularly since the patient has an asthmatic component to his obstructive lung disease.
- In the short-term, design a regimen to taper the patient off of systemic corticosteroids over the next 7 to 14 days.
- Reevaluate the use of theophylline in this patient based on the risk–benefit ratio. He has alcoholic cirrhosis, is a smoker, and is prone to antibiotic use. For these reasons, close monitoring of theophylline levels is necessary.
- He should receive an annual influenza vaccine and the pneumococcal vaccine (if he hasn't received one in the last 5 years) if not contraindicated.

c. *Should home oxygen therapy be considered for the patient at this time?*

- No; the patient should have his medication regimen optimized in the outpatient setting. A decision to use home oxygen therapy would be indicated after medication optimization if the patient had:
    ✓ A resting Pao_2 <55 mm Hg
    ✓ Evidence of right-sided heart failure, polycythemia, or impaired neuropsychiatric function with a Pao_2 <60 mm Hg

d. *Is this patient a candidate for α_1-antitrypsin (Prolastin) therapy?*

- No; Prolastin is generally reserved for patients who suffer from the genetic form of emphysema called α_1-antitrypsin deficiency. These patients develop emphysema in the third to fourth decade of life, thus requiring early intervention and therapy with this expensive human serum-derived product.[3]
- Since the patient has a family history of COLD, it may be advisable to check his serum α_1-antitrypsin level if this has not already been done (reference range, 200 to 400 mg/dL).
- Despite a normal level, cigarette smoke has been shown to oxidize and inactivate this essential antiprotease and therefore permit destruction of alveolar tissue by endogenous proteases.

Optimal Plan

4. *Develop a complete outpatient regimen for the treatment of COLD in this patient, including dose, route, frequency, and duration for therapy.*

- Do not restart nadolol for treatment of HTN. Diuretics are another first-line therapy for HTN, but the patient is already receiving furosemide for his ascites (which may require an increased dose). If additional therapy is needed, consider a calcium channel blocker, a class that does not adversely affect pulmonary function.
- Increase Atrovent to 2 puffs QID. The patient has blurred vision from Atrovent because he uses the "open-mouth technique" and overall

has poor inhaler technique. He should be instructed to use all inhalers with a holding chamber. Proper inhalation technique should be reviewed with him, and he should then be asked to demonstrate it.
- Increase albuterol to 2 puffs QID, which can be alternated with Atrovent or used concomitantly.
- To consolidate the above regimen, the patient could use Combivent inhaler (combined ipratropium and albuterol) at 2 puffs QID to decrease the overall number of inhalations and improve compliance. If applicable, confirm that his insurance plan will cover the cost of this medication.
- The patient demonstrated a reversible component to his current airway obstruction (>12% improvement with FEV_1 after using a bronchodilator) suggesting that his current problems are related to an asthma exacerbation. Therefore, the use of an inhaled corticosteroid should be recommended. Although the use of inhaled corticosteroids in COLD is controversial, his airway symptoms will likely improve by more effectively treating his asthma (refer to the textbook for a discussion of the use of inhaled corticosteroids in COLD). One reasonable choice is fluticasone propionate (Flovent) 110 μg 2 puffs BID (use with a holding chamber and rinse mouth with water after each use). Other products that would be acceptable alternatives include Aerobid (flunisolide), Azmacort (triamcinolone acetonide), budesonide (Pulmicort), and Vanceril or Beclovent (beclomethasone).
- Recommend discontinuing theophylline at this time due to the risk of side effects in this particular patient and questionable effectiveness.
- Consider the use of Serevent (salmeterol) 2 puffs BID at a later time if the patient still has persistent airway symptoms after the above recommendations have been implemented (particularly if the patient has night time symptoms).
- Change IV Solu-Medrol to oral prednisone as soon as the patient is stabilized on the floor (usually within the first 1 to 2 days). At that time, implement a corticosteroid taper over the next two weeks and schedule an outpatient follow-up visit. One sample tapering regimen is as follows:
  Prednisone 60 mg po Q AM × 3 days
  Prednisone 40 mg po Q AM × 3 days
  Prednisone 20 mg po Q AM × 3 days
  Prednisone 10 mg po Q AM × 3 days
  Prednisone 5 mg po Q AM × 3 days, then stop
- The patient requires potassium repletion while in the hospital and may need chronic replacement therapy. Addition of spironolactone to his diuretic regimen would improve his ascites and help conserve potassium.
- Avoid using any oral β-agonists due to the increased risk of cardiac side effects, which include palpitations and dysrhythmias.

Outcome Evaluation

5. *What clinical and laboratory parameters are necessary to evaluate the therapy for achievement of the desired therapeutic outcome and to detect or prevent adverse effects?*

Disease-state Monitoring
- Improve tissue oxygenation to prevent acid–base disturbances and long-term end-organ damage (cor pulmonale). Monitor ABG, resting room air Pao_2, and pulse oximetry during scheduled office visits. The values should be maintained within normal limits. The room air Pao_2 should be used as a gauge for when to initiate home oxygen therapy if necessary.
- Prospectively monitor medical resource utilization with the goal to reduce the rate of hospitalizations and ED visits.
- Reduction in use of PRN bronchodilators for acute symptoms. Monitor patient refills on Atrovent and albuterol during routine office visits to ensure that the patient is using them within prescribed guidelines.
- Prevent rapid decline in pulmonary function over time. Measure DLco and PFTs annually and compare the values to previous years.
- Monitor for other long-term morbidities such as right-sided heart failure (e.g., monitor heart function via ECG) and increased hematocrit at least annually during scheduled office visits.
- Monitor frequency of upper respiratory tract infections over time. Have the patient notify you or his physician in the event of increased sputum quantity, change in sputum color, cough, fever, or other symptoms consistent with pneumonia.
- Monitor tobacco and alcohol consumption, promote cessation of these products, and continue long-term follow-up with cessation plans. Plasma cotinine concentrations can be monitored during routine office visits if compliance with smoking cessation is a concern.
- Monitor peak flows on a daily basis if this patient has persistent asthma (the student should refer to asthma case studies for other information needed to determine severity of asthma).
- Monitor BP during routine office visits.
- Monitor LFTs every 6 months to track the progression of hepatic cirrhosis.

Medication Monitoring
- Prevent thrush (inhaled corticosteroids) by educating the patient how to routinely inspect the oral mucosa for signs of candida infection (e.g., white plaque formation, hoarse voice).
- Measure routine serum potassium levels during office visits to prevent potassium wasting, which can be associated with chronic β-agonist use (particularly in the elderly), and routinely monitor for increased heart rate or tremor which can be associated with β-agonist overuse.
- Avoid HPA axis suppression with systemic corticosteroids and/or excessive doses of inhaled corticosteroids. Routinely monitor for physical signs of adrenal suppression such as electrolyte imbalance, excessive fluid retention, moon facies, and centripetal obesity.

Patient Counseling

6. *What information should be provided to the patient to enhance compliance, ensure successful therapy, and minimize adverse effects?*

- Refer to USP-DI volume II for drug-specific information on the use of ipratropium, albuterol, and fluticasone propionate.
- A complete list of the essential steps that should be used to instruct the patient on metered dose inhaler use follows.[4]

How to Use an MDI Properly (With or Without a Spacer)
- Pre-Dose Stage
  ✓ Remove the cap from the MDI.
  ✓ Shake canister well for 3 to 4 seconds.

✓ Hold MDI upright and exhale normally (to functional residual capacity).
✓ Close lips around mouthpiece of MDI ("closed mouth technique").
✓ Open mouth technique is not recommended for elderly or with spacer devices and holding chambers.
- Dosing Stage
  ✓ Begin to inhale slowly. After one second, discharge 1 puff from the MDI.
  ✓ Continue to inhale deeply and slowly for 5 to 10 seconds.
  ✓ Hold breath for 5 to 10 seconds.
  ✓ Exhale slowly and through the nose if possible.
- Follow-up
  ✓ Wait 1 to 2 minutes before inhaling the next puff (if prescribed). Then repeat the above steps.
  ✓ If the inhaled drug is a corticosteroid, rinse your mouth with tap water when finished and spit the water out; do not swallow it.
- There are numerous holding chambers available. In general, the patient should be instructed to use them as described above, but emphasis on timing of actuation and inhalation is not necessary. Furthermore, many of these devices have a whistle device that sounds if the patient breathes in too fast. This can be useful to further encourage proper technique. Always consult the package insert for the device, since usage directions vary from product to product.
- Educate patients on how to routinely clean their inhaler devices and properly determine the amount of drug in the canister (if necessary).

References

1. Ferguson GT, Cherniack RM. Management of chronic obstructive pulmonary disease. N Engl J Med 1993;328:1017–1022.
2. Nelson HS. Beta-adrenergic bronchodilators. N Engl J Med 1995;333:499–506.
3. MacDonald JL, Johnson CE. Pathophysiology and treatment of alpha 1-antitrypsin deficiency. Am J Health-Syst Pharm 1995;52:481–489.
4. Toogood JH. Helping your patients make better use of MDIs and spacers. J Resp Dis 1994;15:151–166.

Suggested Internet site: Agency for Health Care Policy and Research, http://www.ahcpr.gov/clinic/

21 RESPIRATORY DISTRESS SYNDROME

▶ The Breath of Life (Level II)

Jennifer L. Schoelles, PharmD
Robert J. Kuhn, PharmD

An infant of 34 weeks gestation exhibits signs and symptoms of respiratory distress syndrome and is intubated because of persistent respiratory distress. In addition to ventilatory support, the administration of surfactant therapy is indicated. Students are asked to select an appropriate agent and design a treatment regimen based upon the product chosen. Supportive therapy with sedatives or muscle relaxants is also required to allow optimal ventilator manipulation. The case provides the opportunity for students to describe how they would educate the neonate's caregivers on the potential benefits and adverse effects of surfactant therapy.

▶ Questions

Problem Identification

1. a. *What risk factors does this patient have for developing respiratory distress syndrome (RDS)?*

   - *Prematurity.* Infants born at less than 36 weeks gestational age are at higher risk for RDS. The incidence of RDS increases as the gestational age of the infant decreases. Pulmonary surfactants, found in the lungs of term infants, contain phospholipids that stabilize the air-filled alveolus. At 35 weeks' gestation, the type II alveolar cells, which secrete surfactant, are sufficiently developed and functional. Before 35 weeks' gestation, impaired surfactant production in addition to immaturity of the alveolar lining cells, and the impaired release of surface-active phospholipids are responsible for the increased risk of RDS (refer to the section on Physiology and Pathophysiology in textbook Chapter 26 for more detailed information).
   - Other possible risk factors that the patient does NOT have include:
     ✓ Perinatal asphyxia or hypoxia
     ✓ Cold stress
     ✓ Failure of closure of the ductus arteriosus determined by persistent murmur and/or echocardiogram
     ✓ Diabetes mellitus in the mother
     ✓ Prolonged acidosis

   b. *What signs, symptoms, and other data indicate that this patient needs to be treated for RDS?*

   - The patient exhibits the following signs and symptoms in the first few hours after birth: expiratory grunting, flaring, retractions, and increasing oxygen requirement (need for intubation and increased oxygen).
   - Other signs and symptoms that he *may* have exhibited are: use of accessory neck muscles, paradoxical seesaw retractions, tachycardia, pallor, and cyanosis.
   - Chest x-ray: Diffuse reticulogranular chest x-ray (ground glass pattern) consistent with surfactant deficiency.

- Refer to the textbook section on Clinical Presentation in Chapter 26 for more details.

Desired Outcome

2. What are the goals of treatment in neonates who have RDS?

- The primary goal is to decrease the severity of RDS as evidenced by increased oxygen saturations without supplemental oxygen or ventilatory support.
- Long-term goals are to prevent the development of complications from ventilator and oxygen therapy, which include bronchopulmonary dysplasia, retinopathy of prematurity, and developmental delays.

Therapeutic Alternatives

3. What pharmacologic and non-pharmacologic treatments are available for RDS?

- *Surfactants* are accepted as the most physiologic and cost-effective approach to treatment of RDS. Both natural and synthetic surfactants decrease the severity and duration of RDS, and one product of each type is available in the United States. Other preparations are available in other countries. Although numerous studies have compared various surfactant preparations, a statistically significant difference in outcomes for one product over another has never been consistently shown.[1-3] Average wholesale prices for the two products available in the United States are comparable on a vial-per-vial basis. There are no differences between the two products in rapidity of response.
  - ✓ *Beractant (Survanta)* is a bovine surfactant product that is supplied in a ready-to-administer suspension that must be refrigerated. Beractant should be allowed to warm to room temperature by standing at room temperature for at least 20 minutes or warmed in the hand for at least 8 minutes before administration. Unopened, unused, warmed vials may be returned to the refrigerator within 8 hours of warming and stored for future use. Beractant is a single use vial; any unused drug must be discarded.[4]
  - ✓ *Colfosceril palmitate (Exosurf)* is a synthetic, lyophilized powder formulation that must be reconstituted before administration. Each vial must be reconstituted with the accompanying 10 mL of diluent (preservative-free sterile water for injection). The resulting suspension should be used immediately. Colfosceril palmitate contains no antibacterial preservatives, and any unused drug must be discarded.[4]
- *Mechanical ventilation* is necessary for maintaining adequate oxygenation and ventilation and for the delivery of exogenous surfactant. Arterial blood gas goals are: Pao_2 of 50 to 70 mm Hg and pH of 7.28 to 7.40.
- *Management of acidosis* is critical, because acidosis is associated with increased pulmonary vascular resistance, impaired synthesis of surfactant, reduced cardiac output, and depressed ventilation, all of which increase the severity of RDS. To minimize the risk of acidosis, minimize oxygen consumption and prevent hypoxemia, hypotension, and excessive blood loss. Ventilator management of acidosis may lead to pulmonary and ocular toxicities. Pharmacologic agents that may be needed to correct acidosis include:
  - ✓ *THAM/Tromethamine* (mL of 0.3 M solution to administer = body weight in kg × base deficit in mEq/L)
  - ✓ *Sodium bicarbonate* (mEq to administer = 0.3 × body weight in kg × base deficit in mEq/L)
- *Diuresis* is often necessary to reduce the severity of the disease because pulmonary edema is common in neonates with RDS.
  - ✓ *Furosemide* has been used by some clinicians to decrease the fluid load. Doses from 1 to 2 mg/kg have been used, although the increased risk of patent ductus arteriosus (PDA) and electrolyte imbalances must be weighed against the benefit of using the drug.
  - ✓ Ventilator setting using PEEP (positive end expiratory pressure) may be used to redistribute fluid from air spaces to interstitial tissue and improve gas exchange.
- For additional information on treatment alternatives, refer to the sections on Treatment, Surfactant Therapy, and Tables 26–4 and 26–5 in textbook Chapter 26.

Optimal Plan

4. a. What pharmacotherapeutic drug regimen (including dose and administration information) would you recommend for treating RDS in this patient?

- *Surfactant.* Either of the two commercially available surfactant preparations would be appropriate to use. The choice is usually guided by which product is available on the hospital formulary or by physician preference if both products are available in the institution. Formulary selection often depends on which product is least expensive based on contract pricing. In addition to the dosing information given next, also refer to Table 26–5 and Administration Technique under the Surfactant Section of textbook Chapter 26.
  - ✓ *Colfosceril palmitate.* A dose of 5 mL/kg should be administered immediately. If respiratory distress continues, the dose may be repeated 12 hours later up to 2 times 12 hours apart. Doses should be administered intratracheally. The neonate should be suctioned prior to administration. The dose should be administered in two 2.5-mL/kg aliquots, instilling each slowly over 1 to 2 minutes in small bursts with each inspiration. The infant's head and torso should be rotated 45 degrees to the right for 30 seconds after the first aliquot and to the left after the second.[4]
  - ✓ *Beractant.* A dose of 4 mL/kg should be administered immediately. If respiratory distress continues, the dose may be repeated 6 hours later up to 4 times in the first 48 hours of life. Doses should be administered intratracheally. The neonate should be suctioned prior to administration. The dose should be administered in four 1-mL/kg aliquots, instilling each slowly over 2 to 3 seconds. Each quarter-dose is administered with the infant in a different position.[4]
  - ✓ In clinical practice, physician preference and respiratory therapy practice often determine the administration method employed. Some institutions use the Exosurf FDA-approved administration method regardless of product selection, and other institutions use the Survanta FDA-approved administration method regardless of product selection.

- Mechanical ventilation is necessary in an infant with surfactant deficiency. This infant had the following ventilator settings upon admission to the NICU: Rate = 60, MAP = 8, PAP = 16, PEEP = 4, IT = 0.3, FIO_2 = 100%. Ventilator settings are infant-dependent and should be adjusted according to individual response and the severity of the infant's respiratory distress syndrome.
- Diuresis and management of acidosis are not necessary in this infant. These therapies should be included in the treatment plan for other infants with RDS when necessary. See question 3 for dosing guidelines for furosemide, THAM, and sodium bicarbonate.

b. *What adjunctive care or supportive pharmacotherapy is needed in the management of RDS in this patient?*

- Sedatives or muscle relaxants are sometimes used to allow optimal ventilator manipulation without neonatal resistance. The lowest possible airway pressures are desired to prevent ventilator complications such as pneumothorax. Product selection is institution- and physician-dependent. Potential toxicities must be weighed against clinical benefits. Examples of medications that may be used as sedatives, muscle relaxants, or neuromuscular blockers in the neonate are given here[4] (also refer to the section on Supportive Pharmacotherapy in textbook Chapter 26):
  - ✓ Lorazepam 0.1–0.4 mg/kg IV every 2 to 6 hours PRN
  - ✓ Morphine 0.1–0.2 mg/kg IV every 3 to 6 hours PRN
  - ✓ Phenobarbital 20 mg/kg IV up to 4 doses, then 5 to 10 mg/kg/day with a goal of maintaining a plasma concentration above 60 µg/mL
  - ✓ Chloral hydrate 25 to 50 µg/kg po every 4 to 6 hours PRN
  - ✓ Pancuronium 0.01 to 0.03 mg/kg IV PRN

Outcome Evaluation

5. *What monitoring parameters should be used to evaluate therapy in this infant?*

Acutely
- Monitor acute changes in supplemental oxygen use. Evaluate oxygen saturation and pulse oximetry every 1 to 3 hours. If these parameters do not improve within 6 hours, consider administering a second dose of surfactant.
- Monitor ventilator setting every 3 to 6 hours until the patient is stable. If ventilator pressure can be slowly weaned and neonate maintains adequate oxygen saturations (>95%), neonate is improving and subsequent surfactant doses may not be necessary.

During Hospitalization
- The incidence of PDA should be assessed daily by the attending physician by evaluating for evidence of a heart murmur, and following up with an echocardiogram if necessary.
- Intraventricular hemorrhage is assessed by cranial ultrasound on a regular basis (dependent on institution protocols, which vary for gestational age).
- Pulmonary hemorrhage or pneumothorax is assessed by chest x-ray. The frequency of these x-rays may vary from more than once a day to once every 2 to 3 days depending on the clinical status of the neonate.

Long Term
- Long term need for supplemental oxygen after discharge suggests that the neonate suffered from a severe case of RDS.

Patient Counseling

6. *What information about surfactants should be provided to the infant's parents?*

- Respiratory distress syndrome or RDS can be a very serious problem in neonates like Tanner. In the past, many babies had breathing problems for a long time after developing RDS. A new medicine called surfactant is now available to treat the breathing problem that Tanner has. Now that we have this medication to use, babies like Tanner are getting better much faster and have less difficulty breathing. This medication may help Tanner breathe without the ventilator so that the risk of artificial ventilation will be minimized.
- There are some risks to using surfactant in Tanner. His heart rate may drop, and his blood pressure may increase or decrease while we are giving him the surfactant, but they should quickly return to normal. Since the medication has to be given through the tube that he is breathing through, he may have some difficulty breathing while we are giving the medication, but this will only last for a few seconds. Many studies show that the benefits of using the medication far outweigh the risks of long-term use of artificial ventilation and additional oxygen. Many neonates like Tanner have received this medication before.

▶ Follow-up Question

1. *What measures could have been used prenatally with the patient's mother to prevent or decrease the severity of RDS?*

- Prevention or minimizing maternal hypotension and hemorrhage during labor and delivery, and providing adequate warmth and oxygenation to the neonate at delivery may limit the severity of RDS.
- Delaying delivery to allow for lung maturation can be considered in some cases. See Table 26–2 in textbook Chapter 26 for medications used for this indication.
- Corticosteroids may be given at least 24 hours prenatally to accelerate lung maturation and prevent RDS in the infant. Betamethasone 12 mg IV/IM QD for 2 doses or dexamethasone 5 mg IV/IM Q 12 H for 4 doses may be used.

References

1. Halliday HL. Natural vs synthetic surfactants in neonatal respiratory distress syndrome. Drugs 1996;51:226–237.
2. Ishisaka DY. Exogenous surfactant use in neonates. Ann Pharmacother 1996;30:389–398.
3. Soll RF. Surfactant therapy in the USA: Trials and current routines. Biol Neonate 1997;71(suppl 1):1–7.
4. Taketomo CK, Hodding JH, Kraus DM. Pediatric dosing handbook, 4th ed. Hudson, OH, Lexi-Comp, 1997.

22 CYSTIC FIBROSIS

▶ Blood, Sweat, Lungs, and Gut   (Level I)

Robert J. Kuhn, PharmD

A 9-year-old boy with a long history of cystic fibrosis (CF) is brought to clinic by his mother with worsening symptoms of shortness of breath, pulmonary congestion, and severe fatigue, indicating an acute pulmonary exacerbation of CF. An increased WBC count with left shift and sputum cultures positive for *Pseudomonas aeruginosa, Staphylococcus aureus,* and *Aspergillus* document the presence of an infectious process. When selecting appropriate antibiotic therapy, students should recommend a parenteral drug combination effective against *P. aeruginosa; S. aureus* may be treated satisfactorily with oral anti-staphylococcal agents. A dosage increase in the patient's aerosolized tobramycin may also be employed, but some centers would withhold aerosolized therapy during parenteral treatment. Students are also asked to interpret a set of serum aminoglycoside levels and make an appropriate dosage adjustment. The patient is receiving a number of chronic medications for which educational reinforcement may be beneficial.

▶ Questions

Problem Identification

1. a. Identify this patient's drug-related problems.
- Acute pulmonary exacerbation of CF requiring therapy
- Poor nutritional intake requiring supplementation
- Hyperglycemia

b. What information indicates the disease severity and the need to treat his CF pharmacologically?

- Worsening respiratory symptoms of increased respiratory rate, increased sputum production and color change with decreasing oxygen saturation indicate an acute pulmonary exacerbation of CF.
- The increased WBC count with a left shift and positive sputum cultures demonstrates infection.
- Weight loss and fatigue indicate poor nutritional intake and acute illness requiring supplementation.
- Hyperglycemia may be drug induced or a component of his disease; nearly 15% of CF patients develop this abnormality.

c. Could any of his problems be caused by drug therapy?

Hyperglycemia may be secondary to corticosteroid administration. It is advisable to re-evaluate his fasting blood glucose once he finishes the course of oral prednisone.

Desired Outcome

2. What are the goals of pharmacotherapy in this case?

- Treatment of acute pulmonary exacerbation to restore baseline pulmonary function tests, normalize respiratory rate, and decrease sputum production with antimicrobial therapy.
- Increase nutritional intake or provide supplements to help generate weight gain.

Therapeutic Alternatives

3. a. What non-drug therapies might be useful for this patient?

- *Nutritional assessment and dietary consultation.* A nutritional consultation can determine the caloric goal necessary to maintain growth. It is important that growth and nutritional status be followed closely since pulmonary function seems to be preserved in patients with good nutritional parameters.
- *Percussion and postural drainage.* Most patients require some respiratory therapy treatment to loosen the thick mucus in the CF-affected airways. Aerosol therapy with 0.9% NaCl or an inhaled bronchodilator may be used first, followed by segmental percussion and positional drainage of the lungs. The patient should be given frequent encouragement to expectorate mucus during this 20- to 30-minute procedure. This is often performed two to four times a day to help loosen mucus secretions.

b. What therapeutic alternatives are available for treatment of this patient's acute pulmonary exacerbation?

- *Parenteral antibiotics* for *P. aeruginosa*. Combination IV therapy is mandatory for this organism and may include combinations such as the following:
  ✓ Antipseudomonal penicillin (e.g., ticarcillin, piperacillin) + an aminoglycoside (e.g., tobramycin, gentamicin, or amikacin)
  ✓ Ticarcillin/clavulanic acid (Timentin) + an aminoglycoside
  ✓ Piperacillin/tazobactam (Zosyn) + an aminoglycoside
  ✓ Ceftazidime + an aminoglycoside
  ✓ Imipenem or meropenem + an aminoglycoside
  ✓ Ciprofloxacin alone or + an aminoglycoside
  ✓ Aztreonam + an aminoglycoside

The products containing β-lactamase inhibitors are not used initially because beta-lactamase production is not usually the mechanism of resistance in CF patients. Ticarcillin and piperacillin must be administered every 4 to 6 hours, which may make it more difficult to complete therapy than with agents given less frequently. Ceftazidime is often used in combination with an aminoglycoside and can be dosed every 8 hours in conjunction with the aminoglycoside. Most centers use tobramycin as the aminoglycoside of choice because of its superior effectiveness over gentamicin. Amikacin is usually not more sensitive to *Pseudomonas* than tobramycin and is more expensive. This patient has failed a course of ciprofloxacin prior to hospitalization. There are some data supporting the safety of fluroquinolones in pediatric patients, and they are an option in a 9-year-old patient. Imipenem may precipitate in reservoir-type central venous catheters that are permanently implanted; meropenem is a good alternative.

- *Oral antibiotics for S. aureus.* Patients who are culture-positive for *S. aureus* can be treated with oral antistaphylococcal penicillins (e.g., dicloxacillin, cloxacillin) or with oral first generation cephalosporins. Aggressive dosing with oral agents is usually quite sufficient to eradicate the organism.
- *Aerosolized antibiotics:*
  ✓ A new formulation of aerosolized tobramycin called TOBI (300 mg/5 mL) is now available for CF patients. Doses of 300 mg BID have been used for 28 days (alternating months) as prophylaxis to prevent acute pulmonary exacerbations in CF patients.[1] Some clinicians use other doses ranging from 80 to 600 mg based on clinical experience. No dosage form that will be given by nebulizer should contain preservatives.
  ✓ Colistin 75 mg BID has also been given by inhalation in some patients. There are severe problems with foaming of this solution, and it is very expensive. In Europe, many centers use this drug on a chronic basis. One million units of colistin is equivalent to 75 mg of drug distributed in the United States. A nebulized dosage formulation should be available in the United States within 2 to 3 years.
- *Anti-inflammatory therapy.* During acute exacerbations, parenteral administration of glucocorticoids may also be given to reduce the inflammatory reaction in the airways.
  ✓ *Methylprednisolone 1 to 2 mg/kg/day* has been used and continued for several days. The use of long-term steroids should be discouraged, and patients should be tapered if therapy longer than 10 days is required. Since this patient is steroid dependent, his dose should be increased over his maintenance dose and tapered back down after a few weeks of therapy. Patients with severe disease may become steroid dependent, and long-term problems with linear growth and osteopenia have been reported. Supplemental vitamin D and calcium should be added to his maintenance medications.
  ✓ *Oral prednisone* can also be used to suppress the inflammatory airway reaction in patients with allergic bronchopulmonary aspergillosis. No antifungal therapy is indicated unless there is no clinical improvement on prednisone therapy or symptoms of a systemic fungal infection are apparent.
  ✓ *Ibuprofen* in high doses (25 to 30 mg/kg BID) have been shown to decrease the decline in pulmonary function. Low-dose or PRN doses of ibuprofen[2] may help recruit neutrophil migration to the lung and could exacerbate the inflammatory response. This should be carefully monitored in CF patients, and serum concentrations of the drug should be collected after starting therapy. *Note:* Only a few reference labs do these levels, so the availability of an ibuprofen assay may determine the utility of this therapy.
- *rhDNase therapy (dornase alfa, Pulmozyme)* has been used for long-term therapy in CF patients who demonstrate improvement with decreased hospitalizations or improvement in pulmonary function or other global assessment of improvement. This therapy is usually maintained during an acute exacerbation and a decision to stop therapy should be made with long-term improvement.
- *Pancreatic enzyme replacement* should be evaluated based on a history of steatorrhea or abdominal complaints from the patient.
- *Vitamin supplementation* must be assessed to ensure adequate provision of essential nutrients. Increased supplementation with vitamin K should be used in patients with a recent history of hemoptysis or changes in PT or aPTT levels.

Optimal Plan

4. a. *What drugs, dosage form, dose, schedule and duration of therapy are best for this patient?*

- Combination antipseudomonal therapy with parenteral ceftazidime 150 mg/kg/day divided Q 8 H plus tobramycin 3 mg/kg/dose Q 8 H is a reasonable choice. Appropriate doses of the other combinations described above could also be used, depending upon the sensitivity patterns of the organism.
- For treatment of *S. aureus*, oral cephradine or cephalexin 50 mg/kg/day is usually prescribed because of cost considerations.
- The aerosolized tobramycin may be continued but may need to be increased to 300 mg BID. This recommendation is supported by recent data on the efficacy of TOBI, the new formulation of aerosolized tobramycin. There is controversy over whether aerosolized tobramycin should be continued with parenteral drug. Practices vary among centers, but most would stop aerosolized therapy during parenteral treatment. Refer to Pulmonary System, Antibiotic Selection, in the Treatment section of textbook Chapter 28 for more detailed information.

b. *Based on this new information, evaluate his drug therapy and suggest modification if necessary.*

- Target levels are a peak concentration of 8 to 12 μg/mL and a trough concentration of <2 μg/mL. It is important to note that the peak concentration was drawn late and that the extrapolated peak is approximately 7.8 to 8 μg/mL. The new dose should be approximately 100 mg IV Q 8 H after calculations. To date, there are no studies in pediatric CF patients to support once-daily aminoglycoside therapy. In adults, some patients have been treated with once-daily aminoglycoside therapy with insufficient results at this time to warrant routine use.
- If the patient cannot tolerate oral corticosteroids, then parenteral drug should be administered and doses of 1 to 2 mg/kg/day should be given (e.g., methylprednisolone 15 mg IV Q 6 H). His other medications should be continued for pancreatic insufficiency and vitamin and iron supplementation.

Outcome Evaluation

5. *What clinical and laboratory parameters are necessary to evaluate the therapy?*

- *Pulmonary exacerbation.* Daily temperature charting, respiratory rate, lung exam, energy level, amount of sputum production, and change in sputum color. Biweekly pulmonary function testing to monitor for increases to baseline pre-illness level. Weekly CBC if the patient is not responding to therapy.
- *Nutrition.* Weight gain and increase in appetite, daily assessment of weight.
- *GI tolerance or pancreatic insufficiency.* Continue pancreatic enzymes and monitor for steatorrhea and other GI complaints.
- *Monitoring of toxicity.* Repeat serum tobramycin concentrations are

not indicated unless therapy continues for more than 2 weeks or the patient develops changes in renal function.

Patient Counseling

6. *What information should you provide the patient regarding the administration of aerosolized drug therapy? The patient will be going home on aerosolized tobramycin, dornase alfa, albuterol, and cromolyn sodium.*

- *Dornase alfa (Pulmozyme)* should be stored in the refrigerator and administered with a separate nebulizer and not mixed with any other medication or saline. rhDNase is a protein that will denature when mixed with other aerosols; therefore, its nebulizer should be labeled and not be used for any other treatment with other medications that Eric will get by nebulizer.
- *Cromolyn sodium* should be administered with at least one additional milliliter of saline.
- *Albuterol* should have a volume of at least 3 milliliters when mixed. Note: some centers allow for the mixing of albuterol and cromolyn to help in decreasing the time for nebulization, but few data are available to support this practice.
- The nebulizer tubing needs to be cleaned after each use and changed frequently (every few days), and it is important to keep the compressor clean.

References

1. Saiman L, Campbell P, Burns J, et al. TOBI Consensus Conference. North American Cystic Fibrosis Conference, Nashville, October 1997.
2. Konstan MW, Byard PJ, Hoppel CL, et al. Effect of high-dose ibuprofen in patients with cystic fibrosis. N Engl J Med 1995;332:848–854.

SECTION 3

Gastrointestinal Disorders

Joseph T. DiPiro, PharmD, FCCP, Section Editor

23 GASTROESOPHAGEAL REFLUX DISEASE

▶ More Than Garden-variety Heartburn
(Level I)

Meredith L. Rose, PharmD

A 70-year-old woman with a long history of gastroesophageal reflux disease (GERD) complains of increasing episodes of postprandial heartburn, difficulty swallowing food, and frequent nocturnal awakenings due to reflux symptoms. She requires daily antacid use in addition to her bedtime dose of famotidine 20 mg. Further diagnostic evaluation is required to assess the severity of mucosal damage. Reasonable treatment options include higher-dose acid suppressive therapy using either a proton pump inhibitor (omeprazole, lansoprazole) or an H_2-receptor antagonist (cimetidine, ranitidine, famotidine, nizatidine). Prokinetic agents (bethanechol, metoclopramide, cisapride) would not provide adequate therapy because of the severity of this patient's disease and an increased likelihood of adverse effects. Subsequent upper endoscopy reveals multiple erythematous lesions in the distal esophagus, and the patient is treated effectively. However, she experiences a recurrence of GERD symptoms 3 months after treatment discontinuation. Students are then asked to consider appropriate maintenance therapies for long-term management of this patient's disease.

▶ Questions

Problem Identification

1. a. *Develop a list of this patient's drug-related problems.*

   - Suboptimal dose of H_2-receptor antagonist for the treatment of worsening GERD symptoms.
   - BP inadequately controlled with current medication regimen.
   - Hypokalemia, which is probably the result of diuretic therapy.
   - Constipation most likely secondary to aluminum hydroxide.
   - Constipation being treated with a suboptimal dose of calcium polycarbophil (Fibercon).
   - Absence of therapy for prevention of osteoporosis in this postmenopausal woman.

   b. *What clinical information indicates worsening symptoms of GERD in this patient?*

   - Increasing episodes of postprandial heartburn
   - Patient's complaint of dysphagia
   - Daily use of antacids required for symptom relief
   - Report of nocturnal awakenings secondary to epigastric discomfort
   - Decreased quality of life (QOL) as a result of GERD

   c. *What symptom(s) indicates the possible severity of the patient's GERD? Are the symptoms classic or atypical?*

   - Symptoms associated with GERD are highly variable. Classic or typical symptoms include heartburn, belching, and regurgitation. Hoarseness, asthma, chronic cough, and chest pain that mimics angina are considered atypical symptoms of GERD. Symptoms such as dysphagia and odynophagia indicate the presence of severe disease or complications such as esophageal ulceration, stricture formation, or Barrett's esophagus.

- The severity of mucosal damage in GERD does not correlate well with symptom severity. In fact, approximately 50% of patients with GERD have a normal-appearing esophagus on endoscopy.
- Elderly patients with symptomatic GERD tend to present with more severe mucosal injury and require more aggressive therapy compared to younger patients.[1]
- In this case, the patient's complaint of dysphagia indicates that she may have associated complications of GERD such as erosive esophagitis or esophageal stricture.
- Frequent nocturnal reflux episodes also indicate increasing severity of reflux esophagitis. Nocturnal reflux episodes may cause more mucosal injury due to reduced esophageal acid clearance and salivary acid neutralization during sleep.

d. *What factors may be contributing to the patient's symptoms of GERD? (Refer to Figure 23–2 for a depiction of possible causes of esophagitis.)*

- *Hiatial hernia.* The presence of a hiatal hernia causes a displacement of the lower esophageal sphincter (LES). This displacement removes secondary anti-reflux mechanisms such as diaphragmatic contractions, which normally enhance LES tone. In patients with an already abnormal LES tone, the loss of such secondary anti-reflux mechanisms can result in increasing frequency and duration of esophageal acid exposure.
- *Alcohol consumption.* Alcohol ingestion results in delayed gastric emptying, reduced esophageal clearance (secondary to decreased peristalsis), and reduced LES pressure.
- *Smoking.* Nicotine contributes to increased spontaneous LES relaxations.
- *Verapamil.* Calcium channel blocker therapy reduces LES pressure.

Desired Outcome

2. *What are the goals of pharmacotherapy for this patient's GERD?*

- Relief of symptoms associated with GERD
- Healing of esophageal erosions
- Avoidance of GERD complications
- Prevention of recurrence
- Improvement in QOL

Therapeutic Alternatives

3. a. *What non-pharmacologic therapies or life-style modifications might be useful in the management of this patient's GERD?*

- Patients with GERD are encouraged to implement dietary and life-style modifications in order to reduce the frequency and duration of reflux episodes. Such modifications include:
  - ✓ Elevation of the head of the bed 6 to 8 inches
  - ✓ Remaining upright for 2 to 3 hours after eating
  - ✓ Reduction in dietary fat intake
  - ✓ Reduction in meal size
  - ✓ Avoidance of foods that impair the LES tone (caffeine, chocolate, peppermint)
  - ✓ Avoidance of alcohol
  - ✓ Smoking cessation
  - ✓ Avoiding tight-fitting garments
  - ✓ Weight loss, if obese
- Numerous medications, such as calcium channel blockers and tricyclic antidepressants, can also contribute to the symptoms of GERD by causing a decrease in the LES pressure (refer to Table 30–1 in textbook Chapter 30). When possible, these offending medications should be discontinued in patients with GERD. In this patient's case, consideration could be given to switching her from verapamil to a β-blocker such as propranolol for the treatment of her HTN and prevention of recurrent paroxysmal SVT.
- The clinical efficacy of life-style modifications alone for the treatment of GERD is limited. However, such modifications are an important adjunct to drug therapy to reduce the frequency of reflux and should be encouraged.

b. *What pharmacotherapeutic alternatives are available for the treatment of this patient's GERD?*

- *Antacids* increase the pH of the gastric refluxate by neutralizing gastric acid, thereby decreasing its potential to cause damage to the esophageal mucosa. These agents also increase the LES tone through alkalinization of gastric contents. In patients whose symptoms are relieved with antacids, relief generally occurs within 5 to 15 minutes after administration and may last for 1 to 3 hours, depending upon the rate of gastric emptying. The short duration of action necessitates frequent dosing. Patients taking antacids for relief of GERD symptoms may need 4 to 5 doses throughout the day for adequate symptom relief. Antacids can be used to manage patients with mild intermittent symptoms of GERD without esophagitis. When prescribing or recommending antacid therapy, careful consideration should be given to the adverse effect profile of the agent as well as the potential for drug interactions.
- *Alginic acid* dissociates to form a neutral substance, sodium alginate, which floats on top of the gastric contents, thus creating an anti-reflux layer. Theoretically, the sodium alginate is refluxed instead of gastric acid, and esophageal irritation is minimized. The efficacy of alginic acid for GERD treatment is questionable. Similar to antacids alone, the combination of antacid/alginic acid (Gaviscon) can be used for symptom relief in patients without esophagitis. However, the combination product is more expensive than some antacids alone.
- *Sucralfate* is a mucosal coating agent that forms a protective barrier between esophageal tissue and gastric refluxate. It preferentially binds to ulcerated tissue, preventing penetration of acid. Sucralfate also possesses cytoprotective effects including stimulation of prostaglandin production and enhancing blood flow to the mucosa. Although it does not have FDA approval for the treatment of GERD, sucralfate has been demonstrated to provide symptom relief and esophageal healing. However, its role is limited to cases of mild to moderate esophagitis or to combination therapy. The agent must be administered in a liquid formulation for the treatment of GERD in order to make contact with esophageal tissue. Additionally, sucralfate must be administered

at least 4 times daily (1 hour before meals and at bedtime), making patient compliance difficult.

- *Prokinetic agents* improve esophageal peristalsis and increase LES tone. Through such actions, prokinetic agents enhance luminal clearance and gastric emptying and also reduce the duration and frequency of reflux.
  - ✓ *Bethanechol* is a cholinergic agonist that does not improve gastric emptying. It also has an adverse effect profile that greatly limits its usefulness, particularly in elderly patients. Side effects include abdominal cramps, urinary frequency, malaise, blurred vision, diarrhea, and increased gastric acid secretion.
  - ✓ *Metoclopramide* is a dopamine antagonist that increases LES pressure and accelerates gastric emptying. It is also associated with troublesome side effects, including drowsiness, restlessness, drug-induced Parkinsonism, and tardive dyskinesia. Both metoclopramide and bethanechol are considered to be less effective than H_2-receptor antagonists (H_2RAs) for symptom relief and esophageal healing.
  - ✓ *Cisapride*, on the other hand, has been shown to have similar efficacy to standard dose H_2RAs for symptom relief and healing of mild esophagitis. With higher grades of esophagitis, monotherapy with cisapride is not effective. Careful screening for drug interactions should always be performed when a patient is prescribed cisapride, as potentially life-threatening interactions with drugs that inhibit the cytochrome P450 3A4 isoenzyme have been reported. Because of cardiac events and deaths associated with its use, labeling for cisapride was changed in 1998 to state that it should generally be reserved for patients who do not respond adequately to life-style modifications, antacids, and acid-reducing agents. Labeling also recommends that an ECG be considered before initiating cisapride therapy.

- *H_2-receptor antagonists (cimetidine, ranitidine, famotidine, nizatidine)* are acid-suppressive agents that inhibit stimulation of the gastric parietal cell by histamine. The four commercially available products are equally effective when used in equivalent doses. Although all of the products are available in over-the-counter dosage formulations, such therapy is only effective in patients with mild or infrequent symptoms of GERD without esophagitis. Standard H_2RA regimens administered in divided doses are usually effective for the treatment of mild esophagitis (Savary–Miller I to II). However, the H_2RA dosage regimens employed for healing erosive esophagitis (Savary–Miller III to IV) are higher than those used for the treatment of peptic ulcer disease. Examples of high-dose H_2RA regimens for erosive esophagitis include cimetidine 400 mg po QID; ranitidine 150 mg po QID or 300 mg po BID; and famotidine 40 mg po BID. It is important to consider that these higher doses increase the cost of therapy and may have a negative impact on patient compliance. In addition, tolerance to the effect of H_2RAs may develop over time. Symptom relief is experienced by 32% to 80% of patients treated with H_2RAs, and healing rates of endoscopically confirmed esophagitis range from 0% to 82%.[2] Healing rates with H_2RAs are inversely related to the severity of disease and increase with prolonged duration of therapy (e.g., 12 weeks). Of the available agents, cimetidine is associated with the highest incidence of side effects when used in higher doses or when administered to patients with renal impairment, patients with hepatic impairment, and the elderly. Also, it is a known inhibitor of phase I oxidative metabolism, and therefore is associated with numerous drug interactions.

- *Proton pump inhibitors (omeprazole, lansoprazole)* irreversibly bind to the H+/K+ ATPase pump of the parietal cell, thereby inhibiting the final step of acid secretion. Esophageal healing is related to the degree and duration of gastric acid suppression. Since they inhibit the final common pathway for gastric acid secretion, proton pump inhibitors (PPIs) are more effective at suppressing acid secretion than H_2RAs. As a result, PPIs have been demonstrated to be more effective than H_2RAs for symptom relief and esophageal healing in patients with esophagitis.[3] A PPI is generally considered the drug of choice for patients with moderate to severe erosive esophagitis. The once-daily dosing with the PPIs offers an advantage over high-dose H_2RA therapy in terms of cost and patient compliance.

Optimal Plan

4. Based upon the patient information provided, design an individualized pharmacotherapeutic plan for the management of this patient's GERD.

- It is clear from her presentation that she requires more aggressive therapy for the treatment of her GERD symptoms. However, the patient's complaint of dysphagia may indicate complicated reflux disease and should be diagnostically evaluated to rule out stricture formation or Barrett's esophagus. An endoscopic evaluation of the esophagus and/or a barium swallow is indicated to assess the severity of mucosal damage. Even in the absence of esophagitis on endoscopic evaluation, the patient still warrants more aggressive medical therapy for symptom control.
- Considering the severity of this patient's symptoms, initiation of PPI therapy with omeprazole 20 mg daily or lansoprazole 30 mg daily is warranted. Treatment should continue for 8 weeks, since healing rates are higher at 8 weeks than at 4 weeks.
- Alternatively, high-dose H_2RA therapy for 12 weeks could be initiated. Options include famotidine 40 mg po BID, ranitidine 150 mg po QID, or cimetidine 400 mg po QID. Cimetidine should probably be avoided, considering its potential for adverse effects at higher doses in the elderly and the possibility of drug interactions. Because the patient has normal renal function, there is no need for renal dosage adjustment in this patient.
- The patient's bedtime dose of famotidine should be discontinued. If necessary, the patient can continue antacid use on an as-needed basis for symptom relief. However, the specific antacid that the patient uses should be changed from aluminum hydroxide to magnesium hydroxide or a combination of aluminum hydroxide/magnesium hydroxide to minimize constipation.
- If the endoscopic evaluation reveals severe esophagitis or Barrett's esophagus, high-dose PPI therapy with omeprazole 40 mg daily or lansoprazole 60 mg daily should be recommended.

Outcome Evaluation

5. What clinical and/or laboratory parameters should be evaluated at the patient's next follow-up appointment in order to assess for therapeutic response and to detect or prevent adverse effects?

- *Efficacy.* Ask the patient if she has experienced relief of her symptoms of dysphagia, postprandial heartburn, and nocturnal reflux episodes. If not, determine the frequency and duration of her symptoms. Evaluate patient compliance with the prescribed medication regimen. Determine how often the patient is using antacids for relief of symptoms. Assess for improvement in the patient's quality of life.
- *Adverse effects.* Although PPIs are generally well tolerated, the most common adverse effects are GI (nausea, vomiting, diarrhea, constipation, and abdominal pain), headache, and dizziness. H_2RAs are also commonly associated with GI and CNS (dizziness, headache, drowsiness) side effects. The H_2RAs are also rarely associated with hematologic, cardiovascular, hepatic, and dermatologic abnormalities; routine monitoring for laboratory abnormalities is not considered necessary. Dosage adjustment is required in patients with renal impairment, as all of the agents are primarily renally eliminated. If the patient continues use of antacids containing aluminum or magnesium for symptomatic relief, monitor for altered bowel function (diarrhea or constipation).

Patient Counseling

6. *How will you educate the patient about her GERD therapy in order to enhance compliance, minimize adverse effects, and promote successful therapeutic outcomes?*

General Information
- Implementing life-style and dietary modifications may help to reduce the frequency and severity of your symptoms. Smoking, alcohol, and certain foods (for example, caffeine, fried and fatty foods, and spicy foods) can make your symptoms worse and should be avoided. You should avoid eating within 2 to 3 hours of lying down or going to bed. If possible, elevate the head of your bed 6 to 8 inches using wooden blocks or bricks. This may decrease the amount of symptoms you experience at night. (*Note:* written information that outlines such changes should be given to the patient to reinforce your verbal education.)
- I encourage you to maintain a symptom diary that records the time you have symptoms, the type of symptom that you have, and any things that may have triggered the symptoms. Also record any use of antacids for symptom relief. (*Note:* A diary empowers the patient to become an active participant in the management of her disease and may help her to identify symptom triggers.)

Proton Pump Inhibitor
- This medication is being used to decrease the production of stomach acid, which can reflux up into your esophagus, causing the symptoms of chest pain and difficulty swallowing that you have been experiencing.
- Take this medicine by mouth once a day. It may be easiest for you to remember if you take it in the morning with your other medications.
- Swallow the capsule whole, if possible. Do not crush or chew the capsule. If you have difficulty swallowing it, you may open the capsule and mix the contents with applesauce or with apple, orange, cranberry, grape, or tomato juice.
- You will be taking this medication for at least 4 to 8 weeks. After that time, your doctor will evaluate your need for further therapy.
- Although this medication is usually well tolerated, some patients experience minor side effects such as stomach pain, diarrhea, constipation, and headache.

H_2-receptor Antagonist (e.g., Famotidine 40 mg po BID)
- This medication is being used to decrease the production of stomach acid, which can reflux up into your esophagus, causing the symptoms of chest pain and difficulty swallowing that you have been experiencing.
- The dose of this medication has been increased to achieve better control of your symptoms and to promote healing of any ulcers that may be present in your esophagus. In addition, you will now be taking this medication twice a day (morning and evening) instead of just at bedtime.
- This medication is generally well tolerated, but some patients experience headache, dizziness, and stomach upset.

▶ Follow-up Questions

1. *What is the role of maintenance therapy for the management of this patient's continued GERD symptoms?*

   - Reflux esophagitis is associated with a high rate of relapse following the discontinuation of acid-suppressing therapy. In particular, patients with an initial diagnosis of severe esophagitis, patients who required extended therapy for symptom relief and healing, and patients who experience recurrence of residual symptoms after healing are likely to require long-term medical management to maintain healing and prevent relapse. This patient is a candidate for long-term maintenance therapy, as she has a long history of GERD and recently experienced relapse of her symptoms within 3 months of PPI therapy discontinuation.

2. *What maintenance therapies could be recommended for the long-term management of GERD in this patient?*

   - PPI therapy with either omeprazole 20 mg daily of lansoprazole 15 mg daily is appropriate. PPIs are more effective than H_2RAs in preventing recurrence of esophagitis after healing.
   - Although once-daily administration of famotidine is ineffective in preventing the recurrence of her symptoms, standard or high-dose H_2RA therapy may be more effective as maintenance therapy. The lowest effective dose for the prevention of relapse should be employed to minimize cost and enhance patient compliance.

References

1. Collen MJ, Abdulian JD, Chen YK. Gastroesophageal reflux disease in the elderly: More severe disease that requires aggressive therapy. Am J Gastroenterol 1995;90:1053–1057.
2. DeVault KR, Castell DO. Current diagnosis and treatment of gastroesophageal reflux disease. Mayo Clin Proc 1994;69:867–876.
3. Sandmark S, Carlsson R, Fausa O, et al. Omeprazole or ranitidine in the treatment of reflux esophagitis. Results of a double-blind, randomized, Scandinavian multicenter study. Scand J Gastroenterol 1988;23:625–632.
4. Dimenas E, Glise H, Hallerback B, et al. Quality of life in patients with upper gastrointestinal symptoms: An improved evaluation of treatment regimens? Scand J Gastroenterol 1993:28:681–687.

24 PEPTIC ULCER DISEASE

▶ Stamping Out an Infectious Disease
(Level I)

Marie A. Chisholm, PharmD
Mark W. Jackson, MD, FACG

A 42-year-old woman with hypertension, hypothyroidism, occasional back pain, and type 2 diabetes mellitus complains of epigastric pain, black/tarry bowel movements, and weakness. An EGD revealed a duodenal ulcer, and laboratory evaluation indicated the presence of iron deficiency anemia. In addition to non-pharmacologic interventions, students are asked to recommend pharmacotherapeutic regimens to treat the ulcer and anemia. Infection by *Helicobacter pylori* is subsequently documented, requiring re-assessment of the treatment goals and existing plan. Selection of a combination antimicrobial regimen that will eradicate the organism is a necessary component of the revised plan.

▶ Questions

Problem Identification

1. a. *Create a list of the patient's drug-related problems.*

   - Epigastric pain, GI bleeding, and other findings suggestive of PUD that require appropriate drug treatment.
   - Clinical and laboratory findings of iron deficiency anemia, requiring appropriate replacement therapy.
   - Constipation, which may be caused in part by OTC calcium ingestion (Tums).
   - Tobacco smoking (a drug-related problem if pharmacologic interventions are considered as part of a smoking cessation program; smoking may also affect PUD healing and recurrence rates).
   - Aspirin use for back pain. Aspirin may cause mucosal erosions and ulcerations of the GI tract, especially the stomach and duodenum.
   - The patient's hypertension, hypothyroidism, and diabetes mellitus are chronic stable problems that appear to be well controlled at the present time.

   b. *What information (signs, symptoms, tests, and laboratory values) indicates the presence of peptic ulcer disease?*

   - Localized (non-radiating) epigastric pain that appears to worsen at night and between meals and decreases by ingesting food or antacids often occurs with duodenal ulcer disease.
   - Black, tarry bowel movements (melena) that are heme (+) suggest upper GI bleeding.
   - Iron deficiency anemia can occur with PUD. Signs consistent with iron deficiency anemia include low hemoglobin, hematocrit, MCV, and serum iron; an inappropriately low reticulocyte count in the face of anemia; and the presence of blood detected in the rectal vault.
   - History of NSAID use; NSAIDs are common causes of gastric and (less commonly) duodenal ulcers.

Desired Outcome

2. *What are the goals for treating this patient's PUD?*

   - Relieve pain and discomfort associated with PUD
   - Promote ulcer healing
   - Prevent or treat complications of PUD (GI hemorrhage, anemia, perforation, obstruction, and intractability)
   - Prevent ulcer recurrences
   - Educate the patient about PUD to improve compliance and ensure successful therapy
   - Avoid adverse effects of drugs

Therapeutic Alternatives

3. a. *Considering this patient's presentation, what non-pharmacologic alternatives are available to treat her PUD?*

   - She should be counseled to avoid or decrease smoking, since smoking is strongly correlated with delayed ulcer healing and recurrent disease.
   - Ingestion of foods and liquids that contribute to epigastric pain should be limited or avoided.
   - Since mucosal damage has been reported with the use of aspirin, she should be advised to avoid aspirin and use an acetaminophen-containing pain reliever.
   - Also consider discontinuing the Tums due to its possible contribution to the patient's constipation.

   b. *In the absence of information about the presence of* Helicobacter pylori, *what pharmacologic alternatives are available to treat duodenal ulcers?*

   - Medications used to treat duodenal ulcers include antacids, H_2-receptor antagonists, H^+/K^+-ATPase enzyme (or proton pump) inhibitors, and sucralfate.
   - *H_2-receptor antagonists (cimetidine, ranitidine, famotidine, and nizatidine)* and sucralfate are fairly effective and have similar duodenal ulcer healing rates of 60% to 84% and 82% to 95% after 4 and 8 weeks of therapy, respectively. For active duodenal ulcers, the H_2-receptor antagonists can be taken once or twice daily; sucralfate can be taken two to four times daily.
   - *Proton-pump inhibitors (lansoprazole and omeprazole)* are more effective in healing ulcers than H_2-receptor antagonists and sucralfate, with healing rates >90% within four weeks of therapy. Proton-pump inhibitors are given once daily for a shorter time, thereby providing dosage convenience over most other therapies.
   - *Antacids* may be used adjunctively for pain relief, especially during the initial few days of treatment with other agents. Refer to textbook Chapter 31 for more information on specific agents.

Optimal Plan

4. Based on the patient's presentation and the current medical assessment, design a pharmacotherapeutic regimen to treat her duodenal ulcer and anemia.

- Although the patient's ulcer is not actively bleeding (indicated by the clear ulcer base observed during endoscopy), the ulcer may have been bleeding at some point. This possibility in addition to menstruation likely contributed to her anemia. Therefore, the two primary concerns for this patient are healing her duodenal ulcer and treating her anemia.
- Initial acute therapy with antacids, any of the H_2-receptor antagonists, proton pump inhibitors, or sucralfate is a reasonable choice since the etiology of the peptic ulcer has not yet been determined (refer to the textbook chapter for specific dosages). Because antacid therapy requires large and frequent doses that are associated with inconvenience, noncompliance, and ulcer relapse, antacids have been largely replaced by H_2-receptor antagonists and proton pump inhibitors. Furthermore, antacids decrease absorption of many medications. However, if antacids are to be used early in treatment for pain relief, they should be given at different times than other medications (1 hour before or 2 hours after other medications).
- The duration of treatment for active duodenal ulcer is 4 to 8 weeks with proton pump inhibitor therapy and 6 to 8 weeks with H_2-receptor antagonist and sucralfate therapy. Although generic cimetidine and ranitidine are available at prices about 30% less than their brand name counterparts, the proton pump inhibitors may be less expensive because of the shorter duration of therapy.
- To treat the anemia and replace iron stores, oral iron replacement therapy (e.g., ferrous sulfate 325 mg po TID) for 3 to 6 months should be recommended. Although PUD is a relative contraindication to oral iron replacement therapy, parenteral iron replacement therapy is not justifiable in this patient due to its cost and potential adverse effects.

Outcome Evaluation

5. What clinical and laboratory parameters are necessary to evaluate the therapy for achievement of the desired therapeutic outcomes and to detect or prevent adverse effects?

- Efficacy of treatment is determined by patient symptoms (e.g., resolution of dyspepsia, epigastric pain, and weakness within 4 to 8 weeks of the start of therapy), physical signs of complications (e.g., resolution of bloody stools), and laboratory data (e.g., her reticulocyte count should increase in approximately 1 week and Hgb/Hct levels within 6 weeks).
- In many cases, unless patient symptoms recur, no specific follow-up is necessary for uncomplicated duodenal ulcer disease. However, patients who experience frequent symptomatic recurrences or complications may require endoscopy to determine if ulcers are present or to assess the need for additional therapy.
- Adverse effects of iron therapy are common and may include GI discomfort such as diarrhea or constipation, nausea, vomiting, and discoloration of stools (black stools similar to what is seen with GI bleeding).
- Adverse effects of anti-ulcer agents are uncommon and routine laboratory monitoring solely to detect drug-related adverse effects is usually not performed unless the patient exhibits signs or symptoms of adverse drug effects. Some of the events associated with anti-ulcer agents include:
  - ✓ *Antacids.* Altered bowel function (constipation, diarrhea), rebound hyperacidity, serum electrolyte changes, milk-alkali syndrome.
  - ✓ H_2-*receptor antagonists.* CNS effects (headaches, drowsiness, slurred speech, confusion), dermatologic effects (rash, pruritus, urticaria), gynecomastia (cimetidine), GI upset (abdominal pain, nausea, vomiting, constipation, diarrhea), hematologic abnormalities (thrombocytopenia and pancytopenia), increased liver function tests (AST, ALT, alkaline phosphatase), and increased serum creatinine (due to reduced tubular secretion of creatinine, not renal dysfunction).
  - ✓ *Proton pump inhibitors.* GI upset (abdominal pain, nausea, vomiting, constipation, diarrhea), CNS effects (headaches, dizziness, weakness, numbness, anxiety, confusion), increased liver function tests (AST, ALT), increased serum creatinine.
  - ✓ *Sucralfate.* Constipation, metallic taste, GI upset (abdominal pain, nausea, vomiting), xerostomia, CNS effects (headaches, drowsiness, confusion).

Patient Counseling

6. What information should be provided to the patient to ensure successful therapy, enhance compliance, and minimize adverse effects?

General Information
- Strict compliance with the therapy is important if it is to be effective.
- Contact your doctor if your symptoms do not get better or if they return after initially disappearing.
- Contact your doctor if you develop any severe side effects.
- Avoid or limit use of aspirin or other non-prescription pain relievers containing ibuprofen, naproxen, or ketoprofen; use acetaminophen if you need something for pain.
- Avoid or limit ingestion of foods and liquids that aggravate your abdominal pain.
- Stop or decrease smoking, which can impair ulcer healing and lead to an increased rate of recurrence.
- In light of your family history and anemia, you may consider undergoing an elective colonoscopy to exclude colorectal cancer.

Drug-related Information
- H_2-receptor antagonists (cimetidine, ranitidine, famotidine, and nizatidine) and proton pump inhibitors (lansoprazole and omeprazole) work by reducing the amount of acid secreted by the stomach.
- Sucralfate forms a protective coating that protects the lining against acid in the GI tract. Take sucralfate on an empty stomach, 1 hour before meals or at least 2 hours after meals.
- If taking omeprazole or lansoprazole, swallow the capsules whole; do not chew or crush them. Take lansoprazole before meals.
- Do not take antacids for at least 30 minutes before or after taking sucralfate or an H_2-receptor antagonist.
- Take iron on an empty stomach (food interferes with iron absorption).

Follow-up Questions

1. *What is the significance of this new finding?*

   - Excluding patients taking NSAIDs, at least 95% of duodenal and 80% of gastric ulcers are linked to the presence of *H. pylori*. Furthermore, 90% of the patients who have adenocarcinoma of the distal stomach are seropositive for *H. pylori*.[1,2] Although most patients with duodenal ulcers have this organism, it was important to test for the presence of this organism in this patient because of her history of frequent NSAID use. In light of the many studies that have convincingly linked *H. pylori* to mucosal damage of the GI tract and that ulcer recurrence is greatly diminished as a result of eradicating *H. pylori*, the American College of Gastroenterology recommends that all patients diagnosed with *H. pylori*-associated peptic ulcer disease receive antimicrobial therapy effective against this organism.[3]

2. *Based on this new information, how would you modify your goals for treating this patient's PUD?*

   - In addition to treating the anemia with iron replacement therapy, the primary new goal should be treatment to eradicate *H. pylori* infection. The remainder of the treatment goals are the same as previously discussed in question 2.

3. *What pharmacotherapeutic alternatives are available to achieve the new goals?*

   - Many different antimicrobial regimens have been used to eradicate *H. pylori*. In general, combination antibiotic regimens are more effective than single agents. Because shorter antibiotic therapy and the use of fewer drugs dosed less frequently are desired to increase compliance and decrease cost, there is a trend for practitioners to use shorter course regimens and fewer dosages per day. Research is being conducted to determine the optimal regimen for eradicating this organism (refer to the textbook chapter for more detailed information on therapeutic alternatives).

4. *Design a pharmacotherapeutic regimen for this patient's ulcer that will accomplish the new treatment goals.*

   - Since she is not allergic to any medications, an effective combination antibiotic regimen with or without an antisecretory agent may be used. Three regimens are recommended by the American College of Gastroenterology because they achieve 90% cure rates, usually with 1 week of treatment, and effectiveness appears preserved despite metronidazole resistance:
     - ✓ Bismuth, metronidazole, and tetracycline plus a proton pump inhibitor
     - ✓ Clarithromycin and metronidazole plus a proton pump inhibitor
     - ✓ Clarithromycin and amoxicillin plus a proton pump inhibitor
   - If the patient is not able to afford clarithromycin, the bismuth-metronidazole-tetracycline regimen is a reasonable alternative. Refer to the textbook chapter for specific examples of *H. pylori* eradication therapies.
   - Non-pharmacologic recommendations suggested earlier (refer to question 3) and the need for compliance should be reinforced to prevent eradication failure and to prevent antibiotic resistance.

5. *How should the PUD therapy you recommended be monitored for efficacy and adverse effects?*

   - Efficacy of treatment for *H. pylori* infection is assessed by resolution of the patient's signs and symptoms. Repeat biopsies or other tests to confirm *H. pylori* eradication are generally not performed unless the patient has persistent or worsening symptoms. It is important to remember that serology cannot be used to confirm eradication.
   - Severe adverse effects from *H. pylori* eradication therapies such as drug reactions or pseudomembranous colitis are rare; however, minor adverse effects occur in up to 30% to 40% of patients. These include:
     - ✓ *Amoxicillin*. Diarrhea and candidiasis
     - ✓ *Tetracycline*. Nausea, diarrhea and photosensitivity
     - ✓ *Metronidazole*. Nausea, diarrhea, a disulfiram-like reaction, and metallic taste
     - ✓ *Clarithromycin*. Metallic taste, diarrhea, nausea, and headache
     - ✓ *Bismuth*. Black stools and discoloration of the tongue

6. *What information should be provided to the patient about her therapy?*

   - *H. pylori* is a bacteria that is associated with peptic ulcers. In fact, *H. pylori*-associated peptic ulcer is one of the most common forms of ulcer disease.
   - Treatment with antibiotic regimens, such as the medications you are prescribed, eliminates the organism, results in ulcer healing, and significantly reduces ulcer recurrence.
   - Patient compliance is often poor with *H. pylori* therapy due to adverse effects and complexity of the various regimens. In order to ensure the best outcome for you, it is important to take the medications every day as prescribed for the full course of therapy.
   - Contact your physician if your ulcer symptoms do not resolve or if they recur.

References

1. Peterson WL. *Helicobacter pylori* and peptic ulcer disease. N Engl J Med 1991;324:1043–1048.
2. Graham DY. *Helicobacter pylori*: Its epidemiology and its role in duodenal ulcer disease. J Gastroenterol Hepatol 1991;6:105–113.
3. Soll AH. Consensus conference. Medical treatment of peptic ulcer disease. Practice guidelines. JAMA 1996;275:622–629.

25 STRESS ULCER PROPHYLAXIS/UPPER GI HEMORRHAGE

▶ Prophylaxis Offers No Guarantee (Level I)

Steven V. Johnson, PharmD, BCPS
Christine L. Solberg, PharmD, BCPS, CSPI

Complaints of diffuse abdominal pain and vomiting for 24 hours cause a 57-year-old man to seek treatment in the ED. He is presently taking a number of medications for CAD, CHF, and COPD; he experienced an upper GI hemorrhage due to NSAIDs 5 years ago. Exploratory laparotomy revealed a perforated cecum; he underwent a right hemicolectomy and was returned to the surgical ICU on mechanical ventilation. Students are initially asked to consider which of the patient's medications should be restarted post-operatively in the surgical ICU. The patient should also receive pharmacologic stress ulcer prophylaxis due to respiratory failure requiring mechanical ventilation. Students are asked to discuss possible therapeutic alternatives and select the optimal regimen and route of administration for this patient. Additional interventions must be made when the patient develops a guaiac-positive nasogastric aspirate with gastric pH readings between 2 and 3. The patient's condition later worsens, with bloody NG returns, hypotension, tachycardia, and development of multiple bleeding gastric lesions. Students must also develop a rationale plan to resolve these complications.

Questions

Problem Identification

1. a. *The resident asks for your recommendations about the patient's chronic medications. Specifically, he would like to know which agents should be restarted post-operatively and why. Secondly, he inquires as to which of these agents are available intravenously.*

   - *Furosemide* should be restarted to avoid fluid overload due to the amount of fluid he received in the operating room. He currently has no evidence of being intravascularly depleted (BP, HR, and urine output are acceptable and a CVP of 14 suggests adequate volume status). The furosemide may prevent worsening pulmonary edema and will likely maintain an adequate urine output based on the dose he was receiving as an outpatient.
   - *Atrovent* and *albuterol* inhalers should be restarted based on his COPD history, and because they may prevent prolonged mechanical ventilation.
   - *Enalapril* should be restarted when possible based on the patient's ejection fraction. Its afterload-reducing effects decrease the workload on the heart in CHF patients.
   - *Digoxin* should also be restarted to maintain any positive inotropic effects it may be providing. His admission digoxin level is nearly subtherapeutic. His compliance as an outpatient or the need for a higher dose based on symptoms should be assessed.
   - *Amlodipine* should be withheld at this time and may be restarted if necessary only after assessing the effects of furosemide and enalapril on his BP.
   - *Digoxin, enalapril (enalaprilat),* and *furosemide* are all available intravenously.

   b. *List all of the patient's drug related problems at this point in his hospital course (include both potential and actual drug related problems).*

   Potential Drug-related Problems
   Based on the information provided, the patient has a number of potential drug-related problems that are apparently being addressed adequately. These include:
   - Post-operative pain, treated with morphine continuous infusion.
   - Need for sedation with scheduled doses of lorazepam to help facilitate mechanical ventilation. The morphine allows for smaller doses of lorazepam due to synergy with benzodiazepines (lorazepam) and the sedative properties of morphine.
   - The patient is being treated with furosemide, digoxin, and enalapril to prevent CHF exacerbation.
   - COPD is apparently controlled with Atrovent and albuterol MDIs (given by the Respiratory Therapy Department).

   Actual Drug-related Problems
   The patient has two actual drug-related problems that require attention:
   - The patient is at risk for developing stress ulceration and is receiving no medication to prevent these lesions.
   - The patient is receiving DVT prophylaxis with SQ heparin Q 8 H; one might argue that Q 12 H dosing would be sufficient, especially in a patient at risk of stress gastritis/ulceration.

   c. *What are the risk factors for developing stress gastritis/ulceration in critically ill patients?*

   - Risk factors contributing to stress ulceration include sepsis, shock (hemorrhagic, cardiogenic, anaphylactic, neurogenic), hypotension, head injury, spinal cord injury, respiratory failure, coagulopathy, severe burn injury (>30% TBSA), and multiple organ failure.[1]
   - Respiratory failure requiring mechanical ventilation and coagulopathy were found to be the strongest independent risk factors for developing clinically important bleeding associated with stress ulceration.[2]

   d. *Do the risk factors that this patient has warrant prophylactic therapy to prevent stress ulceration?*

   - The patient has respiratory failure requiring mechanical ventilation and was hypotensive on admission. Therefore, pharmacologic prophylaxis should be initiated.

Desired Outcome

2. *What are the goals of pharmacotherapy for prevention of stress gastritis and ulceration?*

   - Pharmacotherapy in critically ill patients at risk for stress ulceration is given to prevent the development of stress ulcerations and the morbidity associated with them.
   - No difference in mortality has been documented with the use of stress ulcer prophylaxis.

Therapeutic Alternatives

3. *Discuss the pharmacologic options available for the prophylaxis of stress ulceration in critically ill patients.*

- *H₂-receptor antagonists (cimetidine, ranitidine, famotidine)* decrease stomach acidity, which is presumed to be the mechanism of their prophylactic benefit. However, the role that modifying gastric pH plays in determining the success of therapy is still unknown. In a recent multicenter, randomized, blinded comparison of ranitidine and sucralfate in 1200 critically ill patients requiring mechanical ventilation, 1.7% of patients receiving ranitidine and 3.8% of patients in the sucralfate group developed clinically important gastrointestinal bleeding (P = 0.02).[3] There were no significant differences in the rates of ventilator-associated pneumonia, duration of ICU stay, or mortality. However, gastric pH was not measured in this study. Some clinicians feel that H₂-antagonists may not provide any additional benefit in patients who already have a gastric pH >4. There is some evidence that decreasing gastric acidity may increase the risk of developing pneumonia. H₂ antagonists can be given by multiple administration methods (intermittent IV dosing, continuous IV infusions, orally, and as enteral solutions). Dosage adjustments must be made for patients with diminished renal function.
- *Sucralfate* has local protective effects and minimal systemic adverse effects. Although small studies indicated that it was as effective as ranitidine, the large multicenter trial described above showed that it was less effective.[3] It also requires intragastric administration, and its aluminum content may bind with some drugs (e.g., levothyroxine, oral fluoroquinolones) thereby decreasing their absorption. Long-term use in chronic renal failure patients may result in aluminum accumulation.
- *Antacids* are inexpensive agents, but they must be administered frequently (every hour) to be beneficial in stress ulcer prophylaxis. They may also inhibit the absorption of some other drugs.
- *Proton pump inhibitors (omeprazole, lansoprazole)* are the most effective acid suppressants available. However, there are no clinical studies documenting their efficacy for stress ulcer prophylaxis.
- Cost in order of least to most expensive: antacids < sucralfate = po H₂ antagonists < IV H₂ antagonists < proton pump inhibitors.

Optimal Plan

4. What would you recommend for stress ulcer prophylaxis in this patient?

- An H₂-receptor antagonist would be appropriate initial therapy for this patient. His post-operative ileus makes GI absorption unreliable, so IV or topical therapy should be recommended. The H₂-receptor antagonists available are considered to be equally effective. Usual doses are ranitidine 50 mg IV Q 6–8 H, famotidine 20 mg IV Q 12 H, or cimetidine 300 mg IV Q 6 H. Nizatidine is not available parenterally.
- Sucralfate or antacid therapy could also be justified because absorption is not necessary for their effect. Sucralfate is given in doses of 4 to 6 g/day. Antacid dosing is too cumbersome for use as primary agents.

Outcome Evaluation

5. What clinical parameters should be monitored to assess the effectiveness of this regimen?

- The physical characteristics of the NG aspirate should be monitored for the appearance of frank blood or a pinkish color, which may denote bleeding. A guaiac test may also be performed to indicate the presence of occult blood.
- Hemoglobin/hematocrit should be assessed if bleeding is suspected to determine an estimate of blood loss and need for replacement.
- The pH of the NG aspirate should also be tested every 8 hours in patients receiving acid suppressive therapy (not for patients on sucralfate).
- The occurrence of hematemesis is indicative of treatment failure.

▶ Follow-up Questions

1. Based on the above information, what action should be taken to improve the patient's prophylaxis regimen?

- It should first be determined that the patient received the regimen as it was prescribed and that an appropriate amount of time has elapsed to allow for a complete therapeutic effect.
- If these two criteria are met, then changes in the regimen should be considered. The goal is to increase the serum drug concentration of the H₂-receptor antagonist to increase its pharmacologic effect (acid suppression). The following is suggested as an example of a therapeutic continuum for H₂ antagonists: oral H₂ antagonist → IV H₂ antagonist → increase the IV dose → change to continuous infusion → change to proton pump inhibitor. Continuous infusions of H₂ blockers provide a greater and more sustained increase in gastric pH than intermittent administration.[4,5]
- Therapy should be switched to H₂-receptor antagonist therapy (as above) if sucralfate was chosen as the first-line agent for prophylaxis.
- In this situation, the dose of drug that the patient is receiving should be increased (doubled, usually) in an attempt to further decrease gastric acid secretion. Possible regimens include ranitidine 100 mg IV Q 6–8 H, famotidine 40 mg IV Q 12 H, or cimetidine 600 mg IV Q 6 H.
- A continuous infusion would also be an appropriate alternative. Utilize the previous 24-hour dose as the initial 24-hour infusion rate (i.e., ranitidine 50 mg IV Q 8 H = 6.25 mg/hr).

2. If a saline administration were insufficient to restore the patient's baseline hemodynamic status, what therapy should be administered next?

- Blood products (e.g., PRBCs) would probably be indicated in someone like this who has a significant past medical history for coronary dysfunction. Blood would restore necessary oxygen-carrying capacity and decrease his risk for myocardial ischemia.

3. What pharmacologic therapy would you suggest at this time?

- Because of the presence of bleeding gastric lesions, discontinue SQ heparin and change DVT prophylaxis to intermittent pneumatic compression devices (IPCs).
- Continue current H₂-receptor antagonist therapy.
- Continue appropriate supportive care therapies (e.g., adequate vascular support with fluids, PRBCs).
- Perform gastric lavage to assess for continued bleeding.

4. What medication changes, if any, would you recommend at this time?

- All medications can be changed to oral administration, starting at doses that were effective for the patient at admission: furosemide 40 mg po BID, digoxin 0.25 mg po QD, enalapril 10 mg po BID, and Colace 100 mg po BID.
- His risk factors for stress ulceration have resolved, and he should no longer require prophylaxis. However, oral H_2-receptor antagonist therapy at treatment doses for peptic ulcers should continue due to his clinically significant bleeding (requiring blood transfusions). The appropriate duration of therapy following stress ulceration is unknown and is often managed on an individual basis based on the severity and depth of the ulcers present.
- Reasonable regimens include famotidine 40 mg po QD, ranitidine 300 mg po QD, or cimetidine 600 to 800 mg po QD.

References

1. Tryba M, Cook D. Current guidelines on stress ulcer prophylaxis. Drugs 1997;54:581–596.
2. Cook DJ, Fuller HD, Guyatt GH, et al. Risk factors for gastrointestinal bleeding in critically ill patients. Canadian Critical Care Trials Group. N Engl J Med 1994; 330:377–381.
3. Cook DJ, Guyatt GH, Marshall J, et al. A comparison of sucralfate and ranitidine for the prevention of upper gastrointestinal bleeding in patients requiring mechanical ventilation. N Engl J Med 1998;338:791–797.
4. Heiselman DE, Hulisz DT, Fricker R, et al. Randomized comparison of gastric pH control with intermittent and continuous intravenous infusion of famotidine in ICU patients. Am J Gastroenterol 1995;90:277–279.
5. Siepler JK, Trudeau W, Petty DE. Use of continuous infusion of histamine$_2$-receptor antagonists in critically ill patients. Drug Intell Clin Pharm 1989;23(10 suppl): S40–S43.

26 ULCERATIVE COLITIS

▶ The School Teacher's Lament   (Level I)

Nancy S. Yunker, PharmD
Ralph E. Small, PharmD, FCCP, FASHP, FAPhA

An increased frequency of bowel movements, hematochezia, and weakness cause a 31-year-old man with hypertension and sulfa allergy to seek medical attention at the ED. He is given volume and potassium repletion in the ED and referred to the GI clinic for colonoscopy. The results indicate the presence of moderate ulcerative colitis extending from the rectum to the mid-transverse colon. In developing a pharmacotherapeutic plan to achieve disease remission in this patient, students must consider the patient's allergy to sulfa drugs and avoid sulfasalazine. Mesalamine suppositories or enemas are also not viable options due to the extent of the disease process. Corticosteroids should be avoided as first-line therapy in patients with mild to moderate disease. For these reasons, an oral mesalamine product would provide the best initial therapy for this patient. When the patient responds to the recommended therapy, students must consider whether long-term prophylaxis is indicated to prevent disease recurrence.

▶ Questions

Problem Identification

1. a. List all of the patient's drug-related problems, including those existing at his initial presentation to the ED.

- Acute ulcerative colitis, moderate in severity, presently untreated.
- Volume depletion on presentation to ED secondary to increased number of stools and/or hydrochlorothiazide usage.
- Hypokalemia upon initial presentation secondary to increased number of stools and/or hydrochlorothiazide usage.
- Hypertension, currently Stage 1 (140 to 159/90 to 99), risk group B (male). Although the patient is currently under stress with another illness, outpatient BP readings should be investigated and life-style modifications (including weight reduction) should be reinforced in addition to continuing current BP medications.

b. List the signs, symptoms, and laboratory values that indicate the presence and severity of ulcerative colitis; also include pertinent negative findings.

Positive Findings
- The patient is 31 years of age, and the peak incidence of IBD is in the second to fourth decades of life, although infants and the elderly may also develop ulcerative colitis.
- The diagnosis of IBD should be considered when the patient complains of increased numbers of bowel movements (in this case 4 to 5 bowel movements per day), bowel urgency, or blood in the stool.
- Other complaints and physical findings consistent with the diagnosis of IBD in this patient include the chief complaints of BRBPR and weakness, occasional mild abdominal soreness, and the rectal exam demonstrating some tenderness with heme (+) stool.
- The most consistent findings for the diagnosis of ulcerative colitis are the colonoscopy results of edema, erythema, crypt abscesses with mild oozing of blood; continuous lesions from the rectum to the mid-transverse colon with the physician's diagnosis stating that it is consistent with moderate ulcerative colitis. This is supported by the histology report of distorted crypt architecture, mixed acute and chronic inflammation in the lamina propria, and PMNs in the surface epithelium. The absence of granulomas and the continuous lesions from the rectum to mid-transverse colon decrease the likelihood of Crohn's disease.
- The severity of ulcerative colitis can be classified as mild, moderate or severe, based on the clinical signs the patient exhibits. The patient's abdominal exam is NTND with bowel sounds present and no palpable mass, which is consistent with mild to moderate disease.

- The patient's hemoglobin dropped from 10.9 to 10.0 g/dL after receiving 1 liter of IV fluid; this suggests volume repletion. However, the patient appeared pale and his hemoglobin was low prior to the fluid replacement, so causes of blood loss should be investigated.
- Smoking cessation has been associated with the development of ulcerative colitis.

Pertinent Negative Findings
- IBD may occur more commonly if another family member has been diagnosed with the disease. This patient states no family history of IBD.
- In patients with an increased number of bowel movements, infectious causes of the diarrhea should be ruled out. This patient states he has not traveled outside of the city, which eliminates the chance he was exposed to an infectious agent resulting in diarrhea while traveling overseas or to Mexico. The history of no recent antibiotic use or hospitalization decreases the chance of other causes of infectious diarrhea. It would have been appropriate to question the patient about exposure to other people with diarrhea to further investigate causes of infectious diarrhea.
- Ulcerative colitis is a systemic disease with complications including hepatobiliary, joint, ocular, and dermatologic/mucosal manifestations. This patient's LFTs are normal, and he has no skin or eye lesions (no iritis, uveitis, conjunctivitis), or signs and symptoms of arthritis (no joint stiffness/soreness). Refer to textbook Chapter 32 for more detailed information on the systemic complications of ulcerative colitis.

c. *Could the manifestations of the patient's ulcerative colitis have been precipitated by any event?*

- Patients who are ex-smokers have a higher risk of ulcerative colitis than nonsmokers or current smokers. In one study, 20% and 52% of patients developed ulcerative colitis within 1 and 3 years of smoking cessation, respectively.[1] It is possible that this patient's smoking prevented symptoms of ulcerative colitis from appearing earlier.

Desired Outcome

2. *What are the short- and long-term pharmacotherapeutic goals for this patient?*

Short-term Goals
- Resolution of the acute inflammatory process
- Disappearance of symptoms
- Return to normal bowel habits avoiding the use of antidiarrheals if possible
- It does not appear that the patient has developed complications (e.g., arthritis, skin lesions) that need to be addressed at this time.

Long-term Goals
- Prevent relapse
- Prevent complications
- Prevent adverse effects from drug treatment

Therapeutic Alternatives

3. a. *What non-drug therapies might be useful for this patient?*

- Eliminate foods, if any, that the patient feels may exacerbate his symptoms (e.g., milk products in a lactase-deficient patient).
- Provide instructions for a well-balanced, heart-healthy diet that will prevent malnourishment. This should include instructions for weight reduction and contain about 2.4 g of sodium per day because of hypertension.
- Disease-state education is important (e.g., systemic disease manifestations to watch for, and the importance of regular follow-up with the physician).
- Surgical management is not indicated at this time as the patient has no evidence of dysplastic cells noted in the colonoscopy report.

b. *What feasible pharmacotherapeutic alternatives should be considered for the treatment of ulcerative colitis?*

- Drug therapy for ulcerative colitis is usually initiated with one of the following medications: sulfasalazine; a mesalamine derivative (rectal enema or suppository, or oral dosage form); or corticosteroids (oral, parenteral, rectal). The choice of agents is guided by the extent and severity of disease, patient dosage form preference, patient financial status, and perceived patient tolerance of potential adverse drug effects.
- *Sulfasalazine,* a combination of sulfapyridine and mesalamine, is available in tablet and suspension formulations. The mesalamine is cleaved by gut bacteria from the sulfapyridine molecule in the colon. This is the oldest of the mesalamine derivatives used to treat ulcerative colitis and is effective for active mild to moderate, distal and extensive colonic disease. It is also effective for maintenance of remission. The sulfapyridine molecule is not the active component of this drug, but it is responsible for many of the side effects such as nausea, dyspepsia, anorexia, and headache; this medication may not be as well tolerated as the newer agents.[2] Based on the listed AWP price of the tablets, this is the least expensive mesalamine product available. The enteric-coated tablets are more expensive than the regular formulation but may decrease the incidence of dyspepsia. Approximately 80% of patients unable to tolerate sulfasalazine are able to tolerate mesalamine or olsalazine.
- *Oral mesalamine preparations (Pentasa and Asacol)* contain mesalamine in special formulations that allow the drug to reach the site of action in the colon. Asacol tablets have pH-dependent characteristics that release the drug primarily in the distal ileum and colon. Pentasa is a controlled-release capsule that releases drug continuously from the duodenum to the rectum. These drugs are more expensive than sulfasalazine but may be better tolerated and are acceptable alternatives for patients with mild to moderate, distal or extensive disease to achieve and maintain remission.
- *Rectal mesalamine preparations (Rowasa suppository and enema)* are also available. Mesalamine suppositories are effective in the treatment of active proctitis and for maintenance of remission. Mesalamine enemas are effective in inducing and maintaining remission in mild to moderate active disease extending up to the splenic flexure. In appropriate doses, mesalamine enemas have been shown to be more successful than hydrocortisone enemas in inducing remission. Use of topical therapy may be limited by the patient's acceptance of this route.

- *Olsalazine (Dipentum)* is two molecules of mesalamine linked by an azo bond. It has been used to achieve remission in acute disease. This drug requires the presence of colonic bacteria to be effective, and its use for remission induction is limited by dose-dependent diarrhea. It is currently FDA-approved in lower dosages for the maintenance of remission.
- *Balsalazide,* mesalamine linked to an inert carrier, is pending FDA approval for the treatment of acute ulcerative colitis. It should also be an acceptable alternative to sulfasalazine or the other oral mesalamine preparations.
- *Oral, rectal, or parenteral corticosteroids* may be used. The choice of product depends upon the location and severity of the disease. Corticosteroids, regardless of route, are not effective in maintaining remission of the disease and should not be used for this indication.
  - ✓ *Rectal steroids* are available in the United States as a 100-mg/60 mL hydrocortisone retention enema (Cortenema) and 10% hydrocortisone foam (Cortifoam). These products are effective for inducing remission of distal colitis. The foam formulation reaches 15 to 20 cm distally from the rectum and the enema reaches up to the splenic flexure. Therefore, the extent of the disease needs to be taken into account when choosing one of these products. An advantage of topical therapy is often a faster response time, but some patients may feel that this route is unacceptable.
  - ✓ *Oral steroids* are effective for disease throughout the colon but are generally reserved for mild to moderate, extensive, active disease in patients who are resistant to oral mesalamine therapy with or without topical therapy, due to the severity of side effects.
  - ✓ *Parenteral corticosteroids* should be reserved for (1) severe colitis refractory to oral steroids or oral and topical mesalamine products, or (2) patients who present with toxicity, manifested by fever, anemia, tachycardia, or elevated ESR. If the patient responds to 7 to 10 days of parenteral corticosteroids, the patient should be switched to oral therapy.
- *Transdermal nicotine patches* added to mesalamine preparations or low dose corticosteroid therapy have been shown to result in an increased rate of remission and symptom control in patients with active ulcerative colitis.[3]

Optimal Plan

4. a. *Based on your current assessment of the patient's disease severity, recommend an appropriate drug regimen.*

- This patient is classified as having acute disease of moderate severity (more than four stools daily with minimal signs of toxicity) with extensive inflammation (extending proximal to the splenic flexure).[2]
- Due to the patient's allergy to sulfa drugs, sulfasalazine should not be used. In non-allergic patients, daily doses of 4 to 6 g, starting initially with low doses, may be used to achieve remission. This agent is cheaper than the newer mesalamine derivatives and has a long history of use, but it may not be as well tolerated as the newer agents.
- Appropriate initial therapy would consist of an oral mesalamine derivative such as Asacol 800 mg three times a day for 6 weeks or Pentasa 1 g four times a day for up to 8 weeks, depending on patient course and physical exam. Olsalazine tablets may be used, but many practitioners avoid this preparation for remission induction due to dose-related diarrhea that may be confused with a lack of efficacy.
- The mesalamine rectal enema may not provide adequate therapy in this patient because it delivers drug only as far proximally as the splenic flexure; this patient has involvement of the transverse colon. Also, some patients find daily use of an enema to be uncomfortable and inconvenient. Use of the mesalamine rectal suppository is limited to disease reaching approximately 10 cm (i.e., the sigmoid colon and rectum).
- Initial use of systemic corticosteroids should be avoided in moderate, extensive ulcerative colitis because of adverse drug effects.
- Nicotine patches have primarily been investigated in patients who are already receiving mesalamine or corticosteroid therapy. They should probably be reserved for future use in this patient.

b. *What alternatives should be considered if the patient fails to respond to initial therapy?*

- Substitute prednisone 20 to 60 mg orally each morning until significant clinical improvement is observed; 60 mg/day is slightly more effective than 40 mg/day, although the incidence of side effects may be increased.[2] Once improvement is observed, the prednisone should be tapered. The timetable for tapering varies; one suggested regimen is to decrease the dose by 5 to 10 mg weekly until a daily dose of 20 mg is reached. This is then followed by a subsequent dosage decrease of 2.5 mg/week until discontinuation.[2] If the patient is unable to be tapered completely off prednisone without reactivation of the disease, oral azathioprine in dosages of 1.5 to 2 mg/kg/day has been shown to be helpful in controlling the disease process. The onset of azathioprine's effect is slow; up to 3 to 6 months of therapy may be needed to achieve optimal results.
- As an alternative to oral corticosteroids, the patient may be continued on current therapy with the addition of one rectal mesalamine 4 g enema every night for 3 to 6 weeks.
- If the disease worsens, patients with acute, severe, extensive ulcerative colitis have received IV cyclosporine in doses of 4 mg/kg/day after failing to respond to 7 to 10 days of IV corticosteroids. This has not been used for long-term therapy because of side effects.[2]

Outcome Evaluation

5. *What clinical and laboratory parameters are necessary to evaluate the therapy for achievement of the desired therapeutic outcome and to detect or prevent adverse effects?*

Achievement of Desired Outcomes

- The patient should experience resolution of active disease signs and symptoms (return to normal bowel habits, resolution of abdominal tenderness, no blood in the stool). This can be assessed at the patient's next clinic appointment or medication refill. The patient should expect to see significant improvement 2 to 4 weeks after therapy initiation. If symptoms increase or do not significantly improve, the patient should be instructed to contact his physician.

Ulcerative Colitis

- The patient should be able to return to daily functions he may not have been able to perform due to weakness and the increased number of bowel movements. He should be questioned at the next clinic appointment or medication refill.
- The patient's quality of life should be assessed with an appropriate evaluation tool such as the Inflammatory Bowel Disease Questionnaire.[4] The evaluation should be repeated after 4 to 8 weeks of mesalamine therapy.
- The patient should develop no disease complications (e.g., arthritis, abnormal LFTs). The patient should be reexamined after the completion of the initial treatment course of mesalamine. Another physical examination should be performed and AST, ALT, and alkaline phosphatase values should be obtained in the event of a relapse.

Prevention or Detection of Adverse Effects
- Oral mesalamine can cause diarrhea, nausea, dyspepsia, abdominal pain, flatulence, headaches, dizziness, arthralgias, and myalgias. These effects usually disappear with continued treatment; the patient should notify the physician if symptoms worsen or do not improve within 1 to 4 weeks of initiating therapy. Mesalamine can also cause an acute intolerance syndrome (cramping, acute abdominal pain, bloody diarrhea, fever, headache, malaise and rash), skin rash, and itching. The patient should stop taking the medication immediately and notify the physician if these effects occur.
- Rectal mesalamine can cause rectal irritation (bleeding, blistering, pain, burning, itching) in addition to gas/flatulence, fever, and flu-like symptoms.
- Prednisone can cause mood disorders (confusion, hallucinations, depression, or sudden and large mood swings), GI problems (abdominal pain, black tarry stools, bleeding), immunosuppression and infections, increased WBC, hyperglycemia, hypertension, weight gain, sodium and water retention, osteonecrosis, and osteoporosis.

Patient Counseling

6. *What information should be provided to the patient to enhance adherence, ensure successful therapy, and minimize adverse effects?*

Oral or Rectal Mesalamine
- You have been prescribed mesalamine to treat your ulcerative colitis. Please let your physician and pharmacist know if you have ever had an allergic reaction to mesalamine, olsalazine, sulfasalazine, or aspirin. You state that you have an allergic reaction to sulfa drugs; this means that you should not receive sulfasalazine but you should be able to take mesalamine products.
- You must continue to take this medication until your physician either changes your dose or discontinues the medication; this is important even if you feel better. If you miss a dose, take it as soon as you remember, but if it is almost time for your next dose, skip the missed dose. Do not double doses.
- This medicine should be kept out of moist places such as the bathroom. It should also be stored out of direct sunlight and heat. Keep this and all other medications away from children.
- You may experience the following side effects: nausea, gas, mild stomach pain, headache, or rash. Notify your physician if these are severe. Notify your physician immediately if you experience cramping, acute abdominal pain, bloody diarrhea and fever.
  - ✓ *Asacol.* Take two 400-mg tablets three times a day for up to 6 weeks. Swallow these tablets whole; do not break the outer coating, which is designed to protect the active ingredient. Take this medication by mouth before meals and at bedtime with a full glass of water, unless otherwise directed by your physician. You may find what appear to be intact tablets in the stool. This is most likely the empty shell that is left after the medicine has been absorbed. Notify your physician if this occurs repeatedly.
  - ✓ *Pentasa.* Take four 250-mg capsules four times a day for up to 8 weeks. Swallow the capsules whole. Take this medication by mouth before meals and at bedtime with a full glass of water, unless otherwise directed by your physician. You may find what appear to be small beads in your stool. These are most likely empty after the medicine has been absorbed. Notify your physician if this occurs repeatedly.
  - ✓ *Rowasa rectal suspension.* Instill one bottle (4 g) each night at bedtime and try to retain it at least 8 hours to allow maximum contact with the affected area of the colon. It is best if you empty your bowel just prior to instillation. Remove the bottle from the protective foil pouch and the protective sheath from the applicator tip. Follow the instructions for medication administration included with the enema. Shake the bottle to make sure it is thoroughly mixed before using. Do not use the enema if the bottle's contents are dark brown. This product contains sulfites to which some people are allergic. Notify your physician immediately if you notice hives, itching, wheezing, or have trouble breathing. This preparation may stain clothing, painted surfaces, marble, granite, vinyl or any other surface with which it comes in contact.

Prednisone
- You have been prescribed oral prednisone tablets to treat your ulcerative colitis. Take this medicine by mouth with food in the morning, unless otherwise directed by your physician. Do not exceed the dose prescribed by your physician.
- Do not stop taking this abruptly without consulting your physician; this is important even if you feel better. Notify any other health care professional, such as your dentist, that you are receiving prednisone before you undergo any procedures. You may wish to obtain a medical identification bracelet, necklace, or card stating that you are using prednisone.
- If you miss a dose, take it as soon as you remember; if it is almost time for your next dose, skip the missed dose. Do not double doses.
- This medicine should be kept out of moist places such as the bathroom and out of direct sunlight and heat. Keep this and all other medications away from children.
- This medication may increase your susceptibility to infections. Check with your physician as soon as possible if you notice symptoms such as a sore throat, sneezing, fever, or coughing. Do not receive any vaccines without your physician's prior approval.
- This medication may cause water and salt retention, and you should monitor your blood pressure regularly. Your physician may also want you to watch your calories to prevent weight gain in addition to following a low-salt, potassium-rich diet.
- Notify your doctor if you experience any other side effects. Keep all follow-up appointments with your physician.

Follow-up Questions

1. *Considering this new information, what therapeutic intervention(s) do you recommend at this time?*

   - Feasible therapeutic options include: (1) discontinue therapy and monitor the patient for signs and symptoms of recurrence, or (2) institute drug therapy to maintain remission. Three-fourths of patients not receiving therapy will relapse within 1 year. The patient should be involved in the decision-making process; however, initiation of maintenance therapy in this patient should be strongly considered.
   - Sulfasalazine has been shown to be effective, but this is not an option in this patient due to his allergy profile. Acceptable maintenance therapy includes olsalazine 500 mg orally twice a day, Pentasa 4 g daily in divided doses, or Asacol 1.2 to 2.4 g daily in divided doses. It may be preferable to avoid the use of the enema and suppository formulations for patient convenience.
   - Corticosteroids and transdermal nicotine patches should not be used for maintenance of remission.[2,5] Refer to the textbook chapter for more detailed information on maintenance regimens.

2. *What additional information should be provided to the patient?*

   - The mesalamine preparation is now being used to help prevent your disease from relapsing. You will be taking this drug for as long as your physician prescribes it and potentially for the rest of your life. Be sure to take it as directed and refill the prescription on time.
   - Notify your doctor if you experience recurring symptoms of the disease such as diarrhea, abdominal tenderness, or blood in your stool, or if you experience side effects with the drug.
   - Keep all follow-up appointments with your physician, who will evaluate your disease and determine if alternative interventions are necessary.
   - If taking olsalazine: Take this medicine with food to prevent upset stomach.

References

1. Motley RJ, Rhodes J, Ford GA, et al. Time relationships between cessation of smoking and onset of ulcerative colitis. Digestion 1987;37:125–127.
2. Kornbluth A, Sachar DB. Ulcerative colitis practice guidelines in adults. American College of Gastroenterology, Practice Parameters Committee. Am J Gastroenterol 1997; 92:204–211.
3. Sandborn WJ, Tremaine WJ, Offord KP, et al. Transdermal nicotine for mildly to moderately active ulcerative colitis: A randomized, double-blind, placebo-controlled trial. Ann Intern Med 1997;126:364–371.
4. Guyatt G, Mitchell A, Irvine EJ, et al. A new measure of health status for clinical trials in inflammatory bowel disease. Gastroenterology 1989;96:804–810.
5. Thomas GA, Rhodes J, Mani V, et al. Transdermal nicotine as maintenance therapy for ulcerative colitis. N Engl J Med 1995;332:988–992.

27 NAUSEA AND VOMITING

▶ **Jill's Bicycle and Other Cycles**   (Level II)

Amy J. Becker, PharmD

A 36-year-old woman who received her first cycle of CMF chemotherapy for breast cancer 2 days ago returns to the clinic because of nausea and vomiting that started 18 hours after the chemotherapy. Although she had received appropriate pre-chemotherapy antiemetics, she neglected to fill the prescriptions for breakthrough nausea and vomiting. Medical evaluation reveals signs of dehydration and hypokalemia. In addition to fluid and electrolyte repletion, the patient requires adequate treatment of her ongoing vomiting episode, prevention of anticipatory vomiting prior to the next chemotherapy cycle, a more effective pre-chemotherapy antiemetic regimen, and the addition of post-chemotherapy antiemetics for several days after each cycle. The case questions require students to consider the available options for each of these situations and select optimal regimens based on efficacy, side effects, and cost.

Questions

Problem Identification

1. a. *Create a list of this patient's drug-related problems.*

   - Breast cancer, treated with lumpectomy, radiation, and adjuvant CMF chemotherapy.
   - Chemotherapy-related nausea and vomiting due to ineffective antiemetic regimen.
   - Nausea and vomiting requiring acute treatment with antiemetics.
   - Dehydration and hypokalemia secondary to vomiting, requiring fluid and potassium replacement.
   - Migraine headache, inadequately treated, possibly contributing to her nausea and vomiting.
   - Use of phosphate and hydroxyapatite without indication.
   - Sulfa allergy.

   b. *What are this patient's risk factors for nausea and vomiting?*

   - Cyclophosphamide-based chemotherapy; the revised CMF regimen causes emesis in 80% of patients who do not receive pre-chemotherapy antiemetics.[1]
   - Female gender; women experience about 10% more post-chemotherapy nausea and vomiting than men.[2]
   - Young age; women under the age of 50 may experience significantly more post-chemotherapy nausea and vomiting than older women.[3]

- No significant alcohol use; patients with histories of heavy alcohol use generally have much less nausea and vomiting after chemotherapy than patients who report modest or no alcohol use.[3]

Desired Outcome

2. *What are the goals of therapy in this case?*

- Replacement of fluids and electrolytes (primarily sodium, chloride, and potassium)
- Adequate treatment of her acute nausea and vomiting
- Treatment of her migraine headache
- Prevention of acute nausea and vomiting after future chemotherapy doses
- Prevention of anticipatory nausea and vomiting prior to future doses of chemotherapy
- Minimization of adverse effects of antiemetics
- Preservation of quality of life (maintenance of usual performance status, appetite, ability to socialize)
- Provision of cost-effective control of chemotherapy-induced nausea and vomiting

Therapeutic Alternatives

3. a. *What non-drug therapies may be useful to prevent nausea and vomiting?*

- Eating light meals, avoiding spicy or fatty foods, avoiding foods with strong odors
- Diversions such as music, reading, games, and videos
- Relaxation, hypnosis, guided mental imagery

b. *What pharmacologic alternatives may be helpful for the acute treatment of this patient?*

Fluid and Electrolyte Replacement

- This could be accomplished with 2 to 4 L of D5NS with KCl 20 to 40 mEq/L IV over 4 to 6 hours. D5NS with KCl is chosen because it provides fluid in addition to replacing the electrolytes that have been lost (i.e., sodium, potassium, and chloride). The dextrose is included to provide carbohydrates, since this patient has not been eating due to her vomiting.
- The volume of fluid, the composition of the fluid, and the rate of infusion may vary depending on the severity of the patient's signs and symptoms and the extent of her laboratory abnormalities. Because she is vomiting, oral fluid and electrolyte replacement is not an option.

Treatment of Acute Nausea and Vomiting

- The plan for this should take into account the two possible etiologies of this problem: chemotherapy and migraine. Options include a phenothiazine, a butyrophenone, or a substituted benzamide, plus a corticosteroid.[1] 5-HT_3 antagonists are another option, but they have the disadvantages of high cost (at least 10 to 15 times the cost of the other antiemetics), and lack of published data on their use as rescue antiemetics. Examples of treatment plans for this patient include:
  - ✓ Prochlorperazine 10 mg IV + dexamethasone 10 to 20 mg IV, repeated in 6 hours if needed
  - ✓ Droperidol 2.5 to 5 mg IV + dexamethasone 10 to 20 mg IV, repeated in 4 hours if needed
  - ✓ Metoclopramide 1 mg/kg IV + dexamethasone 10 to 20 mg IV, repeated in 2 hours if needed

  Some clinicians would add diphenhydramine 25 to 50 mg IV or lorazepam 1 to 2 mg IV to prevent extrapyramidal reactions from the non-steroid component.

c. *What therapeutic alternatives should be considered prior to her next cycle of chemotherapy to prevent future episodes of nausea and vomiting?*

- This patient may be at risk for anticipatory nausea and vomiting before her next cycle of chemotherapy. Lorazepam 0.5 to 1 mg po prior to coming to the clinic may be beneficial.[1]
- The plan for prevention of acute nausea and vomiting after her next cycle of chemotherapy should involve a review of her pre-chemotherapy antiemetics prior to cycle 1. Since CMF has an emetogenicity rating of 4 (on a scale of 1 to 5, with 5 being the most emetogenic), this patient appropriately received a 5-HT_3 antagonist and a corticosteroid as premedication for cycle 1.[2,3]
- These same agents should be given prior to cycle 2, with the addition of a third agent with a different mechanism of action, such as a phenothiazine or a butyrophenone. Examples of such a combination include:
  - ✓ Granisetron 2 mg po + dexamethasone 10 to 20 mg po + prochlorperazine 10 mg po
  - ✓ Granisetron 10 μg/kg IV + dexamethasone 10 to 20 mg IV + prochlorperazine 10 mg IV
  - ✓ Ondansetron 32 mg IV + dexamethasone 10 to 20 mg IV + prochlorperazine 10 mg IV
  - ✓ Dolasetron 100 mg IV + dexamethasone 10 to 20 mg IV + prochlorperazine 10 mg IV

  Haloperidol 1 to 5 mg po or droperidol 2.5 to 5 mg IV could be used in place of prochlorperazine.

- Another strategy that should be considered is to have her take additional antiemetics on a scheduled basis for several days, starting in the evening of the day she receives her chemotherapy. Examples include:
  - ✓ Metoclopramide 10 mg po + dexamethasone 4 mg po BID–TID for 3 to 5 days
  - ✓ Prochlorperazine 10 mg po + dexamethasone 4 mg po BID–TID for 3 to 5 days
  - ✓ Ondansetron 8 mg po + dexamethasone 4 mg po BID for 3 to 5 days

- She should continue to take propranolol and Midrin for her migraines. She should call the clinic if her headaches increase in frequency or severity.

Optimal Plan

4. a. *Design a plan for the treatment of acute nausea and vomiting in this patient.*

- For control of her acute nausea and vomiting, either the prochlorperazine regimen or the metoclopramide regimen would be preferred because both of these drugs are also effective for the treatment of migraine headache.

- The droperidol regimen or a 5-HT$_3$ antagonist could be used, but additional medication for treatment of her migraine would need to be added.

b. *Design a plan for the prevention of nausea and vomiting in this patient.*

- Benzodiazepines are the drugs of choice for prevention of anticipatory nausea and vomiting. However, she should be cautioned against driving if she takes a benzodiazepine prior to her clinic visit.
- For prevention of nausea and vomiting after her next cycle of CMF chemotherapy, the combination of oral granisetron, oral dexamethasone, and oral prochlorperazine would be preferred over the IV combinations. In this situation, the oral agents are just as efficacious as the IV agents, they are more convenient to administer, and they are less expensive.[4]
- The choice of post-chemotherapy antiemetics to be taken on a scheduled basis may be determined by cost and side effects. The regimens that include a phenothiazine or metoclopramide may cause unacceptable sedation in a patient such as this, who wishes to maintain her work and exercise routine as much as possible. On the other hand, the cost of the regimen that includes the 5-HT$_3$ antagonist may be as much as 50 times the cost of the other regimens.

Outcome Evaluation

5. a. *State how you will determine whether the antiemetic regimen you recommended for her acute treatment has been effective.*

   - After treatment for her acute nausea and vomiting, the patient should be instructed to call the clinic if she has a recurrence of nausea or vomiting that does not respond to the antiemetics that she has at home.
   - After her next course of chemotherapy, a follow-up phone call may help to detect problems early.

   b. *Describe the information you will need to assess the efficacy and adverse effects of the prophylactic antiemetic regimen prior to each future course of chemotherapy.*

   Prior to each course of chemotherapy, her chart should be reviewed for additional information and the patient should be interviewed to assess the following parameters:

   ### Efficacy
   - The presence and severity of anticipatory, acute, or delayed nausea
   - The number of episodes of anticipatory, acute, or delayed vomiting or retching
   - The effectiveness of PRN antiemetics in relieving nausea and/or vomiting
   - Her performance status (better, worse, or the same as it was prior to chemotherapy)
   - Appetite (better, worse, or the same as it was prior to chemotherapy)
   - Her satisfaction with her antiemetic regimen (whether it worked as well as she had hoped, with tolerable side effects)

Adverse Effects
- 5-HT$_3$ receptor antagonists: headache, constipation, diarrhea
- Butyrophenones: sedation, extrapyramidal effects (akathisia, dystonia)
- Metoclopramide: sedation, extrapyramidal effects (akathisia, dystonia), diarrhea
- Phenothiazines: sedation, extrapyramidal effects (akathisia, dystonia)
- Benzodiazepines: sedation, memory disturbances
- Corticosteroids: mood swings, hunger, insomnia

Patient Counseling

6. *How would you counsel this patient on her antiemetic regimen?*

   ### General Information
   - Even though the intravenous medicines that we have given you today have stopped your nausea and vomiting, it will be important for you to continue to take your oral medications whenever you start to feel nauseated.
   - Before and after your next chemotherapy, you will be taking some medications to prevent nausea and vomiting. These medications work best when you take them to prevent the nausea and vomiting from occurring, rather than waiting until you are very uncomfortable.

   ### Lorazepam
   - For each course of your chemotherapy, take one lorazepam tablet before you come to the clinic. This will help to prevent you from getting sick to your stomach before you receive the chemotherapy. You can also take one of these tablets as often as every 4 hours after your chemotherapy if you have nausea or vomiting.
   - Lorazepam may cause drowsiness, so make sure you know how you react to it before you drive, use machines, or do other things that require you to be fully alert. In addition, this medication can sometimes cause short-term memory problems.

   ### Pre-chemotherapy Regimen
   - About 30 minutes before your chemotherapy, we will give you 3 medications to prevent nausea and vomiting. These medications are granisetron (or ondansetron or dolasetron) and dexamethasone (or prednisone) and prochlorperazine (or metoclopramide).
   - You will also be taking the dexamethasone and prochlorperazine (or metoclopramide or ondansetron) on a daily basis for several days after your chemotherapy to help prevent a recurrence of the severe nausea and vomiting you had after your first course.
     - ✓ Granisetron (or ondansetron or dolasetron). This medication sometimes causes headaches. It is okay to take acetaminophen if this occurs. Other side effects that happen infrequently include mild constipation or diarrhea.
     - ✓ Dexamethasone (or prednisone). This medicine can cause mood swings, increased appetite, and hyperactivity. These effects are only temporary and will disappear once you finish the medication.
     - ✓ Prochlorperazine. The main side effect of this medication is drowsiness. Make sure you know how you react to it before you drive, use machinery, or do other things that require you to be fully alert. It may also cause your mouth to be dry. Call

your doctor if you have any uncontrolled movements or unusual restlessness.

✓ Metoclopramide. This medication also causes drowsiness, so the same precautions discussed earlier apply. Diarrhea sometimes occurs, but it is usually not severe. Call your doctor if you have any uncontrolled movements or unusual restlessness.

- If you experience any nausea or vomiting after your chemotherapy, you should take one of your lorazepam tablets or a prochlorperazine (or metoclopramide) tablet. You will also have some prochlorperazine suppositories to use if you are unable to keep the tablets down. You can take the prochlorperazine (or metoclopramide) tablets every 6 hours as needed. The suppositories should only be used every 12 hours as needed.
- Call the clinic right away if you have vomiting despite having taken your medications.
- Just to make sure that I have not left anything out, please tell me about each of your medications for nausea and vomiting.
- If you have any problems with your medications or if you think of additional questions after you get home, please feel free to call me. Here is a card with my name and phone number on it.

References

1. Hesketh PJ, Kris MG, Grunberg SM, et al. Proposal for classifying the acute emetogenicity of cancer chemotherapy. J Clin Oncol 1997;15:103–109.
2. Osoba D, Zee B, Pater J, et al. Determinants of postchemotherapy nausea and vomiting in patients with cancer. Quality of Life and Symptom Control Committees of the National Cancer Institute of Canada Clinical Trials Group. J Clin Oncol 1997;15:116–123.
3. Grunberg SM, Hesketh PJ. Control of chemotherapy-induced emesis. N Engl J Med 1993;329:1790–1796.
4. Nolte MJ, Berkery R, Pizzo B, et al. Assuring the optimal use of serotonin antagonist antiemetics: The process for development and implementation of institutional antiemetic guidelines at Memorial Sloan-Kettering Cancer Center. J Clin Oncol 1998;16:771–778.

28 DIARRHEA

▶ Accentuation of Evacuation (Level I)

Marie A. Abate, PharmD
Charles D. Ponte, BS, PharmD, BCPS, CDE, FAPhA, FASHP, FCCP

A 2-day history of nausea, vomiting, diarrhea, and mild fever causes a 28-year-old woman to seek treatment at an outpatient clinic. Her medications include glyburide and metformin for type 2 diabetes mellitus and OTC Maalox, which she has been taking recently for nausea. Physical exam findings indicate the presence of dehydration, and the patient is hospitalized for several days. The case requires students to ask questions to obtain the additional information needed for a complete patient assessment. Treatment modalities should be directed toward replacement of fluid and electrolyte losses, dietary interventions, discontinuation of any offending drugs, and provision of symptomatic relief with antidiarrheal compounds. Because the patient is also hyperglycemic, attention must be given to proper management of her diabetes during the acute phase of the illness.

▶ Questions

Problem Identification

1. a. *Create a list of the patient's drug-related problems.*

    - Diarrhea, requiring fluids and possibly other symptomatic treatment.
    - Nausea, vomiting, and fever, possibly requiring symptomatic treatment.
    - Orthostasis and dehydration (secondary to diarrhea, vomiting and fever), requiring fluid replacement.
    - Hyperglycemia, possibly requiring medication dosage adjustment.

   b. *What signs and symptoms does this woman have that indicate the presence or severity of the diarrhea?*

    - Six to eight liquid stools since yesterday
    - Cramping with bowel movements
    - Dry mucous membranes
    - Drop in BP, increased pulse upon standing (orthostatic changes); weakness and dizziness upon standing
    - Temperature of 38°C
    - Decreased urination, amber-colored urine, and high urine specific gravity indicating intravascular volume depletion
    - Symptom duration of about 48 hours

   c. *What questions should you ask the patient or members of the medical team to obtain the additional information needed for a complete assessment of this patient?*

   NOTE TO INSTRUCTORS: *The questions that follow also have the answers provided. After you discuss the reason for asking each question with the students, provide them with the response given by the patient or members of the medical team.*

    - Could a parasitic infection be responsible for this patient's diarrhea?

        ✓ This is a possibility. A stool specimen was obtained upon admission for culture and examination for ova, parasites, and WBC/RBC. Eosinophilia may result from parasitic infections but is absent in this case.

    - What else has the patient eaten over the past 48 hours? Has anyone who has dined with her during this time also complained of the same symptoms? This will help you to determine whether bacteria from contaminated food (e.g., *E. coli, Staphylococcus, Salmonella, Shigella*) could be responsible for the diarrhea. If others who ate the same food have similar diarrhea symptoms, then bacteria become a more likely cause.

- ✓ She had cereal for breakfast and a peanut butter sandwich for lunch the day her symptoms began. Her boyfriend ate the pizza with her, and he has felt fine.

- Has she complained of similar diarrhea episodes in the past? This would allow you to determine whether the diarrhea is acute or chronic in nature.

- ✓ She last experienced a diarrhea episode when she had the "flu" about a year ago.

- How frequent is the vomiting? The nausea and vomiting help support an infectious cause (e.g., viral) and could result in a greater risk of fluid depletion and electrolyte abnormalities.

- ✓ She vomited twice yesterday but only once today (earlier in the morning).

- How often has she been using the Maalox? Frequent use or high doses of the antacid could result in diarrhea from the magnesium component.

- ✓ She has taken about two tablespoonfuls per day for the past three days when the symptoms began.

- Is she taking any other OTC medication? It is possible that a patient could be taking a product (e.g., a different antacid) that might cause diarrhea.

- ✓ She is taking no other OTC drugs.

- Does she have a history of lactose intolerance? Since the symptoms began after eating cheese pizza, lactose intolerance could cause diarrhea. However, the other symptoms (e.g., vomiting, fever) are not consistent with lactose intolerance.

- ✓ She has no history of lactose intolerance.

d. *Could any of this patient's problems have been caused by drug therapy?*

- *Maalox* is an antacid containing magnesium hydroxide and aluminum hydroxide. Although it might seem that the GI effects of the magnesium (diarrhea) and the aluminum (constipation) would negate each other, diarrhea tends to predominate with high doses. The magnesium component could be contributing to the diarrhea.
- *Metformin* can also cause GI symptoms including nausea, vomiting, and diarrhea. These are most common during therapy initiation or after dosage increases and tend to resolve with continued therapy. Since this patient's GI symptoms were of acute onset and she had been taking the metformin for 6 months, metformin-induced diarrhea is an unlikely cause of her current complaints.
- The patient does not have a history of recent antibiotic use; antibiotics could cause diarrhea or colitis and should always be ruled out as a cause of these problems.

e. *What are other possible causes of this patient's diarrhea?*

- *Infectious (bacterial or viral)*. Although nothing in her case clearly indicates an infectious cause, this is still a possibility.
- *Chronic underlying disease state*. She has Type 2 diabetes mellitus, which can produce diarrhea in some patients. It is thought to be primarily neuropathic in origin. The diarrhea resulting from diabetes is usually chronic and generally occurs in patients with long-standing diabetes.[1] Thus, since this patient has only had diabetes for 5 years and this was an acute episode of diarrhea, the cause is unlikely to be the diabetes. The possibility of AIDS in a sexually active individual should also be considered since infectious diarrhea can develop in these patients. However, the acute onset of the current problems combined with a single sexual partner rule against AIDS. The HIV status of the patient can be checked to eliminate this as a possibility.

Desired Outcome

2. *What are the goals of therapy for this patient?*

- Rehydrate the patient
- Prevent further excessive water and electrolyte losses and acid-base disturbances
- Provide symptomatic relief
- Manage any underlying causes of the diarrhea
- Provide better control of the diabetes (a secondary goal)

Therapeutic Alternatives

3. a. *What types of non-drug therapy should be considered for this patient?*

- Dietary management (refer to the section on Treatment in textbook Chapter 34 for more detailed information):
  - ✓ Stopping solid foods for 24 hours or eating a digestible, low-residue diet for 24 hours, then gradual resumption of patient's diabetic diet
  - ✓ Rehydration and maintenance of water and electrolytes. Use of IV fluids with electrolytes (e.g., normal saline with KCl) if the patient is dehydrated and in the hospital, or oral rehydration solutions for outpatients; this is critical if the frequency and severity of the diarrhea increase
- Management of any underlying causes
- Discontinuation or dosage reduction of Maalox

b. *What feasible pharmacotherapeutic alternatives are available for treatment of diarrhea in this patient?*

- *Antimotility agents* (e.g., opiates and opioid derivatives including loperamide and diphenoxylate/atropine) are effective in relieving diarrhea and cramping and are easy to administer.[2] However, they may worsen an invasive bacterial infection of colon and may cause drowsiness and constipation.
- *Adsorbents* (e.g., *attapulgite, polycarbophil, kaolin, pectin*) are also effective in relieving diarrhea with minimal side effects. However, dosages required are often large and less convenient to administer. These drugs can also bind other substances such as drugs in the GI tract and may cause abdominal bloating or fullness.

- *Antisecretory compounds* (e.g., *bismuth subsalicylate*) are effective for preventing bacteria-induced diarrhea (e.g., traveler's diarrhea). They are less convenient to administer due to frequent dosing. The salicylate content is a concern in children, patients already receiving large dosages of salicylates, those with aspirin sensitivity, and patients taking other medications that interact with aspirin (e.g., anticoagulants). Bismuth may cause dark-colored stools (which could be confused with melena).
- *Antibiotics* (e.g., *trimethoprim/sulfamethoxazole, fluoroquinolones*) are effective by treating infection if bacteria are responsible for diarrhea. Conversely, they are ineffective if bacteria are not responsible for the diarrhea. Side effects vary depending on the antibiotic used and generally occur more frequently than with the other antidiarrheal agents listed.

Optimal Plan

4. *What non-drug interventions and specific pharmacotherapeutic regimens would you recommend for treating this patient's diarrhea?*

Refer to Textbook Figure 34–1 for more detailed information on treatment recommendations for acute diarrhea.

- *Eliminate contributory factors.* The contribution of drugs to the diarrhea should be considered. If the patient is taking frequent doses of the Maalox, the drug should be discontinued. If antacid use is still desired, consider the use of smaller doses or alternating doses of a magnesium-aluminum hydroxide-containing antacid with a pure aluminum hydroxide product.
- *Change diet temporarily.* Discontinue solid foods for 24 hours since nausea and vomiting are still present, and then begin clear oral liquids and a low residue diet for 24 hours.
- *Replace fluids.* This diabetic patient was admitted to the hospital because of the moderate to severe dehydration that was evident. Replace fluid/electrolyte losses with IV fluid administration (approximately 2 to 2.5 L of normal saline containing KCl 20 to 30 mEq/L adjusted depending upon serum potassium concentration). This volume should be increased if vomiting continues. If the patient remains hospitalized, fluid and electrolyte intake can be maintained with IV fluids until diarrhea stops. An oral rehydration solution should be used cautiously in this patient with close monitoring of blood glucose concentrations, since almost all of the oral rehydration products contain dextrose (although the amount is not usually enough to have a major impact on glucose control).
- *Provide symptomatic relief.* If symptomatic control of the diarrhea is desired (to reduce the discomfort and inconvenience), either loperamide or a polycarbophil product should be recommended. These are equally effective and appropriate for this patient.
  - ✓ *Loperamide* (e.g., Imodium AD caplets or generic versions) 4 mg initially followed by 2 mg after each unformed stool, not to exceed 16 mg/day (8 mg/day when self-medicating) for up to 48 hours
  - ✓ *Polycarbophil* (e.g., Equalactin) 1 g chewed every 30 minutes as needed, not to exceed 6 grams in 24 hours
  - ✓ Products containing *attapulgite* or *bismuth subsalicylate* could be used as alternatives
  - ✓ *Antibiotics* would only be indicated if a bacterial cause is identified

Outcome Evaluation

5. *What clinical and laboratory parameters are necessary to evaluate the diarrhea therapy for achievement of the desired outcome and to detect or prevent adverse effects?*

- Diarrhea is usually a self-limiting symptom of an underlying cause. If Maalox was a contributing factor, discontinuation of the drug should help relieve the diarrhea. Acute diarrhea should generally resolve within 72 hours; thus, the problem should lessen noticeably within the next 24 hours in this patient. Since a fever is present, an infectious cause should be considered and tested for (refer to textbook Figure 34–1). Other specific monitoring parameters include:
  - ✓ Bowel movement frequency and character (e.g., liquid, semi-formed) with each bowel movement
  - ✓ Blood pressure and pulse rate (to assess fluid status) during each hospital shift
  - ✓ Intake and output daily to assess fluid status
  - ✓ Body weight daily (for weight loss and to assess fluid status)
  - ✓ Serum electrolytes daily while diarrhea persists
  - ✓ Other signs of dehydration daily (e.g., dry mucous membranes, weakness or dizziness upon arising)
  - ✓ Body temperature with each hospital shift
  - ✓ Blood glucose concentration finger sticks four times daily (see Follow-Up Questions)

Patient Counseling

6. *What information should be provided to this patient to enhance adherence, ensure successful therapy, and minimize adverse effects?*

General Information
- If anorexia, nausea, vomiting, or diarrhea persist or recur after discharge from the hospital, consult your physician immediately.

Loperamide
- The drug may cause you to become sleepy. Determine how much this affects you before driving or performing other tasks that require you to be fully alert.
- Do not exceed the recommended maximum dosage of 8 mg per day (for self-management without a physician's approval) or use for more than 2 days.
- Do not use this medication if you develop a high fever or if blood appears in the stool.

Polycarbophil
- This product can be used for either diarrhea or constipation treatment. For diarrhea treatment, do not take the tablets with water. Do not exceed the recommended dosage.
- Do not use for more than 2 days; if diarrhea persists, contact your doctor.

▶ Follow-up Questions

1. *How should this patient's diabetes be managed while she is being treated in the hospital?*

- The current poor control of the diabetes could be a result of the acute illness as well as the inability to take (or fully absorb) her usual medications (particularly the glyburide) due to the vomiting.

- The oral glyburide and metformin should be discontinued, and a sliding scale of insulin can be used on a temporary basis for 1 to 2 days while she is in the hospital until the vomiting and diarrhea stop and her diet returns to normal. This can include finger sticks four times daily with regular insulin administered as follows:
  - ✓ 2 units for blood glucose concentrations of 200 to 250 mg/dL
  - ✓ 4 units for blood glucose concentrations of 251 to 300 mg/dL
  - ✓ 6 units for blood glucose concentrations of 301 to 350 mg/dL
  - ✓ 8 units for blood glucose concentrations of 351 to 400 mg/L
  - ✓ 10 units for blood glucose concentrations of >400 mg/dL.
- Her usual medications for diabetes can be resumed when her diet returns to normal.

2. *What interventions would you recommend for her diabetes control if the patient remains hyperglycemic after resolution of this acute illness and resumption of her normal medications?*

- Obtaining a $HgbA_{1c}$ value would provide insight into the patient's long-term glucose control. If this indicates that her disease is indeed poorly controlled, the patient should be questioned about her adherence to her diet and exercise programs as well as compliance with her medication regimen.
- If these programs seem to be in order, an increased drug dosage may be needed because of disease progression or secondary drug failure. Either the glyburide or metformin dose could be increased, as neither is at the maximum recommended daily dose (20 mg and 2550 mg/day, respectively).
- Although other antihyperglycemic agents are available (e.g., other sulfonylureas, acarbose, troglitazone, insulin), it would be premature at this time to recommend changing to an alternative agent.

References

1. Camilleri M. Gastrointestinal problems in diabetes. Endocrinol Metab Clin North Am 1996;25:361–378.
2. DuPont HL, Ericsson CD, DuPont MW, et al. A randomized, open-label comparison of nonprescription loperamide and attapulgite in the symptomatic treatment of acute diarrhea. Am J Med 1990;88(suppl 6A):20S–23S.

29 PEDIATRIC GASTROENTERITIS

▶ Dihydrogen Monoxide and Other Critical Elements (Level II)

William McGhee, PharmD
Basil J. Zitelli, MD, FAAP

A 5-day history of vomiting, diarrhea, and other symptoms causes a young mother to seek medical attention at the ED for her 5-month-old son. The patient has signs of moderate dehydration on physical and laboratory examination. The presumed diagnosis is viral gastroenteritis probably caused by rotavirus. Students should understand that replacement of fluid and electrolyte losses is critical to the effective treatment of acute diarrhea. Oral rehydration therapy with carbohydrate-based solutions is the primary treatment of diarrhea in children with mild to moderate dehydration. Intravenous fluids may be needed for cases of severe dehydration. Early feeding of patients with an age-appropriate diet helps to reduce stool volume after completion of rehydration therapy. Although antidiarrheal products are available, they have limited effectiveness, can cause adverse effects, and may shift attention from appropriate fluid and electrolyte replacement.

▶ Questions

Problem Identification

1. a. *Create a list of the patient's drug-related problems.*

   - This patient has typical viral gastroenteritis, probably rotavirus infection, which is characterized by the acute onset of emesis, progressing to watery diarrhea with diminishing emesis. Rotavirus is the most common cause of pediatric gastroenteritis in the U.S., accounting for 25% of cases. Other common viruses include Norwalk-like viruses and adenovirus.[1] Rotavirus is transmitted by the fecal–oral route. Infection occurs when ingested virus infects enterocytes in the small intestine, leading to cell death and loss of brush border digestive enzymes. Approximately 48 hours after exposure, infected children develop fever, vomiting, and watery diarrhea. Fever and vomiting usually subside in 1 to 2 days, but diarrhea can continue for several days leading to significant dehydration. Approximately 65% of hospitalizations and 85% of diarrhea-related deaths occur in the first year of life.
   - The patient has moderate dehydration (acute weight loss of 8%, from 7.1 kg to 6.5 kg) as well as clinical and laboratory evidence of dehydration with metabolic acidosis.

   b. *What information (signs, symptoms, laboratory values) indicates the presence or severity of gastroenteritis?*

   - By history, the patient had a 5-day history of fever, vomiting, and diarrhea of acute onset; he had a reported decrease in the number of wet diapers; and his lips appeared to be dry. An actual weight loss of 0.6 kg (8%) was documented.
   - He has a social history of day care attendance, where several of his day care mates had similar illnesses recently, as well as a 2-year-old sibling with a recent history of diarrhea for 3 days. This is a typical history in pediatric gastroenteritis.
   - On physical exam, his skin turgor was decreased and the capillary refill was increased at 2 to 3 seconds. His tongue was dry with cracked and dry lips. His anterior fontanelle was sunken and he had sunken eyes, and he was tachycardic and tachypneic.
   - His labs indicated metabolic acidosis (total CO_2 13 mEq/L and Cl 110 mEq/L) and his urinalysis showed a specific gravity of 1.028 (moderate dehydration). His dehydration was isotonic (defined as serum sodium between 130 and 150 mEq/L).
   - See Table 29–1 for clinical assessment guidelines for dehydration.

TABLE 29–1. Clinical Assessment Guidelines for Dehydration in Children of All Ages[2,3]

Parameter	Mild	Moderate	Severe
Weight loss	3–5%	6–9%	≥10%
Body fluid loss	30–50 mL/kg	50–100 mL/kg	>100 mL/kg
Stage of shock	Impending	Compensated	Uncompensated
Heart rate	Normal	Increased	Increased
Blood pressure	Normal	Normal	Normal to reduced
Respiratory rate	Normal	Normal	Increased
Skin turgor	Normal	Decreased	"Tenting"
Anterior fontanelle	Normal	Sunken	Sunken
Capillary refill	<2 seconds	2–3 seconds	>3 seconds
Mucous membranes	Slightly dry	Dry	Dry
Tearing	Normal/absent	Absent	Absent
Eye appearance	Normal	Sunken orbits	Deeply sunken orbits
Mental status	Normal	Normal to listless	Normal to lethargic to comatose
Urine volume	Slightly decreased	<1 mL/kg/hr	<<1 mL/kg/hr
Urine specific gravity	1.020	1.025	>1.035
BUN	Upper normal	Elevated	High
Blood pH	7.40–7.22	7.30–6.92	7.10–6.8
Thirst	Slightly increased	Moderately increased	Very thirsty or too lethargic to indicate

Desired Outcome

2. *What are the goals of pharmacotherapy in this case?*

- Replacement of fluid and electrolyte losses is the critical central element of effective treatment of acute diarrhea.[2] This is necessary to prevent excessive water, electrolyte, and acid–base disturbances.
- Other secondary goals may include providing symptomatic relief and treating any curable causes of diarrhea.

Therapeutic Alternatives

3. a. *What non-drug therapies might be useful for this patient?*

- *Oral rehydration therapy (ORT)* with carbohydrate-based solutions is the mainstay of treatment of fluid and electrolyte losses caused by diarrhea in children with mild to moderate dehydration. ORT can be used regardless of the patient's age, causative pathogen, or initial serum sodium concentration. The basis for the effectiveness of ORT is the phenomenon of glucose-sodium cotransport, where sodium ions given orally are absorbed along with glucose (and other organic molecules) from the lumen of the intestine into the bloodstream.[1] Any of the commercially available oral rehydration solutions can successfully be used to rehydrate otherwise healthy children with mild to moderate dehydration (refer to the table on oral rehydration solutions in textbook Chapter 34 for detailed product information). These products are formulated on physiologic principles and must be distinguished from other nonphysiologic clear liquids that are commonly but inappropriately used to treat dehydration. Clear liquids to be avoided include colas, apple juice, chicken broth, and sports beverages.[3] This patient was inappropriately treated since in addition to an ORT (Pedialyte), her pediatrician recommended a variety of clear liquids including water, Jell-O water, and cola. These liquids have unacceptably low electrolyte concentrations, and cola beverages are hypertonic because of the high glucose concentrations, with osmolalities greater than 700 mOsm.[3]

- *Early feeding of age-appropriate foods.* Although carbohydrate-based ORT is highly effective in replacing fluid and electrolyte losses, it has no effect on stool volume or duration of diarrhea, which can be discouraging to parents. To overcome this limitation, cereal-based ORT has been used investigationally and can reduce stool volume by 20% to 30%. However, there are no commercial products available in the United States. Nevertheless, early feeding of patients as soon as oral rehydration is completed provides similar reductions in stool volume.[3] Therefore, children with diarrhea requiring rehydration should be fed with age-appropriate diets immediately after completing ORT. Optimal ORT incorporates early feeding of age-appropriate foods. Unrestricted diets generally do not worsen the symptoms of mild diarrhea and decrease the stool output compared with ORT alone.

b. *What feasible pharmacotherapeutic alternatives are available for treatment of this patient's diarrhea?*

- *Antidiarrheal compounds* have been used to treat pediatric gastroenteritis. Their use is intended to shorten the course of diarrhea and to relieve discomfort by reducing stool output and electrolyte losses. However, their usefulness remains to be proven, and antidiarrheal compounds generally should not be used to treat pediatric gastroenteritis. These agents have a variety of proposed mechanisms; their possible benefits and limitations are outlined below.

    ✓ *Antimotility agents* (opiates and opiate/anticholinergic combination products) delay GI transit and increase gut capacity and fluid retention. *Loperamide* with ORT significantly reduces the volume of stool losses, but this reduction is not clinically significant. It also may have an unacceptable rate of side effects (lethargy, respiratory depression, altered mental status, ileus, abdominal distention). Anticholinergic agents (e.g., atropine or mepenzolate bromide) may cause dry mouth that can alter the clinical evaluation of dehydration. Infants and children are especially susceptible to toxic effects of anticholinergics. Antimotility agents can worsen the course of diarrhea in shigellosis, anti-biotic-associated pseudomembranous colitis, and *E. coli* 0157:H7-induced diarrhea. Importantly, reliance on antidiarrheal compounds may shift the focus of treatment away from appropriate ORT and early feeding of the child. They are not recommended by the American Academy of Pediatrics (AAP) to treat acute diarrhea in children because of the modest clinical benefit, limited scientific evidence of efficacy, and concern for toxic effects.

- ✓ *Antisecretory agents (bismuth subsalicylate)* may have an adjunctive role for acute diarrhea. Bismuth subsalicylate decreases intestinal secretions secondary to cholera and *E. coli* toxins, decreases frequency of unformed stools, decreases total stool output, and reduces the need for ORT. However, the benefit is modest, and it requires dosing every 4 hours. Also, pediatric patients may absorb salicylate (but the effect on Reye's syndrome is unknown). This treatment is also not recommended by the AAP because of modest benefit and concern for toxicity.
- ✓ *Adsorbent drugs (kaolin & pectin; polycarbophil)* may bind bacterial toxins and water, but their effectiveness remains unproven. There is no conclusive evidence of decreased duration of diarrhea, number of stools, or total stool output. Major toxicity is not a concern with these products, but they may adsorb nutrients, enzymes, and drugs. The FDA recognizes only polycarbophil as an effective adsorbent. These products are not recommended by the AAP because of lack of efficacy.
- ✓ *Colonic microflora replacement products (Lactobacillus acidophilus, L. bulgaricus)* supposedly replace microflora loss secondary to previous antibiotic therapy. They purportedly suppress growth of pathogenic microorganisms, restoring normal intestinal function. There is no consistent evidence that microflora replacement improves diarrhea, and lactobacillus-containing compounds are not recommended by the AAP because of limited scientific evidence of efficacy.

Optimal Plan

4. *What drug(s), dosage forms, schedule, and duration of therapy are best for this patient?*

- Treatment of a child with dehydration is directed primarily by the degree of dehydration present.[1] This patient had diarrhea with moderate dehydration (6% to 9% loss of body weight). There are four treatment situations[3]:
  - ✓ *Diarrhea without dehydration.* ORT may be given in doses of 10 mL/kg to replace ongoing stool losses. Some children may not take the ORT because of its salty taste. For these few patients, freezer pops are available in a variety of flavors. ORT may not be necessary if fluid consumption and age-appropriate feeding continues. Infants should continue to breastfeed or take regular-strength formula. Older children can usually drink full-strength milk.
  - ✓ *Diarrhea with mild dehydration (3% to 5% weight loss).* Correct dehydration with ORT 50 mL/kg over a 4-hour period. Reassess the status of dehydration and volume of ORT at 2-hour intervals. Concomitantly replace continuing losses from stool or emesis at 10 mL/kg for each stool; estimate emesis loss and replace with fluid. Children with emesis can usually tolerate ORT, but it is necessary to administer ORT in small 5- to 10-mL (1 to 2 teaspoonfuls) aliquots every 1 to 2 minutes. Feeding should start immediately after rehydration is complete, using the feeding guidelines described above.
  - ✓ *Diarrhea with moderate dehydration (6% to 9% weight loss).* Since the patient presented to the ED, this treatment was performed there, but it can usually be accomplished at home. Correct the dehydration with ORT 100 mL/kg plus replacement of ongoing losses (10 mL/kg for each stool, plus estimated losses from emesis as above) during the first 4 hours. Assess rehydration status hourly and adjust the amount of ORT accordingly. Close supervision is required, but this can be continued at home. Rapid restoration of blood volume helps correct acidosis and increase tissue perfusion. Resume feeding of age-appropriate diet as soon as rehydration is completed.
  - ✓ *Diarrhea with severe dehydration (≥10% weight loss).* Severe dehydration and uncompensated shock should be treated aggressively with IV isotonic fluids to restore intravascular volume. Poorly treated pediatric gastroenteritis, especially in infants, can cause life-threatening severe dehydration and should be considered a medical emergency. The patient may be in shock and should be referred to an ED. Administer 20-mL/kg aliquots of normal saline or Ringer's Lactate solution over 15 to 30 minutes (even faster in uncompensated shock). Reassess the patient's status after each completed fluid bolus. Repeat boluses of up to 80 mL/kg total fluid may be used. Isotonic fluid replacement may be discontinued when blood pressure is restored, heart rate is normalized, peripheral pulses are strong, and skin perfusion is restored. Urine output is the best indicator of restored intravascular volume and should be at least 1 mL/kg/hr. If the patient does not respond to rapid IV volume replacement, other underlying disorders should be considered, including septic shock, toxic shock syndrome, myocarditis, cardiomyopathy, pericarditis, and other underlying diseases. ORT may be instituted to complete rehydration when the patient's status is satisfactory. Estimate the degree of remaining dehydration and treat according to the above guidelines. The IV line should be kept in place until it is certain that IV therapy will not be reinstituted. After ORT is complete, resume feeding following the guidelines outlined above.

Outcome Evaluation

5. *What clinical and laboratory parameters should be monitored to evaluate therapy for achievement of the desired therapeutic outcome?*

- Vital signs should normalize with appropriate therapy, but they may be unreliable in patients with fever, agitation, pain, or respiratory illnesses. Tachycardia is usually the first sign of mild dehydration (see Table 29–1). With increasing acidosis and fluid loss, the respiratory rate increases and breathing becomes deeper (hyperpnea). Hypotension is a sign usually of severe dehydration.
- Any existing CNS alterations should be reversed. No CNS changes occur in mild dehydration; some patients may appear listless with moderate dehydration, and severely dehydrated patients appear quite ill with lethargy or irritability.
- Skin changes should be normalized. Mucous membranes should appear moist (previously dry in all degrees of dehydration). Capillary refill is normally <2 seconds and usually is not altered in mild dehydration. Capillary refill in moderately dehydrated patients is 2 to 3 seconds and >3 seconds in severe dehydration. Skin turgor (elasticity) should be normal. There is no change in mild dehydration; but it decreases in moderate dehydration, with "tenting" occurring in patients with severe dehydration. The anterior fontanelle should no longer be sunken, which is seen in moderate to severe dehydration.
- The eyes should appear normal. No change occurs in mild dehydration, but in moderate to severe dehydration, tearing will be absent and the eyes will appear sunken.
- Laboratory tests should be assessed appropriately. Most dehydration occurring with pediatric gastroenteritis is isotonic, and serum electrolyte determinations are unnecessary. However, some patients with moderate dehydration (those whose histories and physical examinations are inconsistent with routine gastroenteritis) and all severely dehydrated patients should have serum electrolytes determined and corrected. Urine volume and specific gravity should be normalized. Progressive decreases in urine volume and increases in specific gravity are expected with increasing severity of dehydration. Urine output will be decreased to <1 mL/kg/hr in moderate dehydration and <<1 mL/kg/hr in severe dehydration (see Table 29–1). Specific gravity will be 1.020 in mild dehydration, 1.025 in moderate dehydration, and maximal in patients with severe dehydration. Adequate rehydration should normalize both urine output and specific gravity.

Patient Counseling

6. *What information should be provided to the child's parents to enhance compliance, ensure successful therapy, and minimize adverse effects?*

- Treatment of diarrhea due to gastroenteritis in your child should begin at home.[1] It is a good idea for you to keep ORT at home at all times (especially in rural areas and poor urban neighborhoods where access to health care may be delayed), and to use it as instructed by your doctor. Sometimes doctors instruct new parents about this treatment at the first newborn visit.
- Early home management will result in fewer complications such as severe dehydration and poor nutrition, as well as fewer office or emergency room visits.
- Any of the commercial oral rehydration products can be used to effectively rehydrate your child. However, rehydration alone does not reduce the duration of diarrhea or the volume of stool output. Early feeding after rehydration can reduce the duration of diarrhea by as much as one-half day.
- Effective oral rehydration always combines early feeding with an age-appropriate diet after rehydration. This will correct dehydration, improve nutritional status, and reduce the volume of stool output.
- Vomiting usually does not preclude the use of oral rehydration. Small amounts (1 to 2 teaspoonfuls) of an oral rehydration product can be given every 1 to 2 minutes, providing as much as 10 ounces/hr of rehydration fluid.
- If the child does not stop vomiting after the appropriate administration of oral rehydration (as above) and appears to be severely dehydrated, contact your doctor, who may refer you to the emergency room for intravenous rehydration therapy.
- Oral rehydration is not sufficient therapy for bloody diarrhea (dysentery). Contact your doctor if this occurs.
- Additional treatments, including antidiarrheal compounds and antimicrobial therapy are almost never necessary in the treatment of pediatric gastroenteritis.
- Proper handwashing technique, diaper changing practices, and personal hygiene can help prevent spread of the disease to other family members.

References

1. Duggan C, Santosham M, Glass RI. The management of acute diarrhea in children: Oral rehydration, maintenance, and nutritional therapy. MMWR 1992;41(RR-16):1–20.
2. Provisional Committee on Quality Improvement, Subcommittee on Acute Gastroenteritis. Practice parameter: The management of acute gastroenteritis in young children. Pediatrics 1996;97:424–435.
3. Snyder J. The continuing evolution of oral therapy for diarrhea. Semin Pediatr Infect Dis 1994;5:231–235.

30 CONSTIPATION

▶ **Bound to Be Slow** (Level I)

Barbara L. Kaltenbach, PharmD
Beth Bryles Phillips, PharmD

A 74-year-old woman with a history of hypertension, Parkinson's disease, and heartburn presents to the geriatric clinic with complaints of worsening constipation. She has a number of drug-related problems that students must identify; she is also taking several medications that may be contributing to her constipation. In developing a treatment plan for constipation, students should consider non-pharmacologic approaches such as increased dietary fiber and fluid intake, physical activity, and appropriate bowel habits. Therapeutic agents can be selected from a variety of classes, including bulk-forming agents, hyperosmolar laxatives, surfactants, lubricants, stimulant laxatives, and saline cathartics. Students should be able to identify those agents which are suitable for chronic use and those which should be used only infrequently. Because laxative products are available without a prescription, it is important to provide accurate patient information about their appropriate use.

Questions

Problem Identification

1. a. Develop a list of this patient's drug-related problems.

- Inadequate treatment of constipation.
- Potential exacerbation of constipation by imipramine, Sominex (diphenhydramine), and Permax (pergolide) due to anticholinergic effects.
- Non-adherence to prescribed regimen of imipramine.
- Drug interaction between fluoxetine and imipramine (fluoxetine may increase tricyclic antidepressant levels).
- Inappropriate drug selection of fluoxetine in an elderly patient due to long half-life.
- Inappropriate drug selection of diazepam in an elderly patient due to long half-life.
- Duplicate drug therapy (imipramine and diphenhydramine for insomnia).
- Inappropriate dosing regimen of piroxicam.
- Inappropriate scheduling of triamterene/hydrochlorothiazide.
- Questionable need for Permax (pergolide) as patient exhibits no signs or symptoms of Parkinson's disease.

b. What signs or symptoms in this patient indicate the presence of constipation?

- There is a subjective complaint by the patient of feeling full and constipated.
- She reports going several days (5 to 6 days) at a time without having a bowel movement for the past several months and is straining the majority of the time.
- The rectal exam revealed a large amount of stool in the rectal vault, which is consistent with constipation; she has no evidence of anal fissures, strictures, or hemorrhoids.
- Laboratory tests (TSH, calcium, and potassium) ruled out metabolic causes that could be contributing to the constipation, such as hypothyroidism, hypocalcemia, and hypokalemia.
- Diagnostic tests (barium enema and colonoscopy) in the GI clinic indicate the absence of disorders such as irritable bowel syndrome, diverticulitis, or malignancy, that may be causing the constipation.

c. Does the patient have any medical conditions that could contribute to her constipation?

- Her medical conditions that may contribute to this problem include Parkinson's disease and cerebrovascular disease. Parkinson's disease is associated with autonomic dysfunction that may cause constipation. Cerebrovascular events are associated with neurogenic causes of constipation, but since this patient has no residual deficits (other than possibly tremor) it is unlikely that cerebrovascular disease is a major contributing factor to the presenting symptoms.

d. What information is necessary to adequately assess a report of constipation by a patient?

It would be helpful to obtain the following information:

- What types of food does the patient eat? (i.e., intake of grains, fruits, and vegetables)
- How much fluid intake does the patient have each day?
- What is the patient's level of physical activity?
- Aside from the Metamucil, what has the patient tried in the past, and how well did it work?
- Does the patient have symptoms other than the ones she described, such as thirst, abdominal pain, or bone pain? These may indicate an underlying pathology.

Desired Outcome

2. What are the goals of pharmacotherapy in treating constipation?

- Once underlying conditions have been ruled out, the goals of therapy are to eliminate the symptoms of constipation and prevent future symptoms.
- In this particular patient, increasing the frequency of stools and decreasing her straining are also appropriate goals.

Therapeutic Alternatives

3. a. What non-pharmacologic measures can be used to treat constipation?

- Most patients would benefit from an increase in fiber intake; 14 grams of crude fiber intake is recommended daily. High fiber is found in foods such as cereals, fruits, and vegetables.
- Increasing fluid intake by drinking more water or fruit juices and increasing physical activity will also help.
- Patients should be instructed on appropriate bowel habits, such as setting time aside, particularly after meals, to respond to the need to go the bathroom. Refer to textbook Chapter 34 for more detailed information on non-drug alternatives.

b. What pharmacotherapeutic alternatives are available for the treatment of constipation?

- *Bulk-forming laxatives* are among the safest laxatives available and have very few adverse effects. It may take up to 3 days for a noticeable effect to occur. Patients may experience a feeling of fullness and flatulence for the first few weeks of therapy, but these effects often disappear over time. It is very important to inform patients to take these agents with plenty of water to minimize the risk of GI tract obstruction. Examples of these agents and their usual doses are given below:
  - ✓ *Methylcellulose,* approximately 1 heaping tablespoonful of powder in 8 oz water up to 3 times daily (approximately 2 g per dose)
  - ✓ *Psyllium,* 1 teaspoonful of powder or one packet in 8 oz water 1 to 3 times daily (most formulations contain about 3.5 g of psyllium per dose)
  - ✓ *Polycarbophil* tablets, 1 g up to four times daily as needed
- *Hyperosmolar laxatives* have been shown to be efficacious and safe, particularly in elderly patients, and long-term use has not been found to produce detrimental effects. They generally require 1 to 2 days for noticeable results.
  - ✓ *Lactulose,* 15 to 30 mL of solution daily, as needed; up to 60 mL daily can be used
  - ✓ *Sorbitol,* 15 mL of 70% solution orally, as needed, or 120 mL

of a 25% to 30% solution rectally. Sorbitol is considerably less expensive than lactulose.

- *Emollients (or surfactants)* are relatively safe agents with minimal adverse effects. These agents are stool softeners and have minimal laxative properties. Although they are a good choice for patients who complain of hard stools, they are not very helpful in treating constipation. Their primary use is in preventing constipation. They are often given after surgery or a myocardial infarction to prevent straining. Effects of these agents are not usually seen for several days.
  - ✓ *Docusate sodium* capsules or liquid, 50 to 500 mg orally per day in divided doses
  - ✓ *Docusate calcium* capsules, 240 mg per day in divided doses
  - ✓ *Docusate potassium* capsules, 100 to 300 mg per day in divided doses
- *Lubricants* are useful for the same purpose as the emollient laxatives, but their use is not as common. Mineral oil should not be used routinely for constipation, because it is not as safe as docusate. It can be absorbed systemically and cause a foreign-body reaction, and there is also the danger of lipoid pneumonia due to aspiration in recumbent patients. In addition, malabsorption of fat-soluble vitamins, which can be of particular concern in elderly patients, may occur. As with emollients, effects may not be seen for a few days.
  - ✓ *Mineral oil,* 15 to 45 mL orally as needed
- *Stimulant (or irritant) laxatives.* The diphenylmethane derivative bisacodyl has a rapid onset of action (15 to 60 minutes) when administered rectally. The onset of effect after oral administration is 6 to 12 hours. Bisacodyl is often used as part of a bowel preparation regimen to cause evacuation of the bowel prior to diagnostic examination (e.g., sigmoidoscopy). Its stimulant effect often causes abdominal cramping. When used chronically, stimulant laxatives can cause severe electrolyte abnormalities (i.e., hypokalemia), and cathartic colon may result.[1] For these reasons, bisacodyl is not recommended for regular or chronic use. Phenolphthalein, an agent recently taken off the market, also belongs to this class of laxatives.
  - ✓ *Bisacodyl,* 5 mg tablet or 10 mg rectal suppository, both taken as needed
  Anthraquinone derivatives have a relatively rapid onset of action, up to 2 hours for suppositories and 6 to 10 hours for tablets and granules. They share the same disadvantages as bisacodyl.
  - ✓ *Cascara sagrada,* one tablet or 5 mL of the liquid at bedtime
  - ✓ *Senna,* two tablets at bedtime, up to 8 tablets per day as needed; one rectal suppository as needed; 1 teaspoonful of the granules as needed
- *Saline cathartics* work rather rapidly, producing evacuation of the bowel within 6 hours after an oral dose, and even faster when the rectal form is used. Because of this rapid effect, these agents (like bisacodyl) are useful when complete, acute, evacuation of the bowel is required, such as prior to diagnostic examinations. Accumulation of magnesium and sodium can occur in patients with renal impairment. Hypocalcemia can result in patients using sodium phosphate. In addition, electrolyte depletion and fluid abnormalities can occur with chronic use. Occasional use, such as 10 to 20 mL of magnesium hydroxide (Milk of Magnesia), may be used to treat acute constipation on an as-needed basis, but should not be used more often than every 2 weeks.
  - ✓ *Magnesium sulfate,* 10 to 15 g mixed in a glass of water, as needed
  - ✓ *Magnesium hydroxide,* 30 to 60 mL, or 10 to 30 mL of the concentrated form, as needed
  - ✓ *Sodium phosphate,* 20 to 30 mL mixed with 1/2 glass of water, as needed
- *Miscellaneous agents.* Glycerin is probably the safest choice for laxative use in children. The onset of effect usually occurs within 30 minutes. Glycerin may cause some local irritation.
  - ✓ *Glycerin,* 3 g suppository, intermittently as needed
  - ✓ *Tap water enema,* 200 mL rectally as needed

Optimal Plan

4. *What would be the most appropriate pharmacologic agent, formulation, dose, schedule, and duration of therapy for this patient?*

- The best regimen for this patient, along with the non-pharmacologic interventions, is probably a bulk laxative. Since these agents have relatively few side effects and rarely have systemic effects, they are generally the safest agents to use overall, especially in elderly patients. Since the patient has already tried the powder form of a bulk laxative and did not wish to continue this dosage form, a tablet would be an appropriate dosage form to recommend. A calcium polycarbophil product (e.g., FiberCon, Equalactin, Mitrolan) is a good choice, at a dose of 2 tablets one to four times a day taken with at least 8 ounces of water.
- In addition, medications that can exacerbate constipation (i.e., imipramine, diphenhydramine, and pergolide) should be discontinued.
- In general, laxatives other than bulk forming laxatives should not be used on a regular basis due to the potential problems mentioned above, but they may be used intermittently. Both lactulose, 15 to 30 mL orally each day, or sorbitol, 30 mL daily, would be appropriate alternatives. Bisacodyl 10 mg orally or an anthraquinone derivative (senna or cascara sagrada) may also be chosen for occasional use only. It is recommended that bisacodyl be used as infrequently as once every few weeks. Lastly, glycerin suppositories or a tap water enema may be useful for relieving constipation acutely. Keep in mind that the above regimens should not be used on a regular basis but may be recommended for an occasional bout of constipation.

Outcome Evaluation

5. *What would you monitor in this patient to ensure that the desired therapeutic outcome has been achieved, and to detect or prevent adverse events?*

- She should be reevaluated for signs and symptoms of constipation, as well as for potential adverse effects, depending on the laxative chosen. It would be appropriate to call the patient in one week for follow-up of constipation resolution and/or the presence of adverse drug reactions.
- The patient should also return to the geriatric clinic in one month for follow-up of her medical problems and a physical examination.

Patient Counseling

6. *What information should be provided to a patient receiving a bulk-forming laxative to enhance compliance, ensure successful therapy, and minimize adverse events?*

The following information should be communicated to the patient:
- FiberCon (if this is the brand chosen) is a bulk-forming laxative. It is similar to the Metamucil you tried previously but is in the form of a tablet, which should make it more tolerable for you.
- You are to take two tablets as often as four times each day, spread out throughout the day as much as possible, with a full 8-ounce glass of water with each dose.
- In addition to the full glass of water, you should drink at least six to eight glasses of water or fruit juice each day. The reason for this is that these agents can cause an obstruction in your esophagus or in your stomach if there is not plenty of fluid to wash them down. Adequate fluid intake also helps maintain regular bowel movements.
- If you should happen to miss a dose, just take it as soon as you remember, unless it is almost time for your next dose.
- Some patients get results from this medication in the first day, but most people do not notice a difference for 2 or 3 days, so don't be upset if this doesn't work right away. Just be patient for a few days. Do not be alarmed if you do not begin having bowel movements every day; many people don't. It is normal to have as few as three bowel movements per week.
- Because this medication is not absorbed into your body, it has very few side effects. Initially, you may feel a bit more bloated and may pass more gas than usual, but these effects usually wear off after a few weeks. More severe side effects are rare, but if you do experience symptoms such as difficulty in breathing, a rash on your skin, itching, difficulty in swallowing, or a feeling of having a lump in your throat, notify your doctor right away.
- Lastly, if you have children in your house, keep this medication in a place where they can't reach it. It's best to store the medication away from heat, direct light, and moisture.
- In order to prevent further constipation, along with drinking plenty of fluids, you should also minimize foods that can cause constipation, such as cheese, pastries, cakes, and candies. In addition, try increasing your activity level, perhaps by taking walks throughout the day. All of these things will help maintain regular bowel movements and will help to prevent constipation in the future.

▶ Follow-up Question

1. *Is the patient's current regimen for insomnia appropriate? What recommendations can you make to optimize this regimen?*
   - This patient's insomnia may be easily relieved by non-pharmacologic measures. She reports that she does not sleep very well at night and admits to napping during the day. The medications she has tried have not improved her sleep. She may not sleep very well at night because she is getting too much sleep during the day. She should decrease or eliminate her daytime naps and go to bed at a regular time each evening.
   - As discussed previously, diphenhydramine and imipramine are likely contributing to her complaints of constipation and should be discontinued. In addition to constipation, both of these medications possess other anticholinergic properties and have the potential to cause xerostomia, blurred vision, and urinary retention as well, which may be especially problematic in elderly patients.

Reference

Harari D, Gurwitz JH, Minaker KL. Constipation in the elderly. J Am Geriatr Soc 1993;41:1130–1140.

31 CIRRHOTIC ASCITES

▶ A Pint Is a Pound   (Level I)

Joette M. Meyer, PharmD

A 47-year-old man with diabetes mellitus and cirrhosis is admitted because of abdominal swelling and pain, a 15-pound weight gain, and mental status changes. In addition to a large volume paracentesis, the initiation of sodium restriction and diuretic therapy is required. Students must consider the pathophysiology of ascites formation in the selection of an appropriate diuretic regimen. In addition to assessing parameters to determine the effectiveness of therapy, students must be aware of the need to evaluate the patient carefully to detect and prevent intravascular volume depletion. The case also asks students to consider alternative treatments for preventing spontaneous bacterial peritonitis (SBP), preventing recurrent variceal bleeding, and controlling hepatic encephalopathy in this patient.

▶ Questions

Problem Identification

1. a. *Create a list of the patient's drug-related problems.*
   - Increasing ascites resulting from cirrhosis that requires initiation of diuretic and other therapy.
   - Encephalopathy resulting from liver disease that is inadequately treated with a single daily dose of lactulose.
   - History of SBP without secondary antimicrobial prophylaxis.
   - History of bleeding esophageal varices with no treatment for secondary prevention (e.g., β-blockers with or without nitrates).

   b. *What information (signs, symptoms, laboratory values) indicates the presence or severity of ascites secondary to liver cirrhosis? (See Figure 31–1.)*
   - Objective evidence of abdominal distention, a firm abdomen, and shifting dullness on physical exam
   - Subjectively, the patient reports increasing abdominal girth and a 15-pound weight gain

- Serum-ascites albumin gradient (SAAG) >1.1, which indicates ascites formation is secondary to portal hypertension
- 5 L of fluid removed by paracentesis
- Sodium excretion of 50 mEq/day is less than the 88 mEq/day he is ingesting (if he has been adherent to his diet), so fluid will accumulate. It is also possible that he is not compliant with his diet and the extra sodium intake is contributing to his increasing fluid retention.

Desired Outcome

2. *What are the goals of pharmacotherapy for the management of ascites in this case?*

- The immediate goal is to reduce the ascites and relieve patient discomfort by a large volume paracentesis (as was done in this case). The fluid was appropriately sent for cell count and culture to rule out infection.
- Subsequently, attempts should be made to minimize or eliminate the ascites with diuretics. The goal of diuretic therapy is a slow and gradual diuresis unaccompanied by adverse side effects.
- Ascites develops most frequently as part of the decompensation of liver disease. The goal is to prevent further progression of the disease and to prevent or reduce other complications (e.g., encephalopathy, variceal bleeding, SBP). The patient has received prior treatment with interferon-alfa in an attempt to prevent decompensation due to hepatitis C, and he has abstained from further alcohol consumption. At this stage there is no further pharmacologic intervention available to arrest liver decompensation. The development of ascites in decompensated cirrhosis is a poor prognostic sign, and only 30% of such patients survive 4 years.[1]
- Only liver transplantation can cure ascites by replacing the cirrhotic liver with a normal one. Therefore, the ultimate goal for this patient is to survive until liver transplantation.

Therapeutic Alternatives

3. a. *What non-drug therapies might be useful for this patient?*

- Bedrest to help mobilize fluid and increase response to diuretics
- Enforcement of a sodium-restricted diet (2 g/day) to help achieve a negative sodium balance, treat the ascites, and also to prevent ascites reaccumulation
- Continued abstinence from alcohol to prevent further deterioration of liver synthetic function
- Periodic large volume paracenteses (if drug therapy fails) for symptomatic relief
- Transjugular Intrahepatic Portosystemic Shunt (TIPS) (if drug therapy fails), which will resolve ascites in many patients
- Liver transplantation is the only cure for this disease
- Fluid restriction of 1500 mL/day has been recommended for treatment of ascites since many cirrhotic patients are also mildly hyponatremic. However, sodium retention is the main problem in these patients, and water is retained only passively. Therefore, some hepatologists do not agree with fluid restricting patients unless the serum sodium drops below 120 mEq/L.[2]

b. *What feasible pharmacotherapeutic alternatives are available for treatment of cirrhotic ascites?*

- The purpose of therapy for ascites is to attain a negative sodium balance. Sodium restriction and bed rest (for hospitalized patients), should be employed first line to manage ascites. However, unless the urine sodium excretion is >50 mEq/L, drug therapy with diuretics, in addition to sodium restriction, will likely be necessary to achieve an adequate diuresis.[2]
- *Spironolactone* and *furosemide* are the most widely used diuretics in the management of ascites. Many ascitic patients have activation of the renin-angiotensin-aldosterone system, and spironolactone achieves its diuretic effect by inhibiting aldosterone, which makes it is an especially useful agent. However, the onset of diuresis with this agent alone can take up to 2 weeks,[3,4] and it is associated with hyperkalemia due to its potassium sparing effects. It may be best suited for management of mild to moderate ascites in outpatients. Furosemide acts by inhibiting sodium reabsorption in the ascending limb of the loop of Henle. It has a rapid onset but may require frequent dosage titrations and causes hypokalemia.[4]
- Use of spironolactone as a single agent has been shown to be effective and superior to using furosemide alone in the treatment of ascites.[5] However, the combination of spironolactone and furosemide has been found to be a more effective drug regimen due to a quicker onset of diuresis and fewer problems with potassium imbalance.[4] This regimen is suited for management of ascites in inpatients when hospital days must be minimized and frequent monitoring of electrolytes and renal function is possible, since overdiuresis is more likely to occur with combination therapy than with spironolactone alone.
- Spironolactone is available generically as 25-mg tablets. The 50- and 100-mg tablets are brand only. Patients who pay out-of-pocket can reduce their medication expenses by taking multiple 25-mg tablets to make up their total dose.

Optimal Plan

4. a. *What drug, dosage form, dose, schedule, and duration of therapy are best for this patient?*

- Spironolactone at an initial dose of 100 mg orally once daily in the morning and titrated upwards every 3 to 5 days as necessary to a maximum of 400 mg per day is an option in patients with mild to moderate ascites. This regimen will initiate a gradual diuresis with little potential for overdiuresis. Because spironolactone has a long half-life (3 to 5 days), the steady-state effect of any change will not be seen for up to 4 weeks.
- If the diuretic response is inadequate after a trial of spironolactone, one option is to add furosemide, starting at 40 mg orally once daily and titrating upward. This approach may be sufficient in ambulatory patients.
- Since this patient is in the hospital and has tense ascites, a more appropriate regimen would be to start with a combination of spironolactone 100 mg and furosemide 40 mg orally once daily in the morning. Dosage increases should be made every 3 to 5 days if an inadequate decrease in body weight or an increase in urinary sodium excretion is seen (assuming that the patient tolerates the medications). During dosage titration, it is recommended to keep the ratio of spironolactone to furosemide 100:40.[2,6] The maximum *daily* doses are spironolactone 400 mg

and furosemide 160 mg, which may be given as single daily doses in the morning.

At higher doses no additional effect is obtained. The initial diuretic effects of this regimen should be seen within 3 to 5 days. Therefore, it is appropriate to initiate this regimen in the hospital but, due to the long half-life of spironolactone, dosage titration should be done as an outpatient.

- Treatment with diuretics is associated with a high incidence of azotemia due to intravascular volume depletion, electrolyte disturbances such as hyponatremia and hypo- or hyperkalemia, and hepatic encephalopathy. Therefore, once the ascites has been controlled, diuretic dosages should be re-evaluated and adjusted to the lowest dose that prevents fluid reaccumulation. Diuretics should be continued until transplantation or until the patient's ascites becomes diuretic-resistant or -intractable.

b. *What pharmacologic alternatives would be appropriate if the initial therapy fails or cannot be used?*

- Patients who do not respond to spironolactone 400 mg and furosemide 160 mg daily or who develop adverse effects before reaching an effective dosage are considered to have diuretic resistant or intolerant ascites, respectively. However, before labeling a patient refractory, it is important to rule out dietary non-adherence (either advertent or inadvertent), and use of nonsteroidal anti-inflammatory drugs (NSAIDs).
- Patients who do not respond to a combination of spironolactone and a loop diuretic may benefit from the addition of *metolazone*. However, this agent should be used with caution due to the potential for profuse diuresis and severe electrolyte imbalances. For these reasons, it should be initiated only in hospitalized patients.
- If the patient develops intolerance to spironolactone (e.g., painful gynecomastia), *amiloride* has been suggested as a substitute. The equivalent dose of amiloride is 10% to 20% of the spironolactone dose. Amiloride should be started at 10 mg/day, and the maximum dose is 40 mg/day. However, it is an expensive medication and not often used. Other diuretic agents, such as *hydrochlorothiazide* and *triamterene*, have been used anecdotally, but their routine use in the management of ascites is not recommended.
- If spironolactone is not tolerated, it is acceptable to continue furosemide alone. Other loop diuretics (e.g., *bumetanide*, *torsemide*) can be substituted for furosemide but are more expensive. They have not been studied as extensively and may not offer additional benefit.

Outcome Evaluation

5. *What clinical and laboratory parameters are necessary to evaluate the therapy for achievement of the desired therapeutic outcome and to detect or prevent adverse effects?*

- *Daily weights.* The best way to assess the effectiveness of diuretic therapy is by monitoring body weight. The goal of diuretic therapy is 1 lb/day (0.75 kg/day) of weight loss if patient does not have peripheral edema and 2 lb/day (1 kg/day) in patients with peripheral edema.
- *Daily physical exam of lower extremities for fluid status.* The goal of diuretic therapy is more aggressive in patients with peripheral edema because intravascular volume depletion will rarely occur as long as edema is present. Once edema disappears the extra fluid will be drawn from the intravascular space and complications from volume depletion are more likely.
- *Daily physical exam of the abdomen for fluid.* The goal of diuretic therapy is to reduce the amount of ascites that can be appreciated on physical exam. Monitoring abdominal girth measurements is not routinely done since gaseous distention is common in cirrhotic patients, especially if they are taking lactulose.
- *Daily intake and output.* The goal is for urine output to exceed intake and to correlate with weight loss. Initial fluid restriction is not necessary.
- *Vital signs every 8 hours.* When diuresing a patient, it is important avoid intravascular volume depletion. Cirrhotic patients are usually hypotensive but asymptomatic at baseline. Diuretics should be withheld from any patient whose blood pressure drops below their baseline and they become symptomatic.
- *Electrolyte analysis* at least three times per week (sodium, potassium, BUN, serum creatinine). It is important to avoid changes in electrolytes outside the normal range, especially sodium and potassium. Mild hyponatremia (i.e., serum sodium ≥125 mEq/L) is often seen but is rarely associated with side effects. Therefore, no intervention is necessary unless the level continues to fall. At that time the diuretics should be stopped or reduced and the patient may require fluid restriction. Any increase in serum creatinine above the patient's baseline is of concern and may require a decrease in diuretic dosage. Diuretics should be withheld in patients with a serum creatinine >2.0 mg/dL or with a progressively increasing level.
- *Urine sodium* (ideally a 24-hour urine collection) after initiation or changing the dose of diuretics. The goal of diuretic therapy is a sodium output greater than input (88 mEq for a 2-g sodium diet). Diuretic doses should be titrated to achieve an output greater than input. Under these conditions, the patient will lose weight. If weight loss does not occur, the patient is probably nonadherent to the diet.
- *Daily assessment of mental status* by psychometric testing (i.e., orientation to time, person, place; recall of current events; subtraction of serial 7's) and checking for asterixis. Diuretic therapy can precipitate hepatic encephalopathy. If deterioration in mental status is noted, the patient should be evaluated for other causes of encephalopathy (e.g., infection, GI bleeding), and diuretic therapy may need to be withheld.
- *Note:* Patients do not need to stay in the hospital until the ascites has completely resolved. Once the patient has started to demonstrate daily weight loss and a urinary sodium output greater than dietary intake, the patient may be discharged to follow-up as an outpatient in approximately 1 week. At this visit the blood pressure and weight should be taken and labs obtained for electrolyte analysis and serum creatinine. The patient should be questioned about compliance to diet and medications. A urine sample should also be obtained for spot urine sodium. The frequency of future clinic appointments depends on the overall stability of the patient and his/her renal function and electrolyte balance.

Patient Counseling

6. *What information should be provided to the patient to enhance compliance, ensure successful therapy, and minimize adverse effects?*

- Diuretics, or "water pills," have been prescribed to help control the amount of fluid in your belly. They work by increasing the amount of urine you produce. Furosemide (Lasix) and spironolactone (Aldactone) are the two diuretics that you have been prescribed to take in combination. The furosemide dose is 40 mg and the spironolactone dose is 100 mg.
- Both of these medications are to be taken by mouth once daily. The best time to take these medications is in the morning. There is no need to split the dose and take them more than once daily.
- It is important that you take them every day as directed. If you miss a dose, take it as soon as you remember. However, if it is late in the day skip the dose and resume your regular schedule again in the morning. You will need to remain on the diuretics indefinitely. They work to control the amount of fluid, but as long as your liver is not working properly you will continue to produce fluid. Once you undergo a liver transplant the diuretics will no longer be necessary.
- Both medications are well tolerated. Occasionally spironolactone can cause breast tenderness in men. If this occurs tell your doctor, and he or she can make adjustments to your medications. If you lose too much fluid too rapidly as a result of these medications, you may become dizzy, weak, lightheaded, or confused. Contact your doctor immediately if this occurs. Weigh yourself daily to ensure that you do not begin to gain fluid or lose it too rapidly. About 1 pound per day of weight loss is appropriate initially until the fluid is minimized.
- These medications can be very effective, but you must follow your diet as well. A low-sodium diet will help these medicines work better. Continue to eat a well-balanced diet. Protein from your food can help build up your own internal protein concentrations, and this will also prevent fluid from reaccumulating in your belly.
- Avoid aspirin and other non-steroidal anti-inflammatory drugs (NSAIDs) like generic ibuprofen, Motrin IB, Advil, Aleve, and Orudis-KT. These medications can prevent the diuretics from working, cause sodium to be retained in the body, and may cause ulcers and bleeding. Acetaminophen (Tylenol) can be used safely for pain as long as you do not take more than 4 grams per day.

Additional Case Questions

1. How serious a condition is SBP, and what pharmacologic alternatives are available for its prevention?

- SBP is a serious condition with a prevalence of 10% to 27% among patients with ascites who are admitted to the hospital and is associated with approximately a 50% mortality rate.[7] In addition, recurrence of SBP is a frequent event and is often the cause of death.[8]
- In patients who have survived an episode of SBP, diuretics can be effective in decreasing the amount of ascitic fluid and increasing the concentration of protein and complement (opsonic) fractions in the remaining fluid. SBP is more likely to occur or reoccur in ascitic fluid with low protein concentrations and low opsonic activity. However, patients with progressive liver disease often develop diuretic-resistant or intractable ascites; therefore, other measures are required to prevent recurrence.
- Selective intestinal decontamination with once daily dosing of oral fluoroquinolone antibiotics (e.g., norfloxacin 400 mg po QD) has been proven effective in primary and secondary prevention of SBP. Although antibiotic prophylaxis may decrease SBP recurrences, it has not been shown to improve survival, decrease morbidity, or reduce hospital admissions. Therefore, only high-risk patients should be candidates for use of antibiotic prophylaxis.

2. What pharmacologic alternatives are available for the secondary prevention of variceal bleeding?

- Nonselective β-blockers (e.g., nadolol and propranolol) have been shown to prevent bleeding and decrease the risk of rebleeding in patients with portal hypertension. The beneficial effect is thought to be due to a reduction in splanchnic venous flow caused by a decreased cardiac output (β_1 effects) and by an increase in splanchnic arteriolar resistance (β_2 effects). As a result, portal venous and hepatic arterial flow decreases. Addition of a nitrate (isosorbide mononitrate) has been shown to be superior to a β-blocker alone (nadolol) for primary prophylaxis of variceal bleeding.[9] Although it has not been studied, this combination may also be more effective than monotherapy for secondary prevention of bleeding.

3. How can pharmacologic therapy be optimized to control hepatic encephalopathy in this patient?

- Lactulose is the drug of choice to control hepatic encephalopathy. The optimal dose is patient dependent, and the goal of therapy is to achieve two to three soft bowel movements per day. This patient is only receiving 15 mL orally once daily, which may not be enough. He should be questioned about the number of bowel movements he has been having over the past few days. The lactulose dose should be increased while he is in the hospital and the number of bowel movements should be recorded daily.
- If hepatic encephalopathy (i.e., lethargy, confusion, asterixis) does not resolve despite optimal use of lactulose, an antibiotic to reduce intestinal flora can be added. Oral aminoglycosides, such as neomycin, or metronidazole are commonly used in conjunction with lactulose. These agents are usually reserved for refractory patients and are not used for long-term therapy. In addition, protein restriction (40 g/day) may also be useful in refractory patients.

References

1. D'Amico G, Morabito A, Pagliaro L, et al. Survival and prognostic indicators in compensated and decompensated cirrhosis. Dig Dis Sci 1986;31:468–475.
2. Runyon BA. Refractory Ascites. Semin Liver Dis 1993;13:343–351.
3. Gatta A, Angeli P, Caregaro L, et al. A pathophysiologic interpretation of unresponsiveness to spironolactone in a stepped-care approach to the diuretic treatment of ascites in nonazotemic cirrhotic patients. Hepatology 1991;14:231–236.
4. Fogel MR, Sawhney VK, Neal EA, et al. Diuresis in the ascitic patient: a randomized controlled trial of three regimens. J Clin Gastroenterol 1981;3(suppl 1):73–80.
5. Perez-Ayuso RM, Arroyo V, Planas R, et al. Randomized comparative study of efficacy of furosemide versus spironolactone in nonazotemic cirrhosis with ascites. Relationship between the diuretic response and the activity of the renin-aldosterone system. Gastroenterology 1983;84(5 Pt 1):961–968.
6. Roberts LR, Kamath PS. Ascites and hepatorenal syndrome: pathophysiology and management. Mayo Clin Proc 1996;71:874–881.
7. Bhuva M, Granger D, Jensen D. Spontaneous bacterial peritonitis: An update on evaluation, management, and prevention. Am J Med 1994;97:169–175.
8. Tito L, Rimola A, Gines P, et al. Recurrence of spontaneous bacterial peritonitis in cirrhosis: Frequency and predictive factors. Hepatology 1988;8:27–31.

9. Merkel C, Marin R, Enzo E, et al. Randomised trial of nadolol alone or with isosorbide mononitrate for primary prophylaxis of variceal bleeding in cirrhosis. Gruppo-Triveneto per L'ipertensione portale. Lancet 1996;348:1677–1681.

32 ESOPHAGEAL VARICES

▶ **The Ultimate Price for a Shot and a Beer** (Level I)

Cesar Alaniz, PharmD

A 72-year-old man with a history of alcoholic cirrhosis presents to the ED reporting two episodes of hematemesis, lightheadedness, and weakness.

The patient has had several similar episodes in the past 3 months, and an EGD documented esophageal varices. He has undergone injection sclerotherapy and esophageal band ligation within the past several months. Management of the patient should be directed toward repletion of intravascular volume, control of the current bleeding episode, and prevention of rebleeding. Systemic pharmacologic options to control bleeding include octreotide, vasopressin, or a combination of vasopressin and nitroglycerin. Beta-adrenergic blockers have been used successfully to prevent rebleeding episodes; propranolol has been the most widely studied agent. This is a good teaching case because the patient does not have all of the clinical and laboratory findings usually seen in a patient with alcoholic cirrhosis and esophageal varices. This gives instructors the opportunity to point out that each patient is unique, and that patients do not always fit the "classic" disease state presentation.

▶ Questions

Problem Identification (see Figure 32–1)

1. a. *Create a list of the patient's drug-related problems.*

   - Probable bleeding esophageal varices requiring pharmacologic or other treatment.
   - Cirrhosis (by history) is a potential drug-related problem because it may result in other complications (ascites, hepatic encephalopathy) that may require drug treatment in the future.
   - IDDM (by history); adequacy of chronic glucose control with the present insulin regimen cannot be evaluated given the information presented.
   - Osteoporosis (by history) with no pharmacologic treatment being given.

   b. *What information supports the diagnosis of bleeding esophageal varices, and what indicates the relative severity of disease?*

   Evidence Supporting the Diagnosis of Varices
   - Vomiting blood in a patient with previously documented esophageal varices
   - Recent history of esophageal variceal bleed managed with sclerotherapy and banding
   - Alcoholic liver disease (by history)

   Evidence Indicating the Severity of the Problem
   - Unable to obtain orthostatic BP due to a near syncopal episode (indicating severe intravascular volume depletion)
   - One would expect, given the presence of bleeding esophageal varices, that the patient should have both ascites (shifting dullness, positive fluid wave) and splenomegaly on physical exam. However, this was not the case. The abdominal ultrasound also revealed only a small amount of ascites surrounding the liver and no focal deep fluid collections of ascites. The spleen was not described explicitly as enlarged. Although these are the actual findings from a real patient, instruct the students that they are somewhat atypical of what might be expected in a patient with alcoholic cirrhosis and esophageal varices.

Desired Outcome

2. *What are the goals for managing this patient's clinical condition?*

   - Restore intravascular volume and normalize blood pressure
   - Stop the current GI bleeding episode
   - Maintain hematocrit above 25%
   - Provide airway protection so the patient does not aspirate blood or vomitus
   - Reduce the risk of future GI bleeds (by decreasing portal hypertension)
   - Ensure that the patient continues to avoid alcohol consumption

Therapeutic Alternatives

3. a. *What non-pharmacologic interventions should be considered for this patient (see Figure 32–2)?*

   - *Resuscitation with crystalloid or colloids.* Due to his near syncopal episode upon standing, the patient needs fluid resuscitation with crystalloids, and he may also need blood (e.g., PRBCs). Although his admission hematocrit is near normal, he may be hemoconcentrated. Thus, fluid resuscitation would be expected to decrease his hematocrit.
   - *Control of the bleeding.* As the patient receives fluid, simultaneous efforts should be made to stop the bleeding. There are various interventions that may be tried; none will provide a guarantee that rebleeding will not occur. Once bleeding is controlled, attention is given to options that minimize risk of rebleed (i.e., decreasing portal hypertension).
     ✓ *Saline lavage.* This is used to assess the extent of bleeding and clear the stomach of clots prior to EGD. Iced saline lavage should not be used as it may interfere with local hemostasis or cause hypothermia.
     ✓ *Variceal banding ligation.* This procedure decreases risk of rebleeding, mortality, and the number of interventions re-

quired to eliminate varices when compared to sclerotherapy.[1] Also, there are fewer complications associated with its use compared to injection sclerotherapy, such as esophageal stricture. Band ligation is considered by many to be the intervention of choice in managing bleeding esophageal varices.

✓ *Transjugular intrahepatic porto-systemic shunt (TIPS).* This procedure is recommended by the National Digestive Diseases Advisory Board for the treatment of acute variceal bleeding that is unresponsive to endoscopic or pharmacologic therapy.[2] TIPS appears to be superior to sclerotherapy in prevention of rebleeding. However, TIPS is associated with a higher incidence of encephalopathy. Further, it may be associated with a higher mortality. The patient's age makes him a less desirable candidate for this procedure.

✓ *Balloon tamponade.* This technique applies direct pressure to the varix as a means of hemostasis (see Figure 35–7 in textbook Chapter 35). It is effective in controlling bleeding in the majority of patients but is associated with a high rate of rebleeding. It is generally used in patients who have not responded to other therapy.

✓ *Liver transplant.* This is definitive treatment but is not routinely available for all patients. Multiple considerations are involved in determining if a patient is a candidate for a transplant.

b. *What pharmacologic interventions should be considered for this patient's current condition?*

- *Injection sclerotherapy.* Sclerotherapy with sodium morrhuate, sodium tetradecyl sulfate, or ethanolamine works quickly at the site of bleeding. This form of therapy can be used to stop active bleeding and may be used as prophylaxis for future bleeds. Complications associated with sclerotherapy include ulcer formation, perforation, stricture, and pleural effusions. The patient's previous treatments of banding and sclerotherapy do not preclude repeat sclerotherapy. Consequently, endoscopy with sclerotherapy is a good option.
- *Infusion of octreotide, vasopressin, or a combination of vasopressin and nitroglycerin.* Octreotide and vasopressin have similar mechanisms of action—vasoconstriction of splanchnic beds, thereby reducing portal hypertension to control active bleeding. Both drugs have similar efficacy, but octreotide has gained favor recently because it has been shown to have fewer adverse effects than vasopressin. Side effects of vasopressin are due primarily to systemic vasoconstriction and its antidiuretic hormone (ADH) activity (see the section on sclerotherapy in textbook Chapter 35 for more detailed information). Nitroglycerin is used with vasopressin to minimize the adverse effects of vasopressin. Although octreotide or vasopressin would be reasonable for the patient, octreotide might be favored due to its better side effect profile.
- *A β-blocker (with or without a nitrate).* This should be considered for the long-term management of portal hypertension. Propranolol is the most studied β-blocker and would be a reasonable treatment option for the patient (despite his diabetes). Propranolol has been shown to decrease rebleeding episodes and results in increased survival after 2 years.[3] Addition of a nitrate should be considered in patients who do not respond to β-blocker monotherapy.

Optimal Plan

4. *What pharmacotherapeutic plan should be outlined for managing the patient's current problems?*

- Fluid resuscitation with normal saline should be given immediately. One liter of fluid may be infused at a wide open rate. Subsequently, infusion may be run at 125 mL per hour.
- Blood transfusions (e.g., PRBCs) should be administered in situations when blood loss is determined to be significant (e.g., continued hematemesis, onset of melena, decreased hematocrit after saline resuscitation).
- Octreotide should be initiated with an IV bolus dose of 50 µg followed by a continuous IV infusion of 25 µg/hr. This dose can be increased to 50 µg/hr if necessary. Octreotide has been shown to have similar efficacy to vasopressin with fewer adverse effects. Octreotide should be continued for at least 48 hours because the greatest risk for rebleeding is within 48 hours of presentation.
- Vasopressin may be used instead of octreotide, at a continuous IV infusion rate of 0.3 to 0.9 units/minute. The patient would have a greater potential for adverse effects if vasopressin were used. Nitroglycerin may be given concomitantly with vasopressin to minimize risk of vasopressin-induced side effects and augment the lowering of portal pressure. Nitroglycerin may be started by IV infusion at 10 µg/min and increased by 10 µg/min every 10 to 15 minutes until the systolic blood pressure falls to 100 mm/hg.
- Gastric lavage with normal saline should be used to clear the stomach and assess the rate of blood loss.
- Injection sclerotherapy with sodium morrhuate or a similar agent should be considered if EGD determines the source of the bleeding to be varices.
- Fresh frozen plasma should be administered to correct coagulopathy, if it exists. This patient has only a mildly elevated PT/INR, indicating that FFP is not necessary at this time.
- Platelet transfusions are also not necessary at this time.
- Vitamin K 10 mg SC for 3 days is traditionally given to correct coagulopathy, making it easier to control bleeding and minimize rebleeding.
- A β-blocker should be initiated for long-term management of the patient's esophageal varices. The non-selective β-blockers are preferred, and propranolol has been the most studied agent. Propranolol may be started at 20 mg twice daily.

Outcome Evaluation

5. *What clinical and laboratory parameters should be followed to evaluate therapeutic interventions and to minimize the risk of adverse effects?*

- Vital signs should be conducted hourly in an intensive care setting.
- Frequent monitoring of the hemoglobin and hematocrit is indicated in the actively bleeding patient (every 6 hours).
- Platelet counts should be measured initially. Subsequent measurements should be based on the degree of thrombocytopenia and to determine the need for platelet transfusions.
- The PT, aPTT, and INR should be measured initially and then daily to assess the need for FFP.

- If vasopressin is selected, serum sodium should be followed for hyponatremia secondary to the ADH activity of vasopressin. Patients should be on a cardiac monitor and observed for development of arrhythmias. Ischemic side effects should be evaluated by signs of chest pain, abdominal pain, or skin blanching.
- The propranolol dose should be titrated to decrease heart rate by 25%. The patient should be monitored for symptomatic hypotension, bradyarrhythmias, and heart failure.

Patient Counseling

6. What information should be provided to the patient about his medication therapy?

Propranolol

- The propranolol will help to decrease the chance that you will have another bleeding episode. It is important to take the propranolol exactly as prescribed by your doctor.
- Propranolol may affect how your body regulates glucose and may cause your blood glucose to decrease. Also, it may prevent you from noticing the symptoms of low blood sugar (rapid heart rate, palpitations, shakiness), so it is important that you follow your doctor's instructions for monitoring your diabetes.
- This medication may also cause dizziness, weakness, or difficulty sleeping. Call your doctor if these effects don't go away or are troublesome.
- If you miss a dose, take it as soon as you remember. However, if it is within 4 hours of your next scheduled dose, skip the missed dose and go back to your regular schedule. Don't double up on doses if you miss a dose.

Nitrate (e.g., Isosorbide Dinitrate)

- Take this medication exactly as directed by your doctor.
- Take it with a glass of water on an empty stomach.
- You may experience some dizziness, especially when standing up. Getting up slowly may minimize the dizziness.
- You may experience headaches that last for a short time after taking the medication. These should become less noticeable after you have been on the medication for a while. Contact your doctor if the headaches persist or become more severe.
- If you miss a dose, take it as soon as you remember. However, if the next dose is due within 2 hours, skip the missed dose and go back to the regular schedule. Don't double up on doses if you miss a dose.
- Store the medicine in a dry place (not the bathroom), away from heat and direct light.

References

1. Saeed ZA, Stiegmann GV, Ramirez FC, et al. Endoscopic variceal ligation is superior to combined ligation and sclerotherapy for esophageal varices: A multicenter prospective randomized trial. Hepatology 1997;25:71–74.
2. Grace ND. TIPS: The long and short of it. Gastroenterology 1997;112:1040–1043.
3. Bernard B, Lebrec D, Mathurin P, et al. Beta-adrenergic antagonists in the prevention of gastrointestinal rebleeding in patients with cirrhosis: A meta-analysis. Hepatology 1997;25:63–70.

33 HEPATIC ENCEPHALOPATHY

▶ **People, Places, and Time**   (Level I)

Nancy P. Lam, PharmD, BCPS

Confusion and disorientation in her father prompt a young woman to take him to the ED for evaluation. The patient has end-stage liver disease and has had multiple admissions for hepatic encephalopathy, uncontrolled ascites, and bleeding esophageal varices. In addition to treatment for recurrent hepatic encephalopathy, the patient requires evaluation and treatment for dehydration, hypokalemia, and anemia. Correction of precipitating factors and restriction of dietary protein are the first steps in the treatment of hepatic encephalopathy. Therapeutic alternatives include lactulose, neomycin, a combination of both agents, and branched chain amino acid products. A number of clinical and laboratory parameters must be assessed to determine the effectiveness of the therapy in improving the patient's mental status.

▶ **Questions**

Problem Identification

1. a. Create a list of the patient's drug-related problems.

- Hepatic encephalopathy requiring drug therapy.
- Dehydration possibly resulting from diuretic use.
- Hypokalemia possibly resulting from use of furosemide; potassium supplementation will be required.
- History of noncompliance with medications.
- Use of lorazepam may precipitate hepatic encephalopathy.
- Iron deficiency anemia of unknown etiology that may require further work up to rule out GI bleeding resulting from the use of ibuprofen; also history of esophageal variceal bleeding.

b. What information presented indicates the presence of hepatic encephalopathy in this patient?

- Patient has end-stage liver disease and history of hepatic encephalopathy
- Patient is confused and disoriented to time, place and people
- (+) Asterixis
- High ammonia level in blood, although ammonia level does not correlate with the presence or degree of severity of hepatic encephalopathy

c. *What precipitating factors in this patient could potentially cause hepatic encephalopathy?*

- Noncompliance with his medications (i.e., lactulose)
- Noncompliance with his diet (i.e., excessive protein intake)
- Patient is dehydrated (BUN:creatinine ratio >20) and azotemic, possibly due to the use of diuretics
- Hypokalemia (K 2.8 mEq/L) which can potentially lead to metabolic alkalosis
- Use of lorazepam, a sedative with potential CNS depressant effects

d. *What additional information is needed to satisfactorily assess the hepatic encephalopathy of this patient?*

- Other tests that are routinely done to rule out the presence of additional precipitating factors of hepatic encephalopathy in a patient with liver disease include the following[1,2]:
    - ✓ Cultures of blood and body fluids to rule out infection
    - ✓ Tap of ascites to analyze cell count in ascitic fluid to rule out peritonitis
    - ✓ Obtain a thorough medication history to assess whether the patient has been taking excessive amounts of drugs that can cause CNS depression
    - ✓ Screening (either blood or urine tests) for ingestion of toxins such as alcohol or other drugs that can cause CNS depression; this is particularly important if the patient has a history of alcohol or drug abuse
    - ✓ Rule out GI bleeding (e.g., perform stool guaiac test or NG suctioning to see if there is blood in the stomach). This is important since the patient has a history of esophageal variceal bleeding and has iron deficiency anemia. He also uses ibuprofen, which may potentially cause GI bleed.

Desired Outcome

2. *What are the general principles for the management of hepatic encephalopathy and desired therapeutic outcomes?*

General Principles

- Avoid worsening of hepatocellular function
- Identify, remove, or correct precipitating factors
- Minimize interaction between enteric bacteria and nitrogenous substances
- Promptly treat any complications of liver disease that tend to exacerbate hepatic encephalopathy

Desired Therapeutic Outcomes

- Improve the cognitive function of the patient
- Prevent progression to hepatic coma

Therapeutic Alternatives

3. a. *What non-drug interventions are important before initiating pharmacotherapeutic agents for the treatment of hepatic encephalopathy?*

- Identify and correct all precipitating factors of hepatic encephalopathy:
    - ✓ Hold diuretics, lorazepam, and ibuprofen
    - ✓ Correct potassium deficiency
    - ✓ If infection is present, treat with appropriate antibiotics
    - ✓ If GI bleeding is present and the source of bleeding is identified, stop bleeding by using appropriate interventions; evacuate the bowel; and avoid any gastric irritants
- Dietary protein restriction.[1,2] Depending on the severity of hepatic encephalopathy and the nutritional status of the patient, the intake of protein should be restricted to 20 to 60 g/day. In severe cases, protein intake can be stopped completely for a few days. As the mental status of the patient improves, dietary protein can be gradually increased by 10 to 20 g/day every 2 to 3 days. For this patient, it may be reasonable to restrict the protein to about 20 to 40 g/day initially.

b. *What pharmacotherapeutic alternatives are available for the treatment of hepatic encephalopathy? Include the mechanism of action of each drug in your answer.*

Therapeutic management is aimed at reducing the amount of ammonia in the blood or decreasing production of ammonia from protein metabolism. The two most commonly used agents are lactulose and neomycin.

- *Lactulose* is the drug of choice and is highly effective in the treatment of hepatic encephalopathy.[1,2] It is a disaccharide which is broken down in the colon to form acetic, lactic, and formic acids; this causes acidification of the colon, which converts ammonia to the less readily absorbed ammonium ion, thereby reducing diffusion of ammonia across the gut wall into the circulation. It also induces osmotic diarrhea, which decreases the contact time between gut bacteria and protein, thereby reducing protein breakdown into ammonia. Lactulose can be administered either as an oral solution (or through nasogastric tube) or as a rectal retention enema.
- *Neomycin* is an alternative to lactulose. It is a nonabsorbable antibiotic (only 1% to 3% of the drug is systemically absorbed); it decreases colonic bacteria which leads to less protein breakdown into ammonia.[1,2] It can be administered either as an oral tablet or as a rectal retention enema.
- *Combination of lactulose and neomycin* remains controversial. Theoretically, elimination of colonic bacteria from neomycin can impair degradation of lactulose to organic acids and prevent colonic acidification, which may then decrease the effect of lactulose. Clinically, however, this does not appear to be a problem.
- As a general rule, lactulose should be tried first; if satisfactory results do not occur, switch to neomycin. If both agents fail when used alone, the combination may be beneficial. Stool pH can be monitored; a stool pH <6.0 reflects a synergistic effect of the two agents.
- *Branched-chain amino acids* purportedly restore the altered ratio of branched chain to aromatic amino acids.[3] This should be considered as a last resort—only if patient's encephalopathy worsens despite the use of dietary protein restriction and maximum doses of lactulose and neomycin or the combination of both agents. Products available include an oral solution (Hepatic Aid) and a solution designed for parenteral nutrition (Hepatamine).

Optimal Plan

4. *Outline a pharmacotherapeutic plan that is most suitable for this patient. Include the drug, dosage form, dose, schedule, and duration of treatment.*

- Initiate oral lactulose 30 mL (the dose can vary from 30 to 60 mL) every 1 to 2 hours until catharsis occurs. The dose is then titrated to maintain 2 to 3 soft stools per day or until the symptoms of hepatic encephalopathy resolve (the amount required to achieve this varies from one person to another).[1,2] A response (i.e., improvement in cognitive function) is usually seen within a few days.
- If the patient fails to respond or develops intolerable adverse effects to lactulose, discontinue it and start oral neomycin. Initiate therapy with 0.5 g po QID and titrate the dose upward over a few days based on the patient's mental status and tolerance. The usual daily dose is 2 to 8 g in four divided doses.

Outcome Evaluation

5. How would you monitor the efficacy and adverse effects of the treatment you recommended?

- Improvement in mental status should be seen within 2 to 3 days. Tests that are commonly done on a daily basis to evaluate improvement in cognitive function include the following:
    - ✓ Absence or decrease in asterixis on physical exam
    - ✓ Improvement in confusion and disorientation (e.g., the patient knows his name, his family members, where he is, the current year, who the President of the United States is)
    - ✓ Improvement in simple bedside psychomotor exams, such as serial signatures, number connection test (Reitan test, see Figure 33–1), or drawing a familiar simple figure (e.g., a star, a house)
    - ✓ Assessment of the number of stools per day to make sure that the patient is maintaining 2 to 3 soft stools per day
- Monitoring parameters for adverse effects of lactulose[1,2]:
    - ✓ Signs of dehydration and hypokalemia (both are precipitating factors of hepatic encephalopathy) from excessive diarrhea
    - ✓ The number of stools, serum electrolytes (e.g., potassium), BUN, and serum creatinine
    - ✓ GI symptoms: gaseous distension, flatulence, belching
- Monitoring parameters for adverse effects of neomycin[1,2]:
    - ✓ Serum creatinine may be checked about twice a week when neomycin is started while the patient is in the hospital. It can be checked periodically on an as-needed basis when the patient is on a stable dose as an outpatient.
    - ✓ Hearing loss, primarily with long-term use in patients with renal failure; tell patients to report reduced hearing immediately
    - ✓ Excessive diarrhea

Patient Counseling

6. What medication-related information should be provided to the patient about his therapy upon discharge?

General Information

- One of the complications of your liver disease is confusion. This medication will help to keep you from being confused.
- Keep taking this medicine for as long as your doctor prescribes it. Try not to miss any doses. If you do miss a dose, take it as soon as you remember. However, if it is almost time for the next dose, skip the missed dose and go back to your regular schedule. Do not double doses.

Lactulose

- You can mix the medication with fruit juice or water to reduce the sweetness of the medication.
- It is important for you to maintain bowel movements every day. Any time you become constipated, you can take the medication more frequently until you get a bowel movement, and you should inform your doctor immediately so that he can adjust the dose for you.
- If you experience diarrhea, you may be taking too much of the medication. Contact your doctor immediately so that he can give you instructions on how to decrease the dose of the medication.

Neomycin

- This medication may be taken with or without food.
- The more common side effects of this medication include nausea and vomiting. Notify your doctor immediately if you notice any of these rare side effects: loss of hearing; unsteadiness or weakness; ringing, buzzing, or a feeling of fullness in the ears; greatly decreased urination; or skin rash.
- Store this medication away from heat and direct light and out of the reach of children.

References

1. Cordoba J, Blei AT. Treatment of hepatic encephalopathy. Am J Gastroenterol 1997;92:1429–1439.
2. Riordan SM, Williams R. Treatment of hepatic encephalopathy. N Engl J Med 1997;337:473–479.
3. Fabbri A, Magrini N, Bianchi G, et al. Overview of randomized clinical trial of oral branched-chain amino acid treatment in chronic hepatic encephalopathy. JPEN 1996;20:159–164.
4. Quero JC, Schalm SW. Subclinical hepatic encephalopathy. Semin Liver Dis 1996;16:321–328.

34 ACUTE PANCREATITIS

▶ **Cuts Like a Knife** (Level II)

Charles W. Fetrow, PharmD
Maria Yaramus, PharmD

A 59-year-old man presents to the ED because of complaints of intense mid-epigastric and abdominal pain that has persisted for 3 to 4 weeks. Physical and laboratory examinations indicate the presence of acute pancreatitis. Treatment of the patient involves provision of adequate pain relief, rehydration with IV fluids, correction of hyperglycemia, and temporary institution of parenteral nutrition. The patient subsequently develops steatorrhea, fever, orthostatic hypotension, and leukocytosis with a left shift. Implementation of appropriate empiric antibiotic and pancreatic enzyme replacement therapy is required. The case offers the opportunity to compare the various enzyme replacement products that are available for acute and chronic pancreatitis.

Questions

Problem Identification (see Figure 34–1)

1. a. *What signs, symptoms, and laboratory tests are consistent with the diagnosis of acute pancreatitis?*

    - Nausea and vomiting; weight loss; voluntary guarding; midepigastric abdominal pain; abdominal distention; elevated levels of lipase, amylase, LDH, and AST/ALT.

   b. *What are the likely etiologies that may explain the development of acute pancreatitis in this case?*

    - Choledocholithiasis (gallstone-associated biliary tract disease) is suspected due to the questionable opacity of the common bile duct seen on abdominal ultrasound.
    - Ethanol abuse is possible, but the patient's history is not suggestive of this.

   c. *Construct a drug-related problem list for this patient.*

    - Epigastric pain requiring symptomatic relief
    - Dehydration, requiring volume repletion
    - Glucose intolerance secondary to acute pancreatitis requiring insulin or other treatment
    - Weight loss, necessitating a nutritional assessment and plan

Desired Outcome

2. *What are the desired goals of therapy for this patient?*

    - Alleviate pain
    - Achieve euvolemia and correct underlying hyponatremia and hypokalemia
    - Achieve glucose control
    - Provide adequate nutritional therapy during treatment of acute pancreatitis
    - Prevent potential complications from acute pancreatitis

Therapeutic Alternatives

3. *What therapies may be instituted to achieve the goals outlined above? Provide a rationale for each therapy.*

    - *Supportive care.* Most cases of acute pancreatitis are self-limiting and will resolve after a few days of general supportive therapy, depending on the etiology. Gallstone disease should be excluded in every patient with acute pancreatitis because surgical or endoscopic intervention with subsequent removal of the obstructing stone can minimize further damage and future attacks. Controversy exists as to just how quickly surgical intervention should take place after the diagnosis of a gallstone in the common bile duct has been made.[1] Patients are usually made NPO in the acute phase to minimize exocrine function of the pancreas.
    - *IV fluids and electrolytes.* Repletion with fluids and electrolytes is important to minimize the risk of potential complications such as hypotension, shock, or organ system failure. In severe or recurrent cases, several liters of plasma and blood may be sequestered into peritoneal and retroperitoneal spaces, warranting prompt colloidal supplementation with IV hydroxyethyl starch, albumin, or whole blood to sustain intravascular volume.
    - *IV narcotic analgesics.* Pain control often mandates the use of IV narcotics in an effort to keep the patient pain-free and NPO. Oral analgesics can be instituted once control of the acute phase has been accomplished. Narcotic addiction can become an issue in patients with frequent exacerbations.
    - *Exogenous insulin.* Because endogenous secretion of insulin is temporarily lacking, exogenous insulin, together with appropriate nutrition support, should normalize glucose metabolism even in individuals with minimal remaining pancreatic function.
    - *IV nutrition.* This intervention is most important for patients with acute exacerbations that last more than 3 days. IV nutrition provides the daily caloric substrates needed for energy, maintenance and repletion of body protein stores, while "calming" the pancreas by avoiding the enteral route, and allowing for faster resolution of inflammation.

Optimal Plan

4. *Develop a pharmacotherapeutic care plan for this patient.*

    Analgesia
    - Meperidine PCA, initiated with a loading dose of 100 to 150 mg IV followed by a continuous infusion of 10 to 25 mg/hr, with additional patient-administered boluses of 10 to 20 mg every 15 minutes (maximum, 75 mg/hr).
    - Hydromorphone PCA could also be used, starting with a 2 to 4 mg IV loading dose followed by a continuous infusion of 0.25 to 0.5 mg/hr; the patient may administer additional boluses of 0.1 to 0.25 mg every 15 minutes (maximum 3 mg/hr).
    - Scheduled intermittent narcotic injections may be given if PCA is unavailable; supplemental doses may be given as needed for breakthrough pain. Meperidine 100 to 150 mg IV Q 3 H with an additional 50 to 75 mg IV Q 3 H PRN for breakthrough pain; or hydromorphone 1 to 2 mg IV Q 3 H with an additional 0.5 to 1 mg IV Q 3 H PRN for breakthrough pain. Aggressive analgesia is important. Meperidine is preferred over other narcotic analgesics because it lacks significant effects on the sphincter of Oddi and pancreatic ducts. It should be used cautiously in the elderly and in patients with renal disease because of its potential to cause seizures due to accumulation and toxicity of the metabolite normeperidine.

    IV Fluids
    - Normal saline 1–2 L with 20 mEq KCl at 150 mL/hr. Although of minimal caloric value, crystalloid solutions containing dextrose should be avoided during the acute phase because of the potential to contribute to existing glucose intolerance.

    Sliding Scale SQ Insulin
    - Since this patient will most likely not need to continue on insulin after this admission, a convenient method of providing optimal control of glucose may be the use of a sliding scale insulin approach. One example is given below. For blood glucose:
        - ✓ 200 to 250 mg/dL   Give 2 units regular insulin
        - ✓ 251 to 300 mg/dL   Give 4 units regular insulin
        - ✓ 301 to 350 mg/dL   Give 6 units regular insulin
        - ✓ 351 to 400 mg/dL   Give 8 units regular insulin
        - ✓ >400 mg/dL   Call MD

IV Nutrition

- In most cases this would be withheld for the first few days. In the absence of complications, patients would likely remain in the hospital for only 1 to 2 weeks. However, total parenteral nutrition providing 25 to 30 non-protein kcal/kg/day might be best instituted for patients expected to remain in the hospital for an extended period of time (e.g., patients with morbid complications of pancreatitis or patients with a poor prognosis according to Ranson's criteria (refer to textbook Chapter 37). A standard formula based on weight might include approximately 1.5 g/kg/day of protein in addition to the glucose component. At this time, high triglyceride values contraindicate use of lipid emulsion therapy. In cases of mild or moderate pancreatitis a clear liquid diet can usually be started after 3 to 6 days.

Outcome Evaluation

5. *Outline monitoring parameters for efficacy and adverse effects of therapy for pain management.*

Efficacy

- Clinical interviews conducted with the patient at the bedside will enable assessment of pain relief by use of subjective tests (e.g., numerical scales, color scales, visual analog scales, McGill pain questionnaire).
- Additional information may be gained by examining the patient's vital signs (e.g., blood pressure, respiratory rate, pulse rate), sleep patterns, and requests for additional analgesics.

Adverse Effects

- Monitor the patient for signs of respiratory depression, constipation, excessive sedation, nausea and vomiting, tolerance, and/or narcotic dependence or withdrawal.

▶ Follow-up Questions

a. *What potential etiologies might explain this patient's fever and relapsing acute pancreatitis?*

- Pancreatic necrosis, abscess
- Infected pseudocyst
- Nosocomial pneumonia

b. *What are the new treatment goals for this patient?*

- Control potential infectious process
- Decrease fat malabsorption and steatorrhea
- Achieve and maintain glucose control

c. *Given this new information, what therapeutic interventions should be considered for this patient?*

Antibiotics

- Institution of early empiric antibiotics is controversial for patients with acute pancreatitis who lack documentation of an infectious process.
- When an infected abscess, pseudocyst, or necrosis is suspected, empiric regimens should be designed under the premise that infecting organisms are likely to be enteric gram-negative bacilli (e.g., *E. coli, Proteus* spp. or *Pseudomonas* spp.), enterococci, *Staphylococcus* spp. or anaerobic bacteria.
- Ampicillin 2 g IV Q 6–8 H + gentamicin 3 mg/kg IV Q 24 H + metronidazole 500 mg po Q 12 H is a cost-effective regimen that provides adequate coverage against the most likely implicated organisms.
- Alternatively, ticarcillin/clavulanate (Timentin) 3.1 g IV Q 6–8 H + gentamicin 3 mg/kg IV Q 24 H could be utilized. This regimen is more costly than the previous regimen and lacks adequate coverage of enterococci.
- Other antibiotic regimens utilizing imipenem/cilastatin or meropenem may also be reasonable based on their antimicrobial spectrums. Imipenem/cilastatin has been associated with a reduced incidence of pancreatic sepsis in patients with necrotizing pancreatitis.[2]
- Ultimately, culture and sensitivity data and clinical response should be used to guide antimicrobial therapy.

Pancreatic Enzyme Replacement Therapy

- Fat malabsorption can be managed by a low-fat diet (50 to 75 g/day) and pancreatic enzyme replacement.
- Pancreatic enzyme therapy should be instituted with meals to provide at least 30,000 IU of lipase activity and 10,000 IU of trypsin activity delivered to the duodenum over the 4-hour postprandial period.[3]
- The optimal dosage schedule remains debatable. However, division of the total mealtime dose into before-meal, during-meal, and after-meal portions may further reduce steatorrhea in some situations.
- Initial therapy may be accomplished with 4 Viokase tablets or the equivalent of Viokase powder (approximately 1.4 g) taken with each meal (TID) and with snacks (as needed) every day. This regimen supplies at least 32,000 units of lipase activity. Other therapies may require less tablets or capsules but are likely to be more costly without an associated proven increase in efficacy.[4] For more information on the available products, refer to the table that deals with enzyme content of selected pancreatic enzyme preparations in textbook Chapter 37.

d. *How should these new therapies be monitored for efficacy and adverse effects?*

Antibiotics

- Efficacy is assessed by return of the patient's WBC count and fever toward normal. Patients also tend to report that they are "feeling better" as their infection subsides. Orthostatic hypotension should resolve as appropriate fluid management and antibiotic therapies bring the situation under control. Conversion from IV to oral therapy should be considered as early as 2 to 3 days after initiation of IV antibiotics if patients are clinically improving and markers of infection (e.g., WBC count and temperature) are returning toward normal.
- Adverse effects depend upon the antibiotics chosen; allergic reactions, interstitial nephritis, nephrotoxicity, ototoxicity, disulfiram-like reactions, blood dyscrasias (e.g., neutropenia and thrombocytopenia), and dermatological manifestations are potential side effects of the antibiotics.

Pancreatic Enzyme Therapy

- Efficacy is assessed by examination of the patient's stool daily for fecal fat. A significant increase in fecal fat is usually detected upon gross examination of the stool. The stool usually takes on a "pasty" or "putty-like" appearance. Doses of the pancreatic enzymes should be gradually increased to minimize fat in the stool.

- Adverse effects include impaired folic acid absorption and subsequent folate deficiency. High doses of pancreatic enzymes have resulted in hyperuricosuria, hyperuricemia, nephrolithiasis, and colonic strictures.

Patient Counseling

6. The patient is being discharged today after a prolonged hospital course. The attending physician would like you to talk with the patient about his discharge medications. What information should be provided?

- It is of the utmost importance for you to be compliant with your pancreatic enzyme therapy to minimize return of fat in your stool and reduce the likelihood of recurrent abdominal pain. Be sure to take the required number of doses with each meal or snack every day.
- Swallow these tablets whole with a full glass of water. Do not crush or chew the tablets. Like your disease, these medicines (enzyme therapy) may cause stomach upset, abdominal pain, cramps, and diarrhea. If these problems persist, notify your doctor or pharmacist. Also contact the doctor if you experience any significant changes in the color, odor, or consistency of your stool.
- It is also necessary that you follow a low-fat diet, combined with eating smaller but more frequent meals, instead of large, less frequent meals.
- It is very important that you complete your entire course of antibiotic therapy, as prescribed.

References

1. Steinberg W, Tenner S. Acute pancreatitis. N Engl J Med 1994;330:17:1198–1210.
2. Pederzoli P, Bassi C, Vesentini S, et al. A randomized multicenter clinical trial of antibiotic prophylaxis of septic complications in acute necrotizing pancreatitis with imipenem. Surg Gynecol Obstet 1993;176:480–483.
3. Lankisch PG. Enzyme treatment of exocrine pancreatic insufficiency in chronic pancreatitis. Digestion 1993;54 (suppl 2):21–29.
4. Tenner S, Levine RS, Steinberg WM. Drug treatment of acute and chronic pancreatitis. In: Lewis JH, ed. A Pharmacologic Approach to Gastrointestinal Disorders. Baltimore, Williams & Wilkins, 1994:311–340.

35 VIRAL HEPATITIS

▶ **The Lady With the Ankle Tattoo** (Level I)

Nancy P. Lam, PharmD, BCPS

A 35-year-old woman with a history of hypothyroidism is referred to a liver clinic for assessment of persistently elevated hepatic aminotransferase enzymes. Further laboratory testing and a liver biopsy reveal the presence of chronic hepatitis C virus (HCV) infection. Risk factors for hepatitis in this patient include a remote blood transfusion and an ankle tattoo. Interferon is the treatment of choice for chronic HCV, and students are asked to design a drug regimen using one of the three products currently available. An extensive list of monitoring parameters for efficacy and adverse effects must also be created. Because the patient has no immunity to hepatitis A and B, students are asked to devise vaccination schedules to prevent these diseases. When the patient is classified as a nonresponder after 12 weeks of interferon therapy, therapeutic options include investigational combination drug protocols or a six-month treatment course using increased doses of interferon.

▶ Questions

Problem Identification

1. a. Create a list of the patient's drug-related problems.
- Chronic hepatitis C infection requiring pharmacologic intervention.
- Mild anemia of unknown etiology that may require further workup and treatment.
- Hypothyroidism is a chronic, stable problem that is presently treated adequately with levothyroxine 0.1 mg QD (TSH level within normal limits).

b. What physical findings, laboratory values, or medical history information suggests the presence of chronic hepatitis C virus (HCV) infection?

Physical Findings
- Patient complaint of fatigue (a non-specific finding)
- Tattoo close to the left ankle (tattooing is a risk factor for hepatitis C transmission)

Laboratory Values
- Elevated hepatic aminotransferase enzymes (AST, ALT) indicate the presence of hepatic inflammation
- (+) HCV RNA test indicates the presence of HCV RNA replication
- (+) Anti-HCV indicates either a past or current infection
- (+) HCV genotype 1b has been associated with less favorable response to interferon treatment. A total of six genotypes and over 30 subtypes of HCV have been identified worldwide. Genotype 1a and 1b are the most prevalent HCV types in the United States. This test is not routinely performed, and HCV genotyping is considered an investigational tool at the present time.
- Liver biopsy shows features consistent with chronic hepatitis

Medical History Information
- History of blood transfusion 15 years ago, prior to the availability of hepatitis C screening test of blood products
- History of elevated liver aminotransferase enzymes 2 years ago

Desired Outcome

2. What are the goals of treatment of chronic HCV infection?
- Loss of HCV RNA in serum (indicates loss of HCV replication)

- Normalize liver aminotransferases (indicates resolution of hepatic inflammation)
- Alleviate symptoms
- Decrease progression of liver disease to cirrhosis or hepatocellular carcinoma
- Increase survival

Therapeutic Alternatives

3. a. What non-pharmacologic measures should be considered for this patient?

- No dietary restriction is necessary; a well-balanced and healthy diet is recommended.
- There is no need for restriction of physical activity; the patient can exercise as tolerated.
- Avoid potentially hepatotoxic drugs and chemicals (including alcohol).
- Educate the patient in regard to preventive measures to avoid infecting other people, including (1) refrain from donating blood, organs, tissues, or semen (if male); (2) avoid sharing razors and toothbrushes; (3) cover open wounds; and (4) practice safe sex (use of latex condoms is recommended primarily for persons with multiple sexual partners).

b. What pharmacotherapeutic alternatives are available for treatment of this patient?

- Interferon alfa products are the only agents approved for initial therapy for chronic hepatitis C infection. There are three products approved for this indication:
  ✓ *Interferon alfa-2a (Roferon)*
  ✓ *Interferon alfa-2b (Intron A)*
  ✓ *Interferon alfacon-1 (Infergen)*
- Interferon alfa-2b has been the most extensively studied and has been used for the longest period of time. There are no direct comparative studies to assess the efficacy and adverse effects of the three interferon products. In general, the response rates and the types and incidence of adverse effects with the current approved dosing regimens appear to be similar among the three products.
- Selection of an interferon product is usually based on the clinician's experience with an individual product, accessibility to a particular product, and the cost of each product. The average wholesale price of a 12-month course of treatment is comparable with the three products and ranges between about $4700 and $5100 based on prices available at the time of this writing.
- Patients with compensated liver disease who relapse after receiving initial treatment with interferon alfa may be treated with Rebetron, a combination product containing interferon alfa-2b and ribavirin. The recommended treatment duration is 24 weeks.

c. Does this patient have any concurrent medical conditions that are considered contraindications to receiving the treatments discussed in the previous question?

This particular patient does not have any contraindications to the use of interferon alfa. Contraindications to receiving interferon *in any patient* include:

- Decompensated liver cirrhosis (i.e., history of hepatic encephalopathy, esophageal variceal bleeding, or ascites)
- Severe psychiatric illness (history of hospitalization for depression and suicidal attempts)
- Thyroid disease not controlled by medications (although rare, both hypo- and hyperthyroidism have been associated with the use of interferon). This patient has hypothyroidism but is well controlled with levothyroxine (normal TSH), so there is no contraindication to interferon use. The TSH should be monitored closely during interferon treatment.
- Presence of autoimmune diseases (e.g., autoimmune hepatitis; psoriasis)
- Myelosuppression (WBC $<3.0 \times 10^3/mm^3$) or thrombocytopenia (platelets $<70 \times 10^3/mm^3$)
- Active alcohol or substance abuse
- Immunosuppressed transplant recipients (this is a relative contraindication)

Optimal Plan

4. a. Design a pharmacotherapeutic plan for this patient. Include the drug, dose, schedule, and duration of therapy.

- Since the three different interferon products have similar efficacy and adverse effect profiles, the choice of agent depends upon the experience of the clinician with the individual product and the cost.
- The interferon products are all available in injectable form only, and subcutaneous injection is the recommended route of administration.
- The recommended dosing schedules are as follows:
  ✓ Interferon alfa-2a 3 million units SC three times a week
  ✓ Interferon alfa-2b 3 million units SC three times a week
  ✓ interferon alfacon-1 9 μg SC three times a week
- Based on the recent NIH consensus statement on the management of hepatitis C, the duration of the treatment should be 12 months or longer if the patient responded with normalization of ALT and/or clearance of HCV RNA in serum by 12 weeks of treatment.[1,2]
- It is important to note that the optimal dose and duration of interferon treatment for chronic hepatitis C have not yet been determined.

b. Outline a plan for vaccination against other forms of viral hepatitis for this patient.

- Since the patient does not have antibodies (i.e., no immunity) against hepatitis A or B, she should receive vaccination against hepatitis A and B as recommended in the recent NIH consensus statement on the management of hepatitis C.[1]
- For hepatitis A vaccination, use either Havrix 1440 ELISA units or Vaqta 50 units, both given as an IM injection. A second booster dose should be given 6 to 12 months after the initial dose.
- For hepatitis B vaccination, use either Recombivax HB 10 μg or Engerix-B 20 μg IM now, then repeat at 1 and 6 months after the initial dose. An alternative schedule for Engerix-B is to give injections at 0, 1, 2, and 12 months.
- The hepatitis A and B vaccines can be given at the same time, but each vaccine should be given with a different syringe and at a different injection site.

Outcome Evaluation

5. a. *How should the therapy you recommended be monitored for efficacy and adverse effects?*

    Monitoring Parameters for Efficacy
    - Obtain serum ALT and HCV RNA 12 weeks after the start of treatment to assess whether the patient is responding to therapy. These tests should be repeated at the end of treatment to document the end-of-treatment response. Final testing should be done 6 months post-treatment to determine if a sustained response has been achieved.
    - Inquire about the presence of hepatitis symptoms at each visit.

    Monitoring Parameters for Adverse Effects
    - Flu-like symptoms (e.g., fever, chills, myalgias, and fatigue) are usually most severe with the first dose of interferon.
    - Inquire about symptoms at each visit, including decreased level of performance, mood changes, inability to concentrate, fatigue, muscle aches, loss of appetite, weight loss, diarrhea, headache, and alopecia.
    - Obtain an ALT every 4 weeks.
    - Check a complete blood count weekly during the first 2 weeks of treatment, then monthly thereafter.
    - Obtain a TSH level every 3 months.
    - Inquire about the average amount (per day or per week) of acetaminophen that the patient is taking to reduce adverse effects of interferon.

    b. *Which baseline parameters of this patient have been suggested as predictors of poor response to the treatment you recommended?*

    - Many factors have been suggested as predictors of poor response to interferon treatment. These include long duration of infection, high pretreatment HCV RNA level (>1 mEq/mL), presence of cirrhosis on liver biopsy, genotype 1 HCV, old age, high hepatic iron stores, and coinfection with HIV. The most consistently identified negative factors are cirrhosis, high viral load, and genotype 1.[3]
    - The negative predictive factors of response present in this patient include infection with HCV probably for 15 years, high pretreatment HCV RNA levels (3.4 mEq/mL), and infection with genotype 1 HCV.
    - Although HCV RNA levels and HCV genotype have both been suggested as important factors, the NIH consensus statement pointed out that the decision to treat should not be based on the status of HCV RNA levels (viral load) or HCV genotype.[1]

    c. *What actions can be taken if the patient develops intolerable adverse effects to the treatment you recommended?*

    General Guidelines
    - Premedication with acetaminophen, especially with the first dose, helps to ameliorate the flu-like side effects of interferon.
    - The dosage of interferon should be reduced or the drug temporarily discontinued if moderate to severe adverse effects occur.

    General Dosage Reduction Guidelines for Interferon-alfa
    - Reduce the dose by 50% if any of the following occur: fatigue that interferes with daily routine activities; daily nausea with occasional vomiting; absolute neutrophil count $<0.75 \times 10^3/mm^3$ or platelet count $<50 \times 10^3/mm^3$.
    - Interferon should be stopped if any of the following occur: fatigue that requires bed rest; vomiting more than twice daily; uncontrolled thyroid dysfunction; severe psychiatric complications; absolute neutrophil count $<0.5 \times 10^3/mm^3$ or platelet count $<30 \times 10^3/mm^3$.

    Guidelines for Dosage Reduction With Interferon Alfacon-1 (as Per the Manufacturer)
    - Reduce the dose from 9 µg to 7.5 µg if the patient experiences an intolerable adverse effect.
    - Temporarily stop treatment if the patient experiences severe adverse effects.

Patient Counseling

6. *What information should be provided to this patient regarding her treatment?*

    Interferon
    - This medication is intended to stop the growth of your hepatitis C virus infection. This should help to return your liver function tests to normal and prevent the disease from progressing to more severe forms such as cirrhosis and liver cancer.
    - It is important for you to take this medication exactly as directed by your doctor.
    - Read the patient information sheet carefully and make sure you know how much of your medication should be drawn up into the syringe with each dose.
    - The types and the severity of side effects associated with this medication vary from one person to another. Giving the injection at bedtime may help to reduce some of the symptoms. Four to six hours after the first dose, you may experience very strong flu-like symptoms, such as fever, chills, fatigue, headache, and muscle aches. With continuation of the treatment, most of these side effects will become more tolerable. However, fatigue may persist. Other common side effects that may occur during treatment include thinning of hair, diarrhea, and mood changes. These side effects will disappear when the treatment is stopped. It is important for you to let your doctor know how you feel during the treatment, so that he or she can adjust the dose if necessary.
    - You can take acetaminophen as needed to reduce the headache, muscle or joint aches, and fever. Keep a record of your symptoms and how much acetaminophen you use every day and report them to your doctor or pharmacist at each follow-up visit.
    - It is important for you to keep the follow-up appointments with your doctor, so that your progress can be evaluated during treatment.
    - Never change brands of interferon without informing your doctor first.
    - Do not dispose of your used syringes and needles at home. Bring them back to your doctor's office so they can be disposed of properly.
    - This medicine should be stored in the refrigerator (2 to 8°C or 36 to 46°F).

▶ **Follow-up Question**

1. *Based on this new information, what changes, if any, would you recommend for the treatment of chronic hepatitis C for this patient?*

- Studies have shown that patients who respond favorably to interferon will do so within the first 12 weeks of treatment, as reflected by normalization of ALT and/or loss of HCV RNA in serum. Since the ALT level is still elevated and the HCV RNA test is still (+) at 12 weeks, this suggests that the patient is a nonresponder. According to the NIH consensus statement, it is recommended that interferon be stopped at this point. Nonresponders should be considered for investigational protocols using combination therapy (e.g., ribavirin with interferon) or studies using different dosing regimens of interferon.[1]
- Alternatively, this patient can be tried on higher doses of interferon alfa:
  - Interferon alfacon-1 15 µg three times a week for 6 months has received FDA approval for patients who previously failed to respond to interferon alfa. In the retreatment study which led to the approval of this regimen, a sustained virologic response rate (i.e., HCV RNA remained undetectable in serum 6 months after discontinuation of treatment) of 5% was reported using 15 µg three times a week for 24 weeks.[4] Patients entered into this retreatment study had previously failed to respond to a 24-week course of 3 million units of interferon alfa-2b or 9 µg of interferon alfacon-1 given three times a week.
  - The labeling of interferon alfa-2a also states that retreatment with 6 million units three times a week for 6 to 12 months can be considered for those patients who had only a partial response to initial interferon treatment.
  - Although interferon alfa-2b does not have specific FDA approval for use in higher doses to retreat previous nonresponders, higher doses (5 to 6 million units three times a week) have been studied and used in clinical practice for nonresponders.

Overall, increasing the dose of interferon alfa for retreatment provides only marginal improvement in sustained virologic response. Currently, the equivalent doses of the available interferon products are not known. It should be kept in mind that higher doses of interferon are associated with higher rates of adverse effects. The benefits and risks of using higher interferon doses should be weighed and discussed with the patient prior to making the decision on retreatment.

- In general, chronic hepatitis C infection is a slowly progressive disease. About 25% of patients will develop cirrhosis in 20 to 30 years after the onset of infection. It is not clear whether the remaining 75% of patients will eventually develop cirrhosis. The progression of the disease can be more rapid with concurrent use of alcohol.
- The prognosis of a patient who fails to respond to interferon is not clear. If this patient chooses not to receive further interferon treatment or to participate in investigational trials, she should be encouraged to have follow-up evaluations every 6 to 12 months to assess her liver function and progression of the hepatitis C infection. She should also be reminded to avoid consumption of alcohol.

References

1. National Institutes of Health Consensus Development Conference Panel Statement. Management of hepatitis C. Hepatology 1997;26(suppl 1):2S–10S.
2. Poynard T, Leroy V, Cohard M, et al. Meta-analysis of interferon randomized trials in the treatment of viral hepatitis C: Effects of dose and duration. Hepatology 1996;24:778–789.
3. Davis GL, Lau JY. Factors predictive of a beneficial response to therapy of hepatitis C. Hepatology 1997;26(3 suppl 1):122S–127S.
4. Keeffe EB, Hollinger FB, Consensus Interferon Study Group. Therapy of hepatitis C: Consensus interferon trials. Hepatology 1997;26(3 suppl 1):101S–107S.

SECTION 4

Renal and Genitourinary Tract Disorders

Gary R. Matzke, PharmD, FCP, FCCP, Section Editor

36 DRUG-INDUCED ACUTE RENAL FAILURE

▶ **Unintended Consequences** (Level II)

Mary K. Stamatakis, PharmD

A 71-year-old man receiving his fourth week of a 6-week course of gentamicin plus piperacillin for presumed Serratia marcescens mediastinitis develops elevated renal function tests. He also has other findings consistent with intrinsic acute renal failure (ARF). Students are asked to consider the evidence that supports gentamicin therapy as a contributing factor to the development of ARF. Therapeutic alternatives include fluid restriction and loop diuretic administration to treat volume overload. Replacement of gentamicin with a non-nephrotoxic drug that provides adequate gram-negative coverage should also be considered. The case also requires students to appropriately adjust the dosage of the patient's other medications based on the degree of renal impairment.

▶ **Questions**

Problem Identification

1. a. *Create a list of the patient's drug-related problems.*

   - Acute renal failure (ARF)
   - Volume overload not responding to previous dosages of furosemide
   - Dosage adjustments needed for medications based on the patient's renal function

   b. *What information (signs, symptoms, laboratory values) indicates the presence or severity of each problem?*

   Acute Renal Failure
   - Rise in BUN and serum creatinine from baseline
   - Coarse granular casts on urinalysis
   - Decrease in calculated creatinine clearance. Refer to textbook Table 42–4 for equations to estimate renal function when serum creatinine is stable, and Table 42–5 for equations to estimate renal function when creatinine is changing by more than 10% to 20% per day. In this case, the patient's serum creatinine concentration on admission was stable at 1.3 mg/dL and is currently relatively constant at 3.2 mg/dL with less than 10% to 20% variability. Therefore, an equation such as the Cockcroft–Gault equation, which derives creatinine clearance from ideal body weight (IBW), age, and steady-state serum creatinine concentration, would adequately assess his creatinine clearance. His admission creatinine clearance is estimated as:

$$IBW(kg, male) = 50 + 2.3 \times (\text{every inch in height} > 5 \text{ feet})$$
$$= 50 + 2.3 (8.9)$$
$$= 70.5 \text{ kg}$$
$$CLcr(male) = \frac{(140 - age) \times (IBWkg)}{SCr \times 72}$$
$$= \frac{(140 - 71)(70.5)}{(1.3)(72)}$$
$$= 52 \text{ mL/min (admission creatinine clearance)}$$

Using the same equations, his current creatinine clearance is estimated to be 21 mL/min.

Volume Overload
- 24 hour fluid intake greater than fluid output
- Ankle/sacral edema
- Crackles on respiratory examination
- Shortness of breath

c. *What additional laboratory information would assist in the assessment of this patient?*

- ARF is classified into three categories. Pre-renal ARF is secondary to a reduction in blood delivery to the kidney, such as with hypotension or severe heart failure. Intrinsic renal failure is a result of insult (e.g., nephrotoxic drugs) to the structural tissues of the kidney, and post-renal ARF is due to obstruction of urinary outflow, such as with prostatic hypertrophy. There are additional laboratory tests that can aid in the differential diagnosis of pre-renal renal failure from acute intrinsic renal failure and post-renal renal failure.

Test	Pre-renal ARF	Intrinsic and Post-renal ARF
Fractional excretion of sodium (FE_{Na}) $$FE_{Na} = \frac{(UNa)(SCr) \times 100}{(Ucr)(SNa)}$$ where UNa = urine sodium conc. (mg/dL) SCr = serum creatinine conc. (mg/dL) Ucr = urine creatinine conc. (mg/dL) SNa = serum sodium conc. (mg/dL)	<1%	1–2%
Urinary osmolality (mOsm)	>500	<350
Urinary sodium (mEq/L)	<20	>40
Urine/plasma creatinine ratio	>40	<20
BUN/SCr ratio	>20:1	10–15:1
Urinalysis	(–) Cells, cellular debris	RBCs, WBCs, cellular casts

- With pre-renal ARF, there is a reduction in circulating or effective blood flow to the kidney. To compensate, sodium and water reabsorption by the kidney is increased, with less excreted in the urine. As a result of decreased sodium excretion, fractional excretion of sodium and urinary sodium concentrations are low. The BUN/creatinine ratio is increased due to increased tubular reabsorption of urea secondary to sodium and water reabsorption. Decreased water excretion results in concentrated urine (mOsm >500) and an elevated urine/plasma creatinine ratio.
- In this patient's case, the following results are obtained: FE_{Na} = 2.8%, urine osmolality = 325 mOsm, urine sodium = 77 mEq/L, urine/plasma creatinine ratio = 19.5, and BUN/creatinine ratio = 16:1. The urinary tests indicate that pre-renal renal failure is unlikely. In addition, coarse granular casts on urinalysis are highly suggestive of intrinsic renal failure. Furthermore, symptoms of post-renal disease, such as anuria, periods of anuria alternating with polyuria, flank pain, and infection are absent. Therefore, the patient most likely has an intrinsic cause of his ARF.

d. *Could any of the patient's problems have been caused by drug therapy?*

- Gentamicin therapy is the most likely cause of intrinsic renal failure in this patient. Gentamicin, as with other aminoglycosides, can result in acute tubular necrosis (ATN) due to a direct toxic effect on the proximal tubular cells.[1] Although the patient had a hypotensive episode during surgery which may have resulted in under-perfusion of his kidney, it is unlikely that hypotension was the etiology of ARF due to the delayed rise in creatinine following the hypotensive event. Hypoperfusion of the kidney would typically result in a more immediate decline in renal function. Furthermore, the patient received more than 3 weeks of gentamicin therapy. A prolonged course of aminoglycoside therapy (typically greater than 7 to 10 days) is a risk factor for the development of ARF,[1] especially in a patient with pre-existing chronic renal disease.
- The incidence of gentamicin-induced acute renal failure is greater when cumulative drug exposure is high. Methods to minimize drug exposure include maintaining trough concentrations <2 µg/mL for gentamicin and tobramycin,[2] minimizing duration of therapy, and avoiding repeated courses of aminoglycosides. The association between peak concentrations and nephrotoxicity is less clear; however, consistently elevated peak levels may contribute to toxicity.
- In this case, elevated trough concentrations (>2 µg/mL), peak gentamicin concentrations at the upper limit of normal (8–10 µg/mL), and prolonged duration of therapy (25 days) all contribute to excessive drug exposure.

e. *What risk factors did the patient have for gentamicin-induced acute renal failure?*

- Large total cumulative dose exposure
- Prolonged course of therapy
- Trough concentrations >2 µg/mL
- Pre-existing renal dysfunction (calculated creatinine clearance of 52 mL/min)
- Increased age
- Gram-negative bacteremia

- Concomitant diuretic administration
- Other risk factors for gentamicin-induced ARF include (1) previous course(s) of aminoglycosides, (2) administration of other nephrotoxic medications, (3) co-administration of vancomycin, (4) volume depletion, (5) pre-existing liver dysfunction, and (6) potassium and magnesium depletion.
- For a complete list of potential risk factors for aminoglycoside-induced renal failure, see Table 47-6 of the textbook.

Desired Outcome

2. What are the goals of pharmacotherapy in this case?

- Return renal function to baseline
- Restore volume status to normal
- Resolve the infection
- Optimize other drug regimens

Therapeutic Alternatives

3. a. What non-drug therapies might be useful for this patient?

- A fluid restriction of 1 L/day to promote negative fluid balance (approximately 300 mL/day from IV medications and 700 mL/day from oral intake).

b. What pharmacotherapeutic alternatives are available for treatment of the acute renal failure in this patient?

- *Discontinuing gentamicin and changing to an antibiotic with less nephrotoxic potential* with appropriate gram-negative coverage for the remainder of the six-week course will hasten recovery of renal function. Adjusting the dosage of gentamicin to obtain desirable serum concentrations is an alternative, but his renal function may continue to worsen or fail to improve with prolonged gentamicin therapy. Based on the culture and sensitivity report, ciprofloxacin would be an appropriate alternative.
- *Loop diuretics (furosemide, bumetanide, torsemide, and ethacrynic acid)* are the diuretics of choice for the treatment of volume overload associated with ARF. Loop diuretics inhibit sodium reabsorption in the loop of Henle, a portion of the nephron that accounts for significant reabsorption of the filtered sodium load.[3] In contrast, thiazide diuretics inhibit sodium reabsorption in the distal tubule, which accounts for a small percentage of overall sodium reabsorption. In fact, thiazide diuretics, when used as single agents, are not effective when creatinine clearance is <25 mL/min. The loop diuretics all equally effective when given in equivalent doses. Therefore, initial choice of loop diuretic is often governed by cost, side effects, and pharmacokinetic differences. The incidence of ototoxicity is reported to be highest with ethacrynic acid; therefore, its use is usually limited to patients who are allergic to the sulfa component of the other loop diuretics. Bioavailability of both torsemide and bumetanide is higher and the half-life is longer than that of furosemide. However, furosemide and bumetanide are both available in generic formulations and may be less expensive than torsemide. Although loop diuretics are effective in removing fluid and resolving signs and symptoms related to volume overload, they have not been shown to hasten the recovery process of ATN.
- *Renal-dose dopamine (1–3 µg/kg/min)* stimulates β_1-receptors, resulting in vasodilation of renal vascular beds and increased renal blood flow.[4] Theoretically, renal-dose dopamine used in combination with loop diuretics may enhance delivery of the loop diuretic to its site of action. However, renal-dose dopamine is usually reserved for patients who are oliguric (urine output <400 mL/day) and have failed to respond to an appropriate trial of loop diuretics. Similar to diuretics, renal-dose dopamine has not been shown to hasten the recovery from ARF.[4] Because this patient is not oliguric, a trial of low-dose dopamine is not warranted at this time.

Optimal Plan

4. What drug recommendations are optimal at this point?

- Discontinue gentamicin and initiate oral ciprofloxacin. Secondary references recommend increasing the dosage interval of ciprofloxacin to Q 24 H in patients with a creatinine clearance range of 10 to 50 mL/min. Therefore, an appropriate dosage is 500 mg po Q 24 H.
- Increase the dose of furosemide. The dosage range for a single IV dose of furosemide for the treatment of ARF is 80 to 240 mg. This patient has received 40 mg IV Q 12 H for the past 2 days with little increase in urine output; therefore, it would be appropriate to increase his dosage to 80 mg IV Q 12 H. If his urine output does not increase significantly (increase of >50 mL/hr), the dosage can be increased further or other methods to improve diuresis can be initiated such as (1) shortening the dosage interval; (2) sequential nephron blockage by administering additional diuretics that block sodium reabsorption in different portions of the nephron (e.g., metolazone); and (3) continuous infusion loop diuretic.[3] It is unlikely that the patient would benefit from switching from furosemide to another loop diuretic because of the similarity in mechanism of action.

Outcome Evaluation

5. What clinical and laboratory parameters are necessary to evaluate the therapy for achievement of the desired therapeutic outcome and to detect or prevent adverse effects?

- Daily BUN and serum creatinine concentrations with a goal of returning BUN and creatinine to approximate baseline values of 15 mg/dL and 1.3 mg/dL, respectively.
- Comparison of 8-hour intake and output to assure that fluid intake is not exceeding output and that urine output has increased by >50 mL/hr following furosemide administration.
- Daily weights to assure loss of excess fluid with a goal baseline weight of 78 kg.

Patient Counseling

6. What information should be provided to the patient to enhance compliance, ensure successful therapy, and minimize adverse effects?

- Prior to discharge, the patient should receive discharge counseling on all new medications initiated during his hospitalization. It is likely that he will need to be instructed on the proper administration of oral ciprofloxacin, since he will be completing a 6-week course of antibiotic therapy.

Ciprofloxacin
- Ciprofloxacin may be taken with food or on an empty stomach.
- Avoid taking aluminum- or magnesium-containing antacids within 2 hours of a dose.
- Exposure to sunlight may cause sunburn and skin rash; therefore, avoidance of direct sunlight and the use of protective clothing or sun block is recommended.
- If symptoms of pain in the calves or heel occurs, contact your healthcare provider. Other symptoms that may occur include dizziness and stomach upset.
- It is important that you complete the entire course of antibiotic therapy.

Additional Case Questions

1. Based on the patient's creatinine clearance of 21 mL/min, do any of his medications require dosage adjustment?

- Assess each medication that the patient is receiving to determine if dosage adjustments are necessary based upon his renal function. The degree to which renal failure affects clearance of a given drug depends on the percentage of the drug excreted unchanged by the kidney. Drugs with >50% renal elimination will most likely require a dosage adjustment; those with <50% of the dose excreted unchanged in the urine are less likely to require dosage modification. The most common methods of adjusting a dosage regimen are to reduce the dose, increase the dosing interval, or both reduce the dose and extend the dosage interval. If the desired goal is to obtain the same steady-state concentrations of drug as a person with normal kidney function, it would be most appropriate to extend the dosage interval.[2,5] Standard drug information resources or the primary literature should be consulted to obtain appropriate dosages based on renal function. If specific recommendations are lacking, patient-specific pharmacokinetic parameters can be estimated if the fraction of the drug excreted unchanged by the kidney is known.
- The piperacillin dosage should be decreased, because approximately 75% of a dose is removed unchanged by the kidney. Drug information resources recommend a dosage interval of Q 6–8 H for patients with creatinine clearance values of 10 to 50 mL/min. Because of the wide range in creatinine clearances, a patient-specific dosage can be calculated by determining a dosage adjustment factor.

$$Q = 1 - [fe(1-KF)] \text{ where}$$
Q = kinetic parameter/dosage adjustment factor
fe = fraction of drug excreted unchanged in the urine
KF = ratio of the patient's CLcr to normal CLcr

$$Q = 1 - \{0.75[1-(21/120)]\}$$
$$Q = 1 - \{0.75[1-.175]\}$$
$$Q = 0.38$$

The adjusted dosing interval would be calculated as follows:

$\tau_f = \tau_n/Q$ where τ_f = adjusted dosing interval
τ_n = normal dosing interval

$\tau_f = 4 \text{ hr}/0.38$
$\tau_f = 10.5 \text{ hr}$

The reader is referred to textbook Chapter 47 for a detailed explanation and assumptions of the above equations. Based on the calculations, the optimal dosage regimen of piperacillin for this patient would be to administer 3 g IVPB Q 8 H, rather than selecting an atypical interval of 10 hours.

- For ranitidine, drug information resources recommend administering 50% of the usual recommended dosage for a creatinine clearance range of 10 to 50 mL/min; therefore, an appropriate dosage would be 150 mg po Q 24.
- The digoxin dose may need to be decreased, but it would be prudent to obtain a serum digoxin concentration at this time.
- Furosemide, although eliminated renally, is typically dosed to response and would not warrant a dosage change at this time.
- In addition to altered pharmacokinetics for drugs that are predominantly eliminated by renal excretion, renal disease can also decrease the elimination of metabolites. Metabolites may possess pharmacologic activity and/or toxicologic properties.[2,5] A metabolite of meperidine (normeperidine) has been shown to increase the risk of seizure activity in patients with renal disease. Therefore, meperidine should be discontinued and another narcotic analgesic initiated. Since the patient is taking oral medications, oxycodone 5 mg/acetaminophen 325 mg Q 6 H PRN could be substituted. In the case of allopurinol, the metabolite adds to the efficacy profile, so the current dosage is appropriate based on the patient's renal function.

2. What therapeutic interventions can decrease the likelihood of developing gentamicin-induced nephrotoxicity?

- Maintain trough concentrations less than 2 μg/mL
- Avoid peak concentrations greater than 10 μg/mL (for multiple dosing regimens)
- Avoid prolonged duration of therapy
- Refrain from repeated courses of aminoglycoside therapy, if possible
- Maintain normal volume status
- Select alternative antibiotics in patients at an increased risk of toxicity
- Avoid concomitant nephrotoxic medications

3. When assessing fractional excretion of sodium (FE_{Na}), what influence do previous dosages of furosemide have on interpretation of the results?

- Furosemide administration enhances sodium excretion, which results in an elevated FE_{Na}, limiting the utility of the test. In order to avoid misinterpretation of FE_{Na} results, it is recommended to delay obtaining a FE_{Na} until the effect of a dosage of furosemide is complete. In patients with normal renal function, the duration of action of furosemide is 2 hours and 6 to 8 hours for IV and oral furosemide, respectively. The duration may be prolonged to up to 10 hours in patients with renal disease. In this case, the elevated FE_{Na} of 2.8% may have been the result of previous dosages of furosemide.

References

1. Appel GB. Aminoglycoside nephrotoxicity. Am J Med 1990;88(suppl 3C):16S–20S.
2. Matzke GR, Frye RF. Drug administration in patients with renal insufficiency. Minimizing renal and extrarenal toxicity. Drug Saf 1997;16:205–231.
3. Ellison DH. The physiologic basis of diuretic synergism: Its role in treating diuretic resistance. Ann Intern Med 1991;114:886–894.
4. Chertow GM, Sayegh MH, Allgren RL, et al. Is the administration of dopamine associated with adverse or favorable outcomes in acute renal failure? Am J Med 1996;101:49–53.
5. Lam YW, Banerji S, Hatfield C, et al. Principles of drug administration in renal insufficiency. Clin Pharmacokinet 1997;32:30–57.

37 PROGRESSION OF CHRONIC RENAL DISEASE

▶ The American Patient (Level III)

Reina Bendayan, PharmD
Winnie M. Yu, PharmD, BCPS

A 52-year-old man with hypertension, hyperlipidemia, and type 2 diabetes mellitus requiring insulin is evaluated because of increasing serum creatinine over the past year (from 1.3 to 1.6 mg/dL). A 24-hour urine collection indicates the presence of proteinuria, and the diagnosis of diabetic nephropathy is made. Students are asked to assess the patient's renal function by several different methods and establish treatment goals, consider therapeutic alternatives, and develop treatment and monitoring plans for the renal insufficiency, diabetes, hypertension, and hypercholesterolemia. Dietary protein restriction may be beneficial for preventing renal disease progression in diabetic patients. Antihypertensive drug classes that have been shown to be of benefit for slowing progression of renal disease include ACE inhibitors, nondihydropyridine calcium channel antagonists, and angiotensin-1 receptor antagonists. The patient also requires changes in his present therapy for diabetes, hypertension, and hypercholesterolemia. The case involves a complex interplay among disease states and drug therapies that will provide a challenge to even the most experienced students.

▶ Questions

Problem Identification

1. a. Create a list of the patient's drug-related problems.

- Diabetic nephropathy, a complication of diabetes mellitus and hypertension
- Diabetes mellitus inadequately controlled on current insulin regimen and diet
- Hypertension inadequately controlled by diuretic (hydrochlorothiazide)
- Hydrochlorothiazide may worsen glucose control
- Hypercholesterolemia with poor adherence to diet and not controlled by present dose of pravastatin
- Obesity, with total body weight >30% over ideal body weight

b. What are the signs and symptoms of diabetic nephropathy, diabetes mellitus, hypertension, and hypercholesterolemia in this patient?

- Diabetic nephropathy. Elevated serum creatinine from baseline, overt albuminuria (> 500 mg/24 hr)
- Diabetes mellitus. Positive glucose in urine, high fasting blood glucose, high $HgbA_{1c}$
- Hypertension. Elevated diastolic and systolic blood pressure
- Hypercholesterolemia. Elevated LDL and total cholesterol

c. Calculate this patient's creatinine clearance (CLcr in mL/min) using the following data: 1) baseline CLcr from 1 year ago; 2) current CLcr using the SCr from 2 weeks ago; 3) current CLcr using the data from the 24-hr urine collection. Discuss whether (2) and (3) provide good estimates of the patient's GFR.

- Calculated CLcr from 1 year ago and 2 weeks ago using the Cockcroft and Gault equation:
  ✓ Assume steady state SCr and use ideal body weight since the patient is obese.
  ✓ IBW Male = 50 kg + (2.3 × Height in inches over 5 feet) = 68.4 kg
  ✓ 1 year ago, CLcr = (140 − 51) × 68.4 / (72 × 1.3) = 65.0 mL/min
  ✓ 2 weeks ago, CLcr = (140 − 52) × 68.4 / (72 × 1.6) = 52.3 mL/min
- Calculated CLcr using the data from the 24-hr urine collection:
  1. Calculate daily creatinine production rate to assess if urine collection is adequate.
  ✓ Measured total creatinine production/kg/day = Ucr × Uvol = 60 mg/dL × 21 dL/day = 1260 mg/day = 18.4 mg/kg/day.
  ✓ The usual rate of creatinine production (R, mg/kg/day) can be estimated by the following equation:

  R (Male) = 28 − (0.2 × age)
  R (Female) = 0.8 × R(Male)

  ✓ Therefore, daily creatinine production in this patient should be about 17.6 mg/kg/day (28 − 0.2 × 52). This is close to the measured value of 18.4 mg/kg/day. Thus, the sample is an adequate collection.
  2. Calculate the CLcr based on the following equation:

  CLcr = U × V/P = (60 mg/dL × 21dL/1440 min)/1.6 mg/dL = 54.7 mL/min

  where: U = urine creatinine concentration, V = total urine volume in 24 hours, and P = serum creatinine concentration.
- Discuss whether calculating CLcr using the Cockcroft and Gault equation and using a 24-hour urine collection provide accurate estimates of the patient's GFR:
  ✓ The CLcr is commonly used in clinical practice to evaluate renal function. However, studies have shown that estimated CLcr is an unreliable estimate of GFR. The Cockcroft and Gault equation is designed to predict CLcr rather than GFR. As SCr increases, the equation tends to overestimate GFR, and variability increases.
  ✓ The use of a measured 24-hour CLcr to evaluate renal function is no better than the Cockcroft and Gault equation. Day-to-day variation in creatinine excretion exhibits a coefficient of variation of 3% to 14%. Furthermore, incomplete collection of all urine during the collection interval may result in underestimation of the GFR.

✓ Therefore, neither method provides an accurate estimate of the GFR. Measurement of GFR following the injection of a marker such as inulin or iothalamate is probably the best method to assess the severity of renal insufficiency and renal disease progression. Because these tests are expensive and not routinely available, the measurement of CLcr after an oral dose of cimetidine can be used. Cimetidine blocks tubular secretion of creatinine and the CLcr measured in the presence of cimetidine provides a better estimate of GFR, especially in patients with renal insufficiency.[1]

Desired Outcome

3. *What are the goals of pharmacotherapy for the management of the patient's renal insufficiency, diabetes, hypertension, and hypercholesterolemia?*

- *Renal insufficiency.* His CLcr has declined by about 12 mL/min in the past year. The primary goal is to slow the progression of renal disease. The objective is to reduce the rate of decline in GFR to 1.5 to 2.5 mL/min/year and achieve a 50% reduction in urine albumin excretion rate (≈ 300 mg/24 hr).
- *Diabetes mellitus.* Prevent the development of macrovascular complications of diabetes mellitus such as CAD and slow the progression of diabetic retinopathy. The objectives are to gain strict control of blood sugars to achieve fasting blood glucose of 70 to 120 mg/dL and $HgbA_{1c}$ of < 7% and reduce total body weight by 10% (refer to textbook Chapter 70).
- *Hypertension.* Achieve and maintain BP < 130/85 mm Hg (refer to textbook Chapter 10).
- *Hypercholesterolemia.* He has multiple risk factors for CHD (male > 45 years old, DM, HTN, hypercholesterolemia, and family history of premature heart disease). In this situation, the goal is to maintain an LDL serum concentration <130 mg/dL (refer to textbook Chapter 19).

Therapeutic Alternatives

3. *a. What non-pharmacologic therapies might be useful to control this patient's medical conditions?*

- *Dietary protein restriction.* Although there are some conflicting data, dietary protein restriction may be effective in preventing the progression of renal disease in diabetic patients.[2,3] A meta-analysis of several randomized, controlled trials concluded that protein restriction reduced the overall risk of renal failure or death by 33% and that the effect was not due to differences in blood pressure control between groups. Since this patient is not malnourished and has moderate renal insufficiency, reduction of protein intake to 0.8 g/kg/day should be recommended to reduce the risk of renal failure.
- *American Diabetes Association (ADA) diet.* Because the patient is obese and has uncontrolled DM, he should be on a calorie-restricted diet (500 to 1000 kcal below the daily requirement) as recommended by the ADA, with 55% to 60% of the total calories from carbohydrates, <30% from fat, and 15% to 20% from protein. Artificial sweeteners may also be used.
- *Dietary sodium restriction.* Reduction in sodium intake of 75 to 100 mEq/day has been shown to reduce blood pressure by 6.3/2.2 mm Hg in a meta-analysis.[4] African Americans and patients with DM have also been shown to be more sensitive than others to the effect of sodium. Reduction in salt intake also augments the antiproteinuric and antihypertensive effects of ACE inhibitors. Currently, moderate sodium restriction to no more than 100 mEq/day (i.e., 2.4 g/day) is recommended by the JNC VI.[5]
- *Weight reduction.* Loss of as little as 10 pounds has been shown to enhance the blood pressure lowering effect of antihypertensive medications. Weight reduction by caloric restriction and physical exercise should be beneficial in this patient since he is obese and at high risk for cardiovascular disease.
- *Physical exercise and NCEP Step II diet.* Based on the current NCEP guidelines, physical exercise that involves 30 to 45 minutes of cardiovascular exercise per day and the NCEP Step II diet (<30% total fat, 7% saturated fat, and <200 mg of cholesterol per day) are recommended for high-risk patients with elevated LDL levels. Physical exercise can enhance the effect of diet on lipoprotein levels, but diet or exercise alone may not significantly reduce LDL levels. Exercise should always be used in conjunction with dietary intervention for the management of hypercholesterolemia in high-risk patients.[6]

b. *What are the pharmacotherapeutic alternatives for the prevention of renal disease progression and the management of diabetes mellitus, hypertension, and hyperlipidemia in this patient?*

- *Prevention of renal disease progression.* Albuminuria is not only a surrogate marker for renal disease but also a predictor for disease progression. Excess albumin excretion as a result of glomerular injury may promote the activity of pro-inflammatory molecules that subsequently result in tubulointerstitial injury. Three classes of antihypertensive agents have been shown to retard the progression of diabetic nephropathy; this effect is independent of their antihypertensive effects.
  ✓ *ACE inhibitors (e.g., captopril, enalapril, ramipril)* have been shown to be effective. In normotensive patients with macroalbuminuria and SCr of 2.0 to 2.5 mg/dL, captopril 25 mg three times daily reduced the risk of doubling of SCr and the need for dialysis or transplantation by 50%.
  ✓ *Nondihydropyridine calcium channel antagonists (diltiazem, verapamil)* appear to have efficacy similar to ACE inhibitors.
  ✓ *Losartan, an angiotensin-1 receptor antagonist,* has been shown to reduce proteinuria in non-diabetic hypertensive patients. Large studies to investigate its efficacy in normotensive diabetic patients are ongoing. Results from a short-term study suggest that this class of drugs is as effective as ACE inhibitors in reducing microalbuminuria in normotensive diabetic patients.
- *Diabetes mellitus.* Oral hypoglycemic agents such as sulfonylureas, metformin, troglitazone, and acarbose may be used to optimize glucose control in patients with type 2 diabetes mellitus. This patient has failed therapy with the sulfonylurea glyburide and is currently being treated with two daily insulin doses. The patient's adherence to the insulin regimen should be carefully assessed. He should also perform self-monitoring of blood glucose

at home and report these values at regular clinic visits so that insulin dosing can be optimized.
- ✓ *Metformin (Glucophage)* can be used in some patients to reduce the amount of insulin required, but it should be avoided in this patient because a serum creatinine >1.5 mg/dL increases the risk of lactic acidosis.
- ✓ *Troglitazone (Rezulin)* improves insulin resistance and could be used to reduce the amount of insulin required. Close monitoring of liver function is required because of the potential for hepatotoxicity.
- ✓ *Acarbose (Precose)*, an alpha-glucosidase inhibitor, delays GI absorption of carbohydrates but has only a modest effect on blood sugar control. Patient acceptance is limited by its GI side effects (e.g., flatulence, bloating).
- *Hypertension.* Assuming that the patient has been adherent, his BP is currently not controlled by hydrochlorothiazide 25 mg/day.
  - ✓ *Thiazide diuretics* are not the optimal choice in this patient because they can worsen hyperglycemia, decrease GFR, and increase total cholesterol and triglyceride levels.
  - ✓ *Beta-blockers* have been shown to reduce mortality in the treatment of HTN, but they can mask the signs and symptoms of hypoglycemia in diabetic patients, decrease GFR by reducing renal blood flow, and adversely affect lipid levels by increasing triglyceride and reducing HDL levels.
  - ✓ *ACE inhibitors* and *non-dihydropyridine calcium channel blockers* are reasonable alternatives for this patient. Both drug classes have neutral effects on lipid levels and glucose control. They also have similar efficacy in reducing proteinuria and preventing renal disease progression in patients with diabetic nephropathy. The comparative efficacy of these two classes in reducing cardiovascular morbidity in hypertensive diabetic patients remains unknown and is currently being evaluated in the ALLHAT trial.
  - ✓ *Angiotensin-1 receptor antagonists* are also feasible alternatives in this patient. They have been shown to be better tolerated than ACE inhibitors and have a lower incidence of cough secondary to a neutral effect on bradykinin.
  - ✓ *Direct-acting vasodilators, alpha-2 agonists, and peripheral adrenergic antagonists* should be used as last-line agents due to their poor side effect profile and their inability to prevent renal disease progression.
- *Hypercholesterolemia.* The agents available differ in potency, mechanism of action, and side effect profile.
  - ✓ *HMG-CoA reductase inhibitors (lovastatin, simvastatin, pravastatin, fluvastatin, atorvastatin, and cerivastatin)* are the only class of medication that has been shown to reduce mortality for both primary and secondary prevention of CHD. They are well tolerated with a low incidence of side effects such as dyspepsia, myositis, and liver enzyme elevation. The patient is presently receiving the maximum dose of pravastatin but still requires a 15% reduction in LDL cholesterol to achieve the target level of <130 mg/dL. The patient clearly needs dietary intervention (he regularly has a high cholesterol breakfast). If the LDL level is still high after dietary therapy has been optimized, the patient should be switched to a more potent agent such as simvastatin or atorvastatin; the latter drug is the most potent statin and can reduce LDL by up to 60% in newly treated patients.
  - ✓ *Bile acid binding resins (cholestyramine and colestipol)* have reduced LDL levels by only about 15% to 20%. Compliance is difficult due to GI side effects and the need for frequent dosing. There is no compelling reason to change to this drug class.
  - ✓ *Nicotinic acid (niacin)* is usually used in patients with mixed hyperlipidemia. Its use is limited by side effects of flushing, itching, worsening of peptic ulcer, and elevation of serum glucose and uric acid levels.
  - ✓ *Gemfibrozil* has low efficacy in reducing LDL and can cause dyspepsia and hepatic transaminase elevation. Its use is not recommended in this patient.

Optimal Plan

4. *What drug regimens would provide optimal therapy for this patient's current medical problems?*

- *Diabetic nephropathy.* An ACE inhibitor is probably the best agent for the management of hypertension and diabetic nephropathy. Both captopril and enalapril have been shown to slow renal disease progression in patients with diabetic nephropathy. Ramipril and benazepril have been evaluated primarily in patients with non-diabetic nephropathy. Captopril is contraindicated in this patient because of his history of anaphylactic reaction to sulfa drugs. One can start with enalapril 5 mg po QD and increase the dose in 1 month if necessary to achieve a goal BP of <130/85 and urine albumin excretion rate of ≈300 mg/24 hours. The maximum dose is 40 mg daily. If he develops cough after initiation of enalapril, an angiotensin-1 receptor antagonist such as losartan is an excellent alternative. The starting dose of losartan is 25 mg once daily with a maximum dose of 100 mg/day.
- *Diabetes mellitus.* The patient has a high fasting blood glucose and glycosuria despite the current insulin regimen. Therefore, the dose should be increased to achieve fasting blood glucose of 70 to 120 mg/dL. He should ideally check his blood glucose 4 times daily (before meals and at bedtime) or at least twice daily. He should increase the dose by approximately 1 unit for every 30 mg/dL of glucose above the target range. If his blood glucose is high before lunch and at bedtime, he should probably adjust his regular insulin dose since the effect of regular insulin peaks in 2 to 4 hours. On the other hand, if his blood glucose is high in the morning or before dinnertime, he should increase his Humulin N dose.

  Addition of an oral agent to the insulin regimen is indicated if increasing the insulin dose fails to achieve the target fasting blood glucose level. Since the patient has hyperlipidemia, hypertension, and obesity, the possibility of syndrome X (or hyperinsulinemia syndrome) should be considered. This syndrome is characterized by the presence of excess insulin and insulin resistance. Despite the hepatotoxicity of troglitazone, it is probably the best oral agent for this patient since it is an insulin sensitizer and does not stimulate insulin secretion. Metformin is not a good choice because of his elevated serum creatinine. The low efficacy and side effect profile of acarbose make it a poor choice for this patient.
- *Hypertension.* Discontinue hydrochlorothiazide and start an ACE in-

hibitor such as enalapril 5 mg po QD as described above to manage both hypertension and nephropathy. The dose should be titrated to optimize blood pressure control and to achieve at least 50% reduction in urine albumin excretion.

- *Hypercholesterolemia.* The patient could benefit from a dietary consultation; having eggs and sausages for breakfast on a regular basis complicates management of the disorder. His adherence to the prescribed pravastatin regimen should also be assessed. If the LDL-cholesterol is still above the target level after dietary therapy has been optimized and medication adherence has been assured for several months, he should be changed to a more potent agent such as simvastatin 40 mg/day (maximum 80 mg/day) or atorvastatin 10 mg/day (maximum 80 mg/day). If statin monotherapy should ultimately prove to be inadequate (which is unlikely), one may consider adding a second agent such as a bile acid resin. Niacin could be added, but it may have adverse effects on glucose control; there is also a higher incidence of hepatotoxicity and myositis when niacin is added to statin therapy.

Outcome Evaluation

5. *Outline the clinical and laboratory parameters necessary to evaluate the efficacy and safety of the recommended regimens for the patient's nephropathy, diabetes mellitus, hypertension, and hypercholesterolemia.*

- *Nephropathy.* Measure serum creatinine in 2 weeks and then every 3 months; check serum potassium in 2 weeks, then every 3 months if normal; measure urine albumin excretion every month for 3 months and then every 3 months. Measure GFR annually.
- *Diabetes mellitus.* Perform home blood glucose monitoring 4 times a day (before meals and at bedtime); check $HgbA_{1c}$ every 3 months until <7% (if possible), then at least annually thereafter.
- *Hypertension.* Recheck BP in 2 weeks and then monthly thereafter. Monitor the ACE inhibitor therapy for adverse effects of hyperkalemia, pedal edema, and development of a non-productive dry cough.
- *Hypercholesterolemia.* Check a fasting lipid profile for LDL level after 3 months and then annually if within target range; obtain liver function tests (AST, ALT) if they have not been checked since pravastatin was initiated, recheck in 3 months after changing drugs and then annually.

Patient Counseling

6. *What information should be provided to the patient to ensure successful therapy and minimize adverse effects of the antihypertensive and insulin therapy?*

Enalapril
- This medicine is used to treat your high blood pressure and to prevent further damage in your kidneys.
- Take one tablet (5 mg) once daily. You can take this medicine either with food or between meals, but try to take it at the same time each day.
- If you miss a dose of this medicine, take it as soon as possible. However, if it is almost time for your next dose, skip the missed dose and go back to your regular dosing schedule. Do not double doses.
- This medication is usually well tolerated, but it may cause a non-productive, dry cough that can start within weeks to months after beginning the medication. Other side effects include rash and swelling of your legs; contact your prescriber if these side effects occur.
- You will need to revisit your physician in 2 weeks to check your blood pressure. Because the medication can sometimes increase potassium levels and worsen kidney function, your physician will do a blood test during the visit to make sure that they are normal. Other blood tests will also be performed in a few months to assess your response to the medication.

Insulin
- Check your blood sugar 4 times a day, before meals and at bedtime. Adjust the insulin dose according to your blood sugar results. The desired fasting blood sugar is 70 to 120 mg/dL. The closer your fasting blood sugar value is to the target range, the better you are controlling your disease. Controlling blood sugar can prevent your kidney and eye problems from getting worse. It can also improve your blood pressure.
- In general, for every 30 mg/dL above the target range, increase your insulin dose by 1 unit. The regular insulin is a fast-acting insulin that has a peak effect in 2 to 4 hours. The morning dose of regular insulin will take care of the breakfast meal, and the evening dose of regular insulin will take care of the dinner meal. On the other hand, NPH insulin, the one that has a cloudy appearance, is an intermediate-acting insulin that has a peak effect in 6 to 14 hours. Therefore, the morning dose of NPH insulin will have its effect at noon and the evening NPH dose will provide insulin needs during the night time.
- You may keep your current insulin bottles at room temperature. Discard vials that have not been completely used in 1 month. Unopened insulin vials should be kept in the refrigerator.

Follow-up Questions

1. *What new or persistent drug-related problems does this patient have?*

- Hyperkalemia probably secondary to ACE inhibitor therapy and/or the use of a salt substitute.
- Uncontrolled hypertension despite the new antihypertensive medication and lower sodium intake.

2. *What changes, if any, would you recommend in the patient's drug regimen?*

- *Hyperkalemia.* Cardia Salt is a dietary aid that is designed to reduce the sodium intake of hypertensive patients. The elevated potassium level may be related to the use of this salt substitute. However, his hyperkalemia may also be due to his new ACE inhibitor therapy. In order to determine the precise etiology, he should stop using Cardia Salt, and his potassium level should be rechecked in 2 days. If his potassium level remains elevated, discontinuation of his ACE inhibitor is warranted.
- *Hypertension.* Since his blood pressure remains high despite enalapril 5 mg/day, an increase in the dose would be warranted if he did not have an elevated potassium level. However, in light of the elevated serum potassium, he should continue enalapril at the same dose until his potassium level is rechecked. If his potassium level returns to normal after discontinuation of Cardia Salt, increase the

dose of enalapril to 10 mg/day. However, if his potassium level remains elevated, discontinue enalapril and start a non-dihydropyridine calcium channel blocker (e.g., verapamil SR 120 mg/day or diltiazem CD 120 mg/day).

References

1. Walser M. Assessing renal function from creatinine measurements in adults with chronic renal failure. Am J Kidney Dis 1998;32:23–31.
2. Pedrini MT, Levey AS, Lau J, et al. The effect of dietary protein restriction on the progression of diabetic and nondiabetic renal diseases: A meta-analysis. Ann Intern Med 1996;124:627–632.
3. Klahr S, Levey AS, Beck GJ, et al. The effects of dietary protein restriction and blood pressure control on the progression of chronic renal disease. Modification of Diet in Renal Disease Study Group. N Engl J Med 1994;330:877–884.
4. Midgley JP, Matthew AG, Greenwood CM, et al. Effect of reduced dietary sodium on blood pressure: A meta-analysis of randomized controlled trials. JAMA 1996;275:1590–1597.
5. Joint National Committee on Prevention, Detection, Evaluation, and Treatment of High Blood Pressure. The sixth report of the Joint National Committee on Prevention, Detection, Evaluation, and Treatment of High Blood Pressure. Arch Intern Med 1997;157:2413–2446.
6. Stefanick ML, Mackey S, Sheehan M, et al. Effects of diet and exercise in men and postmenopausal women with low levels of HDL cholesterol and high levels of LDL cholesterol. N Engl J Med 1998;339:12–20.

38 END-STAGE RENAL DISEASE

▶ A Return to the Machine (Level II)

James D. Coyle, PharmD

Resumption of hemodialysis is necessary for a 64-year-old man whose cadaveric renal transplant has recently failed. He manifests many of the complications of uremia, including constitutional and GI symptoms, anemia, hyperphosphatemia, metabolic acidosis, hypertension, and pruritus. Proper management of the patient requires careful consideration of the available therapeutic alternatives for each of these problems. The case provides the opportunity for students to discuss the dosage, administration, monitoring, and patient education required for epoetin alfa therapy.

▶ Questions

Problem Identification

1. a. *Create a list of this patient's medication-related problems.*

   - Anemia without iron deficiency (low hemoglobin, hematocrit, and RBC count; MCV and MCHC low but normal; T. sat. ≥20%, and serum ferritin ≥100 ng/mL)
   - Hyperphosphatemia and secondary hyperparathyroidism (very high PTH). Calculated corrected calcium is 8.9 mg/dL, which is within the normal range and essentially at the lower limit of the targeted concentration range for hemodialysis patients (see below)
   - Hyperchloremic metabolic acidosis (high chloride, low CO_2, and high anion gap)
   - Hypertension (predialysis BP of 170/100 mm Hg [MAP = 123] on an antihypertensive agent [atenolol 50 mg Q HS])
   - Pruritus (dry, itchy skin and observation of dry, scaly skin on arms and legs)
   - Absence of appropriate vitamin supplement
   - Although mild hyperkalemia (K 5.3 mEq/L) might be considered a medication-related problem since it could be addressed using drugs, the clear choice of approaches to this problem is hemodialysis.

   b. *What information (signs, symptoms, laboratory values) indicates the severity of this patient's end-stage renal disease?*

   - The patient presents for staff-assisted hemodialysis exhibiting signs, symptoms, and lab values consistent with uremia including dry, itchy skin; tiredness/weakness; anorexia with nausea and vomiting; constipation; pedal edema; HTN; elevated K, Cl, anion gap, BUN, SCr, phosphorus, aluminum, and PTH; and decreased CO_2, Hgb, Hct, and RBC count.
   - He has a compensated hyperchloremic metabolic acidosis (Cl 110, CO_2 20, and anion gap 18).

Desired Outcome

2. *State the goal of pharmacotherapy with respect to each problem identified.*

   - *Anemia without iron deficiency.* The overall goal is to improve quality of life associated with anemia in ESRD patients. Laboratory results consistent with this goal are achieving and maintaining Hgb between 11 and 12 g/dL and Hct between 33% and 36% within 2 to 4 months.[1] Also need to maintain adequate iron to support hematopoiesis while avoiding iron overload, as evidenced by T. sat. ≥20% (but <50%) and serum ferritin ≥100 ng/mL (but <800 ng/mL).[1]
   - *Hyperphosphatemia and secondary hyperparathyroidism.* The overall goal is to prevent renal osteodystrophy and metastatic calcification by correcting secondary hyperparathyroidism and hyperphosphatemia while maintaining normal calcium. Need to avoid induction of adynamic bone disease by oversuppression of PTH. Laboratory results consistent with this goal are a serum calcium (corrected for albumin) of 9 to 11 mg/dL, serum phosphorus of 4.5 to 6.0 mg/dL (note, still above normal), and an intact or N-terminal PTH of 2 to 3 times normal. For intact PTH (normal range approximately 10 to 60 pg/mL), a targeted range of 100 to 150 pg/mL has been suggested for the dialysis patient. The calcium-phosphorus product (Ca × P with both expressed in mg/dL) should be maintained at ≤70 to minimize risk of metastatic calcification. One equation to correct serum calcium concentration for altered albumin concentration is:

Corrected Ca = measured Ca + [(normal albumin − patient's albumin) × 0.8], where a normal albumin is typically 4.0 g/dL.
- *Hyperchloremic metabolic acidosis.* Acidosis contributes to a variety of conditions that occur in ESRD patients, including renal osteodystrophy, hyperkalemia, enhanced protein catabolism, decreased cardiac inotropy, peripheral vasodilation which may result in hypotension, anorexia, fatigue, and decreased exercise tolerance. The goal of treating metabolic acidosis is to control these conditions, thereby decreasing patient morbidity and mortality and increasing patient quality of life. Optimal goals for controlling metabolic acidosis have not been established for the ESRD patient population. Typical predialysis laboratory values in stable ESRD patients being hemodialyzed using bicarbonate-containing dialysate are total CO_2 21 (range, 17 to 27) mEq/L, anion gap 17 (range, 10 to 24) mEq/L, pH 7.38 (range, 7.37 to 7.39), and arterial Pco_2 37 (range, 34 to 40) mm Hg.[2]
- *Hypertension.* The overall goal is to reduce the morbidity and mortality associated with HTN. Optimal BP goals have not been established for the ESRD patient population. Typical goals include a predialysis MAP <114 mm Hg (corresponding to a BP of ≤140/90); post-dialysis diastolic BP <90 mm Hg; or an interdialytic SBP <160 mm Hg and DBP <95 mm Hg in the absence of end-organ damage or interdialytic SBP <130 mm Hg and DBP <85 mm Hg in the presence of end-organ damage. Elimination of antihypertensive drug therapy is possible in at least 50% of patients with appropriate fluid removal during dialysis. It is also desirable to address other CHD risk factors.[3] In this patient they include age ≥45 (non-modifiable), hyperlipidemia (modifiable), and slightly low HDL cholesterol (modifiable).
- *Pruritus.* The goal is to relieve or at least minimize itching.
- *Absence of appropriate vitamin supplement.* Goal is to prevent water-soluble vitamin deficiency and avoid toxicity due to inappropriate/excessive supplementation. It is usually also necessary to supplement vitamin D in ESRD patients, but that will be considered part of problem 2 (hyperphosphatemia and secondary hyperparathyroidism).

Therapeutic Alternatives

3. *What therapeutic options are available for each of this patient's medication-related problems? Indicate the advantages and disadvantages of each option.*

Anemia Without Iron Deficiency
- *Epoetin alfa* therapy is indicated since there appears to be no cause for anemia other than ESRD (a test for occult blood in stool would be a worthwhile addition to information provided) and the patient is not iron deficient. It may be administered IV or SC (SC is the preferred route according to NKF-DOQI guidelines, but most U.S. patients receive it IV). Advantages of the IV route are that there is no patient discomfort and there is more clinical experience in the United States with this route. Disadvantages include a higher dose usually required and more frequent administration (both leading to higher treatment costs). The initial IV dose is 120 to 180 units/kg/wk (typically 9000 units/wk) given in 3 divided doses.[1] The initial SC dose is 80 to 120 units/kg/wk (typically 6000 units/wk) given in 2 to 3 divided doses.[1] IV and SC doses are adjusted based on hematocrit response to the initial dose (see monitoring plan below).
- *IV iron dextran* 50 to 100 mg per week for 10 weeks is indicated since this patient's T. sat. and ferritin are within acceptable limits.[1] Subsequent dosing is based on T. sat. and ferritin response to the initial dose (see monitoring plan below). Oral iron in doses of at least 200 mg elemental iron per day might be advocated rather than IV iron. While not absolutely inappropriate, oral iron usually fails to maintain adequate iron stores in hemodialysis patients, perhaps due to such factors as decreased iron absorption and poor compliance due to adverse effects (gastric irritation and constipation, the latter of which this patient already has).[1] Potential advantages of the oral route are decreased cost and avoidance of risks of IV iron dextran (anaphylactoid reactions and dose-related arthralgias and myalgias).[4] A variety of oral iron preparations are available including ferrous gluconate (12% elemental iron), ferrous sulfate (20% elemental iron), ferrous fumarate (33% elemental iron), and polysaccharide-iron complex (dosage form strength expressed in terms of elemental iron). None of these agents has any clearly established advantage over the others except for cost; the wholesale cost increases in the order of fumarate, sulfate, gluconate, polysaccharide-iron complex.[1] Use of dosage forms incorporating vitamin C in ESRD patients is generally discouraged due to the lack of data supporting an increase in iron absorption and concern that excessive vitamin C supplementation in this patient population may result in elevated serum oxalate concentrations with increased risk of oxalate tissue deposition.

Hyperphosphatemia and Secondary Hyperparathyroidism
- *Dietary phosphate restriction* should be instituted. High phosphorus content of food generally (but not always) reflects high protein content. Restriction should be used with caution so that the patient's nutritional status is not compromised. The lowest practical intake is 800 to 1200 mg/day. Attempts to limit intake are frequently unsuccessful due to high phosphorus content of many foods in the Western diet, including dairy products, oatmeal, meat/fish/poultry, legumes, nuts, eggs, and many carbonated beverages (especially colas).
- *A phosphate binder (e.g., calcium carbonate or acetate)* should be started. Since this patient's calcium (corrected calcium 8.9 mg/dL) is below the target and the calcium-phosphate product (66.9) is <70, a calcium-containing phosphate binder can be chosen, with calcium carbonate or calcium acetate being the most likely choices. These calcium salts appear to be equally efficacious when dosed appropriately. Although calcium acetate is about twice as potent a phosphate binder as calcium carbonate (per gram of calcium administered), this does not appear to result in a clinically significant advantage since the number of tablets administered per day is approximately the same (calcium acetate requires about half the dose, but each tablet contains only about 62.5% of the elemental calcium as calcium carbonate) and the incidence of hypercalcemia is approximately the same. Calcium acetate has a relatively higher cost and a reported higher incidence of nausea and vomiting compared to calcium carbonate. Typical starting doses are calcium carbonate 1.2 to 3 g elemental calcium (3.0 to 7.5 g calcium carbonate) per day in divided doses with meals, or calcium acetate, 0.6 to 1.0 g elemental calcium (2.4 to 4.0 g calcium acetate) in divided doses with meals. Ideally, the phosphate content of the patient's typical meals is evaluated by a dietician and the phosphate binder doses are divided in proportion to the phosphate content of the meals.

- *Low calcium dialysate* (2.5 mEq/L) is generally used to decrease the incidence of hypercalcemia when calcium-containing phosphate binders are prescribed.
- *Calcitriol* will almost certainly be needed in this patient to control secondary hyperparathyroidism, but its use should be delayed until serum phosphorus is controlled. There are at least two reasons for this approach. First, calcitriol will increase both serum phosphorus and calcium (via increased intestinal absorption). These increases are likely to cause this patient's calcium-phosphorus product to exceed 70, putting him at increased risk of soft tissue calcification. Waiting until the phosphorus is controlled will eliminate or minimize this risk. Second, it has been suggested that calcitriol is unlikely to have a significant impact on PTH concentrations until the serum phosphorus is controlled.[5] This combination of unlikely benefit with increased risk argues against the initiation of calcitriol therapy in this patient at this time. If phosphorus cannot be controlled while maintaining the calcium-phosphorus product below 70 due to increased calcium concentration, short-term use of aluminum- or magnesium-containing phosphate binders until the serum phosphorus is controlled should be considered, with a switch back to only calcium-containing phosphate binders as soon as the phosphorus target is achieved.

Hyperchloremic Metabolic Acidosis

- Metabolic acidosis in ESRD patients is almost always adequately treated by appropriately adjusting the bicarbonate or acetate concentrations in the dialysate. This is clearly the treatment of choice. Calcium carbonate or calcium acetate administered as phosphate binders may also contribute to correction of metabolic acidosis, but this is not typically the purpose of their administration.

Hypertension

- While this patient's BP is clearly elevated, it is not so high that immediate reduction is necessary. Fluid overload is undoubtedly contributing to his HTN. He should be dialyzed to achieve his dry weight over the next 4 to 8 weeks. As HTN is normalized, the atenolol dose should be decreased appropriately with a goal of discontinuation if possible. If an antihypertensive agent continues to be needed, atenolol is probably not ideal for this patient because of its lipid effects, its high degree of dependence on the kidneys for removal from the body, and its high dialyzability. If continued treatment is needed after achieving his dry weight, he should be switched to an ACE inhibitor or a calcium channel blocker. Non-drug approaches to control HTN should be used, especially limitation of sodium and fluid intake (usually done in ESRD patients, although compliance is frequently an issue).

Pruritus

- It is important to rule out and treat non-uremic causes, such as dry skin due to low humidity and hypothyroidism. Effectively treating pruritus due to ESRD is challenging, and no single option is universally effective.[6] Topical emollients, phototherapy with UVB light, oral antihistamines, cholestyramine, and activated charcoal may all be useful in selected patients.

Absence of Appropriate Vitamin Supplement

- Initiate a vitamin supplement containing appropriate amounts of water-soluble vitamins. The exact water-soluble vitamin requirements for ESRD patients have not been established, resulting in significant variation in vitamin supplement content recommendations. Generally, the following content would be considered acceptable: 1.5 mg vitamin B_1 (thiamine), 1.7 mg vitamin B_2 (riboflavin), 10 mg vitamin B_6 (pyridoxine), 6 μg vitamin B_{12} (cyanocobalamin), 1 mg folic acid, 20 mg niacin, 5 to 10 mg pantothenic acid, 0.15 to 0.30 mg biotin, and 60 to 100 mg vitamin C. Daily doses of vitamin C greater than 150 mg are discouraged due to the potential for oxalate (a metabolite of vitamin C) accumulation and soft tissue deposition. Supplementation of fat-soluble vitamins A, E, and K is generally discouraged due to the presence of normal or elevated concentrations of these vitamins in ESRD without supplementation, potential adverse effects related to hypervitaminosis, and/or the absence of an established need for supplementation in the ESRD patient population. Supplementation of vitamin D is based on the needs of the individual patient with respect to the prevention or treatment of secondary hyperparathyroidism and renal osteodystrophy. Many product alternatives exist for supplementation of the water-soluble vitamins with wide variation in cost.

Optimal Plan

4. Which of the available therapeutic options identified in question 3 would you recommend for this patient? Provide a rationale for each recommendation. Include the name, dosage form, dose, schedule, and duration of therapy for any drugs recommended.

Anemia Without Iron Deficiency

- Epoetin alfa 3000 units IV push during each dialysis session. The dose can be injected into either the arterial or venous blood line at any time during dialysis. The acceptable range of initial IV doses based on the above guidelines is about 3000 to 4000 units at each dialysis session treatment. (This recommendation assumes three dialysis sessions per week.) Our center has not converted to SC dosing due to concern that patients will not accept the discomfort associated with the SC route. However, SC dosing is the preferred route in NKF-DOQI guidelines and would be equally acceptable. For duration of therapy, see monitoring guidelines below.
- Iron dextran, 100 mg (2 mL) IV push during each Tuesday dialysis session for 10 weeks. Doses as low as 50 mg per session are also consistent with NKF-DOQI recommendations. The administration rate should be no greater than 1 mL/min. The first dose should be administered as an initial test dose of 25 mg, followed 15 to 60 minutes later by the remaining 75 mg assuming no reaction to the initial 25-mg dose. Drugs, supplies, and equipment required for treatment of anaphylactoid reactions should be immediately available in the dialysis unit when the test dose is administered. The IV route and 100-mg dose were chosen to try to assure adequate iron availability during the initial period of increased hematopoiesis, as discussed above.

Hyperphosphatemia and Secondary Hyperparathyroidism

- Institute phosphate restricted diet as per dietician.
- Start calcium carbonate tablets 3.0 to 7.5 g (1.2 to 3 g elemental calcium) per day in divided doses with meals. For example, Tums E-X Extra Strength (750 mg calcium carbonate [300 mg elemental calcium] per tablet), eight tablets per day with tablets divided among meals and snacks in proportion to their phosphorus content as as-

sessed by the dietician. While a variety of different calcium carbonate products could be recommended, Tums E-X Extra Strength is a reasonable choice because it is a national brand which meets dissolution requirements; it is chewable and flavored, which many patients find acceptable; it is generally competitively priced; and it is not derived from oyster shell calcium, which avoids concerns about heavy metal content of calcium carbonate from that source. Generics may provide the benefit of additional cost savings, although care should be taken to choose products with acceptable dissolution rates. Dose can be titrated upward to 14 g calcium carbonate per day depending on response to the initial dose (see monitoring plan below). Calcium acetate (2.4 to 4.0 g [0.6 to 1.0 g elemental calcium] initially) is also frequently used and acceptable, but calcium carbonate provides equal phosphate binding at a lower cost, with no higher risk of hypercalcemia and possibly a lower incidence of nausea and vomiting, as discussed above.

Hyperchloremic Metabolic Acidosis
- Adequate hemodialysis is the treatment of choice for this problem. No drug therapy is indicated at this time, and it is unlikely to be needed in the future.

Hypertension
- Dialyze the patient to his estimated dry weight over the next 4 to 8 weeks.
- Decrease the atenolol dose as HTN decreases with removal of excess fluid, with the ultimate goal of discontinuation.
- Initiate sodium and fluid restriction. In general, sodium intake in hemodialysis patients without significant residual renal function should be restricted to 40 to 80 mEq/day (approximately 1 to 2 g of sodium or 2.5 to 5 g sodium chloride), and water intake should be restricted to 1 liter/day. These restrictions may be relaxed (e.g., 130 to 170 mEq sodium/day) if the patient has significant residual renal function.
- Switch to either an ACE inhibitor or a calcium channel blocker if HTN is not controlled without drug therapy after the patient has achieved dry weight.

Pruritus
- Topical emollients are the treatment of choice for pruritus, assuming no treatable causes can be identified, especially in this patient who has dry, scaly skin.[6]
- Oral antihistamines are also commonly used (e.g., diphenhydramine hydrochloride 25 to 50 mg every 8 to 12 hours, hydroxyzine 25 to 50 mg every 6 to 12 hours, cyproheptadine 2 to 4 mg every 8 to 12 hours, or clemastine fumarate 1.34 to 2.68 mg every 8 to 12 hours). The patient may only need to take a dose prior to dialysis.
- Pruritus may improve as control of hyperphosphatemia and hyperparathyroidism is established.

Absence of Appropriate Vitamin Supplement
- Nephrocaps, one capsule orally each day, is commonly recommended for supplementation of water-soluble vitamins in hemodialysis patients. It is relatively inexpensive and its content (100 mg vitamin C, 10 mg pyridoxine HCl, 1 mg folic acid, 6 μg vitamin B_{12}, 1.5 mg thiamine, 1.7 mg riboflavin, 20 mg niacinamide, 5 mg pantothenic acid, 0.15 mg biotin) is consistent with the recommendations discussed above.
- Less expensive alternatives might be identified, but caution should be exercised to make sure the content is appropriate for ESRD patients, including adequate amounts of folic acid and pyridoxine, non-excessive doses of vitamin C, and no fat-soluble vitamins.

Outcome Evaluation

5. *What clinical and/or laboratory parameters would you recommend to evaluate the desired and undesired consequences of each of your recommended interventions?*

Anemia Without Iron Deficiency
- Routinely monitor for signs/symptoms of anemia and increased blood loss, including fatigue, weakness, pallor, shortness of breath, and increased frequency or severity of angina.
- Monitor H & H each week until a stable, targeted hematocrit is achieved, then monitor every 2 to 4 weeks.
- Epoetin titration[1]:

If HCT . . .	Then . . .
Increases <2% over 2–4 wk	Increase weekly dose by 50%
Increases >8% over 4 wk but is not at target Hct	Decrease weekly dose by 25%
Increases >8% over 4 wk and Hct is at or near target	Hold epoetin for 1–2 wk, then resume at 75% of weekly dose
Hct >target	Decrease weekly dose by 25%

- If inadequate response to epoetin (defined as failure to achieve target H & H in the presence of adequate iron stores at a dose of 450 units/kg/wk IV or 300 units/kg/wk SC within 4 to 6 months or failure to maintain target H & H subsequently at that dose), the cause should be identified and corrected (if possible). The most common causes of inadequate response are infection/inflammation, chronic blood loss, osteitis fibrosa, and aluminum intoxication.[1] See Chapter 42 of the textbook for an algorithm for identifying causes of inadequate response.
- Monitor for development and/or worsening of HTN by monitoring BP before and after each dialysis.
- Monitor T. sat. and serum ferritin at least every 3 months until targeted H & H are achieved and stable. Monitoring should continue as long as the patient is receiving iron supplementation. T. sat. and ferritin should be measured 2 weeks after the end of any IV iron treatment (typically 10 weeks in duration).[1]
- Once stable H & H are established, adjust the iron dextran dose to the lowest dose (typically 25 to 100 mg each week) required to maintain T. sat. and serum ferritin within acceptable ranges.[1]
- Monitor for adverse effects related to iron dextran. While serious adverse reactions are uncommon, those that do occur are potentially fatal. In a recent retrospective study of 573 hemodialysis patients receiving IV iron dextran (INFeD), 27 patients (4.7%) experienced adverse reactions. Four patients (0.7%) experienced serious reactions (1 cardiac arrest, 3 others requiring hospitalization), while 10 patients (1.7%) experienced anaphylactoid reactions. No deaths or permanent disabilities resulted. The most common adverse effects were

itching (0.5%), swelling (0.5%), dyspepsia (0.5%), diarrhea (0.5%), skin flushing (0.3%), headache (0.3%), cardiac arrest (0.2%), and myalgias (0.2%). Only 5 of the 27 reactions occurred during a test dose, suggesting that monitoring should continue in spite of the absence of an adverse reaction during the test dose.

Hyperphosphatemia and Secondary Hyperparathyroidism

- Evaluate current patient status with respect to renal osteodystrophy and then monitor appropriately. Evaluation of renal osteodystrophy may include assessment of symptoms (bone pain, joint discomfort, and pruritus), which are usually associated with advanced bone disease; signs of hyperparathyroidism (bone tenderness, enlarged parathyroid glands, skin excoriation); laboratory findings (increased serum alkaline phosphatase, variable serum calcium, elevated serum phosphorus, elevated serum PTH); radiologic findings (bone loss or erosion especially in hands, osteosclerosis, or opacities in soft tissues and blood vessels due to metastatic calcification); and, if indicated, bone biopsy.
- To monitor phosphate binder therapy, measure serum calcium and phosphate weekly until stable, then monthly. Note that when calcitriol therapy is started, increases in calcium and phosphate are likely and will require at least weekly monitoring; a need for an increased dose of phosphate binder should be anticipated. Calcitriol therapy, once initiated, should be monitored by measuring PTH every month until stable, then every 3 months. Calcitriol dose adjustments should be based on maintaining a high-normal serum calcium and achieving an intact PTH of 100 to 150 pg/mL.

Hyperchloremic Metabolic Acidosis

- See the Desired Outcomes section earlier.

Hypertension

- Monitor pre- and post-dialysis BP routinely. Consider ambulatory BP monitoring.
- Decrease the atenolol dose as goal BP is achieved.
- Monitor sodium and fluid intake. The best sign of patient compliance with sodium and fluid restriction is the inter-dialysis weight gain, with compliant patients gaining no more than 1 kg/day between dialyses. Patient interviews may also be used to assess compliance.

Pruritus

- Monitor the patient for efficacy and alter the therapy as appropriate.
- If antihistamines are added, monitor for adverse effects, including drowsiness and anticholinergic effects (dryness of mouth, nose, and throat; dysuria; urinary retention; visual disturbances; nervousness).

Absence of Appropriate Vitamin Supplement

- Monitor for compliance and signs/symptoms of vitamin deficiency or toxicity.

Patient Counseling

6. What information should be provided to the patient to enhance compliance, ensure successful therapy, and minimize adverse effects?

- As the pharmacist who works in the dialysis unit, part of my job is to help you get as much benefit from the drugs your doctor prescribes as possible, while minimizing their adverse effects.

Calcium Carbonate

- Today I would like to take a few minutes to discuss one of your new medications with you. If you have any questions while we are talking, please don't hesitate to stop me and ask them.
- One of your new drugs is called Tums E-X Extra Strength. These tablets contain calcium carbonate and are commonly used as an antacid. In your case, Tums E-X is being used for a different purpose—to decrease the concentration of phosphorus in your bloodstream.
- Since Tums E-X works by decreasing the absorption of phosphorus in the food that you eat, you are to take this medication with each meal or snack during the day. This timing is very important because of the way the drug works; if it is going to prevent absorption of phosphorus from food, it has to be in the stomach when that absorption would be taking place. You will be chewing and swallowing 8 Tums E-X tablets per day, some with breakfast, lunch, dinner, and with your evening snack. The number to be taken with each meal is based on the dietician's estimate of the typical phosphorus content of your meals; this will be printed on the bottle label. You will probably be taking these every day indefinitely, although we may need to adjust the number of tablets you take with each meal from time to time.
- The tablets have a chalky taste, and occasionally people complain of mild nausea and rarely vomiting after taking them. There are other possible adverse effects, but we will be checking you carefully to make sure they don't occur. If you notice anything unusual or bothersome after you start taking Tums E-X, please let us know and we will help you decide what to do about it.
- If you happen to forget to take the tablets with a meal, you should chew and swallow the tablets as soon as you remember. I would encourage you to get into some routine for taking these tablets to try to minimize the number of times you forget.

References

1. NKF-DOQI clinical practice guidelines for the treatment of anemia of chronic renal failure. National Kidney Foundation—Dialysis Outcomes Quality Initiative. Am J Kidney Dis 1997;4(suppl 3):S192–S240.
2. Gennari FJ, Rimmer JM. Acid–base disorders in end-stage renal disease. Semin Dial 1990;3:81–85.
3. Summary of the second report of the National Cholesterol Education Program (NCEP) Expert Panel on Detection, Evaluation, and Treatment of High Blood Cholesterol in Adults (Adult Treatment Panel II). JAMA 1993;269:3015–3023.
4. Fishbane S, Ungureanu VD, Maesaka JK, et al. The safety of intravenous iron dextran in hemodialysis patients. Am J Kidney Dis 1996;28:529–534.
5. Felsenfeld AJ. Considerations for the treatment of secondary hyperparathyroidism in renal failure. J Am Soc Nephrol 1997;8:993–1004.
6. Robertson KE, Mueller BA. Uremic pruritus. Am J Health-Syst Pharm 1996;53:2159–2170.

39 RENAL TRANSPLANTATION

▶ Frank's New Kidney   (Level II)

Marie A. Chisholm, PharmD
Tana R. Bagby, PharmD
Laura Mulloy, DO

A 61-year-old man presents to the renal transplant clinic for a routine visit 6 months after receiving a cadaveric kidney transplant. Physical examination and laboratory results indicate the presence of hypertension, post-transplant erythrocytosis, dyslipidemia, and hyperglycemia. The reader is asked to develop therapeutic plans for the resolution of these problems. Angiotensin-converting enzyme inhibitors and angiotensin receptor antagonists have been shown to be effective for post-transplant erythrocytosis. Two months later the patient returns with uncontrollable tremors and an elevated cyclosporine concentration. Concurrent use of nonprescription cimetidine may be responsible for the elevated cyclosporine level, which resulted in tremors. Students are asked to outline a plan for resolving the tremors while maintaining satisfactory immunosuppression.

▶ Questions

Problem Identification

1. a. Create a list of the patient's drug-related problems.

- Status post renal transplantation with satisfactory immunosuppression therapy consisting of cyclosporine, mycophenolate, and prednisone. Normal BUN and SCr indicate that there is no ongoing graft rejection or cyclosporine renal toxicity, and the cyclosporine concentration is within the target range.
- Post-renal transplant erythrocytosis which may be caused in part by cyclosporine.[1]
- Dyslipidemia with no current treatment. Many renal transplant patients have elevated cholesterol and lipid levels prior to transplantation or develop it as a result of postoperative medications. Cyclosporine and prednisone may be contributing to the dyslipidemia. Without obtaining documentation of previous lipid levels, one cannot accurately attribute the dyslipidemia to the renal transplantation or the medications.
- Systolic HTN currently inadequately treated. Although the patient was diagnosed with HTN 25 years ago, cyclosporine and prednisone may be contributing to his elevated BP.
- Slightly elevated fasting blood glucose that may be due in part to prednisone therapy.

b. What information (signs, symptoms, laboratory values) indicates the presence or severity of post-transplant erythrocytosis?

- Post-renal transplant erythrocytosis occurs in 9% to 22% of patients and usually occurs within the first 2 years after transplantation. It is diagnosed when hematocrit levels exceed 50% combined with hemoglobin levels above 17 g/dL in men or 16 g/dL in women.[2,3]
- The etiology of post-transplant erythrocytosis is unclear and is thought to be due to a failure of normal regulation of erythropoietin (EPO) production or an altered sensitivity of erythroid progenitor stem cells to EPO.[2,4]
- Several factors such as graft artery stenosis, graft rejection, and the effects of cyclosporine promoting EPO production have been theorized to contribute to the development of post-renal transplant erythrocytosis.[1]

Desired Outcome

2. What are the goals of pharmacotherapy for this patient?

- Resolve the post-renal transplant erythrocytosis.
- Decrease LDL to <130 mg/dL and total cholesterol to <200 mg/dL. The patient has 2 risk factors for cardiovascular disease (hypertension and male gender over 55 years of age). Refer to textbook Chapter 19, or the guidelines established by the National Cholesterol Education Program,[5] for more information on target cholesterol levels.
- Assure that the patient's glucose level and BP are monitored and controlled.

Therapeutic Alternatives

3. a. What non-drug therapies might be useful for this patient?

- Dietary management should be instituted for dyslipidemia (refer to textbook Chapter 19 for detailed information).
- Dietary intervention, weight reduction, and an appropriate exercise program should be initiated to obtain maximum control of HTN with antihypertensive medications (refer to textbook Chapter 10).

b. What feasible pharmacotherapeutic alternatives are available for treating the post-transplant erythrocytosis?

- *Angiotensin-converting enzyme (ACE) inhibitors* (e.g., captopril, enalapril, lisinopril) in low doses and *angiotensin receptor antagonists* (e.g., losartan) have been shown to successfully treat post-renal transplant erythrocytosis.[2–4,6] The proposed mechanism of action of these agents in resolving post-renal transplant erythrocytosis is believed to be associated with their ability to reduce serum EPO levels.

c. What feasible pharmacotherapeutic alternatives are available for treating the patient's dyslipidemia?

- With an LDL cholesterol of 192 mg/dL and two other cardiovascular risk factors, the patient requires a 32% reduction in LDL to reach the target level of 130 mg/dL.[5] Because dietary therapy alone can only be expected to achieve a 10% to 15% reduction, both diet and drug therapy should be implemented. The management of the patient's dyslipidemia should follow the guidelines established by the NCEP for diet and medication use.[5]

- Conventional agents used for the treatment of dyslipidemia are also effective in treating the disorder in renal transplant patients.
  - ✓ *Niacin* may be used, but liver function tests should be closely monitored if it is used in combination with other hepatotoxic agents (e.g., cyclosporine).
  - ✓ *Bile acid binding resins (cholestyramine or colestipol)* can be used, but doses should be timed so that they do not interfere with the absorption of cyclosporine; the absorption of cyclosporine is dependent on the presence of bile in the GI tract.
  - ✓ *HMG-CoA reductase inhibitors (lovastatin, simvastatin, pravastatin, fluvastatin, atorvastatin, or cerivastatin)* are highly effective in the treatment of dyslipidemia in renal transplant recipients, but they should be used with caution. Rhabdomyolysis resulting in renal failure has been reported when lovastatin is used in combination with cyclosporine. Due to associated hepatotoxicity from reductase inhibitors, close monitoring of liver function is also indicated.
  - ✓ *Gemfibrozil* would not be a drug of choice in this patient because it is primarily indicated for patients with hypertriglyceridemia; it has minimal effects on lowering LDL levels.

Optimal Plan

4. *Based on the patient's presentation and the current assessment, design a pharmacotherapeutic regimen to treat this patient's erythrocytosis and dyslipidemia.*

- In light of the post-renal transplant erythrocytosis, elevated BP, and the large amount of literature supporting their effectiveness, an ACE-inhibitor should be prescribed at a low initial dose (e.g., enalapril 5 mg po daily).
- Because of the need to reduce LDL cholesterol by 32%, an HMG Co-A reductase inhibitor (in conjunction with an NCEP Step I diet) should be started at the usual initial doses. The specific agent chosen may depend upon local formulary considerations and cost.

Outcome Evaluation

5. *What clinical and laboratory parameters are necessary to evaluate the therapy for achievement of the desired therapeutic outcome and to detect or prevent adverse effects?*

Post-transplant Erythrocytosis
- Hematocrit and hemoglobin concentrations should be monitored within the first 4 to 6 weeks of therapy to evaluate the effectiveness of ACE-inhibitor therapy. The erythrocytosis should resolve within a few months of therapy. Additional monitoring may be needed if the post-renal transplant erythrocytosis does not resolve within the first 6 weeks.
- Blood pressure should be monitored at each clinic visit and preferably also frequently at home by the patient.
- The patient should also be asked about the occurrence of rash, abdominal pain, cough, and angioedema that may be associated with ACE-inhibitor therapy.

Dyslipidemia
- After initiating dietary and reductase inhibitor therapy, a follow-up fasting lipid profile (TG, HDL, LDL, and total cholesterol) should be performed at 4 to 6 weeks and again at 3 months. Thereafter, a fasting lipid profile should be performed periodically (at least annually).

- Baseline and follow-up liver function tests should be monitored periodically in patients receiving reductase inhibitors. For most drugs, AST/ALT should be obtained at 6 and 12 weeks into therapy or after dosage increases, and periodically (e.g., semiannually) thereafter. Labeling for pravastatin indicates that testing is needed only at 12 weeks after initiation of therapy or dosage escalation. Labeling for simvastatin recommends testing at the start of therapy and then periodically (e.g., semiannually) for the first year of therapy.
- Because of the risk of rhabdomyolysis, baseline and follow-up CPK measurements should be obtained 6 to 12 weeks after therapy initiation or dosage increases and periodically (e.g., semiannually) thereafter. Monitoring for unexplained muscle pain, tenderness, and weakness is also important in detecting drug-induced rhabdomyolysis.

Patient Counseling

6. *What information should be provided to the patient about his medication therapy to enhance compliance, ensure successful therapy, and minimize adverse effects?*

General Information
- Continue to take your thyroid medication as prescribed (levothyroxine sodium 0.15 mg once daily).
- Continue to take your blood pressure medication as prescribed (Procardia XL 60 mg once daily).
- Continue to take your prednisone 10 mg daily as prescribed.

ACE Inhibitor
- This medication will help to lower your high red blood cell count as well as control your high blood pressure.
- Report any unexplained muscle pain, muscle tenderness, muscle weakness, nausea, vomiting, tremors, dizziness, confusion, cough, or rashes to your physician immediately.

HMG Co-A Reductase Inhibitor
- Refer to the chapter on hyperlipidemia in this casebook for counseling information on these agents.

Cyclosporine
- Continue to take cyclosporine 250 mg twice daily.
- Take each dose at the same time each day. The doses should be taken approximately 12 hours apart (one in the morning and one in the evening).
- On days that you have a clinic visit scheduled, do not take the morning cyclosporine dose until your blood is drawn for laboratory evaluation in the clinic.
- If you miss a dose of cyclosporine, take the missed dose as soon as possible. If it is almost time for your next regular dose when you remember, skip the missed dose. Do not take two doses at the same time.

Mycophenolate Mofetil
- Continue to take mycophenolate 1500 mg twice daily. Take the doses at the same time each day.
- If you miss a dose, take the missed dose as soon as possible. If it is almost time for your next regular dose when you remember, skip the missed dose. Do not take two doses at the same time.

▶ **Follow-up Questions**

1. *Based on this new information, can you propose any potential cause for the patient's tremors?*

   - Tremors can be a symptom of cyclosporine toxicity. The cyclosporine level is above the target range of 400 ng/mL.
   - Taking cimetidine (Tagamet HB) concurrently with cyclosporine is a possible reason for the acute onset of tremors. Cimetidine can inhibit cyclosporine metabolism, resulting in elevated cyclosporine concentrations. This is not a concern when the recommended OTC doses are used (up to 400 mg/day); however, this patient was taking substantially larger amounts (up to 800 mg/day). Other potential causes for the elevated cyclosporine concentration should also be investigated (e.g., excessive cyclosporine ingestion, addition of other interacting drugs to the patient's regimen, dosage administration with grapefruit juice).

2. *Design a pharmacotherapeutic plan to resolve the patient's tremors.*

   - The patient should discontinue cimetidine use immediately.
   - If gastric acid suppression is needed, an alternative agent such as ranitidine or famotidine should be considered.
   - In order to reduce the elevated cyclosporine level, this morning's cyclosporine dose could be withheld and another cyclosporine level obtained later in the day. If the cyclosporine level has decreased to target levels, cyclosporine therapy can be restarted with this evening's dose at his regular dose of 250 mg po BID. This dose is appropriate because his level prior to initiation of cimetidine was within the desired range.
   - An alternative solution is to have the patient discontinue cimetidine use, and instruct him to continue cyclosporine therapy with this evening's scheduled dose.

3. *What clinical or laboratory parameters should be monitored?*

   - Follow-up cyclosporine levels should be taken routinely during outpatient visits.
   - If the patient starts exhibiting symptoms of cyclosporine toxicity, a thorough patient assessment and a trough cyclosporine level should be taken as soon as possible.

4. *What new information should be provided to the patient about his medications?*

   - Many drugs and foods interfere with the metabolism and bioavailability of cyclosporine. Do not take medications other than the ones prescribed without discussing them with your physician or pharmacist.
   - Symptoms such as tremors, nausea, or vomiting may be indications that you are receiving too much cyclosporine. Notify your physician immediately if you develop any of these effects.

References

1. Lezaic V, Djukanovic LJ, Pavlovic-Kentera V, et al. Factors inducing posttransplant erythrocytosis. Eur J Med Res 1997;2:407–412.
2. Gaston RS, Julian BA, Curtis JJ. Posttransplant erythrocytosis: An enigma revisited. Am J Kidney Dis 1994;24:1–11.
3. Perazella MA, Bia MJ. Posttransplant erythrocytosis: Case report and review of newer treatment modalities. J Am Soc Nephrol 1993;3:1653–1659.
4. MacGregor MS, Rowe PA, Watson MA, et al. Treatment of postrenal transplant erythrocytosis. Long-term efficacy and safety of angiotensin-converting enzyme inhibitors. Nephron 1996;74:517–521.
5. Expert Panel on Detection, Evaluation, and Treatment of High Blood Cholesterol in Adults. Summary of the second report of the National Cholesterol Education Program (NCEP) expert panel on detection, evaluation, and treatment of high blood cholesterol in adults (adult treatment panel II). JAMA 1993;269: 3015–3023.
6. Midtvedt K, Stokke ES, Hartmann A. Successful long-term treatment of posttransplant erythrocytosis with losartan. Nephrol Dial Transplant 1996;11: 2495–2497.

40 CHRONIC GLOMERULONEPHRITIS

▶ **Annie Brown's Battle With Lupus (Level III)**

Melanie S. Joy, PharmD

A 23-year-old woman with a history of diffuse proliferative glomerulonephritis (DPGN) secondary to systemic lupus erythematosus presents with hematuria and renal biopsy features characteristic of advanced DPGN. In addition to requiring immunosuppressive therapy for DPGN, she also needs treatment for hypertension, dyslipidemia, and corticosteroid-induced osteoporosis. Cyclophosphamide and azathioprine are potent immunosuppressive agents that may be useful as single agents or combined with prednisone for DPGN. Because she received cyclophosphamide on two previous occasions, it should probably be avoided at this time because of the risk of toxicity. Other potential alternatives include cyclosporine or mycophenolate mofetil. This is a complex case because it requires students to develop pharmacotherapeutic plans for all of the patient's medical problems.

▶ **Questions**

Problem Identification

1. a. *Create a list of this patient's drug-related problems.*

   - DPGN requiring immunosuppressive drug therapy.
   - HTN inadequately treated with present doses of atenolol and clonidine.
   - Hypercholesterolemia which is currently untreated.
   - Osteoporosis/osteopenia in need of treatment to prevent fractures (*Note:* T score is the SD below or above the expected mean peak BMD obtained).
   - Anemia that may be due to renal insufficiency, iron deficiency, or bleeding.

   b. *What information obtained from the medical history, physical examination, and laboratory analysis indicates the presence of glomerulonephritis?*

- Elevated creatinine to 2.2 mg/dL
- Renal biopsy results
- Urinalysis (hematuria, casts, nephrotic range proteinuria)
- Arthralgias and anemia as symptoms of SLE, which is associated with glomerulonephritis
- Gross proteinuria, elevated cholesterol, and decreased albumin are evidence of the nephrotic syndrome

c. *What information indicates complications from the disease itself or long-term treatment?*

- Osteoporosis/osteopenia due to long-term corticosteroid treatment
- Oligomenorrhea secondary to treatment with cyclophosphamide and corticosteroids
- HTN, which may be due to either loss of renal function or corticosteroid therapy
- Dyslipidemia, which may be secondary to corticosteroid therapy and the nephrotic syndrome

d. *Calculate the patient's measured creatinine clearance (CLcr) from the present 24-hour urine collection and compare that to the Clcr 6 months ago to assess the rate of progression of renal failure.*

$$\text{Clcr}_{present} = \frac{\text{Ucr} \times \text{U vol}}{\text{SCr} \times \text{Time collected}} = \frac{54.5 \text{ mg/dL} \times 2151 \text{ mL}}{2.2 \text{ mg/dL} \times 1440 \text{ minutes}}$$

$$\text{Clcr}_{present} = 37 \text{ mL/min}$$

$$\text{Clcr}_{6 \text{ months}} = \frac{81 \text{ mg/dL} \times 1200 \text{ mL}}{1.2 \text{ mg/dL} \times 1440}$$

$$\text{Clcr}_{6 \text{ months}} = 56.3 \text{ mL/min}$$

- With a decline in renal function of 20 mL/min over 6 months, this patient needs aggressive therapy to slow her development to ESRD, given findings on renal biopsy demonstrating continued proliferative glomerulonephritis.

e. *What other risk factors for renal disease progression does this patient have?*

- Uncontrolled hypertension. HTN has been associated with vascular and glomerular damage to the kidneys. The presence of elevated pressure transferred to both renal arterioles and glomeruli leads to sclerosis of the intrarenal arterioles and glomeruli. The ischemia which results from the vascular lesions in the afferent arterioles leads to elevated pressures within the glomerulus and glomerulosclerosis. This results in further basement membrane injury and worsening proteinuria. The MDRD study demonstrated that strict BP control (MAP 92 mm Hg) in patients with baseline proteinuria >1 g/day and GFR of 25 to 55 mL/min had a protective effect against progressive renal disease.[1]
- Hypercholesterolemia. Some data suggest that elevated lipid levels may lead to LDL-cholesterol binding to mesangial cells in the glomerulus. Oxidation of these bound cells by macrophages results in foam cell formation. This oxidized LDL acts as a cytotoxic agent to the glomerulus, causing cell damage.

f. *Describe the possible glomerular lesions attributable to SLE in this patient.*

- Renal disease develops in up to 75% of patients with SLE. Renal biopsy changes may be present in 95% of all lupus patients. Although tubulointerstitial disease may be the only manifestation of renal disease, glomerular disease is more commonly the case. It has been suggested that the glomerular manifestations of the disease occur due to the deposition of IgG anti-double-stranded DNA antibodies in the glomerulus, bound to the antigen. The subsequent glomerular damage occurs due to the activation of complement and damage to tissues. Although the initial damage occurs in the mesangium, increased antigen/antibody complexes lead to enhanced damage to other areas of the glomerulus.
- *Mesangial disease* is the mildest and earliest form of lupus nephritis. It is manifest as increased mesangial proliferation and matrix expansion. Patients present with mild proteinuria, microscopic hematuria, and red cell casts.
- *Focal proliferative disease* involves mesangial and endothelial proliferation in a focal, segmental pattern involving <50% of the glomeruli. Thickening of the basement membrane may occur in the affected areas. Patients present with mild proteinuria, microscopic hematuria, and red cell casts. In addition, nephrotic syndrome, hypertension, or mild renal insufficiency may be present.
- *Diffuse proliferative disease* is more severe than the focal proliferative form. Crescent formation may be present. Immunoglobulins (IgG, IgM, IgA) and complement (C3 and C4) are found in the glomeruli. The mesangial and endothelial deposits are more prominent than in the focal proliferative form. Patients may present similarly to the focal proliferative form. They may also present with acute renal failure, nephritic sediment, nephrotic range proteinuria, edema, and HTN.
- *Membranous disease* is associated with diffuse basement membrane thickening without prominent hypercellularity. Patients usually present with the nephrotic syndrome.[2,3]

g. *What is the typical clinical presentation of SLE, and which attributes are present in this patient?*

- Female to male disposition 9:1; this patient is female.
- Peak onset of disease between ages 15 and 40 years; this patient was diagnosed at age 15.
- Signs and symptoms: arthralgias, arthritis, malaise, malar rash, pleuritis, pericarditis, renal involvement; this patient currently has only arthralgias.
- Laboratory abnormalities: elevated ANA titer, circulating antibodies to double-stranded DNA, hypocomplementemia; this patient has hypocomplementemia and a positive anti-DS DNA.

Desired Outcome

2. *What are the pharmacotherapy goals for this patient's lupus nephritis?*

- Arrest and/or slow the rapid rate of renal function deterioration as demonstrated by improvement in renal biopsy and nephrotic range proteinuria.
- Prevent renal hypertensive complications by achieving a goal MAP of 92 mm Hg in this patient with proteinuria of >3 g/day.
- Treat concurrent hypercholesterolemia to prevent long-term cardiovascular complications. The LDL should be reduced from 204 to 130 mg/dL in a patient without established coronary artery disease but

with two or more risk factors (HTN and decreased HDL) according to the NCEP guidelines.
- Treat the bone complications of long-term corticosteroid therapy in order to show increased and/or stabilized bone mineral density.
- Treat the mild anemia to achieve a hematocrit of 30% to 36% in a premenopausal woman with moderate renal insufficiency.

Therapeutic Alternatives

3. What treatment alternatives are available for achieving the goals related to lupus nephritis and its complications?

Glomerulonephritis

- *High-dose prednisone* (1 mg/kg/day) has been reported to improve renal function in some patients.
- *Cyclophosphamide* may be given orally as 2.5 mg/kg daily or IV as 0.5 to 1.0 g/m^2 BSA monthly for six consecutive months. The IV route may decrease the risk of hemorrhagic cystitis due to less cumulative exposure.
- *Azathioprine* 2 mg/kg daily may be administered in place of cyclophosphamide if cytotoxic therapy is needed for longer than the recommended 6-month period.
- The combination of one of the cytotoxic agents with prednisone is suggested for patients with a presumed poor prognosis (e.g., advanced renal disease on biopsy). When prednisone is used in combination with cyclophosphamide, the prednisone dose is usually decreased to 0.5 mg/kg daily.
- *Methylprednisolone pulse therapy* (250 to 1000 mg IV for 3 days) may be used in patients who present with acute renal failure, with subsequent conversion to standard doses of oral prednisone and cyclophosphamide.
- *Cyclosporine* and *mycophenolate mofetil* have been used to treat steroid-resistant disease in patients who have either failed a course of cyclophosphamide or who are unwilling to receive additional courses of cyclophosphamide.[4,5] For additional discussion of treatment options, refer to textbook Chapter 46 and reference 2.

Hypertension

- The dosage of atenolol and/or clonidine could be titrated to a maximum of 100 mg and 1 mg respectively.
- Alternatively, since this patient is exhibiting progressive renal insufficiency, an agent that has been demonstrated to slow progressive renal disease due to HTN (e.g., ACE inhibitors or the non-dihydropyridine calcium channel blockers diltiazem or verapamil) may be worthwhile alternatives. The ACE inhibitors selectively dilate the efferent arterioles, thus decreasing glomerular capillary pressure and shear forces on the glomerular basement membrane. ACE inhibitors have been shown to reduce urinary protein excretion and decrease the rate of progression of the renal failure, possibly by exerting an independent protective effect on the glomerulus. These agents have been used to prevent progressive renal disease due to nondiabetic as well as diabetic causes.[6] Although initial studies demonstrated renal protective effects of captopril, other ACE inhibitors have been reported to have benefits as well. Initial daily dosages of respective agents include ramipril 2.5 to 5 mg, lisinopril 10 mg, captopril 25 mg, enalapril 5 mg, benazepril 20 mg, fosinopril 10 mg, or quinapril 10 mg. Dosage titration for these agents is based on the BP response, reduction in proteinuria, and elevation in serum creatinine. Although clinical trials have not yet been published, angiotensin receptor blockers may also prove to be protective.
- The patient should be advised to limit usage of NSAIDs due to their antagonism of HTN control, as well as their negative renal effects secondary to inhibition of renal prostaglandins.

Hyperlipidemia

- The patient may benefit from interventions to minimize additional damage to the glomerulus from oxidized LDL and to reduce the risk of premature cardiovascular death. Dietary counseling regarding the avoidance of foods high in fat and cholesterol should be provided in addition to an exercise program.
- Based on the percentage reduction of LDL-C by HMG-CoA reductase inhibitors, their favorable side effect profile, as well as the documented allergy to gemfibrozil in this patient, HMG-CoA reductase inhibitors are the agents of choice.[7] Due to the 36% reduction in LDL-C required, all of the reductase inhibitors except fluvastatin would be adequate. The literature has suggested that lovastatin and atorvastatin are metabolized by the cytochrome P450 3A4 enzyme, and simvastatin is an inducer of this enzyme system. Pravastatin and fluvastatin are not documented to interact with the cytochrome P450 enzymes.
- Niacin is often not well tolerated, and this patient may be predisposed to GI problems due to long-term corticosteroid use.
- Bile acid sequestrants (cholestyramine or colestipol) are also an option, since efficacy is good and they may be preferred in younger patients. Refer to textbook Chapter 19 for a detailed discussion of the treatment of lipid disorders.

Osteoporosis

- Although the patient exhibited osteoporosis of the lumbar spine and osteopenia at the hip, the need for continued long-term corticosteroid administration will predispose to continued worsening of bone density, especially with aging. The patient should be counseled about the need to have an intake of 1500 mg of elemental calcium daily while on chronic corticosteroid therapy.
- If adequate intake is not possible, calcium supplements such as Oscal (500 mg elemental calcium) or Tums (200 mg elemental calcium) should be prescribed.
- In order to enhance calcium absorption, a vitamin D supplement should also be administered. The choice of vitamin D product may be dictated by the need for activated 1,25-dihydroxyvitamin D_3 in patients with chronic renal insufficiency.
- Since the patient has osteoporosis of the spine and osteopenia of the hip, a trial of nasal calcitonin or oral alendronate may help to prevent further bone resorption and help to gain additional bone mass (although the drug is not presently FDA-approved for use in premenopausal women or in men).
- Since the patient is premenopausal, conjugated estrogens or selective estrogen receptor modulators (SERMs) such as raloxifene would not be indicated. Estrogen-containing oral contraceptives would be a reasonable consideration.[8]

Optimal Plan

4. Based on the available therapeutic options, design a pharmacotherapeutic plan for the management of lupus nephritis and its complications.

Glomerulonephritis

- Since this patient has had two courses of cyclophosphamide in the past, she should not receive additional courses due to toxicity, unless other options are unavailable. In addition, since she has had renal disease progression while on maintenance prednisone and exhibits long-term adverse effects, try to decrease her exposure if possible.
- Both azathioprine and mycophenolate mofetil would spare her further deterioration in bone disease. Azathioprine doses of up to 4 mg/kg/day orally have been used. Mycophenolate mofetil must be considered an investigational agent until more efficacy trials are completed. Mycophenolate mofetil dosing can begin at 250 mg twice daily and increased at 2-week intervals to a maximum of 1500 mg twice daily. The slow titration upward will help to establish GI tolerance to therapy.
- A lower dose of prednisone (5 to 10 mg daily) may be possible with combination therapy, thereby limiting its adverse effect potential.
- Cyclosporine therapy would be considered later in the treatment options due to its nephrotoxicity and lack of adequate data demonstrating improved outcomes.

Hypertension

- Due to the additional renal protective benefits of ACE inhibitors in glomerular diseases, one of these agents should be used. The choice may depend on the need for enhanced compliance (i.e., a once daily product). Ramipril 2.5 to 5 mg or lisinopril 10 mg po QD could be initiated. Due to the recent data indicating the protective effects of ramipril in nondiabetic renal disease, it may be the preferred agent in this patient.[6] The need to titrate the dosage upward would depend on the BP reduction demonstrated and the response to proteinuria. The serum creatinine should be monitored to detect continued increases, which is common on initiation of therapy.
- Due to the lack of controlled BP reduction and increased risk of adverse acute cardiovascular outcomes with sublingual nifedipine, this agent should be avoided for the acute reduction in blood pressure.
- If an acute reduction is desired due to the high current level (160/115), a 0.1-mg dose of clonidine would be the recommended oral therapy until the ACE inhibitor begins to reduce the pressure. Clonidine is probably not indicated in this patient, since there is no indication of symptoms or end organ damage.
- Atenolol may be able to be discontinued after the efficacy of the ACE inhibitor therapy is determined. Since the data regarding calcium channel blockers and renal disease progression are not as well established as with ACE inhibitors, these agents would not be considered first-line therapy.

Hyperlipidemia

- Since this patient needs at least a 36% decrease in LDL-C to attain a goal of <130 mg/dL, the bile acid sequestrants are not reasonable choices.
- Any of the reductase inhibitors except fluvastatin would be capable of producing a 36% reduction in LDL-C. The most cost-effective therapy should be instituted. Pravastatin may be the preferred agent due to its lack of activity on the cytochrome P450 3A4 enzymes, although this patient is not currently on medications that may interact. Pravastatin 10 to 20 mg at bedtime could be initiated, with the possibility of increasing the dose to 40 mg for increased efficacy, if tolerated.

Osteoporosis

- The patient should begin therapy with a calcium and vitamin D supplement. Oscal 250 mg with D would be a reasonable combination product option. When administered as two tablets BID, the patient will receive 1000 mg elemental calcium and 500 IU vitamin D daily. With the intake of an additional 500 mg of calcium in the diet, the patient will receive the recommended 1500 mg for patients receiving chronic glucocorticoid therapy.
- Since this patient has progressive renal insufficiency with an estimated creatinine clearance of 37 mL/min, alendronate is not a good option, since it is eliminated primarily in the kidneys and is not recommended for patients with clearances of <30 mL/min.
- Although intranasal calcitonin has only demonstrated a 1-year gain in BMD versus the 3-year gain with alendronate in glucocorticoid-treated patients, it would be a reasonable option in this patient with osteoporosis of the spine and a contraindication to alendronate. Calcitonin is administered once daily in the nostril with one spray delivering 200 IU calcitonin.
- The patient should receive some dietary counseling regarding the amount of calcium present in various foods, as well as some physical activity assessment and counseling to enhance weight bearing exercises to prevent worsening osteoporosis.

Outcome Evaluation

5. *Outline a clinical and laboratory monitoring plan for each of the patient's drug-related problems.*

- The patient should return to nephrology clinic in two weeks for assessment of progressive renal insufficiency and safety and efficacy of mycophenolate mofetil and ACE inhibitor therapy.
- Laboratory assessment should include a CBC, liver enzymes, CPK, and electrolytes. Additional follow-up labs and visits should occur at 4- to 6-week intervals to closely follow this patient's rapidly progressive renal disease and ACE inhibitor and lipid-lowering therapy.
- Urinalysis should be performed at each visit and 24-hour urine collections performed at least every six months.
- Blood pressure measurements will be performed at each clinic visit. In addition, the patient should be taught to take her own blood pressure at home.
- Adverse effect questioning at each subsequent clinic visit and appropriate modification in therapy will enhance patient compliance and disease treatment.
- A repeat DEXA scan should be performed in one year from the implementation of osteoporosis therapy to assess efficacy. A 24-hour urine collection to determine the amount of calcium eliminated may be performed to identify whether a thiazide would be indicated to minimize urinary losses.

Patient Counseling

6. *What should the patient be told regarding the drug therapy she is to receive to treat her condition and its complications?*

Mycophenolate Mofetil (CellCept)

- This drug acts to suppress your immune system in order to control your body's response to lupus. Take one tablet (250 mg) twice daily on an empty stomach for best absorption. The dose may be gradually increased every two weeks to minimize gastrointestinal side effects.
- Use appropriate contraception and avoid becoming pregnant while taking this medication, since it may be harmful to a developing fetus.
- You may experience some gastrointestinal side effects such as diar-

rhea and vomiting; notify your doctor if they become persistent or troublesome.
- The number of white cells in your blood will be monitored monthly because low counts have been reported.

Prednisone
- Prednisone is used to suppress your lupus disease activity. Take your prescribed dose with food to minimize stomach upset.
- Prednisone can cause side effects including increased risk of infection, fluid gain or swelling, increased blood sugar, risk of stomach ulcers, mood swings, and weight gain.

Ramipril (Altace)
- This medication decreases blood pressure, and it may decrease the protein being spilled into your urine.
- Dizziness or lightheadedness may occur if your blood pressure is lowered too much. This will often decrease with chronic therapy. Contact your physician if this persists.
- This drug may increase the concentration of potassium in your bloodstream or cause a nagging cough.
- Contact your physician if you become pregnant because this medication (like mycophenolate mofetil) may harm your unborn child.
- This medication should be taken on an empty stomach for best absorption.

Pravastatin (Pravachol)
- This drug is used to lower cholesterol levels. Take the prescribed 10-mg tablet daily at bedtime. Bedtime is the preferred time to take the drug, since most cholesterol synthesis occurs while you are sleeping.
- Contact your doctor if you experience muscle pain.

Calcium
- Calcium is needed to make the bones strong and to prevent them from breaking. Since you are at high risk of worsening bone disease due to long-term prednisone therapy, you should take 1500 mg of elemental calcium daily. This can be accomplished by taking two Oscal with D tablets twice daily. This will provide you with 1000 mg of your required calcium and 500 I.U. vitamin D. You will need to supplement your diet with high calcium-containing foods such as milk, cheese, beans, yogurt, and ice cream to get the other 500 mg you need. This can be obtained from 2 glasses of milk, 3 to 5 ounces of cheese, 2 cups of yogurt, or 4 cups of ice cream.
- Do not take the calcium with food, since the phosphorus in your diet may reduce its absorption.

Vitamin D
- This vitamin will also prevent your bones from breaking. Since you have been taking prednisone for a long time, you will also require vitamin D. You will receive close to your recommended daily requirement of vitamin D dose of 800 IU by taking the Oscal with D.

Calcitonin (Miacalcin) Nasal Spray
- This medication will prevent continuing bone loss. Administer one spray in one nostril daily. The spray should be alternated between nostrils on a daily basis to prevent irritation.
- Prior to the first dose of medication, the pump should be primed by holding it upright and depressing the two white side arms of the pump until a full spray is produced.
- The opened bottle may be stored at room temperature. Unopened bottles should be stored in the refrigerator.

References

1. Klahr S, Levey AS, Beck GJ, et al. The effects of dietary protein restriction and blood-pressure control on the progression of chronic renal disease. Modification of Diet in Renal Disease Study Group. N Engl J Med 1994;330:877–884.
2. Merkel F, Netzer KO, Gross O, et al. Therapeutic options for critically ill patients suffering from progressive lupus nephritis or Goodpasture's syndrome. Kidney Int Suppl 1998;64:S31–S38.
3. Jennette JC, Falk RJ. Diagnosis and management of glomerular diseases. Med Clin North Am 1997;81:653–677.
4. Levey AS, Lan SP, Corwin HL, et al. Progression and remission of renal disease in the Lupus Nephritis Collaborative Study. Results of treatment with prednisone and short-term oral cyclophosphamide. Ann Intern Med 1992;116:114–123.
5. Steinberg AD, Steinberg SC. Long-term preservation of renal function in patients with lupus nephritis receiving treatment that includes cyclophosphamide versus those treated with prednisone only. Arthritis Rheum 1991;34:945–950.
6. Remuzzi G, Tognoni G, for the GISEN Group. Randomised placebo-controlled trial of effect of ramipril on decline in glomerular filtration rate and risk of terminal renal failure in proteinuric, non-diabetic nephropathy. Lancet 1997;349:1857–1863.
7. Massy ZA, Kasiske BL. Hyperlipidemia and its management in renal disease. Curr Opin Nephrol Hypertens 1996;5:141–146.
8. Recommendations for the prevention and treatment of glucocorticoid-induced osteoporosis. American College of Rheumatology Task Force on Osteoporosis Guidelines. Arthritis Rheum 1996;39:1791–1801.

41 SYNDROME OF INAPPROPRIATE ANTIDIURETIC HORMONE RELEASE

▶ **An Out-of-Body Experience**   (Level I)

Rex W. Force, PharmD, BCPS
Jonathan D. Hubbard, DO

A 48-year-old woman presents to the ED with complaints of body aches, chills, weakness, confusion, and disorientation. She also experienced a tonic-clonic seizure while in the ED. Laboratory evaluation reveals hyponatremia (sodium 115 mEq/L), high urinary sodium concentration, low serum uric acid level, and normal renal function, findings that are consistent with SIADH. The cause of SIADH in this patient is unclear but may be secondary to herbal medications containing licorice and/or to use of her husband's metolazone. In addition to supportive measures, the serum sodium concentration should be gradually normalized over the next 2 to 3 days. Fluid restriction, hypertonic (3%) saline, and furosemide may be required acutely. Patients with chronic SIADH may be treated with demeclocycline. Students should understand that slow repletion of sodium is necessary to prevent the osmotic demyelination syndrome. Changes in neurologic function should be assessed frequently during the recovery period.

Questions

Problem Identification

1. a. *Create a list of the patient's drug-related problems.*

   - Hyponatremia and hypochloremia, apparently caused by SIADH, which will require supplementation and perhaps other treatment.
   - Seizure disorder that required acute treatment with antiepileptic drugs in the ED.
   - Hypokalemia, which will require potassium supplementation.
   - Acute agitation and combativeness requiring sedative treatment in the ED.
   - Use of herbal products for medicinal purposes without medical indication or evidence of effectiveness.

   b. *What information (signs, symptoms, laboratory values) indicates the presence or severity of SIADH as the cause of her hyponatremia?*

   - Hyponatremia is defined as serum sodium concentrations <135 mEq/L. Concentrations <110 mEq/L have been associated with an 8% mortality rate.[1] In addition, the rapid decline in mental status and seizure activity in this patient indicate hyponatremic encephalopathy and thus severe hyponatremia.
   - To identify SIADH in a patient with hyponatremia, the clinician must initially determine the patient's extracellular fluid status. Hyponatremic patients may be *hypovolemic* (due to diuretics or dehydration resulting from vomiting or diarrhea), *hypervolemic* (associated with edema or ascites), or *isovolemic* (refer to textbook Chapter 48 for a discussion of the etiologies of hyponatremia). This patient does not appear to be hypervolemic or hypovolemic (urine sodium >30 mEq/L) and therefore may be classified as having isovolemic hyponatremia.
   - The causes of isovolemic hyponatremia include glucocorticoid deficiency, severe hypothyroidism, thiazide diuretic use, psychogenic polydipsia (excessive water drinking), post-operative hyponatremia, and SIADH. Glucocorticoid deficiency was not thoroughly assessed in this patient, but her clinical picture is not consistent with this diagnosis. She has a normal T4 concentration and no history of diuretic use, water drinking, or recent surgery.
   - SIADH is associated with urinary sodium concentrations >20 mEq/L, high urinary osmolality, low uric acid concentrations, and normal renal function.[2,3] Therefore, SIADH is the most likely diagnosis.

   c. *Could any of the patient's problems have been caused by drug therapy?*

   - With the exception of herbal products, this patient is not known to have taken any medications prior to presentation. Licorice consumption has an aldosterone-like effect and may have caused hypokalemia and predisposed her to hyponatremia.
   - Many drugs, especially thiazide diuretics, have been implicated in causing hyponatremia. Opioids, phenothiazines, chlorpropamide, NSAIDs, carbamazepine, tricyclic antidepressants, clofibrate, vincristine, cyclophosphamide, and oxytocin have caused SIADH either by increasing ADH release or sensitizing the kidney to the effects of ADH.[2,3]

Desired Outcome

2. *What are the goals of pharmacotherapy in this case?*

   - Normalize serum electrolyte concentrations over the next 48 to 72 hours. The serum sodium concentration should not increase faster than 0.5 mEq/L/hr or by 12 mEq/L in first 24 hours to minimize the likelihood of neurologic damage.
   - Prevent seizure recurrence while avoiding adverse events.

Therapeutic Alternatives

3. a. *What non-drug therapies might be useful for this patient?*

   - Supportive therapy in an intensive care unit should be provided for patients with severe hyponatremic encephalopathy. This involves ventilator support, cardiac monitoring, and neurologic care as necessary.
   - In isovolemic patients with hyponatremia, treatment should emphasize water restriction (usually <1 L/day). Typically, patients require about 500 mL/day to achieve obligatory urine output.
   - Treatment of underlying conditions (e.g., hypothyroidism) and discontinuation of possible offending medications should occur.
   - Patients with a history of psychogenic polydipsia should not have free access to water.

   b. *What pharmacotherapeutic alternatives are available for the treatment of hyponatremia?*

   - *Hypertonic saline* (3% NaCl) should be given to patients with severe isovolemic hyponatremia or SIADH in addition to fluid restriction (as described above). Normal saline has no role in the management of isovolemic hyponatremia/SIADH, since the sodium may be excreted rapidly resulting in retention of "free" water.[2]
   - *Furosemide* may be added to hypertonic saline to increase the excretion of free water or if volume overload occurs.
   - *Demeclocycline* 600 to 1200 mg/day po may be given to patients with chronic SIADH if fluid restriction alone does not control the hyponatremia.
   - *Lithium carbonate* has also been used, but its toxicity and somewhat unpredictable response in SIADH have made demeclocycline the drug of choice. Both agents cause diabetes insipidus (insensitivity of the kidney to ADH) over the course of several days. The net result is an increase in serum sodium concentration and tonicity.

Optimal Plan

4. *What drug dosage form, dose, schedule and duration of therapy are most appropriate for initial treatment of this patient?*

   - This patient should receive IV hypertonic saline (3%) 1 to 2 mL/kg/hr.
   - Furosemide in initial doses of 20 to 40 mg IV may be added.
   - Free water restriction to 500 to 750 mL/day is also indicated.
   - The duration of these therapies depends upon the severity of hyponatremia and the rate of correction. In general, to prevent possible neu-

rological damage, the serum sodium concentration should not increase faster than 0.5 mEq/L/hr or by 12 mEq/L in the first 24 hours.
- Demeclocycline and lithium have no role in the treatment of acute SIADH since they require several days to take effect. Patients with stable asymptomatic hyponatremia (usually >120 mEq/L) may not require any treatment.

Outcome Evaluation

5. *What clinical parameters are necessary to evaluate the therapy for achievement of the desired therapeutic outcome and to detect or prevent adverse effects?*

- Initially, serum sodium concentrations should be measured every 2 to 3 hours during treatment. The increase in serum sodium concentration should be kept at 0.5 mEq/L/hr for the first 24 hours. Too rapid repletion of sodium is associated with osmotic demyelination syndrome (or central pontine myelinolysis), which is thought to be caused by rapid fluid and electrolyte shifts within the central nervous system. This syndrome is manifested as quadriplegia, pseudobulbar palsy, mutism, swallowing difficulties, other neurologic symptoms, and even death.
- For this reason, pharmacists should examine patients for changes in neurologic function. These parameters include weakness, paralysis, inability to speak, changes in mental status or sensation, and choking or aspiration. Typical symptoms occur within 5 days of repletion of sodium.[2–4]
- Other electrolytes, including potassium, should be repleted over the next 48 hours.

Patient Counseling

6. *What information should be provided to the patient to enhance compliance, ensure successful therapy, and minimize adverse effects?*

Patients with acute hyponatremia/SIADH may not require any additional therapy. Patients receiving demeclocycline should receive the following information:

Demeclocycline

- Demeclocycline (also known as Declomycin) is used to keep your blood levels of sodium up. Do not change your fluid restriction regimen, dietary intake of sodium, or demeclocycline dosage without your physician's knowledge.
- It is likely that you will be taking this medicine indefinitely. If you miss a dose, take it as soon as you remember. If it is almost time for your next dose, skip the missed dose and go back to your regular schedule. Do not double doses.
- Demeclocycline may cause an exaggerated sunburn. Avoid prolonged exposure to the sun or sunlamps. Wear sunscreen, a hat, and long-sleeved clothing when out in the sun for prolonged periods. If you get a severe sunburn, contact your physician.
- Do not take this medicine within two hours of drinking milk or ingesting dairy products, zinc, magnesium, calcium and/or iron supplements, or antacids.
- If you develop symptoms of low sodium in your blood, consult your doctor or go the emergency department. These symptoms include muscle cramps, weakness, nausea and vomiting, confusion, disorientation, or seizures.
- Never allow your demeclocycline to expire (become outdated). Do not store it in the bathroom and keep it out of the reach of children.

▶ ## Follow-up Question

1. *Does this information alter your assessment of the patient's drug-related problems?*

- Thiazide diuretics have caused *euvolemic* hyponatremia by inhibiting free water excretion by the kidney. This syndrome appears most commonly in elderly women; hypokalemia and polydipsia may play supplementary roles. In addition, it has been reported to occur after as little as one day of treatment.[2,3]
- Licorice consumption, which has an aldosterone-like effect, may have caused hypokalemia, predisposing her to sodium wasting with metolazone (a potent and long-acting thiazide derivative).[2]

References

1. Sterns RH. Severe symptomatic hyponatremia: Treatment and outcome. A study of 64 cases. Ann Intern Med 1987;107:656–664.
2. Fried LF, Palevsky PM. Hyponatremia and hypernatremia. Med Clin North Am 1997;81:585–609.
3. Mulloy AL, Caruana RJ. Hyponatremic emergencies. Med Clin North Am 1995;79:155–168.
4. Laureno R, Karp BI. Myelinolysis after correction of hyponatremia. Ann Intern Med 1997;126:57–62.

42 HYPOKALEMIA AND HYPOMAGNESEMIA

▶ ## Double Trouble (Level II)

Denise R. Sokos, PharmD
W. Greg Leader, PharmD

A 45-year-old woman with a history of alcoholic hepatitis, chronic pancreatitis, and type 2 diabetes mellitus presents to the ED with complaints of dull abdominal pain, weight loss, and generalized weakness. Physical exam is indicative of dehydration, and laboratory evaluation reveals hypokalemia, hypomagnesemia, hyperglycemia, hypocalcemia, and hypoalbuminemia. The patient has multiple possible causes for electrolyte abnormalities, including chronic diarrhea, vomiting, dehydration, and alcohol abuse. Correction of the serum calcium concentration for hypoalbuminemia suggests that no treatment is required for hypocalcemia. Students are asked to develop a cohesive plan to rehydrate the patient and treat both the hypokalemia and hypomagnesemia intravenously on an inpatient basis, with continuing oral treatment in the outpatient setting. Because the patient has chronic medical and social problems that may result in continued electrolyte depletion, patient education on the need for adherence to outpatient oral supplementation is important.

Hypokalemia and Hypomagnesemia

▶ Questions

Problem Identification

1. a. *Create a list of the patient's drug-related problems.*

   - Hypokalemia, hypomagnesemia, and hypocalcemia that are not treated.
   - Type 2 DM inadequately controlled with present treatment
   - Chronic pain that is inappropriately treated
   - Chronic diarrhea that is not treated
   - Ethanol and nicotine addiction that are not treated
   - Inappropriate use of quinine for leg cramps

   b. *What information (signs, symptoms, laboratory values) indicates the presence or severity of hypokalemia, hypomagnesemia, and hypocalcemia?*

   Hypokalemia
   - The normal range for serum potassium concentration is 3.5 to 5.0 mEq/L. Moderate hypokalemia is defined as a serum potassium of 2.5 to 3.5 mEq/L, and severe hypokalemia is defined as a level <2.5 mEq/L. This patient has moderate hypokalemia (2.5 mEq/L). The signs and symptoms of hypokalemia are quite variable, may depend upon the acuteness of the electrolyte loss, and are usually not observed until the serum potassium concentration falls below 3.0 mEq/L. Most symptoms are caused by changes in the cellular resting potential and membrane excitability, which are related to the ratio of intracellular to extracellular potassium. Patients with a chronic loss of potassium may have few symptoms because intracellular potassium moves extracellularly, thus restoring the intracellular to extracellular potassium ratio. This patient does not present with hypokalemic-associated ECG changes (ST segment depression, T wave inversion, and the occurrence of a U wave). However, she does report muscle weakness and is taking quinine for leg cramps (duration and severity unknown). Polyuria and polydipsia may also occur in chronic hypokalemia. The patient is also hypomagnesemic, which often occurs in conjunction with hypokalemia.

   Hypomagnesemia
   - The normal range for serum magnesium is 1.5 to 2.0 mEq/L, with <1 mEq/L being considered hypomagnesemia. Her level of 0.5 mEq/L signifies a severe magnesium deficit; however, serum magnesium is not an accurate indicator of body magnesium stores. Other than some muscle weakness, the patient does not exhibit any signs or symptoms of hypomagnesemia (refer to textbook Table 48–12 for a complete list of the signs and symptoms of hypomagnesemia). The patient also has hypocalcemia, which often accompanies hypomagnesemia.

   Hypocalcemia
   - The normal range for total calcium is 8.5 to 10.5 mg/dL. The occurrence of signs and symptoms of hypocalcemia may be directly related to the time course over which the abnormality occurs. Currently, she is not showing any signs of hypocalcemia (see textbook Table 48–9 for a complete list of the signs and symptoms of hypocalcemia). With a total serum calcium concentration of 7.5 mg/dL, the patient appears to be hypocalcemic, but a serum albumin is necessary to correctly assess total serum calcium concentrations because of calcium's affinity for albumin. A normalized or corrected calcium concentration can be calculated with the following equation:

   Corrected calcium = ([normal albumin − patient's albumin] × 0.8) + total serum calcium

   Corrected calcium = ([4.0 − 2.6] × 0.8) + 7.5 = 8.6 mg/dL

   Because the corrected calcium is within the normal range, this suggests that the patient's ionized calcium is within normal limits and no calcium replacement is necessary.

   c. *What are the potential causes of the electrolyte disorders in this patient?*

   Hypokalemia
   - *Diarrhea* is one of the most common causes of hypokalemia. The normal concentration of potassium and bicarbonate in the stool is very high (about 35 and 40 mEq/L, respectively). Diarrhea may cause both decreased absorption and increased secretion of potassium. The loss of bicarbonate and potassium commonly causes a hypokalemic metabolic acidosis, but acidosis is not present in this patient based on ABGs.
   - *Secondary hyperaldosteronism* may result from dehydration, which is suggested by the patient's history of vomiting, diarrhea and the orthostatic BP changes. Hypovolemia stimulates aldosterone secretion, which in turn increases the renal excretion of potassium, hydrogen, and chloride while retaining sodium and bicarbonate. Although hypokalemic metabolic alkalosis can result, this patient also does not have an alkalosis based on ABGs.
   - *Alcoholism* can contribute to hypokalemia by several mechanisms including poor nutritional status, pancreatitis, emesis, and renal losses activating the renin-angiotensin-aldosterone system.
   - *Vomiting* causes a direct loss of potassium and hydrogen ions. The loss of hydrogen ions may lead to a metabolic alkalosis. To preserve electroneutrality, the body shifts potassium intracellularly. Another mechanism of hypokalemia after emesis is urinary excretion; the loss of hydrogen ions causes an increase in the plasma bicarbonate concentration with concomitant hypovolemia and hyperaldosteronism. This leads to an increase in filtered bicarbonate that exceeds the kidney's capacity to reabsorb it; therefore, more sodium bicarbonate (a nonreabsorbable anion) is delivered to the distal tubule. The kidney reabsorbs sodium to try to preserve volume and electroneutrality by secreting potassium into the urine in exchange for sodium. Normally, this process only occurs for a few days until the kidneys begin to compensate for the increased serum bicarbonate.
   - *Hypomagnesemia* is often a concomitant disorder in alcoholics and in many patients with hypokalemia. Hypomagnesemia may lead to increases in both renal and fecal losses of potassium. The exact mechanism by which hypomagnesemia causes hypokalemia is unclear, but it is thought that magnesium is required for the Na-K-ATPase pump to effectively transport potassium intracellularly.[1] A serum magnesium concentration should always be checked in patients with persistent hypokalemia, especially those resistant to replacement therapy.

Hypomagnesemia
- *Diarrhea* (especially if chronic) can result in significant magnesium losses, as intestinal fluids contain about 14 mEq/L of magnesium.
- *Chronic pancreatitis* can lead to malabsorption and malnutrition resulting in decreased magnesium absorption and intake, respectively. Pancreatic fluids contain an average magnesium concentration of 0.8 mEq/L.
- *Alcoholism and malnutrition* commonly result in hypomagnesemia because of decreased magnesium intake and increased renal elimination of magnesium. Refer to textbook Table 48–11 for other causes of hypomagnesemia.

Hypocalcemia
- *Hypoalbuminemia* is the most common cause of laboratory-reported hypocalcemia. In this case, a corrected calcium concentration should be calculated or an ionized calcium concentration measured. Outside of the ICU setting, calculating a corrected calcium is done more frequently than obtaining an ionized calcium measurement.

Malnutrition could be a contributing factor for all of the electrolyte abnormalities. The patient is a known alcoholic with admitted weight loss, chronic diarrhea, recent vomiting, and a low serum albumin. All of these factors contribute to a clinical diagnosis of malnutrition.

d. *What additional information is needed to satisfactorily assess this patient?*

- For evaluation of the hypokalemia, a urinary sodium, potassium, and osmolality, with concurrent serum values, may be helpful to investigate the source of losses and the patient's volume status.
- If the urinary potassium is <20 mEq/L, then extrarenal losses are more probable (as is suspected from the clinical presentation). Urinary potassium concentrations >20 mEq/L generally indicate renal potassium losses.
- Low urinary sodium concentrations indicate a volume-depleted state.
- Urinary osmolality is normally 900 to 1400 mOsmol/kg. In a hypokalemic state, the osmolality slowly decreases over weeks but generally does not fall below 300 mOsmol/kg. Because of this, urine output normally stays below 3 L/day. Maximal osmolality begins to fall when the potassium deficit exceeds 200 mEq and reaches a minimum with a deficit of 400 mEq (the reflective serum concentration should be below 3.0 mEq/L). This is in contrast to diabetes insipidus where the osmolality may be below 150 mOsmol/kg.

Desired Outcome

2. *What are the goals of pharmacotherapy in this patient?*

Primary Outcomes
- Rehydrate the patient
- Replace potassium and magnesium deficiencies
- Prevent further losses of electrolytes
- Prevent the development of cardiac abnormalities

Secondary Outcomes
- Determine the etiology of diarrhea and treat it appropriately
- Control pancreatitis and abdominal pain
- Control diabetes to prevent end-organ damage
- Assess weight loss and improve nutritional status
- Observe for and treat signs and symptoms of alcohol or nicotine withdrawal; encourage cessation

Therapeutic Alternatives

3. *What feasible pharmacotherapeutic alternatives are available for treatment of dehydration, hypokalemia, hypomagnesemia, and hypocalcemia?*

Dehydration
- *Oral rehydration therapy (ORT)* is an appropriate method of fluid resuscitation for patients who are mildly (3% to 5% deficit) to moderately (6% to 9% deficit) dehydrated, usually because of acute diarrhea. Any one of several oral rehydration products is acceptable in mild to moderate dehydration.
- *Intravenous fluids (IVF)* are indicated in severe dehydration (10% or more deficit, shock, or near shock). Crystalloid solutions include dextrose 5% in water, saline in varying concentrations, dextrose and saline combinations, and Ringer's lactate. Solutions containing only dextrose are considered to be free water (no osmotically active particles) and will not increase the intravascular volume to any great extent. The use of normal saline or Ringer's lactate (both isotonic solutions) will increase the intravascular volume by one-fourth of the infused volume after one hour in healthy individuals. Equilibration with the extracellular space takes place in approximately 20 to 30 minutes. The colloidal solutions dextran, hetastarch, and albumin are not used for simple dehydration and are reserved for shock states.
- This patient is moderately dehydrated, so ORT would normally be appropriate. However, she continues to have diarrhea and was recently seen in the ED for emesis; therefore, IVF are the treatment of choice for this particular patient.

Hypokalemia
- Because the kidneys are the primary regulators of potassium excretion, a patient's renal function should be assessed prior to instituting potassium replacement. In patients with renal insufficiency, potassium replacement should be approached cautiously as hyperkalemia may develop; however, this patient does not have renal insufficiency. Her calculated creatinine clearance is about 133 mL/min by the Cockcroft and Gault equation. However, the patient appears malnourished, and this is likely an overestimation of her true renal function. Rounding her serum creatinine concentration to 1 mg/dL gives a more conservative estimate of 66 mL/minute.
- *Potassium chloride, citrate, and bicarbonate salts* are the available formulations of potassium and are equally efficacious. The oral route is preferred unless there are life-threatening symptoms. Chloride salts are generally used in patients with alkalosis to replenish chloride stores depleted by diuretic use, vomiting, or nasogastric suctioning. Normally, sodium is reabsorbed in the renal tubules with chloride; however, when chloride stores are depleted, hydrogen and/or potassium ions are exchanged for sodium ions. When hypokalemia occurs, hydrogen ions are exchanged for sodium resulting in a metabolic alkalosis. Chloride and fluid replenishment decrease the exchange of hydrogen ions for sodium ions in the renal tubules therefore helping to correct the alkalosis. Citrate, which is metabolized to bicarbonate, or bicarbonate salts are used in metabolic or renal tubular acidosis to replace bicarbonate.

- *Oral potassium* is available in four dosage forms: elixirs, powders, capsules, and tablets. The extended-release tablets are often best tolerated and are the most frequently used. The elixir is the least expensive formulation but has very poor patient adherence during chronic therapy because of its unpleasant taste and resulting nausea.
- *Parenteral potassium* replacement is the preferred route when the patient is unable to take oral medications or when hypokalemia is life-threatening. In general, 10 to 20 mEq/hr can be safely administered and repeated based on serum potassium concentrations. In rare instances for severe hypokalemia with life-threatening symptoms, a rate of 40 to 100 mEq/hr may be used. ECG monitoring is required if potassium is to be administered at a rate of 20 mEq/hr or greater and may be warranted if administration exceeds 10 mEq/hr. The maximum concentration for peripheral administration is 40 to 60 mEq/L or the infusion may be painful and cause venous irritation. When potassium is administered through a central line, 10 to 20 mEq/100 mL may be given over 1 hour with concurrent ECG monitoring. Whenever parenteral therapy is used, frequent laboratory monitoring is necessary.[2,3]

Hypomagnesemia

- *Oral magnesium gluconate* or oxide may be given in most situations. Magnesium gluconate is the preferred agent, because magnesium oxide can cause an osmotic diarrhea.
- *IV magnesium sulfate* is warranted when the serum concentration is less than 1.0 mEq/L or acute symptoms are present. For life-threatening symptoms, give a 2-g IV bolus over one minute followed by an infusion of 0.5 mEq/kg lean body weight (LBW) over 5 to 6 hours. An additional 0.5 mEq/kg LBW should be administered as a continuous infusion over the next 18 hours. For serum concentrations <1.0 mEq/L without life-threatening symptoms, a total of 1.0 mEq/kg LBW should be given over 24 hours. Initially, one-half of the dose (0.5 mEq/kg LBW) should be given as an infusion over 2 to 6 hours (not to exceed 150 mg/min) with the remainder of the dose given as a continuous infusion.

Optimal Plan

4. *Given the above therapeutic alternatives, what therapy would be the most appropriate?*

Rehydration

- Normal saline is the IVF of choice to promote tissue perfusion and to expand the extracellular space. Avoid dextrose-containing solutions because they have a tendency to promote an intracellular shift of potassium and will not appreciably increase extracellular volume. Based on the patient's weight, she will require a minimum of 2700 mL/day to maintain fluid balance. However, since she is dehydrated, additional volume is required to create a positive fluid balance. Maintenance and replacement IV fluids at a rate of 125 mL/hr are the minimum required to meet her needs and provide rehydration. An initial fluid bolus of 500 mL over 1 to 2 hours is appropriate because of the patient's orthostasis (a drop in BP of 20 mm Hg and an increase in pulse of 20 beats/min).

Potassium

- The first step in the assessment of this patient's hypokalemia is to calculate the potassium deficit. In general, a 1-mEq/L fall in serum potassium concentrations represents a 200 to 400 mEq decrease in total body potassium stores. This patient's deficit is approximately 350 to 600 mEq. This implies that a single dose will not be sufficient to correct her serum potassium. For mild deficits, 40 to 80 mEq/day is appropriate. More severe deficits may require up to 100 to 200 mEq/day with frequent monitoring.
- Because the patient needs IV hydration, potassium chloride (40 to 80 mEq/L) should be added to the maintenance IV fluids, obviating the need for oral therapy. Oral therapy as a liquid or tablet could otherwise be used because she is asymptomatic and no longer vomiting. During replacement therapy, intracellular potassium must be restored before changes will be reflected in the serum potassium. Because this patient is also hypomagnesemic, magnesium replacement is necessary for potassium replacement to be successful.

Magnesium

- IV magnesium is indicated since the serum level is <1.0 mEq/L. Give 1 mEq/kg LBW/day; one-half of the dose as a bolus infusion over 2 to 6 hours, then the remainder as a continuous infusion on day 1. On days 2 through 5, give 0.5 mEq/kg LBW/day as a continuous infusion. The reason for the continuous infusion is that up to 50% of an IV dose is excreted in the urine. For this patient, give a 30-mEq (3.75-g) bolus dose, then another 30 mEq (3.75 g) in her maintenance IV fluids.

Treatment Summary

An example regimen for this patient is normal saline 500 mL containing KCl 20 mEq and $MgSO_4$ 30 mEq given over 2 hours with ECG monitoring (because of 10 mEq/hour KCl), followed by normal saline with KCl 40 mEq/L and $MgSO_4$ 10 mEq/L infused continuously at 125 mL/hr. If the fluid bolus is to be administered at a wide-open rate, then no electrolytes should be added to the bolus. They should be started either after the bolus has been infused or in a separate line concurrently with the bolus.

Outcome Evaluation

5. *What clinical and laboratory parameters are necessary to evaluate the therapy for the desired therapeutic outcome and prevention of adverse effects?*

- While hospitalized, serum potassium concentrations should be monitored initially every 4 hours. After initial replacement, potassium should be monitored every 1 to 2 days until stable.
- Magnesium should be monitored twice daily initially, and then every few days after the electrolytes are stable.
- Serum electrolyte concentrations should also be drawn any time signs or symptoms of a hypo- or hyper- electrolyte disorder are noted. These monitoring guidelines are only valid during hospitalization; outpatient monitoring is less intensive and much more difficult. After this patient is discharged, she should return to the clinic in approximately 2 days to have her serum magnesium and potassium concentrations measured. She should then return weekly for serum magnesium and potassium concentration measurements until stable. Given the patient's social situation, this may not be a feasible plan and may need to be altered depending on whether or not the patient is willing to cooperate.
- The patient should be monitored for signs of toxicity from the electrolyte replacement therapy:
    ✓ Potassium therapy should be discontinued if serum levels are

Renal and Genitourinary Tract Disorders   151

>5.0 mEq/L, peaked T waves are noticed on ECG, or for the sudden onset of muscle weakness. The patient should also be monitored for pain and phlebitis with IV therapy and GI irritation when switched to oral therapy.

✓ Magnesium therapy should be discontinued for serum concentrations >2.0 mEq/L, and the patient should be monitored for muscle weakness and cardiac and respiratory abnormalities. The patient should receive the magnesium in a supine position (especially the bolus) and blood pressure should be monitored. The patient may complain of flushing or sweating during IV magnesium administration.

- Serum phosphate and chloride concentrations should also be monitored during potassium and magnesium replenishment. If the serum phosphate concentration drops below 2.5 mg/dL, potassium phosphate can be used instead of potassium chloride. $MgSO_4$ is also compatible with KPO_4 in solution.

Patient Counseling

6. *When the patient is to be discharged on oral potassium and magnesium supplementation, what information should be provided to her to ensure successful therapy and minimize adverse effects?*

Potassium Chloride (e.g., K-Dur Tablets)

- This medication is a potassium supplement called K-Dur. The dose is 20 mEq (one tablet) every day.
- Potassium is essential for the proper functioning of the heart, kidneys, muscles, nerves, and digestive system. Normally, people get enough potassium from their diet; however, because you may not have been eating very well and you have had diarrhea and vomiting, your body is not getting all of the potassium it needs to function properly.
- Take this medicine once a day right after a meal. Take it with a full glass of water or juice and swallow the tablet whole; do not crush it.
- If you forget to take a dose of the medicine, take it as soon as you remember. If it is less than 12 hours until your next dose, skip that dose completely; never take a double dose.
- Side effects of potassium tablets are generally very mild; you may notice some abdominal discomfort, nausea or vomiting, or diarrhea. If you develop confusion or a tingling, burning sensation in your arms or legs, notify your doctor because your dose may be too high. Do not adjust the dose on your own.
- You may be taking this medication for just a few weeks or for several months. Until your stomach, pancreas, and nutritional problems are controlled, it may be difficult to keep the potassium in your blood normal.
- Store this drug at room temperature out of the reach of children.

Magnesium (e.g., Mag-Ox)

- This medication is a magnesium oxide supplement called Mag-Ox 400-mg tablets. Magnesium is essential for the proper functioning of your muscles, heart, and digestive tract.
- Your doctor has asked you to take one tablet twice a day, and you should continue to do so until he tells you to stop taking the drug.
- Swallow each tablet with a full glass of water.
- If you forget to take a dose, take it as soon as you remember and then take any remaining doses at evenly spaced intervals throughout the day. Do not take doses any closer than 6 hours apart; do not take a double dose, simply skip the missed dose and go on with your usual regimen.
- Magnesium tablets may cause diarrhea in some patients. If you have severe diarrhea or diarrhea that lasts for several days, notify your physician.
- Store this drug at room temperature out of the reach of children.

▶ **Follow-up Questions**

1. *What medical options are available for the treatment of this patient's chronic pancreatitis?*

- Medical management of chronic pancreatitis is multifactorial and revolves around proper nutrition and pain control. Adequate pain control is a major requirement that may necessitate narcotic analgesics. The patient should have non-narcotic analgesic doses maximized (e.g., aspirin or acetaminophen) prior to receiving narcotics. In this patient, acetaminophen should be avoided (as a single agent or in combination with a narcotic) because of her alcohol abuse. This patient could be treated with aspirin prior to meals to reduce postprandial gastric pain. The pain medication should be given around-the-clock and not on an as-needed basis.
- Patients should be counseled to adhere to a low fat diet, and the addition of pancreatic enzyme supplementation may also help decrease pain. In general, a starting dose of pancreatic enzymes that provides the equivalent of 30,000 units of lipase and 10,000 units of trypsin with each meal is appropriate, with the dose adjusted to the amount of steatorrhea that occurs. The patient is currently receiving two Pancrelipase capsules with meals, which is below the recommended dosage and should be increased.
- In patients with continued steatorrhea after enzyme replacement therapy and a low intestinal pH, insufficient dissolution of the pancreatic enzyme preparation may lead to treatment failure (most are designed to release their enzymes at a pH of 6.0). In these patients the addition of an agent to increase intestinal pH (e.g., an H_2-receptor antagonist, proton pump inhibitor, or antacid) may increase the effectiveness of the pancreatic enzyme supplementation.
- Parenteral narcotics, ganglionic block, and surgery are options for patients who fail oral therapy.
- See textbook Chapter 37 for a complete description of the treatment of pancreatitis.

2. *What changes should be made in the therapy for the patient's other medical conditions?*

- The patient is currently receiving drug therapy for diabetes mellitus, but her blood glucose is elevated at 305 mg/dL. This could be due to several different factors, including an acute reaction to her illness, poor diet, noncompliance with her medication, alcohol consumption, and hypokalemia. It is possible that her current hyperglycemia is due to the increase in insulin resistance seen with hypokalemia. After correction of her electrolyte disorders, the patient should have the management of her diabetes further evaluated.
- Nicotine and ethanol addiction are both amenable to drug therapy, but the most effective therapies are often a combination of medications and behavioral modification. Nicotine replacement therapy is available in the forms of gum, patch, and nasal spray. Bupropion is

also FDA-approved for smoking cessation. For ethanol addiction, the benzodiazepines are used for detoxification. Disulfiram is also available once detoxification is complete as an avoidance therapy.
- The patient is currently on quinine for the treatment of leg cramps. The patient needs to be questioned about the history of cramps. If appropriate electrolyte replacement causes the leg cramping to disappear, the quinine should be discontinued.

References

1. Dyckner T, Wester PO. Ventricular extrasystoles and intracellular electrolytes in hypokalemic patients before and after correction of the hypokalemia. Acta Med Scand 1978;204:375–379.
2. Kruse JA, Carlson RW. Rapid correction of hypokalemia using concentrated intravenous potassium chloride infusions. Arch Intern Med 1990;150:613–617.
3. Hamill RJ, Robinson LM, Wexler HR, et al. Efficacy and safety of potassium infusion therapy in hypokalemic critically ill patients. Crit Care Med 1991;19:694–699.

43 HYPERKALEMIA, HYPERPHOSPHATEMIA, AND HYPOCALCEMIA

▶ A Lesson in Homeostasis   (Level II)

Brian K. Bond, PharmD
Mary K. Stamatakis, PharmD

A 34-year-old man with type 1 diabetes mellitus, hypertension, and end-stage renal disease on hemodialysis is admitted for treatment of an infected arteriovenous graft site. The patient missed his scheduled hemodialysis session yesterday and presents with hyperkalemia, hyperphosphatemia, and hypocalcemia. The primary focus of the case is on identification of factors that contributed to the electrolyte disturbances and selection of appropriate non-drug and pharmacologic measures to correct them. Appropriate dosing of vancomycin for a probable methicillin-resistant staphylococcus infection of the AV site is also addressed. Items for patient education include dietary interventions to minimize electrolyte disturbances, proper medication administration, and the need for adherence to his hemodialysis appointments.

▶ Questions

Problem Identification

1. a. *Create a list of the patient's drug-related problems.*

   - Hyperkalemia resulting from CRF and missed HD session, requiring pharmacologic or other treatment to prevent complications.
   - Hyperphosphatemia and hypocalcemia secondary to end-stage renal disease requiring pharmacologic treatment.
   - Probable MRSA-infected dialysis graft requiring IV vancomycin therapy.
   - Anemia of chronic renal failure requiring evaluation of current erythropoietin dosage regimen.

Problem 1: Hyperkalemia

b. *What information (signs, symptoms, laboratory values) indicates the presence or severity of hyperkalemia?*

   - Serum potassium concentration of 6.0 mEq/L (mild in severity). Hyperkalemia may be classified as mild (5.5 to 6.5 mEq/L), moderate (6.5 to 8.0 mEq/L), or severe (>8.0 mEq/L).
   - There are no ECG changes suggestive of hyperkalemia, but the potassium concentrations at which the characteristic changes appear are variable; in mild hyperkalemia, one could see peaked T waves and shortening of the QT interval.
   - No complaints of muscle twitching or weakness (asymptomatic hyperkalemia)

c. *Could any of the patient's medications be contributing to his hyperkalemia?*

   - The patient is receiving Metamucil effervescent powder. Each packet contains 310 mg of potassium, so the patient is receiving an additional 930 mg of potassium daily. Since the average hemodialysis patient is restricted to approximately 2 to 3 g of potassium daily, it is likely that his total potassium daily intake is elevated.

d. *What is the pathophysiology of the patient's hyperkalemia?*

   - Potassium homeostasis is regulated by several mechanisms. In patients with normal renal function, potassium balance is primarily regulated through renal excretion of excess potassium. Gastrointestinal excretion of potassium is minimal in patients with normal renal function. However, there is an increase in GI excretion of potassium in ESRD patients which partially compensates for loss of renal excretory function.[1]
   - The second and more rapid process for maintaining potassium homeostasis is an internal shift of potassium from the extracellular to the intracellular fluid compartment. However, total potassium body stores are ultimately regulated through renal and GI excretion. In patients with ESRD who consume excessive quantities of potassium, GI excretion is overwhelmed and hyperkalemia ensues.[1]
   - Finally, missing a regularly-scheduled hemodialysis session most likely contributed to the development of hyperkalemia in this patient by limiting potassium removal.

e. What are the clinical consequences of hyperkalemia?

- Non-cardiac symptoms of hyperkalemia include generalized muscle weakness that frequently progresses from the lower to the upper extremities, muscle twitching, and dyspnea. Non-cardiac symptoms are often absent.
- ECG changes, in order of increasing severity, include peaked T waves and shortening of the QT interval, loss of P waves and prolongation of the QRS complex, and widened QRS interval merging with T waves (sine wave pattern). Cardiac symptoms rarely occur when serum potassium concentration is <6.0 mEq/L and occur more frequently with concentrations >8.0 mEq/L.

Desired Outcome

2. What are the goals for treating this patient's hyperkalemia?

- Reverse hyperkalemia (restore serum potassium concentration in the range of 3.5 to 5.0 mEq/L)
- Identify and correct the reasons why the patient misses HD sessions and implement measures to ensure compliance with sessions

Therapeutic Alternatives

3. a. What non-drug therapies are available for the treatment of hyperkalemia?

- Hemodialysis is an effective method for removing excess potassium from the body. In moderate to severe hyperkalemia, hemodialysis may be indicated in conjunction with drug therapy or when pharmacotherapeutic measures fail. For chronic hemodialysis patients, mild, moderate, and severe hyperkalemia may be treated by routine hemodialysis. Because this patient is a chronic dialysis patient with appropriate hemodialysis access, dialysis is indicated, especially since he missed his regularly scheduled dialysis session.
- Although limiting dietary potassium intake and potassium-containing medications may prevent the development of hyperkalemia, these methods are not useful in acute treatment of hyperkalemia.

b. What feasible pharmacotherapeutic alternatives are available for treatment of hyperkalemia?

Antagonism of the Effect of Hyperkalemia on Cardiac Contractility

- *Calcium chloride or calcium gluconate* given IV is indicated when hyperkalemia is severe (>8 mEq/L) or moderate (>6.5 to 8 mEq/L) when accompanied by significant ECG changes. Calcium antagonizes the effect of hyperkalemia on cardiac tissue, reversing potentially life-threatening changes in conductivity and automaticity in the heart. However, calcium does not enhance elimination of potassium from the body. The dose of calcium chloride is 1 g IV over 5 to 10 minutes; the onset time is 1 to 2 minutes, and the duration is 30 minutes. Additional doses may be repeated if cardiac symptoms recur.

Redistribution of Potassium from the Extracellular to the Intracellular Fluid Compartment

- *Glucose (50 mL of 50% dextrose) and regular insulin (5 to 10 units)* can be given as IV boluses to promote redistribution of potassium from the extracellular to the intracellular fluid compartment, resulting in a decrease in serum potassium concentrations. As with IV calcium, this measure will not remove potassium from the body. Glucose and insulin therapy is indicated in patients with ECG changes and is often administered in conjunction with IV calcium. Redistribution of potassium into the intracellular fluid compartment may delay removal by other means.
- *Sodium bicarbonate 50 to 100 mEq IV* given over 2 to 5 minutes promotes redistribution of potassium into the intracellular fluid compartment. However, its effects are inconsistent and may be delayed for more than 60 minutes. Therefore, sodium bicarbonate is not recommended as a first-line agent for acute redistribution of potassium from the extracellular to the intracellular fluid compartment unless metabolic acidosis is present.
- *Albuterol via nebulized inhalation of 10 to 20 mg* stimulates Na^+/K^+-ATPase pump activity, resulting in redistribution of potassium into the intracellular compartment. As with the other therapies, albuterol does not remove potassium from the body.

Increased Elimination of Potassium from the Body

- *Sodium polystyrene sulfonate (Kayexalate, generic products)* is an ion-exchange resin that increases potassium excretion in the stool by exchanging sodium ions for potassium ions in the colon. Some formulations contain sorbitol, which decreases the incidence of constipation and impaction. Sodium polystyrene sulfonate/sorbitol can be administered orally or as a retention enema. Dosage of the rectal enema is 30 to 50 g and should be retained for 30 to 60 minutes for maximal efficacy. The usual oral dose is a single 15-g dose. A potassium concentration can be rechecked 2 to 4 hours after dosing, and if hyperkalemia persists, repeat dosages can be administered up to 4 times daily.

Optimal Plan

4. What pharmacotherapeutic recommendations are optimal for treatment of this patient's hyperkalemia?

- Since the patient missed his scheduled hemodialysis treatment, it is appropriate that hemodialysis be initiated at this time.
- Pharmacologic therapy that shifts potassium into the intracellular compartment will limit the availability of serum potassium for removal by hemodialysis and is not necessary in asymptomatic hyperkalemia.
- Although sodium polystyrene sulfonate could be administered to enhance potassium elimination, it is not necessary since the patient will be receiving hemodialysis shortly.
- Calcium administration is not warranted because the patient has mild hyperkalemia with no ECG changes.
- Discontinue Metamucil Effervescent Powder due to its high potassium content. Other formulations of psyllium are available with less potassium content. Each packet of Metamucil sugar-free powder contains 31 mg of potassium, one-tenth the content of the effervescent powder. The usual dose is one packet dissolved in 8 ounces of water 3 times a day. Other psyllium-containing products are available (e.g., Konsyl, Hydrocil Instant) that do not contain potassium.

Outcome Evaluation

5. What clinical and laboratory parameters are necessary to evaluate the therapy for achievement of the desired therapeutic outcomes and to detect or prevent adverse effects?

- Measurement of the serum potassium concentration 1 to 2 hours after hemodialysis (goal 3.5 to 5.0 mEq/L).

Patient Counseling

6. *What information should be provided to the patient regarding OTC medications that should be avoided to reduce the risk of hyperkalemia?*

- Check with your pharmacist or physician before starting any OTC medications. Some products that may contain significant quantities of potassium include salt substitutes, multivitamin with mineral supplements, laxatives, and antacids. Examples include, but are not limited to, the following:

Product	Potassium Content
Salt substitutes (Adolph's, Morton)	2165–2640 mg/teaspoonful
Multivitamin with mineral supplements	40–75 mg/dose
Psyllium effervescent formulations (Metamucil)	290–310 mg/dose
Psyllium powder formulations (Metamucil, Konsyl, Hydrocil)	0–31 mg/dose
Potassium bicarbonate (Alka-Seltzer Gold)	312 mg/dose

Problem 2: Hyperphosphatemia and Hypocalcemia

1. b. *What information (signs, symptoms, laboratory values) indicates the presence or severity of hyperphosphatemia and hypocalcemia?*

- Elevated serum phosphorus concentration of 7.4 mg/dL
- Low serum calcium concentration of 7.3 mg/dL

c. *Could any of the patient's medications be contributing to his hyperphosphatemia and hypocalcemia?*

- The patient is not taking any medications known to elevate serum phosphorus concentrations or lower calcium concentrations.

d. *What is the pathophysiology of the patient's hyperphosphatemia and hypocalcemia?*

- The kidney plays a predominant role in phosphorus excretion and activation of vitamin D. As renal function declines, phosphorus excretion decreases. As a consequence of elevated phosphorus concentrations, phosphorus complexes with calcium, resulting in a decrease in both serum phosphorus and calcium concentrations. However, with progressive renal insufficiency, complexation becomes inadequate and hyperphosphatemia and hypocalcemia are maintained.[3]
- In addition, hyperphosphatemia directly inhibits activation of vitamin D, further contributing to decreased renal production of vitamin D. Low concentrations of vitamin D result in decreased GI absorption of calcium with resulting hypocalcemia.
- Hypocalcemia stimulates the release of parathyroid hormone (PTH), which initially decreases phosphorus absorption and increases calcium absorption from the GI tract. However, with progressive renal insufficiency, this adaptive mechanism is no longer maintained, and PTH predominantly stimulates calcium mobilization from bone.

e. *What are the clinical consequences of hyperphosphatemia and hypocalcemia?*

- There are few immediate consequences of hyperphosphatemia. When phosphorus concentrations are markedly elevated (>11 mg/dL), patients may complain of itching. However, the lack of immediate symptoms in patients with ESRD is overshadowed by long-term consequences.
- When the calcium-phosphorus product (calcium concentration in mg/dL × phosphorus concentration in mg/dL) is greater than 70, there is an increased risk of metastatic calcifications in vessels and soft tissues of the body. In addition, chronic PTH secretion with resultant mobilization of calcium from bone leads to a condition known as osteitis fibrosa cystica. Furthermore, osteomalacia can occur due to aluminum accumulation or hypophosphatemia. Both conditions, collectively referred to as renal osteodystrophy, are characterized by symptoms of bone pain and development of skeletal fractures (refer to the section on Renal Osteodystrophy and Secondary Hyperparathyroidism in textbook Chapter 42 for more detailed information).

f. *What is the patient's corrected calcium concentration based on his albumin concentration?*

- Corrected calcium = Observed calcium + 0.8 (normal albumin − observed albumin)
  = 7.3 mg/dL + 0.8 (4.0 mg/dL − 3.2 mg/dL)
  = 7.9 mg/dL

Desired Outcome

2. *What are the goals of pharmacotherapy for treating this patient's hyperphosphatemia and hypocalcemia?*

- Restore serum phosphorus concentrations to near normal concentrations of 4 to 6 mg/dL (low phosphorus concentrations increase the risk of osteomalacia)
- Reverse hypocalcemia (restore corrected serum calcium concentration to the range of 8.5 to 10.5 mg/dL)

Therapeutic Alternatives

3. a. *What non-drug therapies are available for the treatment of hyperphosphatemia?*

- *Dietary phosphorus restriction* is an effective method to prevent development of hyperphosphatemia. The usual daily phosphorus intake in healthy patients is 1000 to 1800 mg.[3] Patients with renal disease who are dialysis-dependent should consume 800 to 1200 mg daily; more severe restrictions should be placed on patients who are not yet dialysis dependent. Foods high in phosphorus include milk, eggs, cheese, beans, meats, chocolate, and carbonated beverages. ESRD patients should receive counseling from a dietitian about their dietary intake of phosphorus.

- *Hemodialysis* removes 500 to 700 mg of phosphorus per session, whereas peritoneal dialysis removes approximately 300 mg daily. Therefore, dialysis alone is ineffective in maintaining normal phosphorus concentrations.

b. *What feasible pharmacotherapeutic alternatives are available for the treatment of hyperphosphatemia?*

- *Phosphate binders* are a class of compounds that bind dietary phosphorus in the GI tract, resulting in decreased phosphorus absorption and increased fecal elimination of the bound phosphorus. Calcium-containing phosphate binders are preferred over aluminum-containing phosphate binders. However, the calcium-phosphorus product should be considered when selecting a phosphate binder. When the product is <70, a calcium-containing product should be selected. When the product is >70, an aluminum-containing product should be initiated to prevent the risk of calcium-phosphorus deposition in tissues. Once the product has been reduced to <70 with an aluminum binder, then a calcium salt can be substituted. Aluminum binders should not be used for long-term therapy due to the risk of aluminum toxicity. However, in cases of hypercalcemia, aluminum binders may be necessary. Refer to the textbook for a phosphate binder titration algorithm.
    - ✓ *Calcium carbonate* (e.g., Tums, generic equivalents) and calcium acetate (e.g., Phoslo) are calcium-containing phosphate binders. Calcium acetate is a more effective phosphate binder compared to calcium carbonate.[4] Usual starting dosages of calcium carbonate range from 650 to 1250 mg po TID. Initial oral doses of calcium acetate range from 667 to 1334 mg po TID. All phosphate binders should be taken with meals to maximize binding of phosphorus in the GI tract. In addition, frequency of administration may need to be adjusted based on the patient's eating habits and meal frequency.
    - ✓ *Aluminum hydroxide* products (e.g., Alutabs, Alucaps, and Amphogel) are highly effective phosphate binders. Initial dosages range from 400 to 800 mg po TID with meals. Since aluminum intoxication is a consequence of long-term use (>1 year), their use should be reserved for cases where the calcium-phosphorus product is >70 or if patients exhibit hypercalcemia.
    - ✓ *Sucralfate* is an aluminum-containing product that has also been shown to lower serum phosphorus concentrations. However, because aluminum toxicity has been demonstrated with sucralfate therapy, long term use is not recommended.
    - ✓ *Magnesium salts* have rarely been used as phosphate binders because they frequently lead to diarrhea and hypermagnesemia. They have been used in conjunction with calcium-containing binders when hyperphosphatemia cannot be controlled on calcium products alone. Magnesium carbonate in combination with a low magnesium dialysate may lead to less GI upset and less hypermagnesemia than other magnesium salts.
    - ✓ *Sevelamer HCl (Renagel)* is a nonabsorbable, calcium- and aluminum-free product that has recently been approved as an alternative phosphate binding agent.

c. *What pharmacotherapeutic alternatives are available for the treatment of hypocalcemia?*

- *Calcium-containing phosphate binders* improve hypocalcemia by increasing calcium absorption and decreasing phosphorus concentrations. Although calcium acetate binds approximately twice the quantity of phosphorus than calcium carbonate, when dosages are adjusted by serum phosphorus concentration, the incidence of hypercalcemia is similar.
- *Oral calcitriol (Rocaltrol)* supplementation is recommended for patients with ESRD who demonstrate hypocalcemia despite treatment for hyperphosphatemia. The usual dose range is 0.25 to 0.5 μg/day.
- *IV calcitriol (Calcijex)* and the calcitrol analog *paricalcitol (Zemplar)* directly inhibit PTH secretion and are used in the treatment of secondary hyperparathyroidism. They may also increase calcium absorption.

Optimal Plan

4. *What drug recommendations are optimal for treatment of this patient's hyperphosphatemia and hypocalcemia?*

- This patient demonstrates hyperphosphatemia despite receiving a phosphate binder (calcium acetate 667 mg po TID). Because he is noncompliant with his HD sessions, it is possible that he is also noncompliant with his phosphate binder regimen. Before recommending a dosage increase, it is important to establish his adherence to his medication regimens. If noncompliant, he needs to be educated about hyperphosphatemia and the proper administration of phosphate binders.
- If it is determined that the patient is compliant with his phosphate binder, then further evaluation of the current regimen is necessary. The patient's calcium-phosphorus product is 59 when using the corrected calcium. Because the product is <70, continued treatment with a calcium salt is appropriate. He has been receiving calcium acetate in the past, and it would be reasonable to continue this salt because of its efficacy compared to calcium carbonate. The dosage should be increased to two tablets (1334 mg) po TID with meals. Alternatively, changing his phosphate binder to calcium carbonate is reasonable if medication costs are an issue.

Outcome Evaluation

5. *How should laboratory parameters be monitored to assess the effectiveness of the therapy for hyperphosphatemia and hypocalcemia?*

- Serum concentrations of phosphorus should be maintained in the range of 4 to 6 mg/dL. Since the patient is hospitalized, a repeat phosphorus level can be obtained in 2 to 3 days. Outpatient monitoring of serum phosphorus and calcium is usually done on a monthly basis.

Patient Counseling

6. *What information should be provided to the patient to help ensure successful therapy and prevent future complications?*

- Always take your phosphate binder with meals and snacks for maximal effectiveness.
- Hyperphosphatemia is an asymptomatic disease. Therefore, you need

to take your phosphate binder even if you don't have any symptoms or complaints related to high phosphate levels.
- Long-term problems that may occur if you don't take your phosphate binder include bone pain and bone fractures.
- In addition to your phosphate binder, you should comply with the phosphorus-restricted diet recommended by your dietician.
- Avoid over-the-counter medicines that contain significant quantities of phosphorus such as multivitamin with mineral supplements and laxatives (such as Phospho-soda liquid, Fleet enema). If you are unsure which medications contain phosphorus, check with your pharmacist or doctor.

Follow-up Questions

1. *What is an appropriate dosage of vancomycin for treatment of presumed MRSA bacteremia in this patient who receives dialysis with a cellulose acetate (low-flux) dialyzer?*

- Vancomycin is not significantly removed during HD with conventional, low-flux dialysis membranes. Because the elimination half-life is prolonged in ESRD, the usual dosage is 15 to 20 mg/kg IV every 5 to 7 days. Based on his weight, an appropriate dosage is vancomycin 1000 mg IV once per week. However, if the patient has residual renal function, it may be necessary to dose more frequently.

2. *What additional information would you need to assess this patient's anemia of chronic renal disease?*

- Iron studies (ferritin and transferrin saturation)
- Previous erythropoietin dosages
- Hematocrit measurements

The target hematocrit for patients with ESRD treated with erythropoietin is 33% to 36%. Although his hematocrit is low, there are several other factors to consider before increasing the dosage of erythropoietin. First, patients must have adequate iron stores in order to utilize erythropoietin. It is recommended that serum ferritin concentrations and percent transferrin saturation be maintained above 100 ng/mL and 20%, respectively. Therefore, it would be prudent to obtain iron studies to assess his iron status. Refer to textbook Chapter 42 for other causes of erythropoietin resistance.

References

1. Allon M. Hyperkalemia in end-stage renal disease: Mechanisms and management. J Am Soc Nephrol 1995;6:1134–1142.
2. Mandal AK. Hypokalemia and hyperkalemia. Med Clin North Am 1997;81:611–639.
3. Delmez JA, Slatopolsky E. Hyperphosphatemia: Its consequences and treatment in patients with chronic renal disease. Am J Kidney Dis 1992;19:303–317.
4. Ben Hamida F, el Esper I, Compagnon M, et al. Long-term (6 months) cross-over comparison of calcium acetate with calcium carbonate as phosphate binder. Nephron 1993;63:258–262.

44 HYPERCALCEMIA

▶ Crazy From the Calcium (Level I)

James S. Lewis II, PharmD
Daniel Sageser, PharmD

Weakness, fatigue, confusion, and vomiting cause the wife of an 80-year-old man with multiple myeloma to seek treatment for her husband. His serum calcium level in the ED is found to be 13.4 mg/dL. Treatment options for normalization of serum calcium in this patient include IV hydration, a loop diuretic (e.g., furosemide), subcutaneous calcitonin, a bisphosphonate (e.g., pamidronate), and perhaps glucocorticoids. Students should be able to recommend appropriate agents for acute calcium reduction and treatments that may be beneficial on a chronic basis. It is also important to understand the mechanism of action, onset time, and duration of action of each therapeutic alternative.

Questions

Problem Identification

1. a. *Create a drug-related problem list for this patient.*

- Multiple myeloma, presently untreated as per the patient's wishes; comfort measures only will be employed.
- Hypercalcemia with symptoms of nausea and vomiting, mental status changes, constipation, bradycardia, and ECG changes. The patient is in need of hydration and other drug therapy.
- Renal failure secondary to multiple myeloma; this is unlikely to improve without treatment for the underlying disease.
- Nausea and vomiting should resolve with correction of hypercalcemia but could also be due to narcotics.
- Mental status changes could be related to the narcotics or promethazine but are more likely to be due to acute onset of hypercalcemia.
- Constipation is possibly related to narcotic use but more likely due to hypercalcemia; it is presently inadequately treated with sorbitol but may resolve with hydration and resolution of hypercalcemia.
- Chronic stable drug-related problems include UTI treated adequately with cephalexin and seizures that are presently controlled with phenytoin levels in therapeutic range.

b. *What signs and symptoms in this patient are consistent with the diagnosis of hypercalcemia?*

- Fatigue, anorexia, bone pain, nausea, vomiting, confusion, lethargy, bradycardia, and ECG changes.

Desired Outcome

2. *What are the goals of pharmacotherapy for hypercalcemia in this case?*

- Normalization of calcium levels (corrected for serum albumin)
- Resolution of cardiac abnormalities
- Clearing of mental status
- Resolution of constipation, nausea, and vomiting

Therapeutic Alternatives

3. *What pharmacotherapeutic options are available for the treatment of this patient's hypercalcemia?*

- *Calcitonin* should be used immediately in this patient. The patient has a corrected calcium of >13 mg/dL and is having ECG changes, which warrants the use of an agent with rapid onset. Calcitonin begins to reduce serum calcium levels within one to two hours. Another benefit of calcitonin in this patient is that it is not nephrotoxic as are some other agents that rapidly decrease calcium (e.g., EDTA).[1] However, tachyphylaxis develops rapidly to calcitonin, and it is not to be used as maintenance medication for hypercalcemia.[2]
- *Hydration with normal saline* is advisable for this patient since he is dehydrated due to repeated bouts of emesis.[1,2] Dehydration results in increased renal calcium reabsorption, further worsening the hypercalcemia. IV infusions of sodium-containing fluids increase the kidney's ability to excrete calcium.
- *Loop diuretics* inhibit the kidney's ability to reabsorb calcium and will increase calcium excretion in the urine. The target for patients with normal kidney function is to achieve a urine output of 200 to 250 mL/hr. This rate may not be feasible in this patient due to his kidney dysfunction. Another key to the successful use of loop diuretics in this patient is to ensure that he is fully hydrated prior to the initiation of the diuretics. Otherwise his GFR may decrease, resulting in less calcium excretion.
- *Bisphosphonates (e.g., pamidronate, etidronate, alendronate)* provide long-term reductions in serum calcium levels.[1] However, they do not provide rapid reductions, and maximum effects are not seen for approximately 5 to 10 days after therapy is initiated.[1,2] Pamidronate is the bisphosphonate of choice since it can be administered as a single dose and has been shown to have a longer duration of action than etidronate.[1,2] Alendronate is not an appropriate choice at present since there is little data to support its use for malignancy-induced hypercalcemia.
- *Glucocorticoids* (e.g., prednisone 40 to 60 mg orally per day or its equivalent) are effective for hypercalcemia related to multiple myeloma and other oncologic conditions. They are not effective as acute therapy, and they will not be maximally effective for 5 to 7 days. A disadvantage to the use of glucocorticoids is immunosuppression which can be particularly disadvantageous in individuals already immunosuppressed due to chemotherapy.
- *Gallium nitrate* could be considered but is probably not a good choice for this patient because of his renal impairment and the nephrotoxicity associated with this agent.[2]
- *IV phosphates* are rarely used in patients with life-threatening hypercalcemia refractory to other treatment measures. Their use is limited because they can cause renal failure, hypotension, and in some cases death. IV phosphates would not be a good choice in this patient due to their nephrotoxic effects.

Optimal Plan

4. *What drug, dosage form, dose, schedule, and duration of therapy are best for reversing this patient's hypercalcemia?*

- Calcitonin and hydration are the two measures that should be undertaken immediately in this patient.
- Calcitonin 325 IU subcutaneously is given every 12 hours for 3 days.[2] Therapy is limited to 3 days because calcitonin has a short duration of action and patients will become refractory after several days of continued use; calcitonin is not suitable for maintenance therapy.[1,2]
- Hydration with normal saline (given cautiously due to renal impairment) should also be undertaken immediately since dehydration increases the kidney's tendency to conserve calcium.[2] In patients with normal kidney function, the usual rate is 200 to 250 mL/hr. In this patient with moderately impaired kidney function the rate should be decreased to 150 mL/hour until it can be determined how well the patient is tolerating the fluid load. Once the patient is completely rehydrated, consider adding potassium to the fluids to maintain normal serum potassium levels.
- Furosemide should be used cautiously due to the patient's mild sulfa allergy. The usual starting dose is 40 to 80 mg IV every 1 to 4 hours to achieve a urine output of 200 to 250 mL/hr. In this patient with chronic renal failure secondary to malignancy, larger doses may be required to achieve adequate diuresis. As stated previously, diuresis should not be initiated until the patient is completely rehydrated since diuresis prior to this point may result in further decline of GFR and increased retention of calcium.[1,2]
- Pamidronate 90 mg IV in one liter of NS × 1 dose should be administered as soon as possible but is chronic maintenance therapy that will not reach full effect for several days.[1]
- Glucocorticoids are an appropriate second-line therapy for this patient since they are considered especially good for hypercalcemia secondary to malignancy. As discussed above, there are several concerns about the use of glucocorticoids, and they are not useful as acute therapy.[1]
- Gallium Nitrate is not an appropriate therapy for this patient due to his chronic renal failure secondary to malignancy.

Outcome Evaluation

5. *What clinical and laboratory parameters are necessary to evaluate the therapy for achievement of the desired therapeutic outcome and to detect or prevent adverse events?*

- Clearing mental status
- Resolution of constipation, nausea, and vomiting
- Improved hydration status
- Decreased serum calcium levels (corrected for serum albumin)
- Decreased SCr and BUN levels to baseline. It is likely that these laboratory values will improve somewhat after the patient has been hydrated
- Resolution of ECG abnormalities and increase in heart rate
- Improved muscle strength
- Laboratory parameters such as calcium, SCr, BUN, potassium, magnesium, and sodium should be obtained 6 hours into the rehydration

process and then daily until calcium levels have been maintained within normal limits for 48 hours. Once the patient has been stabilized, these parameters should be examined every 2 weeks to determine the duration of effect of the long-acting pamidronate.

Patient Counseling

6. What information should be provided to the patient to enhance compliance, ensure successful therapy, and minimize adverse effects?

- Compliance should be a minimal issue since this patient will receive the pamidronate and hydration as an inpatient. Home nursing services will need to be arranged to administer the calcitonin.
- The patient should be made aware that without treatment of the underlying malignancy, hypercalcemia will continue to be a problem, and he and his spouse should be made aware of the symptoms.

References

1. Mundy GR, Guise TA. Hypercalcemia of malignancy. Am J Med 1997;103: 134–145.
2. Chisholm MA, Mulloy AL, Taylor AT. Acute management of cancer-related hypercalcemia. Ann Pharmacother 1996;30:507–513.

45 METABOLIC ACIDOSIS

▶ Of Proximal Tubules, Normal Anion Gaps, and RTA   (Level II)

Melanie S. Joy, PharmD

A 27-year-old woman is referred to the nephrology clinic because of fatigue, dyspnea, somnolence, and muscle weakness. Arterial blood gases and other information indicate the presence of a normal anion gap metabolic acidosis, hypokalemia, hypocalcemia, and hypophosphatemia. Students are asked to consider the possible etiologies of this situation. The available information suggests that the patient has a chronic type II renal tubular acidosis. Correction of the acidosis will require bicarbonate replacement, either as sodium bicarbonate or as sodium or potassium citrate and citric acid. Appropriate potassium, calcium, and phosphate replacement therapies must also be instituted. Because this is a chronic metabolic acidosis, regular follow-up is necessary to ensure continued control of the acidosis and normalization of serum electrolyte concentrations. Patient education on the need for compliance with her therapy is critical to treating the acidosis and preventing further complications.

▶ Questions

Problem Identification

1. a. Identify the type of acidosis (metabolic versus respiratory) this patient exhibits, calculate the anion gap, and identify the potential causes.

Identify the Type of Acidosis

- The ABGs provide information regarding the type of acidosis present in this patient. A metabolic acidosis is present when there is a primary decrease in the concentration of bicarbonate. The normal compensatory change is a decrease in pco_2 of 1.2 mm Hg for every 1 mEq/L fall in bicarbonate.
- In the presence of respiratory acidosis, there would be a primary increase in the pco_2 concentration. The expected compensatory change is an increase in bicarbonate of 1 mEq/L or 3.5 mEq/L for acute or chronic conditions, respectively, for every 10 mm Hg rise in pco_2.
- Based on the arterial pco_2 and plasma bicarbonate levels, this patient is classified as exhibiting a metabolic acidosis. Textbook Chapter 49 reviews the differentiation between metabolic and respiratory (acute and chronic) acidosis and the normal compensatory mechanisms.

Calculate the Anion Gap

- Anion Gap = Na − (Cl + HCO_3) = 143 mEq/L − (119 mEq/L + 12 mEq/L) = 12

Identify the Potential Causes of Acidosis

- The presence of a normal anion gap rules out the possibility of ingestions (e.g., salicylates, methanol, ethylene glycol). Other causes include lactic acidosis, ketoacidosis, and renal failure. The presence of these extra anions increases the value calculated in the anion gap equation.
- The differential diagnosis in determining the reason for the normal anion gap metabolic acidosis includes diarrhea, renal tubular acidosis, renal dysfunction, and hyperalimentation fluids. Since this patient does not report diarrhea or exhibit renal insufficiency and is not receiving hyperalimentation fluids, the most probable cause is a renal tubular acidosis.

b. What medical conditions present in this patient are either untreated or inadequately treated?

- Metabolic acidosis
- Renal tubular acidosis
- Borderline vitamin D deficiency and clinically significant bone disease

c. What information obtained from the patient's symptoms, physical examination, and laboratory analysis indicates the presence of a chronic metabolic acidosis with a renal tubular acidosis component or one of its complications?

- *Symptoms:* Muscle weakness, hip and shoulder pain, somnolence and lethargy.
- *Physical Exam Findings:* Diminished deep tendon reflexes
- *Laboratory Values:* Systemic pH 7.27; reduced serum bicarbonate,

potassium, calcium, and phosphorus; urine pH 5.0; 1,25-dihydroxyvitamin D_3 deficiency; normal anion gap acidosis; fractional excretion of bicarbonate >3%

d. *What are the different types of renal tubular acidosis (RTA), and how do they differ with respect to etiology, mechanisms, and clinical/laboratory findings?*

- *Type II (proximal) RTA.* A reduction in proximal bicarbonate reabsorption is the defect in type 2 RTA. This is due to an increase in the reabsorptive threshold of bicarbonate. The plasma bicarbonate is usually maintained at 26 to 28 mEq/L by reabsorbing approximately 90% of the filtered bicarbonate in the proximal tubule and additional bicarbonate throughout the remaining parts of the nephron. Patients with this disorder generally are able to maintain a plasma bicarbonate concentration of around 12 to 14 mEq/L. Once the filtered load of bicarbonate falls to a level equal to the decreased resorptive capacity, all of the filtered bicarbonate is reabsorbed. In addition to bicarbonate reabsorption, many patients also exhibit Fanconi's syndrome, whereby the reabsorption of phosphate, glucose, amino acids, and urate are also diminished. The mechanisms for this defect include: (1) a defect in the Na^+-H^+ exchanger in the luminal membrane; (2) a defect in the Na^+-K^+-ATPase pump in the basolateral membrane; and (3) a deficiency in the generation of bicarbonate by carbonic anhydrase. Common causes include carbonic anhydrase inhibitors, cystinosis, hypocalcemia, vitamin D deficiency, renal transplant rejection, heavy metal poisonings, consumption of outdated tetracyclines, and multiple myeloma. An increased urinary potassium loss with resultant hypokalemia is also common due to mildly contracted extracellular fluid volume changes resultant to secondary hyperaldosteronism. The phosphate wasting and proximal tubule deficiencies (causing reduced formation of active vitamin D) often lead to osteomalacia in adults and rickets in children.[1,2] Stones are not common in this disorder due to the fact that the urine may be acidified by the distant distal nephron.[3,4]
- *Type I (distal) RTA.* A reduction in the net hydrogen ion secretion in the collecting tubules, causing increased urinary pH (>5.3) is present in this disorder. The reduction in excretion of the dietary acid load leads to hydrogen ion retention. The mechanisms for this defect include (1) a defect in the H^+-ATPase pump; (2) reduction in sodium reabsorption and subsequent decrease in negative charge in the lumen leading to a voltage-dependent defect (e.g., urinary tract obstruction or sickle cell disease); and (3) an increase in membrane permeability allowing the back-diffusion of hydrogen ions (e.g., amphotericin B use). Common causes include urinary tract obstruction, volume depletion, sickle cell disease, autoimmune diseases, renal transplantation, lithium, hyperkalemia, and decreased glomerular filtration rate. Serum potassium levels are usually either reduced or normal but may be increased with the voltage dependent form. In light of the increased urine pH, nephrocalcinosis due to calcium and phosphate deposition can be a complication.[3,4]
- *Type IV RTA.* This type results from either aldosterone deficiency or resistance. Hyperkalemia is a complication of this disease. Plasma bicarbonate levels remain above 15 mEq/L.[3,4]
- Diagnosis of the particular type of RTA can be made on the basis of laboratory analysis, clinical suspicion, and additional testing. Type I and II can be differentiated by administering a sodium bicarbonate infusion (0.5 to 1.0 mEq/kg/hr). The urine pH and fractional excretion of bicarbonate will increase in type 2 RTA since the threshold for reabsorption is exceeded. The urine anion gap (UAG = Na + K − Cl) can also be used as an indicator of ammonium (acid) excretion, whereby a negative UAG indicates appropriate ammonium excretion and a positive UAG represents decreased ammonium excretion (e.g., distal RTA). The UAG may better differentiate between diarrhea and distal RTA in cases where a history cannot be elicited. Fractional bicarbonate excretion can be calculated from the plasma and urine bicarbonate and serum creatinine: [FE = (urine HCO_3 × SCr)/(plasma HCO_3 + urine Cr)].[3,4]

e. *Which type of RTA is most likely present in this patient?*

- A type II RTA is suspected because this patient demonstrates a low urine pH (<5.3), hypophosphatemia, hypokalemia, increased fractional excretion of bicarbonate, decreased vitamin D levels, hypocalcemia, decreased serum bicarbonate, and bone disease.

Desired Outcome

2. *What are the pharmacotherapy goals for this patient?*

- Minimize the degree of acidosis to help ameliorate the symptoms of dyspnea
- Prevent worsening of metabolic bone disease and correct vitamin D deficiency
- Correct potassium, calcium, and phosphate to normal or near-normal levels

Therapeutic Alternatives

3. *What treatment alternatives are available to achieve the desired therapeutic outcomes?*

- *Correction of acidosis.* An alkali (bicarbonate) dose of 10 to 15 mEq/kg per day is usually required in type II RTA to compensate for the amount of bicarbonate excreted in the urine. Bicarbonate can be administered as sodium bicarbonate or as sodium and/or potassium citrate and citric acid, which are metabolized to bicarbonate in the liver. Some available products include:
  - ✓ *Sodium bicarbonate 650-mg oral tablets.* Provides about 7.75 mEq bicarbonate per tablet
  - ✓ *Bicitra oral solution* (500 mg sodium citrate and 334 mg citric acid per 5 mL). Provides 1 mEq bicarbonate per 1 mL of solution
  - ✓ *Polycitra oral solution* (550 mg potassium citrate, 500 mg sodium citrate, and 334 mg citric acid per 5 mL). Provides 2 mEq bicarbonate per 1 mL of solution
  - ✓ *Polycitra-K oral solution* (1100 mg potassium citrate and 334 mg citric acid per 5 mL). Provides 2 mEq bicarbonate per 1 mL of solution
  - ✓ *Oracit oral solution* (490 mg sodium citrate and 640 mg citric acid per 5 mL). Provides 1 mEq bicarbonate per 1 mL of solution

Due to concurrent hypokalemia, an agent containing potassium citrate may be a good option. Bicitra or Polycitra should be better tolerated than bicarbonate since they must be converted to bicarbonate in the liver, thereby eliminating the direct deposition of bicarbonate into the stomach with the production of gastric distention and flatulence. Second-line agents include sodium bicarbonate and sodium citrate. The addition of a thiazide diuretic can increase the proximal reabsorption of sodium and bicarbonate secondary to mild volume depletion.

- *Electrolyte replacement*
  ✓ *Potassium replacement* could be administered orally as potassium citrate (i.e., correcting the acidosis and the potassium depletion). Potassium chloride may be an option in this patient in addition to the potassium citrate if potassium levels are not adequately corrected, especially since weakness and hyporeflexia are present. Since the patient does not exhibit a hyperchloremic metabolic acidosis, this agent is not contraindicated.
  ✓ *Calcium replacement* should be considered due to the presence of somnolence, lethargy, and bone disease. Calcium carbonate supplies more elemental calcium (40%) than the other calcium salts. Thiazide diuretics may decrease calcium elimination in the urine.
  ✓ *Phosphorus replacement* can be administered orally as potassium phosphate. Since this patient exhibits moderate hypophosphatemia and is able to take enteral products, IV therapy may not be indicated. Due to GI intolerance to large oral phosphate doses, administration of more than 1 to 2 packets or capsules twice daily (>1000 mg phosphorus daily) should be avoided. However, the presence of neuromuscular symptoms (e.g., weakness, hyporeflexia), lethargy, and joint arthralgias may indicate the need for a loading dose (oral or IV) and then subsequent maintenance therapy. Oral phosphate products containing potassium phosphate include Neutra-Phos and Neutra-Phos-K.
- *Vitamin D replacement* to correct the deficiency may be accomplished with various forms of oral vitamin D. In the presence of renal insufficiency or proximal tubular dysfunction, the 1,25-dihydroxyvitamin D_3 levels may be decreased, since the kidneys may not be able to 1-hydroxylate the 25-hydroxyvitamin D_3 formed in the liver. Calcitriol (Rocaltrol) may therefore be the preferred agent in this setting. In patients without severely diminished renal function, ergocalciferol (Drisdol) may be appropriate.

Optimal Plan

4. Design a pharmacotherapeutic plan for the management of metabolic acidosis and its complications in this patient.

- *Acidosis.* Since this patient exhibits a proximal RTA, an alkali dose of 10 to 15 mEq/kg daily will be required to overcome the losses in the urine. With a starting dose of 10 mEq/kg/day (750 mEq), approximately 63 g of sodium bicarbonate would be required. Since oral sodium bicarbonate is only available as 650-mg tablets, 97 tablets would be required daily to correct the acidosis. Likewise, large amounts of Bicitra (750 mL daily) would be required to correct the acidosis. Smaller daily amounts of Polycitra and Polycitra-K (375 mL) would be required. Since most patients will not tolerate GI side effects well with this load of solute, the dose of Polycitra should be pushed only as high as tolerated by the patient. If hyperkalemia becomes problematic, some of the bicarbonate replenishment could be administered as Bicitra. Hydrochlorothiazide 25 to 50 mg/day should be added to help with the proximal reabsorption of bicarbonate secondary to sodium by the creation of a mild diuresis.
- *Potassium.* Since this patient exhibits a chronic hypokalemia (serum potassium 3.2 mEq/L), the total body deficit would represent approximately 200 to 300 mEq. In situations of acute hypokalemia, a decrease of 1 mEq would represent a total body deficit of only approximately 100 mEq potassium. The Polycitra-K (2 mEq potassium per mL) or Polycitra (1 mEq potassium per mL) would require approximately 100 mL or 200 mL daily, respectively, to replete potassium stores. Alternatively, if the patient is unable to take these large doses of Polycitra or Polycitra-K, potassium chloride tablets (20 mEq) could be administered to replete the potassium deficit. Amiloride may be reasonable to add by titrating the dose from 10 mg to a maximum of 40 mg daily.
- *Calcium.* The patient should receive calcium carbonate (500 mg elemental calcium) for a total dose of 1.0 to 1.5 g daily. This will ensure adequate intake and may overcome some of the losses of calcium in the urine. The administration of hydrochlorothiazide 25 to 50 mg will also help to increase serum calcium. The partial correction of the acidosis should also facilitate the correction of the hypocalcemia.
- *Phosphorus.* An IV loading dose of 0.16 mmole/kg phosphorus (24 mmoles) would be reasonable due to the serum concentration and patient symptoms. This infusion should be administered over 4 to 6 hours. The patient should then be prescribed an oral phosphate replacement product due to the chronic nature of her disease. Two Neutra-Phos packets or tablets twice daily (250 mg phosphorus and 7.1 mEq potassium) would provide the necessary phosphorus maintenance dose of 1000 mg daily. The potassium would help to replace the chronic potassium losses. In addition, dietary counseling regarding the intake of dairy products for the maintenance of phosphorus and calcium levels should be addressed.
- *Vitamin D.* The 1,25-dihydroxyvitamin D_3 product (calcitriol, Rocaltrol) would be an excellent choice for vitamin D replacement. The presence of Fanconi's syndrome in this patient may indicate the inability of the proximal tubule to activate (1-hydroxylate) the 25-hydroxyvitamin D_3 (hence the low-normal measured levels) necessitating calcitriol therapy. The drug should be instituted at a dose of 0.25 μg daily.

Outcome Evaluation

5. Outline a clinical and laboratory monitoring plan to assess the patient's response to the pharmacotherapeutic regimen you recommended.

- The patient is to return to clinic in 2 weeks. At that point, potassium, phosphorus, calcium and bicarbonate will be rechecked. Serum phosphorus should also be checked at the end of the infusion given in the ED.
- Follow-up laboratory analysis at quarterly intervals should be sufficient to monitor the chronic disease and prevent excessive replacement of electrolytes.
- Urinalysis should be performed at periodic clinic visits to measure excretion of calcium in order to guide in the adjustment of the thiazide.
- The patient should undergo a physical examination at the clinic visits, noting the neurologic findings consistent with electrolyte, calcium, magnesium, and phosphorus depletion.

- Since this patient has been diagnosed with a chronic metabolic acidosis, routine blood gases are not recommended unless acute decompensation occurs.
- Questioning about adverse effects of drug therapy and disease state signs and symptoms should occur at each clinic visit. The resultant appropriate modification in therapy will enhance patient compliance and treatment efficacy. Particular emphasis should be placed on GI side effects (diarrhea, constipation, nausea, and vomiting). In addition, patient questioning for the symptoms of acidosis or electrolyte imbalances (lethargy, muscle weakness, bone pain, and so forth) should be performed at each visit.

Patient Counseling

6. *How should the patient be counseled about the drug therapy to treat chronic metabolic acidosis and renal tubular acidosis?*

- *Potassium Citrate Solution (Polycitra)* will be used to increase the potassium and bicarbonate (base) concentrations in your blood. Side effects may include diarrhea, stomach upset, and symptoms of elevated potassium levels (e.g., palpitations, weakness, and confusion). The solution should be diluted with a glass of water and taken after meals and at bedtime. It may be stored at room temperature or refrigerated.
- *Potassium chloride* will also increase serum potassium levels. Side effects may include diarrhea, stomach upset, and symptoms of elevated potassium levels. Wax matrix tablets or capsules should not be crushed or chewed. Effervescent tablets must be dissolved in water before use, whereas liquids can be diluted or dissolved in water or juice. Take with food to minimize gastrointestinal discomfort. Contact your doctor if you experience irregular heartbeats or confusion.
- *Calcium (Oscal)* is needed to make the bones strong and to prevent them from breaking. Since you are at high risk of bone disease due to chronic acidosis and low calcium levels, you should take 1500 mg of calcium daily. This can be accomplished in part by taking one Oscal 1250 mg tablet (500 mg elemental calcium) three times daily. Side effects may include constipation and stomach upset. Calcium should not be taken directly with meals since absorption will be decreased.
- *Calcitriol (vitamin D, Rocaltrol)* will also help to prevent your bones from breaking. Since you have a disorder in one part of your kidney needed to make vitamin D, you may be at risk for a deficiency in this vitamin. Side effects of vitamin D include elevations in calcium levels causing symptoms of palpitations, weakness, nausea, vomiting, confusion, decreased reflexes, and abdominal pain. Your calcium levels will be monitored closely by your doctor.
- *Potassium phosphate* is used to increase potassium and phosphorus levels. Low levels may cause weakness and blood cell destruction. Side effects include diarrhea, nausea, and stomach pain. Capsules, tablets, or packets should be emptied into 6 to 8 ounces of water, stirred, and swallowed.

References

1. Eiam-ong S, Kurtzman NA. Metabolic acidosis and bone disease. Miner Electrolyte Metab 1994;20:72–80.
2. Oh MS. Irrelevance of bone buffering to acid-base homeostasis in chronic metabolic acidosis. Nephron 1991;59:7–10.
3. Smulders YM, Frissen PH, Slaats EH, et al. Renal tubular acidosis. Pathophysiology and diagnosis. Arch Intern Med 1996;156:1629–1636.
4. Metabolic Acidosis. In: Rose BD, ed. Clinical Physiology of Acid–Base and Electrolyte Disorders, 3rd ed. New York, McGraw-Hill, 1994:540–603.

46 METABOLIC ALKALOSIS

▶ **The ABCs of Acid–Base Chemistry (Level I)**

Jennifer Stoffel, PharmD, BCPS

Shortness of breath and generalized pain cause a 72-year-old man to seek treatment in the ED. He had been discharged from another hospital the day before after being treated for CHF. The patient's other medical problems include s/p liver transplantation (on immunosuppressive therapy), chronic renal insufficiency, and insulin-dependent diabetes mellitus. Abnormal findings during his evaluation include a RLL infiltrate on chest x-ray, electrolyte abnormalities, metabolic alkalosis (probably secondary to overly aggressive diuretic therapy) and respiratory acidosis (possibly related to respiratory tract infection). The initial focus of the case is on identifying and understanding the findings related to the metabolic alkalosis. Treatment measures include discontinuation of the diuretic and administration of normal saline. In some situations, acetazolamide and acidifying agents (e.g., ammonium chloride, arginine) may be used. Students are asked to calculate fluid requirements for the patient and outline a plan for monitoring the success of therapy. In addition to treating metabolic alkalosis, other modifications in the patient's drug regimen are also necessary.

▶ **Questions**

Problem Identification

1. a. *Create a list of this patient's drug-related problems.*

- Possible hospital acquired pneumonia requiring empiric antibiotics.
- Dehydration possibly resulting from diuretic therapy.
- Metabolic alkalosis possibly secondary to diuretic therapy.
- Respiratory acidosis possibly related to respiratory tract infection.
- Renal insufficiency possibly resulting from tacrolimus therapy and/or dehydration.
- Mild hyperkalemia which may be related to captopril and tacrolimus therapy.
- Hyperglycemia (uncontrolled diabetes) requiring modification of insulin therapy.
- Hypermagnesemia likely related to deteriorating renal function and continued supplementation.
- Chronic, stable drug-related problems at the present time include

(1) CHF currently managed with captopril and diuretic therapy; (2) s/p orthotopic liver transplantation requiring immunosuppression without evidence of rejection; (3) increased risk for infection due to immunosuppressive therapy; patient is currently receiving dapsone for *Pneumocystis carinii* prophylaxis.

b. *Describe the clinical findings that are consistent with metabolic alkalosis and those that are not consistent with this acid–base disorder.*

Consistent Findings

- Signs and symptoms of dehydration (decreased skin turgor, dry tongue and mucous membranes, decreased urine output, BUN to serum creatinine ratio >20)
- Administration of furosemide
- Elevated serum bicarbonate
- Decreased serum chloride

Inconsistent Findings

- Normal arterial pH
- Elevated potassium: This patient has renal insufficiency and an impaired ability to eliminate potassium, which helps to explain the absence of hypokalemia that would normally be observed. The elevated potassium may also be secondary to an adverse effect of the ACE inhibitor captopril.
- Urine Chloride >10 mEq/L
- Normal serum sodium
- Hyperventilation

c. *Explain how diuretics such as furosemide can result in a metabolic alkalosis.*

- Furosemide inhibits sodium, chloride, and potassium reabsorption in the ascending loop of Henle, increasing urinary levels of these electrolytes. This results in an increased osmolality in the renal tubule, decreasing water reabsorption by the kidney. When given in excessive amounts, this may cause dehydration, decreased serum chloride, and hypokalemia. In patients not receiving diuretics, dehydration results in a urine chloride level <10 mEq/L.
- Volume depletion causes the release of aldosterone. Aldosterone promotes the retention of sodium in exchange for hydrogen and potassium in the distal renal tubule. The resultant loss of hydrogen and potassium ions contributes to the increased serum pH and hypokalemia that are typically demonstrated in metabolic alkalosis.
- The increased secretion of hydrogen ions into the renal tubule generates bicarbonate. In the presence of hypochloremia, the bicarbonate is reabsorbed with sodium in the distal tubule, thus elevating the concentration in the serum.
- The compensatory response of the body to metabolic alkalosis is hypoventilation and a resultant increase in CO_2 (decreased pH). The predicted increase in pco_2 is 6 to 7 mm Hg for each 10 mEq/L increase in serum bicarbonate.
- In this patient the serum bicarbonate is elevated 10 mEq/L from the normal mean of 25 mEq/L, yet the pco_2 is elevated to 55 mm Hg. The larger than expected increase in pco_2 and the normal pH are likely the result of a coexisting respiratory acidosis despite an increased respiratory rate. The pneumonia the patient has developed is the probable cause of the hyperventilation and poor CO_2 elimination.

Desired Outcome

2. *What are the desired therapeutic outcomes for this patient?*

Metabolic Alkalosis

- Rehydration (eliminate signs and symptoms of dehydration)
- Prevention of symptoms of CHF
- Correction of serum bicarbonate to 21 to 30 mEq/L
- Correction of serum chloride to 95 to 110 mEq/L

Pneumonia

- Elimination of the infecting organism
- Alleviation of the symptoms of pneumonia
- Reversal of CXR findings

Renal Insufficiency

- Decreased serum creatinine and BUN
- Correction of serum potassium to 3.5 to 5.0 mEq/L
- Correction of serum magnesium to 1.4 to 1.8 mEq/L

Diabetes Mellitus

- Correction of serum glucose to 70 to 110 mg/dL

Therapeutic Alternatives

3. *What pharmacologic and non-pharmacologic alternatives should be considered for the treatment of metabolic alkalosis in this patient?*

- The first step in determining a pharmacologic plan is to determine the cause of the metabolic alkalosis and to predict if the alkalosis will be responsive to NaCl. The most likely cause of the alkalosis in this patient is volume depletion secondary to aggressive use of furosemide (see answer to question 1c); this agent should be discontinued.
- *IV fluid resuscitation with sodium chloride* (preferably normal saline) is first-line therapy in sodium chloride responsive cases (urine chloride <10 mEq/L).[1] Normal saline restores proper fluid balance, and administration of chloride improves elimination of bicarbonate by the kidney. Lactated Ringer's solution contains less chloride than normal saline, and the lactate in the solution can produce bicarbonate, which may worsen an existing alkalosis. Fluid therapy should be used cautiously in patients who may have difficulty with excess volume (such as this patient with CHF and renal insufficiency).
- *Potassium supplementation* is needed in most cases because metabolic alkalosis due to diuretic therapy causes potassium depletion. However, this patient has an elevated potassium secondary to drug therapy and renal insufficiency, so supplemental potassium is not indicated.
- *Acetazolamide*, a carbonic anhydrase inhibitor, is an alternative to saline resuscitation in patients who are unable to tolerate increased fluid volume. It should not be used if the patient is experiencing hypokalemia. Often, a one-time IV dose of 250 to 500 mg will result in a return of serum bicarbonate to normal levels.[2]
- *Acidifying agents (e.g., ammonium chloride, arginine, hydro-

chloric acid) may be considered in patients with severe metabolic acidosis (pH greater than 7.55) as well as those intolerant or unresponsive to replacement with volume and sodium chloride.

- ✓ *Ammonium chloride* reverses alkalosis by releasing HCl during its conversion to urea by the liver. Patients with hepatic dysfunction should not receive ammonium chloride, as ammonia may accumulate due to the inability to synthesize urea. High ammonia levels can result in CNS toxicity including confusion, seizures and coma. Ammonium chloride should also be avoided in patients with renal function to avoid worsening of uremia.
- ✓ *Arginine monohydrochloride* also results in the production of hydrogen ion during metabolism to urea by the liver. Arginine also binds to circulating ammonia to produce urea. Arginine may be used in patients with hepatic insufficiency but should be avoided in patients with renal dysfunction to avoid worsening of uremia. Neither ammonium nor arginine is appropriate in this patient because of renal insufficiency.
- ✓ *Hydrochloric acid* can cause serious adverse effects and should be reserved for severe cases in which other acidifying agents are ineffective or contraindicated.[3] Adverse effects of HCl include metabolic acidosis and severe tissue damage with extravasation.

Optimal Plan

4. a. *What drug, dosage form, dose, schedule, and duration of therapy are best for this patient?*

- Diuretic therapy should be suspended until the dehydration and metabolic alkalosis have been resolved.
- Since the patient is hospitalized, intubated, and does not currently have enteral access, IV fluids are a rational first-line therapy. The baseline fluid requirements for an adult with normal organ function are 1500 mL/m^2/day.[4] The patient's body surface area (BSA) estimated by nomogram[5] is 2.28 m^2; thus the baseline fluid requirement is 3.4 L/day (140 mL/hr). Fluid resuscitation should be completed gradually and cautiously to avoid fluid overload in a patient with CHF and renal dysfunction.
- Isotonic saline (0.9%) initiated as a 500-mL bolus over one hour and then as a maintenance infusion of 100 mL/hour is a conservative start. The patient will also receive additional saline as diluent for parenteral antibiotics.
- If normal saline is ineffective in decreasing the serum bicarbonate, a single 500-mg IV dose of acetazolamide may be administered.

b. *What other modifications to the patient's current drug regimen are warranted? Include your rationale.*

- Discontinue magnesium oxide to avoid further accumulation and toxicity that may occur with reduced renal elimination.
- Withhold the scheduled insulin dosing until a feeding regimen is initiated. Regular insulin administered PRN according to a sliding scale based on routine blood glucose measurements will control hyperglycemia resulting from the infectious process and exogenous corticosteroid administration.
- Consider discontinuation of captopril, which may be contributing to hyperkalemia. Consider alternative management for CHF, such as digoxin, angiotensin II receptor antagonists, nitrates, and hydralazine.

Outcome Evaluation

5. a. *What clinical and laboratory parameters are necessary to evaluate the therapy for achievement of the desired outcome and prevention of adverse effects?*

Efficacy

- Measure fluid intake and urine output every 2 hours for 24 hours, then once every shift.
- Assess the patient once each nursing shift (every 8 hours) for physical signs and symptoms of dehydration. Over the next 24 hours there should be clinical improvement in the patient's urine output, skin turgor, and moistness of tongue and mucous membranes.
- Obtain serum electrolytes (sodium, potassium, chloride, bicarbonate), BUN, and serum creatinine every 12 hours for the first 24 hours and then reassess.
- Obtain vital signs every 4 hours.
- Repeat blood gases every 6 hours for 24 hours, then reassess. This is needed because the patient is intubated and has a respiratory infection, not necessarily because of metabolic alkalosis.

Toxicity

- Obtain a chest x-ray in the following morning to monitor for pulmonary edema from excess fluid administration.
- Assess the patient for signs and symptoms of fluid overload (shortness of breath, rales on chest auscultation, peripheral edema).
- Question the patient about possible adverse effects of acetazolamide (e.g., GI distress and fatigue).

b. *What is your assessment of the patient's response to the therapy initiated for treatment of metabolic alkalosis?*

- The infusion of normal saline has resulted in a positive impact on the clinical signs of dehydration (decreased skin turgor, dry tongue and mucous membranes, decreased urine output) and has helped return serum chloride and potassium values to normal.
- There has also been a significant improvement in serum bicarbonate, but the measured concentration and the patient's pH are at the upper limit of the normal range. Further hydration with normal saline should help to improve these values. If hydration is continued at the current rate (4.2 L/day) and urine output does not increase, the patient is likely to develop symptoms of fluid overload (peripheral edema, pulmonary edema, shortness of breath). An empiric decrease in the saline infusion to 75 mL/hr would decrease the daily intake to 3.1 L if other intake remains constant. At this adjusted rate the patient should have a positive fluid balance over the next 24 hours. This intervention should correct the fluid deficit and metabolic alkalosis. As outlined in the answer to question 5a, the patient should be monitored closely for fluid overload.

Patient Counseling

6. *What information should be provided to the patient regarding the isosorbide dinitrate and hydralazine started for the treatment of CHF?*

General Information

- The captopril that you were receiving for heart failure caused the potassium levels in your body to increase. Elevated potassium can cause serious effects including irregular heart rhythms. For this reason, we are stopping the captopril and starting two new agents, isosorbide dinitrate and hydralazine.
- It is important tell your doctor if you develop any symptoms of heart failure as your new medication doses are being adjusted. Inform your doctor if you develop shortness of breath, weight gain, or decreased ability to walk or exercise.
- Store these and all other medications in the original container in a cool dry place out of the reach of children.

Isosorbide Dinitrate

- The dose of isosorbide dinitrate your doctor prescribed is 20 mg three times a day. This drug works best if there are 12 hours between the evening dose and the morning dose. This can be accomplished by taking a dose at the same time in the morning and in the evening with the third dose in the middle of the day.
- The tablet should be taken on an empty stomach with a full glass of water. If you forget to take a dose, take it as soon as you remember. If it is almost time for your next dose, skip that dose and continue with your normal regimen.
- Side effects of this medication include headache, flushing of the face, a fast heart rate, and an upset stomach. This medication may also cause dizziness or lightheadedness, especially when rising from a sitting or lying position. It may be helpful to sit for a moment and dangle your feet when moving from a lying to a standing position.

Hydralazine

- The prescribed dose of hydralazine is 25 mg, which should be taken four times a day. The interval between the doses should be similar but also convenient so you don't forget to take each dose. If you forget to take a dose, take it as soon as you remember. If it is almost time for your next dose, skip that dose and continue with your normal regimen.
- Side effects that may occur with hydralazine include constipation or diarrhea, rapid heart rate, drowsiness, lightheadedness or dizziness, headache, and numbness/tingling in the hands or feet. If these symptoms or others become severe or problematic, please consult your physician.

References

1. Martin WJ, Matzke GR. Treating severe metabolic alkalosis. Clin Pharm 1982;1:42–48.
2. Marik PE, Kusman BD, Lipman J, et al. Acetazolamide in the treatment of metabolic alkalosis in critically ill patients. Heart Lung 1991;20(5 Pt 1):455–459.
3. Brimioulle S, Berre J, Dufaye P, et al. Hydrochloric acid infusion for treatment of metabolic alkalosis associated with respiratory acidosis. Crit Care Med 1989;17:232–236.
4. Cochran EB, Kamper CA, Phelps SJ, et al. Parenteral nutrition in the critically ill patient. Clin Pharm 1989;8:783–799.
5. Anderson PO, Knoben JE. Handbook of Clinical Drug Data, 8th ed. Stamford, CT, Appleton & Lange, 1997:908.

47 BENIGN PROSTATIC HYPERPLASIA

▶ Get Me to the Bathroom on Time (Level II)

Catherine A. Heyneman, PharmD, MS
Richard S. Rhodes, PharmD

Complaints of the recent onset of urinary hesitancy, nocturia, and dribbling cause a 79-year-old man with multiple medical problems to seek treatment. Urologic evaluation leads to the diagnosis of benign prostatic hyperplasia (BPH) with urge incontinence. The patient is taking several medications with anticholinergic activity that may exacerbate BPH symptoms. Consideration should be given to changing these medications. Pharmacotherapeutic alternatives include α_1-adrenergic antagonists (e.g., doxazosin, terazosin, tamsulosin) or finasteride. Surgical procedures may also be performed under certain circumstances. Patients treated for BPH should be questioned about subjective improvement in symptoms about every 3 months.

▶ Questions

Problem Identification

1. a. Create a list of the patient's drug-related problems.

- Anticholinergic side effects of both amitriptyline and trazodone may be exacerbating the patient's BPH symptoms.
- The patient is experiencing symptoms of BPH which could be minimized by pharmacotherapy. Even though this patient's prostate is described as small on ultrasound, it is important for students to recognize that subjective symptoms of BPH do not always correlate well with objective signs.
- Ibuprofen may be causing a GI bleed, and therefore the guaiac-positive stool.
- Amitriptyline and trazodone therapies are not achieving adequate control of his depression.
- Amitriptyline is noted in chart as therapy for headaches. Cimetidine may cause/exacerbate headaches.

b. Describe the natural history and epidemiologic characteristics of BPH.

- BPH is a very common problem in elderly men. Histologic evidence of BPH is apparent in approximately 50% of men 60 years of age and is essentially universal by the ninth decade of life.
- BPH is caused by nonmalignant enlargement (hyperplasia) of

the prostate gland that surrounds the urethra, resulting in bladder outflow obstruction.[1] Approximately 40% of men with histologic evidence of prostatic hyperplasia report lower urinary tract symptoms that may be obstructive or irritative in nature.
- Obstructive symptoms include hesitancy, weak stream, intermittent flow, post-micturition dribble, and incomplete emptying.
- Irritative symptoms include increased frequency of voiding, urgency, nocturia, and urge incontinence.
- Most sequelae of BPH are believed to result from hypertrophy of the bladder detrusor muscle. Analogous to cardiac hypertrophy seen in CHF, detrusor hypertrophy compensates for bladder obstruction by providing an enhanced contractility and thus increased force of contraction to void urine. Hypertrophic detrusor fibers may manifest clinically as symptoms of bladder irritability such as increased frequency, urgency, nocturia, and incontinence.
- Progressive BPH may result in detrusor muscle decompensation, manifesting as hypotonicity, incomplete emptying, and ultimately urinary retention. Complications of urinary retention include recurrent UTIs, uremia, and bladder stones.

c. *Which of this patient's complaints are consistent with obstructive symptoms of BPH? Which are consistent with irritative symptoms?*

The patient complains of urgency with occasional incontinence, nocturia, and terminal dribbling. Urgency, urge incontinence, and nocturia are irritative symptoms, whereas dribbling is an obstructive symptom. The patient also has a history of recurrent UTIs, which is consistent with urinary retention secondary to decompensated BPH.

d. *What steps are recommended in the initial evaluation of all patients presenting with BPH?*

- Detailed GU history. Specifically, the patient should be questioned about (1) both obstructive and irritative symptoms of BPH and which symptoms he finds the most severe; (2) history of UTIs, bladder stones, and hematuria; and (3) any neurological condition which might account for a neuropathic bladder dysfunction.[2]
- Digital rectal exam to rule out prostate or rectal cancer
- Urinalysis to rule out UTI and hematuria
- Serum creatinine because approximately 10% of patients presenting with symptomatic prostatism have renal insufficiency
- PSA (prostate-specific antigen), post-void residuals, and uroflowmetry are optional tests.

e. *What other medical conditions should be ruled out before treating this patient for BPH?*

- A differential diagnosis must rule out those conditions that could mimic the irritative symptoms of BPH: bladder cancer, UTI, neuropathic bladder dysfunction, bladder stones, and urethral stricture unrelated to an enlarged prostate.

f. *Could any of this patient's problems have been exacerbated by drug therapy?*

- Any drug class with prominent anticholinergic side effects (e.g., antihistamines, neuroleptics, tricyclic and heterocyclic antidepressants) has the potential to exacerbate the symptoms of BPH. He is currently taking amitriptyline and trazodone for depression.
- Additionally, cimetidine has the potential to cause/exacerbate headaches.

g. *Are any of this patient's problems amenable to pharmacotherapy?*

- The patient's BPH symptoms and depression are adversely affecting his quality of life. Drug treatment is indicated for patients with moderate or severe symptoms of BPH. Amitriptyline and trazodone have been unsuccessful in lifting his depression and could potentially worsen his BPH symptoms.
- The guaiac-positive stool and normocytic anemia may be the result of an NSAID-mediated upper gastrointestinal bleed. Discontinuation of ibuprofen therapy for osteoarthritis is indicated.

Desired Outcome

2. *What are the goals of pharmacotherapy in this case?*

- Symptoms of BPH that interrupt sleep, create anxiety, and/or cause embarrassment can reduce a patient's quality of life significantly. However, there is considerable variation in the degree to which BPH symptoms bother patients. Thus, the pharmacotherapeutic goals are:
    - ✓ Reduction of the most bothersome BPH symptoms (nocturia, urge incontinence)
    - ✓ Prevention of BPH complications such as urinary retention that could result in even more frequent UTIs
    - ✓ Alleviation of depression
    - ✓ Prevention of further NSAID-induced GI bleeds and resolution of secondary anemia while maintaining adequate analgesia for OA

Therapeutic Alternatives

3. *What are the treatment alternatives for BPH?*

- *Watchful waiting.* This may be particularly valuable in a case such as this where drug therapy may be exacerbating the patient's symptoms of BPH. Discontinuation of anticholinergic medications, if possible, may result in dramatic symptom improvement without further intervention.
- *Alpha-1 antagonists (doxazosin, prazosin, and terazosin)* block α-adrenergic-mediated contraction of prostatic smooth muscle around the urethra. Approximately 60% to 70% of patients treated with an α_1-antagonist experience improvement in BPH symptoms within 1 to 3 months. Because the primary indication for these drugs is the treatment of hypertension (terazosin and doxazosin carry an additional indication for BPH), these agents are often useful for hypertensive patients with BPH. The primary limitation of these agents is orthostatic hypotension.
- *Tamsulosin* is a newer adrenergic blocker with high affinity for the α_{1A} receptor (an adrenoceptor subtype located mainly in the prostate), which results in limited antihypertensive effects and relative selectivity for the genitourinary tract.[3]
- *Finasteride*, a 5-α reductase inhibitor, lowers prostatic dihydrotestosterone levels and can decrease the overall size of the prostate gland.[4] Finasteride has been shown to significantly reduce BPH symptoms, improve urinary flow rates, and reduce the need for prostate surgery and risk of urinary retention by 55% and 57%, respectively.[5] The improvement in symptom scores over placebo, while statistically significant, averaged two points out of a total of 35 points. Thus, the clinical benefits seen with finasteride are modest. Increased prostate size is believed

to be an important determinant of efficacy. Side effects are minimal (reduced sex drive, reduced volume of ejaculate) but it can take 3 to 6 months before patients notice an improvement in symptoms.[6]

- *Surgical interventions,* including transurethral resection of the prostate (TURP), transurethral incision of the prostate (TUIP), balloon dilatation, laser prostatectomy, and open prostatectomy procedures are generally reserved for those patients with refractory urinary retention, recurrent UTIs, recurrent gross hematuria, bladder stones, or renal insufficiency secondary to BPH.[7] These surgical procedures are associated with an 85% improvement in symptoms. While the probability of morbidity directly related to BPH surgery is low, the mean probability of becoming impotent ranges from 12% to 32%, depending on the type of prostatectomy performed.

Optimal Plan

4. What drug, dosage form, dose, schedule, and duration of therapy are best for this patient?

- Because we have identified two drugs in the patient's medication list with anticholinergic activity, watchful waiting after discontinuation of the offending drugs seems to be a rational first step. Replacement of the tricyclic/heterocyclic antidepressants with an SSRI such as sertraline 50 mg po QD, which has minimal anticholinergic activity, may reduce anticholinergic side effects (dry mouth, constipation, tachycardia, confusion, urinary retention).
- If the BPH symptoms are still bothersome after discontinuation of the trazodone and amitriptyline, then drug therapy is recommended. If the patient were hypertensive, a good choice would be terazosin 1 mg po Q HS, gradually titrated up to 10 mg po Q HS, because it is indicated for both hypertension and BPH. Doxazosin (1 mg po QD increasing gradually to a maximum of 8 mg po QD) could also be used in this situation.
- Since he does not have hypertension, perhaps a better choice would be tamsulosin 0.4 mg po QD. It may be preferred over finasteride (5 mg po QD) because finasteride is generally most effective when the prostate is large. This patient's prostate was described as "small." Also, clinical improvement is generally seen more rapidly with α_1-blockers than with finasteride. Tamsulosin is also less expensive than finasteride.
- The patient is taking Capoten (captopril) to prevent diabetic nephropathy; this should not be discontinued and replaced with a traditional α_1-blocker. Addition of a traditional α_1-blocker to the ACE inhibitor would increase the risk of orthostatic hypotension in this patient.
- Prostatectomy remains an option, especially given this patient's history of chronic UTIs.
- Replacement of the NSAID ibuprofen with acetaminophen 500 to 1000 mg po Q 6 H (maximum 4 grams daily) for OA pain is necessary, given the guaiac-positive stool and secondary anemia.

Outcome Evaluation

5. What clinical and laboratory parameters are necessary to evaluate the therapy for achievement of the desired therapeutic outcome and to detect or prevent adverse effects?

- Monitor for subjective improvement in urinary urgency, urge incontinence, increased flow rates and nocturia every 3 months.
- Monitor for subjective/objective improvement in depression, utilizing patient reports, clinical depression scores (such as the Ham-D), and nurses' notes regarding the patient's mood every 3 months.
- Watch for gradual (2 to 4 weeks) resolution of the anemia by monitoring hemoglobin, hematocrit, and RBC for a return to normal values.
- Monitor for improvement/resolution of the UGI bleed by asking the patient for subjective assessment of stomach pain and weekly stool guaiac testing until negative.
- Monitor for improvement in subjective symptoms of OA (pain, limitation of movement).
- Monitor for an increase in headache frequency or intensity. Should this occur, a calcium channel blocker such as verapamil can be considered for HA prophylaxis.

Patient Counseling

6. What information should be provided to the patient to enhance compliance, ensure successful therapy, and minimize adverse effects?

General information

- The medications you have been taking for headache prevention and depression (the amitriptyline and trazodone) may be worsening your urinary symptoms. We would like to discontinue these medications and see if this improves your urinary problems.
- In the meantime, we can prescribe a new antidepressant that may work better for you. It won't interfere with urination and may alleviate your depression as well as the previous drug.
- If your urinary incontinence and getting up at night repeatedly to go to the bathroom don't get better in a week or so, we will consider starting tamsulosin, a new drug specifically designed to treat this problem.
- Please let us know if your headaches become worse. There are other drugs besides amitriptyline that are effective in preventing headaches that won't worsen your urinary symptoms.
- Your guaiac-positive stool and laboratory results suggest that you have blood leaking into your intestinal tract. This is a relatively common side effect of ibuprofen, which you are currently taking for your arthritis. We would like to try switching you to acetaminophen, which will allow the bleeding to stop and your body to begin rebuilding its blood supply.

Tamsulosin

- Tamsulosin is taken once daily by mouth. It is possible for this drug to cause ejaculation problems, dizziness, or headache. Approximately 60% to 70% of patients experience symptom improvement when treated with drugs in this class.

References

1. Lee M, Sharifi R. Benign prostatic hyperplasia: Diagnosis and treatment guideline. Ann Pharmacother 1997;31:481–486.
2. McConnell JD, Barry MJ, Bruskewitz RC, et al. Benign prostatic hyperplasia: Diagnosis and treatment. Clinical Practice Guideline, number 8. AHCPR publication no. 94-0582. Rockville, MD, Agency for Health Care Policy and Research, Public Health Service, U.S. Department of Health and Human Services, February 1994.

3. Wilde MI, McTavish D. Tamsulosin: A review of its pharmacological properties and therapeutic potential in the management of symptomatic benign prostatic hyperplasia. Drugs 1996;52(6):883–898.
4. Lepor H, Williford WO, Barry MJ, et al. The efficacy of terazosin, finasteride, or both in benign prostatic hyperplasia. N Engl J Med 1996;335:533–539.
5. McConnell JD, Bruskewitz R, Walsh P, et al. The effect of finasteride on the risk of acute urinary retention and the need for surgical treatment among men with benign prostatic hyperplasia. N Engl J Med 1998;338:557–563.
6. Wasson JH. Finasteride to prevent morbidity from benign prostatic hyperplasia. N Engl J Med 1998;338:612–613.
7. Tammela T. Benign prostatic hyperplasia. Practical treatment guidelines. Drugs Aging 1997;10:349–366.

48 NEUROGENIC BLADDER AND URINARY INCONTINENCE

▶ **Bladder Matters** (Level III)

Mary Lee, PharmD, BCPS, FCCP

A 74-year-old man develops urinary urgency and frequency six weeks after experiencing a stroke. He has a history of essential hypertension and is taking hydrochlorothiazide and terazosin. Diagnostic tests indicate the presence of urge incontinence due to the stroke and possibly aggravated by his drug therapy. Several non-pharmacologic therapies may be instituted to reduce incontinent episodes. First-line drug treatments include anticholinergic agents (e.g., propantheline bromide) and detrusor muscle relaxants (e.g., oxybutynin). There are also several new drugs approved or about to be approved to treat this common condition. Students will be required to locate and use reference sources other than the textbook to answer the questions in this case.

▶ **Questions**

Problem Identification

1. a. Create a list of the patient's drug-related problems.

- Urge incontinence (also known as detrusor hyperreflexia or detrusor instability) secondary to CVA, but exacerbated by hydrochlorothiazide and terazosin. Hydrochlorothiazide enhances urinary sodium and water excretion, which can increase the volume of urine that must be voided. Since the patient is taking this medication in the evening, it is likely that this is contributing to his nighttime incontinence. Terazosin, an α_1-adrenergic receptor blocking agent, produces relaxation of the internal urethral sphincter and bladder neck, thereby enhancing urinary outflow and leakage.
- Essential hypertension treated with hydrochlorothiazide and terazosin; his blood pressure does not appear to be optimally controlled (but only a single reading is available).
- CVA, 6 weeks ago. The patient is taking low dose aspirin for secondary prevention of recurrent CVA.

b. What information (signs, symptoms, medical history, laboratory values, other test results) indicates the presence or severity of urge incontinence?

- Symptoms of urge incontinence include urinary urgency, frequency, and nocturia. Patients complain of an inability to reach the bathroom on time and soiling of clothing multiple times during the day and night. Patients may resort to wearing diapers and smell of urine.
- This patient has no signs or physical findings of urge incontinence, which is common. In severe cases, patients may develop skin maceration secondary to constant perineal soiling.
- Medical history: He had a CVA 6 weeks ago.
- Laboratory values: Normal BUN and serum creatinine, which suggests that there is no long-term adverse effect of urge incontinence on renal function.
- Urinary flow rate was 16 mL/second (normal, >10 mL/second). This implies that the patient has normal, unobstructed bladder emptying.
- CMG revealed uninhibited bladder contractions at bladder pressures of 40 to 60 cm Hg, which suggests that prior to complete bladder filling, the detrusor muscle is contracting involuntarily. This is the cause of urge incontinence.
- This patient's urge incontinence is interfering with his usual lifestyle. Because he soils himself regularly and smells of urine, he has had to discontinue his usual volunteer activities, use diapers, and has poor quality sleep because of the need to urinate multiple times during the night.

c. Differentiate urge incontinence from stress incontinence, overflow incontinence, and functional incontinence.

- Unlike urge incontinence, stress incontinence refers to urinary leakage which occurs when intra-abdominal pressure is increased in the face of an incompetent internal and/or external urethral sphincter at the bladder neck.[1,2] Thus, activities associated with increased intra-abdominal pressure (e.g., coughing, sneezing, bending over, carrying heavy packages, jogging) produce a similar increase in bladder pressure, which overcomes the weakened bladder neck closure pressure.
- Stress incontinence occurs more commonly in patients with weakened urethral sphincters secondary to childbearing or in

obese patients. It also occurs in postmenopausal women as a result of estrogen deficiency, which is associated with decreased muscular tone of the external sphincter. Stress incontinence also occurs in patients who have had injury or removal of the urethral sphincter following prostatectomy.

- The drug of choice for stress incontinence is an α-adrenergic agonist, which enhances the tone of the internal urethral sphincter. In postmenopausal women, oral and vaginal estrogen replacement have been effective.
- Overflow incontinence results when an anatomic block of the bladder neck obstructs urinary outflow or when the detrusor muscle fails to generate an adequate force of contraction for bladder emptying. As a result, the bladder fails to empty urine completely. Over time, as the bladder outlet obstruction worsens or the detrusor continues to fail, the bladder becomes overdistended. Patients leak urine only when the capacity of the bladder to store urine supercedes the closure pressure at the bladder neck. Urinary dribbling and low urinary stream characterize overflow incontinence.
- The drug of choice for overflow incontinence due to an anatomic block of the bladder neck is an α_1- adrenergic antagonist, which relaxes the bladder neck sphincter, thereby enhancing bladder emptying. The drug of choice for overflow incontinence due to impaired detrusor contractility is bethanechol, a cholinergic agonist that directly stimulates muscle contraction. However, if the patient has severe overflow incontinence, surgical intervention may be necessary.
- Functional incontinence results when a patient is unable to reach the toilet in time to urinate despite the presence of an intact central micturition inhibitory center, good bladder filling and emptying function, and fully functional external and internal urethral sphincters. These patients experience barriers to getting to the toilet. Examples include patients with severe physical incapacitation, severe rheumatoid arthritis, or patients who are restrained in their beds. If given opportunity and access to bathroom facilities, these patients can be fully continent.

d. *In addition to the medications the patient is currently taking, what other drugs could exacerbate urge incontinence?*

- Other drugs known to exacerbate urge incontinence include sedatives and hypnotics. These inhibit the micturition-inhibitory center in the brain, thereby eliminating the usual physiologic suppression of involuntary detrusor muscle contractions in response to small volumes of urine in the bladder. Phenothiazines with dopaminergic receptor blocking activity (e.g., chlorpromazine, fluphenazine, thioridazine), may also cause relaxation of the internal sphincter and exacerbate urge incontinence.

Desired Outcome

2. *What are the goals of pharmacotherapy in this case?*

- Urinary incontinence is a social and a health problem. The goal of pharmacotherapy is to reduce or eliminate the symptoms of urge incontinence (e.g., stop urinary frequency, urgency, and leakage and soiling of clothing) so that the quality of the patient's life can be improved.
- This goal of pharmacotherapy should be achieved with the lowest frequency of adverse effects.

Therapeutic Alternatives

3. a. *What non-drug therapies might be useful for this patient?*

- Non-drug therapies are generally used as sole management of urge incontinence in patients with mild disease or those who cannot tolerate drug therapy.
- With moderate or severe urge incontinence, non-drug therapies are generally combined with more specific drug therapy. For example, timed (prompted) voiding along with oxybutynin has been shown to enhance the responsiveness of some patients to timed voiding procedures.[3]
- Non-drug treatments for urge incontinence include:
    ✓ *Diapers,* which are easy to use and readily available. However, they may not be acceptable to the patient and are expensive when used on a long-term basis. They also do not reduce or eliminate symptoms of urinary leakage.
    ✓ *Timed (prompted) voidings* require the patient to go to the bathroom every 2 to 4 hours around the clock to empty urine from the bladder (even if the bladder is not full).[3] This reduces the amount of urine in the bladder, so less is available to leak from the bladder. This is easy to do during the daytime; at night timed voidings can be reduced to every 4 hours. Nevertheless, this may be inconvenient and bothersome for some patients.
    ✓ *Avoiding fluid intake after 6:00 P.M. and until awakening in the morning* may be helpful. The patient voids before going to bed. Like timed voidings, this reduces the amount of urine in the bladder overnight, so less is available to leak from the bladder.

b. *What feasible pharmacotherapeutic alternatives are available for treatment of urge incontinence?*

- Changing hydrochlorothiazide administration to every morning, instead of every evening, will be beneficial.
- Discontinuing terazosin and switching the patient to an alternative antihypertensive agent with minimal effect on the internal urethral sphincter and bladder neck may be considered. Examples might include an ACE inhibitor (e.g., captopril or enalapril) or an angiotensin II antagonist (e.g., losartan).
- An anticholinergic agent may be added to reduce or eliminate involuntary detrusor muscle contraction. This will increase bladder filling capacity, thereby minimizing or eliminating the symptoms of urgency and frequency. Examples include:
    ✓ *Propantheline bromide (Pro-Banthine)* 15 to 30 mg po Q 6 to 8 H
    ✓ *Hyoscyamine (Cystospaz, Levsin)* 0.125 to 0.25 mg po TID to QID
    ✓ *Glycopyrrolate (Robinul)* 1 to 2 mg po BID to TID
    ✓ *Tolterodine tartrate (Detrol)* 1 to 2 mg po BID

Tolterodine tartrate is a newer high-potency drug that appears to have greater selectivity for inhibiting urinary bladder muscarinic receptors than other peripheral (e.g., salivary gland) receptors. Thus, it may produce a lower incidence of peripheral anticholinergic adverse effects. However, direct comparisons of tolterodine with other anticholinergic agents have not been published.[4] Tolterodine is also more expensive than generic oxybutynin.

- Adding a detrusor muscle relaxant will reduce involuntary muscle contraction. These agents may also have anticholinergic activity.[1] Examples include:
  - ✓ *Oxybutynin (Ditropan)* 5 to 10 mg po BID or 5 mg po QID
  - ✓ *Dicyclomine (Bentyl)* 10 to 40 mg po TID to QID
  - ✓ *Flavoxate (Urispas)* 100 to 200 mg po TID to QID
- *Imipramine* is a tricyclic antidepressant that blocks norepinephrine reuptake, thereby increasing the amount of norepinephrine available in the synapse to stimulate contraction and increase the muscle tone of the internal sphincter. In addition, it has anticholinergic effects that block involuntary detrusor muscle contractions. These dual effects have proven useful in the management of urge incontinence. Low doses of 10 to 25 mg orally three times a day are effective in relieving symptoms of urinary urgency and frequency. Imipramine is not considered first-line therapy for urge incontinence because its pharmacological effects are not specific for, or limited to, urge incontinence. In addition, in larger daily doses imipramine causes sedation, orthostatic hypotension, and anticholinergic adverse effects.

Optimal Plan

4. What drug, dosage form, dose, schedule, and duration of therapy are best for this patient?

- Propantheline bromide is available generically as oral tablets, which is the least expensive of the agents listed above. It can be started at 15 to 30 mg orally every 6 to 8 hours, to a maximum of 120 mg per day. A peak response is expected within a few days of starting the medication. It should be continued as long as the patient's symptoms of urge incontinence respond.
- If propantheline fails or if the patient cannot tolerate the adverse anticholinergic effects of this drug, switching to hyoscyamine or glycopyrrolate would not be a good choice. These agents have been shown to have comparable effectiveness and similar adverse effects. The only clinical benefit of glycopyrrolate or hyoscyamine over propantheline is that they have a longer duration of action and can be dosed two or three times daily. Preliminary noncomparative clinical trial data suggest that tolterodine may produce less dry mouth than propantheline bromide. However, tolterodine has been reported to cause other typical anticholinergic adverse effects. Therefore, it is unclear whether tolterodine is a safer alternative than propantheline.
- A muscle relaxant (e.g., oxybutynin) would be a better alternative in the situation of inadequate response or intolerance to propantheline bromide. Oxybutynin has a direct relaxant or antispasmodic effect on the detrusor muscle, as well as having a mild anticholinergic effect. Therefore, it has a dual mechanism of action in suppressing involuntary detrusor contractions. In addition, oxybutynin has a longer duration of action and can be dosed twice daily. The usual dosage of oxybutynin is 5 mg orally twice a day, to a maximum of 20 mg per day. A peak response is expected within a few days of starting the medication. It should be continued as long as the patient's symptoms of urge incontinence respond.[3]
- Imipramine could be used for the reasons described above if a muscle relaxant such as oxybutynin also fails.

Outcome Evaluation

5. What clinical and laboratory parameters are necessary to evaluate the therapy for achievement of the desired therapeutic outcome and to detect or prevent adverse effects?

Efficacy Parameters for Propantheline Bromide

- Elimination of symptoms including soiling of clothes, nighttime awakenings due to urinary leakage, and odor of urine
- Fewer diapers used each day
- Results of a repeat CMG, which should show reduction or elimination of involuntary detrusor contractions with incomplete bladder filling. However, in usual practice, reduction of a patient's clinical symptoms is considered an adequate measure of clinical response. A repeat CMG is typically done only if the patient fails to respond to a full course of therapeutic doses of medications.

Adverse Effect Parameters for Propantheline Bromide

- Review of systems at each visit to check for dry mouth, heart palpitations, sedation, and constipation.
- If the patient complains of heart palpitations, vital signs should be taken.
- If the heart rate or blood pressure is abnormal or the patient complains of dizziness, an ECG should be done to check for abnormalities.
- If the patient has dry mouth that does not respond to simple palliative maneuvers such as increased water intake or sucking on hard candy, or if the patient has constipation that does not respond to increased fluid (at least 1.5 liters per day) and dietary fiber intake (at least three servings of fiber-rich food daily), or if the patient experiences excessive sedation on usual doses, options include:
  - ✓ Reduce the daily dose of propantheline
  - ✓ Discontinue propantheline and switch to an agent with fewer anticholinergic adverse effects (e.g., oxybutynin)
- If the patient complains of sedation, giving a larger portion of the daily dose at bedtime or taking smaller divided doses throughout the day may be helpful.

Patient Counseling

6. What information should be provided to the patient to enhance compliance, ensure successful therapy, and minimize adverse effects?

Propantheline Bromide

- You are being treated with propantheline bromide, which will prevent muscle spasms of your bladder that are causing your urinary leakage.
- Take one tablet (15 or 30 mg) by mouth four times a day, 30 to 45 minutes before breakfast, lunch, dinner, and at bedtime.
- Each tablet should be swallowed whole and taken on an empty stomach, if possible.
- You should begin to see an improvement in your symptoms within a few days. Continue this regimen as long as you continue to respond to it.
- Do not exceed the prescribed dose. This can lead to side effects such as confusion or excessive drowsiness.
- This medication will decrease sweating, which is one way that your body controls heat. Therefore, be careful not to get overheated in the summer when the weather is hot.
- This medication may cause blurred vision. Be careful when driving until you know how much this affects you.
- Other possible side effects of this medication include rapid heart rate, dry mouth, constipation, and drowsiness. If you feel excessive dizziness or palpitations, contact your doctor as soon as possible.

- Store these tablets in a cool, dry place.
  If you forget to take a dose, take it as soon as you remember. However, if it is close to the time of your next scheduled dose, skip the missed dose. Do not take double doses.

▶ Follow-up Questions

1. *Why has the patient developed new and different voiding symptoms?*

Note to instructors: You may wish to tell students that this patient initially received propantheline 15 mg po every 6 hours. Because of the adverse effects experienced, the patient was changed to oxybutynin 10 mg po twice daily, which he responded to and tolerated well.

- The patient has developed an enlarged prostate, which is now blocking urinary outflow from the bladder neck. The enlarged prostate is likely due to benign prostatic hyperplasia (BPH), which is a noncancerous growth of the prostate that normally occurs as patients age. An enlarged prostate could also be due to prostate cancer. However, based on the rectal exam that revealed no nodules in the prostate and the normal PSA level, it appears that this patient has BPH. The enlarged prostate, which is significantly different from the patient's initial visit to the physician 1.5 years ago, has now produced several complications:
  ✓ Decreased peak urinary flow rate of 7 mL/second
  ✓ Symptoms of slow urinary stream and difficult bladder emptying
  ✓ Relapsing urinary tract infections secondary to prolonged retention of urine in the bladder
  ✓ A large post-void residual bladder volume, which is determined by measuring the volume of urine obtained from the bladder by catheterizing the patient after the patient states that he has just emptied it. A large residual bladder volume predisposes the patient to recurrent urinary tract infections.
  ✓ Loss of detrusor muscle contractility as seen on cystoscopy. This results from decompensation of a hypertrophied detrusor muscle that has exceeded its capacity to contract.
- His difficulty in bladder emptying may be exacerbated by oxybutynin, which blocks detrusor muscle contraction. Therefore, the detrusor muscle is unable to generate sufficient bladder pressure to empty urine from the bladder past the obstructed bladder neck. This is why anticholinergic agents and detrusor muscle relaxants should be used with great caution in elderly men with enlarged prostates.

2. *How should this patient's voiding problem now be managed?*

- The signs and symptoms suggest that the patient has severe obstruction of urinary outflow, exacerbated by oxybutynin. Oxybutynin should be discontinued.

- If the patient's voiding problems persist, the patient could be treated with a 6 or 8-week course of an α_1-adrenergic antagonist (e.g., terazosin, prazosin), which would relax the intrinsic urethral sphincter. If voiding symptoms persist, drug therapy should be stopped.
- The best management for persistent, refractory symptoms would be prostatectomy (surgical removal of the prostate). This can be performed transurethrally by inserting a resectoscope into the urethra or by excising the prostate via an external incision. The latter procedure is known as an open prostatectomy. Both procedures are associated with significant morbidity including impotence, urinary tract infection, stress urinary incontinence, and bleeding.

References

1. Wein AJ. Pharmacologic treatment of incontinence. J Am Geriatr Soc 1990;38:317–325.
2. Resnick NM. Geriatric incontinence. Urol Clin North Am 1996;23:55–74.
3. Ouslander JG, Schnelle JF, Uman G, et al. Does oxybutynin add to the effectiveness of prompted voiding for urinary incontinence among nursing home residents? A placebo-controlled trial. J Am Geriatr Soc 1995;43:610–617.
4. Jonas U, Hofner K, Madersbacher H, et al. Efficacy and safety of two doses of tolterodine versus placebo in patients with detrusor overactivity and symptoms of frequency, urge incontinence, and urgency: Urodynamic evaluation. World J Urol 1997;15:144–151.

49 ERECTILE DYSFUNCTION

▶ A Sensitive Issue   (Level III)

Cara Lawless-Liday, PharmD
Rex W. Force, PharmD, BCPS

A 39-year-old man with diabetes, hypertension, and other medical problems presents to his physician complaining of partial erections that are not sufficient for sexual intercourse. Before treatment is initiated, it is important to perform a complete history to identify and eliminate possible causes of the problem. Nonpharmacologic approaches to the treatment of erectile dysfunction (ED) include psychotherapy, vacuum constriction devices, penile prostheses, and vascular bypass surgery. Pharmacologic alternatives include the alprostadil transurethral suppository; intracavernosal injections of alprostadil, phentolamine, papaverine, or combinations of the three agents; oral yohimbine, transdermal or IM testosterone; and oral sildenafil. The therapy chosen should be one that not only produces successful intercourse but that is also well accepted by the patient, reasonably priced, convenient to use, and associated with a low incidence of adverse effects.

▶ Questions

Problem Identification

1. a. *Create a list of the patient's drug-related problems.*

- ED of unknown etiology without treatment at this time.
- Type 2 DM inadequately controlled (HbA_{1c} 11.8%) on maximum doses of metformin and a small dose of glyburide.
- Diarrhea with no known cause or treatment at this time.
- The patient's weight is substantially above his ideal body weight;

this becomes a drug-related problem if it affects drug therapy or if drug therapy is used as a means of weight reduction.
- Chronic stable problems not requiring intervention at this time include (1) HTN, well controlled on maximum dose of benazepril, low-dose HCTZ, and doxazosin; (2) GERD, apparently well controlled on omeprazole; and (3) COPD, apparently well controlled with PRN use of albuterol.

b. *What risk factors for ED are present in this patient?*

- One of the strongest of the risk factors is DM; men with DM are three times as likely to develop ED as men without the disease.
- Other common risk factors include HTN, smoking, alcohol abuse, hypercholesterolemia, increasing age, anxiety or depression, CAD, hormonal abnormalities, medications, and local trauma or surgery.[1]

c. *What are the etiologies of ED, and what is this patient's most likely etiology?*

- Etiologies of ED include vasculogenic, neurogenic, endocrinologic, psychogenic, drug-induced, or a combination of these.[2] Determining the cause is important for treating the disorder effectively.
- Organic causes of ED are often compounded with psychogenic causes when patient and partner become frustrated and embarrassed.
- The etiology of this patient's ED is most likely a combination of neurogenic and vasculogenic causes due to DM, HTN, and/or antihypertensive medications.

d. *Could any of the patient's problems have been caused by drug therapy?*

- Many antihypertensive medications, including thiazide diuretics, have been implicated in causing sexual dysfunction.
- Although HCTZ may cause a zinc deficiency that could possibly potentiate sexual dysfunction,[3] it is still unclear whether ED is related to the medication or to HTN itself.
- In addition, a single case report implicates omeprazole as a possible cause of sexual disorders among users.[4]

Desired Outcome

2. *What are the goals of therapy in this case?*

- The overall goals are successful intercourse, patient and partner understanding of available treatment options, and satisfaction with the results.
- An additional goal is identifying an individualized treatment modality for this patient that is effective, convenient to use, reasonably priced, and associated with a low incidence of side effects.

Therapeutic Alternatives

3. a. *What non-pharmacologic alternatives are available for the treatment of ED?*

- *Eliminating identifiable causes of ED* should be attempted. Potential measures include smoking cessation, reducing alcohol intake, and discontinuing medications known to cause ED. Obtaining good control of concomitant diabetes, hypertension, and hyperlipidemia is also important.

- *Psychotherapy* may be useful, as there is often a psychologic component to ED. This may include education about the normal sexual response and possible causes of ED, improvement in communication and understanding between sexual partners, and reduction in anxiety and depression in an attempt to improve sexual function.
- *Vacuum constriction devices (VCDs)* are effective for all etiologies of ED. An erection is induced by creating a vacuum around the penis; the negative pressure draws blood into the penis by passively dilating arteries and engorging the corpus cavernosa. The erection is maintained with a constriction band. VCDs have a success rate of >80% for achieving an erection sufficient for intercourse, making them one of the most effective modalities available. Although a VCD has the advantage of a one-time investment, its disadvantages may limit its use. Many patients complain of coldness and lifelessness of the penis, painful ejaculation, lack of spontaneity, and the time involved with its use. VCDs are contraindicated in patients with sickle cell disease, coagulation defects, and those receiving anticoagulant therapy.
- *Penile prostheses* are generally considered when other measures have failed. A semi-rigid or inflatable prosthesis is surgically implanted in the penis to simulate an erection. Although success rates are over 90% and the patient satisfaction rate is fairly high, they are expensive, invasive, and have a significant number of disadvantages, including deterioration (requiring replacement over time), mechanical failure, migration of the device, infection (especially in patients with diabetes), and scarring. Use of a prothesis precludes the use of VCDs and intracavernosal injection therapy.
- *Vascular bypass surgery* is an alternative approach for patients with vascular insufficiency who have failed other less invasive treatments. Revascularization procedures are new, and their effectiveness in returning sexual function is still being investigated.

b. *What pharmacologic alternatives are available for the treatment of ED?*

- *A transurethral alprostadil suppository (MUSE)* is an FDA approved treatment for ED. Alprostadil (or prostaglandin E_1) is absorbed from the urethral mucosa and transferred to the corpus cavernosa where it induces smooth muscle relaxation, resulting in rapid arterial inflow and penile rigidity. The onset of action is within 5 to 10 minutes, and it is effective for 30 to 60 minutes. Although the largest clinical trial to date showed that 66% of men achieved an erection sufficient for intercourse during in-clinic testing,[5] anecdotally it has not been shown to be as effective in clinical practice. Its disadvantages include high cost, significant penile and testicular pain, and hypotension.
- *Intracavernosal injection of medications*
  - ✓ *Alprostadil (Caverject)* is an FDA-approved treatment for ED. As with the product above, alprostadil relaxes corporal smooth muscle leading to vascular engorgement. Monotherapy is initiated with a dose of 2.5 μg for ED of vasculogenic, psychogenic, or mixed etiology. The initial dose is 1.25 (μg for ED of a neurogenic cause (e.g., spinal cord injury). Doses should be titrated to response. The initial dose should be given in the physician's office, and the patient should re-

main until detumescence because of the possibility of priapism. The drug should be given no more than once a day and a maximum of 3 times per week.
✓ *Phentolamine* and *papaverine* are very effective for the treatment of ED, but there are no FDA-approved products at the time of this writing. Like alprostadil, papaverine relaxes smooth muscle leading to engorgement. Phentolamine, an α-blocker, increases arterial inflow by opposing arterial constriction.
✓ *Combination therapy (papaverine plus phenotolamine, or both drugs plus alprostadil)* may be used if alprostadil alone is ineffective or not tolerated. The effects of the drugs may be additive, allowing lower doses of each to be used. Combination therapy may also reduce the risk of adverse effects over monotherapy.

Intracavernosal injection therapy has been shown to have a 90% success rate for all etiologies of ED with the exception of those with severe arterial insufficiency or venous leak. Although success rates are high, a large percentage of patients drop out of home injection therapy. Lack of spontaneity, priapism, pain on injection, penile fibrosis, and high cost are all disadvantages to the use of injection therapies. In addition, the combination preparations must be compounded prior to use.

- *Yohimbine* is a presynaptic α_2-antagonist that appears to have a modest benefit over placebo when given to patients with intermittent, psychogenic ED. Yohimbine can be given as 5.4 or 6 mg tablets orally TID on a continuous basis, or 1 to 3 tablets may be given 45 to 60 minutes before the desired effect. Adverse effects include nausea, irritability, and systolic hypertension.
- *Androgen replacement therapy (testosterone enanthate or cypionate)* is indicated only as treatment for patients with documented deficiencies. Testosterone may be helpful if patients are suffering from hypogonadal disorders or hyperprolactinemia. The usual dose is 200 to 300 mg IM every 2 to 6 weeks. A testosterone transdermal delivery system (e.g., Androderm 2.5 mg/day) may also be used. Adverse effects include moodiness, aggressive behavior, undesirable hair growth, lethargy, hepatotoxicity, dyslipidemia, polycythemia, and prostatic hyperplasia and carcinoma.
- *Sildenafil (Viagra)* is the first oral therapy approved by the FDA for treatment for ED. It is a selective inhibitor of cyclic guanosine monophosphate (cGMP)-specific phosphodiesterase type 5 (PDE5), a substance present in human corpus cavernosal tissue. During erection, nitric oxide is released, which stimulates an increase in cGMP production. This leads to smooth muscle relaxation and erection. By inhibiting the enzyme that breaks down cGMP, sildenafil can enhance penile smooth muscle relaxation and erections as long as sexual stimulation is received to drive the nitric oxide/cGMP system. Improved quality of erections and achievement of erections suitable for intercourse range from 48% to 82% in patients receiving sildenafil depending on dose and etiology of dysfunction. The recommended dose is 50 mg as needed about 1 hour before sexual activity. However, the drug may be taken anywhere from one-half to 4 hours before sexual activity. The dose may be increased to 100 mg if 50 mg is ineffective; doses of 25 mg may be used in patients over the age of 65 or if adverse effects occur with 50-mg doses. The maximum recommended frequency is once daily. The most common adverse effects are headache, flushing, and upset stomach. Visual changes (temporary changes in blue/green color perception) or increased sensitivity to light may also occur. Because it potentiates the hypotensive effect of nitrates, sildenafil is absolutely contraindicated in patients on chronic nitrate therapy or those with CAD who may take sublingual nitroglycerin after exertion or sexual activity. At the time of this writing, the FDA had received 123 reports of deaths associated with sildenafil use. Of 69 evaluable patients, 46 had cardiovascular events (most often MI or cardiac arrest), and 12 men had taken nitrate medications. Almost three-fourths of the patients had one or more risk factors for cardiovascular or cerebrovascular disease. The FDA plans to continue monitoring the safety of the drug and evaluate the need for potential regulatory action.

Optimal Plan

4. *What therapy is most appropriate and effective for initial treatment of this patient? If drug therapy is indicated, list the drug, dosage form, dose, schedule, and duration of therapy.*

- Therapy for ED is largely based on the cause of the dysfunction, and more importantly, on the patient's willingness to try different modalities. Most patients will want to begin with less-invasive treatments, and if ineffective, move on to other therapies. Patients should be given psychological support in addition to medical treatments.
- Initial treatment should be to discontinue the HCTZ and the omeprazole and control his HTN and GERD with other agents.
- If drugs are not the primary causative factor, this patient's ED is most likely due to a neuropathy, but there may be a vascular component as well; therefore yohimbine and testosterone can be excluded as useful agents.
- Vascular surgery and implants should also be excluded until other less invasive measures fail.
- Vacuum therapy, alprostadil suppositories, alprostadil injections, or sildenafil would all be acceptable choices for initial treatment depending on the patient's preference.
  ✓ For alprostadil suppositories (MUSE), the initial dose titration should be carried out in the physician's office to test the patient's responsiveness, demonstrate proper administration technique, and monitor for evidence of hypotension. Titration should begin with lower doses (125 or 250 μg) and then may be increased or decreased until the patient achieves an erection sufficient for intercourse that does not exceed 1 hour. Maximum frequency of use is no more than 2 systems per 24-hour period.
  ✓ Alprostadil injections (Caverject) should also be started with dose titration in the physician's office to insure proper technique and establish an effective dose. Titration should begin with a 2.5-μg dose. If a partial response is observed with the initial dose, the dose may be increased by 2.5 μg, then in 5 to 10-μg increments until an erection suitable for intercourse occurs and a duration of 1 hour is not exceeded. If the initial dose gives no response, the second dose may be increased to 7.5 μg, then increased in 5 to 10-μg increments. After 1 hour of titration, the patient must stop and resume titration in 24 hours. After erection is achieved, the patient must remain in the office until detumescence occurs. Fol-

low-up should occur every 3 months, as additional dose changes may be needed. The recommended frequency of injection is no more than 3 times weekly, with at least 24 hours between doses.
- ✓ VCDs: Patients should be instructed on the use of the vacuums and the different styles available, such as the option between battery-powered or manually operated. There is no recommended maximum number of uses per week, but it is recommended that the constriction band placement be limited to 30 minutes.
- ✓ Sildenafil (Viagra) dosing range is 25 to 100 mg taken orally an hour before anticipated sexual activity, as described above.

Outcome Evaluation

5. *What clinical parameters are necessary to evaluate the therapy for achievement of the desired therapeutic outcome and to detect or prevent adverse effects?*

- Follow-up should occur every 3 months for the first year.
- Question the patient about potential side effects for the chosen treatment:
  - ✓ VCD: Difficulty or discomfort with ejaculation, petechiae
  - ✓ MUSE: Hypotension, priapism, penile pain, partner vaginal itching/burning, possibility of pregnancy in partner
  - ✓ Caverject: Priapism, postinjection penile pain, hematoma
  - ✓ Sildenafil: Headache, facial flushing, dyspepsia, and vision changes
- Assess patient and partner satisfaction with the chosen therapy.

Patient Counseling

6. *What information should be provided to the patient to enhance compliance, ensure successful therapy, and minimize adverse effects?*

General Information
- Your erectile dysfunction may be due to your diabetes, hypertension, or some of your medications.
- Diabetes eventually affects your nerves and blood vessels, including those that supply the penis. Just as your diabetes will not "go away," this problem will probably remain as well.
- The treatments you are trying will not cure your problem but may be effective in helping you to achieve an erection and have a satisfying sexual relationship.
- It is very important that you learn the proper technique for administering this medication (or using the VCD), as improper use may lead to significant adverse effects.
- If you experience an erection lasting longer than 4 hours, contact your physician or go to the emergency room immediately, because this may lead to permanent damage to tissues.
- You should return at least every 3 months while initiating therapy to discuss its effectiveness, possible side effects, and your level of satisfaction with it.

Alprostadil Suppositories (MUSE)
- *Note:* The patient must be instructed on the proper technique for administering the suppository in the physician's office while performing the initial dose titration. He should also be given the manufacturer's patient education booklet and view the instruction video.
- Urinate immediately prior to administration, because a mosit urethra makes administration easier, and the pellet was designed to dissove in a small amount of urine.
- Using a special applicator, place the MUSE inside the urethra. It will then be absorbed into the penis to cause an erection.
- If you suspect that your dose needs to be changed, please call your doctor to determine the new dose.
- Do not use this medication more than twice in 24 hours.
- MUSE should not be used with a pregnant partner unless a condom barrier is also used.
- It is recommended that MUSE be stored in the refrigerator, but it can be kept at room temperature up to 14 days prior to use.
- Possible adverse effects include aching in the penis, testicles, legs, and perineum (area between the penis and anus); warmth or burning sensation in the urethra; minor urethral bleeding or spotting due to improper administration; prolonged erection (priapism); and lightheadedness/dizziness. Your partner may experience mild vaginal burning/itching.
- Factors that may reduce your erection include anxiety, fatigue, tension, too much alcohol, lying on your back too soon after administration, urinating immediately after administration, or using medications that contain decongestants or appetite suppressants.

Alprostadil Injections (Caverject)
- *Note:* The patient must be instructed on proper injection technique in the physician's office while performing the initial dose titration. He should also be given the manufacturer's patient education booklet and view the instruction video.
- The medication is injected into the left or right side of the penis. Avoid visible veins, and alternate the side of the penis injected and the site of the injection.
- If you suspect that your dose needs to be changed, please call your doctor to determine the new dose.
- Do not use Caverject more than 3 times per week, with at least 24 hours between uses.
- Unused vials should be refrigerated, and reconstituted vials should be used immediately.
- Possible adverse effects include penile pain after injection, bleeding or bruising at the site of injection, and erection lasting longer than 4 hours (priapism).

VCD
- *Note:* The patient must be instructed on the proper technique in using the vacuum device. He should also be given the manufacturer's patient education booklet and view the instruction video.
- In general, a plastic cylinder is placed over the flaccid penis and the air in the cylinder is pumped out either manually or with a battery-operated pump.
- Once erect, a constriction band is slipped from the cylinder to the base of the penis to prevent blood drainage. The constriction band should be placed as close to the base of the penis as possible and may be left in place for a maximum of 30 minutes.
- Rigidity can be improved using a double-pumping technique. The vacuum is applied for 1 to 2 minutes, then released for 1 minute, and reapplied for another 3 to 4 minutes.
- Possible adverse effects include bruising around the base of the penis, painful or obstructed ejaculation, and the penis may feel cold after application of the constriction band.

Sildenafil (Viagra)
- Take one tablet (50 mg) 1 hour before anticipated sexual activity. Sildenafil will not spontaneously produce an erection in the absence of sexual stimulation. This tablet can be used only once a day.
- If you suspect that your dose needs to be changed, please call your doctor to determine the new dose.
- Possible adverse effects include headache, facial flushing, upset stomach, and changes in blue/green color perception and sensitivity to light.
- You must not take this drug if you are taking any kind of nitrate therapy (e.g., sublingual or oral nitroglycerin, isosorbide dinitrate or mononitrate) because serious and potentially fatal effects may occur.

References

1. Greiner KA, Weigel JW. Erectile dysfunction. Am Fam Physician 1996;54:1675–1682.
2. Saulie BA, Campbell RK. Treating erectile dysfunction in diabetes patients. Diabetes Educ 1997;23:29–33.
3. Khedun SM, Naicker T, Maharaj B. Zinc, hydrochlorothiazide and sexual dysfunction. Centr Afr J Med 1995;41:312–315.
4. Carvajal A, Martin Arias LH. Gynecomastia and sexual disorders after the administration of omeprazole. Am J Gastroenterol 1995;90:1028–1029. Letter.
5. Padma-Nathan H, Hellstrom WJ, Kaiser FE, et al. Treatment of men with erectile dysfunction with transurethral alprostadil. Medicated Urethral System for Erection (MUSE) Study Group. N Engl J Med 1997;336:1–7.

SECTION 5

Neurologic Disorders

Barbara G. Wells, PharmD, FASHP, FCCP, BCPP, Section Editor

50 MULTIPLE SCLEROSIS

▶ Relapses and Remissions   (Level I)

Barry E. Gidal, PharmD
John O. Fleming, MD

A 24-year-old woman with complaints of sensory loss and fatigue is evaluated and found to have changes on MRI brain scanning that are consistent with multiple sclerosis (MS). The case involves treatment of the acute disease exacerbation and implementation of adjunctive measures to control common complications such as urinary symptoms, difficulty ambulating, and fatigue. When the patient experiences a recurrence 6 months later, measures to modify the disease course are considered, including treatment with interferon beta-1a, interferon beta-1b, and glatiramer. The case provides an opportunity for students to practice educating patients about preparation, self-administration, adverse effects, and storage of disease-modifying agents for MS.

▶ Questions

Problem Identification

1. a. *What information (patient demographics, signs, symptoms, lab values) indicates the presence or severity of multiple sclerosis in this patient?*

   - Her new sensory symptoms suggest a mild exacerbation of MS, probably due to a new lesion deep in her right cerebrum.
   - The patient fits the epidemiologic picture of MS patients. The disease is usually diagnosed between the ages of 20 and 45 years, with the peak incidence occurring in the fourth decade.
   - Women tend to be affected more than men.
   - Patients from northern latitudes, and especially those of Scandinavian ancestry, have a greater prevalence of MS than the general population.
   - Signs and symptoms that support the diagnosis of MS in this patient include fatigue, bladder dysfunction, progressive sensory loss, and gait disturbance.
   - Supportive diagnostic findings include characteristic white matter demyelinating plaques found on MRI.

   b. *What additional information (laboratory tests, diagnostic procedures) may be useful in assessing this patient?*

   - In the case of an uncertain diagnosis, cerebrospinal fluid evaluation for electrophoretic evaluation of IgG bands may be helpful.
   - Electrophysiologic studies such as visual evoked potentials are also useful in confirming the presence of a lesion.

Desired Outcome

2. *What are the goals of therapy for this patient?*

   - The primary goals of therapy are to decrease the severity and intensity of disease exacerbations, prevent or slow the progression of disease, and provide symptomatic treatment for the associated complications of MS. No curative treatment is available at this time.

Therapeutic Alternatives

3. a. *What pharmacotherapeutic options are available to treat this patient's acute exacerbation, and which one would you recommend?*

   - *Methylprednisolone given IV* in high doses is most commonly used to treat severe, acute exacerbations. Typical IV doses range from 250 to 500 mg every 6 hours for 5 days. An alternative regimen is 500 to 1000 mg given IV as a single infusion over 1 to 2 hours; this may be more convenient for clinic- or home-based therapy. Clinical response to IV steroids is usually seen within the first 3 to 5 days of treatment. This option is probably the most appropriate treatment alternative for the patient at this time.
   - *ACTH* given IV or IM in doses of 20 to 100 IU twice daily has also been used, but treatment with methylprednisolone may result in a more rapid and predictable clinical response than ACTH.
   - *Prednisone or methylprednisolone given orally* may be appropriate in milder cases. However, oral corticosteroids are associated with a high rate of relapse and are generally not considered appropriate. Some clinicians use oral prednisone as a taper after IV methylprednisolone.
   - Mild exacerbations that do not result in functional decline may not require treatment.

   b. *What adjunctive treatments may be indicated for this patient?*

   - *Oxybutynin 15 to 30 mg/day* or *flavoxate 300 to 800 mg/day* (anticholinergic agents) may be beneficial if deemed appropriate after urodynamic evaluation. Bowel and bladder problems are common in MS patients.[1]
   - *Baclofen,* a GABA agonist, may be useful if gait problems are due to spasticity. Baclofen is usually initiated slowly (15 mg/day) and titrated upward until the maximum patient response is seen (usually 40 to 80 mg/day).
   - *Tizanidine,* a short-acting centrally acting α_2 agonist, may also be considered for treatment of spasticity. Therapy may be initiated with single oral doses of 4 mg and increased gradually in 2- to 4-mg increments over 2 to 4 weeks until the maximum beneficial effect is observed. The maximum dose is 36 mg/day given in divided doses 3 to 4 times daily.
   - *Antidepressant treatment* may be appropriate in this patient. Depression is a common comorbidity in MS patients, and depressive symptoms should be evaluated and treated appropriately.
   - *Amantadine* (100 to 300 mg/day) may provide some benefit for the patient's complaints of fatigue after an appropriate evaluation is conducted to rule out depression.

   c. *What adverse effects might be anticipated for both first-line and adjunctive treatments?*

   - Methylprednisolone IV is well tolerated, given the short courses of therapy usually employed. GI upset, gastric ulceration, and electrolyte abnormalities such as hypokalemia may occur. Exacerbation of an underlying infectious process is also of concern; for this reason, common infections (such as those of the urinary or respiratory tract) should be ruled out before beginning therapy.
   - Oxybutynin and flavoxate may cause dry mouth, blurred vision, drowsiness, tachycardia, urinary retention, and fever.
   - Amantadine has been associated with dizziness, insomnia, nervousness, anxiety, livedo reticularis, and nausea.
   - Baclofen can cause vertigo, dizziness, and drowsiness.
   - Tizanidine may cause sedation, dizziness, and hepatotoxicity.

   d. *What therapeutic options are available to modify this patient's disease course?*

   - There are presently three agents indicated for reducing the frequency of recurrence of the relapsing–remitting form of MS. These drugs and their usual doses include:
     - ✓ *Interferon beta-1b (Betaseron)* 0.25 mg SC every other day
     - ✓ *Interferon beta-1a (Avonex)* 30 µg IM once weekly
     - ✓ *Glatiramer (Copaxone; also known as Copolymer-1)* 20 mg SC once daily
   - Each of these agents has demonstrated efficacy in reducing the annual MS exacerbation rate.[2–7] Comparative trials between the two interferons or between beta-interferon and glatiramer have not been conducted. However, reductions in annual relapse (exacerbation) rates appear to be comparable. Although MRI data have demonstrated that placebo-treated patients had a significant increase in total lesional area compared with patients receiving interferon beta-1b, no significant differences in clinical disability were noted between the two groups. Data from clinical trials suggest that treatment with interferon beta-1a may slow disease progression. At present, it is unclear whether glatiramer treatment will alter disease progression.
   - Flu-like symptoms including fatigue, headache, fever, myalgias, and malaise occur in a significant number of patients taking interferon beta-1b. Local skin reactions (redness and swelling at the injection site) may also be seen. Depression, suicidal ideation, neutropenia, and elevated liver function tests occur rarely. Interferon beta-1a and glatiramer are associated with significantly fewer local skin reactions and treatment-associated depression than is interferon beta-1b.
   - Ease of administration and cost are other relevant considerations in therapeutic selection. Some patients may be reluctant to receive (or self-administer) the IM injections required for interferon beta-1a and may prefer the SC route used with interferon beta-1b and glatiramer. However, glatiramer requires daily SC injection (versus once weekly with IM interferon beta-1a). Yearly costs of therapy (based on 1998 average wholesale prices) are approximately $13,000 for interferon beta-1b, $11,000 for interferon beta-1a, and $10,500 for glatiramer acetate.
   - *Cyclophosphamide* and *azathioprine* are immunosuppressive agents that represent another therapeutic option. Short-term benefits in disease stabilization with cyclophosphamide have been reported, but the substantial toxicities associated with these agents (e.g., leukopenia, thrombocytopenia) make them less desirable for long-term use.
   - *Cyclosporine* appears to be only modestly effective in slowing disease progression. In addition, patients may develop significant therapy-limiting adverse effects such as nephrotoxicity and hypertension.

Optimal Plan

4. *Design an optimal pharmacotherapeutic plan for reducing the frequency of MS exacerbations in this patient.*

- Selection of a potential disease-modifying therapy should be based upon demonstrated efficacy, adverse effects, convenience of administration, and cost. The patient is concerned about disease progression and appears to be somewhat depressed.
- Because of the patient's depressive symptoms, initial use of interferon beta-1a may be preferred over interferon beta-1b. This agent is also convenient because it only requires self-administration IM once weekly.
- Glatiramer would be an acceptable alternative agent because of the patient's potential depression. However, it requires SC administration daily.

Outcome Evaluation

5. *What clinical and laboratory parameters are necessary for assessment of both efficacy and toxicity?*

Efficacy

- The pharmacologic effect on disease progression can be assessed by (1) decreased annual exacerbation rate and (2) stabilization of the disease state, using disease-specific assessment instruments such as the Expanded Disability Status Scale (EDSS).
- Disease burden and progression may also be assessed by MRI, but its clinical utility in modifying drug therapy is unclear.

Interferon-beta Adverse Effects

- Flu like symptoms are common with both beta-interferon products. These symptoms do not appear to be associated with glatiramer.
- Injection site reactions are common with SC administration of interferon beta-1b and may include skin necrosis. Both weekly IM interferon beta-1a and daily SC glatiramer are associated with fewer local skin reactions.
- Treatment-emergent depression has been reported with interferon beta-1b. During clinical trials, depression was no more common with either glatiramer or interferon beta-1a than with placebo.
- Neutropenia and elevated liver function tests occur rarely with interferon beta-1b; there was no evidence of drug-induced laboratory or hematologic abnormalities attributable to interferon beta-1a during clinical trials. However, patients should have a baseline CBC with differential and a chemistry panel performed prior to receiving either beta-interferon product. Liver function tests (AST, ALT, GGT) and WBC count should be obtained 1 month after treatment and every 6 months thereafter if results are normal. Minor abnormalities that do not affect treatment are commonly seen. However if there is marked neutropenia (ANC <0.750×10^3/mm^3) or an indication of substantial liver dysfunction (liver enzyme elevations >5 times normal), therapy should be discontinued. In some cases therapy can be restarted at one-half the usual dose under careful supervision.
- Caution should be exercised when using interferon beta-1a in patients with seizure disorders. In placebo-controlled trials, four patients receiving interferon beta-1a developed seizures, but no seizures occurred in the placebo group.
- Finally, interferon products should not be used in pregnant women because abortifacient activity has been shown in animal studies.

Glatiramer Adverse Effects

- Approximately 10% of patients experience transient chest tightness, flushing, and dyspnea after glatiramer administration. This reaction appears to be self-limiting and benign.

Patient Counseling

6. *What information would you provide to this patient about her long-term MS therapy?*

General Information

- Patients should be encouraged to learn about the disease and its management. Excellent educational materials and other forms of support are available through the National Multiple Sclerosis Society, a nonprofit organization dedicated to helping patients with this disease and promoting research into the cause and cure of MS.

Interferon β-1a (Avonex)

- *Note:* Prior to initiating treatment, patients should receive instructions in the clinic, and the pharmacist or clinic nurse should help the patient learn how to self-administer the medication. The first injection is usually given in clinic, and antipyretics are given as a precaution.
- This medicine is not a cure for your disease; you may continue to have relapses, but the medicine may make them milder and less frequent.
- It is important to use proper self-injection techniques, including rotation of injection sites.
- If you are not sure how to give yourself an intramuscular injection, have your physician, pharmacist, or other health care provider instruct you on the proper injection technique.
- If you miss a dose, take it as soon as you remember, however two injections *should not* be administered within 2 days of each other.
- This medicine should be stored in a refrigerator both before and after reconstitution. Avoid freezing the medicine.
- Some side effects that you may experience are similar to having the flu; you may feel tired and fatigued. You may also develop a headache or get a fever. In most cases, these side effects go away over time, usually within 24 hours after injection.
- Report any signs of depression or worsening depression to your physician as soon as possible.
- If you become pregnant (or wish to become pregnant) while using this medication, please contact your physician for advice.
- Keep all follow-up clinic appointments with your physician.

References

1. Schapiro RT. Symptom management in multiple sclerosis. Ann Neurol 1994;36(suppl):S123–S129.
2. The IFNB Multiple Sclerosis Study Group. Interferon beta-1b is effective in relapsing-remitting multiple sclerosis. I. Clinical results of a multicenter, randomized, double-blind, placebo-controlled trial. Neurology 1993;43:655–661.
3. Paty DW, Li DK. Interferon beta-1b is effective in relapsing-remitting multiple sclerosis. II. MRI analysis results of a multicenter randomized, double-blind, placebo-controlled trial. Neurology 1993;43:662–667.
4. The INFB Multiple Sclerosis Study Group and the British Columbia MS/MRI Analysis Group. Interferon beta-1b in the treatment of multiple sclerosis. Final outcome of the randomized controlled trial. Neurology 1995;45:1277–1285.
5. Jacobs LD, Cookfair DL, Rudick RA, et al. Intramuscular interferon beta-1a for

disease progression in relapsing multiple sclerosis. The Muliple Sclerosis Collaborative Research Group. Ann Neurol 1996;39: 285–294.
6. Johnson KP, Brooks BR, Cohen JA, et al. Copolymer 1 reduces relapse rate and improves disability in relapsing-remitting multiple sclerosis: Results of a phase III multicenter, double-blind, placebo-controlled trial. The Copolymer Multiple Sclerosis Study Group. Neurology 1995;45: 1268–1276.
7. Hunter SF, Weinshenker BG, Carter JL, et al. Rational clinical immunotherapy for multiple sclerosis. Mayo Clin Proc 1997;72:765–780.

51 COMPLEX PARTIAL SEIZURES

▶ A Lifelong Pattern (Level I)

James W. McAuley, RPh, PhD

A 60-year-old woman with a long history of uncontrolled seizures is referred to the epilepsy clinic for further evaluation and treatment. She has been treated with phenytoin for many years (presently 100 mg po TID) but is experiencing several small seizures per week (complex partial seizures with no secondary generalization) and one large seizure per month (a secondarily generalized tonic-clonic seizure). Because the patient has been unable to tolerate higher phenytoin doses, other alternatives for seizure control must be considered. Options include adding a newer antiepileptic drug to phenytoin (e.g., felbamate, gabapentin, lamotrigine, topiramate, or tiagabine). Switching the patient from phenytoin to carbamazepine could be attempted but would likely not be successful in obtaining seizure control. In addition to giving students the opportunity to compare the advantages and disadvantages of the newer antiepileptic drugs, the case also considers the possible consequences of long-term phenytoin use in this woman.

▶ Questions

Problem Identification

1. a. *Create a list of the patient's drug-related problems.*

   - Seizure disorder, uncontrolled by phenytoin.
   - Potential adverse drug reactions from phenytoin (nystagmus, somnolence, hirsutism).
   - Potential osteomalacia secondary to long-term phenytoin therapy (as evidenced by elevated alkaline phosphatase and decreased serum calcium concentrations).
   - Post-menopausal status and not receiving hormone replacement therapy.

   b. *What information (signs, symptoms, laboratory values) indicates the presence or severity of complex partial seizures?*

   - An abnormal EEG
   - Her current seizure activity of approximately 2 complex partial seizures per week and 1 secondarily generalized tonic-clonic seizure per month.
   - Her low QOLIE-89 scores.[1]
   - She doesn't drive, she fell down the stairs during a seizure, and has a burn on her hand.

Desired Outcome

2. *What are the goals of pharmacotherapy in this case?*

   - The ideal outcome is elimination of seizures; perhaps a more realistic goal is a decrease in seizure frequency and severity.
   - Minimize or avoid drug-related toxicities.
   - Provide an acceptable or improved quality of life.
   - Ensure patient adherence with the prescribed regimen.

Therapeutic Alternatives

3. a. *What non-drug therapies might be useful for this patient?*

   - She should be advised to contact the local Epilepsy Association for further information, support groups, and monthly educational seminars.
   - She and her husband should be given oral and written information on life-style modifications and general safety precautions (e.g., carpeting on floors, microwave cooking instead of cooking on the stove, avoiding ironing).

   b. *What feasible pharmacotherapeutic alternatives are available for treatment of complex partial seizures in this patient?*

   - The patient has uncontrolled seizure activity and there is little room to increase the phenytoin dose because she has a history of "feeling terrible" on higher doses and she has slight lateral gaze nystagmus, indicating substantial serum concentrations of phenytoin. Obtaining a serum phenytoin level would provide little additional useful information, because the patient would probably not tolerate a higher dose, even if the concentration is below the target level (10 to 20 μg/mL). Therefore, adding one of the newer antiepileptic drugs to her current regimen is an appropriate alternative to increasing the phenytoin dose.[2,3] The newer antiepileptic drugs, when used as adjunctive therapy, have the advantage of "attacking" the seizures from a different mechanism of action than the established drugs.
     ✓ *Gabapentin (Neurontin)* has a high tolerability profile and lacks protein binding or other pharmacokinetic interactions with phenytoin, her current treatment. However, it may be less effective than lamotrigine in treatment of complex partial seizures, and it is cleared solely by the kidneys. Therefore, dosage adjustments must be made based on creatinine clearance in patients with renal impairment.

✓ *Lamotrigine (Lamictal)* may be more efficacious than gabapentin in the treatment of complex partial seizures, and there is a vast amount of clinical experience with it compared with the other new agents. It also has no protein binding interaction with phenytoin. However, its clearance will be increased by concomitant phenytoin, which can be compensated for by increased dosages. Its side effects of dizziness, ataxia, and somnolence may be detrimental in this patient's situation. There is also an idiosyncratic side effect of skin rash, which can be severe.

✓ *Topiramate (Topamax)* has advantages of efficacy in many types of seizures and a known ceiling dose. The latter advantage is useful because if benefits are not seen with 400 mg, there is a low likelihood that higher doses will be beneficial. It also has no protein binding interaction with phenytoin. The majority of the drug is cleared by the kidneys, necessitating dosage adjustments based on creatinine clearance in patients with renal impairment. The clearance of topiramate will be increased by concomitant phenytoin, which may increase topiramate dosage requirements. Its dose-related side effects of difficulty concentrating and somnolence may be especially detrimental to this woman. There is also limited clinical experience with topiramate to date.

✓ *Tiagabine (Gabitril)* has the advantage of a known mechanism of action. Theoretically, this is advantageous because it can attack the seizure from a different mechanism. The clearance of tiagabine will be increased by concomitant phenytoin, and there is also a potential protein binding interaction between the two drugs. The clinical implications of the protein binding interaction are unknown. Tiagabine's dose-related side effects include dizziness and somnolence. There is limited clinical experience with this drug to date.

✓ *Felbamate (Felbatol)* has the advantage of being approved for use as either adjunctive or monotherapy for patients with partial seizures, with or without secondary generalization. It will decrease the clearance of phenytoin, and phenytoin will increase the clearance of felbamate. Felbamate has been associated with an increased risk of serious idiosyncratic reactions (aplastic anemia and liver failure) that are not seen with other antiepileptic drugs. For this reason, a case could be made for adding any of the other four agents discussed above to the patient's current phenytoin therapy before considering use of felbamate.

- *Switching to carbamazepine monotherapy* is another option for this patient. She has not tried this agent previously, and its efficacy in treating partial seizures is well documented. A potential disadvantage is that the drug has a similar mechanism of action to phenytoin (which is currently not providing appropriate seizure control); thus, carbamazepine may not control her seizures either.

- *Valproic acid* is a potential alternative (used alone or added to phenytoin), but it is associated with significant side effects (e.g., fine hand tremor, weight gain, hair loss) that would be detrimental to this woman.

- *Phenobarbital* may provide some efficacy for this patient when used alone or added to phenytoin, but the side effects probably outweigh the likely benefits.

Optimal Plan

4. *What drug, dosage form, dose, schedule, and duration of therapy are best for this patient?*

- Adding gabapentin to her current regimen may be the best option (and is the choice of the author), because of the lack of pharmacokinetic interactions with phenytoin and its high tolerability profile. The initial oral dosing scheme should entail 300 mg Q HS for the first day, 300 mg BID for one day, 300 mg TID for the next 3 days, and then 600 mg TID until the next clinic visit.
- If lamotrigine is selected, the initial oral dosing regimen should be 25 mg Q HS for week one, 25 mg BID for week two, 50 mg BID for week three, and then 100 mg BID until the next clinic visit.
- For topiramate, the initial oral dosing scheme is 50 mg Q HS for week one, 50 mg BID for week two, and then 100 mg BID until the next clinic visit.
- Tiagabine's initial oral dosing regimen is 4 mg Q HS for week one, 4 mg BID for week two, 8 mg BID for week three, and then 8 mg TID until the next clinic visit.
- Whichever adjunctive therapy is initiated, phenytoin should be continued at its present dose. However, it should be noted that this postmenopausal woman not receiving hormone replacement therapy is at significant risk for osteoporosis because of the fact that she has been on long-term therapy with an enzyme-inducing antiepileptic drug (i.e., phenytoin). Long-term therapy with these drugs, especially phenytoin and phenobarbital, has been associated with osteomalacia.[4] It is recommended that the patient be informed of these risks and that she receive follow-up evaluation with her primary care physician.

Outcome Evaluation

5. *What clinical and laboratory parameters are necessary to evaluate the therapy for achievement of the desired therapeutic outcome and to detect or prevent adverse effects?*

For Efficacy

- Seizure frequency, as measured by patient's seizure calendar and an interview with the patient and her husband at the next clinic visit.
- QOLIE-89 scores should be obtained at the next clinic visit.
- The frequency of clinic visits will be dictated by the degree of seizure control and the patient's overall medical status.

For Toxicity

- Gabapentin is almost completely renally eliminated, so baseline and periodic evaluation of renal function is necessary. Dosage reductions should be made when the creatinine clearance is less than 60 mL/min. At this point, the patient's calculated creatinine clearance is 78 mL/min, so the dose does not have to be adjusted. Gabapentin is well tolerated, but possible adverse events include somnolence, dizziness, ataxia, fatigue and nystagmus; these effects are transient. Having the patient gradually escalate to the desired dose will further diminish the risk of adverse events.
- Lamotrigine does not require laboratory monitoring, based on the information available at this time. Common adverse effects include

dizziness, diplopia, somnolence, ataxia, fatigue, headache, nausea/vomiting, skin rash, and nystagmus. A gradual escalation to the desired dose will diminish the risk of these adverse events.

- Topiramate is renally eliminated, so baseline and periodic evaluation of renal function is necessary. Dosage reductions should be made when creatinine clearance is less than 70 mL/min/1.73 m^2. Common adverse effects include somnolence, dizziness, ataxia, word-finding difficulties, paresthesias, psychomotor slowing, and nystagmus. Gradually escalating to the desired dose will diminish the risk of adverse events.
- Tiagabine requires no laboratory monitoring, based on the data available to date. Common adverse effects include dizziness/lightheadedness, asthenia/lack of energy, somnolence, nausea, nervousness, irritability, tremor, abdominal pain, and difficulty with concentration or attention. Gradual escalation to the desired dose will reduce the risk of adverse events.

Patient Counseling

6. *What information should be provided to the patient to enhance compliance, ensure successful therapy, and minimize adverse effects?*

- To increase compliance, the patient should be given an instruction sheet with the specifics about how she is to initiate the dosing of her new drug and an explanation that she is to maintain her current dose of phenytoin.

General Information

- Please continue to keep track of your seizures on the calendar. It is important to take your medications as we have discussed. This should make progress toward better seizure control, and the eventual goal is to have you become seizure free.
- Make sure you know how your body will react to this medicine before you do anything that requires being alert and well coordinated.
- It is also important that you do not stop taking your medicines without specific instructions from your doctor.
- If you miss a dose, take it as soon as possible. However, if it is almost time for your next dose, skip the missed dose and go back to your regular dosing schedule. Do not double doses.
- Keep all medicines out of the reach of children. Store them away from heat and direct light. Do not store them in the bathroom, near the kitchen sink, or in other damp places. Heat or moisture may cause the medicines to break down.

Gabapentin

- Do not take a gabapentin dose within 1 hour before or 2 hours after taking an antacid product.
- This medicine sometimes causes fatigue, dizziness, and feeling uncoordinated. Because we are adding this to your current regimen gradually, the chances of these side effects are decreased. If these occur and do not go away within a short period of time, please contact your doctor or pharmacist.

Lamotrigine

- This medicine sometimes causes fatigue, dizziness, double or blurred vision, and feeling uncoordinated. Because we are adding this to your current regimen gradually, the chances of these side effects are decreased. If these occur and do not go away within a short period of time, please contact your doctor or pharmacist.
- Contact your doctor or pharmacist immediately if you develop a skin rash.

Topiramate

- This medicine sometimes causes fatigue, dizziness, difficulty in concentrating, and feeling uncoordinated. Because we are adding this to your current regimen gradually, the chances of these side effects are decreased. If these occur and do not go away within a short period of time, please contact your doctor or pharmacist.
- Make sure you drink plenty of fluids when taking this medicine to prevent kidney stones.

Tiagabine

- This medicine sometimes causes lack of energy, dizziness or lightheadedness, difficulty in concentrating, nausea, and feeling uncoordinated. Because we are adding this to your current regimen gradually, the chances of these side effects are decreased. If these occur and do not go away within a short period of time, please contact your doctor or pharmacist.
- This medicine should be taken with food.

▶ Follow-up Question

1. *Other than non-compliance, what are the potential explanations for this situation?*

- The dose of her new antiepileptic drug is too low.
- She has added interacting medications to her regimen.
- She is not a good historian.

References

1. Vickrey BG, Perrine KR, Hays RD, et al. Quality of life in epilepsy QOLIE-89: Scoring manual and patient inventory. Santa Monica, RAND, 1993:1–16.
2. Marson AG, Kadir ZA, Chadwick DW. New antiepileptic drugs: A systematic review of their efficacy and tolerability. BMJ 1996;313:1169–1174.
3. Dichter MA, Brodie MJ. New antiepileptic drugs. N Engl J Med 1996;334:1583–1590.
4. Hahn TJ. Bone complications of anticonvulsants. Drugs 1976;12:201–211.

52 STATUS EPILEPTICUS

▶ Not Just Another Seizure   (Level I)

Sharon M. Tramonte, PharmD

A 29-year-old man with a history of tonic-clonic seizures is brought to the ED after experiencing a sustained seizure while playing basketball with friends. His wife believes that he stopped his antiepileptic drugs on his own several weeks ago because he has been seizure-free for years and doesn't think he needs the treatment any longer. Students should understand the difference between status epilepticus and other types of seizure disorders and recognize the steps that must be taken immediately to prevent permanent organ-system damage. Drugs used to terminate status epilepticus include benzodiazepines (e.g., diazepam, lorazepam) and phenytoin or fosphenytoin. Second-line agents such as phenobarbital or midazolam may be used for persistent seizures. The case highlights the need for patients with seizure disorders to avoid abrupt discontinuation of their medications.

▶ Questions

Problem Identification

1. a. What are this patient's drug-related problems?

- Status epilepticus requiring immediate pharmacologic therapy.
- Medication non-compliance which may have resulted in this complication.
- Gingival hyperplasia secondary to phenytoin therapy.

b. What steps should be taken when the patient is first seen in the ED?

- Assess cardiopulmonary function, establish an airway if needed, administer oxygen, and monitor with pulse oximetry or blood gases; initiate ECG monitoring.[1]
- Obtain medical history from the chart, friends who are present, and his wife.
- Perform a physical examination, including a full neurologic evaluation.
- Obtain laboratory tests (glucose, electrolytes, BUN, drug screen, serum concentrations of AEDs).
- Insert a heparin lock to provide venous access, and start an IV infusion of normal saline as standard protocol for unconscious patients. The patient also has signs of dehydration (pale nail beds, dry mucous membranes).
- Administer thiamine 100 mg IV (standard ED protocol for unconscious patients to prevent Wernicke's encephalopathy).
- Administer glucose 50% 50 mL IV to treat hypoglycemic seizures, if present. This is probably not the cause in this patient, but it will do no harm.
- Identify any possible precipitating factors
- For more detailed information on acute treatment measures, refer to the section on Treatment in textbook Chapter 53.

Desired Outcome

2. What are the goals of pharmacotherapy in this case?

- Maintain adequate brain oxygenation and cardiopulmonary function. Because of the muscle contraction of the chest, respiration is suspended and patients often become cyanotic as the hemoglobin becomes desaturated and venous return is diminished secondary to increased intrathoracic pressure. The cardiovascular system becomes increasingly stressed from the increased demand of the skeletal system during tonic contractions.
- Terminate seizure activity (both clinical and electrical) using pharmacologic therapy. Termination of electrical seizures must be determined by EEG monitoring. When neuromuscular blockers are used in nonconvulsive status epilepticus, or when the patient is comatose, the use of EEG monitoring is the only mechanism to determine when seizures have stopped.
- Correct metabolic imbalances; glucose and electrolyte imbalances are readily correctable precipitants of seizures. Seizures from hypoglycemia, hyponatremia, and other metabolic complications do not respond to anticonvulsants. This patient has a low glucose, but this is probably a result of the seizure activity and not the cause. Seizures from hypoglycemia generally are caused by a lower glucose concentration than is seen in this case.
- Minimize morbidity and prevent mortality from status epilepticus. Morbidity includes impaired mental capacity or neurologic deficits. Significant complications can occur because of prolonged or repeated seizures. The increased demand on the heart can cause tachycardia or bradycardia depending on the CNS mediated vagal tone. Desaturation and suspended respiration can cause anoxic injury to the CNS and other organ systems. Repeated seizures can cause hypoglycemia and alterations in electrolytes. Serious arrhythmias can occur from hyperkalemia. Repeated contractions can cause muscle damage (rhabdomyolysis), releasing proteins and myoglobin, which can result in renal failure. Although the seizures themselves can cause significant morbidity, the agents used to treat the disorder have serious consequences themselves. Barbiturates can depress the myocardium as well as respiratory drive. Mortality can be caused by prolonged seizure activity, but death is usually due to the underlying cause of the seizures.
- Identify any possible precipitating factors and correct them, if possible.
- Prevent seizure recurrence.

Therapeutic Alternatives

3. What pharmacotherapeutic options are available to treat status epilepticus?

- The perfect drug for treating status epilepticus is one that can be administered rapidly, enters the brain immediately, has an immediate anticonvulsant activity, does not depress consciousness or respiration, has a long half life, and blocks both the somatic symptoms and neuronal discharges. No currently available agent meets all of these criteria.
- *Benzodiazepines* have the advantages of rapid onset of action and ease in administration. The major disadvantages include the short duration of action and CNS depression, which makes assessment of consciousness difficult. Benzodiazepines can also cause respiratory depression, further compromising oxygenation capacity.
    - ✓ *Diazepam* is quick acting and crosses the blood brain barrier rapidly because of its lipid solubility. However, it weakly binds to the benzodiazepine receptor and rapidly redistributes to the more abundant fatty tissue. The duration of effectiveness in the CNS is only 30 minutes. Because of this, use of diazepam necessitates adjunctive therapy with a longer-acting agent such as phenytoin or fosphenytoin.
    - ✓ *Lorazepam* is also quick acting but slower than diazepam. Because it is less lipophilic than diazepam, distribution into and out of the CNS is slower. For this reason the duration of effectiveness is longer than with diazepam.
- *Phenytoin* is an effective anticonvulsant, has a relatively long half life, and lacks CNS depression. However, it has cardiovascular toxicity when given too rapidly, necessitating slow IV administration. Venous sclerosis and skin necrosis at the infusion site may also occur. The injectable Dilantin brand of phenytoin is no longer available, but generic injectable phenytoin is available and may be used for treatment of status epilepticus.
- *Fosphenytoin* has overcome many of the administration difficulties

associated with phenytoin. Fosphenytoin can be administered IV more rapidly than phenytoin and has greatly reduced the incidence of adverse infusion reactions. Fosphenytoin may also be given intramuscularly. Antiarrhythmic effects may be similar to phenytoin, but fosphenytoin does not contain propylene glycol, which allows for more rapid infusion without the cardiovascular complications. Although it is more water soluble and more tolerable than phenytoin, fosphenytoin dosing may cause confusion because it is not ordered in milligrams but "phenytoin equivalents" (1.5 mg fosphenytoin = 1 mg phenytoin). The advantages of fosphenytoin must be weighed against its substantially higher cost; for equivalent doses, fosphenytoin costs at least three times as much as phenytoin.

- *Phenobarbital*[2] or *midazolam*[3] can be used if seizures persist despite administration of diazepam/lorazepam or phenytoin/fosphenytoin. Midazolam is not a first-line agent because of lack of evidence of efficacy. In theory, its efficacy should be similar to other benzodiazepines, but there is not enough data at this time to support that claim.
- *Valproic acid, lidocaine,* and *general anesthetics* are other second-line agents that are less effective.
- *Neuromuscular blockers* are not normally recommended for status epilepticus. They may be used by some practitioners in situations of severe muscle contractions. However, these agents will mask seizures, so the only way to determine if the status epilepticus is stopped is by using an EEG.

Optimal Plan

4. *What is the best pharmacotherapeutic plan for this patient?*

- Administer a benzodiazepine:
  - ✓ Lorazepam 0.1 mg/kg IV given at a rate of 2 mg/minute (may repeat in 5 minutes if necessary). It has a long half-life, so repeated doses may not be necessary.

  OR

  - ✓ Diazepam 0.2 mg/kg IV given at a rate of 5 mg/minute (may repeat in 5 minutes if necessary). Initiate a phenytoin or fosphenytoin infusion to prevent recurrent status epilepticus if diazepam is given because of its short half-life:
    - Phenytoin 15 to 20 mg/kg IV at a rate of 50 mg/minute. Repeat doses of 100 to 150 mg/dose may be given at 30-minute intervals to a maximum of 1500 mg (in 24 hours). A daily maintenance dose of 300 mg (or 5 to 6 mg/kg) may then be given in 3 divided doses.
    - Fosphenytoin 15 to 20 phenytoin equivalents (PE)/kg at a rate of 100 to 150 PE/minute. A maintenance dose of 4 to 6 PE/kg/day IM or IV should be initiated after the loading dose.
- If status epilepticus persists after administration of a benzodiazepine and phenytoin/fosphenytoin, give:
  - ✓ Phenobarbital 20 mg/kg IV at a rate of 100 mg/minute

  OR

  - ✓ Midazolam 0.2 mg/kg loading dose, followed by an infusion of 0.1 to 0.4 mg/kg/hr

Outcome Evaluation

5. *What clinical and laboratory parameters are needed to evaluate the therapy to ensure the best possible outcome?*

- Clinical and/or electrical evidence that seizures have been stopped must be obtained. If neuromuscular blockers have been used, electrical evidence with an EEG is needed.
- If lorazepam or diazepam is used, the patient should be monitored for CNS depression (which is impossible in an unresponsive patient) and respiratory depression. Respiratory depression is monitored by obtaining vital signs (specifically the respiratory rate) every 15 minutes and by monitoring gas exchange (by arterial blood gases or pulse oximetry). If reversal of the benzodiazepine is necessary, flumazenil 0.2 mg (2 mL) may be administered. If the desired effects of flumazenil are not seen after 45 seconds, additional doses of 0.2 mg may be given at 1-minute intervals to a maximum dose of 1 mg (10 mL).
- Fosphenytoin does not cause many infusion site reactions, but the patient should be monitored for possible phlebitis and/or burning (if the patient is conscious). A serum phenytoin level should be obtained 12 to 24 hours after the initiation of the infusion. Vital signs, especially blood pressure, should be obtained while the infusion is running.

Patient Counseling

6. *What information should the patient receive to ensure successful therapy and to minimize adverse effects?*

The single most important issue is patient education. In adults, the most likely etiology of status epilepticus is withdrawal of anticonvulsants. It is imperative to stress the importance of medication compliance. The presence of an abnormal baseline EEG is predictive of recurrent seizures and is an added risk in this patient. Also, counseling on recreational drug and alcohol use may be needed.

General Information

- It is important to take your medications as directed every day to prevent seizures.
- It is a good idea to carry identification stating your medical condition. A wallet card should state the medications and doses you are taking.

Phenytoin

- Take this medication with food to decrease GI discomfort.
- This may cause dizziness or drowsiness.
- Phenytoin may cause increase in gum growth. Routine dental care consisting of brushing your teeth two to three times a day, flossing, and regular check-ups with your dentist will help prevent this adverse effect.
- Do not change brands or dosage forms of this medication before checking with your physician.
- Small blood samples will need to be collected periodically for laboratory testing.

Carbamazepine

- Take this medication with food to minimize the stomach upset it sometimes causes.
- This medication may cause drowsiness or dizziness.
- Notify your physician if there is any unusual bleeding or bruising, abdominal pain, fever, chills, sore throat, or ulcers in the mouth.
- Small blood samples for periodic laboratory testing will need to be drawn.

References

1. Weise KL, Bleck TP. Status epilepticus in children and adults. Crit Care Clin 1997;13:629–646.
2. Lowenstein DH, Aminoff MJ, Simon RP. Barbiturate anesthesia in the treatment of status epilepticus: Clinical experience with 14 patients. Neurology 1988;38:395–400.
3. Kumar A, Bleck TP. Intravenous midazolam for the treatment of refractory status epilepticus. Crit Care Med 1992;20:483–488.

53 ACUTE MANAGEMENT OF THE HEAD INJURY PATIENT

▶ Bowled Over (Level III)

Denise H. Rhoney, PharmD
Mark S. Luer, PharmD

A 25-year-old unresponsive man is brought to the emergency department after a motor vehicle accident. Physical examination reveals respiratory distress, and a head CT shows evidence of an intracranial hemorrhage. The patient is ultimately transferred to the neurotrauma unit for monitoring after surgical evacuation of the subdural hematoma and ventriculostomy placement for monitoring of intracranial pressure (ICP). The patient requires appropriate fluid resuscitation and management of increased ICP. The comprehensive pharmaceutical care plan must also include measures to prevent the medical complications of hyperglycemia, seizures, protein breakdown and resultant malnutrition, stress ulceration, electrolyte abnormalities, alcohol withdrawal, and venous thromboembolism. Close monitoring of the patient is required because of the multiplicity of medical complications that may occur.

▶ Questions

Problem Identification

1. a. *What information (signs, symptoms, laboratory values) indicates the severity of this patient's head injury?*

   - Corneal reflexes, pupillary response to light, and eye movement abnormalities are important parameters to evaluate brain stem involvement. This patient had one dilated pupil and pupils that were nonreactive to light bilaterally. This indicates possible brain stem involvement of his injury.
   - The evidence of Battle's sign (postauricular ecchymoses), raccoon eyes (periorbital ecchymoses), and hemotympanum are evidence of a basilar skull fracture.
   - ABGs indicates poor oxygenation and hyperventilation necessitating intubation of the patient.

   b. *What is the Glasgow coma score for this patient?*

   - The Glasgow coma score (GCS) is the most widely used scoring system to define the level of consciousness. It is based on eye opening, motor response, and verbal response (see Table 54–1 in textbook Chapter 54). The GCS ranges from 3 to 15, with 15 corresponding to a normal neurologic examination.
   - The GCS for this patient is E = 1 M = 2 V = 1 for a total of 4. It is important to note that if a patient is intubated the examiner is unable to determine the verbal response; this is usually indicated as V = 1T.
   - The classification of this patient's head injury is severe since the GCS is in the range of 3 to 8 (refer to the textbook chapter for more detailed information).

   c. *Does this patient have any factors that may complicate assessment of the neurologic examination?*

   - Studies have found that a blood alcohol concentration >200 mg/dL significantly depresses the GCS.
   - The administration of sedatives and neuromuscular blocking agents may also affect the neurological examination; assessment of their administration times in relation to the timing of the examination must be considered.

Desired Outcome

2. a. *What are the goals of therapy for this patient?*

   Goals for the management of this patient are known as "cerebral resuscitation" and include the following:
   - Establish an adequate airway along with maintenance of breathing and circulation (ABC)
   - Maintain adequate CNS perfusion and oxygenation
   - Abolish and prevent seizure activity
   - Modify or reverse mechanisms of secondary injury (refer to the textbook chapter for a complete discussion of secondary injury)
   - Protect uninjured tissue that is vulnerable to a secondary insult
   - Maintain a balance between cerebral oxygen delivery (CDo_2) and cerebral metabolic rate of oxygen consumption ($CMRo_2$)
   - Prevent and/or treat associated medical complications

   b. *What are the goals of fluid resuscitation and hemodynamic monitoring for this patient?*

   - Although fluid restriction was recommended in the past, recent data suggest that this approach may cause systemic hypotension, which is associated with increased ICP and worse neurologic outcome. Therefore the goal of fluid therapy is to expand the pa-

tient's circulatory volume without reducing the plasma osmolarity (euvolemia). The target CVP = 5 to 10 mm Hg and PCWP = 10 to 14 mm Hg.
- Head injury patients require maintenance of systemic hemodynamics as well as attention to cerebral hemodynamics. Most head injury patients have increased metabolic oxygen consumption, mild hypertension, and increased cardiac indices. A CI of 4 to 5 L/min/m² may be seen as normal due to an increased metabolic rate. This patient has BP 175/85 and a heart rate of 140. The goals of hemodynamic monitoring are to:
  ✓ Optimize volume status and cardiac function
  ✓ Maximize tissue perfusion (including the brain)
  ✓ Avert complications of fluid management and pharmacologic hemodynamic therapy
  ✓ Preserve cerebral perfusion pressure (CPP), calculated as CPP = MAP − ICP. Patients who have a sustained CPP >70 mm Hg have been shown to have a decreased morbidity and mortality.
  ✓ Maintain systemic oxygen availability, since hypotension and hypoxia are major factors contributing to secondary injury. A single episode of hypotension with SBP <90 mm Hg has been reported to result in a mortality rate of 85%.[1]

Therapeutic Alternatives

3. a. *What therapeutic alternatives are available for fluid resuscitation, and which would be the most appropriate for this patient?*

- *Isotonic solutions (0.9% NaCl = 308 mOsm/kg)* are the most appropriate solutions for TBI patients. This patient should receive 0.9% NaCl with 20 mEq of KCl at a rate of 100 mL/hr initially. Urinary output should be monitored and maintained at 30 to 50 mL/hr.
- *Hypo-osmolar solutions (D_5W, 0.45% NaCl)* reduce serum sodium and increase brain water and ICP. Lactated Ringer's solution is more hypo-osmolar than its calculated 273 mOsm/kg and should not be used in patients with TBI.
- *Hypertonic solutions (3% NaCl)* can decrease brain water content and ICP and have been evaluated for fluid resuscitation with conflicting results; they are currently used in Europe. Concerns over hypertonic therapy with 3% NaCl include hypernatremia and central pontine myelinolysis due to an over-correction of sodium too rapidly.
- *Colloids (albumin, hetastarch)* have increased molecular weight with low vascular permeability, resulting in a longer intravascular retention time and more sustained effect. However, they offer very little benefit over isotonic crystalloids and are higher in cost.
- *Packed red blood cells* are beneficial in patients with decreased Hgb/Hct (hemorrhagic shock) in order to maximize cerebral oxygen delivery.

b. *What non-drug therapies may be useful in preventing or treating increased ICP?*

- *Head Position.* Elevation of the head of the bed between 15 and 30 degrees from horizontal is effective in lowering ICP by decreasing cerebral venous outflow resistance. However, euvolemia must be established first to prevent decreases in MAP and CPP. The neck must be maintained in a neutral position and external compression of the jugular venous system (i.e., tight cervical orthosis or endotracheal tube stabilization tape) must be avoided.
- *Cerebrospinal fluid (CSF) drainage.* The CSF may be drained if a ventriculostomy is inserted as the ICP monitor as long as the ventricles are not compressed.
- *Prevention of hyperthermia.* ICP will increase by several mm Hg for every 1°C increase in body temperature. Therefore, aggressive use of cooling blankets and/or antipyretic agents is indicated. The goal is maintenance of core body temperature <37.5°C. Brain temperatures often are higher than body temperatures, so optimal temperature measurement should include monitoring brain temperature when possible. Ventricular catheters with temperature sensors are now available, but their high cost is a limiting factor.
- *Hyperventilation.* This is an established and effective mechanism for decreasing ICP. Cerebral blood flow changes approximately 2% to 3% for every 1 mm Hg change in CO_2 from a pco_2 of 40 mm Hg. However, recent evidence suggests that inappropriate or excessive hyperventilation can produce or exacerbate cerebral ischemia.[2] The Brain Trauma Foundation treatment guidelines recommend that pco_2 be maintained near 35 mm Hg, especially during the first 24 hours, and then in the range of 30 to 35 mm Hg if ICP control is inadequate.
- *Hypothermia.* Recent studies have shown that moderate hypothermia (32 to 33°C) when begun within 6 hours of the injury resulted in better outcome. However this treatment modality is still considered investigational and limited to patients with refractory ICP.
- *Surgery.* Decompressive craniotomy with lobectomy and craniectomy (i.e., leaving the skull plate off so the brain has room to expand) are methods of "giving room to the swelling brain." This is usually reserved for patients who are resistant to pharmacologic therapy for increased ICP.

c. *What pharmacotherapeutic alternatives are available for the treatment of increased ICP?*

- *Sedation/Analgesia*
  ✓ *Propofol* is a 1% solution in a 10% lipid carrier emulsion. Propofol decreases CBF, $CMRo_2$, ICP, MAP, and CPP in a dose-dependent fashion. It has a rapid onset of effect due to high fat solubility, so it crosses the blood–brain barrier (BBB) rapidly and has a rapid termination of sedation (5 to 10 min) after short-term infusions. Longer infusions may be associated with prolonged sedation due to its large Vd and accumulation in the tissues. The dose ranges from 5 to 50 μg/kg/min. Nutrition support must be adjusted to compensate for the amount of lipid infused in propofol (1 kcal/mL) and monitoring should include triglycerides.
  ✓ *Benzodiazepines (e.g., lorazepam, midazolam)* decrease CBF and $CMRo_2$. Decreases in CBF following benzodiazepine infusions are not associated with substantial changes in cerebral blood volume, which suggests that these agents are less effective in decreasing ICP in patients with low intracranial elastance but may be effective in patients with high intracranial elastance. The most commonly used agents are lorazepam (1- to 5-mg bolus doses or 0.5 to 5 mg/hr infusion) and midazolam (1- to 5-mg bolus doses or 1- to 20-mg/hr infusion). Midazolam has been reported to become long-acting after continuous infusion for >24 hours. Rever-

sal with flumazenil is not advocated because of the possible risk of seizure activity and the risk of increasing ICP.
- ✓ *Opioids* have no effect or decrease CBF and $CMRo_2$. There has been controversy regarding the effects of opioids on ICP. Any ICP changes that may be seen can be explained by autoregulatory responses to decreased MAP.
- ✓ *Etomidate* (0.1 to 0.3 mg/kg IV bolus) decreases ICP by decreasing CBF and $CMRo_2$. It has limited hemodynamic effects similar to the other sedative/analgesic agents, but it is not suitable for prolonged infusion due to inhibition of adrenal corticosteroid synthesis. Prolonged infusions should be avoided unless steroids are concomitantly administered.

The effects of these agents on the neurologic examination must be considered, and there may be a need to coordinate daily baseline neurologic exams with sedative administration and/or use short-acting agents. Cost is another consideration when choosing a sedative agent.

- *Neuromuscular blockade.* Paralysis is useful when added to sedation in patients with refractory increased ICP, in patients who have ICP spikes with posturing, or in patients resisting ventilatory support. Prophylactic paralysis is not recommended due to an increased risk of complications and ICU length of stay.[3]
- *Diuretics*
  - ✓ *Mannitol* is the most commonly used diuretic for reducing ICP. Repeated doses will increase serum osmolarity and reduce its effectiveness and possibly precipitate acute renal failure. Doses of 0.25 g/kg appear to be as effective as doses of 1 g/kg, although the duration of action is shorter. Serum osmolarity should be monitored and maintained below 320 mOsm/L.
  - ✓ *Furosemide* is also effective in lowering ICP but to a lesser extent than mannitol. There is some evidence that furosemide (0.5 to 1 mg/kg) may work synergistically with mannitol to lower ICP and may be useful when there is no response to mannitol alone.
- *Corticosteroids* are commonly used in patients with structural brain lesions. Use of steroids in patients with head injury results in an increased risk of complications, causing the Brain Trauma Foundation guidelines to recommend that corticosteroids not be used in these patients.
- *Barbiturates* in high doses have been used since the 1970s for refractory ICP control since they reduce $CMRo_2$ and CBF by as much as 50%. The response rate ranges from 27% to 80% with a significantly increased mortality in nonresponders. Blood pressure may need to be supported during barbiturate therapy, and patients must be ventilated before instituting therapy.
  - ✓ *Pentobarbital* is the most common agent used because of predictable metabolic clearance ($t_{1/2} = 24$ hours), availability of serum concentrations, and lack of active metabolites. Patients should be normovolemic prior to initiating therapy. Pentobarbital administration can begin with a 10 mg/kg loading dose over 30 minutes followed by 5 mg/kg/hr for the next 3 hours. The loading dose is followed by a maintenance infusion of 1 to 3 mg/kg/hr. Supplementation with 200 mg of pentobarbital may be necessary to achieve burst suppression.
  - ✓ *Thiopental* may also be used. Since it is more lipid soluble, it achieves rapid brain concentrations. However, it also redistributes rapidly and thus may have a shorter duration of coma. Thiopental also has active metabolites, one of which is pentobarbital. The dose of thiopental is 20 mg/kg over 1 hour, then 2 to 12 mg/kg/hr.

Optimal Plan

4. a. *Develop an optimal pharmacotherapeutic plan to treat the patient's increased ICP.*

   - Ventriculostomy opened to drain CSF
   - Elevation of the head of the bed from 15 to 30 degrees horizontal and head in midline position
   - Acetaminophen 500 to 1000 mg po for T >37.5°C
   - Mannitol 0.25 g/kg IV Q 4 H if serum Osm <320 mOsm/kg
   - Sedation, titrated until the patient is no longer agitated using one of the options listed below:
     - ✓ Propofol IV infusion given initially at 5 µg/kg/min
     - ✓ Lorazepam 1 mg IV push Q 6–8 H PRN
     - ✓ Remifentanil IV infusion at 0.1 µg/kg/hr
     - ✓ Morphine 1 mg IV push Q 1–2 H PRN

   b. *Outline a pharmacotherapeutic plan for prevention of medical complications that may occur in this patient.*

   - *Hyperglycemia* occurs commonly after TBI, and small clinical trials suggest that glucose concentrations >200 mg/dL worsen neurologic outcome after TBI by worsening secondary damage. This patient's glucose is already over 200 mg/dL, so administration of insulin may be warranted.
   - *Seizure prophylaxis* is recommended even though the overall incidence of posttraumatic seizures (PTS) is relatively low (<5%) because seizures greatly increase $CMRo_2$. PTS may be categorized as early (≤1 week postinjury) or late (>1 week postinjury). The majority of early PTS occur in the first 24 hours. A randomized, placebo-controlled trial documented a significantly lower incidence of early PTS in patients receiving prophylactic phenytoin (3.6%) versus placebo (14.2%).[4] No difference in the incidence of late PTS was observed between the two patient groups, suggesting that prophylaxis beyond the first week is not warranted. The Brain Trauma Foundation guidelines do not recommend use of prophylactic antiepileptic agents beyond 7 days. This patient should receive a loading dose of 20 mg/kg IV of phenytoin, followed by a maintenance dose of 200 mg IV Q 12 for 7 days. Aggressive therapy is recommended for patients having documented seizures.
   - *Nutritional intervention* is necessary because moderate or severe head injury results in a generalized hypermetabolic and hypercatabolic state. In the absence of adequate nutritional support the resulting hypercatabolic state causes endogenous protein breakdown to amino acids ultimately resulting in multiorgan dysfunction and an immunocompromised state. Enteral nutrition results in improved mesenteric blood flow and prevents gut atrophy and mucosal breakdown that promotes bacterial translocation. Head injury patients are reported to have gastric hypomotility following injury that may last for 4 to 5 days. In this setting, early gastric feeding may be poorly tolerated. On the other hand, early jejunal feedings can begin shortly after injury even when bowel sounds are absent. Ideally, feeding should begin

within 24 to 48 hours of injury. Most critically ill TBI patients expend 25 to 35 kcal/kg/day and need 1.5 to 2 g/kg/day of protein. Patients with abdominal trauma or who are unable to tolerate enteral feedings should receive TPN. This patient should receive jejunal feedings if possible or administration of gastric feedings while monitoring for residuals. The patient should be fed about 2000 to 2500 kcal/day and 120 to 160 g of protein. The appropriate enteral formula with additional protein added should be chosen to meet these goals.

- *Stress ulcer prophylaxis* is routinely given with either sucralfate or H_2-receptor antagonists because erosive gastritis and GI bleeding are common complications after head injury.[5] Options include:
  - ✓ Sucralfate 1 g Q 6 H per NG tube (give only if the patient has a source of gastric administration)
  - ✓ Cimetidine 900 to 1200 mg/day either orally or by continuous or intermittent infusion
  - ✓ Ranitidine 150 mg/day IV either by continuous infusion or intermittent infusion; or 150 mg po Q 12 H
  - ✓ Famotidine 40 mg/day either orally or by continuous or intermittent infusion
  - ✓ Omeprazole 20 mg per NG tube QD
- *Electrolyte abnormalities* are common after head injury.
  - ✓ *Hyponatremia* lowers seizure threshold and can exacerbate cerebral edema. The most common cause is the administration of hypotonic fluids. Other causes include SIADH and cerebral salt wasting (CSW), which are characterized by low serum sodium and serum osmolality and high urine sodium and urine osmolality in a setting of normal renal, adrenal, and thyroid function. Treatment of SIADH is fluid restriction to 500 to 1000 mL/day until serum sodium normalizes. Refractory or severely low sodium may respond to 3% NaCl infusion and occasionally demeclocycline. Treatment of CSW includes fluid and salt supplementation. Accurate diagnosis is important as treatments differ and improper fluid restriction in the presence of CSW can result in additional morbidities.
  - ✓ *Hypernatremia* is another common electrolyte disorder, and it is frequently a manifestation of hypovolemia but may be caused by diabetes insipidus (DI). Diabetes insipidus is more common with cranial base fractures with resultant hypothalamic and/or pituitary stalk injuries and is frequently a terminal event in severely brain-injured patients. The diagnosis of DI is made when serum sodium is >145 mEq/L, serum osmolality is >290 mOsm/L, urine specific gravity is <1.003, and urine output exceeds 300 mL/hr. Free-water deficit should be corrected slowly. Treatment is ADH replacement with vasopressin 5 to 10 units SC Q 6–8 H (or 1 to 2 units/hr as a drip) or DDAVP. This patient's sodium and urine output need to be monitored carefully since his serum sodium is at the upper limit of normal.
  - ✓ *Hypomagnesemia* lowers seizure threshold, complicates alcohol withdrawal, and (in experimental head injury) hinders neurologic recovery. It appears reasonable and safe to maintain serum magnesium levels in the upper range of normal. This patient's magnesium level is already low and needs supplementation. Replace this patient's magnesium with magnesium sulfate 2 g IV.
- *Alcohol withdrawal prevention* measures should be instituted, as agitation secondary to alcohol withdrawal may contribute to intracranial hypertension. Benzodiazepines can be administered but may affect the neurologic exam. In the patient who chronically ingests alcohol, it may also be necessary to administer thiamine, multivitamins, folic acid, and magnesium.
- *Prophylaxis of thromboembolism* (DVT/PE) should be initiated, as the incidence of thromboembolic complications is 29% to 43% in head injury patients. Prophylactic options include:
  - ✓ Pneumatic compression boots, which resulted in clinically evident DVT in 2.3% and PE in 1.8%.[6]
  - ✓ Low-dose heparin (5000 U SC Q 12 H) has been studied for prophylaxis starting on postoperative day one or post-injury day one, but there is no universal standard in clinical practice.
  - ✓ Low-molecular-weight heparin (e.g., enoxaparin, dalteparin) is another option and theoretically should be associated with fewer hemorrhagic complications. However, this effect has been minimal in clinical trials, and its efficacy in head injury patients has not been established.
  - ✓ If full anticoagulation with IV heparin is needed, the ideal timing for safe anticoagulation is unclear but should be at least 7 to 14 days post-injury.

  This patient should be started on pneumatic compression devices along with either heparin 5000 U SC Q 12 H, enoxaparin 30 mg SC Q 12 H, or dalteparin 2500 IU SC QD.
- *Coagulation abnormalities* are common after TBI. A proposed mechanism involves the release of tissue thromboplastin from the injured brain tissue either locally or into the bloodstream. The peak incidence is during the first 3 post-traumatic days. Evaluation should include analysis of platelet function along with studies of clotting factors and bleeding time. This patient has low platelets and further investigation may be warranted. Exercise caution in administering other agents (e.g., heparin) that may decrease platelets or have antiplatelet properties.

Outcome Evaluation

5. *What monitoring parameters should be instituted to ensure efficacy and prevent toxicity for the therapy recommended for treating increased ICP?*

- *Maintain CPP.* Implement continuous monitoring of ICP and MAP for maintenance of CPP ≥70 mm Hg. ICP can be measured either by an intraventricular catheter or fiberoptic intraparenchymal device. MAP can be monitored by an intra-arterial catheter. Drugs may have to be titrated to achieve the desired effect on ICP, or vasoactive agents may have to be added in addition to IV fluids for BP support.
- *Prevent hypovolemia and acute renal failure associated with mannitol therapy.* Monitor serum osmolality every 6 hours and do not administer mannitol if osmolality is >320 mOsm/L. Continuously monitor fluid status (CVP or PCWP) and fluid intake/output. Also measure serum electrolytes, BUN, and creatinine at least once daily but optimally every 6 hours until the patient's ICP is stabilized.
- *Prevent prolonged neuromuscular blockade with neuromuscu-*

lar blocking agents. Peripheral nerve stimulation using Train-of-Four stimulation should be performed every 6 hours. The goal is to titrate therapy to clinical end point (i.e., ICP <20 mm Hg, CPP >70 mm Hg) while trying to prevent achieving complete blockade (0 out of 4 twitches).

- *Monitor barbiturate coma.* Continuous monitoring of EEG to evaluate for burst suppression is necessary to guide titration of therapy. Serum pentobarbital concentrations may be evaluated every 24 hours. Serum concentrations of 25 to 40 μg/mL are associated with barbiturate-induced coma, electrically silent EEG, and a maximal reduction in metabolic rate. One to three bursts per minute are common at serum levels of 30 to 40 μg/mL. Supplementation with 200 mg of pentobarbital may be necessary to achieve burst suppression. CPP may decrease, especially during loading dose administration due to decreases in cardiac output and systemic vasodilation. The loading infusion may need to be slowed if CPP falls below 70 mm Hg. Blood pressure may need to be supported during barbiturate therapy, and patients must be ventilated before instituting therapy. Vasoconstrictors, inotropes, and volume expansion may be required to support the patient. Cardiac output monitoring is recommended particularly in patients with a history of cardiac disease. Continuous assessment of body temperature is necessary since pentobarbital may cause hypothermia.
- *Monitor sedation/analgesia*
  - ✓ Propofol. Daily triglyceride levels should be monitored to evaluate for increasing trends from baseline.
  - ✓ Long-term etomidate. Adrenal suppression can persist 6 to 8 hours after a single bolus of etomidate. Therefore, cortisol levels should be evaluated every morning if continuous etomidate therapy is utilized. Glucocorticoid supplementation may be necessary.
- *Monitor hyperventilation.* ABGs should be monitored at least every 6 hours to specifically look at pco_2, which should be maintained near 35 mm Hg if ICP is adequately controlled and should always be maintained ≥ 35 mm Hg in the first 24 hours following injury. Thereafter, pco_2 may be lowered to 30 to 35 mm Hg if ICP is not controlled.
- *Monitor nutrition.* During feedings, monitor blood glucose and serum electrolytes to prevent hyperglycemia and electrolyte deficiency or excess.
- *Monitor seizure prophylaxis.* Assess for factors that may decrease seizure threshold (i.e., electrolyte abnormalities, drugs, hypoxia, infection).
- *Monitor stress ulcer prophylaxis.* Check gastric pH, output from NG tube, Hct, Hgb, and other signs and symptoms of GI hemorrhage (i.e., melena, hematemesis).

Patient Counseling

6. *What medication counseling should this patient receive if he is discharged on phenytoin?*

   - This medication is used to control seizures.
   - It is extremely important that you do not miss a dose and that you do not start or stop taking other medicine without talking to your doctor, because other drugs may affect the way this drug works.
   - Do not change brands or the amount of this drug you take without first checking with your pharmacist or doctor.
   - This medication will add to the effects of alcohol and cause you to have more drowsiness.
   - Check with your doctor if you notice any of the following symptoms while you are taking this medication: bleeding, tender, or enlarged gums; clumsiness or unsteadiness; confusion; continuous uncontrolled back-and-forth and/or rolling eye movements; skin rash; slurred speech or stuttering; muscle weakness or pain; seizures; nervousness or irritability; blurred or double-vision; and fever.
   - Good oral hygiene with frequent brushing/flossing and regular dental cleanings is essential during phenytoin therapy to prevent gum overgrowth.

References

1. Chesnut RM, Marshall LF, Klauber MR, et al. The role of secondary brain injury in determining outcome from severe head injury. J Trauma 1993;34:216–222.
2. Muizelaar JP, Marmarou A, Ward JD, et al. Adverse effects of prolonged hyperventilation in patients with severe head injury: A randomized clinical trial. J Neurosurg 1991;75:731–739.
3. Hsiang JK, Chesnut RM, Crisp CB, et al. Early, routine paralysis for intracranial pressure control in severe head injury: Is it necessary? Crit Care Med 1994;22:1471–1476.
4. Temkin NR, Dikmen SS, Wilensky AJ, et al. A randomized, double-blind study of phenytoin for the prevention of post-traumatic seizures. N Engl J Med 1990;323:497–502.
5. Reusser P, Gyr K, Scheidegger D, et al. Prospective endoscopic study of stress erosions and ulcers in critically ill neurosurgical patients: Current incidence and effect of acid-reducing prophylaxis. Crit Care Med 1990;18:270–274.
6. Black PM, Baker MF, Snook CP. Experience with external pneumatic calf compression in neurology and neurosurgery. Neurosurgery 1986;18:440–444.

54 PARKINSON'S DISEASE

▶ **On Shaky Ground** (Level II)

Mary Louise Wagner, MS, PharmD

A 73-year-old man with Parkinson's disease (PD), BPH, and hypothyroidism presents for a routine evaluation with complaints that indicate worsening of some PD symptoms. The patient is currently receiving selegiline and carbidopa/levodopa; several alterations in the patient's current medication regimen could be made to improve disease control. A dopamine agonist (pergolide, bromocriptine, pramipexole, or ropinirole) or a COMT inhibitor (tolcapone) could also be added. Only one change in the regimen should be made at a time, and doses of new agents should be increased slowly. The case highlights the importance of individualizing drug therapy for PD by timing medication administration with the reappearance of the patient's symptoms.

188 Parkinson's Disease

▶ Questions

Problem Identification

1. a. Create a list of the patient's drug-related problems.

- Progression of Parkinson's disease that is not being adequately controlled on the current medication regimen.
- The patient's insomnia can most likely be attributed to his selegiline (Eldepryl) dosing as well as to disease progression. Selegiline can cause insomnia when administered too close to bedtime.
- In addition, depression could be a contributing factor to the patient's insomnia and should be more carefully evaluated.
- Primary sleep abnormalities often occur in PD and may contribute to insomnia.
- Chronic stable problems that do not appear to require interventions at this time include (1) BPH treated with terazosin (Hytrin) with no current urinary complaints; and (2) hypothyroidism treated with levothyroxine (Synthroid) with a TSH within the normal range and no signs/symptoms of hypo- or hyperthyroidism.

b. What signs and symptoms of PD are present in this patient?

- The cardinal motor signs of PD are resting tremor, rigidity, bradykinesia (akinesia), gait problems, and postural instability. This patient manifests all of these signs; however, only his gait and postural stability have worsened since his last UPDRS exam. His resting tremor, bradykinesia, and rigidity remain stable.
- His masked facies and decreased eye blinking are signs of bradykinesia.
- Micrographia is due to bradykinesia and rigidity.
- He is also experiencing end-of-dose wearing off, which he describes as trouble walking and apathy in the afternoon, a shorter duration of effect of Sinemet, and morning dystonia (foot cramp).
- Non-motor symptoms that may be seen in PD (not all are observed in this patient) include psychological disturbances (i.e., psychosis, dementia, depression, behavioral problems), sleep disorders, autonomic dysfunction (i.e., drooling, constipation, sexual dysfunction, urinary problems, sweating, orthostatic hypotension, seborrhea), speech disturbances, and sensory changes. This patient reports decreased speech volume, depression, apathy, and seborrhea.

c. According to the Hoehn–Yahr Scale, what stage is his disease?

- The patient exhibits early signs of Stage III PD. He has bilateral symptoms and postural instability but is still able to walk and stand unassisted. Refer to Table 55–3 in textbook Chapter 55 for more detailed information.

Desired Outcome

2. What are the goals of therapy for PD?

- Currently, there is no cure for PD or therapies that are proven to delay disease progression.
- Therefore, the goals of treatment are to reduce the incidence and severity of motor and non-motor symptoms, improve activities of daily living, and minimize complications of drug therapy.

Therapeutic Alternatives

3. a. What non-pharmacologic alternatives may be beneficial for the treatment of PD in this patient?

- An *exercise program* and increased activity during the day should decrease the amount of daytime sleep and, hopefully, improve his sleep at night. Maintaining a daily routine that allows PD patients to remain as independent as possible is of psychological and physical importance.
- *Physical therapy* could teach him skills that would improve his motion and reduce his risk of falling. This is important since his risk of falling is increased due to balance and gait problems.
- *Occupational therapy* can provide information about adaptive equipment for the home, specialized clothing, and personal training that can maximize his independence, safety, and activities of daily living.
- *Speech therapy* may be helpful, but the effects in this patient probably will not be impressive.
- *Dietary modification* can improve nausea, erratic drug absorption, and minimize the risk of aspiration. However, these problems are not currently a concern for this patient.
- *Surgical procedures* have been used, but this patient is currently not a candidate for surgery because there are several medication options that have not yet been tried.

b. Based upon the patient's signs and symptoms, which pharmacotherapeutic alternatives are viable alternatives for him at this time?

- The following agents can be used to improve the motor symptoms of PD. Note that dyskinesias, insomnia, constipation, orthostatic hypotension, and psychological disturbances are common PD symptoms and may be difficult to differentiate from drug effects.
- *Anticholinergics* may be good for tremors and drooling, but they are not a good option in this patient because of his advanced age and BPH history. These agents are usually avoided or used with caution in those >60 years of age because of an increased risk of cognitive problems and hallucinations. Side effects include dry mouth, blurred vision, constipation, memory or cognition problems, urinary retention, and sedation. They also are not as good as other drug classes in controlling rigidity, bradykinesia and gait problems. Some of the available products include:
  - ✓ *Trihexyphenidyl (Artane)*
  - ✓ *Benztropine mesylate (Cogentin)*
  - ✓ *Procyclidine (Kemadrin)*
- *Dopamine agonists* are good to add to Sinemet because they are longer acting than Sinemet, decreasing off-time and improving his wearing-off symptoms. Products available include:
  - ✓ *Pergolide (Permax)*
  - ✓ *Bromocriptine (Parlodel)*
  - ✓ *Pramipexole (Mirapex)*
  - ✓ *Ropinirole (Requip)*
  - ✓ *Cabergoline (Dostinex)*

Pergolide and bromocriptine are ergot derivatives; pramipexole, ropinirole, and cabergoline are non-ergot derivatives. Cabergoline is effective for PD, but the manufacturer sought an indication for hyperprolactinemia instead of PD. Ergot side effects include pleuropulmonary and retroperitoneal fibrosis, coronary vasoconstriction, and erythromelagia (all uncommon). Non-ergot side effects include nausea, dyskinesias, somnolence, hallucinations, nightmares, confusion, postural hypotension, and transient nasal stuffiness. Dyskinesias due to dopamine agonists can be improved by decreasing the Sinemet dose.

- *Sinemet CR (levodopa/carbidopa sustained release)* is a good choice for this patient because it is longer acting than Sinemet, decreasing off-time and improving wearing-off symptoms. Bedtime administration may improve off-symptoms during the night. Some patients may need to also take standard release Sinemet when they want a quicker onset of effect such as the first morning dose. Side effects include dyskinesias, orthostatic hypotension, confusion, nausea, and psychological effects (hallucinations, nightmares, and altered behavior).
- *COMT inhibitors* include *tolcapone (Tasmar)* and *entacapone* (investigational at the time of this writing). These drugs are used in conjunction with Sinemet to prolong the action of levodopa by decreasing the peripheral catabolism of levodopa. They are also being used as adjunctive therapy to promote continuous dopamine stimulation, potentially minimizing long-term complications associated with intermittent therapy. Entacapone inhibits peripheral COMT activity, whereas tolcapone inhibits both peripheral and central COMT activity. The significance of this pharmacological difference is unknown. Side effects include GI disturbances (diarrhea, nausea, vomiting), anorexia, dyskinesias, sleep disorders, and hallucinations. Dyskinesias should improve with decreasing the Sinemet dose. COMT inhibitors are a good choice for this patient because they increase the half-life of Sinemet, decreasing off time and improving his wearing-off symptoms. Tolcapone has been associated with several cases of severe liver failure, including fatalities. For this reason, it should be reserved for use only in patients who can't take or don't respond to other drugs. AST and ALT should be monitored at baseline and then every two weeks for one year, then every four weeks for the next 6 months, and then every 8 weeks for the remainder of therapy.
- *Selegiline (Eldepryl)* is a selective, irreversible inhibitor of monoamine oxidase type B, which increases dopaminergic activity. It may also act through other mechanisms. It delays the need to start Sinemet therapy an average of 9 months in *de novo* patients. It decreases off time and improves wearing-off symptoms in patients with motor fluctuations. Side effects include nausea, confusion, hallucinations, insomnia, orthostatic hypotension, dyskinesias. Dyskinesias should improve with decreasing the Sinemet dose.
- *Amantadine* is an option of last resort in this patient because its benefits are modest. In addition, its anticholinergic properties may worsen the patient's BPH and cognitive state. Its stimulant action may worsen insomnia. Other side effects include nausea, dizziness, insomnia, livedo reticularis, peripheral edema, orthostatic hypotension, hallucinations, and confusion.

Optimal Plan

4. What drug, dosage form, dose, schedule, and duration of therapy are best for this patient?

- Discontinue selegiline because it is not helping the motor fluctuations (wearing off) in this patient. Some physicians would continue the selegiline for its theoretical effect of minimizing "oxidative stress" (slowing disease progression). There is no clinical proof, however, to support this theory. In fact, one study indicated that adding selegiline to levodopa increased mortality.[1] However, this study may be flawed for numerous reasons but primarily because patients in the selegiline group may have had a higher risk of mortality independent of the drug.
- If selegiline is continued, the dose can be decreased to 5 mg once daily. Evidence suggests that 5 mg/day is clinically as effective as 10 mg/day in patients receiving Sinemet. Furthermore, the patient's insomnia can probably be attributed to his selegiline dosing as well as to disease progression. Eliminating the evening selegiline dose could improve the insomnia.
- Change the Sinemet to Sinemet CR to address his Parkinson's symptoms and wearing-off symptoms. This dosing conversion can be made by increasing the total daily dose by 10% to 30% and decreasing the dosing frequency by one-third to one-half depending on whether the patient is stable or having wearing-off symptoms. Some practitioners double each individual dose. Then assess how long each Sinemet dose lasts, double this interval, and subtract 1 hour for the longer time to peak effect of Sinemet CR. For example, this patient receives Sinemet every 4 hours and claims that each dose does not last the full interval. Assuming the effect lasts about 3 hours in this patient, double the interval to 6 hours and subtract 1 hour to make 5 hours. Thus, this patient would receive Sinemet CR 50/200 every 5 hours while awake.
- Adding a dopamine agonist or COMT inhibitor may also be considered to achieve improved symptom control:
  ✓ *Pergolide.* Start with 0.05 mg/day and increase by 0.05 to 0.15 mg/day every few days over several weeks to a usual maintenance dose of 2 to 3 mg/day in three divided doses (the maximum dose is usually 5 mg/day; rarely, doses of 6 to 10 mg/day are used).
  ✓ *Bromocriptine.* Start with 1.25 mg/day given at bedtime for one day, then 1.25 mg BID for one week. On week 2, increase the dose to 2.5 mg BID, then increase by 2.5 mg/day every 2 to 4 weeks up to 15 to 75 mg/day (doses above 30 mg/day are rarely necessary).
  ✓ *Pramipexole.* Start with 0.125 mg TID, then increase gradually every 5 to 7 days up to 4.5 mg/day. Some practitioners use a lower starting dose of 0.125 mg QD and increase over a 2-week period to 0.125 mg TID to minimize adverse effects. Rarely, patients may use up to 6 mg/day. Use a reduced dose if the patient's creatinine clearance is less than 60 mL/min.
  ✓ *Ropinirole.* Start with 0.25 mg TID, increasing weekly by 0.25 mg/dose to an average dose of 1 to 8 mg TID. Some practitioners use a lower starting dose of 0.25 mg/day increased over a 2-week period to 0.25 mg TID to minimize adverse effects.
  ✓ *Tolcapone.* Start with 100 mg TID and decrease the daily levodopa dose if needed based on occurrence of dopamine side effects such as dyskinesias. Based on the dosing from clinical trials, the first dose of tolcapone is administered with the first dose of the day of Sinemet or Sinemet CR. The second dose is given 6 hours later, and the third dose is given 6 hours after the second dose. Some patients may take 200 mg TID, but daily doses

greater than 600 mg/day have not been adequately evaluated. Some practitioners use a lower starting dose of 100 mg once daily increased over a 2-week period to 100 mg TID to minimize adverse effects.
- It would be appropriate to either change to Sinemet CR *or* add a dopamine agonist and COMT inhibitor. However, only one change should be made at a time. Considering the patient's age, it may be prudent to reserve the dopamine agonists and COMT inhibitors for use if additional disease control is needed after reducing the dose or discontinuing selegiline and changing to Sinemet CR.
- The patient may require an antidepressant (one with low anticholinergic properties, such as paroxetine or sertraline) to control his depression if the depression does not improve when adding a PD agent that will decrease his off-time.
- The patient's seborrhea is mild enough not to treat. It often improves as the PD symptoms improve. OTC dandruff shampoos often help.

Outcome Evaluation

5. *What monitoring parameters should be used to evaluate the patient's response to medications and to detect adverse effects?*

- The sub-parts of the UPDRS and patient diaries are used to measure the patient's response to therapy and disease progression.[2] The UPDRS is a six-part scale in which each question is assigned a score ranging from 0 to 4 (none to severe). It evaluates mentation, mood, and behavior (part 1, total score of 16), activities of daily living (part 2, total score of 52), PD motor symptoms (part 3, total score of 108), complications of therapy (part 4), and stage of disease (parts 5 and 6).
- The occurrence of side effects from all medications should be assessed at each visit. Patients who experience side effects or unresolved PD symptoms between visits should call their physician. Because patients often have difficulty driving, they may be evaluated via telephone interviews.

Patient Counseling

6. *How would you counsel this patient to ensure successful therapy, enhance compliance, and minimize adverse effects?*

General Information
- Try to stay as physically active as possible.
- It is normal to have good days and bad days; do not be anxious to increase medication doses too quickly.
- It is a good idea to stay active in Parkinson's disease support groups.
- Keep a diary of symptoms and medication times just before and after clinic visits. This will help the clinicians make dose adjustments and evaluate changes that were made.

Medication Information
- Describe the adverse effects of Sinemet CR, dopamine agonists, or COMT inhibitors, depending on the agent(s) selected.
- Sinemet CR: Do not crush or chew the sustained-release formulation. The timing of doses will be based on the symptoms you are having.
- Selegiline: Do not take this medication close to bedtime. If you are taking two doses a day, take the second dose no later than 6 P.M. If insomnia is still a problem then take the second dose in the early afternoon.
- Dopamine agonists: The dosage of this medication needs to be increased slowly to minimize adverse effects. Timing of the doses will be based on the symptoms you are having.

▶ Follow-up Questions

1. *What side effects of therapy does the patient now manifest?*

- Hallucinations are dose-related side effects of all dopaminergic drugs. The relative selectivity of dopamine agonists for each of the dopamine receptor subtypes is variable. Therefore, the newer non-ergot dopamine agonists may be associated with fewer side effects. However, all dopamine agonists can induce psychiatric adverse effects, including vivid dreams, personality changes, confusion, hallucinations, paranoid thoughts, and encephalopathy. Thus, they should be used with caution in older patients and patients with a history of psychiatric illness.
- Nausea is a dose-related side effect of dopaminergic drugs.

2. *What adjustments in drug therapy do you recommend at this time?*

- The pergolide dose was too high; it should have been started at a lower dose and increased more gradually. Decrease the pergolide dose to 0.1 mg BID and observe the patient's PD symptoms and adverse effects. If his PD symptoms worsen, slowly increase the dopamine agonist dose by 0.05 to 0.15 mg per day over several weeks until the symptoms are well controlled.
- If he continues to experience nausea, decrease the dose by 50% and titrate the dose upward more gradually.
- If adjusting the pergolide dose does not improve the nausea and hallucinations, the pergolide dose should be tapered downward over several days and discontinued. A different dopamine agonist may be tried since a dopamine agonist dramatically improved the patient's PD symptoms. If the second dopamine agonist also causes hallucinations, other dopamine agonists should probably be avoided in this patient.
- Switch to Sinemet CR if the patient does not tolerate dopamine agonists.
- Another alternative that could be considered is to add a COMT inhibitor.
- If the patient continues to hallucinate after adjusting his PD medications, the following medications can be added (note that traditional antipsychotics, such as haloperidol, worsen PD symptoms and are contraindicated)[3]:
    - ✓ Clozapine (Clozaril). Start with 6.25 or 12.5 mg/day and increase the dose slowly (doses >100 mg/day are rarely needed). Weekly blood tests are required since it can decrease the WBC count. This agent also has strong anticholinergic effects that could worsen the patient's BPH symptoms and cognitive function.
    - ✓ Quetiapine (Seroquel). Although additional studies are needed, efficacy should be similar to clozapine; studies in patients with PD are currently ongoing. Unlike clozapine, it has no anticholinergic properties and no need for special monitoring.
    - ✓ Ondansetron (Zofran). This drug is a serotonin antagonist with no anticholinergic effects that may be effective in treating psychosis without worsening PD symptoms.[4] Its expense may prohibit extensive use.
    - ✓ Risperidone (Risperdal) and olanzapine (Zyprexa). These antipsychotics may worsen PD symptoms at the doses needed to control psychotic symptoms.

3. What new patient education should be provided to the patient?

- The patient should be told that the "friendly" hallucinations that he is experiencing are due to his drug therapy and should resolve once the medication dose is adjusted slowly over several weeks.
- The patient's wife should be told not to worry about the hallucinations, but to monitor his behavior for any change, such as unfriendly hallucinations and violent or unusual responses to them. In such instances, the neurologist should be contacted so that the appropriate adjustments are made to the drug therapy.

ACKNOWLEDGMENT

The author would like to thank Jacob I. Sage, MD, and Margery H. Mark, MD, for providing the patient case and for their editorial comments.

References

1. Lees AJ. Comparison of therapeutic effects and mortality data of levodopa and levodopa combined with selegiline in patients with early, mild Parkinson's disease. Parkinson's Disease Research Group of the United Kingdom. BMJ 1995;311:1602–1607.
2. Lang EA. Clinical rating scales and videotape analysis. In: Koller WC, Paulson G. eds. Therapy of Parkinson's Disease, 2nd ed. New York, Marcel Dekker, 1995: 21–46.
3. Olanow CW, Koller WC. An algorithm (decision tree) for the management of Parkinson's disease: Treatment guidelines. American Academy of Neurology. Neurology 1998;50(suppl 3):S1–S57.
4. Corboy D, Wagner ML, Sage JI. Apomorphine for motor fluctuations and freezing in Parkinson's disease. Ann Pharmacother 1995;29:282–288.
5. Zoldan J, Friedberg G, Livneh M, et al. Psychosis in advanced Parkinson's disease: Treatment with ondansetron, a 5-HT3 receptor antagonist. Neurology 1995;45:1305–1308.
6. Pappert EJ, Goetz CG, Niederman F, et al. Liquid levodopa/carbidopa produces significant improvement in motor function without dyskinesia exacerbation. Neurology 1996;47:1493–1495.

55 PAIN MANAGEMENT

▶ A Pain in the Iliac (Level II)

Karen Beauchamp, BPharm, RPh
Daniel Sageser, PharmD

Constant back pain causes a 68-year-old woman with multiple myeloma to seek medical attention. Diagnostic studies reveal the presence of compression fractures that may be due to her malignancy, to osteoporosis, and/or to her current corticosteroid regimen. Therapeutic alternatives for analgesia include opioid agonists, NSAIDs, acetaminophen, or combination products. Calcitonin, corticosteroids, and bisphosphonates may also have roles in this particular patient's treatment. After initiation of an individualized regimen, the patient should be assessed carefully for adequacy of pain relief and the presence of adverse effects. Readers of the case are asked to make further interventions after the patient develops constipation, nausea, and increased renal function tests four weeks after starting an analgesic regimen.

▶ Questions

Problem Identification

1. a. Create a list of all of the patient's drug-related problems.

- Multiple myeloma, presently treated only with corticosteroids.
- Compression fractures of unknown etiology causing pain that requires treatment.
- Diabetes mellitus is a chronic, stable problem that is apparently treated adequately with glyburide.

b. What are the possible causes of spinal fracture in this patient, and what additional diagnostic tests might be helpful in determining their etiology?

- Multiple myeloma is the most likely etiology of this patient's fractures. It is a malignant plasma cell disorder in which patients often present with hypercalcemia, bone pain, or acute renal failure. Most of this patient's laboratory values are within normal limits for her age. It is interesting that her calcium is not elevated as might be expected in multiple myeloma.
- Postmenopausal osteoporosis could be a contributing factor to her fractures. The patient is well past the onset of menopause, but she began taking estrogen just 3 years ago. Most of the bone-preserving benefits of estrogen replacement are seen in the first 5 years post-menopause.
- Long-term, high-dose corticosteroid therapy is a treatment of choice for myeloma. However, one side effect of long-term corticosteroid use is a decrease in bone density, which may also be a contributing factor in this patient.
- The patient has already undergone MRI, DEXA scan, and radiographic studies. MRI is useful in evaluating vertebral body involvement in epidural spinal cord compression and in identifying brain metastases. MRI is one of the most useful diagnostic procedures in evaluating cancer patients.
- Plain radiographic films are useful screening procedures, but a negative film should not overrule a clinical diagnosis of pathologic fracture. Radiographic films can vary in quality, and bone shadows can make pain location assessment difficult.
- Bone scans are sensitive for detecting abnormalities in bone structure and density but if positive do not establish a diagnosis of metastatic disease. Patients with osteoporosis and collapsed vertebral bodies will have positive bone scans without metastatic disease.
- CT scanning is an additional test that may have been helpful in pain diagnosis. CT can produce three-dimensional studies of bone and soft tissue lesions. CT studies can be helpful in diagnosis, assessing disease severity, and in planning surgical procedures.

c. List appropriate questions and the tools you would use in assessing pain severity and foci in this patient.

- Take a careful history of the patient's pain. This history should include a description in the patient's own words of the following:

- ✓ Site of pain
- ✓ Quality of pain
- ✓ Exacerbating and relieving factors
- ✓ Temporal pattern, if any
- ✓ Exact onset of pain
- ✓ Associated signs and symptoms
- ✓ Extent of interference with activities of daily living
- ✓ Impact on the patient's psychological state
- ✓ Response to current or previous analgesics
- Pain intensity scales are valuable tools for assessment and can include:
  - ✓ Simple descriptive pain intensity scales that range from "no pain" to "worst possible pain"
  - ✓ Numeric pain intensity scales that rank the degree of pain from 0 (no pain) to 10 (worst possible pain)[1,2]
  - ✓ Visual analog scales on which the patient marks pain severity on a blank line between "no pain" and "pain as bad as it could possibly be"
  - ✓ The Brief Pain Inventory developed by the Pain Research Group, Department of Neurology, University of Wisconsin-Madison includes qualitative and quantitative measure of patient pain. It covers pain location, effect on ADL, effect on mood, and relations with other people, among other parameters.[2]
  - ✓ Other assessment tools that may be used include the Memorial Symptom Assessment Scale, Rotterdam Symptom Checklist, and Symptom Distress Scale.[2]

Desired Outcome

2. What are the goals for pain management in this patient?

- Keeping the patient free of pain and as comfortable as possible are the primary goals. However, it may not be possible to entirely eliminate a patient's pain.
- Maintaining the patient's quality of life and ability to function as normally as possible within her family and society is also important.[3,4]

Therapeutic Alternatives

3. Compare the pharmacotherapeutic alternatives available for treatment of this patient's pain.

- *Opioid agonists* (e.g., morphine, morphine controlled release, fentanyl, hydromorphone, meperidine) provide effective pain control in moderate and severe pain, and there are no dosage ceilings. However, the opioids cause sedation; affect CNS function; cause mood changes; can cause nausea, vomiting, and urinary retention; decrease gastric motility causing constipation; and can lead to tolerance and escalating doses. Meperidine is not considered appropriate for cancer pain due to its short duration of action and the potential accumulation of its neurotoxic metabolite, normeperidine. The opioids also cause physical dependence and tolerance and must be tapered if doses are decreased.
- *Combination analgesic products* (e.g., codeine, hydrocodone, oxycodone with aspirin or acetaminophen) are effective in mild to moderate pain and can be effective in pain with an inflammatory component. However, they have defined dosage ceilings based on the aspirin/acetaminophen dosage, patient tolerance develops over long-term treatment, they can slow gastric motility and cause nausea and stomach upset, and aspirin can damage gastric mucosa and cause ulcer disease.
- *Acetaminophen* (APAP) is an effective analgesic in mild to moderate pain and is also an effective antipyretic. APAP does not inhibit platelet aggregation, affect prothrombin response, or produce GI ulceration. APAP may cause severe hepatic toxicity with high dose chronic use and in acute overdose.
- *Nonsteroidal anti-inflammatory drugs* (NSAIDs) include aspirin, choline magnesium trisalicylate, ibuprofen, diflunisal, etodolac, ketoprofen, ketorolac, naproxen, and others. They are effective analgesic agents in mild to moderate pain and have antipyretic and anti-inflammatory properties. However, each agent has daily dosing limits. All of these agents can cause adverse GI events, disrupt platelet function, and precipitate changes in renal function.
- *Calcitonin* can slow the progression of the patient's osteoporosis by inhibiting osteoclastic bone resorption, and it has also been used in the treatment of neuropathic pain. The drug can be given IM, SC, or intranasally. Calcitonin's major side effect is nausea, which can be avoided by slow escalation of the dose. Urticaria, erythema at the injection site, and intestinal cramping have been reported.
- *Corticosteroids* have been used in bone pain, neuropathic pain from compression of neural structures, and many types of cancer pain. Corticosteroids have been shown to improve appetite, decrease nausea, and reduce pain. Dexamethasone, methylprednisolone, and prednisone have all been used employing a variety of doses with success. The disadvantages associated with these agents are well known and include insomnia, nervousness, weight gain, indigestion, hypertension, osteoporosis, hyperglycemia, and increased risk of infection. This patient is currently on cyclic steroid therapy for her myeloma. Increasing the total steroid dose by adding steroids to her pain control regimen would be of questionable benefit to the patient.
- *Bisphosphonates* inhibit osteoclast activity and can reduce bone resorption, reducing the likelihood of adverse disease-related outcomes. Patients taking pamidronate and alendronate can experience fever, esophagitis, nausea, and electrolyte abnormalities.

Optimal Plan

4. Design a pharmacotherapeutic pain management plan specific for this patient.

- This patient's pain is moderate to severe in nature. The key components of the chosen regimen should be around-the-clock dosing, appropriate agents for long-term use, and a definitive plan with timelines for re-evaluation of the patient and regimen.[1,2] Generally, a step-wise approach is used in an effort to keep the regimen simple and to allow for selection of additional agents as the patient becomes tolerant or as the disease state progresses.
- Based on what the patient has used with success in the past and using tools such as the WHO analgesic ladder for cancer pain, choose agents that are effective in moderate to severe pain. Following the WHO guidelines, options include an opioid agonist, a non-opioid analgesic, and/or add an adjuvant such as an NSAID or corticosteroid.[1]
- Commonly used oral opioid agonists include morphine, morphine controlled-release, and hydromorphone. Since this patient is not currently receiving opioids, an extended-release morphine product at 15

mg every 12 hours would be an adequate starting point. She will also need a short-acting opioid for breakthrough pain or transient increases in pain. Oxycodone 5 mg every 4 hours as needed can be used initially.

- Use of an NSAID in this patient's regimen is recommended because the source of her pain is believed to be bone. NSAIDs commonly used for this purpose include aspirin, ibuprofen, choline magnesium trisalicylate, etodolac, ketoprofen, indomethacin, naproxen, and naproxen sodium. All of these agents carry some risk of adverse GI events, so the minimum effective dosage should be used. Starting doses in this patient should be conservative due to her age and potentially impaired renal function resulting from multiple myeloma.
- Acetaminophen may also be considered. A combination of an opioid with an NSAID or acetaminophen would also be an appropriate choice for breakthrough pain. For example, this patient could be started on oxycodone 5 mg/acetaminophen 500 mg tablets every 4 hours instead of oxycodone alone.

Outcome Evaluation

5. Identify monitoring parameters both for efficacy and adverse effects of your pain management plan.

- Some patients can be very stoic, whereas others may have emotional or social barriers to effective pain control. It is important to continually reevaluate pain control through interview techniques or assessment tools listed previously.[4]
- It is appropriate to call the patient or a family member the day after starting a new regimen to assess pain control. Pain assessment can be evaluated by the patient's appetite, level of activity, and overall mood as well as pain control.
- Plan to follow up or have a family member keep in contact at least weekly during the first 4 weeks of treatment and after every dosage change. After an effective regimen is established, contact can be reduced to monthly with the patient and family members doing careful, consistent self-monitoring including changes in blood pressure, stool color, appetite, respiratory rate, mood, and cognitive status.
- The patient should be seen after the first 2 to 3 weeks of treatment for objective monitoring tests: blood pressure, CBC, liver function tests (AST, GGT), BUN, and serum creatinine. Once a regimen is established and if the patient remains stable, lab tests can be reduced to every other week or even monthly.[2]

Patient Counseling

6. Outline pertinent medication information you would provide to this patient and her family regarding her pharmaceutical care plan.

Opioids

- Opioids are strong pain relievers that can be used alone or together with other drugs such as aspirin or acetaminophen (Tylenol). Using two drugs that relieve pain by different mechanisms can sometimes provide better relief than using a single drug.
- When opioids are used for a long time, your body may get used to them so that larger amounts are needed to relieve pain. This is called tolerance to the medicine. For this reason, it is important to have frequent visits or consultations with your doctor or other caregivers. Frequent communication will ensure that your medicine is working the way it should to relieve your pain and that you are not experiencing unpleasant, preventable side effects.
- This medicine may cause you to become drowsy, dizzy, lightheaded, or to have a false sense of well-being. Make sure you know how you react to this medicine before you do anything that requires your complete concentration or that may be dangerous if you are drowsy.
- You may experience dizziness or lightheadedness when getting up suddenly from a sitting or lying position. Rise slowly after sitting or lying down to prevent falls.
- Nausea or vomiting may occur, especially after the first few doses. Reclining or lying down after taking the medicine can lessen the feeling of nausea. Taking your medication with a small amount of food or after eating can also reduce nausea. Notify your doctor if nausea and vomiting persist or are severe.
- This medication may cause dryness of the mouth. Persistent dryness of the mouth may increase the chance of dental disease, including tooth decay, gum disease, and fungal infections. For temporary relief, chew sugarless gum or candy, melt bits of ice in your mouth, or use a saliva substitute.
- This medicine may cause constipation. Drinking lots of fluids will help prevent this problem. Notify your doctor if this becomes troublesome or severe.
- Avoid taking alcohol or other drugs that cause drowsiness when taking this medication.
- Signs of excessive doses of this medicine may include convulsions, confusion, severe nervousness or restlessness, severe dizziness or drowsiness, shortness of breath or labored breathing, and severe weakness.

▶ Follow-up Questions

1. How would you alter your care plan for this patient?

- If you placed the patient on an opioid, she should be receiving a bowel regimen. Regimens can vary but should be effective and safe for long-term use. As an example, docusate 100 mg po BID and milk of magnesia 10 to 30 mL po Q HS could be initiated with the narcotic. Other options include increasing dietary fiber and adding mild laxatives (senna or casanthranol) or osmotic cathartics (sorbitol or lactulose) to her regimen.
- Since this patient already has constipation, her plan would include a more aggressive approach with either frequent sorbitol or lactulose (e.g., 30 mL every 4 hours until response) or a stimulant laxative (e.g., senna) every 6 to 8 hours.
- The patient's pain is not controlled. It is important to ensure that the patient is compliant and using the medication around-the-clock. If you are convinced she is using her medications appropriately, you may elect to change her regimen. One option is to shorten the dosing schedule of the extended-release opioid (from an every-12-hour to an every-8-hour schedule). One can also increase the opioid dose. If these strategies do not achieve adequate pain control or the patient develops intolerable adverse effects, another option is to change to a different opioid, perhaps using hydromorphone, switching first to an equianalgesic dose and then adjusting the dose as needed.
- Determine whether the patient's nausea is caused by the uncontrolled pain or the pain medication. This information will help you decide whether to treat the nausea.

- The cause of the elevated renal function tests should be determined. Progressive myeloma may adversely affect renal function. Alternatively, the patient may be dehydrated because of vomiting. Fluid replacement may be needed.
- In patients with declining renal function, avoid using agents with toxic metabolites and those excreted primarily by the kidneys (e.g., meperidine). Switch from NSAIDs to acetaminophen if a non-opioid agent is still warranted.
- Renal impairment does not preclude opioid therapy, but even greater care must be taken to detect side effects by continually re-evaluating the dose, route, and efficacy.

2. *What additional monitoring parameters should you consider in an immobilized patient?*

- An immobilized patient is at increased risk for edema, hypotension, respiratory infections, bladder infections, DVT, PE, cellulitis, decubitus ulcers, electrolyte abnormalities, and depression. Frequent monitoring of vital signs, cognitive function, serum electrolytes, and creatinine are advised.

References

1. Agency for Health Care Policy and Research. Management of cancer pain: Adults. Am J Hosp Pharm 1994;51:1643–1656.
2. Portenoy RK, Ingham J. The measurement of pain and other symptoms. In: Doyle D, Hanks GWC, MacDonald N. Oxford Textbook of Palliative Medicine, 2nd ed. New York, Oxford University Press, 1993:203–219.
3. Daut RL, Cleeland CS, Flanery RC. Development of the Wisconsin Brief Pain Questionnaire to assess pain in cancer and other diseases. Pain 1983;17:197–210.
4. Ferrell BR. The impact of pain on quality of life: A decade of research. Nursing Clin North Am 1995;30:609–624.

56 HEADACHE DISORDERS

▶ Streaks of Light (Level II)

Mark S. Luer, PharmD
Susan R. Winkler, PharmD, BCPS

A 28-year-old woman with a history of migraine presents to a walk-in clinic with complaints of nausea and aura, which for her signal an impending migraine headache. The patient has received various treatments in the past and has responded well to subcutaneous sumatriptan. However, she refuses to self-administer the medication and requires medical assistance for her treatment. Effective treatment of the nausea and vomiting that often accompany migraines is as important as treating the headache itself. When selecting abortive therapy for this patient, consideration should be given to using a medication that can be given by a route that the patient can administer herself. Intranasal sumatriptan or DHE are reasonable therapeutic approaches for this patient. Use of a headache diary is an effective means of monitoring the patient's response to therapy.

▶ Questions

Problem Identification

1. a. *Create a list of the patient's drug-related problems related to this clinic visit.*

- Migraine with aura requiring abortive therapy; the most effective abortive therapy (sumatriptan) is not prescribed in a formulation that the patient is willing to self-administer.
- Non-compliance with prophylactic migraine agent (carbamazepine).
- Chronic stable problems include (1) depression which seems to be adequately treated with sertraline, and (2) endometriosis, with symptoms controlled with an oral contraceptive.

b. *What information indicates the presence or severity of the migraine headache?*

- The patient is experiencing a classic aura for her (nausea and flashing lights) which typically precede her severe migraine attacks.

c. *Could any of the patient's problems have been caused or exacerbated by her drug therapy?*

- Patients with excess estrogen have experienced migraine headaches, and those with a prior history of migraine can have an increased incidence or severity of attacks during oral contraceptive therapy.[1] Although oral contraceptives have been associated with migraine headaches, this patient is taking a low-dose estrogen product which she requires for endometriosis.
- The use of SSRIs in migraine therapy has not been well addressed in the literature. Although fluoxetine has demonstrated some benefit in preventing migraines, it has also been implicated as a possible cause of migraine with aura. Since this patient's headaches have occurred for the past 15 years and she only began taking sertraline last year, it is unlikely that the sertraline is adversely affecting her headache status.
- However, she intermittently takes sumatriptan, which enhances serotonin activity. There is considerable opportunity for a pharmacodynamic interaction, as both sertraline and sumatriptan enhance serotonergic neurotransmission. Signs and symptoms of excess serotonergic activity include nausea, weight loss, ataxia, sexual dysfunction (predominantly in males), alterations in cognition (e.g., disorientation, confusion), behavioral changes (e.g., agitation, restlessness), autonomic dysfunction (e.g., diarrhea, diaphoresis), and neuromuscular activity (e.g., myoclonus, hyperreflexia). Patients experiencing serotonergic overload (serotonin syndrome) usually respond to discontinuation of the implicated drug(s) along with supportive care. In extreme cases, treatment with antiserotonergic agents such as propranolol may be necessary.

- The patient has received effective prevention of her headaches with carbamazepine. Unfortunately, she has a history of noncompliance that can be related to the onset of her migraines.

Desired Outcome

2. *What are the initial and long-term goals of therapy for this patient?*

Initial Goals
- Reduce the severity and duration of the impending headache
- Relieve the nausea associated with the migraine attack

Long-term Goals
- Reduce the frequency of migraine attacks by improving compliance
- Identify an abortive agent that not only alleviates her pain, but one that she is willing to self-administer
- Identify trigger factors that may be exacerbating her migraines
- Enhance her quality of life, allowing her to return to normal daily activities

Therapeutic Alternatives

3. a. *What pharmacotherapeutic alternatives are available for treatment of the patient's nausea, and how will they impact potential abortive therapies?*

For some patients, the extreme nausea and vomiting associated with the headache can be more disabling and demoralizing than the headache pain itself and can directly affect the effectiveness of subsequent abortive agents. The following items need to be considered when evaluating options for relieving nausea and/or vomiting associated with migraine:
- Is an aura present or has the headache pain started? Not all people experience or can identify an aura. Although the presence of an aura may signal impending migraine pain, it may also limit or affect the timing of abortive drug administration.
    - ✓ In some instances, symptoms experienced during an aura may limit treatment if nausea and/or vomiting are a component. These may preclude the administration of an oral abortive agent early during the attack without first using an antiemetic.
    - ✓ See sumatriptan in question 4 for information on how an aura may also affect drug selection or the timing of administration of abortive drug therapies.
- Will the gastroparesis associated with the migraine attack be problematic for the administration of abortive therapies?
    - ✓ Gastroparesis can limit the bioavailability of some oral abortive agents. Both simple analgesics and the oral NSAIDs have reduced absorption during the migraine attack.
- Can the antiemetic be administered by a method other than the oral route?
    - ✓ If nausea and/or vomiting are present, administration of an antiemetic via parenteral or rectal routes may be necessary.

For this patient in whom nausea is a problem both during her aura and with her migraine, an ideal agent could be administered immediately without the limitation of her nausea.

Treatment Options and Concerns
- *Antihistamine antiemetics (e.g., dimenhydrinate, hydroxyzine)* can be given orally or parenterally. These agents cause sedation, which may or may not be advantageous. While this class of drugs might be a reasonable choice to alleviate the patient's nausea, they will not treat and may worsen gastroparesis which could limit the bioavailability of some oral abortive therapies.
- *Phenothiazine antiemetics (e.g., chlorpromazine, prochlorperazine, or promethazine)* can be administered parenterally, rectally, and orally. Each may effectively relieve the nausea and provide some direct headache relief but will likely cause sedation. In general, they do little to alleviate gastroparesis if an oral abortive agent is desired.
- *Cisapride* can be used to enhance gastric motility and improve the efficacy of some oral abortive agents but is ineffective in treating the nausea and vomiting.
- *Metoclopramide* is a good adjunctive therapy to many abortive therapies not only to treat the nausea, but also to provide some direct headache pain relief. Added benefits of metoclopramide are that it can be administered orally or parenterally and it enhances gastrointestinal motility, increasing the efficacy of some oral abortive agents. Parenteral metoclopramide can rapidly reverse gastroparesis, but oral dosage forms do not provide immediate relief.

b. *What pharmacotherapeutic alternatives are available for aborting her current migraine attack?*

In general, migraine attacks that have a fast onset (<1 hour) or are associated with severe nausea or vomiting may not respond to oral agents. Commonly prescribed agents used for abortive therapy include those listed below. This list should not be considered all-inclusive.
- *Acetylsalicylic acid* (oral)
- *Acetaminophen* (oral)
- *Ibuprofen* (oral)
- *Naproxen* sodium or *naproxen* (oral; naproxen sodium is absorbed faster than naproxen)
- *Isometheptene/dichloralphenazone/acetaminophen* (e.g., oral Midrin; limit use to ≤2 days per week)
- *Aspirin/butalbital/caffeine* (e.g., oral Fiorinal; limit use to ≤2 days per week)
- *Acetaminophen/butalbital/caffeine* (e.g., oral Fioricet; limit use to ≤2 days per week)
- *Metoclopramide* (e.g., Reglan oral or IV; risk of dystonic reaction)
- *Indomethacin* (e.g., Indocin rectal)
- *Serotonin 5-HT$_1$ receptor agonists* (limit use to ≤2 days per week; screen patients for asymptomatic cardiac disease; do not use if an ergotamine derivative has been administered within 24 hours)
    - ✓ *Sumatriptan* (Imitrex 25 and 50 mg oral tablets, 12 mg subcutaneous injection, or 5 and 20 mg nasal spray)
    - ✓ *Naratriptan* (Anerge 1 or 2.5 mg oral tablets)
    - ✓ *Zolmitriptan* (Zomig 2.5 and 5 mg oral tablets)
    - ✓ *Rizatriptan* (5 mg and 10 mg conventional oral tablets [Maxalt] and rapidly dissolving mint-flavored wafers [Maxalt-MLT] that can be placed on the tongue and taken without water)
- *Ergotamine +/− caffeine* (e.g., Cafergot oral tablets, Ergostat sublingual tablets, Wigraine rectal suppository; Medihaler Ergotamine inhaler; addition of caffeine to oral products improves absorption; pretreatment with antiemetic may be required; limit use to ≤2 days per week; administer at onset of migraine attack; contraindicated for patients with prolonged auras [>1 hour])

- *Dihydroergotamine* (D.H.E. 45 IM injection, Migranal 4 mg nasal spray; pretreatment with antiemetic is not necessary; administer at onset of migraine attack; contraindicated for patients with prolonged auras (>1 hour))
- *Ketorolac* (Toradol IM injection; useful when triptans or ergotamine derivatives are contraindicated or have failed)
- *Meperidine* (IM; useful when standard abortive therapies are contraindicated or have failed; narcotics are the preferred agents during pregnancy)
- *Butorphanol* (Stadol NS nasal spray; useful when triptans or ergotamine derivatives are contraindicated or have failed; limit use to ≤2 days per week; may cause sedation)

Optimal Plan

4. Considering this patient's past successes and failures in treating her migraine attacks, design an optimal pharmacotherapeutic plan for aborting her headaches now and in the future.

Although simple analgesics or NSAIDs are the preferred first-line pharmacologic alternatives for aborting a migraine attack, they have not proven efficacious for this patient in the past. Ergotamine tartrate caused severe nausea and should be avoided unless she is going to be pretreated with an antiemetic agent. Available options with proven efficacy or which have not yet been tried include the following:

- Sumatriptan (Imitrex SC or nasal spray). This agent has proven beneficial in the past and would be a good option. Although it is common practice to administer sumatriptan as early in the course of a migraine as possible, it has been suggested that sumatriptan not be administered until after the aura of the migraine has stopped and the headache pain has begun.[2] The symptoms of an aura are thought to relate to arterial vasoconstriction with possible ischemia resulting in neurologic dysfunction. This vasoconstrictive phase is theorized to precede the cerebral vasodilation and neurogenic inflammation responsible for the subsequent headache pain. Sumatriptan is contraindicated in conditions of ischemia. Standard practice generally dictates that the earlier the drug is given, the more effective it is in relieving headache symptoms.

   Extreme caution should always be exercised when administering sumatriptan (and probably all similar agents with vasoconstrictive properties) if the prodromal phenomena are severe (e.g., aphasia or hemiparesis). In these circumstances, waiting until the aura abates would always be prudent. For this patient, sumatriptan has been used previously without difficulties related to her aura and thus would be a good choice.

   While subcutaneous sumatriptan could be used, it will not provide this patient with an agent that she is willing to self-administer. She would have to continue to rely on visits to the physician's office. She would, however, be a good candidate for intranasal sumatriptan.[3]

   Sumatriptan nasal spray provides significant relief as early as 15 minutes after administration, which is faster than oral sumatriptan but slower than the parenteral formulation. Dosing should be individualized and can range from 5 mg to 20 mg per dose (the usual dose is 20 mg). Two unit-dose spray devices are available and can deliver either 5 mg or 20 mg per spray. A 10-mg dose can be delivered by a single 5-mg spray into each nostril. For headaches that return, a repeat dose may be administered no less than two hours after the first dose (maximum dose 40 mg/24-hour period). A second dose should not be administered if there was no symptom relief with the first dose. It should not be used to treat more than 4 migraine headaches during any 30-day period. Safety with more frequent administration has not been established. The same contraindications for SC and PO sumatriptan also apply to intranasal sumatriptan (e.g., uncontrolled hypertension, heart disease, pregnancy, or the administration of ergotamine, dihydroergotamine, or methysergide within the past 24 hours).

- Naratriptan, rizatriptan, and zolmitriptan are other triptans which produce effects statistically similar to sumatriptan in both efficacy and apparent adverse effects.[4-6] Because each new triptan is currently only available in an oral formulation, none is likely to be a good choice for this patient unless an antiemetic is first administered. The rapidly disintegrating rizatriptan oral wafer formulation (Maxalt-MLT) must still be swallowed (although with saliva, not water). It has a slower onset of action than the regular tablet and the time to reach the maximum serum concentration is longer. Refer to textbook Chapter 57 for detailed information on these agents.

- Dihydroergotamine (Migranal) nasal spray has never been used by this patient and is a viable option. The vomiting that she experienced with ergotamine tartrate is not as prevalent with the DHE nasal spray. The recommended dose is 2 mg. The dose is administered as 1 spray in each nostril, which is repeated after 15 to 30 minutes (4 sprays total). The same contraindications for parenteral DHE also apply to intranasal DHE (e.g., uncontrolled hypertension, heart disease, pregnancy, or use in combination with other vasoconstrictors).

Outcome Evaluation

5. What clinical and/or laboratory parameters should be assessed regularly to evaluate the therapy for achievement of the desired therapeutic outcome and to detect or prevent adverse effects?

Prophylactic Therapy

- Efficacy is assessed by the incidence and intensity of headaches and associated symptoms.
- Tolerance/safety is related to the potential side effects of carbamazepine (refer to textbook Chapter 52 for more detailed information).

Abortive Therapy

- Efficacy is evaluated by the intensity and duration of headaches and associated symptoms.
- Tolerance and safety depend upon the therapy chosen.
   ✓ Sumatriptan (Imitrex) nasal spray. The primary adverse effects reported include bad or bitter taste, malaise, fatigue, drowsiness, flushing, nausea, vomiting, nasal or throat irritation (i.e., burning, numbness, paresthesia, discharge, pain or soreness), tingling, dizziness, and vertigo. Additional adverse effects reported with parenteral or oral sumatriptan therapy include chest pain; wheezing; rash or hives; facial swelling; heaviness, pressure, or tightness in the chest, jaw, or neck; flushing; and ECG abnormalities. For patients with a history of chest tightness or pain who do not have a contraindicated diagnosis (e.g., angina pectoris or a history of myocardial infarction), a baseline ECG would be prudent to help rule out a cardiac conduction abnormality.
   ✓ Dihydroergotamine (Migranal) nasal spray. The major adverse effects relate primarily to the route of administration and in-

clude nasal congestion, rhinorrhea, sneezing, nasal edema, throat discomfort, nausea, taste perversion, and dizziness. Additional adverse effects reported with parenteral dihydroergotamine include numbness and tingling in the fingers and toes, muscle pain, weakness in the legs, precordial distress and pain, tachycardia, bradycardia, and vomiting.

Patient Counseling

6. What information should be provided to the patient regarding her new abortive therapy?

General Information on Use of Nasal Sprays for Migraine

- Abortive therapy is intended to relieve the effects of acute migraine and does not reduce the incidence of attacks.
- If you become pregnant or intend to become pregnant, notify your physician so that the risks and benefits of using this drug during pregnancy can be discussed.
- Disturbances in taste (unpleasant, bitter) and nasal irritation are common adverse effects and should be expected.
- If you experience persistent or severe chest pain; wheezing; heart throbbing; pain or tightness in the throat; rash; lumps; hives; or swollen eyelids, face, or lips; stop using the drug and contact your physician immediately.
- General directions for use:
    ✓ While sitting down, clear nasal secretions.
    ✓ With head in an upright position, close one nostril with index finger and exhale through mouth.
    ✓ With the opposite hand, place the nozzle of the nasal spray about one-half inch into the open nostril.
    ✓ Tilt your head back slightly and close your mouth.
    ✓ Begin inhaling through open nostril and while taking the breath, push the plunger on the nasal spray bottle.
    ✓ Remove the nozzle from nostril, keeping the head slightly tilted back for an additional 10 to 20 seconds.
    ✓ Continue to inhale through the nose and exhale through the mouth during this time.
    ✓ If you are using the dihydroergotamine (Migranal) nasal spray, repeat the dosing procedure in the opposite nostril. When the individual dose to be administered is more than 1 mg (two sprays), wait at least 10 minutes between consecutive administrations into the same nostril.

▶ Follow-up Question

1. Describe how a headache diary could help the treatment of this patient's migraine headaches (see Figure 56–1).

- Headache diaries or activity logs may be used to refine headache treatments. A headache diary is simply a document that accurately describes the headache profile and the medications taken for an attack. Each entry into the diary should include the date of attack, duration of attack, presence of aura, description of aura (if present), intensity of attack, description of pain, associated symptoms, precipitating factors (e.g., exercise, food), non-drug therapy instituted and its effect, abortive therapy required and its effect, side effects of medications, and overall impact of each headache on lifestyle or daily activities. Additional information to include in the calendar is the date and time of daily prophylactic medication administration. The information gained in a headache calendar can assist in identifying trigger factors including the overuse of abortive agents, assessing current drug efficacy and tolerance, and acts as a reminder for the patient to take the prophylactic medications as prescribed. A sample of a headache diary is included in Figure 56–1. Diaries should accompany the patient each time they visit the physician's office.

References

1. Silberstein SD. The role of sex hormones in headache. Neurology 1992;42(3 suppl 2):37–42.
2. Moore KL, Noble SL. Drug treatment of migraine: Part I. Acute therapy and drug-rebound headache. Am Fam Physician 1997;565:2039–2048.
3. Ryan R, Elkind A, Baker CC, et al. Sumatriptan nasal spray for the acute treatment of migraine. Results of two clinical studies. Neurology 1997;49:1225–1230.
4. Mathew NT, Asgharnejad M, Peykamian M, et al. Naratriptan is effective and well tolerated in the acute treatment of migraine. Results of a double-blind, placebo-controlled, crossover study. Neurology 1997;49:1485–1490.
5. Edmeads JG, Millson DS. Tolerability profile of zolmitriptan (Zomig; 311C90), a novel dual central and peripherally acting 5HT1B/1D agonist. International clinical experience based on >3000 subjects treated with zolmitriptan. Cephalalgia 1997;17(suppl 18):41–52.
6. Visser WH, Terwindt GW, Reines SA, et al. Rizatriptan vs sumatriptan in the acute treatment of migraine. A placebo-controlled, dose-ranging study. Arch Neurol 1996;53:1132–1137.

SECTION 6

Psychiatric Disorders

Barbara G. Wells, PharmD, FASHP, FCCP, BCPP, Section Editor

57 ATTENTION-DEFICIT HYPERACTIVITY DISORDER

▶ **The Keys to My Success** (Level I)

William H. Benefield, Jr, PharmD, BCPP, FASCP
Donna M. Jermain, PharmD, BCPP

A 33-year-old woman seeks a psychiatric evaluation for symptoms of attention-deficit hyperactivity disorder (ADHD). Although ADHD is usually considered to be a disorder of childhood, many patients have symptoms that persist into adulthood. First-line pharmacologic treatment generally consists of one or more trials of stimulant drugs (methylphenidate, dextroamphetamine, or amphetamine mixture). The initial dosage should be increased gradually based upon patient response and tolerance. Pemoline is considered to be an option of last resort because of concerns related to hepatotoxicity. A number of second-line treatments are available for patients who fail to respond satisfactorily to trials of two or more different stimulants. These options include clonidine, guanfacine, tricyclic antidepressants, selective serotonin-reuptake inhibitors, venlafaxine, bupropion, and monoamine oxidase inhibitors.

▶ Questions

Problem Identification

1. a. *Create a list of the patient's drug-related problems.*

   - Symptoms of ADHD presently not controlled and untreated. Approximately 50% to 70% of children have ADHD symptoms that persist into adulthood.

   b. *What information (signs, symptoms, laboratory values) indicates the presence or severity of ADHD?*

   - The patient displays numerous symptoms of ADHD which interfere with her activities of daily living. These include:
     ✓ Failure to give close attention to details
     ✓ Inattentiveness when spoken to directly
     ✓ Difficulty organizing tasks
     ✓ Forgetfulness in daily activities
     ✓ Easy distractibility
     ✓ Tendency to misplace things
     ✓ Failure to finish duties in the workplace
     ✓ Inability to meet deadlines
   - Adult ADHD may differ from childhood ADHD. Adults generally have fewer signs of excessive motor activity such as not remaining seated or running around. The hyperactivity symptoms may be seen as fidgeting or as an inner feeling of restlessness. Restlessness in the adult may lead to difficulty doing sedentary activities such as desk jobs.

Desired Outcome

2. *What are the goals of pharmacotherapy in this case?*

   - The goals of therapy are to ameliorate symptoms of ADHD, avoid drug-induced adverse effects, and restore function and stability to her day-to-day activities in both the office and home setting.

Therapeutic Alternatives

3. a. What non-drug therapies might be useful for this patient?

- Keeping an appointment book or purchasing an electronic calendar with alarm reminders may be helpful in attempts to provide structure and organizational skills on a daily basis.
- Most nonpharmacologic treatment strategies have been studied in children and include behavioral interventions such as identifying problematic behaviors and establishing interventions that use a point or token system to reward good behavior. Decreasing sensory stimulation and reducing noise may improve hyperactivity in children.

b. What feasible pharmacotherapeutic approaches are available for treatment of ADHD in this patient?

- Refer to textbook Chapter 59 for a complete discussion of the proposed biochemical abnormalities that are believed to contribute to ADHD. This will provide the background needed to understand the rationale for the pharmacotherapeutic interventions that are useful in ADHD.
- *Stimulants (e.g., methylphenidate, dextroamphetamine, and amphetamine mixture)* are usually considered the drugs of first choice unless there is such significant comorbidity that a different class of agents should be used first line. Some patients will respond to one and not to another. If a trial of one stimulant does not improve symptoms significantly, it is recommended to try a second and even a third stimulant. The sustained-release products are useful since they may be taken once daily, but there is no difference in efficacy.[1,2]
- *Clonidine* is also effective for ADHD but is more beneficial for hyperactivity symptoms. It would not be a first-line agent for this patient because hyperactivity is not a significant presenting complaint. The most common adverse effect is sedation. Clonidine is relatively contraindicated if depressive symptoms are present.
- *Guanfacine* has also been effective in the treatment of ADHD. The drug is expensive and longer-acting than clonidine. It may also have fewer adverse reactions. It appears to be less sedating and cause less mood lability than clonidine.
- *Tricyclic antidepressants* may be less effective than stimulants for ADHD. Drug tolerance has been noted after several months. Anticholinergic and cardiac effects such as orthostasis may limit their use.
- *Selective serotonin-reuptake inhibitors* (SSRIs) such as fluoxetine, sertraline, and paroxetine may be effective but may aggravate hyperactivity, especially in children.
- *Venlafaxine* has been noted to improve ADHD symptoms, but additional research is needed to define the drug's role in treatment. Some investigators believe it may replace tricyclic antidepressants in the future.
- *Bupropion* was shown to be superior to placebo for hyperactivity but not for conduct. It should be avoided if the patient has concomitant seizures or an eating disorder. Bupropion may also exacerbate tics.
- *Monoamine oxidase inhibitors (phenelzine, tranylcypromine)* may be as effective as dextroamphetamine. However, dietary restrictions and drug interactions limit the use of these drugs.
- *Pemoline* is now considered a treatment of last resort because of its potential hepatotoxicity. The hepatotoxicity is usually mild and reversible, but there have been cases of fatal liver failure and cases requiring liver transplantation.

Optimal Plan

4. a. What drug, dosage form, dose, schedule, and duration of therapy are best for this patient?

- A stimulant is a good first choice for this patient. Options and initial doses include:
  - ✓ Methylphenidate 5 to 10 mg po Q AM. If using the immediate-release preparation, the dose may be divided and given as often as morning, noon, and 4:00 PM.
  - ✓ Dextroamphetamine 5 to 10 mg po Q AM
  - ✓ Amphetamine mixture 10 mg po Q AM
- The initial dosage should be titrated based upon clinical response. Although the effect of the stimulant is noted within hours, it is best to wait 3 to 4 days before increasing the dose. If one stimulant does not work try another. Trials of several different stimulants should be recommended (except for pemoline) before changing to another pharmacologic class. Stimulants should be dosed in the morning and/or early afternoon and avoided after 4:00 p.m. to minimize insomnia.

b. What alternatives would be appropriate if the initial therapy fails or cannot be used?

- Alternative agents may be appropriate first-line therapy depending on comorbidities of the patient and clinical preference. In this patient with no comorbidity, alternative agents would be used after a trial of at least 2 stimulants. The alternative agents include:
  - ✓ Bupropion 100 to 450 mg/day
  - ✓ Venlafaxine 75 to 375 mg/day
  - ✓ Clonidine 0.05 to 0.4 mg/day
  - ✓ Guanfacine 1 to 6 mg/day
  - ✓ Tricyclic antidepressants (dosing is generally 25 to 150 mg/day)
  - ✓ SSRIs (e.g., fluoxetine 20 mg/day, sertraline 50 mg/day, paroxetine 20 mg/day)

Outcome Evaluation

5. What clinical and laboratory parameters are necessary to evaluate the therapy for achievement of the desired therapeutic outcome and to detect or prevent adverse effects?

- Onset of response from stimulants usually occurs within a few hours. It is generally recommended to wait several days before increasing the dose. Doses may need to be increased if the target symptoms indicate that she has not responded to the medication.
- After initiating therapy, the patient should return to the clinic in one week to assess for adverse reactions. One should monitor for loss of appetite, insomnia, nervousness, headache, and the onset of tics. The onset of tics may occur later, and she should be advised that this is a possibility. She should be advised that tics may present as more frequent eye blinking, shoulder shrugging, or clearing her throat more than normal.

Patient Counseling

6. What information should be provided to the patient to enhance compliance, ensure successful therapy and minimize adverse effects?

Stimulants

- It is important to take this medication exactly as prescribed.
- If you miss a dose, take it as soon as you remember. However, if it is after 4:00 PM, do not take the missed dose.
- This medicine may cause headache and nausea early in the course of treatment.
- It may also keep you awake at night, so avoid taking it after 4:00 PM. It is also advised that you take the medication with a meal or after you eat to minimize any appetite suppression.

▶ Follow-up Question

1. Given this new information, what interventions, if any, would you recommend at this time?

- Because she has had minimal response to methylphenidate 20 mg/day, one may consider increasing the dose, since studies show that methylphenidate doses up to 1 mg/kg in adults may be needed for full effect.[3] However, a dosage increase may worsen the tachycardia. Limiting her intake of coffee may be suggested, as caffeine may be contributing to her tachycardia.

References

1. Spencer T, Biederman J, Wilens T, et al. Pharmacotherapy of attention-deficit hyperactivity disorder across the life cycle. J Am Acad Child Adolesc Psychiatry 1996;35:409–432.
2. Popper CW. Antidepressants in the treatment of attention-deficit/hyperactivity disorder. J Clin Psychiatry 1997;58(suppl 14):14–29.
3. Spencer T, Wilens T, Biederman J, et al. A double-blind, crossover comparison of methylphenidate and placebo in adults with childhood-onset attention-deficit hyperactivity disorder. Arch Gen Psychiatry 1995;52:434–443.

58 ANOREXIA NERVOSA

▶ **Sweet Sixteen** (Level I)

Rae Ann Maxwell, RPh, PhD

A 16-year-old female referred to the Eating Disorders Clinic from the local ED complains of decreased energy and a "need to lose weight." The patient has multiple signs and symptoms of anorexia nervosa with a depressive component, but she has not engaged in any purging activities, such as ipecac ingestion or forced vomiting. Psychotherapy to modify eating habits, nutritional support, and group therapy involving family members are the primary methods of treatment. Antidepressants may be required if depression persists after refeeding and weight gain begin. Selective serotonin-reuptake inhibitors, especially fluoxetine, have been shown to be successful in some patients with this disorder. The primary outcome parameters include changes in eating habits, demonstrated weight gain, and elevation of mood. Overall, pharmacotherapy plays a limited role in the treatment of anorexia nervosa.

▶ Questions

Problem Identification

1. a. Create a list of this patient's drug-related problems.

- Anorexia nervosa, presently untreated.
- Malnutrition secondary to anorexia nervosa, which requires nutritional intervention.
- Depression, presently untreated.
- Constipation, possibly secondary to anorexia nervosa, presently untreated.

b. What information from the history and physical exam is consistent with a diagnosis of anorexia nervosa?

- The patient is obsessed with being thin; she perceives herself as being "pudgy" or not normal in weight.
- She has restricted her own food intake. She collects recipes of low-fat dishes and likes to prepare food for others but not herself.
- She is approximately 10 kg underweight (22 lbs or 18% below ideal body weight), which is her lowest weight to date.
- She has abused OTC weight-loss products (Dexatrim) and Lasix.
- She exercises every day to the point of excess.
- She complains of dizziness and has a history of fainting, decreased energy, and fatigue. She has an intolerance to cold.
- She is constipated, and her last menses was 1 year ago.
- She has low blood pressure.
- Her physical exam is remarkable for dry, scaly skin and hypoactive bowel sounds.
- She is 16 years old. The condition typically begins in adolescence to early adulthood (ages 14 to 18, mean onset age 17) and is more common in girls than boys.
- She is a high achiever (a straight "A" student who wants to attend Princeton).
- She prefers sports that are individual based rather than team based (track versus volleyball).
- Her home life is stressful. She has a brother with ADHD, her parents divorced when she was young, and she doesn't care for her mother's current boyfriend.
- There is a history of psychiatric disorders in her family (mother and uncle with depression, brother with ADHD).
- She comes from an upper-middle-class American family (the dis-

order is more common in industrialized countries and in middle to upper-class families) and appears to be somewhat of a loner (she does not speak of any friends).
- She has some signs of depression (decreased energy, fatigue, irritability, crying for no reason, suicidal ideation with no plan). Co-morbidity with depression, OCD, and social phobias is common in these patients.[1]

c. *What signs and symptoms of malnutrition often seen in anorexia nervosa are not exhibited by this patient?*

- Discolored skin; the skin may have a yellow hue due to hypercarotenemia from high levels of retinol and retinyl esters that may be the result of diminished conversion of beta-carotene to vitamin A
- Downy lanugo hair may be seen on the sides of the face, back or arms
- Peripheral edema
- Osteoporosis (patients may have history of fractures)
- Anemia (normochromic, normocytic type)

d. *Classify the subtype of anorexia that this patient has. How severe is the disorder at this point?*

- This patient has the restrictive subtype; she does not binge/purge and only restricts calories and intake.
- She has no history of using ipecac or vomiting (dentition is intact; no sore throat, epigastric or abdominal pain).
- Her laboratory and physical exam data do not suggest purging (she is not hypochloremic, hypokalemic, or dehydrated).
- She is in an early stage of development of the disorder.

Desired Outcome

2. a. *What are the goals of treatment for this patient?*

- Set a target weight for her to achieve in a defined period of time.
- Employ behavior modification to change eating habits so as to achieve and maintain the target weight.
- Provide education on the disorder and psychotherapy for both the patient and family members to help with underlying problems.[2,3]
- Overcome the patient's denial of the problem and her perception of self and self-worth.
- The ultimate goal is to prevent death by starvation or secondary complications.

b. *What secondary complications do you want to avoid in this patient?*

- Further cardiac involvement, including bradycardia (<60 bpm), hypotension (<90/60 mm Hg), overt changes in the ECG (prolonged QT/QTc interval, A-V junctional block), decreased cardiac size
- Renal impairment, manifested by decreased concentrating ability, dehydration, polyuria, and edema
- Hematologic complications of leukopenia, thrombocytopenia, and anemia
- Osteoporosis
- Glucose intolerance
- Immunosuppression

Therapeutic Alternatives

3. a. *What non-pharmacologic interventions must be considered for this patient?*

- *Psychotherapy* is the primary treatment for this disease rather than medications. Cognitive-behavioral and group psychotherapy may be employed. Both the patient and family members need to be involved.[3]
- *Nutritional support* is important. Patients may delete foods from their diet to reduce caloric intake or become finicky eaters. Patients need to be refed; the oral route is preferred, but tube feeding may be needed if the GI tract is not functional. TPN may be needed for non-compliant patients. Good eating habits need to be developed and reinforced through both positive techniques if she gains weight (granting of privileges or activities such as television or visitors if she is an inpatient) and negative techniques if there is no weight gain (isolation, use of tube feedings, no granting of privileges).[2]

b. *What pharmacologic interventions may be considered for this patient?*

- *Antidepressants* may be needed if depression persists after refeeding and weight gain begin. They may be helpful in preventing relapse in weight-restored patients, but data that support this contention are limited.[4]
- *Bulk-forming laxatives (e.g., psyllium)* may help to ease constipation.
- *Vitamin supplementation* may be given along with increased caloric intake.[2,4]
- *Cyproheptadine* (12 to 32 mg po daily in divided doses) is an antihistamine and serotonin antagonist that has been used with minimal success for weight gain by stimulating appetite.[4] Therapy may be initiated at 4 mg po TID and adjusted based on response. It may take 3 to 12 weeks to achieve weight gain. Once the drug is discontinued, patients usually lose the weight they have gained from the medication.
- *Prokinetic agents* (metoclopramide 10 mg po QID, cisapride 10 to 20 mg po QID) and *cholinergic agents* (bethanechol 10 mg po QID) may be used to improve delayed gastric emptying and subjective feelings of bloating. They may be helpful initially but are not beneficial for long-term use in these patients.[4]
- *Benzodiazepines* (e.g., alprazolam 0.125 to 0.25 mg or lorazepam 0.25 to 0.5 mg) are sometimes given in low doses 30 minutes before meals to decrease excessive anxiety surrounding mealtimes; their use is discouraged.

Optimal Plan

4. *Design an optimal therapeutic regimen for this patient.*

- Set a target weight for weight gain; 0.2 kg/day is appropriate.
- Provide nutritional rehabilitation by consulting a dietitian and employing behavioral modification.
- Implement feeding of frequent small meals.
- Educate the patient and family on good nutrition, eating habits, and food selection. Meal times should be a time of social interaction with family and friends and not a point of confrontation.

- Begin psychotherapy for disturbance of self-image, depression, and family conflicts. The goal is to lessen her obsession with food.
- Patients should be confined to sedentary activities, and those who purge should be denied access to bathrooms after meals to prevent purging (not a concern at this point in this patient).[2]
- Antidepressant therapy may be necessary if depression persists once the target weight has been reached. Antidepressants are usually avoided until weight is regained because (1) depression usually disappears when normal weight is approached and (2) anorexia nervosa patients do not tolerate the medications well because of side effects.
  - ✓ An SSRI is a good first choice because the patient has had suicidal ideation but no plan. Tricyclic antidepressants are not appropriate in this situation because overdoses are commonly used in attempted suicides. Cardiovascular effects, respiratory depression, and mental status changes are common signs of a tricyclic overdose. Fluoxetine is the SSRI that has been used the most widely in this population, and open-label studies support its use.[4] Doses range from 20 to 60 mg/day. It is prudent to begin at 10 mg/day for 1 week to assess for side effects and then increase to 20 mg/day. This dose should be maintained for 4 to 6 weeks for an antidepressant effect to be achieved. If depression continues after this time, the dose may be increased (especially if weight has remained stable). Treatment for depression could continue for 6 months to a year using the most effective maintenance dose. Withdrawal of fluoxetine can be attempted if the patient is maintaining her weight and has no signs of depression. A slow taper is suggested, since cases of SSRI withdrawal syndrome have been reported. The dose can be reduced by 10 mg every 4 to 6 weeks.
  - ✓ Any other SSRI (fluvoxamine 50 to 250 mg, paroxetine 10 to 40 mg, or sertraline 50 to 250 mg daily) could be used for the depression or if the patient has underlying obsessive-compulsive traits (which may coexist in these patients). However, these agents have not been as fully evaluated as fluoxetine for stimulating appetite or weight gain in anorexia nervosa patients.
  - ✓ Few patients are treated with clomipramine as first-line therapy.
  - ✓ Tricyclic antidepressants are not first-line agents due to their side effects of sedation and anticholinergic and α-adrenergic effects.

Outcome Evaluation

5. How should the therapy you recommended be monitored for efficacy and side effects?

- Monitor weight gain daily as an inpatient and as an outpatient at home. Inpatients need to maintain goal weight for 14 consecutive days prior to discharge. Weight gain should be gradual to prevent gastric dilation, pedal edema, and congestive heart failure.
- Scheduled appointments for outpatient weigh-ins at the EDC will vary from weekly to monthly, depending on the clinical situation. Weigh-ins must be standardized, using the same scale, the same day of the week, and the same clothing.
- Two minimum weights should be prospectively established prior to initiation of an outpatient behavior program.[3] Since body weight fluctuates, two weights (the lowest acceptable) for a particular patient are determined. For example, in this patient the minimum weights might be 120 and 124 pounds (approximately her ideal body weight). Outpatient monitoring is continued until the patient has maintained weight above the higher of the two minimum weights (e.g., 124 pounds in this case) for at least 6 months of consecutive weigh-ins. This would be considered successful treatment.
- Monitor electrolyte balance throughout treatment (weekly if an inpatient; outpatient assessment is initially bimonthly, then monthly, and then every 6 months as the patient's recovery continues).[2,3]
- For depression, monitor mood (which encompasses sustained feelings); change in affect (the overall emotional tone of the patient); decrease in crying spells; increased energy; and no fatigue, suicidal thoughts, or actions. Assess the patient's actions (i.e., whether she is more involved with people and is going out with friends). Several scales can be used to evaluate depression: the HAM-D, which is clinician-rated, and the Beck Depressive Inventory, which is patient rated.
- If there appears to be an obsessive-compulsive overlay to her diagnosis, YBOCS may be appropriate to perform during the treatment phase; this would help rule out any obsessions or compulsions.
- The pharmacist may monitor the purchase of disallowed OTC items (laxatives, ipecac, diet aids).

Patient Counseling

6. What information should be provided to the patient about her non-drug and drug therapies?

Note: The pharmacist should work with the physician, nurse, and dietitian to reinforce the dietary and nutritional aspects of therapy. Provide medication counseling on the proper use of laxatives (not a concern with this patient at this point); the dangers associated with chronic ipecac use (emetine toxicity), if appropriate; and warn her about the risks involved in using another person's medication (such as her mother's Lasix).

Fluoxetine (Prozac)

- This medication can be taken with or without food.
- If you take two doses a day (which may happen if the dose is 40 mg or above), it is best taken in the morning and early afternoon (before 2:00 or 3:00 PM).
- If you forget to take a dose, take the missed dose as soon as you remember. However, if it is almost time for your next dose, skip the missed dose and go back to your regular schedule. Do not take two doses at once.
- This medication make may make you sleepy or dizzy during the first week and for several days after dosage increases. These effects should go away or become less troublesome as you continue the medication. Stand up slowly from a lying or sitting position to decrease the likelihood of dizziness.
- Contact your doctor if you experience side effects such as fast heart rate, skin rash, hives, wheezing or trouble breathing, feelings of agitation or anxiety, shakiness, nervousness, or headache.
- Tell your clinician of any other medications that other doctors prescribe so that possible drug interactions are avoided.
- It may take 2 to 6 weeks before your mood begins to improve. Do not stop taking the medication on your own; whether it is because you don't feel the benefit immediately or because you feel completely better and think you don't need it any longer.

▶ **Follow-up Question**

1. *What is the likelihood of relapse or resistance to therapy?*

   - The prognosis is poor in these patients.[2-4] Denial and the need to control their perceived weight problem are the biggest obstacles to overcome in treatment.
   - Weight restoration is successful in 80% to 85% with supportive therapy; however, relapse is common.
   - Most patients have the illness for years and have recurrent exacerbations interspersed with periods of normal weight.
   - Mortality varies from 5% to 20%; death occurs from starvation, electrolyte abnormalities, or suicide.

References

1. Jarry JL, Vaccarino FJ. Eating disorder and obsessive-compulsive disorder: Neurochemical and phenomenological commonalities. J Psychiatry Neurosci 1996;21:36–48.
2. Rock CL, Curran-Celentano J. Nutritional management of eating disorders. Psychiatr Clin North Am 1996;19:701–713.
3. Walsh BT, Devlin MJ. Psychopharmacology of anorexia nervosa and bulimia nervosa and binge eating. In: Bloom FE, Kupfer D, eds. Psychopharmacology: The Fourth Generation of Progress. New York, Raven Press, 1995:1581–1589.
4. Jimerson DC, Wolfe BE, Brotman AW, et al. Medications in the treatment of eating disorders. Psychiatr Clin North Am 1996;19:739–754.

59 ALZHEIMER'S DISEASE

▶ **Irreversible, But Not Untreatable   (Level I)**

Cynthia P. Koh-Knox, PharmD
Virginia L. Stauffer, PharmD, BCPS

A 67-year-old woman with complaints of memory loss, lack of interest in daily activities, tearful periods, and difficulty sleeping is diagnosed with Alzheimer's disease (AD) and mild depression. Therapy with tacrine and sertraline is initiated. After 1 year of therapy, the patient's cognitive symptoms of AD remain unchanged, but her depressive symptoms have improved. Alternative AD therapy is considered because the patient is having difficulty remembering how to take the tacrine regimen and because elevated liver function tests are reported. Donepezil is an alternative cholinesterase inhibitor that has a once-daily administration schedule and requires no laboratory monitoring. Periodic evaluation of the patient's mental state should be performed to assess the cognitive and behavioral symptoms and progression of AD. Improvement in symptoms may not be seen for several months after the initiation of therapy.

▶ **Questions**

Problem Identification

1. a. *Create a list of the patient's drug-related problems.*

   - Unchanged MMSE score and global deterioration scale since the original diagnosis.
   - Elevated liver enzymes/hepatic impairment probably due to tacrine therapy.
   - Recent weight loss.
   - Glaucoma of unknown severity, presently untreated.
   - Depression, with symptoms improved on treatment with sertraline.
   - GERD is a chronic stable problem not requiring intervention at this time; this problem may resolve with tacrine discontinuation.

   b. *What information (signs, symptoms, laboratory values) indicates the presence or severity of Alzheimer's disease?*

   - Cognitive deficits and noncognitive/behavioral symptoms are unchanged as reported by family members.
   - Folstein MMSE score (20/30) is slightly increased from the initial clinic visit.

   c. *Could any of the patient's problems have been caused by drug therapy?*

   - Tacrine use has been associated with elevated liver enzymes, anorexia/weight loss, and GI problems (nausea, vomiting).
   - Elevated liver enzymes may lead to hepatic dysfunction. Impaired hepatic function can lead to increased sertraline levels due to decreased metabolism.
   - Weight loss can be a symptom of depression. This may indicate that the antidepressant therapy has not been completely effective or that sertraline is causing GI irritation.
   - Compliance is difficult for the patient and family members due to the complexity of the alternating tacrine doses and the QID regimen.
   - Folstein MMSE score reveals that cognitive status is unchanged or stable with the current tacrine regimen, and the global deterioration scale is unchanged.

Desired Outcome

2. *What are the goals of pharmacotherapy in this case?*

   - Provide palliative treatment of existing cognitive and noncognitive/behavioral symptoms (AD is incurable)
   - Slow or retard the progression of AD
   - Prevent harm/danger to the patient
   - Delay nursing home placement
   - Prevent further weight loss

Therapeutic Alternatives

3. a. *What non-drug therapies might be useful for this patient?*

   - Family education and counseling about AD and the importance of their support as caregivers in the treatment of the patient.
   - Recognizing nutritional problems and maintaining adequate

nutrition. Cognitive problems, (e.g., forgetting to buy or cook food and eat meals, swallowing difficulties) may lead to malnutrition.
- Wander-guard devices are available to protect the patient from harm or danger.[1]

b. *What feasible pharmacotherapeutic alternatives are available for the treatment of Alzheimer's disease?*

Treatment of Cognitive Deficits
- *Donepezil (Aricept)* is a reversible cholinesterase inhibitor approved for the treatment of AD. Its advantages over tacrine (Cognex) include once-daily dosing, minimal adverse effects, and lower cost of therapy. Efficacy and safety have been demonstrated by statistically significant improvement in cognitive assessment scales when compared to placebo. There have been no trials directly comparing donepezil and tacrine. The incidence of treatment-emergent adverse effects with donepezil is comparable to placebo. Once-daily dosing increases patient compliance, and donepezil has no clinically significant effects on vital signs, biochemical tests, or hematology tests. It is not associated with hepatotoxicity as seen with tacrine use. Donepezil and tacrine are comparable in drug cost, but the overall cost of donepezil is less due to lack of need for liver enzyme monitoring.[2]
- *Estrogen* has been studied for the treatment of AD, mainly for its antioxidant effect and potential neuroprotective effects on the brain. There have been reports of improvement in attention, calculation, memory, mood, orientation in time and space, social interaction, and daily activities.[3] Estrogen has not yet received FDA approval for this indication.
- *Ginkgo biloba* is approved in Germany (but not in the United States) for treatment of dementia. It has been reported to improve cognitive performance and social functioning for 6 months to 1 year. One study used Ginkgo biloba extract 40 mg po 3 times daily with a low incidence of adverse effects.[4]
- *Alpha-tocopherol (vitamin E)* has been studied in patients with AD. Sano et al reported that 2000 IU per day resulted in positive effects on cognitive function and in slowing the progress of disease.[5]

Treatment of Noncognitive Symptoms and Behaviors
- Pharmacologic therapy may be considered when patients display symptoms and behaviors such as depression, disruptive behavior, or aggression.[1] Agents commonly used to treat these symptoms include:
  - ✓ *Antidepressants* (e.g., desipramine, nortriptyline, fluoxetine, paroxetine, sertraline, and trazodone)
  - ✓ *Antipsychotics* (e.g., haloperidol, risperidone, olanzapine)
  - ✓ *Anticonvulsants* (e.g., carbamazepine, valproic acid)
  - ✓ *Miscellaneous agents* (selegiline, buspirone, oxazepam, lorazepam)

c. *What economic, psychosocial, racial, and ethical considerations are applicable to this patient?*

- This patient is fortunate to have many children who are able and willing to share the caregiving responsibilities.
- Simplification of her medication regimen will enhance their continued desire to keep her at home rather than placing her in a nursing home.

Optimal Plan

4. a. *What drug, dosage form, dose, schedule, and duration of therapy are best for this patient?*

Treatment of Cognitive Deficits
- Tacrine (Cognex) can be discontinued because of its apparent lack of efficacy and the emergence of elevated hepatic enzymes.
- Donepezil (Aricept) can be initiated 2 to 3 days after stopping tacrine, with 5 mg po at bedtime daily for four weeks, then increased to 10 mg daily. Therapy should be continued for 3 to 6 months before assessing effectiveness of treatment.
- Estrogen and vitamin E may be considered to improve cognitive and social functioning. Gingko biloba may not be a desirable addition to therapy due to its dosing regimen. These three agents are not FDA approved, and (as with other unlabeled uses) the clinician should assess the risks versus benefits before initiating therapy.

Treatment of Noncognitive Symptoms/Behaviors
- The patient has been on sertraline for more than a year. Depressive symptoms appear to be improved or resolved based on reports of increased family interaction and happier, less tearful periods. Therefore, discontinuation of antidepressant therapy may be considered. Although she is taking the lowest recommended daily dose, tapering over 1 to 2 weeks before discontinuing medication will reduce the risk of recurrent depressive symptoms and possible withdrawal effects, such as GI symptoms.

b. *What alternatives would be appropriate if the initial therapy fails or cannot be used?*

- At the time of this writing, there are no other approved options for treating the cognitive deficits. If further treatment is desired after failure of approved therapies, the patient/caregivers may opt to try an investigational agent. However, the risks and benefits should be carefully assessed. It is important for the patient and family to understand that AD is not curable.
- If agitation or psychotic behaviors occur, consider antipsychotics that do not affect cognitive behavior.[1]

Outcome Evaluation

5. *What clinical and laboratory parameters are necessary to evaluate the therapy for achievement of the desired therapeutic outcome and to detect or prevent adverse effects?*

- Progression of AD and cognitive decline should be assessed regularly. The Folstein MMSE or other mental state tests can be given to assess the cognitive and behavioral symptoms and progression of AD. It is best to use the same tests for consistency in assessment methods.
- A positive response to donepezil therapy can be observed by improvements in symptoms, an unchanged or maintained level of functioning, or a slower rate of decline.
- AD continues to progress during therapy, and donepezil does not alter the underlying disease. Therefore, improvement of symptoms may not be noted for several months.[2]

- The most common adverse effects associated with donepezil are diarrhea, insomnia, nausea, and vomiting. The rate of discontinuation from donepezil treatment due to adverse events is not significantly different from placebo.
- Donepezil therapy does not require laboratory monitoring.

Patient Counseling

6. What information should be provided to the patient to enhance compliance, ensure successful therapy, and minimize adverse effects?

- Family and caregivers should be included in counseling and instruction because of their strong involvement in the care of the AD patient. Interviews with caregivers and patients are useful when assessing the patient's response to therapy.

Donepezil

- This medication, called donepezil or Aricept, is in the same drug class as tacrine (Cognex), but the regimen is simpler to take.
- Take (or give) one tablet (5 mg) orally once daily at bedtime for 4 weeks. We will assess your response after about 4 weeks and may increase your dose at that time.
- This medication may be taken with or without food.
- Effects may not be seen for several weeks or even longer, so have patience and continue taking it as prescribed.
- Do not stop taking this medication or increase the dose unless your doctor instructs you to do so.
- If you miss a dose and you remember before you go to bed, take the dose. If you remember in the morning, skip the dose and take the next dose as scheduled. Never take double doses.
- Nausea, vomiting, and diarrhea are common side effects that may appear in a few days. They will resolve as therapy continues. Inform your physician or pharmacist if these effects are unbearable.
- Always ask your doctor or pharmacist about new prescribed medications to make sure that it is all right to take them with this medicine.
- Avoid using over-the-counter anti-inflammatory drugs such as ibuprofen (Motrin-IB, Advil), naproxen (Aleve), or ketoprofen (Orudis-KT). Using these types of medications with Aricept may lead to stomach irritation.

Sertraline Discontinuation

- Because your depression has improved, you can stop taking the sertraline (Zoloft), but this has to be done gradually. Take one-half tablet (25 mg) once daily at the same time each day for 1 week. Taking it at bedtime with Aricept may make it easier for you to remember. After 1 week at the lower dose, you can stop taking it altogether.
- Contact your doctor if you experience any problems such as upset stomach, diarrhea, nervousness, feeling sad, or decreased energy.

References

1. Filley CM. Alzheimer's disease: It's irreversible but not untreatable. Geriatrics 1995;50:18–23.
2. Rogers SL, Friedhoff LT, and the Donepezil Study Group. The efficacy and safety of donepezil in patients with Alzheimer's Disease: Results of a US multicentre, randomized, double-blind, placebo-controlled trial. Dementia 1996;7:293–303.
3. Paganini-Hill A, Henderson VW. Estrogen in the treatment and prevention of Alzheimer's disease. Int J Pharmaceutical Compounding 1998;2:24–29.
4. Le Bars PL, Katz MM, Berman N, et al. A placebo-controlled, double-blind, randomized trial of an extract of Gingko biloba for dementia. North American EGb Study Group. JAMA 1997;278:1327–1332.
5. Sano M, Ernesto C, Thomas RG, et al. A controlled trial of selegiline, alpha-tocopherol, or both as treatment for Alzheimer's disease. The Alzheimer's Disease Cooperative Study. N Engl J Med 1997;336:1216–1222.

60 ALCOHOL WITHDRAWAL

▶ **No More Drinking and Driving (Level I)**

Jill Slimick-Ponzetto, PharmD, BCPS

A 69-year-old man presents to the emergency department seeking help to stop drinking. He has just been released from jail after serving a 2-day sentence for driving while intoxicated. He reports drinking about 750 mL of vodka per day for the past 7 to 8 years. Because the patient has been required to abstain from alcohol for at least 2 days, he displays signs and symptoms of alcohol withdrawal upon examination. He ultimately becomes agitated, experiences auditory hallucinations, and must be physically restrained. The treatment of choice for acute alcohol withdrawal symptoms is a benzodiazepine; some clinicians prefer long-acting agents (diazepam or chlordiazepoxide), whereas others prefer shorter-acting agents (e.g., lorazepam). This patient also requires thiamine, magnesium repletion, and fluid and electrolyte replacement with dextrose-containing IV solutions.

▶ Questions

Problem Identification

1. a. Create a list of the patient's drug-related problems.

- Alcohol dependence and withdrawal, requiring treatment.
- Post-traumatic stress disorder, presently untreated.
- History of depression, currently untreated.
- Hypertension, uncontrolled on present felodipine regimen (which may be due to acute alcohol withdrawal).
- Benign prostatic hyperplasia, symptoms currently treated with prazosin.
- Unspecified GI upset, self-treated with Gaviscon.

b. What information (signs, symptoms, laboratory values) indicates that the patient is going through alcohol withdrawal?

- *Signs:* Sweating, tremor, tachycardia, elevated BP, elevated body temperature, exaggerated reflexes.

- *Symptoms:* Complaints of vomiting, sweating, shaking, auditory hallucinations, nervousness, and anxiety
- *Laboratory values:* The fact that his alcohol level was negative is consistent with alcohol withdrawal. The elevated GGT is consistent with recent alcohol ingestion.

c. *What signs and symptoms are consistent with delirium tremens?*

- *Signs:* Confusion, fever, agitation, tachycardia, diaphoresis, occasional premature heartbeats.
- *Symptoms:* Auditory hallucinations.

d. *What signs, symptoms, and history are consistent with alcohol dependence in this patient?*

- 8-year history of drinking 750 mL of vodka/day
- Recent conviction for driving while intoxicated
- History of alcohol abuse and failed rehabilitation attempts in the past

e. *What laboratory abnormalities may be expected in a patient with a history of alcohol abuse?*

- Elevated AST, ALT, GGT, alkaline phosphatase, and bilirubin levels are consistent with liver toxicity
- Low magnesium levels (as seen in this patient) indicate electrolyte imbalance
- Other laboratory abnormalities associated with alcoholism, but not exhibited in this patient, include low hemoglobin, hematocrit, and albumin; and elevated MCV and MCH (due to folate and/or vitamin B_{12} deficiency).

Desired Outcome

2. *What are the short-term and long-term goals of pharmacotherapy in this case?*

Short-term Goals
- Achieve rapid control of withdrawal symptoms and delirium tremens (DTs)
- Prevent withdrawal complications (e.g., seizures, hallucinations)
- Prevent complications of alcohol dependence such as Wernicke's encephalopathy
- Correct fluid, electrolyte, and vitamin abnormalities

Long-term Goals
- Prevent or control alcoholic liver disease
- Maintain abstinence from alcohol
- Treat coexisting psychiatric disorders that complicate recovery

Therapeutic Alternatives

3. *What pharmacotherapeutic alternatives are available for the treatment of alcohol withdrawal and to prevent further alcohol withdrawal complications?*

- *Benzodiazepines* have anticonvulsant activity and demonstrated effectiveness in controlling the signs and symptoms of alcohol withdrawal and DTs. They are favored over barbiturates because they are safer at higher doses, have fewer adverse effects on the liver, and less respiratory depression. When choosing a benzodiazepine, one must consider the pharmacokinetic differences between them. The duration of the desired effect and the patient's liver and renal function are also important factors to consider. Agents with a shorter duration of action have the advantage of easier dosage adjustment and less risk of excessive sedation. Agents with longer durations of action have the advantage of smoother withdrawal from alcohol. One of the four benzodiazepines available in parenteral forms may be selected for initial therapy:
  - ✓ *Diazepam* and *chlordiazepoxide* are long-acting drugs that are preferred by some clinicians because they effectively control withdrawal symptoms with few rebound effects after they are discontinued. However, both drugs are metabolized in the liver to active metabolites, so they have the potential to accumulate in elderly patients and in patients with hepatic dysfunction. IM injections of these two drugs are erratically and poorly absorbed.
  - ✓ *Midazolam* has a very short half-life and duration of action, but its clinical experience in treating DTs is limited. There is no oral form for continuation of therapy.
  - ✓ *Lorazepam* and *oxazepam* are short-to intermediate-acting drugs that have no active metabolites, are less affected by liver dysfunction, and have few residual sedative effects after discontinuation. Lorazepam has the advantage of being available in both parenteral and oral dosage forms.
- *Barbiturates* also have anticonvulsant activity and may be effective in controlling the signs and symptoms of alcohol withdrawal and DTs. However, controlled trials documenting efficacy for treatment of alcohol withdrawal or DTs are lacking. For this reason and the other reasons outlined above, they not considered to be first-line agents.
- *Carbamazepine* has only been studied for use in alcohol withdrawal in the United States on a limited basis; it also is not recommended as a first-line therapy.
- *Sympatholytics (e.g., β-blockers)* may be useful in controlling symptoms of marked autonomic nervous system hyperactivity that is associated with withdrawal. However, they may mask or block the signs and symptoms of withdrawal, therefore clouding the picture of withdrawal, which may lead to DTs and seizures. The sympatholytics may be useful in decreasing blood pressure and heart rate, which may be beneficial in many patients. They should not be used as monotherapy because they do not have anticonvulsant activity.
- *Clonidine* is an α_2-agonist that has a negative feedback inhibitory effect on noradrenergic discharge. Activation of this negative feedback system decreases adrenergic activity and produces relief of withdrawal symptoms. However, studies of its use for alcohol withdrawal are inconclusive, and it may not prevent severe withdrawal symptoms, such as seizures. Until further data are available that document its efficacy and safety, clonidine should not be considered a first-line agent.
- *Supportive nutritional, electrolyte, and fluid replacement therapies:*
  - ✓ *Thiamine* is given to replace thiamine stores and to prevent Wernicke's encephalopathy. A common supportive therapy regimen is thiamine 100 mg IM for one dose, followed by 100 mg orally each day thereafter.
  - ✓ *Magnesium* needs to be given because the patient is hypomagnesemic; replacing his deficit may increase the seizure thresh-

old. This may be accomplished by giving magnesium IM (e.g., 1 g) daily for 1 to 3 days. Oral supplementation may be continued thereafter if necessary.
- ✓ *Fluid and electrolyte replacement* is necessary to correct dehydration and electrolyte disturbances. Dextrose 5% in 0.45% saline solution is given if the serum sodium is normal. If the patient has hyponatremia, then correction with dextrose 5% in 0.9% saline is appropriate. The serum glucose concentration should be monitored. Hypoglycemia may occur and add to the patient's confusion and agitation. Hypoglycemia should be corrected with 50% dextrose after thiamine has been administered.
- ✓ A *multivitamin supplement* may be given daily to replete other vitamins that may be deficient due to chronically poor dietary intake.

Optimal Plan

4. *Design an optimal pharmacotherapeutic plan to rapidly control withdrawal symptoms in this patient and to prevent further withdrawal complications. Explain the rationale for your selections.*

- Benzodiazepines are the drugs of choice for alcohol detoxification (the treatment of acute withdrawal from alcohol).[1-3] Treatment should be initiated with parenteral therapy to obtain rapid control of withdrawal symptoms and DTs. Lorazepam is a good option because it has a rapid onset of action, and rapid control of this patient's agitation and hallucinations is desirable. One sample regimen is lorazepam 2 mg IM, repeated after 2 hours if necessary. This may be followed by a detoxification taper schedule as follows: lorazepam 2 mg QID × 2 days, then 2 mg TID × 2 days, then 2 mg BID × 2 days, then 2 mg QD × 1 day, then discontinue. An as-needed dose of lorazepam 2 mg IM may also be added to the regimen for seizures, hallucinations, and agitation. Refer to the associated textbook chapter for the typical dosage regimens of other benzodiazepines.
- Give thiamine 100 mg IM × 1 dose and then 100 mg po daily thereafter.
- Give magnesium supplementation (e.g., 1 g IM the first 1 to 3 days) followed by oral supplementation each day thereafter if necessary.
- Give an oral multivitamin preparation daily.
- Administer fluid and electrolyte replacement therapy (e.g., dextrose 5% in 0.45% saline solution by continuous IV infusion).

Outcome Evaluation

5. *What clinical and laboratory parameters are necessary to evaluate your chosen therapy for the achievement of desired outcome and to detect or prevent adverse effects?*

Efficacy Parameters

- The Clinical Institute Withdrawal Assessment Scale for Alcohol revised (CIWA-Ar) is a validated tool for the measurement of symptom severity in alcohol withdrawal.[4] Monitoring should be done frequently initially while the patient is symptomatic, such every hour. As the symptoms become under control, they can be monitored less frequently, such as 3 times a day.
- Specific signs and symptoms of withdrawal to be observed include nausea and vomiting, paroxysmal sweats, agitation, headache, anxiety, tremor, visual disturbances, tactile disturbances, auditory disturbances, orientation and mental status, blood pressure, pulse, seizures, and fevers. Vital signs should improve, and the signs and symptoms of withdrawal should improve. Worsening of withdrawal symptoms may be exhibited as worsening vital signs and increased hallucinations, agitation, and tremors.

Adverse Effect Parameters

- The adverse effects of benzodiazepines to monitor for include drowsiness, lethargy, ataxia, confusion, dizziness, amnesia, and respiratory depression.

Patient Counseling

6. *What information should be provided to the patient to enhance compliance, ensure successful therapy, and to minimize adverse effects?*

- Educate the patient about the current treatment regimen and inform him that the withdrawal signs and symptoms will go away after several days.
- Educate the patient about alcoholism and encourage him to participate in some type of treatment program for the alcohol dependence.
- Encourage the patient to report any adverse effects of therapy.

References

1. Mayo-Smith MF. Pharmacological management of alcohol withdrawal: a meta-analysis and evidence-based practice guideline. The American Society of Addiction Medicine Working Group on Pharmacological Management of Alcohol Withdrawal. JAMA 1997;278:144–151.
2. Saitz R, O'Malley SS. Pharmacotherapies for alcohol abuse: Withdrawal and treatment. Med Clin North Am 1997;81;881–907.
3. Moskowitz G, Chalmers TC, Sacks HS, et al. Deficiencies of clinical trials of alcohol withdrawal. Alcohol Clin Exp Res 1983;7:42–46.
4. Sullivan JT, Sykora K, Schneiderman J, et al. Assessment of alcohol Withdrawal: The revised clinical institute withdrawal assessment for alcohol scale (CIWA-Ar). Br J Addict 1989;84:1353–1357.

61 NICOTINE ADDICTION

▶ **Kicking Mr. Butts** (Level I)

Julie A. Cold, PharmD, BCPP

A 55-year-old woman with emphysema, hypothyroidism, and osteoporosis presents to the community pharmacy with complaints of increased difficulty breathing. She currently smokes two packs of cigarettes per day and has smoked for 40 years. In this situation, the pharmacist should ask about her smoking status and educate her about the adverse effects that smoking has upon the body. When the patient is ready to stop smoking, several non-drug therapies should be implemented, such as discarding tobacco-related items and joining a smoking cessation support group. There are numerous OTC and prescription products available to help the smoker become abstinent, including nicotine replacement products (gum, transdermal patches, nasal spray, and oral inhaler) and bupropion. An OTC transdermal system is a good initial option because it does not require a visit to a physician. When this patient develops a skin rash and reports other problems with a nicotine transdermal system, several options are available, including changing to a different patch. When the patient relapses after trying the patch for 8 weeks, a trial of bupropion therapy may be a reasonable therapeutic option.

▶ Questions

Problem Identification

1. a. *Create a list of this patient's drug-related problems.*

   - Chronic cigarette smoking resulting in symptomatic chronic obstructive lung disease (COLD); lack of the Atrovent inhaler for the past 2 weeks has left the emphysema untreated.
   - Hypothyroidism treated with levothyroxine; the adequacy of treatment is unknown because of the lack of physical examination and laboratory data.
   - Post-menopausal status treated with Premarin (conjugated equine estrogens).
   - Osteoporosis treated with Fosamax (alendronate); the effectiveness of treatment cannot be evaluated with the available data.

   b. *What information in the patient's history can be identified as disease or symptomatology that is probably directly related to the consumer's smoking history?*

   - Emphysema
   - Early-onset menopause
   - Osteoporosis
   - Increased incidence of skin wrinkling
   - Smoking-related illnesses can affect many different systems in the human body. In addition to this consumer's own smoking history (2 ppd × 40 years = 80 pack-years), she was exposed to environmental tobacco smoke (ETS) as she was growing up, so her cumulative exposure to tobacco smoke is great. ETS exposure is more toxic than cigarette smoke directly inhaled from her own cigarettes. ETS is not filtered and introduces all of the toxins created at the burning end of the cigarette into the environment. Tar and nicotine exposure is significantly higher with ETS than with the mainstream smoke (i.e., what the smoker inhales from the cigarette).

   c. *What stage of change for smoking cessation is the consumer in at this time?*

   - This consumer is in the contemplation stage of change that is noted in smokers who are trying to quit. The process for a smoker to achieve a smoking abstinent state is dynamic, consisting of 5 stages which the smoker may move between during the attempt to quit smoking.[2]
     1. In the *precontemplation stage* the smoker has not seriously considered quitting. However, the pharmacist should ask about smoking status at each contact and clearly state to the consumer that smoking is causing adverse effects upon the body.
     2. In the *contemplation stage* the smoker has considered seriously quitting but has not made any commitments to become smoking abstinent. At this stage the pharmacist should educate the smoker about the adverse effects of smoking and the positive effects of living a smoke-free life. The smoker should be encouraged to make the decision to quit smoking (with the pharmacist's help), set a date to quit smoking within 2 weeks of the contact, and prepare to quit and be educated about the available options (both pharmacologic and non-pharmacologic) to help the smoker quit.
     3. The *action stage* occurs when the smoker has tried to quit smoking or has recently quit smoking. At this stage, the pharmacist is a resource to support the former smoker in his or her decision to quit smoking and to provide education about nicotine withdrawal and coping skills.
     4. In the *maintenance stage* the smoker has quit smoking and the pharmacist should support the abstinent state and encourage recognition of the many obstacles the smoker overcame to accomplish this smoke-free life.
     5. The fifth stage is *relapse*—a time when the smoker has had a "slip" (smoked one or two cigarettes) or has resumed smoking at the previous level. The pharmacist should encourage this person to try to quit smoking again and never use this situation to shame the consumer.
   - Despite the stage of change that the smoker is currently in (except if maintenance has been achieved for many years), the consumer should always be queried about current smoking status, and the pharmacist should provide stage-appropriate smoking cessation intervention that is relevant to the consumer and includes education about the risks of continued smoking. Even a 3-minute intervention may be enough stimulus to cause some smokers to quit smoking.

   d. *What signs or symptoms in this consumer's presentation indicate the severity of this consumer's nicotine addiction?*

   - She continued smoking despite the smoking-related illnesses that she is exhibiting. In this scenario, the emphysema is the most acute problem being displayed.

   e. *List other questions that you can ask the consumer to determine her dependence upon nicotine.*

   - The Fagerstrom test for nicotine dependence has six questions that are used to assess the degree of nicotine dependency displayed by a person.[3] Two questions are easily asked and can help the pharmacist evaluate the degree of nicotine dependency.
     1. The consumer should be asked about the total of number of cigarettes smoked per day. Consumers who smoke more than 20 cigarettes/day have a higher nicotine dependency.

2. The consumer should also be queried about which cigarette would be the hardest to give up. If the consumer states it would be the first cigarette of the day, then this response also indicates a high degree of nicotine dependence. The consumer with a high degree of nicotine dependence may be more likely to achieve smoking abstinence when pharmacotherapy is part of the comprehensive plan to quit smoking.

Desired Outcome

2. What are the goals of smoking cessation pharmacotherapy in this case?

- Achieve and maintain smoking abstinence with minimal nicotine withdrawal symptoms.
- Delay the progression of smoking-related illnesses, particularly emphysema.
- Permit a better response to pharmacotherapy for other diseases after smoking cessation.

Therapeutic Alternatives

3. a. Describe non-drug therapies that may help this consumer quit smoking.

- *Skills building* involves implementing coping skills to address nicotine craving and being around others who continue to smoke.
- *"Readying the environment"* includes discarding all tobacco paraphernalia (i.e., lighters, ashtrays, clothing with tobacco advertisements) and thoroughly cleaning the home, vehicle, and workstation.
- *Social support* means that the smoker informs family, friends, and acquaintances that an attempt to quit smoking is being made. Positive support from this social group is very beneficial.
- *Joining a smoking cessation support group* should also be considered. Alternatively, the patient can rely upon his or her pharmacist or other health care provider for support and positive feedback.

b. What feasible pharmacotherapeutic alternatives are available for the treatment of the nicotine dependence?

- *Nicotine replacement products* that are available OTC should be explored first with this consumer because she can start using a product immediately without taking the time for a physician visit.
  - ✓ *Nicotine gum* is available in 2 and 4-mg doses.
  - ✓ *Nicotine transdermal systems* (NTS) such as Nicoderm-CQ and Nicotrol differ primarily by their dosing schedules. Nicoderm-CQ is worn 24 hours a day for 8 weeks, and Nicotrol is worn for 16 hours a day for 6 weeks.
  - ✓ All nicotine replacement products (both OTC and prescription) are equally effective; approximately 25% of smokers quit with each product. Even with these relatively low success rates, the AHCPR guidelines recommend that the nicotine patches be considered first-line treatment.
- *Some NTS, nicotine nasal spray, nicotine oral inhaler, and bupropion* are prescription products that are FDA-approved for the treatment of smoking cessation.[4] The cost of these products is equal to the cost of 1½ pack of cigarettes per day. All of the nicotine replacement products are helpful in preventing nicotine withdrawal because they provide a limited quantity of nicotine to the smoker who is trying to quit. In contrast, bupropion specifically works by decreasing nicotine craving.
  - ✓ Nicotine gum, nasal spray, and oral inhaler provide a bolus nicotine dose to abate withdrawal symptoms. The nicotine dose is self-regulated by the smoker. These products provide oral pleasure for the smoker that may help him or her cope with the loss of oral stimulation from the cigarette. However, detailed instructions must be provided concerning proper use; they provide variable nicotine concentrations; nicotine dependence has been reported; and the gum is contraindicated in denture wearers or those with temporomandibular joint disease. Nasal spray administration can be observed by others and causes mucosal stinging.
  - ✓ Nicotine transdermal systems (OTC and prescription) are associated with fewer compliance problems. Limited clinician time is needed to explain proper use of product; they are available in once-a-day dosing regimens and they avoid variability in nicotine concentrations. However, sensitivity to nicotine or the adhesives in the patch may occur.
  - ✓ Bupropion decreases nicotine craving and has an antidepressant effect. Continued smoking is allowed while a therapeutic bupropion level is titrated during the first week of treatment. It has a simplified dosing schedule compared to nicotine gum, spray, or inhaler. However, it does not provide nicotine to help curb other withdrawal symptoms. Bupropion is contraindicated in persons with seizure disorders (either active or a past history). It is also contraindicated in persons with a current eating disorder.
- *Antidepressants* (e.g., doxepin, imipramine, fluoxetine), *antianxiety medications* (i.e., benzodiazepines and buspirone), *clonidine,* and *weight reduction products* are alternative agents used to encourage smoking cessation. Combination therapy is usually reserved for the consumer who has repeatedly tried to quit smoking; different aspects of the relapse process necessitate this type of treatment. Since this is the consumer's first attempt to quit smoking, the prescription products would be considered a second-line approach.
- All smoking cessation products help the smoker by decreasing the exposure to the toxic components of cigarettes and can be used in settings where smoking is prohibited.

c. What economic, psychosocial, racial, and ethical considerations are applicable to this consumer?

- *Economic.* The first-line recommendation for helping the consumer quit smoking is an NTS. If she has insurance that will cover a prescription NTS product she may want to consider a prescription medication rather than an OTC product that she would pay for out of her own pocket.
- *Psychosocial.* Most of this consumer's family members smoke cigarettes and she will need to learn coping skills to address this situation. Smokers who quit smoking often become depressed when they try to quit smoking. If a smoker has a history of depression, then antidepressant therapy may be necessary to help

210 Nicotine Addiction

the smoker quit. Alcohol use should be discouraged during an attempt to quit smoking, since the use of alcohol has been identified as a risk factor that may cause the consumer to relapse and start smoking.
- *Race and gender.* White women have a greater incidence of skin wrinkling when they smoke.
- *Ethical considerations.* Clinicians should provide smoking cessation intervention to every smoking consumer they contact in their practices.

Optimal Plan

4. What drug, dosage form, dose, schedule, and duration of therapy are best for this patient?

- Recommend a NTS that is available OTC because the product is readily available without a visit to the physician. The product should be used at the highest dose for 8 weeks. The two patches available OTC are Nicoderm-CQ 21 mg/day worn for 24 hours/day for 8 weeks and Nicotrol 15 mg/day worn for 16 hours/day for 6 weeks. Using the Nicoderm-CQ in this smoker may be advantageous because the 24-hour patch delivers nicotine over a 24-hour period, avoiding a decrease in the nicotine blood level that could potentiate nicotine craving and ultimately cause relapse. The patch should be removed each day and replaced with a new patch.
- Prescription NTS that are worn for 24 hours/day for 8 weeks could be considered and include Habitrol 21 mg/day or ProStep 22 mg/day.
- Nicorette gum is available in 2 and 4-mg doses. Nicorette 4 mg would be appropriate for the smoker who is highly dependent upon nicotine (i.e., smokes more than 20 cigarettes/day, those who smoke within 30 minutes of awakening, or those who find it difficult to refrain from smoking in places where smoking is forbidden). The nicotine gum is not an option in this patient because she wears dentures.
- If the Nicotrol nasal inhaler is considered, the dosing regimen is one spray (0.5 mg) in each nostril, not to exceed 5 doses per hour or 40 doses per day. This nasal spray is used in this manner for 6 to 8 weeks and then the dose is gradually reduced over 4 to 6 weeks.
- Each Nicotrol oral inhaler contains 10 mg of nicotine. Six to 16 cartridges are used initially during a 24-hour period. The smoker should decrease the inhaler use 12 weeks after initiation, with a maximum of 6 months' use recommended.
- Bupropion is dosed 150 mg per day for the first 3 days and then increased to BID dosing for 7 to 12 weeks. The smoker should use the medication for one week prior to their smoking quit date.

Outcome Evaluation

5. What clinical and laboratory parameters are necessary to evaluate the therapy for achievement of the desired therapeutic outcome and to detect or prevent adverse effects?

- Sustained smoking abstinence is monitored clinically, most frequently by the consumer's report of smoking status.
- Laboratory tests that could be conducted to confirm smoking abstinence include measuring nicotine, cotinine (nicotine's major metabolite), thiocyanate, or carboxyhemoglobin in the consumer's blood, saliva, urine, hair, or expired air. However, these biological assessments are expensive and are not commonly performed to monitor smoking status.

Patient Counseling

6. What information should be provided to the patient to enhance compliance, ensure successful therapy, and minimize adverse effects?

- Inform your physician(s) that you are trying to quit smoking and that you are using a nicotine patch. The patch maintains a constant level of nicotine in your system so that you will not experience severe nicotine withdrawal symptoms, such as anxiety, decreased concentration, and irritability, and so that you can enlist coping skills in your environment to address risk factors that would potentiate relapse.
- The patch should be applied to a hairless area of the body and should be removed each day before a new patch is applied. Apply the patch to different areas of the body each day. This patch should be used at this dose for 8 weeks and then discontinued. No cigarettes should be smoked while on this treatment.
- You will notice an improvement in some areas immediately (i.e., clothes will not smell of nicotine, food will taste better, your breath will not have a bad odor, and you will experience increased physical endurance). However, if you have a smoker's cough, the cough will worsen during the first few weeks while your body is detoxified of the nicotine. This cough will go away over time.
- Decrease your intake of caffeine by one-half, because when you quit smoking the caffeine is not eliminated from your body as quickly.
- The most common side effect of the patch is irritation at the application site. However, insomnia, nightmares, stomach upset, and headaches may also occur. Call me if you have any of these problems.

▶ Follow-up Questions

1. What is the risk of smoking relapse at this point?

- The consumer is at a high risk of relapse since she has not been on pharmacotherapy for long and her resolve to quit smoking may be weakening. Smokers using the patch who smoke a cigarette within the first 2 weeks of therapy are at greater risk of not being successful in becoming smoking abstinent.
- Cutaneous irritation may cause the consumer to stop using the patch.
- Insomnia, which may be a side effect from the patch or a nicotine withdrawal symptom, may set this patient up for relapse.
- Concerns about weight gain need to be addressed.

2. Has the treatment goal changed at this point?

No.

3. Evaluate the consumer's complaints and recommend alternative treatments that should be reinforced at this point.

- About 10% of persons exposed to the NTS will have an allergic reaction to the adhesive components of the patch. Attempt to determine how significant the rash is in causing her to stop therapy. If the rash is mild, then it can be treated with OTC hydrocortisone cream.
- Provide suggestions about how to improve her sleep hygiene (e.g., increased exercise, no heavy meals at the end of the day, relaxing music).

- Discuss the fact that smokers can gain 10 pounds when they quit smoking. Therefore, provide suggestions about proper diet, use of sugarless gum or candy, and increased exercise. Quickly reinforce that the benefits from smoking cessation greatly overshadow this weight gain.
- Reinforce the need to continue to stay off of the cigarettes.

4. *Design an alternative pharmacotherapeutic plan to address the consumer's nicotine addiction.*

- Insomnia can be a side effect from the NTS and, in conjunction with other complaints, may be a reason to try the 16-hour NTS. Switch this consumer to the Nicotrol patch to determine if she can tolerate this patch.
- Recommend that she talk with her support system about the difficulties she is experiencing in her quest to quit smoking.
- Recommend a smoking cessation support group in the community.

5. *Describe clinical monitoring parameters for the consumer at this point in treatment.*

- Evaluate her tolerance to this patch.
- Reinforce, in the consumer's mind, your availability as a support person.
- Have her self-report about her smoking status.

▶ Follow-up Questions

1. *To determine what pharmacotherapy may be beneficial at this point, list the positive and negative factors that are important in determining whether the patient is ultimately able to become smoking abstinent.*

Positive Factors
- Desire to quit smoking and willingness to try again
- Quit smoking for 8 weeks earlier this year
- The fact that smoking has exacerbated smoking-related disease may be further stimulus to stop
- Pharmacist is willing to reinforce need for smoking cessation and act as a reference person for education about coping skills

Negative Factors
- Feeling of failure
- Possible onset of depression
- Entire family smokes
- High degree of craving even with the use of the nicotine replacement product

2. *Evaluate the consumer's complaints and recommend alternative treatments that should be reinforced at this point.*

- Discussion of other pharmacotherapy options to help the smoker quit
- Need for a smoking cessation support group
- Possible feelings of depression may warrant antidepressant therapy in combination with another nicotine replacement system

3. *Design an alternative pharmacotherapeutic plan to address her nicotine addiction.*

- Consider combination therapy of bupropion sustained release 150 mg po QD for the first 3 days, then 150 mg po BID for 7 to 12 weeks and Nicotrol nasal spray.
- The bupropion will help to decrease the depressive symptoms and the nicotine craving. The nasal inhaler will help the smoker avoid the nicotine withdrawal symptoms and allow her more control over the administration of the nicotine dose. The nicotine plasma concentration achieved with the nasal spray is similar to that with NTS but allows the consumer to manipulate the dose to try to avoid withdrawal symptoms. The spray will probably be needed at full dose for the first 8 weeks with a downward titration for 4 to 6 weeks afterwards.

4. *What information should be provided to the patient to enhance compliance, ensure successful therapy, and minimize adverse effects?*

Bupropion
- The dose of medicine will be increased after 3 days of treatment, and then you will take this medication twice a day for 7 to 12 weeks.
- Quit smoking during the second week of bupropion therapy.
- The side effects of this medication include headache, insomnia, runny nose, dry mouth, and anxiety.
- At this dose of medication, most consumers do not gain as much weight when they quit smoking.

Nicotine Nasal Spray
- Use one spray in each nostril as needed to reduce nicotine craving; do not exceed 5 doses per hour (or 40 doses per day). This product should not be used for more than 6 months.
- The spray should only be used after you have stopped smoking and only if you experience a great deal of nicotine craving.
- The most common side effects include headache, insomnia, runny nose, and dry mouth.

References

1. Nunn-Thompson C, Barr CC, Tommasello AC, et al. APhA Special Report: A Review of the New Smoking Cessation Strategies for the Agency for Health Care Policy and Research. Washington, DC, American Pharmaceutical Association, 1996.
2. Hudmon KS, Berger BA. Pharmacy applications of the transtheoretical model in smoking cessation. Am J Health-Syst Pharm 1995;52:282–287.
3. Wongwiwatthananukit S, Jack HM, Popovich NG. Smoking cessation: Part 1—an overview. J Am Pharm Assoc 1998;38:58–70.
4. Setter SM, Johnson MD. Smoking cessation and drug therapy. US Pharmacist January 1997:91–102.

62 SCHIZOPHRENIA

▶ !Yo Quiero Taco (I Want a Taco)   (Level I)

William H. Benefield, Jr., PharmD, BCPP, FASCP
Lawrence J. Cohen, PharmD, BCPP, FASHP, FCCP

A 35-year-old woman is brought to the state hospital by police after causing a disturbance at a fast-food restaurant. The patient's speech exhibits symptoms consistent with schizophrenia (paranoid type), including delusions and paranoid ideations, grandiose ideations, and disorganized speech. The goals of therapy are to achieve and maintain control of her target symptoms of schizophrenia. Non-pharmacologic therapy such as medication education classes, vocational training, and group therapy are useful adjunctive measures. Although any antipsychotic agent could be used for this first episode of schizophrenia (except clozapine), newer atypical antipsychotics (risperidone, olanzapine, or quetiapine) are commonly used as first-line therapy because they carry a lower risk of extrapyramidal symptoms, tardive dyskinesia, and cognitive impairment than traditional antipsychotics (e.g., phenothiazines, thioxanthines, and butyrophenones). A benzodiazepine such as lorazepam may be used during the first two weeks to treat aggressive behavior while the antipsychotic is taking effect. It may take several months for the full effect of the atypical antipsychotics to be seen.

▶ Questions

Problem Identification

1. a. *Create a list of the patient's drug-related problems.*

   - Untreated indication: She requires stabilization of her psychotic symptoms with antipsychotic medication.

   b. *What information (signs, symptoms, laboratory values) indicates the presence or severity of an acute exacerbation of schizophrenia, paranoid type?*

   Target Symptoms
   - Delusions and paranoid ideations: These may be multiple but revolve around a coherent theme (worms and snakes in her stomach, being raped, ideas given to communists, someone impersonating her, feet were cut off, children killed by the government, transmitters in her body).
   - Grandiose ideations: She believes that she was a surgeon, she took part in signing the treaty with Germany, and she owns gold and great wealth.
   - Disorganized speech as stated in the mental status exam.

   Laboratory Values
   - There are no laboratory values that can be used to diagnose or assess the severity of an acute exacerbation of schizophrenia.

Desired Outcome

2. *What are the goals of pharmacotherapy in this case?*

   - Achieve and then maintain control of the target symptoms of schizophrenia.
   - Promote patient adherence to the prescribed regimen.[1]
   - Minimize side effects from medications.
   - Improve the patient's quality of life, thereby permitting her to function as a contributing member of society.
   - Provide effective treatment that will decrease long-term hospitalizations and perhaps avoid suicide.

Therapeutic Alternatives

3. a. *What non-drug therapies might be useful for this patient?*

   - *Medication education classes* to promote compliance and understanding about the illness (once she is stabilized)
   - *Vocational training* to promote independence
   - *Group therapy* for support once symptoms are under control with medication

   b. *What pharmacotherapeutic alternatives are available for the treatment of this patient?*

   - *Phenothiazines, thioxanthines, butyrophenones,* or any other traditional ("typical") antipsychotic may be used for "first-break" (the first episode of) schizophrenia (see textbook Chapter 64 for a complete list of drugs and dosage regimens). Typical antipsychotics are inexpensive, and generic products are available for most drugs. Some forms are available for IM use. These agents are useful in treating aggressive target symptoms. However, they have the potential to cause cognitive impairment and have a high incidence of extrapyramidal symptoms (EPS), including dystonias, pseudoparkinsonian symptoms (drooling, cogwheeling, pill-rolling tremor), akathisia (e.g., pacing), and tardive dyskinesia.
   - *Atypical antipsychotics* are newer agents that are usually regarded as first-line therapy because they have a lower risk for EPS, minimal risk for tardive dyskinesia, and a lower incidence of cognitive impairment than traditional neuroleptics. In addition, pharmacoeconomic evaluations have shown that atypical agents may be more cost-effective despite their higher acquisition cost than traditional agents.[2,3] No therapeutic serum concentration ranges have been established for any of these newer agents.
     - ✓ *Risperidone (Risperdal)* does have a lower incidence of EPS than traditional antipsychotics, but EPS can occur at lower doses (<6 mg/day) and may require treatment with benztropine or diphenhydramine.
     - ✓ *Olanzapine (Zyprexa)* is less effective for initial aggression in the acute phase of the illness, thus requiring concomitant agents and perhaps coadministration of a traditional neuroleptic. The full effect of the drug may not be seen for several months.
     - ✓ *Quetiapine (Seroquel)* is also less effective for initial aggression in the acute phase, which may require treatment with concomitant agents, including a traditional neuroleptic. Annual ophthalmologic examinations are required because lens changes have been observed with long-term therapy. As with olanzapine, full effectiveness may not be observed for several months.
   - *Clozapine (Clozaril)* was the first atypical antipsychotic approved for use in the United States. It shares the advantages of the other atypical agents with respect to minimal EPS and a lower incidence of cognitive impairment than traditional agents.[4] There have been no reports of tardive dyskinesia directly attributable to the drug. Clozapine is also effective in treating the negative symptoms of schizophrenia and may be effective in cases that are re-

fractory to other agents. There is no official established therapeutic serum concentration range. Cautious dosage titration is needed to minimize the risk of hypotension, seizures, and sedation. Clozapine is also associated with agranulocytosis that is potentially fatal, requiring weekly or twice weekly monitoring of the WBC count. The drug also has a high acquisition cost. For these reasons, it should be reserved for refractory patients who have failed two or more antipsychotic agents from different classes using adequate doses and for an adequate duration.

- *Benzodiazepines* (e.g., lorazepam po or IM) may be used as adjunctive medication during the first few weeks of the illness to treat aggression, agitation, or combativeness while the antipsychotic is taking effect. It should be tapered slowly once symptoms have remitted.

Optimal Plan

4. a. What drug, dosage form, dose, schedule, and duration of therapy are best for this patient?

- As stated above, an atypical antipsychotic (except clozapine) would represent the optimal therapy for this patient. Reasonable regimens include any of the following:
    ✓ Risperidone 1 mg po BID initially. Further dosage adjustments should generally occur at intervals ≥1 week. When dosage adjustments are necessary, small dosage increments of 1 to 2 mg are recommended. Dosages >6 mg/day greatly increase the risk of EPS.
    ✓ Olanzapine 5 to 10 mg po QD with a target dose of 10 mg/day by the seventh day. Further dosage adjustments can then be made as indicated at 1-week intervals. Typical doses range from 10 to 15 mg/day. Doses >10 mg/day should only be made after appropriate clinical assessment. Doses >20 mg/day have not been evaluated in clinical trials and are not recommended.
    ✓ Quetiapine 25 mg po BID, increasing by 25 to 50 mg per day on the second or third day as tolerated. The target range is 200 to 400 mg/day by day 4 of therapy, given in 2 or 3 divided doses. Any further dosage adjustments should be made at intervals of at least 2 days.
- Lorazepam 0.5 to 1 mg po TID (or PRN) may be used adjunctively as needed for agitation or aggression.

b. What alternatives would be appropriate if the initial therapy fails or cannot be used?

- The patient could be started on another atypical drug. For example, if she received risperidone initially, a trial of olanzapine or quetiapine could be started.
- A trial of a traditional or typical antipsychotic (e.g., haloperidol, fluphenazine, thiothixene, loxapine) at the usual doses can also be attempted (see textbook chapter).
- Clozapine would be considered in this patient only after she has failed adequate trials of 2 or more antipsychotics from different classes.

Outcome Evaluation

5. What clinical and laboratory parameters are necessary to evaluate the therapy for achievement of the desired therapeutic outcome and to detect or prevent adverse effects?

Efficacy Parameters

- Each atypical agent (risperidone, olanzapine, or quetiapine) should be given an adequate trial for at least 6 to 8 weeks at a therapeutic dose. In some instances, full response may not be seen for several months.

Adverse Effect Parameters

- A Dyskinesia Identification System: Condensed User Scale (DISCUS) or Abnormal Involuntary Movement Scale (AIMS) scale should be completed prior to starting the medication and then quarterly for the assessment for tardive dyskinesia.
- Risperidone may cause EPS (about 2% incidence), anxiety, somnolence, dizziness, constipation, nausea, and dyspepsia. Orthostatic hypotension may occur, especially during initial dosage titration.
- Olanzapine therapy may cause EPS, somnolence, agitation, dizziness, and constipation. Orthostatic hypotension may also occur, especially during initial dosage titration.
- Quetiapine can cause dizziness, postural hypotension, dry mouth, and dyspepsia. Somnolence occurs frequently, especially during the initial dosage adjustment period. Periodic eye examinations are recommended because of the lens changes that have been observed during long-term therapy.

Patient Counseling

6. What information should be provided to the patient to enhance compliance, ensure successful therapy and minimize adverse effects?

General Information for Risperidone, Olanzapine, and Quetiapine

- *Note:* During the first few weeks, counseling may be limited due to lack of comprehension. Once stabilized, the patient should be encouraged to take the medication as prescribed and to have examinations quarterly to detect any abnormal movement disorders. Newer atypical agents have been shown to improve cognition and improve compliance.[1]
- This drug may cause drowsiness, dizziness, anxiety, constipation, and nausea.
- Lowered blood pressure causing dizziness or fainting may occur upon arising from a lying or sitting position. This is more likely to occur early in therapy when we are increasing your dosage. You can minimize this problem by arising slowly after sitting or lying down.
- Because this medication may cause drowsiness or otherwise affect your ability to perform tasks such as driving a car, be careful when driving until you know how much this affects you.
- Contact your doctor if you become pregnant or intend to become pregnant while taking this medication.
- Tell your doctor if you are taking or plan to take any new prescription or nonprescription medications during therapy with this drug.
- It is best to avoid drinking alcoholic beverages while taking this medication.

References

1. Marder SR. Facilitating compliance with antipsychotic medication. J Clin Psychiatry 1998;59(suppl 3):21–25.

2. Revicki DA. Methods of pharmacoeconomic evaluation of psychopharmacologic therapies for patients with schizophrenia. J Psychiatry Neurosci 1997;22: 256–266.
3. Glazer WM. Olanzapine and the new generation of antipsychotic agents: Patterns of use. J Clin Psychiatry 1997;58(suppl 10):18–21.
4. Sharma T, Mockler D. The cognitive efficacy of atypical antipsychotics in schizophrenia. J Clin Psychopharmacol 1998;18(suppl 1):12S–19S.

63 MAJOR DEPRESSION

▶ A Life Worth Living   (Level I)

Brian L. Crabtree, PharmD, BCPP

A 38-year-old woman presents to her family physician with complaints, signs, and symptoms indicative of a recurrent major depressive episode with melancholic features. She is involved in an abusive relationship with her husband; they have been separated for 3 months. Non-drug therapies such as psychotherapy and a support group should be initiated concurrently with pharmacotherapy. Feasible drug treatment options for this patient include tricyclic antidepressants, selective serotonin reuptake inhibitors, and a number of other agents with mixed reuptake inhibition pharmacology. Efficacy is determined by evaluating target signs and symptoms; standardized rating scales may also be used. It is important to question the patient about adverse effects at each visit and to encourage adherence to the prescribed therapy.

▶ Questions

Problem Identification

1. a. *Create a list of this patient's drug-related problems.*

   - Recurrent depression, presently untreated with conventional therapy.
   - Current use of St. John's wort, with possible implications for other medication therapy.
   - Stable problems not requiring treatment at this time include occasional allergies treated with antihistamines and decongestants; headache and menstrual cramps treated with ibuprofen; and constipation treated with MOM.

   b. *What signs, symptoms, and laboratory values indicate depression in this patient?*

   - Sleep disturbance (difficulty falling asleep and premature nocturnal awakenings)
   - Fatigue
   - Loss of appetite with weight loss
   - Concentration impairment
   - Feeling down and sad
   - Anxiety (commonly comorbid with depression), "racing heartbeat," muscle tension
   - Crying spells
   - Anhedonia
   - Passive suicidal ideas (no active plan, but wants to "go to sleep and not wake up")
   - Frequent headaches
   - Declining self-care (appearance and hygiene)
   - Mental status exam findings help to determine drug therapy target symptoms
   - Normal physical and laboratory exams help to rule out non-psychiatric causes of depression

   c. *What factors in the family history support a diagnosis of depression?*

   - The mother is depressed and anxious and takes antidepressant medication. One sister committed suicide.

   d. *Why is this patient's depression considered to be recurrent even though this is her first psychiatric treatment?*

   - The PMH indicates a life-long history of periods of intense sadness of several weeks' duration and associated with a disturbance in occupational and social function such as missing school or work.

   e. *Is there anything in the patient's medication history that could cause or worsen depression?*

   - Oral contraceptives can, but this is unlikely in this case due to her long history of recurrent episodes and the fact that she hasn't taken them for 2 months prior to this presentation.

Desired Outcome

2. *What are the goals of pharmacotherapy in this case?*

   - Eliminate or significantly reduce symptoms
   - Restore functioning to premorbid levels
   - Prevent depressive relapse
   - Minimize medication side effects
   - Ensure adherence with the prescribed regimen

Therapeutic Alternatives

3. a. *What non-pharmacologic treatments are important in this case? Should non-pharmacologic treatments be tried before beginning medication?*

- Psychotherapy, supportive counseling, and support groups are important non-drug therapies. Because of the severe psychosocial aspects of this patient's depression, including the stormy and violent relationship with the husband, it is important for her to work through issues in her life with a therapist and support group for at least a few months in addition to medication. Different types of psychotherapy vary in cost, but support groups are usually free of charge.
- Pharmacotherapy should be initiated concurrently with nonpharmacologic therapy.

b. *What pharmacotherapeutic options are available for the treatment of depression?*

- Antidepressant medications are generally considered equally effective. Choice is based on factors such as side-effect profile, ease and frequency of dosing, and cost.
- *Tricyclic antidepressants* (TCAs) are the oldest antidepressant agents and may be particularly useful in patients with melancholic features of depression,[1] but they require especially careful dosage adjustment to find the correct dosage and commonly cause bothersome side effects, particularly sedation, anticholinergic effects, and orthostatic hypotension. They also are problematic in patients with comorbid non-psychiatric disease such as cardiovascular disease or benign prostatic hyperplasia.
- *Selective serotonin reuptake inhibitors* (SSRIs; fluoxetine, fluvoxamine, paroxetine, sertraline) are often more easily tolerated than the TCAs[2] and have the advantages of single daily dosing and efficacy with the usual starting dosage. Disadvantages include their side-effect profile and a propensity for drug–drug interactions.
- *Antidepressants with mixed reuptake inhibition pharmacology,* such as trazodone, nefazodone, venlafaxine, bupropion, and mirtazepine have their own advantages and disadvantages. The reader is referred to textbook Chapter 65 for a complete discussion.
- *Monoamine oxidase inhibitors* (MAOIs; phenelzine, tranylcypromine) are not usually used as first-line agents because of necessary dietary restrictions and the associated risk of a hypertensive reaction.

Optimal Plan

4. a. *What drug regimen (drug, dosage, schedule, and duration) is best for this patient?*

- If the patient could tell us the name of the mother's medication and how she responds to it, this information could possibly serve as the basis for an initial choice of treatment for this patient. In the absence of such information, the choice is less clear.
- Use of a medication that can be given once daily and is likely to be effective with the initial dosage is desirable. The SSRI antidepressants fit this description well.
- An example initial regimen would be fluoxetine 20 mg po QD in the AM. The dosage can range up to 80 mg per day. Fluoxetine is usually given in the morning in order to minimize the risk of insomnia.
- Other SSRIs, TCAs, or mixed pharmacology antidepressants would all be appropriate for initial treatment. Refer to textbook Chapter 65 for a listing of usual starting dosages.
- Venlafaxine is available in a sustained-release dosage form that allows single daily dosing once a maintenance dosage is established by the initial titration.
- Bupropion is also available in a sustained-release formulation, but divided dosing is still indicated if the total daily dosage exceeds 150 mg per day.
- Trazodone, nefazodone, and immediate release formulations of venlafaxine and bupropion usually require more than one dose per day.
- TCAs often cause side effects that increase the likelihood of noncompliance, but prescription costs are lower for TCAs than many other antidepressants. Some TCAs, including imipramine, desipramine, and nortriptyline can be monitored with serum concentrations as an additional parameter in assessing and adjusting therapy.
- If the patient responds satisfactorily, antidepressant therapy should be continued for at least 6 to 12 months before an attempt is made at tapered reduction. In a patient such as this with a history of recurrent episodes, it would be appropriate to continue medication even longer, perhaps on an indefinite maintenance basis.[3]

b. *How should the patient be advised about the herbal therapy, St. John's wort?*

- She should be advised to stop taking the St. John's wort. Research on efficacy is inconclusive,[4] standardization of the formulation is often unreliable, she has taken it for a month with no apparent benefit, and it could interact adversely with antidepressant medication that will be recommended.

c. *What alternatives would be appropriate if the patient fails to respond to initial therapy?*

- In the absence of significant side effects, initial therapy should be optimized with dosage increases and a trial of at least 4 weeks. If a switch to a different agent is advisable, a drug from a different chemical class may be considered. The SSRIs are not a chemical class, however, and many patients respond to one SSRI after failing another.
- If an SSRI was used initially, other options include bupropion, trazodone, nefazodone, venlafaxine, and the tricyclic antidepressants. MAOIs are usually reserved for more difficult patients or patients with atypical depression because of dietary restrictions.

Outcome Evaluation

5. *What clinical and laboratory parameters are necessary to evaluate the therapy for efficacy and adverse effects?*

- The principal drug therapy outcomes are the target signs and symptoms identified in the history, ROS, and physical exam, particularly the mental status exam findings. Some clinicians also use standardized rating scales such as the Hamilton Depression Rating Scale. Patient self-rated scales include the Beck Depression Inventory.
- Monitoring of potential adverse effects should be specific to the antidepressant agent being used. With fluoxetine, common side effects

include GI disturbance such as nausea and diarrhea; CNS effects such as irritability, jitteriness, and headache; sleep disturbance such as insomnia; and sexual dysfunction including erectile impotence, anorgasmia, and loss of libido. Side effects are assessed primarily on the basis of the clinical interview.
- Side effects should be assessed at each clinical interaction, since side effects are the most common reason for noncompliance with antidepressant therapy. Patients can be interviewed briefly during clinic visits or visits to the pharmacy for prescription refills. A general question such as, "Are you having any problems with your medication?" can be asked within the context of reassurance that some side effects are common but may be temporary. If side effects are particularly bothersome or interfere with daily function or quality of life, the patient should be encouraged to report these so that appropriate adjustments in therapy can be made.
- Laboratory data monitoring is not always indicated with antidepressant therapy. The SSRIs can cause hyponatremia in some patients and electrolyte monitoring at 6 months and annually may be prudent. The TCAs are well known for their cardiac effects; ECG monitoring at baseline and annually is advisable, especially in patients over 40 years of age.

Patient Counseling

6. *What information should be provided to the patient to enhance compliance, ensure successful therapy, and minimize adverse effects?*

Patient counseling should be individualized to patient needs and the agent being used. Important points with this case include the following items.
- The name of this medication is Prozac. It is used for your depression.
- Take this medication every day in the morning.
- Medication for depression often takes up to 4 weeks, or even longer, to be optimally effective. Don't be discouraged if you don't feel better in the first few days.
- Some symptoms may improve before others. Sleep, energy, and appetite sometimes get better before the depressed feeling goes away.
- If you miss a dose, take it as soon as you remember. If you forget until the next day, skip the missed dose and continue with the regular schedule.
- Common side effects to watch for with this medication include upset stomach, a jittery feeling, headaches, and sleep disturbance. These don't occur with every patient and some of these side effects are similar to the symptoms of depression. If they are due to depression, they should improve as the medication works. If they are due to medication, the symptoms may linger or get worse.
- If you have questions or problems with your medication, contact your physician or pharmacist for more information and assistance.

References

1. Perry PJ. Pharmacotherapy for major depression with melancholic features: Relative efficacy of tricyclic versus selective serotonin reuptake inhibitor antidepressants. J Affect Disord 1996;39:1–6.
2. Preskorn SH. Comparison of the tolerability of bupropion, fluoxetine, imipramine, nefazodone, paroxetine, sertraline, and venlafaxine. J Clin Psychiatry 1995;56(suppl 6):12–21.
3. Frank E, Kupfer DJ, Perel JM, et al. Three-year outcomes for maintenance therapies in recurrent depression. Arch Gen Psychiatry 1990;47:1093–1099.
4. Linde K, Ramirez G, Mulrow CD, et al. St. John's wort for depression—an overview and meta-analysis of randomised clinical trials. Br Med J 1996;313:253–258.

64 BIPOLAR DISORDER

▶ **Love at First Bite**   (Level II)

Andrea Eggert, PharmD, BCPP
William H. Benefield, Jr., PharmD, BCPP, FASCP

The police bring a 25-year-old man to the hospital after neighbors complain about his bizarre behavior and vocal ranting. The patient has a previous history of psychiatric admissions for acute mania. Although he has been prescribed lithium, his current serum concentration is subtherapeutic (0.1 mEq/L). After a physical examination and extensive interview, the patient is diagnosed with bipolar disorder, current episode mixed. In addition to psychotherapy and counseling, pharmacotherapeutic options include lithium (if noncompliance resulted in relapse), valproate, or carbamazepine. Adjunctive benzodiazepine or antipsychotic medication is advised to promote sleep and reduce agitation.

▶ **Questions**

Problem Identification

1. a. *From the case information and patient interview, write a mental status examination for this patient.*

- *Appearance.* 25 yo mildly obese, disheveled, malodorous, Caucasian male, inappropriately dressed in bathrobe and wearing a garlic necklace. Patient is alert, distractible and hyperactive, with unusual mannerisms (pacing, and waving his arms in the air). Excessive eye-blinking and grimacing are present. He is cooperative with the interview, occasionally showing disdain or anger toward the interviewer. The patient is hypertalkative with loud, pressured speech. Speech is also significant for flight of ideas with some clanging (preaching about the light, might, right; republicans redeeming the public for the republic).
- *Neologisms.* Demoncrat.
- *Mood.* Patient describes his mood as "playful," but also refers to feeling miserable at points during the interview. Affect is labile, alternating between elation, anxiety, tears, and anger.
- *Sensorium.* Not formally assessed; patient appears to be oriented

to person, place, and time. Memory appears intact though not formally assessed.
- *Intellectual functioning.* Not formally assessed. Estimated intelligence is average to above average based on education, employment, and vocabulary.
- *Thought processes/content.* Delusions (religious, grandiose, and persecutory); patient believes vampires are in the city and are out to get him; God and the republicans are persecuting him.
- *Insight and judgment.* Poor (trying to bite police, throwing furniture on lawn).
- No laboratory abnormalities are associated with the disease itself except possibly mild dehydration; elevated WBC may be due to very recent lithium use.

b. *Create a list of this patient's drug-related problems.*

- Bipolar disorder, current episode mixed requiring treatment.
- Migraine headaches apparently adequately treated with occasional ergotamine and ibuprofen.

c. *What information (target symptoms, laboratory values) indicates the presence and severity of bipolar disorder, mixed episode?*

- *Target symptoms.* Abnormally elevated, expansive and irritable mood; decreased sleep; pressured speech; racing thoughts; increased activity and agitation (psychomotor agitation); persecutory and grandiose delusions; depressed mood (talk of misery/tearfulness); guilt (must perform penance, God is punishing him, "I'm sorry"); possible thoughts of death (he will be the next to die).

Desired Outcome

2. *What are the goals of pharmacotherapy in this patient?*

- Achieve and then maintain control of the target symptoms of mania and depression
- Promote compliance with the prescribed regimen
- Avoid drug interactions with migraine therapy
- Minimize side effects and improve quality of life
- Decrease the risk of suicide and long-term hospitalization by giving appropriate treatment

Therapeutic Alternatives

3. a. *What non-drug therapies might be useful for this patient?*

- Ongoing psychotherapy to help the patient understand and accept his diagnosis, as well as come to terms with his sexual orientation.
- Counseling on possible precipitating factors for relapse of bipolar symptoms (irregular or poor sleep, change in employment or residence, bereavement) and the need for long-term medication therapy.
- Counseling about the potential for refractory disease incurred by repetitive noncompliance and relapse.
- Support and education about bipolar disorder for the patient's family, emphasizing the importance of minimizing family stress. Poor family support has been associated with increased risk of relapse.

b. *What feasible pharmacotherapeutic alternatives are available for treatment of bipolar disorder?*

- *Lithium* is a reasonable choice if it can be shown that lithium noncompliance resulted in relapse. It has been effective in treating prior episodes in this patient and is generally effective as maintenance therapy to prevent manic and depressive episodes. It is also an inexpensive agent, and there is more than 40 years' clinical experience with this medication. However, it may be less effective than other choices in mixed mania. Also, based on the information given, it is unclear whether lithium noncompliance precipitated the present episode or whether noncompliance occurred after the onset of mania (which would indicate lithium failure). The patient may be experiencing lithium-related adverse effects such as GI upset, loose stools, psoriasis (which can be secondary to or worsened by lithium), weight gain, and possible interference with thyroid function (TSH is on the high end of the normal range). Ibuprofen, which the patient takes for migraines, can interfere with lithium clearance, presenting the potential for lithium toxicity if he uses ibuprofen on a regular basis. Another disadvantage of using lithium is that it has a narrow therapeutic index, and periodic serum lithium concentration monitoring is required.
- *Valproic acid* or *divalproex sodium* may be more effective than lithium in mixed mania.[1,2] The response to valproate is independent of previous lithium response. This drug may also decrease the frequency of migraine headaches in the patient. The loading dose is easy to calculate and usually places patients within the desired therapeutic range. Using a loading dose may also provide more rapid onset of clinical effect.[3] However, there are no controlled studies of valproate for prophylaxis of mania or depression; although open studies suggest benefit. Adverse effects of valproate include GI side effects, transient sedation, fine hand tremor, impaired platelet function (easy bruising), thrombocytopenia, pancreatitis or hepatotoxicity (rare), hair loss (2.6% to 12%), weight gain (common 44%), and abnormal thyroid function tests.
- *Carbamazepine* has acute antimanic effects similar to lithium based on the results of clinical studies. It may be more effective than lithium in treating mixed episodes. Efficacy does not appear to be affected by previous nonresponse to lithium.[4] However, carbamazepine has been less well studied in prophylaxis of bipolar disorder than lithium. Adverse effects include rash (5% to 15%), photosensitivity, potential for severe skin reactions (Stevens–Johnson syndrome), neurologic effects (dizziness, sedation, fatigue, blurred vision, ataxia, nystagmus), GI upset, and rare cases of agranulocytosis, SIADH, and altered thyroid tests. Carbamazepine also has numerous drug interactions with other hepatically metabolized drugs.

Optimal Plan

4. a. *What drug, dosage form, dose, schedule, and duration of therapy are best for this patient?*

- Because this patient may have relapsed despite ongoing lithium therapy, and there is evidence (albeit controversial) that lithium is not as effective as anticonvulsants in mixed mania, use of val-

proate or carbamazepine may be preferable to continued use of lithium monotherapy.
- Starting the patient on an anticonvulsant in addition to lithium with plans to taper lithium after a positive response has been achieved would also be an acceptable strategy.
- Since valproate might be more effective in mixed mania, is easy to titrate using a loading dose, and may serve the dual purpose of treating migraine headaches, valproate would likely be the drug of first choice for this patient.
- Valproic acid or divalproex sodium may be initiated with a loading dose of 20 mg/kg/day (94 kg × 20 mg/kg = 1880 mg).[5] Based on capsule strength, a load of either 1750 mg/day or 2000 mg/day is convenient and acceptable. Divided dosing TID with meals is suggested to reduce the potential for GI upset with initial dosing. Alternatively, valproate can be initiated at 250 mg TID with meals in accordance with package insert instructions. The dose of valproate should be titrated (generally increased in increments of 250 to 500 mg) every 5 to 7 days until a satisfactory response is seen. It is suggested that valproate serum concentrations be maintained in the range of 50 to 125 μg/mL initially to increase the likelihood of achieving a response while avoiding adverse reactions.
- Divalproex is more expensive than generic valproic acid but is associated with less GI upset. However, if generic valproic acid is given with food, GI upset is minimized and tolerability approximates that of divalproex in many patients.
- If lithium is selected, the clinician should check prior records to determine which dose resulted in serum concentrations > 0.8 mEq/L. The dose predicted by pharmacokinetic equations ranges between 1500 mg/day to 2000 mg/day; whereas the recommended package insert starting dose is 900 mg/day. Since we know the patient's previous dose was 1500 mg/day, he should be restarted on this dose. *Note:* Patients who are acutely manic may benefit from higher lithium levels initially to achieve more rapid symptom control. Therefore, dosing at 1800 mg/day initially with careful monitoring with dosage reduction to 1500 mg as the patient responds is also acceptable. A lithium level should be obtained in 5 days, and the patient should be monitored closely for signs and symptoms of toxicity.
- Carbamazepine is an alternative drug of choice that can be initiated at a dose of 200 mg po Q HS, or 200 mg po BID with meals or snack. The dose should be increased every 3 to 5 days based on patient tolerance, until a dose of 600 to 1200 mg daily is reached. Doses should be divided BID–QID. Serum concentrations of 8 to 12 μg/mL are suggested, but there is little literature support correlating serum concentrations with response. A serum concentration is recommended weekly during dose titration, then every 2 weeks for the first 6 to 8 weeks of therapy. Dosage increases may be needed, because auto-induction occurs during the first month of therapy.
- Whichever agent is selected, therapy should be continued indefinitely (lifelong) based on the presence of the following risk factors, which predict high probability of morbidity and recurrence.
    ✓ The patient has experienced two prior episodes.
    ✓ Episodes of mania significantly limit this patient's function and quality of life.
    ✓ There is a family history of affective disorders.
- Adjunctive use of a benzodiazepine or antipsychotic is advised to promote sleep and reduce agitation. If the patient has not discontinued his haloperidol, this should be continued until symptoms have remitted, then a slow taper can be instituted. If the patient has discontinued his haloperidol, a trial of benzodiazepine augmentation may be preferred. For example, lorazepam 1 to 2 mg po/IM every 2 to 8 hours may be given initially, with titration based on response. The presence of psychotic symptoms during the manic episode does *not* signal the need for ongoing antipsychotic use once symptoms have remitted. Benzodiazepines and antipsychotics can be tapered and discontinued when the mania subsides. Patients with affective disorder are at a higher risk for tardive dyskinesia. This patient already shows signs of tardive dyskinesia secondary to neuroleptic use (or possibly withdrawal dyskinesias if haloperidol was recently discontinued).

b. *What alternatives would be appropriate if the initial therapy fails or cannot be used?*

- If two attempts at monotherapy with different agents are unsuccessful, combined use of two agents may be attempted (lithium plus carbamazepine, lithium plus valproate, or carbamazepine plus valproate). About 50% of patients will respond to this strategy.
- Other alternative regimens (in approximate order of preference) include electroconvulsive therapy (ECT), clozapine, atypical antipsychotics in combination with mood stabilizers, lamotrigine, gabapentin, or the calcium channel blocker verapamil. These recommendations are primarily based on case reports or small studies, few of which were done in refractory patients. ECT shows a high likelihood of response in refractory bipolar disorder and clozapine has about a 65% efficacy rate. Evidence for the efficacy of verapamil is limited to acute mania responsive to lithium.

Outcome Evaluation

5. *What clinical and laboratory parameters are necessary to evaluate response to therapy and to detect or prevent adverse effects?*

General Efficacy and Adverse Effect Parameters
- Assess response through patient interviews and observation. The first symptoms to respond are generally agitation, uncooperativeness, and decreased need for sleep. Assess speech (rate, volume, degree of tangentiality or flight of ideas), thought content (preoccupation with sexual or religious themes, expansiveness, delusions), appropriateness of appearance and dress, and behavior on the inpatient unit. Rating scales such as the Schedule for Affective Disorders in Schizophrenia may also be used to assess treatment response.
- Monitor for adverse effects using a review of systems and observation of the patient's appearance. Parameters for individual drugs are included in the information below.

Valproic Acid
- Serum valproic acid concentrations are suggested weekly during dose titration. Thereafter, serum concentrations may be monitored to assess compliance or to evaluate potential toxicity. If the patient does not respond to therapy, the dose may be increased to concentrations of 125 to 150 μg/mL, or higher if tolerated.
- Approximately 50% of patients will experience a 50% decrease in

symptoms within 3 weeks of starting therapy. Onset is generally within the first 2 weeks, with faster response seen when loading doses are used (occasionally within 48 hours).
- Laboratory monitoring should include LFTs and platelet counts at baseline and every 2 weeks during dose titration. Thereafter, the routine monitoring of laboratory values is unnecessary unless physical signs or symptoms of adverse reactions develop.

Carbamazepine
- Carbamazepine concentrations are suggested weekly during dose titration, then every 2 weeks for the first 6 to 8 weeks of therapy. Thereafter the routine monitoring of laboratory values is unnecessary unless physical signs or symptoms of adverse reactions develop. Limited data are available concerning serum concentration response relationships. One study indicates that levels > 8 µg/mL may be more likely to achieve efficacy.
- About two-thirds of patients have an onset of effect within 10 days.
- Laboratory monitoring should include a CBC with differential, electrolytes, and LFTs every 2 weeks for the first 6 to 8 weeks of therapy. Thereafter, routine monitoring of laboratory values is unnecessary unless interacting medications are prescribed or discontinued, or if physical signs or symptoms of adverse reactions develop.

Lithium
- Serum lithium concentrations should be monitored weekly for the first month of therapy. Thereafter, monitoring is at the discretion of the clinician. Periodic monitoring may enhance compliance.
- The onset of response is generally within 1 to 2 weeks.
- Baseline laboratory monitoring should include CBC with differential, serum creatinine and BUN, electrolytes, urine specific gravity, thyroid function tests, and ECG. Laboratory monitoring should be repeated one month after stabilization on lithium, and then annually (TSH may replace full thyroid function monitoring), or if the patient becomes ill or adverse effects suggest monitoring is warranted.
- Female patients should have a pregnancy test prior to initiating therapy.

Patient Counseling

6. What information should be provided to the patient to enhance compliance, ensure successful therapy, and minimize adverse effects?

- Patients and their families require ongoing education regarding bipolar illness and the need for long-term medications. Referral to local community support groups such as the Alliance for the Mentally Ill or the National Depressive and Manic-Depressive Association can help families and consumers receive ongoing support.
- Regarding medications, a single counseling session when the patient is acutely ill is not satisfactory. Most patients will not be able to withstand long counseling sessions at this point in their illness, and it is not uncommon for patients to be irritable, suspicious of your motives, or uncooperative. Most patients with acute mania will require hospitalization; therefore, the opportunity for ongoing counseling should not be neglected.
- Patients must provide informed consent prior to starting therapy. In many cases, this is an opportune time to address any concerns regarding medications (perform initial counseling) and outline the proposed therapeutic plan. Patients may be more likely to comply with therapy if they are allowed to provide input into medication decisions, and if they believe that their opinions about therapy are important to the clinician. If there is no compelling reason to use a specific medication, it may be helpful to allow the patient to choose among the two or three therapies of choice.
- If the patient will not consent to therapy and is acutely agitated, most states provide avenues to medicate the patient on an emergency basis (PRN) for a limited time; in some states, a court order must be obtained to medicate the patient against his or her will. Hiding the medication in food or drink or surreptitiously administering medication is illegal, unethical, and does not foster a trusting relationship with the patient.
- After asking the patient what they already know about the prescribed medication, information can be presented addressing missing information including goals of therapy, drug dosage, adverse reactions and how to minimize their occurrence, and methods to deal with missed doses, acute or concomitant medical illness, and drug interactions. Students should fill in these data from their answers to the above questions. Written information and a mechanism for the patient to receive ongoing counseling after discharge are critical. Information on lithium is given below as an example.

Lithium Carbonate Film-coated Tablets (e.g., Lithobid)
- This is a medication that you have taken before. It is intended to help even out your mood swings; it may take 1 or 2 weeks until you feel better.
- Take this medication exactly as directed by your doctor; do not take more of it or take it more frequently than your doctor ordered.
- It is important that you take the lithium every day, even if you feel well.
- Swallow the tablets whole; do not break, crush, or chew them before swallowing.
- If you miss a dose, take it as soon as you remember; if it is within about 6 hours of your next dose, skip the missed dose and continue on your regular schedule.
- This medicine sometimes causes dizziness or drowsiness; make sure you know how you react to it before performing any activities that require you to be fully alert.
- Avoid altering the daily salt intake in your diet; this can affect the lithium level in your blood.
- Drink adequate fluids (2 to 3 quarts per day) to maintain adequate hydration; avoid prolonged exposure to the heat during the summer months.
- Avoid alcohol while taking this medication or limit your alcohol intake to one or two drinks per day.
- Do not take any over-the-counter or prescription medications without telling your doctor or pharmacist.
- It is important that you keep all follow-up appointments with your doctor.

References

1. Swann AC, Bowden CL, Morris D, et al. Depression during mania: Treatment response to lithium or divalproex. Arch Gen Psychiatry 1997;54:37–42.
2. Freeman TW, Clothier JL, Pazzaglia P, et al. A double-blind comparison of valproate and lithium in the treatment of acute mania. Am J Psychiatry 1992;149:108–111.

3. Goldberg JF, Garno JL, Leon AC, et al. Rapid titration of mood stabilizers predicts remission from mixed or pure mania in bipolar patients. J Clin Psychiatry 1998;59:151–158.
4. Algorithm for patient management of acute manic states: Lithium, valproate, or carbamazepine? J Clin Psychopharmacol 1992;12:57S–63S.
5. McElroy SL, Keck PE, Tugrul KC, et al. Valproate as a loading treatment in acute mania. Neuropsychobiology 1993;27:146–149.

65 GENERALIZED ANXIETY DISORDER

▶ The Worrywart (Level I)

Chad M. VanDenBerg, PharmD
Michael W. Jann, PharmD, FCP, FCCP

Complaints of constant worrying, insomnia, fatigue, restlessness, and lack of ability to concentrate cause a 23-year-old woman to seek medical attention. She is ultimately diagnosed with generalized anxiety disorder (GAD). She has been treated with buspirone 10 mg po TID for 2 months without relief of symptoms. She then received psychotherapy and behavioral therapy along with maximal doses of buspirone (20 mg po TID) with no relief of anxiety. Although benzodiazepines are usually considered the treatment of choice for GAD, they are not a reasonable alternative for this patient because she has a history of alcohol abuse. Low doses of an SSRI or tricyclic antidepressant and trazodone are acceptable alternatives that may be effective in this situation. The non-pharmacologic measures already implemented should be continued, and the patient should be advised to reduce her tobacco and caffeine intake.

▶ Questions

Problem Identification

1. a. Create a list of the patient's drug-related problems.

- Karen has previously been prescribed alprazolam for her anxiety symptoms, but she is apprehensive about taking this medication due to the potential for addiction. Also, her history of alcohol abuse shows a predisposition to substance dependence that should be taken into account when considering the use of a benzodiazepine. Her current prescription for buspirone has not given her relief from her symptoms and she has discontinued taking it for 2 months.
- Cigarette smoking at the rate of 1 to 2 packs of cigarettes per day. This would be considered a drug-related problem if pharmacologic treatments are used in an attempt to help her stop smoking.
- Caffeine intake consisting of 4 to 5 cups of coffee per day; this may be aggravating her GAD.
- A chronic stable problem is occasional heartburn that appears to be adequately self-treated with occasional OTC cimetidine 200 mg on a PRN basis.

b. What information indicates the presence or severity of GAD?

- She has been experiencing restlessness, insomnia, fatigue, and has had difficulty concentrating more days than not over the past year, and her symptoms seem to be increasing both in intensity and frequency.
- Her constant anxiety and worry over school, money, and her family are troubling her to the point where she believes she may have a mental illness.
- Karen appears to be an otherwise healthy female with no additional psychiatric illnesses.

Desired Outcome

2. What are the goals of pharmacotherapy in this case?

- Relieve the symptoms of anxiety (eliminate fatigue and restlessness, improve concentration and sleep pattern)
- Reduce time spent worrying and improve overall functioning (enhance school and job performance)
- Minimize future exacerbation of the illness and future interactions with the health care system
- Avoid adverse drug effects

Therapeutic Alternatives

3. a. What non-drug therapies might be useful for the patient to consider?

- *Cognitive therapy* is considered one of the most effective psychological therapies for GAD patients. Supportive psychotherapy, short-term counseling, behavioral therapy, and group therapy may benefit the patient and help her effectively control her anxiety.
- *Stress management* and *relaxation therapy* (biofeedback, relaxation exercises, and meditation) may also be useful in the management of GAD.
- *Nicotine cessation* and *reduced caffeine* intake would also be of benefit for this patient.

b. What feasible pharmacotherapeutic alternatives are available for the treatment of GAD?

- *Benzodiazepines* are considered the treatment of choice for GAD, although buspirone has been shown to be equally effective.[1]
- *Beta-adrenergic antagonists* (e.g., propranolol) are less effective anxiolytics than benzodiazepines but may be useful in patients with physical symptoms (cardiovascular complaints) that do not respond adequately to benzodiazepine therapy.

Psychiatric Disorders   221

- *Tricyclic antidepressants* (e.g., imipramine, nortriptyline), *nefazodone, trazodone,* and *low-dose SSRIs* (e.g., paroxetine 10 mg) have also been shown to be effective in treating GAD.[2–3]
- *Antihistamines* (e.g., hydroxyzine) have sedative effects that may also be beneficial in treating GAD.

Optimal Plan

4. a. *What drug, dosage form, dose, schedule, and duration of therapy are best for this patient?*

- Buspirone is given in initial doses of 5 mg po TID, increasing by 5 mg/day every 2 to 3 days up to 30 mg/day in divided doses. At a dose of 30 mg/day, the patient did not experience any improvement and had stopped taking the medication. Subsequently, she was prescribed the maximum dosage of buspirone (60 mg/day) and still did not experience improvement in her symptoms despite 4 weeks of treatment compliance. Although the maximum response may take 4 to 6 weeks, initial relief of symptoms should begin within 2 to 3 weeks of initiation or dosage increase.
- Benzodiazepines are not a reasonable alternative in this patient due to past alcohol abuse.
- Antidepressant therapy is an appropriate alternative for those in whom it is desirable to avoid benzodiazepines and who have failed treatment with buspirone.[3,4] Refer to the treatment algorithm for the general management of GAD in textbook Chapter 67 for a detailed approach to treatment. Comorbid depression is common in patients with GAD, so the use of an antidepressant can serve a dual purpose.
  ✓ Choice of an antidepressant is dependent upon patient-specific factors (e.g., concomitant disease states, financial constraints), potential adverse events, and physician/patient preference.
  ✓ Due to their potential to cause increased agitation and anxiety, initial doses of antidepressants in patients with anxiety disorders are generally less than those used to treat depression.
  ✓ Paroxetine would be a good choice for this patient, as it may be less likely to cause agitation than either fluoxetine or sertraline. It should be initiated as a single oral daily dose of 10 mg, usually given in the morning.
  ✓ Low-dose fluoxetine (10 mg) or sertraline (25 mg) are alternative SSRIs that are also acceptable for the treatment of GAD. Titration is indicated after establishing initial safety and tolerability. Optimal daily doses for GAD have not been established but if dose changes are necessary, they should occur in minimal increments and at intervals of at least 1 week.
  ✓ Tricyclic antidepressants (TCAs) are also acceptable alternatives for this patient. Initial doses of imipramine and nortriptyline are low (10 mg po TID for both), and may be increased gradually according to clinical response and the occurrence of adverse events. TCAs are often associated with more prominent adverse events than SSRIs but may impart a significant reduction in cost of therapy.
  ✓ Trazodone could also be used; its common adverse event of sedation is potentially advantageous for GAD patients with sleep disturbances. Trazodone may be initiated at 50 mg po Q HS and titrated up to 150 mg po Q HS. The effects of all antidepressants are not immediate but occur after several weeks of therapy.
- Beta-adrenergic antagonists are not recommended for this patient, but, they may useful for patients with more prominent cardiovascular symptoms.
- Antihistamines have weaker anxiolytic effects and may produce marked adverse events at effective doses. They induce drowsiness, sedation, and impair psychomotor performance at high doses.[2]
- Both antihistamines and beta adrenergic antagonists have rapid onset of clinical effect and can be taken either as a single dose or on a regular basis.
- Non-pharmacologic measures are also an important part of the overall treatment plan.
  ✓ In addition to continuing the program with her cognitive and behavioral therapist, relaxation training, stress reduction techniques, regular exercise, and referral to self-help literature or groups can be beneficial in managing GAD.
  ✓ The patient should also be instructed to decrease (preferably discontinue) caffeine intake to minimize the potential for increased GAD symptoms.
  ✓ Discontinuation of tobacco use is advisable for all patients due to its many adverse effects. However, stabilization of the anxiety disorder could be difficult if the patient attempts to stop smoking and/or discontinue caffeine intake at the same time. It may be advisable to initiate a smoking cessation plan after the new medication has begun to show a positive effect.
- Effective treatment should continue for 2 to 6 months before considering discontinuation of the medication. Medication withdrawal should be gradual and guided by the patient's symptoms and ability to function. Most GAD patients do not require long-term medication treatment, but those who relapse should be allowed to continue effective pharmacotherapy. Continuation of non-pharmacologic therapy is appropriate during both medication withdrawal and after discontinuation.

b. *What pharmacotherapeutic alternatives would be appropriate if the optimal plan fails?*

- If the patient fails to respond after 4 weeks of the maximally tolerated dose of SSRI, consideration should be given to switching to an alternative medication from a different pharmacologic class. In this patient, a TCA, trazodone, or nefazodone are appropriate alternatives. Initiation of a TCA may not be appropriate for a patient with suicidal potential. For patients with no contraindication to benzodiazepines, combination therapy with SSRIs, buspirone, or nefazodone may be beneficial when there is incomplete response to maximal monotherapy. Nefazodone and SSRIs, however, can inhibit the metabolism of some benzodiazepines resulting in more pronounced adverse effects, so caution should be exercised when combination therapy is initiated. The monoamine oxidase inhibitor phenelzine is an option of last resort.

Outcome Evaluation

5. *What clinical and laboratory parameters are necessary to evaluate the therapy for achievement of the desired therapeutic outcome and to detect or prevent adverse effects?*

- At all follow-up evaluations, the patient should be questioned about the type, frequency, and severity of her anxiety symptoms. Relief of her symptoms should begin within 2 or 3 weeks of the initiation of SSRI therapy, while maximal response may take 4 to 6 weeks.
- There are no specific laboratory tests recommended during SSRI therapy.
- The main adverse events associated with SSRI therapy are GI symptoms (nausea, vomiting, diarrhea), nervousness, somnolence, dizziness, insomnia, and sexual dysfunction. These adverse events are usually mild and dissipate with continued use of the medication.
- TCA therapy is associated with anticholinergic effects, sedation, orthostatic hypotension, seizures, and cardiac conduction abnormalities. Anticholinergic effects such as dry mouth, constipation, blurred vision, urinary retention, dizziness, tachycardia, and memory impairment may influence patient tolerance and compliance.
- Trazodone has minimal anticholinergic effects but can cause sedation, orthostatic hypotension, and cognitive slowing.

Patient Counseling

6. *What information should be provided to the patient to enhance compliance, ensure successful therapy, and minimize adverse events?*

- SSRIs should not be taken if you are currently taking a monoamine oxidase inhibitor (e.g., Parnate, Nardil). If another physician has prescribed a monoamine oxidase inhibitor, please notify them immediately.
- This medication can be taken with food if it upsets your stomach.
- The benefits of this medication may not be seen for 2 to 3 weeks, and it may take 4 to 6 weeks to achieve maximum benefit. You are encouraged to continue therapy until advised by your physician to stop.
- Take this medication only as directed by your doctor; do not take more of it or take it more often than your doctor has ordered.
- Make sure you know how you react to this medication before you drive or engage in other activities that require you to be fully alert.
- Avoid drinking alcohol while taking this medication.
- Please consult with your physician or pharmacist whenever you are using other medications, especially over-the-counter medications, since there may be interactions.
- If this medication causes sedation, it is possible to take the dose at bedtime; consult with your physician or pharmacist.

References

1. Schweizer E, Rickels K. Strategies for treatment of generalized anxiety in the primary care setting. J Clin Psychiatry 1997;58(suppl 3):27–31.
2. Hoehn-Saric R. Generalised anxiety disorder: Guidelines for diagnosis and treatment. CNS Drugs 1998;9:85–98.
3. Rocca P, Fonzo V, Scotta M, et al. Paroxetine efficacy in the treatment of generalized anxiety disorder. Acta Psychiatr Scand 1997;95:444–450.
4. Nutt D. Management of patients with depression associated with anxiety symptoms. J Clin Psychiatry 1997;58(suppl 8):11–16.

66 PANIC DISORDER

▶ **Another Trip to the ER** (Level I)

W. Alexander Morton, PharmD, BCPP

Recurrent sudden episodes of fearfulness, crushing chest tightness, shortness of breath, heart palpitations, and other symptoms cause a 33-year-old woman to respond to an advertisement for a research program on anxiety. After a complete medical and psychiatric evaluation, the patient is diagnosed with panic disorder with agoraphobia and generalized anxiety disorder. Supportive therapy and cognitive behavioral therapy may be indicated in addition to pharmacotherapy. Therapeutic alternatives include benzodiazepines and antidepressants, either alone or in combination, depending upon the patient's presentation. The fact that panic disorder is often misdiagnosed and inappropriately treated is an important aspect of the case for students to remember.

▶ Questions

Problem Identification

1. a. *Create a list of the patient's drug-related problems.*

- Panic disorder with agoraphobia, not optimally treated with a PRN benzodiazepine. Low-dose diazepam is not indicated and only portrays someone as a hypochondriac or drug seeker; if benzodiazepines are to be used, an adequate amount should be prescribed.
- History of depression, currently untreated. Patients with undertreated panic disorder often have comorbidity. Depression, GAD, social phobia, PTSD, and OCD are common comorbid conditions.[1]
- GAD, inadequately treated. This patient was using alcohol to relax and sleep. Alcohol is a fast acting, relatively effective antianxiety drug associated with tachyphylaxis, tolerance, physical dependence, and numerous side effects. Patients often self-medicate with this drug.
- Balance disorder, probably secondary to anxiety and inappropriately treated with Antivert.
- Irritable bowel syndrome, probably secondary to anxiety and inappropriately treated with Librax.
- Antivert and Librax are sometimes prescribed inappropriately for symptoms that may be part of a panic attack or a limited symptom attack (less than 4 symptoms).[2]
- Headaches, probably secondary to anxiety, and inappropriately treated with ibuprofen.
- Herbal remedy use may be inappropriate and excessive. These products may contribute to symptoms and cause potential drug interactions.

b. *What information indicates the presence or severity of panic disorder in this patient?*

- There is no currently available laboratory test or procedure to demonstrate the presence of panic. It is established by an accurate history usually in the absence of abnormal laboratory and physical findings.
- The classic presentation of panic disorder includes chest pain, shortness of breath, dizziness, sweating, nausea, and fear of dying.
- During evaluation, the following items should be characterized: 1) the number of attacks; 2) the severity of attacks; 3) level of agoraphobia (avoidance); 4) utilization of health services (office visits, ER visits, labs, prescriptions); 5) presence and severity of depression and/or other comorbid symptoms; 6) use of alcohol to treat symptoms.
- Her episodes occur spontaneously; panic attacks do not have to have a psychological stimulus to occur and can occur while a patient is asleep or totally relaxed.
- Patients usually seek treatment in an ER initially. They may wear out their welcome once no physical abnormality is detected.
- This 33 yo woman is seeking treatment with a familiar presentation of how anxiety disorders are overlooked, misdiagnosed, and undertreated. Anxiety disorders are serious biologic disorders that have profound effects on people's lives with respect to quality of life, productivity, utilization of health care services, and comorbidity of other medical and psychiatric disorders.[1]
- Patients may not seek treatment because they: 1) think no one will understand them; 2) think they will be made fun of and embarrassed; 3) are embarrassed; 4) think they should get over it themselves; 5) have no words to describe the experience; 6) are afraid they will be told they are crazy; 7) are afraid they are going crazy; 8) are afraid they will be committed to a mental hospital; 9) have had poor experiences with health care professionals in the past; 10) think this experience is normal; 11) think there is nothing that can be done for their problem; 12) have been given ineffective medication in the past; 13) think it's their imagination.
- Health care practitioners are likely to discount a patient's experience. Both patients and practitioners may see hypochondria as an issue. If ineffective or no treatment is given, patients will continue to experience physical symptoms and the disorder will worsen.
- Patients with panic attacks often seek treatment for the following problems with the following practitioners: 1) alcoholism, drug abuse (psychiatrists); 2) strokes, seizures (neurologists); 3) hypoglycemia (endocrinologists); 4) asthma, shortness of breath (pulmonologists); 5) heart attack, angina (cardiologists); 6) cancer, tumors (oncologists); 7) "something's wrong" or "I need a complete physical" (internists, family medicine); 8) hot flashes, change of life (gynecologists); 9) irritable bowel syndrome (gastroenterologists); 10) inner ear or balance problem (otolaryngologists).

c. *What medications would be expected to make this problem worse?*

- Alcohol-rebound hyperactivity
- Stimulants (OTC decongestants, cocaine, caffeine)
- Xanthines

Desired Outcome

2. *What are the goals of pharmacotherapy in this case?*

- Ideally, the primary goals of pharmacotherapy are for the patient to have no panic attacks, no anticipatory anxiety, and no avoidance of previously feared situations.
- An acceptable goal is for the patient to have a significant decrease in the number and severity of panic attacks along with decreased anticipatory anxiety.
- There should be elimination of primary avoidance behaviors that interfere with the patient's functioning and enjoyment of life. This might be seen by a return to work or starting a new job as well as return to normal social activities.
- The patient needs to have current depression treated as well as prevent depression from recurring.
- An overall goal is to decrease the utilization of health care services by the patient.

Therapeutic Alternatives

3. a. *What non-drug therapies might be useful for this patient?*

- *Information.* People feel and get better when they know what is going on with their body. Many people are surprised that this disorder has a name, other people also have it, treatment is available, and they can be helped. Information can be supplied verbally and reinforced with educational literature.
- *Supportive therapy.* Information and encouragement can be given by you or other health professionals.
- *Cognitive-behavioral therapy (CBT).* This can be done by the patient; you can get them started if you have the information, the time, and the desire. More effective CBT is available through a referral to a clinical psychologist. While it may be initially expensive, concomitant CBT and pharmacotherapy is indicated and usually more effective than either one alone.

b. *What feasible pharmacotherapeutic alternatives are available for treatment of panic disorder?*

- Treatment pathways are not simple for panic disorder. The following considerations are important in selecting appropriate therapy: 1) desired time of onset of effects; 2) side effects; 3) cost; 4) avoidance symptoms and behaviors; 5) presence of other anxiety disorders and depression; 6) risk of suicide and lethality of medication; and 7) history of chemical dependence.
- Benzodiazepines and antidepressants may be indicated alone and in combination at different times in the treatment. Ideally, one medication is started initially based on the above information. A single medication may be easier for a patient to initiate, comply with, and tolerate. The initial regimens that follow should be titrated slowly as tolerated. Both classes of medication, benzodiazepines and antidepressants, may be used indefinitely (for life) in some patients. Some of these low-dose regimens may require pharmacy reformulation to arrive at this dosage form.

Benzodiazepines
- Alprazolam 0.5–1 mg po TID
- Clonazepam 0.25–0.5 mg po BID
- Lorazepam 0.5–1 mg po TID

Selective Serotonin Reuptake Inhibitors
- Fluoxetine 5 mg po QD
- Paroxetine 5 mg po QD
- Sertraline 12.5 mg po QD
- Venlafaxine 37.5 mg po QD

Tricyclic Antidepressants
- Desipramine 10 mg po QD
- Imipramine 10 mg po QD

Monoamine Oxidase Inhibitors
- Phenelzine 7.5 mg po QD
- Tranylcypromine 10 mg po QD

- Because benzodiazepines work so quickly and effectively, patients may be reluctant to discontinue them because of experiencing such a positive response.
- All antidepressant medications are generally effective in treating panic disorder. Patients and practitioners may have trouble with the term "antidepressant," as these medications also have antianxiety activity.
- SSRIs are probably the class of choice due to a lower side-effect profile than the other antidepressant classes. However, tricyclic antidepressants (TCAs) and monoamine oxidase inhibitors (MAOI) are quite effective if used carefully and adequately.
- TCAs offer plasma level monitoring if a patient is non-responsive. Effective levels have been established for desipramine and imipramine in the treatment of panic disorder.
- MAOIs also have a place in pharmacotherapy, and the diet is not too difficult to follow.
- Cost and likely compliance with the regimen are important. Many patients cannot tolerate the side effects of the older and less expensive medications. The costs of the drug versus the economic effects of increased illness, decreased work, more visits to the ER, increased heath care visits, unnecessary laboratory tests, depression, and suicide need to be considered in developing a treatment plan.

Optimal Plan

4. a. *What drug, dosage form, dose, schedule, and duration of therapy are best for this patient?*

- This patient may respond best to a combination of a SSRI and adequate doses of a benzodiazepine due to the comorbid conditions of panic disorder, depression, and GAD. The combination would have the added benefits of a fast onset from the benzodiazepine as well as blocking some of the potential initial anxiety produced by the SSRI.
- An example regimen is alprazolam or lorazepam 0.5 mg po TID increased to 1 mg po TID as tolerated. At the same time, sertraline 12.5 mg po QD or paroxetine 5 mg po QD (very low-dose) could be initiated and increased by gradually titrating up as tolerated over 1 to 4 weeks to 50 to 100 mg and 20 to 40 mg/day, respectively.[3]

- Treatment should be initiated slowly to avoid hyperstimulatory effects from the antidepressants and oversedation from the benzodiazepines.
- If the patient has never been treated with a benzodiazepine, discuss initial length of treatment and ease fears of "addiction." Some patients may need treatment with a benzodiazepine for several months, whereas for others, this may be the best treatment and will be used indefinitely.

b. *If initial treatment fails, what alternatives should be considered?*

- Assess the initial length of treatment: allow 8 to 12 weeks.
- Determine whether an adequate dose was given.
- Consider an adequate trial of another SSRI, then a TCA, then a MAOI.
- Consider using CBT and other psychotherapies.
- Determine whether the patient has used other substances that may exacerbate anxiety, panic, or depression.

Outcome Evaluation

5. *What clinical and laboratory parameters are necessary to evaluate the therapy for achievement of the desired therapeutic outcome and to detect or prevent adverse effects?*

Efficacy

- Assess overall quality of life by patient interview to determine if the panic attacks, avoidance, and anticipatory anxiety are affecting her life at home, work, and socially.
- Have the patient keep a written account or panic diary. Count the number of panic attacks and the intensity (mild, moderate, severe). Ideally, patients will be panic-free; however, a change from 10 panic attacks a week to one every other week may be clinically significant.
- Ask the patient if she continues to avoid situations and activities that she wants or needs to do, such as shopping, driving, socializing, and leisure activities. Find out whether she is staying at home because of fear.
- Assess levels of anxiety and depression using the Hamilton Rating Scale for Anxiety and Depression (HAM-A and HAM-D) if she is not responding adequately. Scores of 20 or more (HAM-A) and 16 or more (HAM-D) are clinically significant and deserve attention.
- Assess the patient's level of suicidal ideation by interviewing the patient, initially asking, "Are there times you wish you weren't alive?" or "Have you thought you would be better off if you were dead?" or "Have you thought of taking your life?"

Adverse Events

- *SSRIs.* Sedation and insomnia; GI symptoms including cramps, nausea, and diarrhea; sexual dysfunction including decreased libido and lack of orgasm in women and retarded ejaculation in men; CNS effects such as headache, anxiety, and restlessness.
- *Benzodiazepines.* Sedation, ataxia, lethargy, cognitive defects.

Patient Counseling

6. *What information should be provided to the patient to enhance compliance, ensure successful therapy, and minimize adverse effects?*

- The response to this medication is usually slow and gradual, but it

will work. You will likely see a decrease in your panic attacks and anxiety over the next 3 to 8 weeks with maximum effects seen as late as 12 weeks. The positive effects will be like watching spring occur—like watching leaves on a tree appear as you move from winter into spring.
- Side effects may occur before you see the beneficial effects. Fortunately, they are often few, mild, tolerable, and resolve with continued treatment. Many people do not even notice they are taking any medication.
- Please give me a call on the phone a few hours after the first dose of this medication (antidepressant). I would like to know how you feel.
- Initial treatment for panic disorder usually lasts at least 6 to 12 months after having a good response and being panic free. Then you gradually taper the medication under your physician's supervision.
- Please read these written materials on panic and anxiety.
- Remember, a panic attack is a medical, biologic event. Panic disorder can be a successfully treated medical disorder. Most people would have had the same symptoms if they had a panic attack.
- *Teach simple cognitive therapy.* When you feel an attack coming on, slowly and repeatedly say to yourself, "This is a panic attack. It will soon go away. I have had them before and I always get over them."
- When you are having a panic attack, you breathe too fast and change your body chemistry. Sit down, take a deep breath on the count of 1, 2, 3, 4 and then slowly exhale, on the count of 1, 2, 3, 4. Breathe from your diaphragm.
- I want you to ask questions and take an active role in your treatment. This is usually a long-term disorder and you may have it for life.
- All of these medications can be used safely on a long-term basis, sometimes for life. When you take a benzodiazepine for several months, your body can become physically dependent on it. This is not usually a problem if the medication is helping you, not causing you any side effects, and you don't have to increase the dose. However, you can't just stop it abruptly; you will need to taper the dose down over several months.
- If you do develop physical dependence, that doesn't mean you have become an addict. It means your body needs the medication on a regular basis for normal functioning as well as to control your panic disorder. An addict is someone who uses medication for an unapproved use, in an uncontrolled manner, usually taking very high doses and trying to get high.
- Short-acting SSRIs (paroxetine, sertraline, venlafaxine) should be tapered gradually to avoid any withdrawal effects.

References

1. Kessler RC, McGonagle KA, Zhao S, et al. Lifetime and 12-month prevalence of DSM-III-R psychiatric disorders in the United States. Results from the National Comorbidity Survey. Arch Gen Psychiatry 1994;51:8–19.
2. Lydiard RB. Anxiety and the irritable bowel syndrome: psychiatric, medical, or both? J Clin Psychiatry 1997;58(suppl 3):51–58.
3. Giesecke ME. Overcoming hypersensitivity to fluoxetine in a patient with panic disorder. Am J Psychiatry 1990;147:532–533.
4. Katschnig H, Amering M, Stolk JM, et al. Long-term follow-up after a drug trial for panic disorder. Br J Psychiatry 1995;167:487–494.

67 OBSESSIVE-COMPULSIVE DISORDER

▶ The Little Girl on the Swing   (Level II)

Lyle K. Laird, PharmD, BCPP

A 31-year-old man is referred to an anxiety disorders clinic because of persistent obsessions and compulsions that are negatively impacting his quality of life. The patient has been treated with the maximum dose of clomipramine (250 mg/day) for 6 weeks but has ECG changes that may indicate an adverse effect of the drug. Although the patient has not received an adequate 8- to 12-week trial of clomipramine, it may be prudent to consider other pharmacotherapeutic options such as an SSRI (fluvoxamine, fluoxetine, paroxetine, or sertraline). Cognitive-behavioral therapy is also an important part of the therapeutic plan. The response to therapy should be assessed periodically by an objective instrument such as the Yale–Brown Obsessive-Compulsive Scale (Y–BOCS). Patients with OCD generally require long-term treatment to prevent symptom recurrence.

▶ Questions

Problem Identification

1. a. *Create a list of the patient's drug-related problems.*

- Diagnosis of OCD treated with an anti-OCD medication at the maximum dose (clomipramine 250 mg/day) for at least 6 weeks without resolution of the condition.
- Possible comorbid depressive disorder.
- ECG abnormalities that may be a result of his present medication(s).
- Need for proper medication selection for the patient's conditions.

b. *What signs, symptoms, or laboratory parameters indicate the presence of OCD in this patient?*

- The diagnosis of OCD is made after careful consideration of presenting symptoms and the patient's history. The specific diagnostic criteria for this disorder are outlined in the DSM-IV.[1] Refer to textbook Chapter 68 for complete information.
- This patient has several key symptoms that are critical in making the diagnosis.
    - ✓ He has repeated intrusive thoughts that are disturbing to him. These obsessions consist of thoughts that his handiwork with a swing has resulted in a child being injured and that the police will be coming to arrest him. Also, he obsesses that he might have run over someone with his car.

- ✓ He is aware that his thoughts are abnormal.
- ✓ He has some compulsions, such as repeatedly checking the mail and driving around the block.
- ✓ The obsessions and compulsions are time-consuming and significantly interfere with his daily functioning, especially impacting his job.
- ✓ On physical exam, his skin shows signs of excessive washing and perhaps scrubbing.
- The patient has recent signs of a possible coexisting depressive disorder (e.g., poor appetite, insomnia, and a helpless or hopeless sense that includes fleeting suicidal ideation). Refer to textbook Chapter 65 for more information.
- OCD cannot be diagnosed by any laboratory assessments.

Desired Outcome

2. What are the goals of the pharmacotherapy for OCD in this case?

- Decrease the patient's overall level of anxiety and specifically the frequency of obsessive thoughts. Complete suppression of the obsessions is unlikely to be achieved.
- Reduce the time spent performing compulsive behaviors and rituals (e.g., to stop searching for bodies when his car hits a bump in the road).
- Enable him to return to his job and maintain a reasonably normal quality of life.
- Minimize adverse reactions to his medication regimen; medication doses tend to be high in OCD cases, and patients can experience dose-related side effects.

Therapeutic Alternatives

3. a. What non-drug therapies might be useful for this patient?

- Cognitive-behavioral therapy (CBT) consists of exposure and/or response prevention.
    - ✓ *Exposure* is a technique in which the patient is carefully introduced to situations where the stimuli that evoke the anxiety are present. Over time and with continued controlled exposure to the stimuli, the patient's anxiety is gradually dampened (habituation) and lessened.
    - ✓ *Response prevention* is a technique whereby the patient is taught to resist performing the compulsive behavior. Over time, there is less of a need to perform it and less uncomfortable anxiety.
- These techniques are known to be useful and effective therapeutic interventions in OCD. They are time-consuming (e.g., with a session lasting up to 90 minutes), and as with medications, they can take 3 months or more to be maximally effective.
- Combining either or both of these CBT techniques with pharmacotherapy may be of more benefit to the patient than either one of the treatment modalities alone.[2]
- His overall level of anxiety (i.e., not including his obsessive-compulsive symptoms) might be improved if he cut down on his daily consumption of caffeine.

b. What feasible pharmacotherapeutic alternatives are available for the treatment of OCD?

- *Option one.* Continue the clomipramine for another 4 to 6 weeks with careful follow-up of the ECG. The use of a rating scale such as the Y–BOCS is strongly encouraged. This will assist in better tracking of the clinical outcome and is useful in justifying the therapeutic intervention.
- *Option two.* An alternative strategy is to change to one of the SSRIs such as fluvoxamine, fluoxetine, paroxetine, or sertraline and give an 8- to 12-week trial while following the patient for adverse effects as well as for clinical improvement on a rating scale (e.g., Y–BOCS).
- CBT should be combined with the pharmacotherapy option selected, if possible.

Optimal Plan

4. What drug, dosage form, dose, schedule, and duration of therapy are best for this patient?

Option One: Continue Clomipramine

- The patient has been receiving clomipramine 250 mg daily (the maximum recommended dose) for 6 weeks. An adequate trial of an anti-OCD medication requires 8 to 12 weeks. This tricyclic antidepressant (TCA) was the first medication that gained FDA approval for the treatment of OCD. It is quite effective for this indication; indeed, the experience and research with this medication in OCD resulted in the "serotonin hypothesis" for OCD, a possible explanation for the pathophysiologic basis of the disorder. However, the patient needs to be assessed for the presence of adverse effects from clomipramine. As a TCA, clomipramine has a high incidence of anticholinergic effects (e.g., dry mouth, blurred near vision, constipation) and sedation. Daily doses in excess of 250 mg have been associated with an increased incidence of seizures. The patient's ECG shows a borderline A-V block; although the QTc interval is not yet dangerously prolonged (0.436 sec), it should be carefully followed if the TCA is continued. With the availability of medications such as the SSRIs that do not seem to lengthen the QT interval, a switch to one of these medications may be prudent.[3] The SSRIs lack significant affinity for cholinergic, histaminic, and α-adrenergic receptors and hence do not result in the same adverse-effect profile as the TCA clomipramine.

Option Two: Start an SSRI and Discontinue Clomipramine

- *Fluvoxamine.* A reasonable fluvoxamine regimen is to start with 50 mg orally at bedtime, followed by increases of 50 mg/day every week as tolerated until maximum benefit is achieved. The dosage titration might be faster if the patient were an inpatient. Clinical response is indicated by improvement in the obsessive-compulsive symptoms and not necessarily complete resolution of the illness. If doses are 100 mg/day or greater, the regimen should be divided into two doses with the larger dose being given at bedtime. The dosage range generally associated with therapeutic effectiveness is 100 to 300 mg/day.
- *Fluoxetine.* The initial dose of fluoxetine is 20 mg/day with dosage increases every other week until clinical response is observed. Fluoxetine is often given once daily in the morning. When it is given as a BID regimen, the doses are typically taken in the morning and at noon to reduce the likelihood of insomnia that has been reported with SSRIs. Some patients actually experience sedation on this medication; if this occurs, it can be given at bedtime. The dosage range

for fluoxetine generally associated with effectiveness is 20 to 80 mg/day.
- *Paroxetine*. If paroxetine is selected, the starting dose is 20 mg (usually in the morning), and this is titrated by 10 mg/day every week as tolerated until clinical response is observed. The usual therapeutic dosage range is 40 to 60 mg/day.
- *Sertraline*. This SSRI is also indicated for OCD, and it may be started at 50 mg once daily, either in the morning or at bedtime. It should be titrated upward in 25- to 50-mg increments every week. The usual therapeutic dosage range for OCD is 50 to 200 mg/day.
- This patient does not have a history of taking multiple other medications. Nevertheless, when any of the SSRIs are used, it is necessary to be aware of potential drug–drug interactions. For example, fluvoxamine affects other medications that are metabolized by the cytochrome P450 liver enzymes such as theophylline, caffeine, haloperidol, and astemizole. Fluoxetine and paroxetine can affect drug levels of the TCAs, and haloperidol and sertraline can affect some of the benzodiazepines.
- For any of the medications used to treat OCD, a reasonable trial is considered from 8 to 12 weeks. If an SSRI or clomipramine does not effect a clinical improvement after a reasonable trial, then another SSRI might be tried.
- The use of a CBT program in combination with the pharmacotherapy is extremely important in attaining a successful treatment regimen for this OCD patient.
- In addition to trials of other monotherapies, various augmentation strategies are available should the patient prove to be treatment-resistant.[4,5] Examples include the addition of buspirone, lithium, or even the atypical antipsychotic risperidone.
- Long-term effectiveness of any of these medications in OCD has not yet been conclusively established. Because of the chronic nature of OCD and the almost certain resurgence of symptoms if a regimen is stopped prematurely, it is reasonable to expect that these medications will be used for extended periods in the patient who has responded adequately to a given regimen. The clinician should work diligently with the patient to find the lowest effective dosage. Treatment regimens need to be periodically reevaluated for effectiveness and adverse effects and adjusted accordingly.

Outcome Evaluation

5. *What clinical and laboratory parameters are necessary to evaluate the therapy for achievement of the desired therapeutic outcome and to detect or prevent adverse effects?*

- Because the goal of pharmacotherapy is to minimize and/or resolve symptoms, the clinician should carefully document the symptoms at baseline (description, frequency, and severity) and then follow them over time for resolution.
- Ideally, the effectiveness of pharmacotherapy should be monitored by a valid OCD rating scale such as the Yale–Brown Obsessive-Compulsive Scale (Y–BOCS).[6,7] This 10-item, clinician-administered questionnaire allows the clinician to assess on a regular basis how specific obsessive thoughts and/or compulsive behaviors are responding to the therapy. It is specific for OCD in that it excludes questions regarding depression or anxiety not related to the obsessive-compulsive symptoms. The results of a Y–BOCS can range from 0 to 40. A score of 0 corresponds to a lack of symptoms and 40 shows an extremely severe case of OCD. It should be mentioned that the Y–BOCS is used primarily for following response to therapy and is not a valid diagnostic tool.
- Clinical progress cannot be assessed by the use of any laboratory test or procedure. Thus, blood concentrations of the current anti-OCD medications are not presently clinically useful in assessing therapeutic effectiveness.
- The patient should be informed of the significant and common adverse effects associated with the pharmacotherapy. At follow-up visits, patients receiving SSRIs should be assessed for the presence of nausea, vomiting, headache, irritability, tremor, and sexual dysfunction (such as impotence or abnormal ejaculation). Clomipramine can cause tremor, dry mouth, dizziness upon standing, drowsiness and sedation, sexual dysfunction, and dose-related seizures (do not exceed 250 mg/day).

Patient Counseling

6. *What information should be provided to the patient to enhance compliance, ensure successful therapy, and minimize adverse effects?*

General Instructions
- Take this medicine daily only in the manner prescribed for you.
- Use caution in driving until you know how the medication affects you.
- This medication will be started at low doses and gradually increased as indicated by your response.
- If you miss a dose, take it as soon as you remember unless it is past 3:00 PM. If it is past 3:00 PM, skip the dose and take the next scheduled dose at its regular time. Do not double doses.
- Medications used in the treatment of OCD are generally used on a long-term basis. Relapse of symptoms is common if the medications are discontinued prematurely. Do not stop taking the medication unless directed by your prescriber or unless you have discussed it with him or her.
- Inform the prescriber of all other drugs, vitamins, or herbal products that you are taking.
- Contact your prescriber if you notice or suspect side effects.
- Keep all scheduled follow-up appointments with your prescriber.

Fluoxetine
- Take this medication in the morning (if once a day) or in the morning and at noon (if twice daily).
- It may be taken with or without food or on a full or empty stomach.

Fluvoxamine
- At first, you will take this medication once a day (e.g., at bedtime); as you need higher doses, you may be instructed to take it twice a day.
- This may be taken with or without food or on a full or empty stomach.

Paroxetine
- At first, you will take this medication once a day (e.g., in the morn-

ing or in the evening); as you need higher doses, you may be instructed to take it twice a day.
- This may be taken with or without food or on a full or empty stomach.

Sertraline
- At first, you will take this medication once a day (e.g., in the morning or in the evening); as you need higher doses, you may be instructed to take it twice a day.
- It may be taken with or without food or on a full or empty stomach.

Clomipramine
- This medication is initially taken in small doses several times daily with meals or food to prevent it from upsetting your stomach or causing nausea.
- Since you are already taking a maintenance dose, you may continue to take the single 250-mg dose once a day. Taking it at bedtime is helpful because it is sedating and can make you drowsy.

▶ Follow-up Questions

1. Why is it important to taper the clomipramine?

- Clomipramine has a significant anticholinergic component; once a patient has been stabilized on such a medication, abrupt withdrawal could result in a cholinergic rebound withdrawal syndrome. This syndrome may consist of signs of general discomfort such as flu-like symptoms, anxiety, insomnia, and GI distress.
- A taper of the clomipramine prior to starting the fluvoxamine also serves to avoid a clinically significant drug–drug interaction; the fluvoxamine could raise the level of the TCA, which may result in an increase in adverse effects or toxicity.
- In addition to precipitating a possible withdrawal reaction, abrupt discontinuation of the clomipramine could foster a sense of distrust from the patient toward the therapist or prescriber. It is generally wise to taper TCAs unless otherwise clinically indicated (e.g., in cases of acute toxicity or if the patient is in imminent danger of a severe adverse drug reaction).

2. Why is it important to minimize the use of the hypnotic?

- The SSRIs can interact with benzodiazepines, causing an increase in the serum benzodiazepine concentration and an increase in its adverse effects, including excessive sedation.
- Also, the need for the sleeping medication should lessen as the OCD and/or depression is adequately treated.
- Furthermore, long-term efficacy of benzodiazepine hypnotics is in question.

3. Why was he apparently so intolerant of coffee when he was placed on fluvoxamine?

- Fluvoxamine can inhibit the metabolism of caffeine and thereby increase caffeine levels resulting in accentuated caffeine side effects (e.g., feeling "buzzed").

4. When is a decrease in the Y–BOCS score considered clinically significant?

- When the Y–BOCS is used in clinical drug trials, a decrease of 35% from baseline is operationally considered "significant." Clinically speaking, a significant reduction in the Y–BOCS could be any decrease in the Y–BOCS.
- An "acceptable" reduction in symptomatology needs to be recognized not only by the clinician but also be accepted by the patient. It should be remembered that complete remission of OCD symptoms is a rarity in clinical practice and that recurrence of symptoms upon premature medication discontinuation is commonplace.

References

1. American Psychiatric Association. Diagnostic and Statistical Manual of Mental Disorders (DSM-IV), 4th ed. Washington, DC, American Psychiatric Association, 1994.
2. Greist JH. An integrated approach to treatment of obsessive compulsive disorder. J Clin Psychiatry 1992;53 (suppl):38–41.
3. Laird LK, Lydiard RB, Morton WA, et al. Cardiovascular effects of imipramine, fluvoxamine, and placebo in depressed outpatients. J Clin Psychiatry 1993;54: 224–228.
4. Laird LK. Issues in the monopharmacotherapy and polypharmacotherapy of obsessive-compulsive disorder. Psychopharmacol Bull 1996;32:569–578.
5. McDougle CJ. Update on pharmacologic management of OCD: Agents and augmentation. J Clin Psychiatry 1997;58 (suppl 12):11–17.
6. Goodman WK, Price LH, Rasmussen SA, et al. The Yale–Brown Obsessive Compulsive Scale. I. Development, use, and reliability. Arch Gen Psychiatry 1989;46: 1006–1011.
7. Goodman WK, Price LH, Rasmussen SA, et al. The Yale–Brown Obsessive Compulsive Scale. II. Validity. Arch Gen Psychiatry 1989;46:1012–1016.

68 INSOMNIA

▶ In Search of Safe and Restful Sleep (Level II)

Penny S. Shelton, PharmD, BCPP, FASCP
Mollie Ashe Scott, PharmD, BCPS

A 67-year-old man with a history of anxiety disorder, BPH, osteoarthritis, and dyslipidemia reports with his daughter to an ambulatory care clinic seeking treatment for insomnia. He reports difficulty falling asleep, early morning awakening, and other symptoms. His anxiety and insomnia have worsened since the death of his wife 3 months ago. He has attempted self-treatment with Sominex (diphenhydramine 50 mg) without relief and has recently been taking St. John's wort upon the recommendation of his daughter. The patient has a number of underlying contributing causes of insomnia that should be corrected before initiating pharmacotherapy. Nonpharmacologic approaches such as education on good sleep hygiene and relaxation techniques should also be considered. Pharmacologic alternatives include benzodiazepines, zolpidem, tricyclic antidepressants, trazodone, antihistamines, chloral hydrate, barbiturates, and melatonin. Careful attention must be paid to patient-specific factors when selecting the optimal pharmacotherapy for this patient.

Questions

Problem Identification

1. a. Create a drug-related problem list for the patient.

- Insomnia (sleep onset and sleep maintenance deficits) that may ultimately benefit from pharmacologic and/or nonpharmacologic interventions.
- Anxiety (GAD versus panic disorder) presently untreated.
- Right hip and knee pain and stiffness secondary to osteoarthritis, presently untreated.
- Symptomatic BPH, possibly aggravated by the anticholinergic effects of Sominex (diphenhydramine 50 mg) and presently untreated.
- Iatrogenic hyperthyroidism (decreased TSH and elevated free T_4) due to excessive levothyroxine dosage.
- Hypercholesterolemia inadequately treated with present Pravachol (pravastatin) dose (goal LDL ≤100 mg/dL with known CHD).
- Nicotine addiction that may benefit from pharmacologic and/or psychological intervention.
- Use of an herbal remedy (St. John's wort) without a medical indication and which may be contributing to insomnia.

b. What information (signs, symptoms, laboratory values) indicates the presence or severity of insomnia?

Duration
- The patient has had difficulty with sleep for at least 3 months, which is indicative of chronic insomnia. Refer to the section on "Insomnia" in textbook Chapter 69 for more detailed information.

Sleep Disorder
- The patient has difficulty getting to sleep and maintaining sleep.

Insomnia
- Typically a symptom of a psychiatric or medical problem, as in this case (refer to Table 69–2 in the textbook). Contributing factors include:
  - ✓ *Anxiety.* The patient has episodes of shortness of breath, palpitations, a feeling of overwhelming doom, and choking sensations. He expressed an overwhelming fear of dying and excessive worrying. His current hyperthyroid status may contribute to anxiety (see below).
  - ✓ *Mental stressors* (e.g., the recent death of his spouse, financial difficulties since working only part-time).
  - ✓ *Pain* can interfere with getting to sleep and maintaining sleep. He did complain of mild to moderate joint pain upon awakening and after sitting for extended periods of time.
  - ✓ *Nocturia* can disrupt sleep. The patient is awakening 2 to 3 times a night with the need to urinate. He is exhibiting symptoms of urinary retention and difficulty with initiating a urine stream.
  - ✓ *Iatrogenic hyperthyroidism* (low TSH and high T_4).

c. Could any of the patient's problems have been caused by drug therapy?

Agents That May Contribute to Insomnia
- Recent use of alcohol to aid in sleep may be worsening the problem by reducing the quality of sleep.
- Nicotine from smoking can increase catecholamine activity, which can cause insomnia.
- The Synthroid dose is too high, causing iatrogenic hyperthyroidism.
- St. John's wort (an herbal remedy used for depression and anxiety); its mechanism of action is believed to inhibit monoamine oxidase, which can cause restlessness and insomnia in some individuals).[1]

Agents That May Contribute to Anxiety
- Excessive Synthroid dose
- Nicotine use
- St. John's wort

Agents Contributing to Urinary Retention
- Sominex contains diphenhydramine (an antihistamine with anticholinergic properties), which can reduce detrusor activity leading to urinary retention, bladder distention, pain, and overflow incontinence, particularly in older men with BPH.

d. What additional information is needed to satisfactorily assess this patient?

- Specific information regarding the patient's sleep hygiene and diet are needed (refer to Table 69–3 in the textbook). For example:
  - ✓ How often does he nap during the day?
  - ✓ Is his sleep schedule the same every evening, or is it different on days he works compared to days he is off?
  - ✓ How much caffeine does he consume each day?
  - ✓ Does he eat late at night or right before going to bed?
  - ✓ Does he use his bedroom only for sleep or is he working or watching television in the same room?
- Assessment of the patient's anxiety disorder by a psychiatrist is recommended.

Desired Outcome

2. What are the goals of pharmacotherapy in this case?

- Treat the underlying causes or contributors to insomnia.
  - ✓ Since the majority of sleep disorders are associated with psychiatric problems, and since this patient's clinical picture suggests some type of anxiety disorder, he should be referred to a psychiatrist to have his anxiety disorder appropriately identified and treated (i.e., GAD, given the patient's history, versus panic, due to the overwhelming sense of impending doom, the duration of discrete "attacks," and his physical symptoms such as tachypnea, tachycardia, and sweating).[2] The insomnia may improve after appropriate treatment for anxiety is initiated.
  - ✓ Thyroid function should be normalized and stabilized.
  - ✓ Osteoarthritis pain should be treated.
  - ✓ Potential contributing OTC medications should be discontinued (i.e., St. Johns wort and Sominex).
- Reduce daytime napping and increase nocturnal sleep to > 5 hours each night.

Therapeutic Alternatives

3. a. *What non-pharmacologic therapies might be useful for this patient?*

    - Patient education regarding normal age-related changes in sleep.
    - Patient education regarding good sleep hygiene. Refer to textbook Table 69–3 for more complete information.
    - Counseling or psychotherapy may be of benefit, particularly due to the recent death of his spouse.
    - Relaxation and stress-reducing techniques may also be of benefit since stress and anxiety can exacerbate and maintain insomnia.
    - Discontinue drinking the glass of wine at bedtime.
    - Educate the patient on the importance of a smoking cessation program.

    b. *What feasible pharmacotherapeutic alternatives are available for treatment of insomnia?*

    - *Benzodiazepines* have been found to be effective in the short-term management of insomnia. However, due to this patient's history of substance abuse and currently elevated liver transaminases, these agents should be avoided at this time. In addition, benzodiazepines have been shown to increase the risk of falls and cognitive impairment in the elderly.[3] This pharmacologic class could, however, potentially benefit his anxiety disorder.
    - *Zolpidem* has been found to be similar in efficacy to the benzodiazepines for both acute and chronic insomnia. Like the benzodiazepines, zolpidem works by increasing GABA activity; however, it selectively binds to one benzodiazepine receptor (ω1). It also appears to have fewer deleterious effects on sleep architecture and fewer cognitive and psychomotor side effects when compared to benzodiazepines.[4] Because the GABA-receptor complex activity theoretically carries the risk for dependence like benzodiazepines, this agent may be less than ideal for this patient based on his history. Zolpidem is also expensive, and this patient is concerned with finances and is on a limited budget. Therefore, avoiding this agent as first-line treatment would be prudent.
    - *Tricyclic antidepressants* (TCAs) can be useful in insomnia associated with depression due to their sedative properties. However, TCAs have significant adverse effects, including anticholinergic effects, orthostatic hypotension, lowering of the seizure threshold, and cardiac arrhythmias. Therefore, these agents would be less than ideal in this patient who currently has a history of symptomatic BPH, constipation, and left BBB.
    - *Trazodone*, a serotonin-specific antidepressant, is a good alternative for insomnia in patients who should not take benzodiazepines or TCAs.[5] The advantages of trazodone include its availability in a generic form, lack of tolerance or dependence, and lack of anticholinergic and arrhythmogenic side effects. However, orthostatic hypotension is a potential problem, particularly in the elderly.
    - *Antihistamines* are less effective than benzodiazepines in the management of insomnia. These agents should be avoided in this patient due to anticholinergic side effects that can potentially worsen his symptomatic BPH.
    - *Chloral hydrate* should be avoided since it offers no clear advantage over other agents and can cause significant gastrointestinal irritation.
    - *Barbiturates* are strongly associated with abuse and dependence. These agents also increase the risk for falls and cognitive impairment in the elderly. Barbiturates are no longer recommended for treatment of insomnia due to their side-effect profile and potential for enzyme induction interactions. In addition, they would not be a good choice given this patient's history of Seconal (secobarbital) addiction.
    - *Melatonin* may be a viable alternative for the management of insomnia in elderly patients with melatonin deficiency, according to the results of several small controlled trials.[6] However, melatonin is not an FDA-approved product and consumer products have not been thoroughly assessed for product impurities or long-term adverse effects.

Optimal Plan

4. a. *What drug, dosage form, dose, schedule, and duration of therapy are best for this patient?*

    - Trazodone 25 to 75 mg po Q HS PRN is the best option because other therapeutic alternatives have distinct disadvantages for this particular patient. It should be prescribed for short-term use (4 weeks only).
    - The non-pharmacologic therapy described above should also be implemented.
    - A benzodiazepine would benefit his anxiety as well as provide relief from insomnia. However, with his substance abuse history, using buspirone for anxiety and trazodone for insomnia is a safer way to initiate therapy for GAD. This patient requires a psychiatric assessment prior to initiation of an anxiolytic, particularly since first-line treatments for panic disorder differ from GAD.

    b. *What alternatives would be appropriate if the initial therapy fails or cannot be used?*

    - The patient has difficulty with sleep latency and early morning awakening; therefore, an agent with an intermediate duration taken 1 hour before bedtime would be most appropriate.
    - Benzodiazepines that are glucuronidated are not affected by age-related changes in pharmacokinetics. An intermediate-acting glucuronidated benzodiazepine such as temazepam 7.5 to 15 mg po Q HS PRN is a reasonable choice.
    - If used, the lowest possible dose of temazepam should be prescribed due to the increased pharmacodynamic sensitivity to these drugs in the elderly.
    - Temazepam is a second-line choice due to the potential for addiction in this patient with a history of barbiturate addiction.
    - Long-acting benzodiazepines (e.g., chlordiazepoxide, diazepam, flurazepam) should be avoided in the elderly. An intermediate-acting agent carries less risk of oversedation. However, all benzodiazepines have been found to increase risk of falls in the elderly.

Outcome Evaluation

5. *What clinical and laboratory parameters are necessary to evaluate the therapy for achievement of the desired therapeutic outcome and to detect or prevent adverse effects?*

    - For clinical outcomes, obtain follow-up information about his insomnia and contributing factors in 2 weeks. You should specifically

assess time to sleep onset, nocturnal awakenings, number of hours of sleep each night, and quality of sleep. Also evaluate the severity of OA pain and stiffness and the presence of BPH symptoms after the discontinuation of the anticholinergic Sominex. Recommendations from psychiatry regarding anxiety management should be followed.
- Laboratory tests that should be performed include a follow-up TSH in 4 weeks after Synthroid dosage reduction and repeat of the lipid profile in 3 months after an increase in the Pravachol (pravastatin) dose.
- Adverse effects to be monitored include assessment of oversedation and orthostatic blood pressure monitoring in 2 weeks at his scheduled follow-up visit. However, the patient should be instructed to call his physician or pharmacist if problems with morning grogginess, dizziness, or unsteadiness develop.

Patient Counseling

6. What information should be provided to the patient to enhance compliance, ensure successful therapy, and minimize adverse effects?

Trazodone
- The name of your new medicine for insomnia is trazodone. You are to take one-half tablet, which is 25 mg, by mouth an hour before you go to bed. If you find that this amount is ineffective, you may try 50 mg, which is one whole tablet. If one tablet is ineffective, you can take up to a maximum of 1.5 tablets, or 75 mg. Most patients get relief from their insomnia between 25 and 75 mg. Start with 25 mg and find the dose that works for you. It may take a few nights to find the right dose. Do not take more than 1.5 tablets (75 mg) a night without first consulting your physician. (*Note:* The clinician should check to see if the patient understands the directions and can break the tablets correctly.)
- Use this medication only when you need it and take the smallest amount necessary to help you sleep. Also, use this medication every 2 or 3 nights, rather than every night; this will help it work better and minimize side effects. You will take the medicine for up to 4 weeks.
- You may find that you are sleepy when you wake up in the morning. Use caution when you are driving or using machinery at work until you know how this drug affects you. Be careful when you stand up after sitting or lying; rise slowly to avoid getting dizzy.
- Monitor how you sleep at night and let your doctor know at your next visit if you are sleeping better.
- Be sure to store the medicine away from children and pets.

▶ Follow-up Question

1. What other medication adjustments should be made at this time?

- D/C St. John's wort.
- D/C Sominex due to its anticholinergic properties, which may be worsening the patient's BPH.
- This patient's symptomatic BPH (as evidenced by difficulty initiating a urine stream) appears to have become problematic following the use of Sominex. Therefore, no specific BPH treatment is recommended at this time. However, the BPH symptoms should be reevaluated after the discontinuation of Sominex at the follow-up visits in 2 and 4 weeks.
- Decrease the Synthroid dose to 100 μg po QD due to the patient's suppressed TSH and elevated T_4. As stated above, reevaluate the thyroid panel in 4 weeks at the second follow-up visit.
- Treat OA with a scheduled regimen of acetaminophen (up to a maximum of 4 grams per day). Monitor LFTs after 4 weeks of therapy. Counsel the patient to avoid OTC combinations containing acetaminophen.
- Increase Pravachol (pravastatin) to 20 mg po Q HS with a goal LDL of ≤ 100 mg/dL.

References

1. Woelk H, Burkard G, Grunwald J. Benefits and risks of the hypericum extract LI 160: Drug monitoring study with 3250 patients. J Geriatr Psychiatry Neurol 1994;7(suppl 1):S34–S38.
2. Nowell PD, Buysse DJ, Reynolds CF III, et al. Clinical factors contributing to the differential diagnosis of primary insomnia and insomnia related to mental disorders. Am J Psychiatry 1997;154:1412–1416.
3. Lechin F, van der Dijs B, Benaim M. Benzodiazepines: Tolerability in elderly patients. Psychother Psychosom 1996;65:171–182.
4. Roger M, Attali P, Coquelin JP. Multicenter, double-blind, controlled comparison of zolpidem and triazolam in elderly patients with insomnia. Clin Ther 1993;15:127–136.
5. Scharf MB, Sachais BA. Sleep laboratory evaluation of the effects and efficacy of trazodone in depressed insomniac patients. J Clin Psychiatry 1990;51(suppl):13–17.
6. Chase JE, Gidal BE. Melatonin: Therapeutic use in sleep disorders. Ann Pharmacother 1997;31:1218–1226.

SECTION 7

Endocrinologic Disorders

Robert L. Talbert, PharmD, FCCP, BCPS, Section Editor

69 TYPE 1 DIABETES MELLITUS

▶ Carolyn Carter's Ketoacidosis (Level II)

Scott Jacober, DO, CDE
Linda A. Jaber, PharmD

A 33-year-old woman with type 1 diabetes mellitus presents with complaints of vomiting, weakness, and dizziness. Physical examination and laboratory evaluation reveal the presence of diabetic ketoacidosis (DKA) probably precipitated by viral gastroenteritis. The primary goals of therapy are to appropriately rehydrate the patient, correct the acidosis, replete the electrolyte deficiencies, and gradually correct the hyperglycemia. Intravenous insulin should be used initially, as subcutaneous or intramuscular absorption may be impaired in DKA patients who are dehydrated. As the DKA resolves, students are asked to reestablish a subcutaneous insulin regimen that will ultimately lead to normoglycemia in the patient.

▶ Questions

Problem Identification

1. *What problems beyond hyperglycemia are encountered in DKA that may require intervention?*

   - *Insulin deficiency.* Hyperglycemia results from the relative or absolute deficiency of insulin. Free insulin levels on presentation of DKA are usually measurable, and therefore an absolute deficiency of insulin is not necessary (as in this case) for the development of DKA. Ketogenesis is promoted by an altered glucagon (increased) to insulin (decreased) ratio. Hypertriglyceridemia and elevated free fatty acid levels are also present as the insulin deficiency decreases the activity of lipoprotein lipase and overall promotes lipolysis. Insulin also regulates Na^+-K^+-ATPase activity, and hyperkalemia may be present initially as a result of a leak of intracellular potassium into the bloodstream.
   - *Dehydration.* As a result of the osmotic diuresis initiated by the hyperglycemia, patients with DKA typically have a free water deficit approximating 10% of body weight, depending on the severity and duration of the pathophysiologic process. Symptoms may range from minimal to severe orthostasis with extreme dizziness to complete cardiovascular collapse with shock.
   - *Acidosis.* Ketoacids accumulate not only because of excess production but because the dehydration has decreased GFR and reduced renal clearance. The resulting metabolic acidosis is partially compensated by a respiratory alkalosis (i.e., Kussmaul's ventilatory pattern). The acidosis may be further complicated by vomiting, which causes a metabolic alkalosis.
   - *Hyperosmolality.* As the dehydration becomes more and more severe, hyperglycemia can become very extreme in the face of a significantly reduced GFR. The reduced GFR compromises the renal clearance of glucose (i.e., glycosuria). The hyperosmolality in addition to the cardiovascular collapse are mechanisms that cause mental obtundation.

- *Electrolyte abnormalities.* Hyperkalemia may be present initially, but with therapy for DKA, hypokalemia may predominate as the total body potassium deficit becomes apparent. Other electrolytes are depleted with the osmotic diuresis and typically include phosphorus, magnesium, and calcium. Serum sodium levels must be corrected for the degree of hyperglycemia to determine the severity of the abnormality (potential hypernatremia). This formula is

$$Na_{corrected} = Na_{measured} + (1.6 \times [BG - 100]/100).$$

Desired Outcome

2. What are the goals of therapy for this patient?

- The therapeutic goals are to rehydrate the patient, correct the acidosis, replete the electrolyte deficiencies, and reestablish a subcutaneous insulin regimen that will restore ketogenesis to normal levels and lessen the severity of hyperglycemia.
- Normoglycemia need not be achieved prior to discharge, but a long-term goal should be to optimize glucose levels.

Therapeutic Alternatives

3. What therapies are available to correct the presenting metabolic derangements of DKA?

- *Normal saline* should be the IV fluid given on preliminary evaluation, since isotonic saline is optimal for resuscitating the intravascular compartment. This should be infused rapidly (1 to 2 L/hr).
- *IV regular insulin* should be administered as the diagnosis of DKA becomes established. If insulin is given in a hypoperfused subcutaneous or intramuscular compartment, absorption may be significantly impaired with little therapeutic benefit. Once these compartments become adequately perfused, absorption may occur at an inappropriate time causing hypoglycemia. Insulin may be given as an IV bolus of 10 to 20 units (0.2 units/kg) followed by a continuous infusion of 5 to 10 units/hr (0.1 units/kg/hr). Fifty mL of the insulin solution should be used to prime the IV tubing to saturate binding to the polymer.[1-2]
- *Sodium bicarbonate* should be administered to correct for severe acidosis (pH 6.9 to 7.1). This may be administered as a bolus or as a continuous infusion (e.g., two 50-mL ampules of sodium bicarbonate 8.4% [50 mEq/ampule] added to 0.45% NaCl solution to approximate isotonic saline).[1-3]
- Emergent treatment of the presenting hyperkalemia (other than insulin) should be reserved for instances where the effects of hyperkalemia are apparent on ECG tracings.

Optimal Plan

4. Outline your specific plan for providing the IV fluids and medications that should be administered to this patient.

- Normal saline should be administered at a rate of at least 500 mL/hr (preferably 1 liter in the first 30 minutes unless there are cardiac or renal constraints).
- This patient may receive an IV bolus of 15 units of regular insulin followed by an infusion of 8 units/hr of insulin in a convenient concentration that would not require frequent replacement (e.g., 100 units/L). These insulin infusion rates are empiric, and the precise rate is not critical. One could typically administer 5 units/hr for a small person (~50 kg) and 10 units/hr for a large person (~100 kg) and a number in between for an individual of intermediate size. Concentrated solutions should be reserved for patients with renal failure who do not develop significant volume depletion. Although the patient has been treated with lispro insulin subcutaneously, there is no difference between the IV action of human regular or lispro insulins.
- Sodium bicarbonate need not be given with this pH (7.05). However, some clinicians may administer bicarbonate if a threshold of pH 7.1 is used. Presently, there is a tendency to use a more acidotic pH threshold (6.9 or 7.0).
- Treatment of the hyperkalemia is adequate with insulin alone.
- After sufficient cardiovascular resuscitation has been provided, the rate of IV fluids may be decreased to 200 to 400 mL/hr and the fluid may be replaced with 0.45% NaCl.[1-3]

Outcome Evaluation

5. a. What monitoring of therapy is necessary for the plan that you outlined for the patient?

- Blood glucose should be measured hourly and electrolytes should be measured every 2 to 8 hours depending upon the severity of the volume depletion, acidosis, symptoms, and electrolyte abnormalities.
- Repeat measurements of ABGs are unnecessary unless there is compromised oxygenation. The acidosis can be monitored by measuring the anion gap and CO_2 levels.
- Serial measurements of acetone may be misleading unless β-hydroxybutyrate is measured directly. The ratio of acetoacetate to β-hydroxybutyrate (not measured by the nitroprusside test) may shift during therapy favoring acetoacetate, where acetoacetate levels may stabilize or increase despite an overall drop in ketoacids.

b. What changes in the therapeutic regimen should be considered when the blood glucose drops below 300 mg/dL or the potassium drops into the low normal range?

- Therapeutic decision points exist when glucose levels drop below 300 mg/dL and when potassium levels drop into the low normal range.
- When the blood glucose levels decrease to less than 300 mg/dL, the IV solution is changed to one containing 5% dextrose to maintain elevated blood glucose levels and not correct the hyperosmolality too quickly. Too rapid correction of the hyperosmolality may cause fatal cerebral edema (which is more common in children and the elderly). Other electrolytes are replaced on an as-needed basis and ultimately are readily corrected when the patient resumes a normal diet.
- If the patient is not oliguric, potassium replacement may be anticipated before the patient becomes hypokalemic. Potassium can be replaced as the chloride or phosphate salt. Non-renal failure patients in DKA frequently are hypophosphatemic and may benefit from replacement with potassium phosphate. However, controlled trials show no overt benefit with regard to outcome when using this form of potassium unless the patient is severely hypophosphatemic (< 1.0 mg/dL). Potassium should not be administered at rates greater than 10 mEq/hr.[1-2]

c. *When is the DKA considered to be resolved, and when can IV insulin therapy be converted to subcutaneous therapy?*

- The DKA is considered to be corrected when the anion gap has been normalized. This may occur before the CO_2 level returns to normal because many patients have a hyperchloremic metabolic acidosis. This bicarbonate-loss acidosis results from ketonuria during the development of the ketoacidosis and not from excess chloride administration (during IV fluid resuscitation) as previously thought. Therefore, resolution of the DKA occurs when the anion gap is corrected and not when the CO_2 levels or pH return to normal. The patient may still have residual ketonuria and ketosis at this point but is not ultimately ketoacidotic.
- Conversion from IV to subcutaneous insulin is important for decreasing the length of stay in hospital for patients with DKA. It is critical to understand that the initial use of IV insulin is preferable to other routes because it assures more predictable circulating levels when hypoperfusion of the subcutaneous and intramuscular compartments is uncertain with severe dehydration. Ketosis may be treated with additional insulin using any route of administration. Therefore, transition from IV to subcutaneous insulin may be made when the patient is adequately rehydrated.

d. *Outline a plan for converting the patient from IV to subcutaneous insulin after resolution of the DKA.*

- The half-life of IV insulin is less than 10 minutes, and the insulin drip must be continued for a period of time after subcutaneous short-acting regular or lispro insulin is given. Since patients are insulin resistant at this time, it may be preferable to allow the short-acting subcutaneous insulin to "peak" before discontinuing the IV insulin.
- Because it is difficult to estimate how much insulin is required at atypical times of the day (such as in the middle of the night), subcutaneous insulin is best resumed at the usual administration times and at the usual dose when the patient is able to resume their usual diet.
- For new patients, estimates of the subcutaneous insulin dose can be made by giving 0.5 units/kg/day (actual weight) divided as follows ("rule of thirds"): $2/3$ in the AM, $1/3$ in the PM, with $2/3$ of each dose given as intermediate-acting insulin and $1/3$ given as short-acting insulin. Older methods that estimate insulin requirements using regular insulin four times daily, summing the total dose administered, and reconfiguring according to the rule of thirds, prolong hospital stay and are no longer cost-effective.

Patient Counseling

6. *How should patients be counseled about self-management on a "sick day" (i.e., when they are anorectic, nauseated, or vomiting)?*

- Patient education is an essential preventative measure, including recognition and treatment of hypoglycemia and hyperglycemia, although an intercurrent illness may obscure their usual warning symptoms.
- Patients should be counseled when to monitor urinary ketones (e.g., when feeling ill or when the blood glucose exceeds 300 mg/dL) and what action to take (take additional insulin or contact a health care provider).
- Patients should also be instructed when feeling ill not to omit insulin if they are unable to eat. Frequently, the illness is associated with insulin resistance that is severe enough to cause hyperglycemia to persist despite reduced carbohydrate consumption.
- Patients should also learn how to convert the carbohydrate portion of their meal plan to liquid carbohydrate for episodes of nausea and vomiting.
- Importantly, patients must be instructed to maintain hydration.

References

1. DeFronzo RA, Matsuda M, Barrett EJ. Diabetic ketoacidosis: A combined metabolic-nephrologic approach to therapy. Diabetes Rev 1994;2:209–238.
2. Foster DW, McGarry JD. The metabolic derangements and treatment of diabetic ketoacidosis. N Engl J Med 1983;309:159–169.
3. Morris LR, Murphy MB, Kitabchi AE. Bicarbonate therapy in severe diabetic ketoacidosis. Ann Intern Med 1986;105:836–840.
4. Ennis ED, Stahl EJB, Kreisberg RA. The hyperosmolar hyperglycemic syndrome. Diabetes Rev 1994;2:115–126.

70 TYPE 2 DIABETES MELLITUS

▶ Establishing Optimal Control   (Level II)

Milissa A. Rock, RPh, CDE
Jean-Venable (Kelly) R. Goode, PharmD, BCPS

A 68-year-old man with type 2 diabetes mellitus, hypertension, and hyperlipidemia presents to a diabetes clinic for a regular check-up. Blood glucose and cholesterol levels have improved since his last visit, but laboratory evaluation indicates that neither condition is under optimal control. Blood pressure also remains above desirable levels. Pharmacologic options for obtaining better glucose control include increasing the dose of his present medications (glyburide and metformin); discontinuing metformin and adding acarbose, troglitazone, or bedtime insulin/daytime sulfonylurea (BIDS) therapy; discontinuing glyburide and adding repaglinide; or discontinuing all oral medications and initiating insulin therapy. Based on this patient's characteristics, use of glyburide and troglitazone is the most reasonable initial choice. Liver enzymes must be monitored periodically while on troglitazone therapy. The case offers students the opportunity to practice providing comprehensive counseling to a patient with type 2 diabetes. Students are also asked to develop treatment plans to optimize control of the patient's hypertension and hyperlipidemia.

Questions

Problem Identification

1. a. *What are this patient's drug-related problems?*

   - Type 2 DM inadequately controlled on the present regimen of diet, exercise, and medication.
   - Hypertension uncontrolled on a moderate dose of an ACE inhibitor.
   - Hyperlipidemia inadequately treated with non-pharmacological therapy alone (target LDL-C for a patient with two or more risk factors is < 130 mg/dL).

   b. *What findings indicate poorly controlled diabetes in this patient?*

   - Fasting blood glucose and pre-dinner glucose in the range of 140 to 175 mg/dL.
   - Random blood glucose of 289 mg/dL.
   - HbA_{1c} 8.2% (indicating suboptimal long-term control).
   - Blurred vision.

Desired Outcome

2. a. *What are the goals of treatment for the management of type 2 diabetes in this patient?*

   - Control blood glucose with the goal parameters being FBG 80 to 120 mg/dL, bedtime BG 100 to 140 mg/dL, and $HbA_{1c} < 7\%$[1]
   - Improve the patient's quality of life
   - Prevent or relieve symptoms and acute complications
   - Decrease the risk factors for chronic complications (i.e., retinopathy, nephropathy, neuropathy, peripheral vascular disease, and cardiovascular disease) by maintaining BP < 130/85 and LDL-C < 130 mg/dL[1-3]

   b. *What individual patient characteristics should be considered in determining the goals of treatment?*

   - Setting individual goals should be based on the patient's ability to understand and carry out the treatment regimen, his risk for severe hypoglycemia, and other factors such as age and comorbidities that may increase risks or decrease benefits.[1]

Therapeutic Alternatives

3. a. *What non-pharmacological interventions should be recommended for this patient?*

   - Continue education and support for adherence to the treatment plan
   - Continue the regular exercise regimen
   - Attempt to reduce alcohol consumption
   - Encourage weight reduction
   - Refer to the dietitian for continued nutrition therapy

   b. *What pharmacologic interventions could be considered for this patient?*

   - *Increase metformin (Glucophage) dose.* The maximum dose of metformin (2550 mg/day) is generally not recommended in the elderly. Although lactic acid levels were not monitored in this patient, the risk for lactic acidosis may be significant, considering his reported symptom of leg pain and the level of alcohol consumption (which may be an underestimate of actual intake). His response to metformin was less than anticipated (usually up to 60 to 80 mg/dL), suggesting that liver glucose production may not be the major factor contributing to his hyperglycemia.
   - *Increase glyburide (Glynase) dose.* The maximum dose of the Glynase product is 12 mg/day given in divided doses. This may result in improved glycemic control initially and is relatively cost effective, but the magnitude of benefit may be small. Maximum effective doses of sulfonylureas are lower than previously assumed, and continued exposure to high concentrations may down-regulate beta-cell sensitivity.[4] It would also pose increased risks for adverse effects, including hypoglycemia, hyperinsulinemia, and weight gain.
   - *Discontinue metformin and add acarbose.* This combination is unlikely to produce a satisfactory response since acarbose decreases postprandial BG levels with minimal effect on FBG levels. Addition of acarbose as a third agent is generally unacceptable due to additive GI adverse effects, poor adherence prospects, and additional costs.
   - *Discontinue metformin and add troglitazone.* Troglitazone represents a therapeutic approach for this patient that addresses insulin resistance as its primary mechanism of action. Since the patient presents with classic syndrome X characteristics (refer to the section on oral hypoglycemics in textbook Chapter 70), this regimen may improve glycemic control through improved glucose utilization without increasing (and by possibly decreasing) insulin requirements. However, this medication is costly and requires intensive monitoring of liver enzymes prior to and during therapy.
   - *Discontinue Glynase and add repaglinide.* Repaglinide is a nonsulfonylurea in the meglitinide class that stimulates phase I insulin secretion. It has a rapid onset and short duration of action, which allow for flexible adjustable dosing of 0.5 to 4 mg with meals, given 2, 3, or 4 times a day. The maximum dose is 16 mg/day. Repaglinide is approved for use as monotherapy or in combination with metformin. Its rapid elimination may lessen the risks of prolonged hypoglycemia and downregulation of beta-cell sensitivity.[4] Adjustable dosing schedules may allow for more flexible and individualized drug therapy management plans for patients on oral agents. However, it is difficult to predict its place in therapy since limited published data are available at the time of this writing.
   - *Discontinue metformin and initiate BIDS therapy (bedtime insulin/daytime sulfonylurea).* This therapy has been increasingly successful when initiated before titration to maximum doses of sulfonylureas and while there is still sufficient beta-cell function intact. It provides for a period of interim insulin use with only one daily injection needed. Bedtime administration of insulin enhances the suppression of nocturnal hepatic glucose production that occurs in the fasting state. BIDS should be reserved for use after treatment failure with oral agents alone or if the cost of oral combination therapy is prohibitive. It does pose

increased risks for weight gain, hypoglycemia, and hyperinsulinemia. Increased frequency of self-monitoring of blood glucose (SMBG) and patient acceptance may be limiting factors (refer to the section, "Correcting Hyperglycemia With Insulin" in textbook Chapter 70).
- *Discontinue oral medications and initiate insulin therapy.* This may simplify the drug regimen and control hyperglycemia, but patient acceptance of more frequent SMBG and more than one daily injection along with the increased risks associated with insulin use suggest that this option is premature. It should be reserved for use after treatment failure with combination oral therapy.

Optimal Plan

4. a. *What pharmacotherapeutic regimen would you recommend for this patient?*

- The use of troglitazone and Glynase is the most logical choice for this patient. Insulin resistance appears to be a major contributing factor to hyperglycemia as evidenced by his classic syndrome X characteristics, obesity, and insufficient response to the metformin/Glynase combination.
- Most patients with type 2 diabetes exhibit a 60% to 80% decrease in glucose uptake. Troglitazone's primary site of action is in skeletal muscles, where 80% to 90% of glucose uptake occurs. Troglitazone also exhibits an insulin-sparing effect, reducing elevated insulin levels by as much as 50%.[5]
- Increasing glucose utilization with troglitazone may preclude or delay the need to increase the sulfonylurea dose (and possibly allow for a decrease in the dose), thereby preserving pancreatic function and avoiding exacerbation of hyperinsulinemia. Manufacturer claims for the efficacy of the metformin/Glynase combination are a decrease in HbA_{1c} of up to 1.7%, whereas claims for the troglitazone/Glynase combination are a decrease in HbA_{1c} of up to 2.7%. Instituting a troglitazone/Glynase regimen offers an approach that more specifically addresses insulin resistance as the primary contributing factor and may prove more efficacious.
- Baseline liver function tests should be performed before initiation of therapy with troglitazone due to the rare but serious risk of liver injury, including liver failure. If the baseline ALT is > 1.5 times the upper limit of normal, troglitazone should not be used.
- Metformin should be discontinued and troglitazone initiated at 200 mg once a day. The dose may be increased at 2- to 4-week intervals to a maximum of 600 mg once a day. If patients do not respond adequately to 600 mg/day after 1 month, the drug should be discontinued.

b. *What alternative therapies might be appropriate if the initial plan fails?*

- If the desired outcomes are not achieved with Glynase 6 mg and troglitazone 600 mg after 6 to 8 weeks, BIDS therapy should be initiated.
- If the patient is resistant to initiation of insulin therapy, the Glynase dose could be increased (as a last resort) by 1.5 mg/day at weekly intervals to a maximum of 12 mg/day in 2 divided doses. This option should be discouraged since it will probably have limited success.

Outcome Evaluation

5. *What parameters should be monitored to evaluate the efficacy and possible adverse effects associated with the optimal regimen you selected?*

Efficacy
- The patient's SMBG logbook (with twice-daily testing) should be evaluated every 2 to 4 weeks while adjusting drug therapy.
- FBG should be obtained at every office visit.
- HbA_{1c} should be measured after 2 to 3 months, then every 3 months until stable, then 2 to 4 times a year thereafter.
- Fasting lipid profile should be checked after 4 to 6 weeks, then at least annually thereafter.
- BP should be monitored at every visit.

Adverse Effects
- Troglitazone can cause headache, peripheral edema, dizziness, diarrhea, and liver dysfunction.
  ✓ Liver enzymes should be measured prior to troglitazone therapy, every month for the first 8 months, every-other-month for the remainder of the first year, then periodically thereafter or if the patient develops symptoms such as nausea, vomiting, abdominal pain, fatigue, anorexia, dark urine, or jaundice. If patients experience moderate ALT increases at any time (1.5 to 2 times the upper limit of normal), then weekly monitoring must be instituted until the ALT returns to normal. Therapy should be discontinued if the ALT rises to > 3 times the upper limit of normal.
- Glynase (glyburide) can cause hypoglycemia, a disulfiram-like reaction with alcohol, headache, dizziness, skin rash, pruritus, photosensitivity reactions, hematologic effects (leukopenia, thrombocytopenia, hemolytic anemia, agranulocytosis), arthralgias, and paresthesias.
  ✓ Patients receiving Glynase should be monitored for symptoms of hypoglycemia and blood disorders (e.g., fever, sore throat, rash, and unusual bruising or bleeding). Liver and kidney function should also be monitored periodically.

Patient Counseling

6. *What information should be given to the patient regarding diabetes mellitus and his treatment plan to increase adherence, minimize adverse effects, and improve outcomes? Include information on use of a glucagon emergency kit (see Figure 70–1).*

General Information
- *Note:* Patient education regarding diabetes mellitus should be comprehensive and delivered over a series of visits. Determine what the patient knows and what information other members of the health care team are providing.
- Diabetes is a condition in which your body cannot properly use glucose or sugar from digested food. It builds up in the blood and doesn't get into the muscles and other organs that need it as a source of energy. Insulin allows the glucose to move from the blood into the muscles. In type 1 diabetes, the pancreas doesn't produce any insulin, so insulin injections are needed. In type 2 diabetes, the pancreas doesn't produce enough insulin or the insulin released doesn't work properly. Many people with type 2 diabetes will also eventually need to use insulin.

- You can control your blood glucose levels by following a treatment plan designed for you that includes meal planning to fit your needs and preferences, regular exercise, and medication.
- The amount of glucose in your blood depends on the amount and types of food you eat, the timing of your meals, the amount and timing of activity or exercise (which pulls more glucose out of the blood for energy), and the amount and timing of your medication. High or low blood glucose levels can result if all of these actions are not coordinated appropriately.
- Maintaining your blood glucose levels as close to normal as possible may prevent or delay complications such as blindness, kidney disease, limb amputations, heart disease, and strokes.
- High blood sugar (or hyperglycemia) can cause symptoms such as increased thirst; hunger and increased urination; dry, itchy skin; more frequent infections that are difficult to cure; nausea; fatigue; blurry vision; and numbness or tingling in the fingers or toes. If untreated, it can lead to coma and death.
- It is important to monitor your blood glucose levels twice a day as instructed to know if your diabetes is in control or if you need to work toward better control. Would you show me how you check your blood glucose so we can make sure everything is accurate and still working properly?
- Check your blood glucose more often if you are sick or under any other physical or emotional stress that could cause your levels to rise. Always ask for advice if any of these problems occur and before taking any non-prescription medicines.
- You can also get low blood sugar (or hypoglycemia) due to delayed or missed meals, increased activity or exercise, alcohol consumption on an empty stomach, or taking too much diabetes medicine. The warning signs of hypoglycemia include increased heart rate, weakness, dizziness, headache, shakiness, sweating, numbness or tingling around the mouth, irritability, drowsiness, coldness, and unconsciousness, which can progress to seizures, coma, and death.
- When any symptoms of low blood sugar occur, check your blood glucose, if possible. If it is low, treat it immediately with a quick-acting source of sugar such as $1/2$ cup of juice or regular soda, 3 to 4 glucose tablets, glucose gel, or 1 cup of milk. Check your blood glucose again in 15 minutes and repeat the treatment if necessary; then follow with a snack if a meal is not planned within $1/2$ to 1 hour.
- Glucagon injections may be needed to treat low blood sugar if you cannot swallow or if you are unconscious. Someone else should be instructed on how to give this injection. If you do not recover sufficiently, call an ambulance or have someone take you to the emergency room. Always notify your physician when a severe reaction occurs.
- Ideally, your fasting blood glucose should stay between 80 and 120 mg/dL. Some people do not experience any symptoms when their blood glucose is low. Always carry some form of quick-acting sugar with you and wear a medical alert bracelet or necklace.
- It is also important to check your feet daily since simple irritations, calluses, or infections can progress quickly to ulcers and infections that do not heal well. Apply lotion to the calluses on your feet every day, and wear socks and shoes that fit properly. If any redness or discomfort develops, or the condition worsens, consult a podiatrist.
- Good oral hygiene is important to prevent periodontal disease. Poor glucose control can make infections very difficult to cure.
- Your blood pressure should be maintained below 130/85 and your LDL cholesterol below 130 mg/dL. We will check your blood pressure and cholesterol regularly. You should have an annual dilated eye exam and a yearly urine test for protein and albumin to check for kidney disease.
- It is important to ask for advice if any problems arise, or if you have any questions, because it is possible to control your diabetes if everyone works together to help you learn how to manage it.

Glynase
- Glynase (a form of glyburide) is used to treat type 2 diabetes. It causes the pancreas to release more insulin, which helps the glucose move from the blood into the muscles and other organs where it is used for energy.
- You will continue to take one Glynase 6-mg tablet by mouth each morning with breakfast.
- This medicine may cause nausea, vomiting, headache, or dizziness, especially when taken with alcohol. It may also cause a change in taste, constipation or diarrhea, heartburn, and decreased appetite.
- Less commonly, it may cause skin rash, itching, sensitivity to the sun, fever, sore throat, or unusual bruising or bleeding. Notify your physician if you experience any of these symptoms.
- If hypoglycemia occurs, treat it immediately as we discussed and try to determine the cause so it will not happen again. Seek advice on preventing future episodes and notify your physician.
- As with all of your medicines, store Glynase in a cool, dry place, not in the refrigerator or bathroom.
- If you miss a dose, take it as soon as you remember. If it is almost time for the next dose when you remember, skip the missed dose and continue your regular schedule.

Troglitazone
- Troglitazone (or Rezulin) is your new medication to replace the Glucophage. This works in the muscles and organs to help the insulin pull the glucose out of the blood and lower your blood glucose levels.
- You will start by taking one 200-mg tablet daily with breakfast. You can take this at the same time as your other medications. It is important that you take it with food.
- If you miss your dose you can take it at the next meal. If you forget to take it, do not double your dose the next day; just take your next scheduled dose.
- Your physician will be checking your logbook to see how effective this medicine is and may increase the dose if needed. It is very important to keep testing and recording the results in your logbook so that the correct dose can be determined.
- You may experience some side effects such as headache, dizziness, diarrhea, or swelling of the hands or feet. Notify your physician if they occur.
- It is also very important that you have blood tests prior to starting therapy, every month for 8 months, then every other month for the remainder of the first year to check for any changes in your liver function. If you experience nausea, vomiting, abdominal pain, fatigue, decreased appetite, dark urine, or jaundice, notify your physician immediately.

Follow-up Questions

1. *What are the measurable objectives and long-term goals for treating hypertension and hyperlipidemia in this patient?*

   - The measurable objectives are to achieve and maintain BP < 130/85 mm Hg, total cholesterol < 200 mg/dL, HDL-C > 35 mg/dL, LDL-C < 130 mg/dL, and triglycerides < 200 mg/dL.
   - The long-term goals for treating hypertension and hyperlipidemia are to reduce the risk factors for developing cardiovascular disease, thereby preventing the development or progression of the complications of target organ disease (including nephropathy and retinopathy in the case of hypertension).
   - Hypertension, dyslipidemia (specifically high LDL-C and low HDL-C), and diabetes are all independent risk factors for cardiovascular disease. Management and goals of therapy are determined in part by the stage or severity of the disease and the presence of various risk factors. Aggressive management of blood pressure and hyperlipidemia in patients at high risk can significantly reduce morbidity and mortality.
   - It is further suggested that optimal benefits may be seen by maintaining blood pressure at 120/80 mm Hg if possible, LDL-C < 100 mg/dL, and HDL-C > 45 mg/dL. In general, women tend to have higher HDL levels than men. Therefore, it may be beneficial for women to maintain HDL levels > 45 mg/dL. HDL cholesterol levels > 60 mg/dL are considered to be a negative risk factor for cardiovascular disease for both men and women.[1,2,3]

2. *What non-pharmacological and pharmacological interventions would you consider to reach these goals?*

   Non-pharmacological Interventions
   - *Hypertension.* Decrease salt intake to < 2.4 g of sodium/day; maintain adequate intake of dietary potassium, calcium, and magnesium; continue the exercise regimen; continue efforts to lose weight.[3]
   - *Hyperlipidemia.* Continue to work with the dietitian to incorporate the recommendations of the NCEP Step II diet, which limits saturated fats to < 7% of total calorie intake and cholesterol intake to < 200 mg/day. Regular exercise, moderate alcohol consumption, and weight loss are also important lifestyle modifications to address.

   Pharmacological Interventions
   - *Hypertension.* Several potential options for gaining blood pressure control are available.
     - ✓ Increase the dose of Zestril (lisinopril) by 5 mg/day in 1- to 2-week intervals up to a maximum of 40 mg/day given in a single daily dose or divided doses.
     - ✓ Add a second drug to lisinopril 20 mg/day, such as hydrochlorothiazide 12.5 mg/day. Combination therapy at low doses will minimize the potential adverse effects of either agent when used alone at higher doses. A low dose of hydrochlorothiazide will probably have minimal adverse effects on glycemic control. Many studies have shown a reduction in morbidity and mortality with the use of diuretics. In addition, this would be the most cost-effective option.
     - ✓ Addition of a calcium channel blocker to lisinopril may also be considered.

   There is no compelling reason to choose one of these or one of several other options, but possible adverse effects and cost should be considered. However, β-blockers are relatively contraindicated.[3] They may mask some symptoms of developing hypoglycemia and adversely affect recovery from it.
   - *Hyperlipidemia.* Initiation of therapy with any of the HMG-CoA reductase inhibitors could be considered. A reduction in LDL-C of at least 23% is desired and may be accomplished with the lowest dose of most agents. The possible choices include single daily doses of simvastatin 5 mg (24% reduction), pravastatin 10 mg (22% reduction), lovastatin 10 mg (21% reduction), fluvastatin 20 mg (19% reduction), atorvastatin 10 mg (39% reduction), and cerivastatin 0.2 mg (25% reduction). When choosing the appropriate dosage for the desired reduction (23%), fluvastatin and cerivastatin are the most cost-effective options. If desirable cholesterol levels cannot be achieved with these agents, simvastatin, pravastatin, and atorvastatin are equally cost effective and less expensive than lovastatin. Atorvastatin provides the most cost-effective therapy when an LDL-cholesterol reduction of > 30% is desired.

References

1. American Diabetes Association. Standards of medical care for patients with diabetes mellitus. Diabetes Care 1998;21(suppl 1):S24–S39.
2. Expert Panel on Detection, Evaluation, and Treatment of High Blood Cholesterol in Adults. Summary of the second report of the National Cholesterol Education Program (NCEP) Expert Panel on detection, evaluation, and treatment of high blood cholesterol in adults (Adult Treatment Panel II). JAMA 1993;269:3015–3023.
3. Joint National Committee on Prevention, Detection, Evaluation, and Treatment of High Blood Pressure. The sixth report of the Joint National Committee on Prevention, Detection, Evaluation, and Treatment of High Blood Pressure. Arch Intern Med 1997;157:2413–2446.
4. Melander A. Oral antidiabetic drugs: An overview. Diabet Med 1996;13 (9 suppl 6):S143–S147.
5. Saltiel AR, Olefsky JM. Thiazolidinediones in the treatment of insulin resistance and type II diabetes. Diabetes 1996;45:1661–1669.

71 HYPERTHYROIDISM: GRAVES' DISEASE

▶ Gland Central (Level I)

Kristine E. Santus, PharmD
Tara L. Posey, PharmD

Symptoms of palpitations, difficulty swallowing solid food, insomnia, leg swelling, and weight loss despite a good appetite cause a 58-year-old woman to seek treatment at an ambulatory care clinic. Physical examination, laboratory evaluation, and ECG indicate that the patient has hyperthyroidism and atrial fibrillation. The thioureas propylthiouracil (PTU) and methimazole are generally used to induce and maintain a remission of the hyperthyroid state. Beta-adrenergic blockers (e.g., propranolol) or calcium channel blockers (e.g., diltiazem) may also be used adjunctively to relieve symptoms of tremor, anxiety, and palpitations and to control ventricular response in patients with atrial fibrillation. Warfarin should also be initiated in this patient to prevent thromboembolism due to atrial fibrillation. The case offers the opportunity to discuss appropriate monitoring of thyroid replacement therapy using thyroid function tests.

Endocrinologic Disorders

▶ Questions

Problem Identification

1. a. Create a list of the patient's drug-related problems.

- Symptomatic hyperthyroidism requiring treatment.
- Atrial fibrillation (probably secondary to hyperthyroidism) presently untreated.
- Microcytic, hypochromic anemia, possibly due to iron deficiency, that requires further evaluation and treatment.
- Postmenopausal status and the patient apparently has not been considered for estrogen therapy.
- Symptomatic peptic ulcer disease versus gastroesophageal reflux disease requiring treatment.

b. What signs, symptoms, and laboratory values indicate the presence or severity of hyperthyroidism?

- *Signs.* Tachycardia; thinning hair; warm, moist, hyperpigmented skin; proptosis, lid lag, and lid retraction; enlarged thyroid; pulsating neck vessels; hyperreflexia; brittle nails.
- *Symptoms.* Weight loss despite good appetite; increased heart rate and palpitations; nervousness and behavior described as "hyper."
- *Laboratory values.* Decreased TSH; increased total T_4, free thyroxine index, total T_3, and T_3 uptake.
- *ECG.* Rapid atrial fibrillation and sinus tachycardia.

Desired Outcome

2. What are the goals of pharmacotherapy in this case?

- Control the signs and symptoms of hyperthyroidism
- Induce and maintain remission of the hyperthyroid state as determined by thyroid function tests
- Reduce ocular symptoms
- Attempt to "cure" the disease; patients can become hypothyroid by radioactive iodine and be "cured" of Graves' disease

Therapeutic Alternatives

3. a. What non-drug therapies might be useful for this patient?

- There are no non-drug therapies available to control hyperthyroidism.
- Patients should be advised to avoid medications containing sympathomimetic and anticholinergic drugs (e.g., antihistamines) to prevent exacerbations of sinus tachycardia.
- Patients should avoid iodine-containing medications (e.g., amiodarone and some cough syrups) or substances and foods that may cause goiters (e.g., cabbage). The patient's iodine intake should be assessed.
- Surgery can also be used to reduce thyroid size in patients in whom breathing or swallowing is a problem (i.e., due to obstruction). Drug therapy is used prior to surgery to reduce thyrotoxicosis and decrease vascularity of the gland.

b. What feasible pharmacotherapeutic alternatives are available for the treatment of hyperthyroidism in this patient?

- *Propylthiouracil (PTU)* and *methimazole* are antithyroid drugs (thioureas) that prevent organification of iodine and iodotyrosines, thereby preventing the synthesis of thyroid hormones. PTU is often given initially because it also inhibits the peripheral conversion of thyroxine (T_4) to triiodothyronine (T_3). This causes a more rapid onset of action that can decrease clinical signs and symptoms due to circulating hormones. Initial doses are PTU 300 to 600 mg daily or methimazole 30 to 60 mg daily. The drugs may be given as a single daily dose; however, one study showed that 3 to 4 divided daily doses are optimal for achieving euthyroidism within 3 months.[1,2] The onset of action is not seen until stored hormone is depleted, which may take 4 to 8 weeks. When clinical symptoms begin to diminish and thyroid function tests begin to decline, the dose should be decreased to a maintenance dose of PTU 50 to 100 mg daily or methimazole 5 to 10 mg daily. Antithyroid medications should be continued for 12 to 24 months until the patient is in remission.
- Some clinicians favor supplementing antithyroid drugs with levothyroxine (100 to 200 μg/day) to prevent iatrogenic hypothyroidism and to decrease the relapse rate. Levothyroxine suppresses thyrotropin secretion and presentation of thyroid antigens, which can, in turn, minimize an autoimmune response.[1,3]
- *Beta-adrenergic antagonists (e.g., propranolol, atenolol, nadolol)* are used as adjunctive agents to treat some of the symptoms of hyperthyroidism (tremor, anxiety, and palpitations) and to control ventricular response in atrial fibrillation. These drugs have no effect on thyroid function. Propranolol is often the preferred agent because it inhibits the peripheral conversion of T_4 to T_3.
- *Calcium channel blockers (diltiazem or verapamil)* are used in patients in whom β-blockers may not be an ideal choice, such as patients with asthma or heart failure with systolic dysfunction.
- *Iodine* may be used for a few days or weeks to inhibit the release of thyroid hormones. Iodine is sometimes used prior to surgery to decrease the vascularity of the thyroid gland but should not be used prior to radioactive iodine.
- *Radioactive iodine* is used in a single dose to destroy thyroid tissue and cause a hypothyroid state. It is contraindicated in pregnancy and in children under 17 years of age.

Optimal Plan

4. What drug, dosage form, dose, schedule, and duration of therapy are best for this patient?

- One option is PTU 300 to 600 mg/day given in 4 divided doses.
- An alternative is methimazole 30 to 60 mg/day given in 3 to 4 divided doses.
- PTU may be a better choice than methimazole because it inhibits the peripheral conversion of T_4 to T_3 and provides more rapid relief of symptoms. However, the maximal effect of either drug is not seen for 2 to 4 weeks.
- A β-blocker should also be given to decrease heart rate and palpitations. Propranolol may be an ideal choice as it inhibits the peripheral conversion of T_4 to T_3, although other β-blockers are also appropriate. The dose of propranolol is 80 to 320 mg/day in 2 to 4 divided doses (the usual dose for thyrotoxicosis is 10 to 40 mg every 6 hours). Atenolol (50 to 100 mg/day in 1 to 2 divided doses) and nadolol (40 to 80 mg/day) have also been used.

- Calcium channel blockers are an alternative in patients who cannot tolerate β-blockers. Agents with negative inotropic effects, such as verapamil (240 to 480 mg/day) or diltiazem (240 to 360 mg/day), are the best selection in patients with hyperthyroidism.
- Warfarin should also be initiated in this patient with atrial fibrillation to prevent thromboembolism. The dose should be adjusted to maintain an INR between 2.0 and 3.0. Atrial fibrillation may be caused by hyperthyroidism and may resolve once the patient achieves a euthyroid state. If this occurs, the warfarin can be discontinued. If atrial fibrillation does not resolve when the patient becomes euthyroid, warfarin must be continued, and the patient should receive a cardiovascular evaluation with consideration of electrocardioversion or chemical conversion, if appropriate.

Outcome Evaluation

5. *What clinical and laboratory parameters are necessary to evaluate the response to therapy and to detect or prevent adverse effects?*

- Symptoms of hyperthyroidism should begin to resolve within a few days; however, maximal effects are not seen for 2 to 4 weeks or longer, depending on intrathyroidal stores.
- Thyroid function tests (TFTs), including TSH and free T_4, should be evaluated after 4 weeks of therapy. If TSH remains suppressed at that time, the dose of the thiourea should be increased.
- TFTs should be checked 1 month after a dosage adjustment and then repeated every 2 months when the patient is taking a stable dose.
- The patient should be evaluated early in treatment (after 2 to 4 weeks) to determine how well the therapy is being tolerated.
- Approximately 10% of patients taking a thiourea develop a mild, transient leukopenia that does not require drug discontinuation.
- More serious toxicities of thioureas include agranulocytosis and aplastic anemia. Therefore, a baseline CBC with differential should be obtained prior to initiating therapy.
- Periodic evaluations of CBC will not aid in predicting the onset of leukopenia, agranulocytosis, or aplastic anemia. Consequently, subsequent CBCs and differentials should be obtained only when necessary (e.g., if the patient reports signs or symptoms consistent with leukopenia, agranulocytosis, or aplastic anemia).
- If the absolute neutrophil count drops below $1.5 \times 10^3/mm^3$, the thiourea should be discontinued.
- The incidence of agranulocytosis is 0.5% to 6% and may be dose-related. If the patient develops agranulocytosis, switching to another thiourea is not an option. These patients must be treated with either radioactive iodine or surgery for ablation.
- In this patient taking warfarin, the PT and INR should be monitored regularly (every 2 to 4 weeks), as changes in the thyroid function of the patient can cause fluctuations in the INR. A hyperthyroid state can cause an increase in the activity of warfarin and an increase in the INR. Hyperthyroidism can also decrease the protein binding of warfarin, which can also increase the INR. As the patient becomes euthyroid or hypothyroid, the activity and protein binding of warfarin are decreased and the INR can fluctuate.[4]

Patient Counseling

6. *What information should be provided to the patient to enhance compliance, ensure successful therapy, and minimize adverse effects?*

Propylthiouracil or Methimazole
- This medication will decrease the production of thyroid hormone.
- The symptoms of rapid heart rate and nervousness should decrease as the medication begins to work.
- The medicine should be taken 3 times a day at regular intervals. You may find it easier to remember to take your medicine if you take a dose with each meal.
- The medication can decrease the number of white blood cells in your body, which can increase the risk of infections, and it can decrease the number of red blood cells, causing anemia. Contact your doctor immediately if you develop a sore throat or a fever, become very fatigued, or notice unusual bleeding or bruising.
- Some patients develop a rash while on this medication. Contact your doctor if this occurs.

Beta-blockers or Calcium Channel Blockers
- This medication helps to control heart rate and decrease palpitations associated with hyperthyroidism.
- If taking propranolol, this medication should be taken at regular intervals three times a day. Taking the medication with meals may help you remember to take each dose.
- If taking atenolol, nadolol, verapamil, or diltiazem, take the medication at the same time every day.
- These medications may cause shortness of breath, dizziness, weakness, or headaches. Try to make slow changes in posture (from lying to sitting to standing) to minimize dizziness.

Warfarin
- Your heart is beating in an abnormal rhythm called atrial fibrillation. Because of this, blood does not flow through the heart as well as it does normally, which can cause a clot to form in your heart.
- This medication helps to protect the heart from forming a blood clot.
- Take this medication once a day at the same time every day.
- Do not take aspirin, ibuprofen, naproxen, ketoprofen, or other nonsteroidal anti-inflammatory agents while taking this medication.
- Many other medications can interact with warfarin. Consult your doctor or pharmacist any time you start a new medication or if one of your current medications is changed.
- Several foods, such as green leafy vegetables (e.g., broccoli, spinach) and beef liver, contain vitamin K, which can counteract the effects of warfarin. Maintain a consistent diet while taking warfarin to minimize alterations in the effects of warfarin.
- This medication requires frequent monitoring of bleeding time (PT and INR) to adjust the dose of warfarin. Make sure you have your blood drawn at the regular intervals that your doctor advises.

▶ Follow-up Questions

1. *What interventions, if any, would you suggest at this point?*

- Continue the thiourea (PTU or methimazole), because the patient's TFTs reflect continued hyperthyroidism. When TFTs do not indicate improvement, the thiourea dose should be increased (PTU maximum dose 1200 mg/day; methimazole maximum dose 120 mg/day). If TFTs indicate worsening hyperthyroidism, more aggressive thyroid ablation with ^{131}I or thyroidectomy may be indicated.
- Continue the adrenergic antagonist (e.g., propranolol), as the patient still shows signs of atrial fibrillation.

- Recheck thyroid function tests in 1 month. At that point, if TSH and T_4 are normal (which indicates a euthyroid state), decrease the dose of PTU or methimazole.
- The INR is low. Assess the patient for missed doses, changes in diet, or changes in other medications. If there have been no missed doses or dosage changes, increase the dose of warfarin by 10% to 20%. Recheck the INR in 1 to 2 weeks.

2. *If the patient subsequently becomes hypothyroid but clinical signs indicate that the patient still has Graves' disease, what plan should be implemented?*

- The patient should remain on thioureas until remission occurs.
- If the patient becomes hypothyroid, levothyroxine (50 to 100 μg po QD) should be started to maintain a euthyroid state and allow continuation of the thiourea until the patient is in remission. Levothyroxine suppresses TSH, which prevents thyroid hormones from being produced and released into circulation, thereby preventing hyperthyroidism from recurring and decreasing the rate of relapse when the thiourea is discontinued.[3]
- The optimal length of thiourea therapy to induce a remission of Graves' disease is at least 12 months and can be as long as 24 months. Remission occurs in 50% to 60% of patients taking thioureas.
- Most patients relapse after discontinuation of the thiourea. Patients who relapse should receive radioactive iodine for thyroid ablation and then be given levothyroxine for supplementation.
- Levothyroxine is highly protein bound and can interact with warfarin. If this patient is started on levothyroxine, the INR must be monitored closely until the patient is stabilized.

References

1. Vanderpump VMJ, Ahlquist JA, Franklyn JA, et al. Consensus statement for good practice and audit measures in the management of hypothyroidism and hyperthyroidism. BMJ 1996;313:539–544.
2. Kallner G, Vitols S, Ljunggren JG, et al. Comparison of standardized initial doses of two antithyroid drugs in the treatment of Grave's disease. J Intern Med 1996:239:525–529.
3. Hashizume K, Ichikawa K, Sakurai A, et al. Administration of thyroxine in treated Grave's disease: Effects on the level of antibodies to thyroid-stimulating hormone receptors and on the risk of recurrence in hyperthyroidism. N Engl J Med 1991;324:947–953.
4. Self TH, Straughn AB, Weisburst MR. Effect of hyperthyroidism on hypoprothombinemic response to warfarin. Am J Hosp Pharm 1976;33:387–389.

72 HYPOTHYROIDISM

▶ The Battle to Control the Thermostat
(Level II)

Tara L. Posey, PharmD

A 53-year-old woman with hypertension and a recent history of iron-deficiency anemia presents to her primary care physician with complaints of persistent fatigue, dry skin, and cold intolerance. The results of laboratory evaluation are consistent with the diagnosis of hypothyroidism. Although several natural and synthetic thyroid replacement products are available, levothyroxine is considered to be the drug of choice. Therapy should be initiated with low doses that are gradually increased over time to an individualized maintenance dose. After thyroid function has been normalized, annual evaluation of therapy with TSH measurements is sufficient to monitor the therapy. Overreplacement of thyroid hormone should be avoided, as it may lead to hyperthyroidism, which can result in decreased bone density and increased fracture risk, especially in postmenopausal women.

▶ Questions

Problem Identification

1. a. *Identify this patient's drug-related problems.*

- Hypothyroidism not receiving drug therapy.
- Borderline-high cholesterol not receiving intervention with dietary or drug therapy (further assessment is required; see follow-up question).
- Chronic stable problems not requiring intervention at this time include: 1) HTN appropriately treated with a β-adrenergic antagonist (Goal BP < 140/90); and 2) iron-deficiency anemia appropriately replaced with ferrous sulfate.

b. *What information (signs, symptoms, laboratory values) indicates the presence of hypothyroidism?*

- *Signs.* Trace periorbital edema; dry skin and scalp.
- *Symptoms.* Itchy skin and scalp; fatigue; cold intolerance. Inability to cope with job-related stress and body aches may also be attributed to hypothyroidism.
- *Laboratory values.* Elevated TSH and low total and free serum T_4 levels. Hypercholesterolemia may be worsened by existing hypothyroidism.
- *Other.* The patient is a 53-year-old Caucasian woman. The incidence of hypothyroidism increases with age and is more common in women than men and in whites than blacks.

c. *Could any of the patient's problems have been caused by drug therapy?*

- None of the patient's current medications would contribute to hypothyroidism. Exposure to internal or external radiation can precipitate hypothyroidism. Iodine excess and deficiency can interfere with TSH synthesis and result in hypothyroidism, but this is very rarely seen in adults.

Desired Outcome

2. *What are the goals of pharmacotherapy in this patient?*

- Alleviate the clinical signs and symptoms of hypothyroidism.
- Normalize thyroid concentrations in the tissues (normalization of TSH and free T_4 will render the patient euthyroid).

Therapeutic Alternatives

3. a. What non-drug therapies might be useful for this patient?

- Dry and itchy skin can be ameliorated by using a non-allergenic lotion to provide moisture until thyroid concentrations are normalized.
- The patient can also avoid using dyes or harsh shampoos and conditioners to avoid adding to the itchiness and dryness.

b. What feasible pharmacotherapeutic alternatives are available for treatment of hypothyroidism?

- There are several natural or synthetic thyroid preparations that may be used (refer to Table 71–3 in textbook Chapter 71 for a complete listing).
- *Thyroid USP* and *thyroglobulin* are natural products that may have an unpredictable biologic response, may be allergenic, and can be expensive. Different generic formulations of natural products may not be bioequivalent.
- *Levothyroxine* (T_4) is the drug of choice for thyroid replacement therapy because it is a synthetic formulation that is chemically stable, has more uniform bioavailability and potency, is not allergenic, and is relatively inexpensive. Although there has been concern that synthetic generic formulations may not be bioequivalent with the branded product Synthroid, a recent study suggests that certain generic formulations are bioequivalent.[1] However, as a general rule, it is not wise to switch between formulations or manufacturers, and consistency is recommended.
- *Liothyronine* (T_3) is also a synthetic product, but it has clinical disadvantages that include a higher incidence of cardiac side effects, difficulty in monitoring with conventional laboratory tests, and higher cost than levothyroxine.
- *Liotrix* (a combination product containing T_4:T_3 in a 4:1 ratio) is a high-cost product that lacks therapeutic rationale because T_4 is converted to T_3 in the periphery.

Optimal Plan

4. What drug, dosage form, dose, schedule, and duration of therapy are best for this patient?

- The gold standard for thyroid replacement is levothyroxine. Its advantages include once daily dosing, stability, predictable potency, and a variety of dosage strengths to allow for easy dosage titration.
- Levothyroxine therapy should be initiated with 50 μg once daily. The TSH should be reevaluated in 6 to 8 weeks. If it has not normalized, the dose should be increased by 25 μg and the TSH rechecked in another 6 to 8 weeks. This process may be repeated until the patient is euthyroid.[2]
- In elderly patients and patients with cardiac disease, therapy should be initiated with a dose of 25 μg daily and titrated slowly upward.[2] Clinical and biochemical evaluation should be performed 6 to 8 weeks after initiation of treatment. If the TSH is still elevated, the dose may be increased by 25 μg and the therapy then reevaluated as described.[2]
- Studies suggest that the average maintenance dose for most adults is 110 to 120 μg/day.
- This patient will likely require life-long thyroid replacement.

Outcome Evaluation

5. What clinical and laboratory parameters are necessary to evaluate thyroid replacement therapy to achieve euthyroidism and prevent adverse effects?

- Clinical and biochemical reevaluation should be performed at 6- to 8-week intervals with dosage increased until the serum TSH and free T_4 concentrations are normalized.
- Once serum thyroid concentrations are normalized, annual evaluation of therapy with TSH measurements should be performed.[2]
- The patient should obtain relief of her symptoms of fatigue within 2 to 3 weeks of beginning therapy. However, dry, itchy skin and scalp may take several months to subside.[2]
- The primary risk with dosage elevation is cardiotoxicity (angina, MI, arrhythmia, CHF) especially in patients with undiagnosed cardiac disease.
- Overreplacement of thyroid hormone can lead to signs and symptoms of hyperthyroidism. Long-term overreplacement can lead to reduced bone density, which can increase the risk of fractures, especially in elderly postmenopausal women.
- Patients with bipolar disorder may experience exacerbations of this disorder with thyroid hormone replacement.

Patient Counseling

6. What information should be provided to the patient to enhance compliance, ensure successful therapy, and minimize adverse effects?

Levothyroxine

- Take this medication once a day exactly as your doctor directed.
- Space this medicine from your iron tablets by at least 2 to 4 hours. The iron tablets may reduce the amount of thyroid hormone your body will absorb.
- If you miss a dose, take it as soon as you remember, unless it is within 12 hours of your next dose. If it is too close to your next dose, forget about the dose you missed and continue with your regular regimen. Do not double doses.
- You should begin to feel better within 2 to 3 weeks of starting this medication.
- Blood tests will need to be checked periodically (every 6 to 8 weeks) until your doctor determines the appropriate dose for you. After that, you will only need to have a blood test once a year.
- If the dose of your medication is too high, you may experience diarrhea, sweating, tremors, or intolerance to heat. Call your doctor if you notice these side effects.
- Call your doctor immediately if you experience any chest pain, palpitations, or irregular heart beats.
- Because your thyroid gland is not producing enough thyroid hormone, you will likely need to take this medication for the rest of your life.
- It is very important to keep regular appointments with your doctor to monitor your therapy so that you can gain the full benefit of this therapy while avoiding potential side effects.

▶ **Follow-up Questions**

1. *How should this patient's elevated cholesterol be handled at this point?*

   - Hypercholesterolemia can be effectively treated with dietary management or pharmacotherapy. However, treatment should be withheld at this time. Hypercholesterolemia may be associated with hypothyroidism, but this is less likely in this patient with strong family history for CAD. This issue should be reassessed after normalization of her thyroid function.

2. *Assume that the patient returns for a routine exam in 6 months and her cholesterol is still elevated. How should this be assessed?*

   - A fasting lipid panel should be obtained to further assess her risk factors for CAD. The panel should include measurement of HDL-cholesterol, LDL-cholesterol, triglycerides, and total cholesterol.
   - This patient's other risk factors for CAD include a family history of CAD (mother with MI before 65) and HTN. If the results of the lipid profile show an HDL > 60 mg/dL (positive risk factor), the patient's risk for CAD is somewhat reduced, and the goals for hypercholesterolemia in this patient include total cholesterol < 200 mg/dL and LDL < 160 mg/dL. Drug therapy should be initiated if the LDL is > 190 mg/dL.
   - If the patient does not have a high HDL level, more aggressive cholesterol goals are warranted, including total cholesterol < 200 mg/dL and LDL < 130 mg/dL. Drug therapy should be initiated if the LDL is > 160 mg/dL.

References

1. Dong BJ, Hauck WW, Gambertoglio JG, et al. Bioequivalence of generic and brand-name levothyroxine products in the treatment of hypothyroidism. JAMA 1997;277:1205–1213.

2. Singer PA, Cooper DS, Levy EG, et al. Treatment guidelines for patients with hyperthyroidism and hypothyroidism. Standards of Care Committee, American Thyroid Association. JAMA 1995;273:808–812.

73 CUSHING'S SYNDROME

▶ **When One Gland Affects Another (Level II)**

Jerry D. Smith, PharmD
John G. Gums, PharmD

A 31-year-old woman presents with complaints of fatigue, weakness, a 50-pound weight gain over the past 2 years, and depression with insomnia. The patient has Cushingoid features on physical examination, and laboratory evaluation reveals hyperglycemia and dyslipidemia. An MRI performed after referral to an endocrinologist indicates the presence of an enlarged pituitary gland, but a discrete tumor cannot be localized. Specific laboratory testing for plasma and urinary steroids confirms the diagnosis of Cushing's disease. Transphenoidal surgery to remove a clearly circumscribed pituitary microadenoma would be the treatment of choice if the tumor could be localized. In this patient's case, the tumor cannot be localized, and subtotal resection of the anterior pituitary would normally be the recommended treatment. However, this patient wishes to have children in the future, which makes pituitary irradiation with adjunctive drug therapy a feasible option. Drugs used with radiation therapy to lower circulating cortisol levels include ketoconazole, metyrapone, aminoglutethimide, mitotane, cyproheptadine, and others.

▶ **Questions**

Problem Identification

1. a. *Create a list of this patient's drug-related problems.*

   - Cushing's disease (pituitary mass) requiring drug or other treatment.
   - Elevated blood pressure probably due to Cushing's disease, but could also be due to levonorgestrel component of Triphasil-21.
   - Hirsutism probably due to Cushing's disease, but could also be due to levonorgestrel.
   - Elevated plasma glucose probably due to Cushing's disease.
   - Elevated total cholesterol and triglycerides probably due to Cushing's disease.
   - Weakness and fatigue probably due to Cushing's disease, but could also be due to levonorgestrel.
   - Depression (self-treated with St. John's wort) probably due to Cushing's disease, but could also be due to levonorgestrel.
   - Headaches (possibly due to pituitary mass), which may require treatment.

   b. *What information (signs, symptoms, laboratory values) indicates the presence or severity of Cushing's syndrome?*

   - *Signs.* Truncal obesity, rounding face (moon facies), hirsutism, thin skin, purple striae, elevated BP.
   - *Symptoms.* Fatigue, weakness, sadness/depression with insomnia, weight gain, easy bruising, blurred vision, occasional back pain.
   - *Laboratory values.* Elevated plasma glucose, total cholesterol, and triglycerides; mild hypokalemia; positive response on low- and high-dose DST; and elevated plasma ACTH, indicating probable ACTH-dependent Cushing's syndrome.
   - Lack of menstrual irregularities goes against the diagnosis, but the patient is receiving exogenous estrogen/progesterone (Triphasil-21).

Desired Outcome

2. *What are the goals of pharmacotherapy in this case?*

   - Elimination of hypercortisolism
   - Prevention of associated disorders (depression, diabetes, cardiovascular disease, and electrolyte disturbances)
   - Reduction of morbidity and mortality from untreated disease
   - Cure of disease by removal of the tumor is a surgical goal

Therapeutic Alternatives

3. a. *What non-drug therapies might be useful for this patient?*

   - Transphenoidal surgery (80% cured)
   - Pituitary irradiation (45%–85% cured)
   - Total bilateral adrenalectomy (100% cured, but there is a 10%–15% risk of Nelson's syndrome[1])

   b. *What feasible pharmacotherapeutic alternatives are available for the treatment of Cushing's disease?*

   - *Steroidogenic inhibition* involves inhibiting adrenal synthesis of cortisol to decrease circulating cortisol levels.[2] Therapy with all of these drugs is continued indefinitely, as long as the patient has Cushing's disease. They are not curative, and their effects are reversible on discontinuation. Drug therapy is indicated to lower cortisol secretion under specific circumstances, such as in patients waiting for radiotherapy to be effective, when surgery is ineffective, after chemotherapy, or when there are severe consequences of hypercortisolism.
     - ✓ *Ketoconazole (Nizoral)* lowers cortisol in Cushing's disease, resulting in normal corticosteroid values in 84% of patients with an additional 11% of patients reporting improvement. It can also lower plasma testosterone values, which may be useful in this patient who has hirsutism. The most common adverse effects of ketoconazole are reversible elevation of hepatic transaminases, gynecomastia, and GI upset. The usual dose is 600 to 800 mg po twice daily.
     - ✓ *Metyrapone (Metopirone)* may initially cause an increase in plasma ACTH concentrations because of a sudden drop in cortisol. It lowers serum cortisol levels in about 80% of patients but only normalizes it in about 25%.[2] Adverse effects include GI complaints (nausea, vomiting, abdominal discomfort), CNS effects (somnolence, vertigo, headache, dizziness), and allergic rash. The usual dose is 250 mg po QID.
     - ✓ *Aminoglutethimide (Cytadren)* is indicated for short-term use in inoperable Cushing's disease with ectopic-ACTH syndrome as the suspected underlying etiology. It is used more as an actual treatment than as adjunctive therapy and is usually initiated in the hospital. Plasma cortisol concentrations are reduced by up to 50% after aminoglutethimide therapy. However, it normalizes elevated serum cortisol in only about 10% of patients and causes side effects in about 60%.[2] Side effects include severe sedation, nausea, hypothyroidism, ataxia, and skin rashes. Most of these reactions are dose-dependent and limit its use in the majority of patients. The usual dose is 250 mg every 6 hours, which may be increased by 250 mg/day at 1- to 2-week intervals; the maximum dose is 2 g/day.
     - ✓ *Aminoglutethimide in combination with metyrapone* allows for smaller doses of both drugs to be used, thereby minimizing the toxicity associated with each agent. The combination appears to be effective for various etiologies of Cushing's disease and is useful in the inoperable patient.
   - *Adrenolytic agent*
     - ✓ *Mitotane (ortho, para, dichloro-diphenyldichloroethane; o,p'-DDD, Lysodren)* decreases cortisol secretion rate, plasma cortisol concentrations, urinary free cortisol, and plasma concentrations of the 17-substituted steroids. It appears to selectively inhibit adrenocortical function without causing cellular destruction and is considered the drug of choice for inoperable adrenocortical carcinoma. Mitotane produces a measurable tumor reduction in 50% of patients; 75% of patients have > 30% reduction in urinary excretion of 17-OHCS. Because mitotane can severely reduce urinary excretion of 17-OHCS, the patient should be hospitalized before initiating therapy. If necessary, steroid replacement therapy can be given. Approximately 80% of mitotane-treated patients develop GI side effects such as nausea, vomiting, anorexia, or diarrhea. Lethargy, somnolence, and other CNS adverse reactions occur in approximately 40% of patients. The usual dose is 9 to 10 g/day given in divided doses 3 or 4 times daily. Mitotane can be discontinued 1 year after irradiation if UFC has normalized. It can be reinitiated if hypercortisolemia recurs.
   - *Neuromodulators of ACTH release* decrease ACTH secretion in patients with Cushing's disease as a means of decreasing cortisol concentrations.
     - ✓ *Cyproheptadine (Periactin, various generics)* should be reserved for nonsurgical candidates who fail more conventional therapy. Morning plasma cortisol concentrations, as well as 24-hour UFC concentrations should be monitored. Side effects are minor and include sedation and hyperphagia. The response rate is < 30%, and patients should be followed closely for relapses. The initial dose is 4 mg twice daily, titrated upward gradually to 24 to 32 mg/day.
     - ✓ *Bromocriptine (Parlodel)* has been used, but most patients exhibit little or no response. The usual dose is 1.25 to 2.5 mg 2 to 4 times/day.
     - ✓ *Valproic acid (Depakote, Depakene)* has also been used. However, one study has shown that long-term therapy with sodium valproate is not useful in the therapeutic management of Cushing's disease either as alternative or as adjunctive therapy to surgery. The dose is individualized and usually ranges from 250 to 500 mg 3 times daily.
     - ✓ *Octreotide (Sandostatin)* does not suppress ACTH release in most patients with untreated Cushing's disease. This finding is supported by *in vitro* studies. However, octreotide (or the natural hormone somatostatin) inhibits pathologic ACTH secretion in Nelson's syndrome. Doses range from 50 to 100 mg 1 to 3 times/day; the usual dose is 50 mg once or twice daily.
   - *Glucocorticoid receptor-blocking agent*
     - ✓ *Mifepristone (RU-486)* blocks cortisol action at the receptor site, and is therefore useful in all etiologies of hypercorti-

solism. It is highly effective in reversing the manifestations of hypercortisolism. As a receptor antagonist, it leads to higher cortisol and ACTH levels; therefore, the diagnosis of treatment-induced glucocorticoid insufficiency must rest on clinical signs only. The efficacy and long-term adverse effects of RU-486 remain to be determined. It is not commercially available at the time of this writing.

Optimal Plan

4. a. What drug, dosage form, dose, schedule, and duration of therapy are best for treating this patient's Cushing's disease?

- The optimal plan would be to perform transphenoidal microadenomectomy, if a clearly circumscribed microadenoma can be identified and resected.
- Otherwise, patients should undergo 85% to 90% resection of the anterior pituitary, unless they wish to have children, in which case they should receive pituitary irradiation. If the latter therapy fails, bilateral total adrenalectomy should be performed.
- This patient has an enlarged pituitary gland, but no focal inhomogeneity that would suggest an isolated adenoma. She does not wish to have surgery and desires to have children. Therefore, irradiation and adjunctive therapy are the best options at this time.
  - ✓ During the 3 to 12 months required to achieve maximum benefit from irradiation, the hypercortisolism can be controlled with adrenal enzyme inhibitors (as single agents or in combination). Irradiation and adjunctive mitotane therapy results in a remission rate of 80% in the first year, which increases further in later years.[1] Discontinuing mitotane drops the sustained remission rate to about 50% to 70%. Mitotane can be discontinued after 1 year if the urinary cortisol has normalized and can be reinitiated if hypercortisolism occurs. By 3 years, 80% to 90% of patients will have achieved biochemical remission and will no longer require mitotane. Four to 6 weeks of therapy with mitotane is usually required before a benefit is seen.
  - ✓ Ketoconazole is useful to treat the symptoms of hypercortisolism during the time it takes for the radiation and mitotane to take effect.
  - ✓ Therefore, the best treatment option is probably to treat this patient with irradiation and mitotane and to control her symptoms with ketoconazole. The radiation is used to cure the disease, and mitotane is used to augment the radiation therapy. The mitotane should be started at 1 g po 3 times daily and increased by 2 to 4 g/day every 3 to 7 days if a response is not seen. The ketoconazole should be started at 200 mg po once daily and increased at 4- to 7-day intervals until urinary cortisol concentrations become normal. Mitotane and ketoconazole are Pregnancy Category C drugs. Therefore, the risks and benefits of the use of these drugs must be evaluated before the patient contemplates pregnancy or if she becomes pregnant.
  - ✓ Other agents could be used as adjunctive therapy if the patient does not respond to mitotane or ketoconazole, but as outlined in the answer to question 3.b., most of the other agents are not as effective.

b. In addition to treatment for Cushing's disease, what other changes in this patient's drug therapy may be beneficial?

- The patient may be having androgenic effects associated with her Triphasil (ethinyl estradiol/levonorgestrel). Levonorgestrel has the most androgenic properties of the currently available progestins. Although this may be a minor effect compared to the Cushing's disease, it could be easily avoided by switching to another progesterone with less androgenic effects such as a norgestimate-containing oral contraceptive (e.g., Ortho-Novum).
- After the patient's Cushing's disease is controlled, her blood pressure, fasting blood sugar, fasting lipid profile, headaches, weakness/fatigue, and depression should be reevaluated and treated if necessary.

Outcome Evaluation

5. What clinical and laboratory parameters are necessary to evaluate the therapy for achievement of the desired therapeutic outcome and to detect or prevent adverse events?

- To monitor for adrenal insufficiency, daily monitoring of serum cortisol levels (target value of < 5 μg/dL, while an inpatient) and 24-hour UFC levels (target value of < 20 μg) are essential with all types of adrenal blocking medications.
- Liver function tests should be monitored at baseline, at 1 to 2 weeks, biweekly for 2 months, then bimonthly for the next 4 months during ketoconazole therapy. Ketoconazole should be discontinued if the ALT or AST rise to > 3 times the upper limit of normal.
- To monitor for successful treatment with radiation (which may take from 1 to 18 months), the patient should be without symptoms and have a plasma cortisol of 5 to 25 μg/dL and/or 24-hour urinary excretion of 17-hydroxycorticoids of 4 to 12 mg and UFC of 20 to 100 μg while not on concomitant drug therapy for Cushing's disease. Retesting should be performed based on patient symptoms and response. It is reasonable to recheck these tests during the course of therapy, at the end of therapy, and again within the first 3 to 6 months.

Patient Counseling

6. What information should be provided to the patient to enhance compliance, ensure successful therapy, and minimize adverse events?

Ketoconazole (Nizoral)

- This drug is often used to treat fungal infections, but it is also useful in treating the symptoms caused by Cushing's disease.
- You will take one 200-mg tablet by mouth 2 times per day and increase the dose only if instructed to do so by your physician.
- If you miss a dose, take it as soon as you remember; however, if it is almost time for the next dose, just take the next dose at the regularly scheduled time and skip the missed dose.
- Take this tablet with food to decrease stomach upset and to increase the amount that gets into your system.
- Some possible side effects include nausea, vomiting, and abdominal pain, which should be minimized by taking it with food.
- If you are allergic to this drug, you may develop a rash or another reaction. If this occurs, do not take any more of the drug until you

speak with your physician. If the reaction becomes severe or if you have trouble breathing, get someone to take you to the emergency room.
- This medicine also causes liver damage rarely, but your physician will be monitoring your liver enzymes to be sure this does not occur. Contact your physician if you develop a loss of appetite, nausea and/or vomiting, yellowing of your skin or eyes, very dark urine, or pale feces after taking this drug for a few days.

Mitotane (Lysodren)
- This medicine is used to reduce the amount of corticosteroid hormones produced by the adrenal glands in patients with Cushing's disease.
- Take two 500-mg tablets by mouth 3 times each day. Your physician will be increasing this dose every 3 to 7 days if you do not respond to the initial doses.
- Take the very first dose at bedtime with a light snack.
- If you miss a dose, take it as soon as you remember; however, if it is almost time for the next dose, skip the missed dose and just take the next dose at the regularly scheduled time.
- The most common side effects of mitotane include nausea, vomiting, diarrhea, and loss of appetite, which may be reduced by taking each dose with food.
- It is also common for people to become drowsy, fatigued, and/or dizzy when taking this medication, especially in the beginning of therapy.
- Therefore, avoid drinking alcohol or taking other drugs that may make you drowsy while taking this medication. Use caution when driving or operating machinery until you know how this medicine affects you.
- Some patients also get a rash; inform your physician if this occurs.
- There is not enough information available to establish whether mitotane and ketoconazole are safe or dangerous during pregnancy. It is important to discuss the continued use of these medicines with your doctor before you try to become pregnant or if you become pregnant.

▶ **Follow-up Question**

1. How do the dexamethasone dosage and procedures for collecting urinary/plasma steroid levels differ in the 2-day versus the overnight dexamethasone suppression test for the diagnosis of Cushing's syndrome?

Two-day Low-dose DST
- Give dexamethasone 0.5 mg po every 6 hours for 8 doses (48 hours).
- Collect a 24-hour urine collection beginning with the second 24-hour period.
- Urinary cortisol levels >10 μg per 24 hours or 17-hydroxycorticosteroid levels > 2.5 mg per 24 hours indicates Cushing's syndrome.
- In place of or in addition to the urine collection, a plasma cortisol level may be drawn 6 hours after the last dexamethasone dose. A level > 3 μg/dL indicates Cushing's syndrome.

Overnight DST
- Give dexamethasone 1 mg po at 11 PM or midnight.
- Draw plasma cortisol levels at 8:00 AM
- Plasma cortisol > 5 μg/dL indicates Cushing's syndrome.
- Collect a 24-hour urine collection beginning at 8:00 AM; urine 17-hydroxycorticosteroid levels > 4 mg per 24 hours indicates Cushing's syndrome.

References
1. Tsigos C, Chrousos GP. Differential diagnosis and management of Cushing's syndrome. Annu Rev Med 1996;47:443–461.
2. Engelhardt D. Steroid biosynthesis inhibitors in Cushing's syndrome. Clin Investig 1994;72:481–488.

74 ADDISON'S DISEASE

▶ The Unintentional Tan   (Level II)

Cynthia P. Koh-Knox, PharmD
Bruce C. Carlstedt, PhD

A 42-year-old woman with hypothyroidism presents with progressive fatigue, nausea, anorexia, a recent unintentional weight loss, and hyperpigmentation. Orthostatic hypotension, hyponatremia, a low random morning cortisol level, and an elevated ACTH level confirm the diagnosis of primary adrenal insufficiency, or Addison's disease. Although the patient exhibits some early signs of acute adrenal crisis, she does not require IV hydrocortisone and fluid replacement. Oral hydrocortisone and fludrocortisone therapy are the treatment of choice in this situation. Patient education regarding strict adherence and the lifelong need for therapy is important. Another ACTH level post-initiation will determine if therapy is adequate or if more extensive tests on the patient's pituitary–adrenal axis are needed. Recent adjustments of the patient's thyroid replacement therapy presents a concern for the development of the polyglandular failure syndrome.

▶ **Questions**

Problem Identification

1. a. *Create a list of the patient's drug-related problems.*

- Addison's disease requiring pharmacologic replacement therapy.
- Hypothyroidism presently treated with excessive doses of levothyroxine. The low TSH value indicates the need to reduce her thyroid replacement therapy to achieve appropriate TSH concentrations. Hypothyroidism is not normally seen with adrenal insufficiency, but it can be associated with autoimmune diseases or polyglandular failure syndrome.[1,2]

b. *What information (signs, symptoms, laboratory values) indicates the presence or severity of Addison's disease?*

- *Symptoms.* Profound fatigue, nausea, anorexia, unintentional weight loss.
- *Signs.* Increased pigmentation, including nonexposed areas and skin creases of palms; hypotension.
- *Laboratory values.* Hyponatremia, low cortisol level in AM, high ACTH level.[1–4]

Desired Outcome

2. *What are the goals of pharmacotherapy in this case?*

- The intended outcome is to establish cortisol and aldosterone replacement therapy to mimic normal circadian adrenal rhythm (refer to the section "Addison's Disease" in textbook Chapter 72 for more detailed information).
- Elimination of symptoms and prevention of addisonian crisis are desirable to improve the patient's quality of life.
- Patient education to reinforce adherence is important, as this will be lifelong therapy.
- Preventing or minimizing adverse effects of the medications.

Therapeutic Alternatives

3. a. *What non-drug therapies might be useful for this patient?*

- Non-drug therapies include stress management, proper diet and sodium intake, and regular monitoring of blood pressure and serum glucose levels. These strategies will be explained to the patient to minimize or prevent undesirable side effects.
- Avoidance of exposure to sunlight and extreme temperatures will minimize sunburn and dehydration.
- Patient education on recognizing when an adrenal crisis may be occurring and what to do in that situation is important.
- A medical alert bracelet or necklace stating her condition is advisable in case of an emergency.[1–3]
- A local or state support group may be helpful for patients and families with Addison's disease. The National Adrenal Diseases Foundation is a support group that can be accessed via the Internet.[2]

b. *What feasible pharmacotherapeutic alternatives are available for the treatment of Addison's disease?*

- *Cortisol replacement therapy with oral corticosteroids* is necessary to replace that which is no longer being produced by the adrenal glands. The available corticosteroids differ in duration of action as well as glucocorticoid, mineralocorticoid, and sodium-retaining potencies. The cost of therapy for most products is low, and dosing regimens are simple. The lowest effective dose should be used, and dosing schedules should mimic the normal diurnal adrenal rhythm.
    ✓ *Hydrocortisone, prednisone,* and *cortisone* are the agents of choice for cortisol replacement therapy. Usual morning doses are hydrocortisone 20 mg, prednisone 5 mg, and cortisone 25 mg; evening doses of each agent given at 50% of the morning dose will usually be adequate to duplicate the normal circadian rhythm of cortisol production.
    ✓ *Fludrocortisone acetate (Florinef)* may be added for mineralocorticoid replacement if the glucocorticoid used does not provide sufficient mineralocorticoid potency, and a deficiency of aldosterone is apparent by the continued presence of hyponatremia and hyperkalemia.[1–3,5] The usual dose is 0.05 to 0.2 mg orally once daily.
    ✓ *Prednisolone, triamcinolone, methylprednisolone, betamethasone,* and *dexamethasone* are alternative agents. However, they offer no advantage over the previously listed options and may be more expensive. Furthermore, use of any of the latter four agents, which have little or no sodium-retaining potency, may make the addition of fludrocortisone necessary.
    ✓ The rapid ACTH-stimulation test may be obscured if the patient is taking cortisone, hydrocortisone, methylprednisolone, or prednisone. Therefore, steroid therapy should be initiated after this test is performed. Dexamethasone can be used initially until laboratory tests are done.

c. *What psychosocial considerations are applicable to this patient?*

- Adrenal insufficiency therapy is chronic, and the ability to deal with the lifelong risk of developing adrenal crisis must be present with strong family support. The patient's quality of life can be maintained with proper education and medication adherence.[3]

Optimal Plan

4. *What drug, dosage form, dose, schedule, and duration of therapy are best for this patient?*

- Hydrocortisone 20 mg orally in the morning and 10 mg in the evening provides cortisol replacement therapy adequate to mimic the normal circadian adrenal rhythm in many patients. Prednisone 5/2.5 mg or cortisone 25/12.5 mg daily would provide equivalent replacement therapy.
- If necessary, mineralocorticoid loss can be replaced with an oral morning dose of 0.05 mg fludrocortisone acetate. The dosage can be increased to a maximum of 0.2 mg as necessary to control hyponatremia and hyperkalemia.
- Duration of therapy will be lifelong, and individualized dosage adjustments must be made according to the patient's response to therapy based on diminished clinical symptoms and normalization of serum laboratory tests.[1–3]

Outcome Evaluation

5. *What clinical and laboratory parameters are necessary to evaluate the therapy for achievement of the desired therapeutic outcome and to detect or prevent adverse effects?*

- Although hyperpigmentation is not a universal marker in all patients with Addison's disease, a reduction in the patient's pigmentation is a good clinical indicator of response to therapy.
- Confirmation of the patient's compliance with therapy and an assessment of her overall sense of well-being are also important parameters.[1,3,4]
- Other monitoring parameters include body weight, blood pressure measurements, blood and urine glucose concentrations, ophthalmo-

logic exams, serum and urine electrolytes, and stool testing for occult blood. The frequency of monitoring these parameters varies depending on the resolution of signs and symptoms. Body weight, blood pressure, and glucose monitoring are relatively easy for self-monitoring and less costly than the other parameters.
- Clinicians may opt to perform annual adrenal function studies, such as the ACTH stimulation test.
- The patient's hypothyroid condition should also be monitored after initiation of cortisol and mineralocorticoid therapy.

Patient Counseling

6. *What information should be provided to the patient to enhance compliance, ensure successful therapy, and minimize adverse effects?*

General Information
- The names of your medications are hydrocortisone and fludrocortisone. Their intended action is to replace the hormones normally produced by your adrenal gland. You will need to take these medicines for the rest of your life.
- Take both of your medications with food to minimize upset stomach.
- Stressful situations, such as surgery, infection, or trauma can trigger what is called an "adrenal crisis." This means that your body is not producing or receiving the amount of steroid hormones needed to maintain normal body functions. Signs and symptoms of adrenal crisis include muscle soreness, general malaise, vomiting, fever, fainting, and decreased blood pressure. If you experience any of these symptoms, seek immediate medical attention. Do not hesitate to call 911.
- It is important to wear or carry identification stating that you are taking chronic corticosteroid therapy in case of a serious illness or other emergency situation.
- Always ask your doctor or pharmacist about new medications that are prescribed to ensure that they are compatible with these medications.

Hydrocortisone
- You will be taking a larger dose of this medication in the morning with breakfast and a smaller dose in the evening. This is intended to mimic the way your body normally produces the natural steroid hormone. Try to take the two doses approximately 12 hours apart.
- Never stop taking this medication or change your dose unless your doctor instructs you to do so. This medication requires gradual tapering if you need to stop therapy.
- If you miss a morning dose and you remember in the morning, take the missed dose. If you remember in the afternoon, skip the morning dose and take the evening dose as scheduled.
- If you miss the evening dose and remember before going to bed, take the missed dose. Otherwise, skip the dose and take the next morning dose as scheduled. Never take double doses.
- Side effects of hydrocortisone include stomach irritation, increased risk of infections, sodium retention and leg swelling (edema), loss of body potassium and magnesium, cataracts, delayed wound healing, and easy bruising. Your health care providers will minimize these side effects by using the lowest dose necessary to control your disease.

Fludrocortisone (Florinef)
- This medication helps to normalize the amount of sodium and potassium in your body.
- Take this medicine just once daily. Choose a time that is convenient for you, such as in the morning, and maintain consistency with the time.
- Side effects are minimal but may include upset stomach, leg edema, and low blood potassium levels.

References

1. Corrigan EK. Addison's disease. NIH publication no. 90-3054. Internet website: http://wellweb.com/INDEX/qaddison.htm
2. Margulies P. Addison's disease: The facts you need to know. Internet website: http://medhlp.netusa.net/www/nadf3.htm
3. Stoffer SS. Addison's disease: How to improve patients' quality of life. Postgrad Med 1993;93(4):265–266, 271–278.
4. McDermott MT, Georgittis WJ, Asp AA. Adrenal crisis in active duty service members. Mil Med 1996;161:624–626.
5. Cronin CC, Callaghan N, Kearney PJ, et al. Addison disease in patients treated with glucocorticoid therapy. Arch Intern Med 1997;157:456–458.

75 HYPERPROLACTINEMIA

▶ **Preconceived Ideas** (Level I)

Amy M. Heck, PharmD
Karim A. Calis, PharmD, MPH, BCPS, BCNSP, FASHP

A 31-year-old woman with a history of oligomenorrhea since menarche (age 14), GERD, and occasional migraine headaches presents to her gynecologist with symptoms of amenorrhea and galactorrhea and a concern that she may not be able to become pregnant. The patient began treatment with a dopamine agonist, and after 4 weeks of therapy, she experienced significant adverse effects without clinical improvement or substantial reduction in serum prolactin concentrations. There are several potential causes for the patient's initial poor response to therapy, and an alternative treatment option must be considered in order to achieve the treatment goals.

▶ **Questions**

Problem Identification

1. a. *Create a list of this patient's drug-related problems.*

- Hyperprolactinemia (amenorrhea, galactorrhea, and infertility) requiring drug therapy to normalize serum prolactin concentrations and relieve the associated symptoms.

- Chronic stable problems requiring no intervention at this time include: 1) GERD treated effectively with omeprazole; and 2) occasional migraine headaches well controlled with sumatriptan.

b. *What signs, symptoms, and laboratory values indicate the presence of hyperprolactinemia?*

- Amenorrhea
- Galactorrhea
- Infertility
- Serum prolactin concentration >20 μg/L measured on different days
- *Note:* Because prolactin is released in a pulsatile fashion and many physiologic factors (e.g., sleep, exercise, coitus, eating) may cause transiently elevated prolactin serum concentrations, it is critical to document increased prolactin concentrations on multiple occasions to confirm the diagnosis of hyperprolactinemia.

c. *Could this patient's hyperprolactinemia be drug-induced?*

- Although many pharmacologic agents have been reported to cause hyperprolactinemia, this patient does not appear to be taking any of these medications (refer to textbook Chapter 73 for a complete list of these medications).
- Moreover, a known cause of hyperprolactinemia (i.e., microprolactinoma) has been identified in this patient.

Desired Outcome

2. *What are the goals of treatment for a woman with hyperprolactinemia?*

- Normalize prolactin serum concentrations (i.e., to < 20 μg/L)
- Relieve symptoms (galactorrhea and amenorrhea)
- Restore fertility

Therapeutic Alternatives

3. a. *What non-drug therapies can be considered for the treatment of hyperprolactinemia?*

- Non-drug therapies include transsphenoidal surgical removal of the prolactin-secreting adenoma and radiation treatment.
- Because drug therapy with dopamine agonists is often more effective than surgery or radiation, it is usually the preferred treatment option for hyperprolactinemia (refer to the section "Hyperprolactinemia Treatment" in textbook Chapter 73 for a more detailed discussion).

b. *What pharmacotherapeutic options are available for the treatment of hyperprolactinemia in this woman?*

- *Dopamine agonists* are the mainstay of therapy for hyperprolactinemia. Three dopamine agonists currently available in the U.S. have been used for the management of hyperprolactinemia:
  - ✓ *Bromocriptine (Parlodel, generics)* was the first D_2-receptor agonist to be used for the treatment of hyperprolactinemia. Bromocriptine has been shown to normalize prolactin serum concentrations, restore gonadotropin production, and shrink tumor size in approximately 90% of patients with prolactinomas.[1] Usual therapeutic doses range from 2.5 to 15 mg/day given in 2 to 3 divided doses. The most common adverse effects include headache, lightheadedness, dizziness, nervousness, fatigue, and GI effects such as nausea, abdominal pain, and diarrhea. Although most of these adverse effects diminish with continued treatment, about 12% of patients discontinue treatment due to intolerable side effects.[1]
  - ✓ *Pergolide (Permax)* is a dopamine receptor agonist with affinity for both D_1 and D_2 receptors. In the United States, pergolide is not FDA approved for the treatment of hyperprolactinemia and is most commonly prescribed for the treatment of Parkinson's disease. However, pergolide is recognized as a safe and effective alternative to bromocriptine and offers the advantage of once-daily dosing. The average dose of pergolide that achieves optimal suppression of prolactin serum concentrations is 50 μg/day given as a single dose. Its adverse effects are similar to those of bromocriptine and include nausea, vomiting, headache, and dizziness.
  - ✓ *Cabergoline (Dostinex)* is a long-acting dopamine agonist with high selectivity and affinity for dopamine D_2 receptors. This agent is approved by the FDA for the treatment of hyperprolactinemia and has been shown to effectively reduce serum prolactin concentrations in 80% to 90% of hyperprolactinemic patients.[2] Cabergoline may also be effective for patients who are intolerant of or resistant to bromocriptine. The usual dose is 0.5 to 1 mg twice weekly; however, higher doses have been used. The most common adverse effects are nausea, vomiting, headache, and dizziness. These effects are similar to those associated with bromocriptine and pergolide. In a large comparative study, cabergoline was associated with fewer adverse effects than bromocriptine.[3] As with other dopamine agonists, adverse events usually occur early in therapy and subside with continued treatment (refer to the section on hyperprolactinemia treatment in textbook Chapter 73 for further discussion of these agents).
  - ✓ Other dopamine agonists available in the United States (pramipexole, ropinirole) have not been studied for the management of hyperprolactinemia.

Optimal Plan

4. *What medication regimen would you recommend for this patient?*

- Bromocriptine, cabergoline, and pergolide are all effective for the initial treatment of hyperprolactinemia and any of the three agents would be an appropriate choice for initial therapy.
- Most clinical experience in the treatment of hyperprolactinemia is with bromocriptine. To minimize adverse effects, the initial dose of bromocriptine should be 2.5 mg given with food at bedtime. The dose should be increased in 1.25-mg increments every week and given in 2 to 3 divided doses.
- Pergolide offers the advantage of once-daily dosing and is considerably less expensive than bromocriptine or cabergoline ($1/7$ to $1/10$ the cost). Pergolide should be initiated at a dose of 25 μg given once daily at bedtime.
- Cabergoline therapy may be initiated at a dose of 0.5 mg given once weekly or 0.25 mg given twice weekly. This dose may be increased in increments of 0.25 mg twice weekly at 4-week intervals based on serum prolactin concentrations.

Outcome Evaluation

5. a. *What clinical and laboratory parameters are necessary to monitor the patient's response to therapy?*

- Serum prolactin concentrations should be monitored every 3 to 4 weeks (target concentration < 20 µg/L).
- Symptoms of galactorrhea should resolve within 3 months. Some patients may experience complete resolution within a few days, whereas others may require more than 6 months of therapy for complete cessation of galactorrhea.
- Menstrual cycles should return to baseline within 6 months.
- The size of the pituitary adenoma should decrease, as assessed by MRI after 6 months of therapy.
- The patient should be questioned about the adverse effects of dopamine agonist therapy as discussed previously.

b. *If the initial therapy you recommend is effective, how soon can the patient hope to become pregnant?*

- Fertility is restored in 57% to 100% of hyperprolactinemic women who receive medical therapy with dopamine agonists. Ovulation and menstruation generally resume within 6 to 8 weeks of treatment.[4,5]

Patient Counseling

6. *What information should be provided to the patient to enhance compliance, ensure successful therapy, and minimize adverse effects?*

Bromocriptine

- This medication is known as a dopamine agonist. It works by blocking the release of prolactin from the pituitary gland and decreasing the amount of prolactin in your blood.
- Bromocriptine may cause an upset stomach. The dose should be taken with food and just before bedtime to decrease the nausea and stomach pain.
- This medication may make you feel drowsy or dizzy. You should not take part in any activities that require you to be alert (such as driving) until you know how you react to this medication.
- Bromocriptine may also cause a dry mouth. You can use sugarless candy, ice chips, or a saliva substitute for temporary relief of this side effect.
- While taking bromocriptine, you should use a barrier method of birth control (e.g., condom, diaphragm) because the effects of this medication on a developing baby are not completely understood.
- When your menstrual cycle returns to normal, tell your doctor so that you can both decide the best time for you to stop using birth control and attempt to become pregnant. It may take many weeks for bromocriptine to restore your normal menstrual cycle, but do not stop taking this medication without first discussing it with your doctor or pharmacist.

▶ Follow-up Questions

1. *Identify the possible reasons for the patient's poor initial response to therapy.*

- *Poor compliance.* Dopamine agonists may cause significant GI adverse effects, including nausea, abdominal pain, and diarrhea. Taking the medication with food can minimize these effects. Lack of compliance due to significant adverse effects may have caused her poor response to therapy, and this possibility should be investigated further.
- *Suboptimal dose.* Inadequate dosing of dopamine agonists can result in a poor response. For example, although the average daily dose of bromocriptine for the treatment of hyperprolactinemia ranges from 2.5 to 15 mg/day, some patients require doses as high as 40 mg/day. The maximum reduction in serum prolactin concentration generally occurs after 4 weeks of continuous bromocriptine therapy. Assuming that this patient was compliant and that her bromocriptine dose was slowly increased to 7.5 mg/day over a 4-week period, a modest reduction in serum prolactin concentration would have been expected. Therefore, the initial doses that this patient was receiving may have been insufficient for adequate reduction in serum prolactin concentrations.
- *Treatment-resistant prolactinoma.* Dopamine agonist-resistant prolactinomas have been described in a small number of patients. Poor response to bromocriptine in such patients may be due to receptor defects or a reduced number of dopamine receptors on the pituitary lactotroph cell membrane.[6]

2. *Given the new patient information, what alternative therapies should be considered?*

- Clinical response to an individual dopamine agonist may vary from patient to patient; although all three drugs are effective, some patients may respond better to one agent than to another.
- Cabergoline may be effective for patients who do not respond to or are intolerant of bromocriptine. Cabergoline may also have fewer adverse effects than bromocriptine and may improve compliance due to the flexibility of twice-weekly dosing.[1]
- Pergolide may also be an appropriate alternative. It is significantly less expensive than both bromocriptine and cabergoline and offers the advantage of once-daily dosing.[1]

3. *How long will this patient require drug treatment for the prolactinoma?*

- Many patients require life-long therapy with dopamine agonists to maintain normal serum prolactin concentrations and to relieve the symptoms of hyperprolactinemia. However, recent studies suggest that some patients with hyperprolactinemia due to pituitary microadenomas enter remission during treatment with dopamine agonists. Therefore, discontinuation of therapy after 2 to 3 years should be considered to assess the need for continued therapy.[7]

References

1. Webster J. A comparative review of the tolerability profiles of dopamine agonists in the treatment of hyperprolactinaemia and inhibition of lactation. Drug Saf 1996;14:228–238.
2. Webster J, Piscitelli G, Polli A, et al. The efficacy and tolerability of long-term cabergoline therapy in hyperprolactinaemic disorders: An open, uncontrolled multicentre study. European Multicentre Cabergoline Study Group. Clin Endocrinol 1993;39:323–329.

3. Webster J, Piscitelli G, Polli A, et al. A comparison of cabergoline and bromocriptine in the treatment of hyperprolactinemic amenorrhea. Cabergoline Comparative Study Group. N Engl J Med 1994;331:904–909.
4. Yuen BH. Etiology and treatment of hyperprolactinemia. Semin Reprod Endocrinol 1992;10:228–235.
5. Cunnah D, Besser M. Management of prolactinomas. Clin Endocrinol 1991;34: 231–235.
6. Molitch ME. Pathologic hyperprolactinemia. Endocrinol Metab Clin North Am 1992;21:877–901.
7. Sarapura V, Schlaff WD. Recent advances in the understanding of the pathophysiology and treatment of hyperprolactinemia. Curr Opin Obstet Gynecol 1993;5: 360–367.

SECTION 8

Gynecologic Disorders

Barbara G. Wells, PharmD, FASHP, FCCP, BCPP, Section Editor

76 CONTRACEPTION

▶ I Need the Pill (Level II)

Carla B. Frye, PharmD, BCPS

A 17-year-old female who has a seizure disorder treated with carbamazepine presents to a family practice clinic requesting a prescription for birth control pills. The patient has no absolute contraindications to oral contraceptives (OCs) but has a family history of cardiovascular disease and diabetes mellitus. Non-drug contraceptive methods include male or female condoms with vaginal spermicide, diaphragm with spermicide, cervical cap, and intrauterine devices. Pharmacotherapeutic methods of contraception include monophasic or triphasic estrogen/progestin combinations, progestin-only OCs, levonorgestrel implants, and medroxyprogesterone acetate suspension for IM injection. In order to make an informed choice, the patient needs to be educated on the risks and benefits of each contraceptive type, typical failure rates, the importance of compliance, and proper methods of use. The fact that carbamazepine may reduce the effectiveness of OCs in this patient should be considered. When this patient complains of never having a menstrual period 3 months after starting an OC, possible causes and potential treatments must be evaluated carefully.

▶ **Questions**

Problem Identification

1. a. *Create a list of this person's potential drug-related problems.*

   - Carbamazepine can cause somnolence, fluid retention, bone marrow suppression, rashes, and GI distress. The patient should be assessed for these disorders before adding another medication that could mask or worsen some of them. Nausea is the most common side effect of OCs. Estrogen can also cause melasma (facial hyperpigmentation) and fluid retention.
   - Carbamazepine induces the hepatic metabolism of hormonal contraceptives, potentially resulting in decreased contraceptive effectiveness.

   b. *What medical problems are absolute contraindications to hormonal contraceptive use, and do any of those conditions apply to this patient?*

   - Active thrombophlebitis or thromboembolic disorder (does not apply)[1]
   - Cerebrovascular accident or history thereof (does not apply)
   - Coronary artery or ischemic heart disease (does not apply)
   - Known or strongly suspected estrogen-dependent neoplasia (does not apply)
   - Pregnancy (urine pregnancy test negative)
   - Benign hepatic adenoma or liver cancer (does not apply)
   - Markedly impaired liver function (need more information, but this is highly unlikely)
   - Diagnosis of AIDS (the patient has not had an HIV test, and the risk of contracting HIV from her boyfriend is difficult to assess, given the limited information about him; she needs a barrier contraceptive method to prevent disease transmission)

Gynecologic Disorders   253

c. *What medical problems are relative contraindications to hormonal contraceptive use, and do any of these apply to this patient?*

- Migraine headaches (positive family history may be a potential problem)[1]
- Hypertension (family history of cardiovascular disease may be a potential problem)
- Diabetes mellitus (positive family history may be a potential problem)
- Elective major surgery requiring immobilization planned in the next 4 weeks (does not apply)
- Undiagnosed abnormal vaginal/uterine bleeding (does not apply)
- Sickle cell disease (does not apply)
- Lactation (does not apply)
- Gestational diabetes (does not apply)
- Active gallbladder disease (does not apply)
- Over 50 years of age (does not apply)
- Family history of hyperlipidemia (positive family history may be a potential problem)

d. *What other information should be obtained before finalizing a pharmacotherapeutic plan?*

- *Test for HIV,* Chlamydia, *gonorrhea and syphilis.* The patient admits to unprotected sex with her boyfriend for a few months, therefore her risk of sexually transmitted disease (STD) or AIDS should be evaluated with tests for *Chlamydia,* gonorrhea, syphilis, and HIV.
- *Lipid profile.* She has a strong family history of cardiovascular disease and lipid disorders. This would be a good time to evaluate her fasting lipid profile, obtaining total cholesterol, HDL-C, LDL-C, and triglyceride values. The progestin component of combined OCs can cause a dose-related decrease in HDL-C and an increase in LDL-C. If her lipid profile suggests cardiovascular risk (e.g., total cholesterol > 200 mg/dL, LDL-C > 160 mg/dL, TG > 400 mg/dL, or HDL-C < 35 mg/dL), consideration should be given to the progestin component of the OC. It has been suggested that norgestimate and desogestrel have the least effect on plasma lipids.[2]
- *Fasting blood sugar.* She also has a family history of diabetes mellitus. At a minimum, a fasting blood sugar level should be obtained. According to the 1998 Clinical Practice Recommendations from the American Diabetes Association, testing should be considered at a younger age or be carried out more frequently in individuals who have a first degree relative with diabetes.[3] A fasting blood glucose is also generally recommended for all women started on OCs.
- *Liver function studies.* Carbamazepine can cause abnormalities in liver function tests, as can OCs. It is debatable whether elevated transaminases (ALT/AST) in this individual would preclude use of an OC, but baseline values would be valuable.

Desired Outcome

2. *What are the goals of pharmacotherapy in this case?*

- Prevention of pregnancy using a contraceptive method that has a reasonable cost, a low failure rate, convenience, and minimal adverse effects
- Prevention of STDs
- Patient understanding of how the methods work and participation in the choice of a method that is both acceptable to her and most appropriate for her contraceptive goals

Therapeutic Alternatives

3. a. *What non-drug methods of contraception might be useful for this patient, considering the advantages and disadvantages of each?*

- Refer to Table 76–1 in textbook Chapter 76 for more detailed information on these devices.
- *Male or female condoms with vaginal spermicide/foam.* These methods provide protection against STDs and HIV but are not as reliable as hormonal methods for the prevention of conception. Both are potentially unacceptable to the user, as they are considered "unnatural" or "messy" and not as convenient since their use must be planned in advance.
- *Diaphragm with spermicide or cervical cap.* These methods provide protection against STDs and HIV but require a physician office visit and are less reliable than hormonal methods with typical use.
- *Intrauterine devices or IUDs (either hormonal or non-hormonal).* These devices provide long-term contraception (12 months to 10 years) and are extremely reliable forms of contraception. However, there is an increased risk of ectopic pregnancy, they are expensive, and they require a physician for placement.

b. *What pharmacotherapeutic alternatives are available for prevention of pregnancy in this patient, and what are the advantages or disadvantages of each (see Table 76–1 and Figure 76–1)?*

- Refer to Table 76–1 in textbook Chapter 76 for more detailed information on contraceptive products.
- *Monophasic or triphasic estrogen/progestin OC combinations.* The most desirable products in this class are either lower dose estrogen/progestin combinations or the triphasic combinations. If using combined hormonal OCs, the initial dose should be the lowest dose of ethinyl estradiol that is effective (generally 35 μg). The lower doses of estrogen and progestin have the least effect on plasma lipids, blood glucose, and blood pressure. OCs provide protection against ovarian and endometrial cancer, iron deficiency anemia, fibrocystic breast disease, and ovarian cysts. However, OC combinations do not provide protection against STDs and have an increased risk of benign hepatocellular adenomas. They are reliable when taken correctly but have a high failure rate in adolescents and teenagers due to noncompliance and/or adverse effects.
- *Progestin-only OCs.* These products can be used in women who are breastfeeding and avoid estrogen-related side effects (e.g., bloating, nausea, breast tenderness). Progestin-only dosage forms do not provide protection against STDs, have an increased risk of ectopic pregnancy, and cause frequent spotting and amenorrhea.
- *Levonorgestrel implants (Norplant).* This product provides ef-

fective contraception for 5 years, and its effects are quickly reversed with removal of the inserts. It does require a surgical procedure, causes irregular bleeding, does not protect against STDs, and has progestin side effects. Most patients are hesitant to use this product.
- *Medroxyprogesterone acetate IM suspension (Depo-Provera).* This product for IM injection provides effective contraception for 3 months, has few drug interactions, and is a "passive" contraceptive method. However, it can decrease HDL-C, has progestin side effects, does not protect against STDs, and requires an office visit.

Optimal Plan

4. What method, dose, schedule, and duration of therapy will be best for this patient?

- Contraceptive choice is very dependent on patient preference. In order to make an informed choice, patients need to be made aware of the risks and benefits of each type of contraceptive available. They should be informed of the failure rates, the importance of compliance, and how each method should be used to ensure efficacy.
- Textbook and Casebook Table 76–1 provide comparative information on first-year failure rates with typical use versus perfect use of the various contraceptive methods.[1]
- This individual came to the clinic requesting OCs; she may not be aware of the other forms of contraception. She needs to be questioned about her willingness to take a pill every day. She needs to be informed that OCs will not protect her from STDs.
- She also needs to be aware that the medication (carbamazepine) she takes for seizure control can potentially render OCs less effective at preventing pregnancy. Depo-Provera or levonorgestrel implants are less affected by carbamazepine and could be better choices for her. She has no absolute contraindications to any of the contraceptive methods.
- If she has only one sexual partner, is made aware of her risks for contracting an STD, understands that her anticonvulsant may interact with OCs, and still chooses OCs as her contraceptive method, several options are available.
  ✓ In general, the clinician should start most patients on a product that contains 35 μg or less of ethinyl estradiol and a low dose of a progestin.
  ✓ In a teenager, and in view of this person's menstrual irregularity, it would also be desirable to start her on a combination product that contained a progestin with low androgen activity. Teenage pill users may be more likely to stop taking an OC due to minor side effects such as spotting or nausea (symptoms of estrogen excess) and are more likely to have irregular menstrual periods. Acne is also a particular problem in this population. Using lowest dosages of estrogen and a low-dose progestin with low androgen activity (such as norgestimate, desogestrel, norethindrone, or ethynodiol diacetate) would appear to be the best choices. Products containing these minimally androgenic progestins include Ortho-Cyclen, Desogen, Tri-Cyclen, Ovcon-35, Brevicon, and Modicon.
  ✓ Her treatment with carbamazepine may require the use of a higher dose of estrogen for contraceptive effectiveness. Norlestrin 1/50 or Ovcon-50 might be necessary if a 35-μg estrogen combination is not effective. The patient could experience breakthrough bleeding if the carbamazepine induces the metabolism of the estrogen component of her pill; she could develop spotting if the metabolism of the progestin is induced. Either symptom should cause the clinician to reevaluate therapy. The patient could also experience contraceptive failure (pregnancy) from this interaction.
  ✓ Because this individual is 2 weeks from the date of her last menses, the clinician must decide whether to start the OC immediately or wait until onset of her next menses. Since her pregnancy test was negative, the OC can be started as soon as possible. Discussion with the patient will determine when to start the medication. Most patients prefer to start OCs on a Sunday to avoid weekend periods.

Outcome Evaluation

5. What clinical and laboratory parameters are necessary to evaluate the therapy for efficacy and adverse effects?

Efficacy
- *Lack of pregnancy.* If she continues to have menstrual irregularity or misses a period, another urine pregnancy test should be performed.

Adverse Effects
- She may continue the pill indefinitely and should have pelvic exams and PAP smears annually.
- The American Cancer Society recommends that women begin monthly self breast exams at age 20 and have a clinical exam by a health professional every 3 years from ages 20 to 39. Mammography is recommended every 1 to 2 years after age 40. She should be instructed on self-breast exams and should begin them on a monthly basis with the initiation of contraceptive therapy.
- The National Cholesterol Education Program II (NCEP-II) report recommends that serum total cholesterol should be measured in all adults ≥ 20 years of age at least once every 5 years; HDL-C should be measured at the same time if accurate results are available.[4] This young woman is only 17, but many authorities recommend a serum lipid profile before initiation of OC therapy and then follow the NCEP recommendations thereafter.
- Since she has a family history of diabetes mellitus, a fasting blood sugar and/or glucose tolerance test should be performed. The American Diabetes Association recommends that all individuals should have an oral glucose tolerance test or a fasting plasma glucose test by age 45, repeated at 3-year intervals if normal.[3] Persons who have first-degree relatives with diabetes should have testing at a younger age and have it repeated more frequently. Combination OCs may affect carbohydrate metabolism, and most authorities recommend baseline testing in women who might be at risk for the development of diabetes mellitus. No definite recommendation for subsequent testing is available, but a fasting plasma glucose could be recommended annually due to its ease of performance, low cost, convenience, and widespread availability.
- Blood pressure, assessment of any new medical complaints, headaches, weight gain, edema, signs of thromboembolic disease, depression, and nausea/emesis should be evaluated at least annually.

Patient Counseling

6. *What information should be provided to the patient to enhance compliance, ensure successful therapy, and minimize adverse effects?*

   General Information for Hormonal Contraception
   - There is a delay of several weeks in the onset of contraceptive effectiveness. Therefore, you should use a barrier method (e.g., condom) throughout the first menstrual cycle.
   - You may notice a change in your usual pattern of menses or new vaginal bleeding during your cycle, including cycle irregularity (too long or too short), breakthrough bleeding (between usual menses), or lack of bleeding (called amenorrhea), especially in the first several months of use. Contact your prescriber if you are bothered by any of these bleeding changes.
   - Watch for any of the following effects, which you can remember by the word ACHES. A = abdominal pain, C = chest pain or shortness of breath, H = headaches (severe, throbbing headaches on one side of the head), E = eye problems (blurred vision, double vision, blindness), S = swelling or severe leg pain. If any of these problems develop, contact your physician or clinic as soon as possible or seek immediate medical care if the problem is severe.
   - If you have or will have more than one regular sexual partner, or if you believe that your partner has or had more than one partner, you may be at risk of contracting a sexually transmitted disease (including HIV infection). You should use a condom or other barrier form of contraception. You cannot generally tell who has or does not have an STD or HIV when you have sex, even with a "faithful" partner.
   - This medication can interact with the carbamazepine (Tegretol XR) that you are taking. The result of this interaction may be that the combination OC is not effective. Contact your doctor immediately if you miss a period. Also, contact your doctor or pharmacist before taking any new prescription or non-prescription medication.
   - Diarrhea or vomiting may reduce the amount of the pill that is absorbed into your system and may result in breakthrough bleeding or even pregnancy. If nausea or vomiting continues more than 1 or 2 days, it is advisable to call your doctor and/or use a barrier method for the remainder of your cycle.
   - Birth control pills can cause weight gain, nausea, worsening of acne, facial skin darkening or rash, and depression. Call your doctor if any of these symptoms become troublesome.
   - Take this medication every day as directed. If you miss a single dose, take the pill as soon as you remember (i.e., take two pills in one day). If you have missed pills for 2 days, take double doses for the next 2 days and use a barrier method (condom) for the remainder of the cycle. If you have missed doses for 3 days, call your doctor. Missing 3 days may cause you to have a period, and you will need to discard that month's pack, starting a new one on day 8 from the time of your last dose. In any case, use an alternative method of birth control for the remainder of the cycle.

▶ **Follow-up Questions**

1. *What are the most likely causes of amenorrhea in this patient?*

   - Pregnancy
   - Inadequate build-up of the endometrium due to use of a low-dose OC product
   - Intensive exercise schedule associated with cross-country running
   - Endocrine causes (e.g., pituitary tumor, hypothyroidism)

2. *How could this problem be evaluated?*

   - Administer a pregnancy test.
   - Give a progestin-challenge test (medroxyprogesterone acetate 10 mg orally daily for 5 days). If bleeding occurs after stopping the medroxyprogesterone, the diagnosis is anovulation, which may be treated with medroxyprogesterone acetate 10 mg orally once daily for 10 days every month.
   - Obtain a prolactin level; if it is elevated, the patient must be evaluated for pituitary tumor.
   - Check a TSH level; if elevated, the patient may be hypothyroid, and appropriate replacement with a thyroid preparation (e.g., levothyroxine) should restore the normal menstrual cycle.

3. *If her pregnancy and other diagnostic tests are negative, what are the pharmacotherapeutic alternatives for treating the amenorrhea?*

   - Give additional estrogen (ethinyl estradiol 20 μg/day or conjugated estrogens 0.625 mg/day) taken 12 hours after the OC (to avoid nausea) for 1 to 2 cycles.
   - Alternatively, use a product with higher progestin activity (e.g., Norinyl 2 or Norlestrin 2.5/50; both of these have higher estrogen amounts as well).
   - Another option is to change to a different form of birth control. In view of her concomitant carbamazepine treatment and her family history of diabetes mellitus, breast cancer, and migraines, a progestin-only form of birth control such as Depo-Provera would be a good alternative.

4. *If she had developed breakthrough bleeding when she initiated her OC, what could be some of the possible causes?*

   - Missed pills or the patient did not take them at the same time every day
   - Ectopic pregnancy
   - Pelvic inflammatory disease
   - Cervical lesions (cervicitis, polyps, cancer, condylomas)
   - Endometrial lesions (polyps, cancer)
   - Uterine fibroids
   - Endometriosis
   - Decreased OC bioavailability

5. *If breakthrough bleeding is not caused by a concomitant medical condition, how can it be managed?*

   - Take the pills at the same time each day
   - Increase the estrogen content if the breakthrough bleeding is early in the cycle
   - Increase the progestin content if the bleeding is late in the cycle
   - If using a biphasic or triphasic pill, switch to a monophasic product with greater progestin activity
   - Add supplemental estrogen for 1 week
   - Add supplemental estrogen for 1 to 3 cycles (taken 12 hours after the pill)

References

1. Hatcher RA, Guillebaud J. The pill: Combined oral contraceptives. In: Hatcher RA, Trussell J, Stewart F, et al, eds. Contraceptive Technology, 17th ed. New York, Ardent Media, 1998:405–465.
2. Lewis MA, Spitzer WO, Heinemann LA, et al. Third generation oral contraceptives and risk of myocardial infarction: An international case-control study. Transitional Research Group on Oral Contraceptives and the Health of Young Women. BMJ 1996;312:88–90.
3. American Diabetes Association. Report of the expert committee on the diagnosis and classification of diabetes mellitus. Diabetes Care 1998;21(suppl 1):S5–S19. Also see www.diabetes.org/diabetescare/supplement198.
4. National Cholesterol Education Program: Second report of the National Cholesterol Education Program (NCEP) Expert Panel on detection, evaluation, and treatment of high blood cholesterol in adults (Adult Treatment Panel II). Circulation 1994;89:1329–1445.

77 PREMENSTRUAL DYSPHORIC DISORDER

▶ Dual Identity (Level II)

Donna M. Jermain, PharmD, BCPP

A 38-year-old woman is referred to the PMS clinic by her gynecologist because of emotional symptoms including irritability, inability to concentrate, depression, confusion, mood swings, chocolate cravings, and suicidal ideation that begin several days prior to the onset of menses. She also experiences physical symptoms of fatigue, incoordination, weight gain, bloating, backaches, cramps, breast tenderness, and headaches. After a complete medical history, physical exam, and laboratory tests are obtained, the diagnosis of premenstrual dysphoric disorder (PMDD) is made. Selective serotonin reuptake inhibitors (SSRIs) are first-line pharmacologic treatment for PMDD and are effective for both physical and emotional symptoms. Alprazolam may be effective for anxiety and depressive symptoms. These agents have been effective when given only during the luteal phase (the two weeks prior to the onset of menses). Other antidepressants, spironolactone, and bromocriptine may be useful for selected symptoms. It is important for patients to maintain a calendar of their symptoms before treatment begins and after treatment is initiated so that an objective measure of treatment success may be obtained.

▶ Questions

Problem Identification

1. a. *What are the patient's drug-related problems?*

   - Premenstrual dysphoric disorder (PMDD), currently untreated.
   - Elevation in fasting total cholesterol and LDL-cholesterol, currently untreated.
   - Headaches, which may not have been adequately assessed and treated.

   b. *What pattern of symptoms does this patient have that are consistent with PMDD requiring treatment?*

   - Cyclic pattern of fatigue, poor coordination, feeling out of control, crying, headache, anxiety, aches, irritability, mood swings, bloating, food cravings, nervous tension, cramps, depression, breast tenderness, insomnia, and confusion.
   - Once her menses begins, her symptoms begin to resolve, and she relates no symptoms at present.

   c. *Which symptoms does this patient have that are amenable to drug therapy?*

   - Ideally, drug therapy for PMDD will help with all the symptoms she is experiencing.
   - Her elevated cholesterol panel is more amenable to non-pharmacologic therapy such as a low-fat diet and exercise. Other than elevated LDL-cholesterol, the only potential risk factor she has for coronary heart disease is a possible family history of premature CHD (the age of onset of her father's CHD is unknown). For patients with 0 to 1 risk factor, the goal LDL-cholesterol is ≤ 160 mg/dL. She requires about a 9% reduction in LDL-cholesterol to achieve this goal, which can be achieved with dietary therapy and exercise.

Desired Outcome

2. *What are the goals of treatment for PMDD in this case?*

   - Reduce both the physical and emotional symptoms of PMDD
   - Decrease the emotional stress on the family by addressing her symptoms
   - Enable her to be more productive at work during the PMS time frame
   - Improve her overall quality of life
   - Minimize adverse reactions to drug therapy

Therapeutic Alternatives

3. *What non-pharmacologic and pharmacotherapeutic choices are available for persons with PMDD?*

- *Exercise* has been noted to be beneficial for PMDD and would also be beneficial for her obesity and elevated cholesterol levels.
- *Selective serotonin reuptake inhibitors (SSRIs)* have been shown to be beneficial for both the physical and emotional symptoms of PMDD with minimal adverse reactions. Sertraline has been studied for luteal phase dosing and appears to be effective when given only during the luteal phase (the 2 weeks prior to menses).[1]
- *Alprazolam* has been effective for the anxiety and depressive symptoms. It has also been dosed just during the luteal phase and is tapered once menses begins.[2]
- *Nefazodone* was shown to be helpful for physical and emotional symptoms in one study, but the study had an open-label design.[3]
- *Clomipramine* and *desipramine* have been studied and appear to reduce emotional symptoms but have anticholinergic side effects that may limit their use.
- *Danazol* and *gonadotropin-releasing hormone agonists (leuprolide)*, which are agents that inhibit ovulation, have been successful but are not used because of high cost, androgenic side effects, and the potential long-term risks of osteoporosis and heart disease.[4,5]
- *Spironolactone* is the only diuretic shown to be effective for bloating, weight gain, and edema related to PMDD.
- *Bromocriptine* has been effective for edema, weight gain, bloating, and breast tenderness.
- *Oral contraceptives* may worsen, lessen, or have no appreciable effect on PMDD.
- *Progesterone suppositories* have not been shown to be beneficial.
- *Pyridoxine (vitamin B_6)* has not been shown to be beneficial.

Optimal Plan

4. *Outline a pharmacotherapeutic plan to treat this patient's PMDD.*

- A drug in the SSRI class is the most reasonable first choice since they have the most convincing data supporting efficacy for both physical and emotional symptoms. Any SSRI would probably be helpful, and recommended dosing is typical of antidepressant doses. For example, fluoxetine 20 mg/day, sertraline 50 to 100 mg/day, or paroxetine 20 mg/day may be used.
  - ✓ With the encouraging data on luteal phase dosing with sertraline, however, this would be a good first choice. Luteal phase dosing, by definition, is given for only 2 weeks out of the month. Therefore, the exposure to the drug is more limited than giving an SSRI daily. This may minimize the risk of adverse reactions and decreases the cost of pharmacotherapy significantly.
  - ✓ A woman whose menstrual cycle is not controlled by hormones such as birth control pills will have a luteal phase of 14 days. In order to accomplish luteal phase dosing, one must determine when to begin the sertraline. A relatively easy way of doing this is to determine her normal cycle length (the number of days from the start of one period to the start of the next period) and subtract 14 days.
  - ✓ For example, if this patient had a 30-day menstrual cycle, she would start sertraline on day 16 of her cycle. Since day 1 of her cycle is the day she starts her period, she would count 16 days forward and mark that day on her calendar to begin sertraline. She would take the sertraline until the onset of menses and then stop the drug. The typical starting dose of sertraline is 25 to 50 mg/day during the luteal phase. Some women may require a higher dose (100 mg/day) during the luteal phase.
- Luteal phase dosing of alprazolam may also be used. A typical starting dose is alprazolam 0.25 mg po TID. At the onset of menses, the alprazolam can be tapered by 25% per day. The taper can generally be completed over 3 days.

Outcome Evaluation

5. *What clinical parameters are necessary to evaluate the therapy for achievement of the desired therapeutic outcome and to detect or prevent adverse effects?*

- Have the patient continue to fill out daily ratings of her PMS symptoms. Compare the ratings while taking the drug to the ratings when she was not on medication.
- Beneficial effects from pharmacotherapy will be seen quickly. Unlike the treatment of depression, women will note improvement in symptoms within days of starting medication.
- SSRI adverse effects to monitor include headaches, nausea, jitteriness, irritability, dizziness, insomnia, tremor, and sexual dysfunction (e.g., anorgasmia in women).
- Alprazolam adverse effects to monitor include sedation, ataxia, confusion, disorientation, and anterograde amnesia.

Patient Counseling

6. *What information should be provided to the patient to enhance compliance, ensure successful therapy, and minimize adverse effects?*

Sertraline

- This medication is called sertraline (Zoloft); it is intended to improve both the physical and emotional symptoms you are suffering during the 2 weeks prior to your menstrual period.
- Take this medicine only as prescribed. Sertraline (usually 50 mg once daily) is generally started during the luteal phase (the 2 weeks before the onset of your period). This dose may be increased in subsequent menstrual cycles if your symptoms have not appreciably decreased. You will take this medicine for only about 2 weeks out of the month; you are to stop taking it once your period begins.
- If you miss a dose, take it as soon as you remember. However, if it is almost time for your next dose when you remember, skip the missed dose and go back to your regular schedule. Do not take two doses at once or very close together.
- This medication may cause changes in your sleep patterns (either insomnia or sleepiness). If it makes you sleepy, take it at bedtime or with dinner. If it causes insomnia, take it in the morning with breakfast.
- Sertraline can also cause nausea. Take each dose with a meal to minimize the chance of this side effect.
- Another side effect is sexual difficulties, such as not being able to achieve orgasm. The incidence of this problem is not well defined. Contact your physician if sexual problems occur. There may be recommendations to alleviate the problem.
- If you are having any difficulty with the medicine, ask your pharmacist or doctor before discontinuing the drug.
- Keep all scheduled follow-up appointments with your physician.

Follow-up Questions

1. What is your assessment of the patient's response to the intervention?

- She has responded well to the luteal phase dosing of sertraline. She and her family note marked improvement in symptoms.
- One ongoing monitoring parameter will be the nausea that she experienced when initiating the drug. Since she will be going on and off the drug each month, she may find it difficult to tolerate that side effect. However, the nausea may improve as she learns techniques to minimize its occurrence.
- Some patients with adverse effects that recur each month prefer to remain on the drug all month long. This is an acceptable alternative, but the cost of therapy and the likelihood of adverse effects will increase.

2. How long would you recommend that she continue therapy?

- This is a difficult question, as there are no clear guidelines for treatment duration of PMDD. At the present time, some clinicians are recommending that patients stay on the medication for 6 months to 1 year.
- In reality, many patients are reluctant to stop the medication because of the significant improvement they experience. Further research in the area of optimal treatment duration may bring answers to this important question.

References

1. Halbreich U, Smoller JW. Intermittent luteal phase sertraline treatment of dysphoric premenstrual syndrome. J Clin Psychiatry 1997;58:399–402.
2. Freeman EW, Rickels K, Sondheimer SJ, et al. A double-blind trial of oral progesterone, alprazolam, and placebo in treatment of severe premenstrual syndrome. JAMA 1995;274:51–57.
3. Freeman EW, Rickels K, Sondheimer SJ, et al. Nefazodone in the treatment of premenstrual syndrome: A preliminary study. J Clin Psychopharmacol 1994;14:180–186.
4. Halbreich U, Rojansky N, Palter S. Elimination of ovulation and menstrual cyclicity (with danazol) improves dysphoric premenstrual syndromes. Fertil Steril 1991;56:1066–1069.
5. Mezrow G, Shoupe D, Spicer D, et al. Depot leuprolide acetate with estrogen and progestin add-back for long-term treatment of premenstrual syndrome. Fertil Steril 1994;62:932–937.

78 HORMONE REPLACEMENT THERAPY

▶ Reaching the Climacteric (Level II)

Alka Z. Somani, PharmD

A 50-year-old woman with a history of hypertension and hypercholesterolemia was started on conjugated estrogen and cyclic medroxyprogesterone several months ago to treat perimenopausal symptoms of hot flashes and nausea. She discontinued this medication on her own because of difficulty in remembering when to take each medication; she also developed vaginal spotting. Stopping the therapy caused a return of her symptoms of hot flashes. Because of the beneficial effects of estrogen for her menopausal symptoms, cardiovascular protection, and osteoporosis prevention, a more tolerable estrogen/progestin combination should be sought. Estrogen alone is undesirable in this woman with an intact uterus because of an increased risk of endometrial cancer. Several other cyclic regimens may be attempted that will be easier for the patient to remember. A continuous daily combined estrogen/progestin regimen is also easy to remember, and many patients cease vaginal spotting after several months of therapy. One possible concern with the latter regimen is that continuous progesterone may blunt the cardioprotective effects of estrogen.

▶ Questions

Problem Identification

1. a. Create a list of the patient's drug-related problems.

- Vasomotor symptoms of menopause (hot flashes and nausea) requiring treatment with a regimen the patient can tolerate.
- Troublesome side effects (breakthrough bleeding) with the current HRT regimen, resulting in patient non-adherence.
- Use of acetaminophen in unknown quantities for joint pain after exercise.
- Hypertension is well controlled on the present dose of nifedipine (Procardia XL), but the choice of nifedipine (a calcium channel blocker) is suboptimal; only β-blockers and thiazide diuretics have been shown to reduce mortality in hypertension.
- The patient's hypercholesterolemia is well controlled without drug therapy. With two risk factors for CHD (hypertension and family history of premature CHD), her goal LDL-cholesterol level is < 130 mg/dL.

b. What information (signs, symptoms, laboratory values) indicates the presence or severity of this patient's problems as she begins menopause?

- *Signs.* GU atrophy (pelvic exam showed mucosal atrophy and was painful).
- *Symptoms.* Vasomotor instability (complaints of hot flashes and nausea).
- *Laboratory values.* FSH > 30 mIU/mL.
- *Other.* Her age is 50, her last menstrual period was 3 months ago, and she had a negative pregnancy test.

Desired Outcome

2. What are the benefits and risks of hormone replacement therapy for this patient?

Benefits
- Relief of perimenopausal symptoms,[1] cardioprotective effects of estrogen (increase HDL and decrease LDL),[2] and prevention of osteoporosis (the risk of fractures reduced by 50% to 60%).[3] Estrogen replacement therapy may also reduce dementia,[4] Alzheimer's disease,[5] decrease the risk of colon cancer,[6] and decrease macular degeneration.[7]

Risks
- Increased risk of breast and endometrial cancer and risk of venous thrombosis.[8]

Therapeutic Alternatives

3. a. *What non-drug therapies might be useful for this patient?*

   - Maintaining ideal body weight, an appropriate exercise regimen, and a calcium-rich diet will help control her hyperlipidemia and prevent osteoporosis.

   b. *What feasible pharmacotherapeutic alternatives are available for treatment of menopause (see Figure 78–1)?*

   - *Estrogen with no progesterone.* Unopposed estrogen is not desirable as it can increase the risk for endometrial cancer since she has an intact uterus.
   - *Estrogen with cyclic progesterone.* Regimens vary and can be complex, so compliance may be an issue (refer to textbook Chapter 78 for more detailed information on specific cyclic regimens). This patient was having difficulty being compliant with cyclic progesterone, so this may not be the best option for her.
   - *Continuous combined estrogen and progesterone.* This regimen is the simplest to take, and compliance may be enhanced. A proprietary product is available that contains conjugated estrogens 0.625 mg and medroxyprogesterone acetate 2.5 mg in a single tablet (Prempro). The disadvantage to this method is that continuous progesterone may limit the cardioprotective effects of estrogen.
   - *Estrogen vaginal cream.* Vaginal creams help relieve symptoms of senile vaginitis but will not decrease the vasomotor symptoms she is experiencing.
   - *Estradiol transdermal system.* Several different products are available; two of the patches are replaced twice weekly and one is replaced once weekly. However, no studies have been performed to assess the efficacy of estrogen patches on preventing osteoporosis or cardiovascular disease.

Optimal Plan

4. *What drug, dosage form, dose, schedule, and duration are best for this patient?*

   - This patient can be tried on a different cyclic estrogen and progesterone regimen. However, when a cyclic regimen was previously prescribed, she was not able to be compliant. She may be compliant with a simpler regimen such as continuous combined estrogen and progesterone.
   - Continuous combined estrogen and progesterone (e.g., Prempro) will decrease or eliminate breakthrough bleeding (spotting) and requires taking only a single tablet once a day, every day. If desired, the estrogen and progesterone can also be taken separately rather than using the combination proprietary product Prempro.
   - Refer to the previous answer for reasons why the other potential regimens are not optimal for this patient.

Outcome Evaluation

5. *What clinical and laboratory parameters are necessary to evaluate the therapy for achievement of the desired therapeutic outcome and to detect or prevent adverse effects?*

Efficacy Parameters
- At each encounter, ask the patient about the adequacy of relief from hot flashes, vaginal pain, and nausea.

Adverse Effect Parameters
- At each encounter, ask the patient whether she has experienced cramping, bloating, headache, irritability, and vaginal bleeding.
- Each year, the patient should have a mammogram to screen for breast cancer and a pelvic exam and Pap smear to detect endometrial cancer.
- The patient should perform monthly breast self-examinations to check for breast cancer.
- Cholesterol and triglycerides should be checked at least annually to prevent cardiovascular disease.

Patient Counseling

6. *What information should be provided to the patient to enhance compliance, ensure successful therapy, and minimize adverse effects?*

Conjugated Estrogens and Medroxyprogesterone Acetate (Prempro)
- This medicine contains conjugated estrogens 0.625 mg and medroxyprogesterone acetate 2.5 mg in each tablet. As such, it is called a continuous combined hormone replacement product.
- This medication is used for hormone replacement therapy (or HRT) in postmenopausal women. It will help decrease your symptoms of hot flashes and nausea. Estrogen is also useful in preventing heart attacks, osteoporosis, and perhaps other medical conditions.
- Take one tablet each day at the same time every day.
- You may experience nausea, bloating, cramps, breast tenderness, irritability, or weight gain. Contact your physician if changes in vaginal bleeding, breast pain, or breast lumps occur.
- Rarely, this medication can cause clots in the veins in your body. Notify your doctor immediately if you develop leg swelling or pain, chest pain, or shortness of breath.
- There may be a slight increase in breast cancer in women who take estrogen. For this reason, it is important to perform monthly breast examinations. Also schedule regular gynecological follow-up exams and doctor appointments.
- Store this medicine in a cool, dry place.
- If you forget to take a dose, take the missed dose as soon as you remember. However, if it is almost time for your next dose, skip the missed dose and go back to your regular schedule. Do not take two doses at one time to make up for the missed dose.

Follow-up Question

1. *What changes in the patient's therapy, if any, should be considered at this point?*

   - Her triglyceride level is borderline-high (200 to 400 mg/dL). Although no change in therapy is currently needed, her fasting triglycerides should be monitored every 3 to 4 months. If the triglycerides increase to > 500 mg/dL, then transdermal estrogen should be considered. Elevations in triglycerides do not occur as frequently with transdermal estradiol. However, estrogen patches have not been proven to provide the same benefits as oral estrogen.[9]

References

1. Belchetz PE. Hormonal treatment of postmenopausal women. N Engl J Med 1994;330:1062–1071.
2. Writing group for the PEPI Trial. Effects of estrogen or estrogen/progestin regimens on heart disease risk factors in postmenopausal women. The Postmenopausal Estrogen/Progestin Interventions (PEPI) Trial. JAMA 1995;273:199–208.
3. Weiss NS, Ure CL, Ballard JH, et al. Decreased risk of fractures of the hip and lower forearm with postmenopausal use of estrogen. N Engl J Med 1980;303:1195–1198.
4. Birge SJ. Is there a role for estrogen replacement therapy in the prevention and treatment of dementia? J Am Geriatr Soc 1996;44:865–870.
5. Paganini-Hill A, Henderson VW. Estrogen replacement therapy and risk of Alzheimer's disease. Arch Intern Med 1996;156:2213–2217.
6. Calle EE, Miracle-McMahill HL, Thun MJ, et al. Estrogen replacement therapy and risk of fatal colon cancer in a prospective cohort of postmenopausal women. J Natl Cancer Inst 1995;87:517–523.
7. Vingerling JR, Dielemans I, Witteman JC, et al. Macular degeneration and early menopause: A case-control study. BMJ 1995;310:1570–1571.
8. Lobo RA. Benefits and risks of estrogen replacement therapy. Am J Obstet Gynecol 1995;173:982–989.
9. Lufkin EG, Ory SJ. Relative value of transdermal and oral estrogen therapy in various clinical situations. Mayo Clin Proc 1994;69:131–135.

SECTION 9

Immunologic Disorders

Gary C. Yee, PharmD, FCCP, Section Editor

79 SYSTEMIC LUPUS ERYTHEMATOSUS

▶ More Than Just Skin Deep   (Level II)

Thomas W. Redford, PharmD
Ralph E. Small, PharmD, FCCP, FASHP, FAPhA

A 46-year-old woman with a 2-year history of systemic lupus erythematosus (SLE) is admitted with worsening renal function and an erythematous rash on her arms. Renal biopsy indicates progression of segmental proliferative glomerulonephritis due to SLE. Aggressive therapy is needed to prevent renal failure and further kidney damage. The treatment of choice is either IV pulse cyclophosphamide or IV pulse methylprednisolone. Concomitant oral prednisone therapy is also given. Antimalarials (hydroxychloroquine or chloroquine) are the treatment of choice for the cutaneous manifestations of SLE.

▶ Questions

Problem Identification

1. a. Create a list of the patient's drug-related problems.

- Worsening lupus nephritis, requiring therapy.
- Prednisone dosage subtherapeutic and inadequate to control lupus nephritis.
- Possible drug toxicity with enalapril (elevated serum creatinine).

b. What information indicates worsening lupus nephritis?

- Renal biopsy demonstrates progression of proliferative glomerulonephritis.
- Increased BUN, serum creatinine, uric acid.
- RBCs, RBC casts, 3+ proteinuria on urinalysis.
- Elevated erythrocyte sedimentation rate.
- Decreased serum complement (C3, C4) and elevated anti-double-stranded DNA antibodies.

Desired Outcome

2. What are the goals of pharmacotherapy for lupus nephritis in this patient?

- Prevent renal failure
- Arrest further kidney damage
- Alleviate signs of lupus nephritis
- Prevent future exacerbations of disease

Therapeutic Alternatives

3. a. What nonpharmacologic therapies might be useful in this patient?

- Avoid factors that can exacerbate SLE (e.g., UV light, viral or bacterial infection).
- Use sunscreens and protective clothing in sunlight and ensure that vaccinations are up-to-date. Do not vaccinate after IV cyclophosphamide therapy; this may increase the risk of infection from the vaccinating agent.

b. *What pharmacotherapeutic alternatives are used to manage patients with lupus nephritis?*

- Although the prognosis for SLE patients with renal involvement has improved, lupus nephritis remains a significant cause of morbidity and mortality.
- At the time of presentation, serum creatinine >1.5 mg/dL, hypertension, and a WHO histological classification Class IV (diffuse proliferative nephritis) are associated with poorer life-supporting renal function 10 years after the diagnosis.
- Others have found proteinuria > 3 grams in a 24 hour urine, duration of renal disease before biopsy, vasculitis, and C3 (complement) levels to be significant markers for renal insufficiency, renal failure, and death due to renal SLE.
- Due to the increasing creatinine and worsening renal histology in this patient, a trial of aggressive immunosuppressive therapy is necessary.
- *IV pulse cyclophosphamide* has been used in several lupus nephritis trials even though it is more of a cytotoxic than immunosuppressive drug. Regimens including cyclophosphamide better preserved renal function than those containing prednisone or azathioprine alone, and IV pulse cyclophosphamide proved less toxic than daily oral cyclophosphamide.[1]
- *IV pulse methylprednisolone* has been used due to the beneficial effects observed in controlled and uncontrolled studies.[2]
- *Azathioprine* may be less effective for lupus nephritis than cyclophosphamide, but it has been found to be beneficial in treating multisystemic active disease.[3]
- *Plasmapheresis* has been used for patients with SLE to reduce the number of autoantibodies and circulating immune complexes that are inadequately cleared by a saturated reticuloendothelial system. However, a controlled trial demonstrated that the addition of plasmapheresis did not show any beneficial effects beyond the standard regimen of cyclophosphamide and prednisone.[4]

Optimal Plan

4. *Outline a specific pharmacotherapeutic plan for treating lupus nephritis in this patient.*

- This patient with worsening renal indices should receive IV pulse cyclophosphamide, based on previous studies.[1] The initial dose of cyclophosphamide is usually 0.5 g/m^2 × 1 every month and is increased 25% monthly if the WBC count does not fall below 2.0 × 10^3/mm^3. The WBC count is determined 7 and 14 days after infusion. Cyclophosphamide is infused over 30 minutes to 1 hour with adequate hydration to prevent hemorrhagic cystitis. Antiemetic regimens consisting of dexamethasone, metoclopramide, or serotonin antagonists (e.g., ondansetron, granisetron, dolasetron) are used to help control nausea and vomiting. The duration of therapy is dependent on improvement in renal function, including decreased creatinine and urinary sediments. Proteinuria may not resolve if glomerular damage is sclerotic. IV cyclophosphamide given for longer than 6 months may increase the risk of gonadal failure.
- IV pulse methylprednisolone is a secondary choice if the patient cannot tolerate cyclophosphamide. The usual dose is 1.0 g/day methylprednisolone sodium succinate IV for 3 consecutive days; repeat doses can be given monthly for up to 6 months if active disease persists.
- Pulse therapy with cyclophosphamide and methylprednisolone is usually accompanied by oral prednisone 0.5 mg/kg per day for 4 weeks with tapering to alternate-day therapy by 8 weeks. Patients may stay on alternate-day prednisone indefinitely in an attempt to prevent recurrences.

Outcome Evaluation

5. *How should this patient be monitored for efficacy and adverse effects?*

The patient should be assessed at monthly visits with the following parameters.

Disease Monitoring

- Ask the patient about symptoms of fatigue and joint pain at each return visit.
- Evaluate the patient for signs of erythematous rash and vasculitic lesions at each return visit.
- Perform a urinalysis monthly for the first 6 months to assess the degree of proteinuria (24-hour protein), red blood cells, and casts. Testing may be reduced to 4 times a year thereafter.
- Obtain blood tests, including CBC and RBC indices, monthly for the first 6 months. Thereafter, testing may be reduced to 4 times a year.
- Check serology (including complement levels, anti-double-stranded DNA, C-reactive protein, and ESR) every 6 months.

Drug Monitoring

- *IV pulse cyclophosphamide*
  ✓ Ask the patient about nausea and vomiting.
  ✓ Detect hemorrhagic cystitis by monitoring for hematuria.
  ✓ Assess the degree of leukopenia by obtaining WBC count at 7 and 14 days after cyclophosphamide.
  ✓ Monitor thrombocytopenia by assessing platelet count, bruising, and hemoglobin/hematocrit.
  ✓ Detect infection (particularly herpes zoster) by checking CBC with differential and temperature.
- *IV pulse methylprednisolone and prednisone*
  ✓ Monitor blood glucose (particularly in diabetics).
  ✓ Check serum electrolytes after methylprednisolone injection and at follow-up visits.
  ✓ Obtain hemoglobin/hematocrit and stool cards to assess potential GI bleeding.
  ✓ Monitor for infection as for cyclophosphamide.
  ✓ Evaluate for cataracts and osteoporosis with long-term therapy.

Patient Counseling

6. *What information should be provided to the patient regarding her drug therapy?*

IV Cyclophosphamide

- This medicine is being given to control your kidney disease. We will give you other medications to prevent nausea and vomiting from this drug.
- Before you are given cyclophosphamide, it is important that you drink extra fluids and empty your bladder frequently. This will help prevent kidney and bladder problems.
- Report any bruising, bleeding, or black tarry stools to your doctor. If you can, avoid people with infections and let other doctors know that you are receiving monthly injections of cyclophosphamide.

IV Pulse Methylprednisolone and Oral Prednisone

- This medication is being given to control your kidney disease.
- Tell your doctor if you have other conditions such as diabetes before receiving this medicine.
- Like cyclophosphamide, avoid contact with persons who have an infection, and report any bruising, bleeding, or black tarry stools.
- Prednisone may cause bone disease (osteoporosis) with long-term use, and we will attempt to reduce the prednisone dose to prevent this side effect. Other side effects include cataracts, diabetes, elevated cholesterol, and stomach ulcers. These conditions may occur more frequently because you have systemic lupus erythematosus.

▶ Follow-up Question

1. *What other medications can be used to control this patient's non-renal disease manifestation (i.e., erythematous rash)?*

    - Antimalarials are the mainstay for treatment of cutaneous SLE, especially in those patients with accompanying systemic manifestations. Hydroxychloroquine (200 to 400 mg/day) and chloroquine (250 to 500 mg/day) are used to treat chronic, subacute, and acute cutaneous manifestations. Patients should receive an ophthalmologic examination every 6 months to assess for hydroxychloroquine-induced maculopathy.
    - The use of cyclosporine for treatment of SLE has yet to be defined. Cyclosporine has potent immunosuppressive properties and is used in organ transplantation. A low dose (< 5 mg/kg/day) is used to minimize the nephrotoxicity observed in cyclosporine trials for other autoimmune diseases. Side effects such as hypertrichosis, hypertension (responds to antihypertensive therapy), gingival hyperplasia, and increased BUN levels need to be monitored. Although it is unknown whether pre-existing renal disease precludes the use of cyclosporine, the drug appears to be useful in controlling the non-renal manifestations of SLE.

References

1. Austin HA III, Klippel JH, Balow JE, et al. Therapy of lupus nephritis. Controlled trial of prednisone and cytotoxic drugs. N Engl J Med 1986;314:614–619.
2. Liebling MR, McLaughlin K, Boonsue S, et al. Monthly pulses of methylprednisolone in SLE nephritis. J Rheumatol 1982;9:543–548.
3. Sztejnbok M, Stewart A, Diamond H, et al. Azathioprine in the treatment of systemic lupus erythematosus. A controlled study. Arthritis Rheum 1971;14:639–645.
4. Lewis EJ, Hunsicker LG, Lan SP, et al. A controlled trial of plasmapheresis therapy in severe lupus nephritis. The Lupus Nephritis Collaborative Study Group. N Engl J Med 1992;326:1373–1379.

SECTION 10

Bone and Joint Disorders

L. Michael Posey, RPh, Section Editor

80 OSTEOPOROSIS

▶ **These Brittle Bones** (Level II)

Carla B. Frye, PharmD, BCPS

A 72-year-old woman presents to an ambulatory clinic for a routine follow-up visit for hypertension and osteoporosis. Her only complaint is nausea from her calcium supplementation product. A DEXA scan 4 months prior revealed severe osteoporosis, and the patient reports a 2-inch loss in height since she was 35 years old. More aggressive osteoporosis treatment is needed. Estrogen replacement therapy should be withheld initially in this patient because she has a history of breast cancer. Feasible treatment alternatives include oral alendronate, oral raloxifene, and subcutaneous or intranasal calcitonin. The patient should also receive 1500 mg of calcium daily through diet and/or supplementation. Vitamin D (calcitriol) may also be considered because many elderly patients are deficient in this vitamin. Non-pharmacologic interventions such as dietary modification, reduced caffeine intake, and implementation of a weight-bearing exercise program play an important role in the management of osteoporosis.

▶ Questions

Problem Identification

1. a. Create a list of the patient's drug-related problems.

- *Antihypertensive therapy.* Beta-blockers can provoke bronchospasm. This patient is taking a β_1-selective β-blocker (atenolol), but the risk of bronchospasm should be weighed against the benefits. Beta-blockers are a good choice in this post-MI patient and have been shown to reduce mortality in patients with hypertension. However, the onset of COPD coincided with her MI. Beta-blockers can also cause or worsen hypertriglyceridemia, can decrease HDL, and can cause cold intolerance. Calcium channel blockers (Procardia XL or nifedipine) are effective but are not necessarily first line therapy in this patient group; this patient seems to be tolerating the drug. There is some evidence that thiazide diuretics can improve bone density.[1] Use of a thiazide should be reconsidered in this patient.
- *Hyperlipidemia therapy.* Because this patient has known coronary artery disease, her goal LDL-cholesterol is <100 mg/dL.[2] Her lipid levels are responding to therapy, but the atorvastatin (Lipitor) dose should be increased to 20 mg/day. The patient should also receive diet and lifestyle modification information, if not already done. Beta-blockers can raise triglycerides by 15% to 50%.
- *Osteoporosis therapy.* Because of the nausea caused by the calcium carbonate (Oscal), a different calcium supplement should be tried. Also, in view of patient's DEXA results, age, loss of height, and back pain, more extensive osteoporosis therapy is needed.
- *Hypothyroidism therapy.* TSH is normal, indicating that the levothyroxine therapy is adequate; however she is experiencing cold intolerance. This could be worsened by β-blocker therapy.
- *COPD therapy.* As stated above, β-blocker therapy should be reevaluated.

b. *What information (signs, symptoms, laboratory values, risk factors) indicates the presence or severity of the patient's osteoporosis? Also identify her risk factors for developing osteoporosis.*

- The DEXA scan results indicate severe osteoporosis. Criteria for interpreting the results of a DEXA scan are:[3]
  - ✓ Normal: within one standard deviation (SD) of young adult mean value
  - ✓ Osteopenia: between 1.0 and 2.5 SD below the mean, repeat scans in 2 years
  - ✓ Osteoporosis: > 2.5 SD below the mean value
  - ✓ Severe osteoporosis: > 2.5 SD below the mean and one or more fragility fractures exist

  This patient is >3 SD from the young adult mean value, and she has one or more fragility fractures (back pain and loss of height).
- Risk factors that she has for osteoporosis are fair complexion, early menopause, smoking history, postmenopausal status, increased age, and prolonged use of thyroid hormone replacement therapy.

c. *What additional information would be useful in determining the extent of the patient's osteoporosis and the need for aggressive therapy?*

- Serum calcium, phosphorus, alkaline phosphatase; possibly PTH level, vitamin D level, and serum cortisol. Consider 24 hour urinary calcium and creatinine.
- Biochemical markers of bone remodeling are not readily available at present but may be useful in the future.[4] Markers of bone formation include serum osteocalcin, bone-specific alkaline phosphatase, and carboxy-terminal extension peptide of type I procollagen. Markers of bone resorption include urine pyridinoline, deoxypyridinoline, *N*-telopeptide of the cross-links of collagen, and *C*-telopeptide of the cross-links of collagen.

Desired Outcome

2. *What are the goals of pharmacotherapy for osteoporosis in this case?*

- Increase bone mass
- Prevent or decrease the incidence of fractures
- Prevent further bone loss and loss of height
- Maintain normal bone structure
- Prevent falls that can result in debilitating fractures
- Provide calcium supplementation and other drug therapy that is well tolerated.

Therapeutic Alternatives

3. a. *What non-drug therapies might be useful for this patient's osteoporosis?*

- Ensure adequate calcium and vitamin D intake through diet and/or supplementation (see Table 82–6 in textbook Chapter 82 for the calcium content of various foods).
- Perform regular weight-bearing exercise.
- Decrease caffeine intake.
- Eliminate opportunities to fall by removing throw rugs and extension cords, adding handrails to the bathtub and other areas, and obtaining non-skid mats for slippery surfaces such as bathtubs.

b. *What feasible pharmacotherapeutic alternatives are available for treatment of the osteoporosis?*

- *Adequate calcium ingestion* will help decrease the rate of bone loss. Daily intake should be at least 1500 mg/day of elemental calcium in patients not taking estrogen and 1000 mg/day in patients taking estrogen (see Table 82–7 in the textbook for the content of elemental calcium in oral calcium supplementation products). Calcium supplements should be taken between meals to improve absorption. Constipation is the most common side effect. Therapy should be lifelong.
- *Vitamin D* enhances calcium absorption in the small intestine. The recommended daily allowance (RDA) for adults over 24 years of age is 200 IU/day. The estimated RDA for postmenopausal women is 400 to 800 IU/day. Dairy products are the best source of vitamin D; most diets provide adequate amounts of vitamin D. However, elderly patients are the most likely to have vitamin D deficiency due to inadequate or limited exposure to sunlight.
  - ✓ *Calcitriol* (oral Rocaltrol; injectable Calcijex) is a synthetic vitamin D analog. The recommended dose is 0.5 to 2 μg/day orally or 0.5 μg injected 3 times/week. Calcitriol is not FDA approved for the treatment of osteoporosis and is generally used only in patients who have had vertebral fractures. Vitamin D or calcitriol replacement will most likely be given for the rest of the patient's life.
- *Estrogen replacement therapy* is the treatment of choice for osteoporosis. It inhibits bone resorption by decreasing the rate of the bone activation cycle. Estrogen also decreases the risk of cardiovascular disease. It decreases total cholesterol and LDL levels and increases HDL levels. In women with an intact uterus, unopposed estrogen increases the risk of endometrial hyperplasia; it should be given with a progestin (e.g., medroxyprogesterone acetate 2.5 mg/day) in those patients to decrease the risk of endometrial cancer. Estrogen is relatively contraindicated in patients with breast cancer; the benefits of estrogen replacement may outweigh risks in breast cancer patients who have been clinically "cured" and especially in those who did *not* have estrogen sensitive tumor types. Adverse effects include fluid retention, abdominal pain, headache, and increased risk of thromboembolic events. Examples of estrogen products that could be used include:
  - ✓ *Conjugated equine estrogens* (Premarin) 0.625 mg/day (the most studied and widely used product)
  - ✓ *Estropipate* (Ogen) 0.625 mg/day
  - ✓ *Estradiol* (Estrace) 0.5 mg/day
  - ✓ *Estradiol transdermal system* (Estraderm) 0.05 mg/24 hours (patch replaced twice weekly)
- *Bisphosphonates* block osteoclast resorptive activity with no effect on osteoblasts.
  - ✓ *Alendronate* has been shown to reduce vertebral fractures and increase bone mineral density in the spine, femoral neck, trochanter, and total body. It has poor oral absorption and must be taken on an empty stomach, which increases side effects. The most common adverse effects are abdominal pain, constipation, diarrhea, musculoskeletal pain, headache, and esophagitis. The treatment dose is 10 mg once daily; the dose for prevention of osteoporosis is 5 mg once daily.

- *Fluoride* replaces hydroxyl groups in hydroxyapatite, stimulating osteoblasts to form new bone. However, new bone may be more brittle than normal bone, and trabecular bone development may be at the expense of cortical bone. Fluoride should be used cautiously in patients with renal failure. The usual dose of fluoride is 10 to 20 mg daily (75 mg sodium fluoride = 32 mg fluoride).
- *Calcitonin* inhibits bone resorption by inhibiting osteoclast function. It also provides some pain control in patients with fractures. Salmon calcitonin is available as a nasal spray or subcutaneous injection; the usual dose is 100 to 200 IU/day. When using the nasal spray, the patient should alternate nostrils daily. The nasal spray can cause rhinitis, epistaxis, and headache. Calcitonin is an expensive agent.
- *Selective estrogen receptor modulators or SERMs (e.g., raloxifene)* have estrogen-like effects on cortical bone and antiestrogen-like effects on breast tissue and the endometrium. Raloxifene increases bone mineral density, but to a lesser extent than estrogen. Its effects on fracture risk were unknown at the time of this writing. Also, the drug is presently indicated only for prevention of osteoporosis, not for treatment of existing osteoporosis. Raloxifene decreases serum total- and LDL-cholesterol concentrations with no effect on HDL or triglycerides. It is unknown whether the lipid changes provide cardioprotection similar to estrogen. Raloxifene is safe in patients with breast cancer or a history of breast cancer because it is an estrogen antagonist in uterine and breast tissues. There is an increased risk of thromboembolic events similar to estrogen; the risk is greatest during the first 4 months of treatment. The most common side effects are hot flashes and leg cramps. The usual dose of raloxifene is 60 mg/day. It should be combined with calcium supplementation.

Optimal Plan

4. a. *What drug, dosage form, dose, schedule, and duration of therapy are best for treating this patient's osteoporosis?*

- The patient should be started on alendronate 10 mg po on an empty stomach every morning.
- Avoid the use of estrogen at this time because of her history of breast cancer. It may be considered later if the response to alendronate is inadequate.
- Raloxifene 60 mg po daily is another potential option for this patient. However, the drug is presently indicated only for prevention of osteoporosis, and its effects on reducing fracture risk are unknown.
- There is no information on the use of both alendronate and raloxifene. Although there is no reason to think that this combination would be unsafe, there are also no data to support use of the two drugs concurrently. Therefore, one drug or the other should be chosen. Raloxifene may be preferred in this patient due to its positive effects on the lipid profile and lack of GI side effects.
- Use a different calcium salt to decrease nausea. Sufficient calcium intake is essential to increasing bone density. The patient should take 1500 mg of calcium daily. Citracal (calcium citrate) 950 mg (200 mg elemental calcium) 6 to 8 tablets per day or Posture (tricalcium phosphate) 1565 mg (600 mg elemental calcium) 2 to 3 tablets per day are examples of appropriate products and dosages for this patient.
- Stress the importance of ingesting calcium and vitamin D through the diet.
- Decrease caffeine intake.
- Begin a weight-bearing exercise program for 30 minutes 3 to 5 times weekly.

b. *What alternatives would be appropriate if the initial therapy fails or cannot be used?*

- Add calcitonin injection (100 IU/day) or nasal spray (200 IU/day). It is generally used as alternative therapy due to its expense. It should be given in conjunction with adequate calcium and vitamin D.
- Calcitriol (0.5 to 1 µg po QD or Calcijex 0.5 µg injected thrice weekly) or sodium fluoride (75 mg/day) could be added. These agents are not FDA approved for the prevention or treatment of osteoporosis and should be used only when standard therapy fails or is contraindicated. Fluoride therapy should be accompanied by calcium and vitamin D supplementation.
- The combination of alendronate and raloxifene could be given. Combination therapy has not been studied and should not be attempted unless maximal therapy with either agent individually is unsatisfactory.
- Supplementation with estrogen and progesterone (e.g., 0.625 mg conjugated estrogens with 2.5 mg medroxyprogesterone daily) should be reserved for use only if other therapies fail, due to the patient's history of breast cancer. However, since her breast cancer occurred over 30 years ago and she has had no subsequent recurrences, her risk is low.

Outcome Evaluation

5. *What clinical and laboratory parameters are necessary to evaluate the therapy for achievement of the desired therapeutic outcome and to detect or prevent adverse effects?*

Efficacy Parameters
- Repeat the DEXA scan in 6 months. Target a significant improvement in lumbar spine or femoral neck density. Since her previous DEXA scan was > 3 SD from the young adult mean, the target could be to stabilize her at this level (i.e., no further bone loss for the next 6 months) or to improve her bone density to not more than 2.5 SD below the mean after 6 months of therapy.
- Biochemical markers described above could be obtained, if available. These markers continue to improve in availability and reliability. Check the local laboratory for availability and cost. If a biochemical marker is available, obtain a baseline value now and repeat the test at 3, 6, and 12 months.
- Evaluate the patient for pain relief using a standardized pain questionnaire or visual analog scale. Establish baseline pain at this time and reevaluate at each subsequent clinical encounter.
- The patient should not experience more fractures or any additional loss of height. Question the patient at each subsequent visit, and evaluate any sudden onset of bone pain radiologically. Measure the patient's height at this appointment and at each subsequent visit.

Toxicity Parameters
- *Alendronate.* Check serum calcium, serum creatinine, and BUN every 3 months and question the patient about side effects such as

esophagitis, abdominal pain, nausea, vomiting, or diarrhea at each subsequent office visit.
- *Raloxifene.* Question the patient about side effects such as pain in the legs, leg swelling, or hot flashes at each office visit.

Patient Counseling

6. What information should be provided to the patient to enhance compliance, ensure successful therapy, and minimize adverse effects?

Alendronate (Fosamax)

- Your physician has prescribed alendronate (Fosamax) to help strengthen your bones and prevent any further bone fractures in your spine.
- Take alendronate 10 mg every morning at least 30 minutes before any other food, beverage, or medication. Take the tablet with a full 8 ounces of plain tap water. Do not lie down for at least 30 minutes afterward *and* until after your first food of the day; stay standing or seated upright.
- This medicine may cause stomach upset and headache; tell your prescriber if these effects become bothersome.
- Stop taking the drug and contact your doctor if you develop difficulty or pain on swallowing, chest pain, or new or worsening heartburn.
- If you forget to take a dose until after you have eaten, do *not* take it later in the day. Skip the dose entirely and resume your normal dosing schedule the following morning. Do not double doses.
- It is important to ingest enough calcium by eating foods rich in calcium such as yogurt, milk, and cheese, or by taking calcium supplementation.
- Be sure to keep all follow-up appointments with your doctor.

Raloxifene (Evista)

- Raloxifene (Evista) is a medication prescribed to prevent further weakening of your bones. This medication acts like estrogen on your bones but does not have as great an effect as estrogen. It does not act like estrogen on the breast or uterus and is therefore safe for you to use, even though you have had breast cancer. It will not cause you to have menstrual periods like estrogen could.
- Take one Evista tablet each day, preferably at the same time each day. You may take it with or without food.
- If you miss a dose, take the medicine as soon as you remember. If you don't think of it until the next day, skip the missed dose and just resume taking it once a day.
- Raloxifene may cause leg cramps and hot flashes. Tell your prescriber if these side effects become troublesome.

- A rare but serious side effect of Evista is blood clots in the veins. If you have pain in your calves, leg swelling, sudden chest pain, shortness of breath, coughing of blood, or change in your vision, contact your physician immediately.

References

1. Cauley JA, Cummings SR, Seeley DG, et al. Effects of thiazide diuretic therapy on bone mass, fractures and falls. The Study of Osteoporotic Fractures Research Group. Ann Intern Med 1993;118:666–673.
2. Summary of the second report of the National Cholesterol Education Program (NCEP) Expert Panel on Detection, Evaluation, and Treatment of High Blood Cholesterol in Adults (adult treatment panel II). JAMA 1993;269:3015–3023.
3. Assessment of fracture risk and its application to screening for postmenopausal osteoporosis. Report of a WHO Study Group. World Health Org Tech Rep Ser 1994;843:1–18.
4. Ebeling PR, Atley LM, Guthrie JR, et al. Bone turnover markers and bone density across the menopausal transition. J Clin Endocrinol Metab 1996;81:3366–3371.

81 RHEUMATOID ARTHRITIS

▶ Joint Project (Level II)

Ralph E. Small, PharmD, FCCP, FASHP, FAPhA
Thomas W. Redford, PharmD
Amy L. Whitaker, PharmD

A 58-year-old woman with a 6-year history of rheumatoid arthritis (RA) presents to her rheumatologist with complaints of increasing joint pain, knee swelling, and morning joint stiffness. She is currently being treated with the NSAID nabumetone (Relafen) and low-dose prednisone. Because her disease is inadequately controlled, a disease-modifying antirheumatic drug (DMARD) should be added. Methotrexate has emerged as the DMARD of choice for treating RA. Other DMARDs include hydroxychloroquine, sulfasalazine, gold salts, penicillamine, and immunosuppressive agents (e.g., azathioprine, cyclophosphamide, cyclosporine). The patient should receive a short course of high-dose steroids during the time it takes for the beneficial effect of the DMARD to be seen. The NSAID therapy should be continued. A number of parameters should be evaluated regularly to assess the efficacy of therapy. Most DMARDs are associated with potentially serious toxicities, and periodic clinical and laboratory evaluation is necessary to detect and prevent adverse effects.

▶ Questions

Problem Identification

1. a. List the patient's drug-related problems.

- The patient is experiencing a flare of RA that is inadequately treated with the current regimen of prednisone and nabumetone (Relafen).
- Swelling in the left knee may benefit from fluid drainage and an intra-articular corticosteroid injection.
- The patient is a postmenopausal female who should be evaluated for hormone replacement therapy and osteoporosis prevention with calcium and vitamin D supplements.

b. What information (signs, symptoms, laboratory values) indicates the presence and severity of rheumatoid arthritis?

- *Signs.* Decreased ROM in joints, Boutonniere deformities, ulnar deviation, decreased grip strength, and muscle atrophy.
- *Symptoms.* Joint pain, swelling, morning stiffness, and fatigue.
- *Laboratory values.* Decreased hemoglobin (anemia of chronic disease), ANA negative, RF titer positive, elevated Westergren ESR, presence of white cells in synovial fluid.

c. *What additional information is needed to assess the patient?*

- Examine the RBC indices and an iron panel to confirm anemia of chronic disease.
- Obtain x-rays of joints to detect joint space narrowing and bone erosion.
- Determine 50-foot walking time to assess the patient's agility and ease of movement.
- Administer a quality of life survey to aid in determining the impact of RA on the patient's life and activities of daily living.
- Perform a complete fasting lipid profile since the patient has 2 risk factors for CHD (female > 55 yo, HTN) and a total cholesterol > 200 mg/dL.

Desired Outcome

2. *What are the goals of pharmacotherapy in this case?*

- Relief of pain
- Decrease in inflammation and swelling
- Preservation of muscle strength
- Prevention of disease progression
- Decrease in the progression of irreversible bone erosion and joint deformity
- Maintenance of the patient's quality of life and ability to perform activities of daily living

Therapeutic Alternatives

3. a. *What non-pharmacological modalities may be beneficial to this patient?*

- *Physical therapy* is beneficial for patients with RA since it helps to maintain ROM in joints and prevent muscle atrophy. A proper balance of rest and exercise is essential. Proper rest decreases the systemic inflammatory response and protects the joints, to permit repair. Proper exercise moves the joints through their full range of motion and maintains strength, to minimize instability.
- *Occupational therapy* teaches patients how to manage activities of daily living and properly use supportive devices such as canes or splints, which may become necessary as RA advances.
- *Support services and patient/family education* play an important role in helping patients and their families cope with a potentially debilitating disease. Patients need to feel empowered to manage their own disease and maintain their quality of life.
- *Nutritional consultation* about a proper diet is important since the patient has an elevated cholesterol level and her weight is above her ideal body weight.

b. *What pharmacologic alternatives are available for the treatment of RA?*

- *Non-steroidal anti-inflammatory drugs (NSAIDs)* are the initial treatment of choice for the management of RA since they work via prostaglandin inhibition to reduce joint pain and swelling and improve function.[1] The onset of analgesic effect is rapid, but the anti-inflammatory effect may not be complete for 4 to 6 weeks. If a patient fails therapy with a particular NSAID at the maximum recommended dose, another NSAID from a different chemical class should be tried.
- *Corticosteroids* work rapidly in reducing inflammation and relieving symptoms of RA. They may be administered intra-articularly or orally. Injections directly into the joint restore range of motion and quickly control symptoms. Oral steroids are beneficial in acute flare situations where the patient's ability to perform activities of daily living has been impacted, or during the period of therapy after a DMARD has been initiated but not yet reached full effect. Chronic low-dose steroids may be needed for some patients to manage symptoms. However, long-term use should be avoided if possible to minimize side effects (HPA axis suppression, osteoporosis, cataracts, glaucoma, increased susceptibility to infection) seen with long-term therapy. It may not be necessary to taper the dosage in patients receiving high-dose steroid bursts for only 1 to 2 weeks. In patients who have received steroids for more than 1 month, it is necessary to taper the steroid gradually over a period of time proportional to the length of time that the patient has been receiving steroids. Slow tapering allows the body to resume its natural cortisol production, which has become suppressed since the patient has been taking exogenous steroid. It may be necessary to decrease the dose by 1 mg every 1 to 2 weeks if the patient experiences symptoms or has other complaints.
- *Disease modifying anti-rheumatic drugs (DMARDs)* are designed to reduce joint damage, preserve joint integrity and function, and prevent disease progression.
  - ✓ *Methotrexate* has become the DMARD of choice for managing RA. The convenient once-weekly dosing greatly improves patient adherence, and the onset of effect may be seen within 1 month of starting therapy. Patients on methotrexate also tolerate treatment well, with more than 50% remaining on therapy for more than 5 years, the longest time for any DMARD. Methotrexate can cause hematologic, pulmonary, and hepatic toxicities, and it is important to carefully monitor for these effects. The drug is contraindicated in pregnant or lactating females and patients with chronic liver disease, immunodeficiency, leukopenia, thrombocytopenia, or a creatinine clearance < 40 mL/min.
  - ✓ *Hydroxychloroquine* is advantageous because it lacks the myelosuppressive, hepatic, and renal toxicities associated with other DMARDS. The twice-daily dosing schedule is also convenient for patients, and it is available in a generic formulation, which helps to decrease cost. Monitoring for ocular toxicity such as retinopathy and visual blurring is important. As is the case with most DMARDS, onset of effect is slow, and benefit may not be seen for 2 to 6 months.
  - ✓ *Sulfasalazine* has limited usefulness due to adverse reactions such as nausea, vomiting, diarrhea, and anorexia. It is also associated with the development of leukopenia and thrombocytopenia. Sulfasalazine also has a number of potential drug interactions. Its absorption may be decreased by antibiotics that destroy natural gut flora. Iron-containing

preparations decrease the absorption of sulfasalazine by binding the drug in the GI tract. Sulfasalazine may increase the INR in patients receiving warfarin therapy because sulfasalazine decreases the protein binding of warfarin. Patients should be closely monitored for changes in the INR when initiating or changing doses of sulfasalazine therapy. The onset of effect with sulfasalazine is slow, and benefit may not be seen for 2 to 6 months.

✓ *Gold salts* were once the "gold standard" for managing RA. The use of these agents has declined due to their increased toxicity and decreased efficacy compared to other DMARDS. Gold may be administered either orally (auranofin) or IM (aurothioglucose or gold sodium thiomalate). Although patients prefer the oral preparation, it is poorly absorbed from the GI tract and often causes diarrhea. The IM preparation is administered weekly at first and then once monthly; it delivers higher synovial fluid concentrations than the oral preparation. Toxicities are similar for both oral and IM administration and include skin rash, stomatitis, proteinuria, hematuria, leukopenia, and thrombocytopenia. The onset of effect is slow and may take 3 to 6 months.

✓ *Penicillamine* is another agent with limited usefulness because of adverse effects. Skin rash, metallic taste, hypogeusia, stomatitis, nausea, vomiting, diarrhea, and glomerular nephritis may occur. Penicillamine has the potential to induce other autoimmune disorders such as myasthenia gravis and systemic lupus erythematosus. Because of this effect, penicillamine use is restricted to patients for whom other therapies have failed. The onset of effect may be from 1 to 3 months, but the maximum effect is usually seen after 6 months of therapy. Ten percent of patients who have an allergic reaction to penicillin will have a hypersensitivity to penicillamine. This is not an absolute contraindication to therapy, but caution should be used.

✓ *Immunosuppressive agents (azathioprine, cyclophosphamide, and cyclosporine)* are used to manage more severe cases of RA.[2] Toxicities associated with these agents include thrombocytopenia, leukopenia, nephrotoxicity, alopecia, and GI intolerance. Although the onset of effect is fairly rapid (from 1 to 3 months), long-term toxicities limit the use of these agents.

c. *What economic and psychosocial considerations are applicable to this patient?*

- Cost of medication and associated laboratory monitoring is a factor since this patient may be living on a fixed income. Medications that are available in generic formulation help to decrease costs. Depending on the medication chosen, the patient may have to pay for monthly doctor visits and associated laboratory charges if her insurance does not cover such services. Coverage of durable medical equipment by the patient's insurance company may become an issue. The cost of supportive devices such as canes, splints, crutches, wheelchairs, and collars adds to the patient's out of pocket expense if they are not covered. Medicare will pay for these devices, but the patient must be 65 years of age or older to qualify.

- Psychosocial considerations for this patient include the ability of the patient to ambulate, do volunteer work, maintain her quality of life, and perform activities of daily living. Therapy chosen for this patient should positively impact all of these areas. It is important to identify areas of the patient's life that are important and clarify the goals and expectations of therapy. Patients should fully understand what is involved in their treatment and play an active role in managing their disease.

Optimal Plan

4. *What drug, dosage form, dose, schedule, and duration of therapy are best for this patient?*

- The patient's current therapy with prednisone and nabumetone are not effective. The patient should be started on a DMARD since she has a confirmed diagnosis of RA and has continued joint pain, morning stiffness, fatigue, active synovitis, and an elevated ESR despite adequate treatment with an NSAID.[3]

- The optimal therapy is to begin methotrexate 2.5-mg tablets, 3 tablets at once, one time per week. Should the patient develop GI upset with this dosing, 1 tablet may be taken every 12 hours for 3 doses, once a week. If GI problems persist, methotrexate may be administered SC or IM. Therapy should be evaluated after 1 month, at which time the dosage may be changed. If the patient is not experiencing relief, the methotrexate dose may be increased up to 15 mg/week.

- The patient should also be given a "steroid burst" to help her through the acute flare and to cover the period of time before methotrexate begins to take effect. For example, prednisone 60 mg po QD should be given for 2 weeks followed by a slow taper with the goal to have the patient completely off the corticosteroid if possible. Tapering may consist of a 10-mg decrease every 4 days. Once the dose is at 10 mg daily, further decreases should be by 2½ mg every 4 days, with the goal to ultimately discontinue therapy if possible. Example: 60 mg QD × 2 weeks, 50 mg QD × 4 days, 40 mg QD × 4 days, 30 mg QD × 4 days, 20 mg QD × 4 days, 10 mg QD × 4 days, 7½ mg QD × 4 days, 5 mg QD × 4 days, 2½ mg QD × 4 days, then D/C if possible.

- Monitor the patient for signs/symptoms of infection since she will be receiving steroid therapy.

- The patient should be given an intra-articular injection of triamcinolone acetate 40 mg into her left knee. This will help with the acute flare and relieve the pain she is experiencing in her knee.

- Since the patient will be receiving methotrexate therapy, it will be necessary to also start folic acid 1 mg po QD. This will help to minimize side effects that the patient may experience and help to prevent folate deficiency that may develop with extended use of methotrexate.

- Nabumetone therapy will be continued at the current dosage prescribed. Although NSAIDs will not impact on prevention of flares, the patient did not complain of any side effects, and the medication is probably helping to control pain and inflammation.

- A physical therapist should be consulted to develop an appropriate exercise program that will maintain muscle strength and range of motion.

- The patient should be referred to her primary care physician to discuss and consider hormone replacement therapy, have her lipid pro-

- file evaluated, and discuss osteoporosis prevention. The benefits and risks associated with these therapies should be discussed along with any concerns that the patient may have.
- Education about a heart-healthy diet should also be reinforced since this will impact her blood pressure and cholesterol levels.

Outcome Evaluation

5. *What clinical and laboratory parameters are necessary to evaluate the patient's drug therapy?*

Efficacy

- Ask the patient at every prescription refill about any changes in her medication regimen (prescription, non-prescription, herbal, home remedies). Also ask about how she feels (increase or decrease in pain, ability to move around, fatigue, morning stiffness, swelling in joints) and if there have been any changes or new areas where she is experiencing pain or discomfort.
- At each physician visit, repeat the above items along with a 50-foot walking time, joint exam, grip/muscle strength, and range of motion. The patient should be evaluated in all areas where RA may impact her life (physical, mental, social) so that a complete understanding of patient management may occur.
- Obtain a Westergren ESR every 6 months to monitor efficacy and reduction of inflammation.
- Perform joint x-rays every 6 to 12 months to evaluate disease progression and the efficacy of therapy.

Methotrexate Adverse Effects

- Perform a complete assessment of hepatic function (AST, ALT, alkaline phosphatase, serum albumin, total bilirubin, hepatitis B and C studies, coagulation studies) and a CBC with platelets, electrolytes, and serum creatinine prior to initiating therapy.[4] Obtain LFTs, electrolytes, and CBC with platelets monthly thereafter. These tests are necessary to detect hematologic (thrombocytopenia, leukopenia) and hepatic (elevated enzymes, cirrhosis) toxicities.
- Obtain a chest x-ray at baseline and every 6 to 12 months thereafter while the patient is receiving methotrexate to monitor for pulmonary changes (fibrosis, pneumonitis).
- The laboratory tests collected for methotrexate therapy would also monitor for the development of renal dysfunction associated with NSAID therapy.
- Ask the patient about the presence of GI upset and the development of a dry, non-productive cough.

Hydroxychloroquine Adverse Effects

- Monitoring parameters include a baseline ophthalmologic exam and a repeat exam every 6 to 12 months to detect the development of ocular toxicities.

Sulfasalazine Adverse Effects

- Ask the patient about the presence of nausea, vomiting, diarrhea, and anorexia.
- Obtain a CBC with platelets every week during the first month of therapy, and then monthly thereafter to monitor for leukopenia and thrombocytopenia.

Gold Salt Adverse Effects

- Evaluate patients for the development of rash and stomatitis.
- In order to detect proteinuria, hematuria, leukopenia, and thrombocytopenia, obtain a urinalysis and CBC with platelets at baseline and then once monthly for the oral preparation and with each IM injection.

Penicillamine Adverse Effects

- Evaluate patients and ask about the presence of skin rash, metallic taste, hypogeusia, stomatitis, nausea, vomiting, and diarrhea.
- In order to detect glomerular nephritis, obtain a urinalysis and CBC with platelets at baseline and once every week for 1 month, then monthly thereafter and with dosage changes.

Immunosuppressive Agent Adverse Effects

- Ask the patient about GI intolerance and evaluate for alopecia.
- In order to detect thrombocytopenia, leukopenia, hepatotoxicity, and nephrotoxicity, periodically evaluate CBC with platelets, LFTs, urinalysis, and serum creatinine.

Patient Counseling

6. *What information should be provided to the patient to enhance adherence, ensure successful therapy, and minimize adverse effects?*

Methotrexate

- This drug is known as a disease modifying anti-rheumatic drug that works to decrease the activity of arthritis in your body and improve your symptoms. It works differently from the steroid (prednisone) and NSAIDs (Relafen) that you have been taking.
- Unlike the steroid and NSAID, it takes some time for this medication to begin working. You should begin to see benefit within 1 month, but it may take up to 2 or 3 months. In order to make sure that you are comfortable in the interim, we will continue your steroid and Relafen so that you will have symptom control.
- It is important to take methotrexate only as directed by your physician. Take 3 tablets all at once, 1 day a week. Take the medication on the same day each week. It may be helpful to mark a calendar for the days you are to take the tablets.
- Do not take MTX more than once a week, since serious side effects may develop. Taking more tablets will not make you feel better any faster.
- If you miss a dose, do not double your next dose. Resume taking your medication on your regular dosing schedule. If you have any questions, call your doctor or pharmacist.
- Side effects may include nausea, vomiting, diarrhea, loss of appetite, and mouth sores. Notify your doctor if any of these become troublesome, persist, or become worse over time. It may be necessary to change the dosage of your medication or how you take your medicine.
- You will be taking folic acid 1 mg daily to help minimize these adverse effects.
- Other side effects that are less common but may be serious include liver abnormalities or changes in your lungs. To minimize liver changes, avoid drinking any alcohol while you are taking methotrexate. If you develop a dry, hacking cough, notify your physician so it may be evaluated.
- Regular laboratory tests are needed to help your doctor detect and prevent side effects. It is important to have this blood work done as requested by your doctor.

- Keep your scheduled follow-up appointments with your doctor so that your progress can be monitored.
- Be sure to tell both your doctor and pharmacist about any changes in medications you may have for prescription, non-prescription, and herbal or home remedies. This information will be helpful in avoiding dangerous drug interactions.

Prednisone
- This medication is a corticosteroid that works to decrease inflammation in your knee and decrease the pain and swelling you have been experiencing.
- It does not take a long time to notice the effect of prednisone, and you should see benefit within several days.
- The dosage of prednisone has been increased above what you had been taking. This is called a "steroid burst," which is used to treat acute flares of RA.
- Take the prednisone only as directed by your doctor. The number of tablets you will be taking will decrease as you gradually taper off the medication.
- Take all of your tablets at once at the same time each day. Be sure to take the medication after you have eaten a meal.
- If you miss a dose, do not double your next dose. Resume taking the medication on your regular dosing schedule; call your doctor or pharmacist if you have any questions.
- Some side effects include nausea, an increase in appetite, nervousness, and easier bruising. Taking the prednisone with food will minimize the nausea. The other effects should subside as your dosage is decreased. If any of these effects become bothersome or persist, contact your doctor or pharmacist.

Triamcinolone Acetonide
- The triamcinolone injection that you are receiving is also a corticosteroid. It is being injected directly into your knee and should rapidly help to decrease the inflammation and pain in your joint.
- After receiving the injection, you may experience pain at the injection site. This is normal, but notify your doctor if you experience severe pain or swelling that persists.

Nabumetone
- Continue to take your nabumetone (Relafen) as you have been. This medication will work with the other medications you are taking to help decrease the pain and inflammation you experience with arthritis.

References

1. American College of Rheumatology Ad Hoc Committee on Clinical Guidelines. Guidelines for the management of rheumatoid arthritis. Arthritis Rheum 1996;39:713–722.
2. Cash JM, Klippel JH. Second-line drug therapy for rheumatoid arthritis. N Engl J Med 1994;330:1368–1375.
3. Brick JE, DiBartolomeo AG. Rethinking the therapeutic pyramid for rheumatoid arthritis. When are NSAIDs alone not enough? Postgrad Med 1992;91:75.
4. American College of Rheumatology Ad Hoc Committee on Clinical Guidelines. Guidelines for monitoring drug therapy in rheumatoid arthritis. Arthritis Rheum 1996;39:723–731.

82 OSTEOARTHRITIS

▶ **Murder by Joints** (Level II)

Michael A. Oszko, PharmD, BCPS

Complaints of increasing lower back, hip, and knee pain cause a 49-year-old woman with a long history of osteoarthritis (OA) to seek attention at a family medicine clinic. She had been treated previously by a rheumatologist who eventually told her to find another doctor after she began demanding large quantities of opioids for pain relief. The first step in the proper management of this patient is to obtain an accurate history of her past analgesic and anti-inflammatory drug use. Acetaminophen given in scheduled doses (0.5 to 1 gram po QID) is the treatment of choice for OA unless it has definitely been shown to be ineffective for her disease. NSAIDs are also effective analgesics, but inflammation is often not a component of OA; NSAIDs should be reserved for second-line therapy due to their potential for GI and renal adverse effects in older patients. Opioid analgesics should generally be used only on a short-term basis for control of breakthrough pain. Non-pharmacologic therapies such as weight loss, exercise, physical therapy, and occupational therapy also play an important role in the management of OA.

▶ Questions

Problem Identification

1. a. *Create a list of the patient's drug-related problems.*

   - Analgesic regimen for osteoarthritis is inadequate or suboptimal.
   - Antihypertensive regimen is potentially inadequate or suboptimal; the present BP of 164/94 mm Hg is above the goal level of < 130/85 mm Hg in diabetic patients.
   - Probable suboptimal antidiabetic regimen; the current random, non-fasting glucose is high (248 mg/dL).
   - Hypercholesterolemia (total cholesterol 354 mg/dL), presently not fully evaluated and untreated.
   - Possible opioid dependence or abuse.
   - Loratadine (Claritin) use for unknown indication.

   b. *What information (signs, symptoms, laboratory values) indicates the presence or severity of the primary problem (osteoarthritis)?*

   Symptoms
   - Lower back, hip, and knee pain.

   Signs
   - *Physical exam.* Back pain radiating to right buttock with

straight leg raising at 60°; right hip pain with flexion > 90° and with internal and external rotation > 45°; both hips tender to palpation; right knee crepitus.
- *X-rays.* Degenerative changes consistent with osteoarthritis are noted in the lumbar spine, hips, and right knee.

Laboratory Values
- ESR 46 mm/hour (a non-specific indicator of inflammation).

c. *What additional information is needed to satisfactorily assess this patient?*

- This patient's presentation is typical of many patients in the outpatient setting—multiple medical problems, multiple medications, and an unclear history of the use of, indications for, and safety and efficacy of these medications. Perform a careful, thorough medication history to acquire the necessary additional information.
- Ask the patient which analgesics she has taken in the past as well as their frequency and duration. Determine which ones were most effective and which ones were least effective or caused adverse effects.
- Clarify the adverse effects of past pain medications. Find out which one(s) caused nausea. Assess whether the nausea was dose-related. Find out whether it occurred when the drug was taken with food or on an empty stomach. Determine whether any of these medications were effective in relieving pain, even though they caused nausea.
- Ask the patient about the OTC medicines (including herbal and non-traditional therapies) she is taking or has taken in the past.
- Determine whether there is evidence of opioid abuse or dependence. Questions to ask include:
  - ✓ Do you ever take a Vicodin for something other than pain (e.g., sleep, anxiety)?
  - ✓ Are you taking more than the prescribed dose of Vicodin?
  - ✓ Do you become anxious or experience symptoms such as excessive tearing of the eyes or diarrhea when you don't take the Vicodin for a period of time?
- The diagnosis of osteoarthritis is primarily based on clinical and radiologic findings. Further tests do not appear to be indicated. A number of biochemical markers for osteoarthritis are being studied[1] but none is in routine clinical use.
- Although it appears that the patient's blood pressure is not adequately controlled, additional readings are necessary to verify this; the patient's compliance should also be assessed.
- A hemoglobin A_{1c} level will help to assess the severity of this patient's hyperglycemia over the past 3 months.
- Fractionation of this patient's cholesterol (e.g., a fasting lipid panel) will assist in directing pharmacotherapy for this disorder. This is important for her because she possesses at least two other risk factors for CHD (HTN and DM).

Desired Outcome

2. *What are the goals of pharmacotherapy for each of this patient's drug-related problems?*

- *Osteoarthritis.* Control pain, improve mobility (or limit immobility), avoid adverse drug effects.

- *Hypertension.* Improve blood pressure control (goal BP in diabetic patients is <130/85 mm Hg).
- *Diabetes.* Improve blood glucose control (goal is HbA_{1c} < 7%, if possible).
- *Hypercholesterolemia.* After obtaining a fasting lipid profile, initiate an appropriate regimen of dietary therapy for at least 6 months. Begin drug therapy if dietary therapy alone is insufficient to achieve target LDL levels of < 130 mg/dL (assuming the patient has high LDL-cholesterol and ≥ 2 other risk factors for CHD).
- Facilitate weight loss (as an adjunct to diet and exercise) to help control hypertension, diabetes, and hypercholesterolemia.

Therapeutic Alternatives

3. a. *What non-drug therapies might be useful for this patient?*

- *Weight loss* should be achieved in this morbidly obese patient. Obesity has been associated with an increased prevalence of osteoarthritis.[2,3] However, it is unclear whether weight loss slows the progression of the disease. Weight loss will certainly be beneficial in treating this patient's hypertension, diabetes mellitus, and hypercholesterolemia.
- *Exercise, physical and occupational therapy, and the use of a cane* may help to maintain or improve this patient's mobility. Exercise, combined with a proper diet, will also assist in weight loss. Aquatic exercise programs are particularly suitable for patients with osteoarthritis.
- *Local application of heat, ultrasound, and massage therapy* may be beneficial for muscle spasms occurring around affected joints.

b. *What feasible pharmacotherapeutic alternatives are available for treatment of this patient's osteoarthritis?*

- *Non-opioid analgesic therapy* is the cornerstone of pharmacotherapy in patients with osteoarthritis.
  - ✓ *Acetaminophen* is the first-line drug for treatment of osteoarthritis. It provides effective analgesia, is generally well-tolerated, and is inexpensive.
  - ✓ *Non-steroidal anti-inflammatory drugs* in analgesic (not anti-inflammatory) doses are as effective as acetaminophen. Although they are typically more expensive and cause more GI and renal side effects, they may be used when acetaminophen is not effective.
  - ✓ *Non-acetylated salicylates (e.g., choline magnesium salicylate, salsalate)* may also be effective with fewer adverse GI effects than traditional NSAIDs.
- *Opioid analgesics* should be reserved for unremitting or breakthrough pain only. Their use in the chronic management of osteoarthritis should be avoided because of the potential for abuse.
- *Capsaicin cream* is a topical adjunct or alternative to systemic analgesics. It is particularly useful when only a few joints are involved. In this patient, application of capsaicin cream to the right knee, pretibial area, and ankle may be helpful.
- *Tricyclic antidepressants* may be helpful in relieving pain in patients with OA of the spine who have nerve involvement (e.g., sciatica). This patient complains of "shooting pains" radiating from her back to her buttocks and groin; it is unclear at this point whether or not this pain is due to nerve involvement. In this

situation, a tricyclic antidepressant may be helpful; she is already receiving amitriptyline (Elavil) to treat her depression.
- *Muscle relaxants (e.g., cyclobenzaprine, methocarbamol)* may be beneficial for muscle spasms occurring around the affected joints.
- *Antioxidant micronutrients (vitamins A and E, beta-carotene)* have been suggested by preliminary studies to slow the progression of osteoarthritis.[4] However, supplementation is not recommended at this time until more definitive data become available.
- *Oral or intra-articular corticosteroids* may improve symptoms. However, steroids should be reserved for cases where an inflammatory process is clearly present because this disease is usually non-inflammatory in nature and because long-term, systemic steroid use has serious detrimental effects.
- Because this patient is a poor historian with regard to which analgesics she has used in the past, it is best to "start over" and systematically try and evaluate individual analgesics for their efficacy and tolerability.

Optimal Plan

4. a. What drug, dosage form, schedule, and duration of therapy are best for treating this patient's osteoarthritis?

- Acetaminophen 0.5 to 1 g po QID (scheduled, not PRN) is the treatment of choice for this patient, unless it has definitely been shown to be ineffective in the past.
- An opioid analgesic, such as oxycodone 2.5 to 10 mg po QID PRN may be used for acute exacerbations ("breakthrough" pain) only. Avoid combination opioid analgesic products containing acetaminophen while she is receiving acetaminophen as her primary analgesic.
- Adjunctive therapy can include capsaicin cream (e.g., Zostrix) 0.025% applied to the right knee, pretibial area, and ankle up to 4 times/day.

b. What alternatives would be appropriate if the initial therapy fails or cannot be used?

- An NSAID, started at the lowest dose and titrated upward, is as effective as acetaminophen.[5]
- Non-acetylated salicylates (choline magnesium salicylate, salsalate) may also be used (refer to textbook Chapter 84 for specific dosage regimens).
- Opioid analgesics are inappropriate for long-term use, except when all other pharmacologic and surgical options have been tried and have failed, due to their adverse effects (e.g., "narcotic bowel") and their propensity to result in physical dependence.

Outcome Evaluation

5. What clinical and laboratory parameters are necessary to evaluate the therapy for achievement of the desired therapeutic outcome and to detect or prevent adverse effects?

Efficacy

- This patient will most likely require life-long analgesic therapy, but it should be assessed periodically. Initially, assess the efficacy of the analgesic regimen every 1 to 2 weeks and every 1 to 3 months thereafter.

- Pain relief is the most important end point in this patient. Ask the patient about the adequacy of the analgesic regimen at each clinical encounter. A pain rating scale may be helpful to quantify the efficacy of the regimen and to track the patient's progress over time.
- Ask the patient about the frequency of her opioid analgesic use as well. If possible, this information should be corroborated by refill records. Alternatively, prescriptions for opioids can be made non-refillable, thereby requiring the patient to contact the physician for additional doses. Excessive use of opioids necessitates reassessment of the efficacy of the primary analgesic regimen as well as possible abuse.

Adverse Effects

- Both acetaminophen and NSAIDs can result in hematologic, hepatic, and renal dysfunction. A CBC, AST, ALT, BUN, and serum creatinine determination should be performed periodically (e.g., every 6 to 12 months) while the patient is taking these drugs.

Patient Counseling

6. What information should be provided to the patient to enhance compliance, ensure successful therapy, and minimize adverse effects?

Acetaminophen

- Acetaminophen is the primary drug that we are going to use to treat your arthritis. Start by taking one extra-strength tablet (500 mg) 4 times daily on a regular basis. If this does not control your pain, you can increase the dose to 2 tablets (1000 mg). Do not take more than 8 tablets in one day.
- Do not drink alcohol while you are taking acetaminophen.
- Do not take any over-the-counter products (including cough and cold products) that contain acetaminophen.

Oxycodone

- Use the oxycodone ($^1/_2$ to 2 tablets or 2.5 to 10 mg) only when you are in severe pain and when the acetaminophen does not seem to be working. Do not take more than 4 tablets a day. If you find that you are using the oxycodone on a regular basis, contact your physician.

Capsaicin Cream

- Apply a small amount of this cream to those joints that are particularly painful. Initially, you may experience a burning sensation, but afterward you should experience pain relief.
- You may reapply the cream up to 4 times daily.
- Be sure to wash your hand thoroughly after handling the cream.

Additional Case Questions

1. What risk factors for coronary artery disease does this patient have? Should she be placed on aspirin as a cardioprotectant in light of the fact that she is taking either acetaminophen or an NSAID?

- Her risk factors for CAD include diabetes mellitus, hypercholesterolemia, and hypertension.
- Yes, this patient can safely take aspirin (81 to 325 mg/day) without it adversely affecting her analgesic therapy. Although the data on use of aspirin for the primary prevention of CAD in women are inconclusive,[6] the potential benefits outweigh the risks in this patient.

2. What effect might NSAID therapy have on this patient's antihypertensive therapy?

- NSAIDs can attenuate the diastolic blood pressure-lowering effects of many antihypertensives by 3 to 6 mm Hg.[7] ACE inhibitors such as benazepril (Lotensin) can be affected in this manner. This effect is clinically significant, since the risk of stroke is markedly reduced when blood pressure is lowered by as little as 5 mm Hg.

3. *Is this patient a candidate for pharmacotherapy to treat her morbid obesity?*

- Yes. Her body mass index (BMI) is 35.7 kg/m^2, which is potentially life threatening. In addition, her morbid obesity may be a contributing factor to her osteoarthritis, hypertension, hypercholesterolemia, and diabetes mellitus.
- Although fenfluramine and dexfenfluramine are no longer available in the United States, phentermine (Adipex), sibutramine (Meridia), and orlistat (Xenical) are available at the time of this writing. One of these agents should be considered for this patient in addition to diet, exercise, and behavior modification.

References

1. Kraus VB. Pathogenesis and treatment of osteoarthritis. Med Clin North Am 1997;81:85–112.
2. Anderson JJ, Felson DT. Factors associated with osteoarthritis of the knee in the first national Health and Nutrition Examination Survey (HANES I). Am J Epidemiol 1988;128:179–189.
3. Felson DT, Zhang Y, Anthony JM, et al. Weight loss reduces the risk for symptomatic knee osteoarthritis in women. The Framingham Study. Ann Intern Med 1992;116:535–539.
4. McAlindon TE, Jacques P, Zhang Y, et al. Do antioxidant micronutrients protect against the development and progression of knee osteoarthritis? Arthritis Rheum 1996;39:648–656.
5. Bradley JD, Brandt KD, Katz BP, et al. Comparison of an antiinflammatory dose of ibuprofen, an analgesic dose of ibuprofen, and acetaminophen in the treatment of patients with osteoarthritis of the knee. N Engl J Med 1991;325:87–91.
6. Rich-Edwards JW, Manson JE, Hennekens CH, et al. The primary prevention of coronary heart disease in women. N Engl J Med 1995;332:1758–1766.
7. Pope JE, Anderson JJ, Felson DT. A meta-analysis of the effects of nonsteroidal anti-inflammatory drugs on blood pressure. Arch Intern Med 1993;153:477–484.

83 GOUT AND HYPERURICEMIA

▶ The Professor's Lament   (Level II)

Page H. Pigg, PharmD
Ralph E. Small, PharmD, FCCP, FASHP, FAPhA

Complaints of severe pain in the left great toe cause a 44-year-old man to seek medical attention. In addition to swelling, warmth, erythema, and tenderness in that digit, the patient also has a mildly elevated temperature, an elevated serum uric acid level (11.5 mg/dL), leukocytosis, and soft tissue swelling on x-ray of the affected joint. A synovial fluid aspirate contains white blood cells and monosodium urate crystals, documenting the diagnosis of gout. The patient is taking hydrochlorothiazide for the treatment of hypertension, which may contribute to hyperuricemia. Pharmacotherapeutic alternatives for treatment of this initial attack of acute gout include prescription-strength NSAIDs and colchicine. NSAIDs such as indomethacin are generally preferred because of their high efficacy and low-toxicity profile when used for the short-term treatment of acute gout. When this patient presents 6 months later after having several additional acute attacks, students are asked to consider whether chronic uric acid-lowering therapy with probenecid or allopurinol should be initiated.

▶ Questions

Problem Identification

1. a. *Create a list of the patient's drug-related problems.*

- Initial presentation of acute gouty arthritis requiring drug treatment.
- Chronic, stable problems requiring no intervention at this time include hypertension and seasonal allergic rhinitis.

b. *What information (signs, symptoms, laboratory values) indicates the presence or severity of an acute gouty attack?*

- *Symptoms.* Excruciating pain in a single digit of the lower extremity (left great toe), interrupting sleep and mobility.
- *Signs.* Physical examination of the affected joint reveals swelling, warmth, erythema, and tenderness.[1] The patient has a mildly elevated temperature.
- *Laboratory values.* Elevated WBC, ESR, and serum uric acid concentration. Microscopic examination of the joint aspirate reveals PMNs and monosodium urate crystals.
- *Other.* Positive history of excessive EtOH use the 2 nights before the attack. The patient is in the typical age range/gender for the initial presentation of gout.

c. *Could any of the patient's problems have been caused by drug therapy?*

- Hypertension/hydrochlorothiazide may predispose patients to uric acid-based diseases; thiazide diuretics can inhibit renal excretion of uric acid by inhibiting tubular secretion, contributing to high serum and tissue concentrations.
- Low dose salicylates (daily aspirin) may predispose to uric acid-based disease by inhibiting renal excretion of uric acid.

Desired Outcome

2. *What are the goals of pharmacotherapy in this case?*

- Relief of the pain and discomfort of the acute gouty attack
- Prevention of future acute gout attacks and uric acid deposition disease
- Provision of alternative therapy for hypertension

Therapeutic Alternatives

3. a. What non-drug therapies might be useful for this patient?

- *Avoid alcohol and purine-rich foods* such as organ meats and anchovies.[2]
- *Exercise and hydration* with lots of fluids, especially when exercising.
- *A controlled weight-loss program* would provide positive effects on joint symptoms and overall cardiovascular health.

b. What feasible pharmacotherapeutic alternatives are available for treatment of the acute attack of gouty arthritis?

- *NSAIDs* (any of the prescription agents) have become the drugs of choice for the treatment of acute gouty arthritis because of the toxicity profile of colchicine. Although NSAIDs also have adverse effects (e.g., GI distress, nausea, vomiting, peptic ulceration, GI bleeding, reduced renal blood flow), these problems seldom cause serious harm when used for the short-term treatment of acute gout. Some examples of effective NSAID regimens include:
    - ✓ *Fenoprofen* (Nalfon, generics) 800 mg po Q 6 H
    - ✓ *Flurbiprofen* (Ansaid) 100 mg po QID for 1 day, then 50 mg po QID
    - ✓ *Ibuprofen* (Motrin, generics) 600 to 800 mg po QID
    - ✓ *Indomethacin* (Indocin, generics) 50 mg po TID
    - ✓ *Ketoprofen* (Orudis, generics) 50 mg po QID or 75 mg po TID
    - ✓ *Meclofenamate* (Meclomen, generics) 100 mg po TID to QID
    - ✓ *Naproxen* (Naprosyn, generics) 750 mg po initially, then 250 mg po Q 8 H
    - ✓ *Piroxicam* (Feldene, generics) 40 mg po QD
    - ✓ *Sulindac* (Clinoril, generics) 200 mg po BID
    - ✓ *Tolmetin* (Tolectin) 400 mg po TID to QID

    Any NSAID may be used, but many clinicians prefer indomethacin because of its long history of effectiveness for the disorder.

- *Colchicine* (po or IV) is also highly effective for the treatment of gout. The usual dose for treatment of an acute attack is 0.4 to 1.2 mg as the initial dose, followed by 0.5 to 0.6 mg every hour (or 1 to 1.2 mg every 2 hours) until there is improvement, GI side effects, or a total of 8 to 10 mg has been given. Colchicine causes potentially serious GI effects in many patients prior to resolution of the acute attack. Diarrhea can be particularly harmful when it results in dehydration and electrolyte disturbances. IV colchicine avoids these GI effects but may result in local extravasation injury. As a result, many clinicians would avoid colchicine for treatment of this initial attack and initiate it if attacks before more frequent. Colchicine can also be used for prophylactic therapy after resolution of the attack. The usual initial dose is 0.5 to 0.6 mg po BID; additional colchicine may be taken at the first sign of a new attack. Prophylactic colchicine is generally considered only for those patients who have frequent gouty attacks, urate tophi, evidence of renal damage, or hyperuricemia from required medications.

- *Corticosteroids* could be used in cases resistant to first-line therapy. They would not be used in this patient since this attack represents the initial presentation of disease.

- Uric acid-lowering therapy should be avoided during treatment of the acute attack because of potential complications, the possibility of exacerbating the disease, and the present lack of documentation of the patient's status as an overproducer or underexcretor of uric acid.

Optimal Plan

4. What drug, dosage form, dose, schedule, and duration of therapy are best for this patient?

- Any prescription-strength NSAID would provide acceptable treatment for this patient; relatively high doses are required, as shown in the list outlined previously. As stated, clinicians prefer indomethacin for acute gouty attacks. Although various dosage schedules have been used, a common regimen is indomethacin capsules (not the sustained-release dosage form) 50 to 75 mg po for 1 dose, followed by 50 mg Q 6 H for 48 hours, then 50 mg Q 8 H for 28 to 72 hours (depending on response). All NSAIDs should be taken with food to minimize GI complaints.

- Although colchicine could be used, its use has generally been superseded by NSAIDs because of their high degree of efficacy and low toxicity when used for the short-term treatment of an acute gout attack.

- Because of its potential contribution to hyperuricemia, the hydrochlorothiazide should be discontinued and alternative therapy for HTN should be initiated. Beta-blockers (e.g., propranolol, atenolol, metoprolol) are the only other class of agents that have been shown to reduce mortality in HTN to date. However, other drug classes, such as ACE inhibitors (e.g., captopril, enalapril) or calcium channel blockers (e.g., nifedipine, diltiazem, verapamil) are commonly used as initial single-drug therapy for HTN.

Outcome Evaluation

5. What clinical and laboratory parameters are necessary to evaluate the therapy for achievement of the desired therapeutic outcome and to detect or prevent adverse effects?

- Telephone the patient after 2 days and ask him about the degree of reduction in pain, swelling, warmth, redness, and fever. Symptoms should decrease in 1 to 2 days with total relief achieved in 3 to 6 days.

- Because of the short-term nature of NSAID treatment, laboratory testing for toxicity is generally not necessary.

- Monitor CBC with differential if long-term colchicine therapy is used; the drug can cause bone marrow toxicity. With prophylactic colchicine, perform these tests in 2 weeks and then as often as every 4 weeks, based on the clinician's judgment.

- Repeat a serum uric acid level to evaluate the disease process 2 to 3 weeks after the acute attack. However, symptomatic therapy with an NSAID or colchicine will not reduce serum uric acid levels.

- Two to 3 weeks after resolution of the acute attack, place the patient on a low-purine diet for 3 to 5 days; then obtain a 24-hour urine collection to determine the amount of uric acid excreted in the urine in 24 hours. The goal is to document whether the patient is an overproducer or underexcretor of uric acid (refer to textbook Chapter 85 for more detailed information on how to interpret this test). This information can be used to guide future treatment.

- For the patient's HTN, monitor BP in 1 month and then quarterly thereafter with the goal of achieving and maintaining a BP of < 140/90 mm Hg.
- Because of the patient's obesity, monitor weight in 1 month and then quarterly thereafter with the goal of achieving weight loss through dietary intervention.

Patient Counseling

6. *What information should be provided to the patient to enhance compliance, ensure successful therapy, and minimize adverse effects?*

   Example NSAID: Indomethacin Prompt-Release Capsules
   - This medication is related to the drug Motrin or Advil that you may have heard about. The medications in this class are very useful for treating gout and other joint problems.
   - This medicine will only be needed for several days. The directions are to take 1 capsule (50 mg) every 6 hours for 48 hours, then 1 capsule every 8 hours for 1 to 5 days (depending on how well you respond to the medication).
   - Take each dose with food to help avoid stomach upset.
   - You should begin to see relief of your toe pain and swelling within 1 to 2 days; your symptoms should be completely resolved within 3 to 6 days.
   - If you forget to take a dose, take the missed dose as soon as you remember. However, if it is almost time for the next dose, skip the missed dose and go back to your regular schedule. Do not take a double dosage.
   - Do not take aspirin, ibuprofen (e.g., Advil), naproxen (e.g., Aleve), ketoprofen (e.g., Orudis KT), or other similar non-prescription agents or combination products that contain these agents while you are taking indomethacin.
   - This medication is usually well tolerated when used for short periods, but there are several possible side effects that you need to be aware of.
     - ✓ Indomethacin can cause upset stomach, nausea, vomiting, and stomach ulcers. These effects can be minimized or prevented by taking each dose with food. Stomach ulcers are very uncommon when the drug is used for short courses such as the one you are receiving.
     - ✓ Drowsiness occurs in some people; use caution when driving or performing other tasks that require you to be fully alert until you know how much this affects you.
     - ✓ Headache may also occur; contact your doctor if this becomes troublesome so that an alternative medication may be selected.
     - ✓ Bruising and bleeding occur rarely with indomethacin; discontinue the medication and contact your doctor if these effects occur.
   - As with any prescription medicine, do not share this medication with any person for whom it has not been prescribed.

▶ Follow-up Questions

1. *Provide an interpretation of the urine uric acid value.*

   - Normal individuals excrete < 600 mg of uric acid in the urine daily. Persons who excrete > 600 mg of uric acid per 24 hours on a purine-free diet (as seen in this patient) are defined as overproducers of uric acid. Hyperuricemic individuals who excrete < 600 mg/24 hours on a purine-free diet are considered to be underexcretors of uric acid. Therefore, this individual is categorized as an overproducer of uric acid.

2. *What recommendations do you have for further management of this patient?*

   - Because the patient is an overproducer, allopurinol should be used as the prophylactic therapy.[3]
   - It is given in doses of 100 to 300 mg once daily, depending on the renal function of the patient.

References

1. Agudelo CA, Wise CM. Gout and hyperuricemia. Curr Opin Rheumatol 1991;3: 684–691.
2. Star VL, Hochberg MC. Prevention and management of gout. Drugs 1993;45: 212–222.
3. Edwards NL. Drugs to lower uric acid levels. How to avoid misuse in gouty arthritis. Postgrad Med 1991;89:111-113, 116.

SECTION 11

Eyes, Ears, Nose, and Throat Disorders

L. Michael Posey, Section Editor

84 GLAUCOMA

▶ **Another Silent Disease**　　　　　　(Level II)

Tien T. Kiat-Winarko, PharmD, BSc

A 34-year-old man with a 9-year history of advanced open-angle glaucoma presents with fogging and distortion of vision in the left eye. Physical examination reveals worsening of glaucoma despite pharmacologic treatment with a number of topical agents. Students are asked to consider additional and alternative therapies that will decrease and maintain lower intraocular pressures to prevent further vision loss, minimize adverse reactions, and facilitate patient adherence to the multidrug regimen. The case includes discussion of new therapeutic agents and novel approaches to the treatment of glaucoma. The presentation also offers the opportunity for students to practice educating patients on the proper administration of ophthalmic medications.

▶ Questions

Problem Identification

1. a. Provide a list of this patient's drug-related problems.

- Chronic open-angle glaucoma inadequately treated with present regimen.
- Depression due to his chronic disease state.
- Nephrolithiasis associated with oral acetazolamide usage is a problem that has apparently resolved with discontinuation of acetazolamide.

b. What risk factors for primary open-angle glaucoma (POAG) are present in this patient?

- High myopia
- Father, mother, and sister have glaucoma
- Accident/trauma-induced glaucoma is also a possibility; nerve damage could occur due to increased IOP, resulting in decreased visual acuity and visual fields
- Refer to textbook Chapter 86 for additional risk factors not present in this patient

c. What information (signs, symptoms) indicates the presence or severity of this patient's glaucoma?

- POAG in its early stages does not present with noticeable symptoms. It is a chronic, slowly progressive disease and is usually diagnosed during a routine ophthalmologic examination. In this patient, it was diagnosed during his hospital stay after a skydiving accident.
- Presence of tunnel vision indicates that nerve damage is extensive.
- C/D ratio of 0.99 in OS and 1.0 in OD; the right disk appeared whitish, fully cupped (normal C/D ratio ≤ 0.33). This patient suffers from advanced stage chronic open-angle glaucoma. The optic nerves in this patient are severely damaged.

- Decreased visual fields. This patient can only see hand motion in his right eye standing 3 inches away from the examiner. The patient complained of fogging and distortion of vision in the left eye for the last 3 months, occasionally progressing to tunnel vision and central area visual blurring (refer to the section "Primary Open-Angle Glaucoma" in textbook Chapter 86 for more detailed information).

Desired Outcome

2. *What are the goals of pharmacotherapy in this case?*

- Decrease and maintain IOP in the low teens (10 to 14 mm Hg) to prevent deterioration of vision due to further damage of the optic nerve, thereby preventing further loss of visual fields.
- Maximize topical medications from different classes with different mechanisms of action.
- Minimize adverse drug reactions. Reserve oral carbonic anhydrase inhibitors (CAIs) as a last resort due to history of kidney stone formation from acetazolamide.
- Increase blood flow to the eye and optic nerve to maintain its current state and to prevent further optic nerve damage.

Therapeutic Alternatives

3. a. *What non-drug therapies might be useful for this patient?*

- Eye massage (also called digital ocular pressure) is performed by applying a constant, moderate digital pressure to the inferior sclera through the lid for 10 seconds using the broad portion of the index finger. Repeat the massage after a 10-second rest for 2 to 3 times.[1]
- Eye massage 4 to 8 times daily will help this patient lower IOP by 2 to 3 mm Hg, especially during the time when diurnal variation in IOP is at its peak.[2,3] Generally, human IOP is high in the late morning and low in the afternoon and evening. This patient experienced a peak IOP of 28 mm Hg at 10:40 AM and a trough IOP of 11 mm Hg at 3:30 PM (data not shown in patient presentation). This follows the generally accepted theory that IOP fluctuates in a sigmoidal pattern relative to circadian rhythm.[2]

b. *What feasible pharmacotherapeutic alternatives are available for treatment of the patient's glaucoma?*

- The treatment for POAG is usually initiated in a stepwise manner. Therapy starts with medications of lower strength and the least side effects that are compatible with patient characteristics, the presence of other disease states, economic considerations, as well as physician preference.
- Initial therapy typically consists of a *parasympathomimetic* (e.g., *pilocarpine*), with the addition of *sympathomimetics (or alpha-adrenergic agents)* for additive effects. Oral agents such as CAIs are reserved as second-line therapy because they are associated with increased systemic adverse drug reactions.
- Topical adrenergic agents such as *epinephrine* and *dipivefrin* are not commonly prescribed because they are less effective in reducing IOP and have increased adverse effects when compared to β-blockers, miotics, and other newer agents.
- This patient's current topical medications for glaucoma include betaxolol (Betoptic) 0.5% ou BID, apraclonidine (Iopidine) 0.5% os TID, and dorzolamide (Trusopt) 2% os TID.
  ✓ *Betaxolol (Betoptic)* is preferred over timolol and other β-blockers due to its cardioselective property. Betaxolol is more desirable in this patient who has a history of childhood asthma, which may relapse when the patient is under extreme stress.
  ✓ *Apraclonidine (Iopidine)* is a potent α-agonist and is dosed TID. Apraclonidine 0.5% is not FDA approved for long-term use. In some patients, apraclonidine has demonstrated a loss in effectiveness in IOP control after a few months. It is being used in this patient for its additive effects with the β-blocker and topical CAI.
  ✓ *Dorzolamide (Trusopt)* is a topical CAI. This agent is relatively costly when compared to other topical agents. In light of this patient's history of developing kidney stones associated with systemic use of acetazolamide, the topical CAI dorzolamide is preferred, if a CAI is to be used.
- Other alternative agents that may be considered for this patient include the following products.
  ✓ *Cosopt* is a combination ophthalmic solution containing dorzolamide 2% and timolol maleate 0.5%. The recommended dosage is one drop in the affected eye(s) twice daily. This product might be useful if both individual drugs are the optimal agents for a particular patient. However, the cost for the combination product may be more expensive than giving each agent individually (since timolol is available generically).
  ✓ *Brinzolamide (Azopt)* ophthalmic suspension is another topical CAI that has demonstrated similar efficacy to dorzolamide in a 3-month comparative trial. It may be associated with less eye irritation and a better tolerability profile, which may enhance patient adherence. It offers another option for patients who are unable to tolerate dorzolamide or other ocular antihypertensive agents.
  ✓ *Latanoprost 0.005% (Xalatan)* is a prostaglandin $F_{2\alpha}$ analog that is thought to reduce IOP by increasing the uveoscleral outflow of aqueous humor. It is indicated for reduction of elevated IOP in patients who are intolerant of or insufficiently responsive to other IOP-lowering medications. Administration of latanoprost in the evening offers nocturnal IOP control. Clinical trials and post-marketing surveys have shown latanoprost to be as efficacious as timolol. It also has an excellent side-effect profile, except for the possibility of brown iris pigmentation in patients with green or blue eyes. Patients should be assessed regularly, and treatment should be discontinued if increased pigmentation occurs. The increase in brown iris pigment does not progress once latanoprost is discontinued.
  ✓ *Brimonidine 0.2% (Alphagan)* is an α-2 adrenergic agonist indicated for long-term use; it lacks the tachyphylactic property associated with apraclonidine. This is an important advantage, as long-term apraclonidine therapy may become costly when additional agents are needed for IOP control.
  ✓ *Cholinesterase inhibitors (echothiophate, physostigmine, demecarium bromide)* are not used as frequently as they

were in the past. They have a long duration of action but also many adverse drug reactions and drug–drug interactions. Extreme caution is advised before or during general anesthesia because of possible respiratory and cardiovascular collapse. They should be discontinued at least 2 weeks before surgery if succinylcholine is to be used. In addition, the effects of cholinesterase inhibitors may be enhanced in persons who are exposed to substances such as organophosphate insecticides, which may be absorbed through the respiratory tract or skin. In this particular patient, cholinesterase inhibitors are not the agents of choice due to the risk of asthma precipitation and the possibility of potentiation of depression.

Optimal Plan

4. a. Devise an optimal pharmacotherapeutic regimen for the treatment of this patient's glaucoma.

- The Betoptic 0.5% solution given BID is recommended to be replaced by Betoptic S 0.25% suspension given Q AM. The Betoptic S suspension has a longer duration of action, thereby allowing once-daily dosing. Betoptic S suspension or Timoptic-XE gel Q AM will improve the convenience of therapy and increase patient compliance. Retaining the β-blocker will permit additive effects with other topical agents that work by different mechanisms of action.
- Adding latanoprost 0.005% Q HS would help to maximize the patient's topical therapy. Latanoprost has a unique mechanism of action that will complement those of the other medications. Because this patient has a previous history of kidney stones from acetazolamide, it may be prudent to avoid systemic and topical CAIs in this patient. For this reason, gradually taper dorzolamide from TID to BID with the addition of latanoprost. Discontinue dorzolamide after 2 weeks while maintaining a desirable IOP. Once-daily dosing of latanoprost at bedtime will increase the patient's compliance compared to TID dosing with dorzolamide.
- Brimonidine 0.2% given BID is also a recommended addition to optimize this patient's therapy. Because of its lack of tachyphylaxis, it should be used in place of apraclonidine.
- Nimodipine (Nimotop) 30 mg po TID and pentoxifylline (Trental) 400 mg po TID are to be continued as prescribed by the neuro-ophthalmologist. These drugs are used for unlabeled indications. Pentoxifylline is used for eye circulation disorders; nimodipine is used to increase blood flow to the brain and optic nerve. Nimodipine is one of the most useful calcium channel blockers for brain ischemia because of its high permeability across the blood–brain barrier.[4,5] This may retard or prevent further damage to the optic nerve, which is interconnected with the brain.
- Discontinue eye massage to enable more accurate assessment of the effectiveness of the new therapy.
- Continue Paxil 20 mg po QD. This patient is a young and ambitious PhD who was athletic and had an active life. Paxil is beneficial to prevent him from becoming progressively depressed.

b. What alternatives would be appropriate if the initial therapy fails or cannot be used?

- Repeat surgical intervention such as a filtering procedure with drainage tube implantation. The filtering surgery, also called trabeculectomy, involves the creation of a channel through which aqueous humor can flow from the anterior chamber to the subconjunctival space. The tube implant decreases IOP by mechanically draining aqueous humor from the eye to the subconjunctival space, where it is reabsorbed by the vasculature. Antimetabolities such as 5-fluorouracil and mitomycin C are used in glaucoma filtering surgery to improve surgical success by retarding fibroblast formation, which will close the surgically created channel or opening (refer to the textbook section on antiproliferatives used in glaucoma surgery). Complication of this procedure may include total loss of the vision remaining. However, surgical intervention is indicated when this patient has exhausted all the medical interventions and is still complaining of vision distortion and fogging, progressing to tunnel vision and unstable IOP that lead to throbbing band-like headaches.

Outcome Evaluation

5. What clinical and laboratory parameters are necessary to evaluate the therapy for achievement of the desired therapeutic outcome and to detect or prevent adverse effects?

- Regular follow-up of IOP every 1 to 2 weeks after the start of therapy. IOP measurement and follow-up may be reduced to every 6 to 8 weeks after stabilization of IOP.
- Visual field and funduscopic examination should be performed at least every 6 months in this patient. These examinations should be performed more frequently if there are drug or dosage changes.
- Simplifying this patient's drug therapy regimen minimizes side effects. Compliance is maximized with the use of Betoptic S 0.25% Q AM, latanoprost 0.005% Q HS, brimonidine 0.2% BID.
- Monitor BP, HR, any cardiac irregularity or arrhythmia, chest pain, drowsiness, and dizziness with the use of nimodipine and pentoxifylline. Hypotension is not uncommon with concurrent use of pentoxifylline and the antihypertensive agent nimodipine.
- Observe for any eye color changes with the use of latanoprost. Increase in brown pigmentation of the iris may not be noticeable for several months to years. Monitor this patient every 4 to 6 weeks, and ensure that the patient is also doing self-monitoring for the development of iris pigmentation. The brown pigmentation around the pupil usually spreads concentrically toward the periphery. Therapy should be discontinued if increased pigmentation continues. The long-term effects from increased iris pigmentation are unknown.

Patient Counseling

6. What information should the patient receive about the disease of glaucoma, proper medication administration technique, and possible side effects of treatment?

- It is important that you contact your doctor or pharmacist and seek prompt treatment if aura, flashing lights, eye discomfort, or headache occurs.
- Inform your doctor or pharmacist if changes in the color of the iris occur. Discontinue use of latanoprost when this happens.
- Latanoprost does not need to be refrigerated after it leaves the pharmacy. However, it is only stable for 6 weeks at room temperature.

- The combination of Trental and Nimotop can cause effects on the heart and lower blood pressure. I will be happy to teach you how to self-monitor your heart rate and blood pressure at home. These medications may also cause chest pain, dizziness, and abnormal heart rhythms.
- Educate the patient on the technique of nasolacrimal duct occlusion to improve ocular bioavailability and minimize systemic absorption and side effects (see the textbook chapter section on patient education).
- Refer to the textbook chapter for information on educating the patient about the sterile technique for eye drop instillation.

References

1. Kane H, Gaasterland DE, Monsour M. Response of filtered eyes to digital ocular pressure. Ophthalmology 1997;104:202–206.
2. Liu JH. Circadian rhythm of intraocular pressure. J Glaucoma 1998;7:141–147.
3. Sacca SC, Rolando M, Marletta A, et al. Fluctuations of intraocular pressure during the day in open-angle glaucoma, normal-tension glaucoma and normal subjects. Ophthalmologica 1998;212:115–119.
4. Ichihara S, Tsuda Y, Hosomi N, et al. Nimodipine improves brain energy metabolism and blood rheology during ischemia and reperfusion in the gerbil brain. J Neurol Sci 1996;114:84–90.
5. Herbette LG, Mason PE, Sweeney KR, et al. Favorable amphiphilicity of nimodipine facilitates its interaction with brain membranes. Neuropharmacology 1994; 33:241–249

85 ALLERGIC RHINITIS

▶ Reining in Rhinitis   (Level I)

W. Greg Leader, PharmD

A 32-year-old woman with a long history of seasonal allergic rhinitis presents to clinic with complaints of postnasal drainage, throat irritation, and an occasional non-productive cough. She has been taking the second-generation antihistamine astemizole for 3 years with inadequate control of her symptoms. Before changing pharmacotherapy, a more complete history should be obtained to identify and eliminate specific allergen triggers. Avoidance therapy (e.g., removing potential allergen sources and the use of air filters and products to kill dust mites) is an important part of the management of this disorder. Pharmacotherapeutic alternatives include other oral antihistamines, oral or nasal decongestants, oral antihistamine/decongestant combinations, intranasal mast cell stabilizers, intranasal corticosteroids, intranasal ipratropium bromide, and immunotherapy. Monitoring parameters should be directed toward relief of symptoms and adverse effects of the medications used.

▶ Questions

Problem Identification

1. a. *Create a list of the patient's drug-related problems.*

   - Allergic rhinitis that is inappropriately treated (undertreated).
   - Eczema is a chronic, stable problem that appears to be adequately treated with PRN hydrocortisone and does not require any intervention at this time.

   b. *What information (signs, symptoms, laboratory values) indicates the presence or severity of allergic rhinitis?*

   - The patient exhibits classic symptoms of seasonal allergic rhinitis, including frequent sneezing, pruritic eyes and ears, pink conjunctivae, and post-nasal drip. The symptoms are similar in perennial allergic rhinitis, but there is usually more nasal blockage and less ocular itching. The occurrence of post-nasal drip and sore throat may be indicative of nasal blockage. The patient presents with a history of year-round symptoms that are exacerbated in the spring, indicating components of both perennial and seasonal allergic rhinitis.
   - She does not have fever, purulent nasal discharge, persistent or productive cough, or sinus pain, indicating that sinusitis or other infectious diseases are probably not contributing to her problem.

   c. *Could any of the patient's problems have been caused by drug therapy?*

   - The estrogens contained in oral contraceptives may cause vasodilation and congestion by inhibiting acetylcholinesterase, thereby increasing muscarinic activity. Although the patient should be questioned about whether or not her symptoms began or worsened with the initiation of oral contraceptive use, she is exhibiting signs other than congestion (sneezing, pruritus). While it is possible that the oral contraceptive is contributing to her problem, it is extremely unlikely that it is the primary causative agent.
   - Tolerance occurs with the first-generation antihistamines, and cross-tolerance also occurs to agents in other classes.[1] To date, this phenomenon has not been reported with second-generation antihistamines.[2]
   - The patient's increase in symptoms may also be caused by non-adherence to the drug regimen, seasonal exposure to a new allergen, or worsening of the disease state.

   d. *What additional information from the patient history is needed to satisfactorily assess this patient?*

   - Seasonal and perennial allergic rhinitis can be caused by a variety of different allergens. A more complete history designed to elicit this type of data may be helpful in designing a more specific treatment plan. Questions should include:
     ✓ What type of environment do you live in?
     —Is the home in an urban, suburban, or rural area?
     —What type of heating and cooling system does the home have?
     —Are there pets in the home?
     —Does anyone in the home smoke?

—What types of furnishings are in the home (carpet, drapes, feather pillows and/or mattresses)?
—How old is the home?
✓ What type of environment do you work in?
—Are you exposed to tobacco smoke on the job?
—Are you exposed to chemicals on the job?
—Do any coworkers suffer from "sick building" syndrome?
✓ How do you spend your free or recreational time?
—Are you involved with pets or animals (horseback riding, animal shows, time with pets)?
—Do you spend time gardening?
✓ What is the pattern and severity of the symptoms?
—How often do the symptoms occur (daily, seasonally, continuously)?
—What factors (tobacco smoke, mowing the lawn, gardening, household cleaners) precipitate the symptoms?
—Do the symptoms interfere with your normal lifestyle?
—Are you less active than you would like to be?
—Do you avoid certain activities because of your disease state?
—Do you miss work or school (if applicable) because of rhinitis symptoms?
—Does the disease affect your sleep patterns or habits?
✓ Have you undergone skin testing for allergen identification in the past? If so, what were the test results?

Desired Outcome

2. What are the goals of pharmacotherapy in this case?

- Relieve current symptoms of allergic rhinitis
- Prevent the future occurrence of symptoms associated with allergic rhinitis
- Provide optimal pharmacotherapy with minimal or no adverse effects
- Meet the patient's expectations of and satisfaction with allergic rhinitis care

Therapeutic Alternatives

3. a. What non-drug therapies might be useful for this patient?

- *Avoidance therapy* plays an important role in the management of allergic rhinitis. Information gained from a more thorough patient history designed to elucidate information specific to the patient's allergic rhinitis allows for formulation of an avoidance therapy plan specific for this patient. To be effective, avoidance therapy must be initiated and maintained in an aggressive manner. This process can often be tedious and expensive. Specific avoidance measures include:
  ✓ *Pollen avoidance.* Monitor the pollen forecast; avoid high pollen areas; stay indoors when the pollen count is high; keep windows and doors closed when the pollen count is high; use high-efficiency particulate air (HEPA) filters; wear a mask when gardening, mowing the lawn, or raking hay or grass.
  ✓ *House dust mite control.* Use plastic covers on mattresses and pillows; avoid feather pillows and mattresses or wool blankets; wash bed linens in hot water (> 60°C) weekly; remove carpet from the bedroom; vacuum upholstered furniture frequently and use a vacuum with disposable paper bags and a filter or a vacuum with a water reservoir; wear a mask while vacuuming; wipe all surfaces weekly; remove items from the bedroom that collect dust (e.g., picture frames, figurines); stuffed or furry toys should be vacuumed, tumbled dried, or put in the deep freeze (−20°C) overnight or removed; use of acaracides may decrease dust mite populations.
  ✓ *Pet avoidance.* Do not have furry or feathered pets in the home; remove current pets from the home; if pets cannot be removed, wash them regularly, and do not allow them in the bedroom.
  ✓ *Miscellaneous measures.* Decrease humidity in the home to < 50% to decrease mold growth; do not allow tobacco smoke in the home; if there is a cockroach problem, use commercial insecticides to control the problem.

b. *What feasible pharmacotherapeutic alternatives are available for treatment of allergic rhinitis?*

Decongestants

- $Alpha_1$-adrenergic agonists are effective in decreasing or eliminating the congestion associated with rhinitis when applied intranasally or given systemically, but they have no effect on itching, sneezing, or rhinorrhea. However, combinations containing decongestants and antihistamines are effective in alleviating all of the symptoms of allergic rhinitis.
  ✓ *Intranasal decongestants* have a quick onset of action, and some products have a duration of action approaching 12 hours (see Table 87–5 in textbook Chapter 87). However, use of these agents for more than 3 to 4 days can cause rebound congestion leading to overuse of the drug.
  ✓ *Systemic oral decongestants* are also effective but may cause an increase in blood pressure, heart rate, and intraocular pressure as well as insomnia and nervousness. Care should be taken when using these agents in patients who have cardiovascular disease, diabetes, glaucoma, hypertension, or prostatic hyperplasia.

Antihistamines

- Antihistamines continue to be the agents of choice for treating seasonal allergic rhinitis. They are effective in relieving the itching, sneezing, and rhinorrhea associated with allergic rhinitis, but they have little effect on congestion.
- *First-generation oral antihistamines* often cause sedation or anticholinergic effects, but they are an inexpensive alternative for the treatment of allergic rhinitis in patients who can tolerate them. Table 87–3 of the textbook compares the relative side-effect profiles of these agents. Tolerance to the sedative effect occurs in approximately 1 to 2 weeks.
- *Second-generation or non-sedating oral antihistamines* are more selective for peripheral H_1-histamine receptors and are less likely to cross the blood–brain barrier, resulting in a lower incidence of sedation. These agents also have a lower incidence of anticholinergic effects (see textbook Table 87–3). One major drawback to these agents is their price; therapy can cost as much as 50 times more than with first-generation agents. They are also

available by prescription only. Some of these drugs are associated with potentially fatal drug interactions.

- ✓ *Astemizole (Hismanal)* is metabolized by the hepatic cytochrome P450 3A4 enzyme. Coadministration of drugs that inhibit this metabolic pathway (e.g., erythromycin, ketoconazole, itraconazole) may lead to the accumulation of the parent compound and certain metabolites, causing a prolongation of the QT interval and a ventricular dysrhythmia known as torsades de pointes. (*Note:* In June 1999, the manufacturer announced its intention to voluntarily withdraw astemizole from the U.S. market because the antihistamine class includes agents that have not been associated with these abnormalities.)
- ✓ *Loratadine (Claritin)*, which is also metabolized via CYP3A4, has not been associated with this phenomenon.
- ✓ *Fexofenadine (Allegra)* and *cetirizine (Zyrtec)* are primarily eliminated renally and are not problematic when administered with enzyme inhibitors.

Most antihistamines have a rapid onset and are effective when given approximately two hours prior to exposure. Astemizole is an exception, and it may require administration for several days before an effect is seen.[3]

- *Azelastine (Astelin)* is an intranasal antihistamine that appears to be effective in the treatment and prevention of seasonal allergic rhinitis and may be as effective as topical steroids.[4] Azelastine has a rapid onset of action and is devoid of many of the adverse effects associated with first-generation antihistamines as well as the drug interactions associated with the second-generation agents. The most common adverse effects are bitter taste, headache, and somnolence.
- *Levocabastine (Livostin)* is an ophthalmic antihistamine available for topical treatment of ocular symptoms.

Mast Cell Stabilizers

- *Cromolyn sodium (Nasalcrom)* is an intranasal mast cell stabilizer used for the prophylaxis of mild to moderate allergic rhinitis. Cromolyn appears to block both the early and late phase response of allergic rhinitis. Its biggest disadvantages are the prolonged amount of treatment time required before the drug is effective (2 to 4 weeks) and the need for administration 4 times a day. This may lead to poor patient adherence. Cromolyn is more effective in preventing rhinitis associated itching, rhinorrhea, and sneezing than congestion. Patients should begin therapy 2 to 3 weeks prior to allergy season. The nasal spray is now available as a nonprescription preparation.
- *Cromolyn sodium (Crolom)* and *lodoxamide tromethamine (Alomide)* are mast cell stabilizers available as ophthalmic solutions to treat ocular symptoms of allergic rhinitis.

Intranasal Corticosteroids

- These agents are the most effective for the treatment of allergic rhinitis. Intranasal corticosteroids block both the early and late phase response in allergic rhinitis. They also decrease all of the nasal symptoms of allergic rhinitis. Although intranasal steroids probably do not directly affect ocular symptoms of allergic rhinitis, these symptoms may improve because of steroid-induced improvements in nasal drainage. Many patients may begin to have symptom relief in 1 to 3 days after initiating treatment, but the maximal effect is not seen for 2 to 3 weeks. Intranasal corticosteroids are relatively safe; the most common adverse effects are nasal stinging, bleeding, and burning. These effects tend to occur more commonly with the aerosol propellant systems than the aqueous solutions; however, some patients may dislike the distinctive smell of the aqueous solution and the tendency for the aqueous solution to drain into the pharyngeal area after use. Although concern exists over systemic toxicities associated with intranasal steroids, newer agents have a very high therapeutic ratio, and systemic toxicities rarely occur at normal dosages. Because of relatively high systemic absorption and the potential for significant systemic effects, dexamethasone (Dexacort Phosphate Turbinaire) is not recommended.

Ipratropium Bromide (Atrovent) Nasal Spray

- This agent works by blocking cholinergic receptors. When administered intranasally, ipratropium may be effective in relieving rhinorrhea, but it does not affect sneezing, nasal itching, or nasal congestion. Adverse effects are minimal.

Immunotherapy

- Subcutaneous administration of standardized allergen extracts may suppress the allergic response (e.g., IgE antibody levels and basophil and lymphocyte responsiveness to allergens). Controlled trials of specific allergen extracts have proven the benefit of immunotherapy, but there is a real risk of anaphylaxis. The injections should be given only in controlled environments under appropriate medical supervision with the appropriate rescue drugs available. Immunotherapy should be limited to allergens to which the patient has demonstrated both a clinical and an IgE-mediated sensitivity.

Optimal Plan

4. a. *What drug, dosage form, dose, schedule, and duration of therapy are best for this patient?*

- The patient has a history of both perennial and seasonal allergic rhinitis that has failed a long trial of astemizole. If the sneezing, itching, and rhinorrhea were adequately controlled with the antihistamine, a systemic decongestant could be added to help control the congestion or assumed nasal blockage. However, the patient is still complaining of itching and sneezing.
- The efficacy of intranasal cromolyn is similar to that of the antihistamines, and intranasal corticosteroids appear to be more efficacious than intranasal cromolyn. Therefore, assuming the patient has been compliant, the next step in the patient's care should be a trial of an intranasal steroid. Also, if the patient is having continuous symptoms (this is not clear from the patient's history), intranasal steroids would be the agents of choice.[5] An aqueous-based spray given once daily is an effective regimen, given its potential for enhanced compliance and less nasal irritation than the CFC-based propellants. Examples of acceptable regimens include:
  - ✓ Beclomethasone 84 μg/actuation (Vancenase AQ Double Strength) 1 to 2 sprays in each nostril QD
  - ✓ Fluticasone 50 μg/actuation (Flonase) 2 sprays in each nostril QD

✓ Mometasone 50 µg/actuation (Nasonex) 2 sprays in each nostril QD
✓ Triamcinolone 55 µg/actuation (Nasacort AQ) 2 sprays in each nostril QD

Because the half-life of astemizole is so long, it can be discontinued at the initiation of the intranasal corticosteroid. A systemic decongestant (e.g., pseudoephedrine 30 to 60 mg po Q 6 H) or local decongestant (e.g., oxymetazoline 1 spray each nostril Q 12 H) can be used during the initial 3 to 5 days of steroid therapy.

b. *What alternatives would be available if the initial therapy fails?*

- Although little additive or synergistic effect has been shown in clinical trials, an oral antihistamine can be added to the intranasal corticosteroid to help relieve breakthrough symptoms.
- Because cromolyn appears to be less effective than intranasal corticosteroids, switching the patient to intranasal cromolyn is not likely to prove beneficial.
- If nasal symptoms are controlled but ocular symptoms continue to be bothersome, levocabastine (an ophthalmic antihistamine), lodoxamide tromethamine or cromolyn sodium (ophthalmic mast cell stabilizers), ketorolac tromethamine (Acular, an ophthalmic NSAID), or ophthalmic corticosteroid preparations may be used to control ocular symptoms.
- Patients failing an adequate trial of intranasal corticosteroids and avoidance therapy should be considered for immunotherapy. Patients should be informed that relief may not occur for at least 6 months and that therapy will need to continue for at least 3 years. Patients who respond are sometimes able to discontinue therapy after 3 years and maintain a reduction in symptoms or other medication use. Patients with coronary artery disease, severe hypertension, asthma, or atopic dermatitis are at an increased risk of death should anaphylaxis occur. Additionally, patients receiving β-blockers or monoamine oxidase inhibitors may not respond to epinephrine if anaphylaxis occurs. Finally, immunotherapy should not be started in a pregnant patient; however, if a patient receiving immunotherapy becomes pregnant, therapy may be continued.

Outcome Evaluation

5. *What clinical and laboratory parameters are necessary to evaluate the therapy for achievement of the desired therapeutic outcome and to detect or prevent adverse effects?*

- Monitoring parameters should be matched to the goals of therapy. In general, laboratory parameters are not used to monitor rhinitis therapy.
- Ask the patient to monitor for a decrease in symptoms over the short term. She should see some relief in 2 or 3 days. The patient should continue to monitor for a decrease in symptoms for another 3 to 4 weeks.
- Also have the patient monitor for potential adverse effects to the drugs used (see "patient counseling" section).
- At each return visit to the pharmacy or clinic, ask the patient about the symptoms she has had since the last visit as well as if she has had any nasal burning, stinging, or bleeding.
- Ask her whether or not she has had to use any non-prescription cough and cold preparations, antihistamines, or decongestants. Frequent or increased use of these agents should prompt a referral to her physician for further evaluation.
- Question the patient about how satisfied she is with the degree to which her allergic rhinitis is being controlled.

Patient Counseling

6. *What information should be provided to the patient to enhance compliance, ensure successful therapy, and minimize adverse effects?*

Example Information for Fluticasone Nasal Spray

- Your doctor has prescribed Flonase (fluticasone) nasal spray. This drug is a cortisone-like medication that belongs to the corticosteroid family. The drug is sprayed into the nose to help relieve the irritation, itching, and congestion caused by hay fever or allergies of the nose. These "steroid" drugs are different from the steroids that people use to build muscles, and unlike the non-prescription nose sprays, you cannot get "hooked" on steroid nose sprays.
- The directions are to spray 2 sprays in each side of your nose once a day. Use the drug every day, not just when your nose is itching or running or when you feel congested. Continue using this medication as directed until your doctor tells you to stop taking the drug.
- If you miss a dose of this medication and you remember it within 1 to 3 hours of when the dose is supposed to be given, you may take it at that time. Otherwise, wait until your next scheduled dose.
- The first time you use your nasal inhaler, it is important to make sure that there is drug in the spraying device. First, shake the bottle gently, then take the green cap off of the container. With the white spraying tip pointed away from you, hold the bottle with your thumb on the bottom and your index and middle finger on each side of the part that goes into your nose. Press down and release the pump 3 or 4 times until a nice spray appears. You should repeat this process if you do not use your inhaler for several days, but you do not have to do this every day.
- Let me demonstrate to you the correct way to use this nose spray.
    ✓ Before using your sprayer, blow your nose to clear any mucous or liquid from it.
    ✓ First, shake the bottle gently, then take the green cap off of the container.
    ✓ Hold the bottle with your thumb on the bottom and your index and middle finger on either side of the part that goes in your nose.
    ✓ Close one nostril with your finger, tilt your head slightly forward, and keeping the bottle upright, insert the white tip (called the nasal applicator) into the open nostril. Be sure the nasal applicator is pointed toward the corner of your eye and not toward the inner portion or septum of your nose.
    ✓ Start to breathe in through the open nostril, and while breathing in, press down on the white portion while supporting the bottom of the bottle with your thumb. Breathe in gently through the open nostril.
    ✓ Breathe out through your mouth.
    ✓ Repeat these steps for the same nostril, then repeat them twice for the other side of the nose.
    ✓ The green cap is a dust cover and should be put back on the bottle when you are through using it.
- Along with the good effects of this medicine, some undesired side effects may occur. These effects are uncommon and include nasal

burning or irritation and sneezing. Continued or excessive nasal stinging or irritation should be reported to your doctor. Rarely, a bloody discharge or crusty sores on the inside of the nose will occur; call your doctor if this happens. Also call your doctor if you have trouble breathing, tightness in the chest, persistent sore throat or cough, or swelling of the hands, face or feet.

- Store this drug with the cap on and out of the reach of children. Keep it stored in a place that has comfortable temperatures so that the drug does not freeze or become too hot. Do not use this drug if the date is past the date shown on the label or the box.
- Clean your nasal sprayer at least once a week. Remove the green cap and gently pull upward on the white nasal applicator portion of the sprayer to remove it from the bottle. Wash the white applicator and dust cover in warm tap water and allow them to dry at room temperature. Replace the white applicator portion on the bottle and replace the green cap. If the nasal applicator becomes blocked, remove the applicator and let it soak in warm water. Do not use a pin, knife, or other sharp object to unblock the nasal applicator.

References

1. Long WF, Taylor RJ, Wagner CJ, et al. Skin test suppression by antihistamines and the development of subsensitivity. J Allergy Clin Immunol 1985;76:113–117.
2. Simons FE, Watson WT, Simons KJ. Lack of subsensitivity to terfenadine during long-term terfenadine treatment. J Allergy Clin Immunol. 1988;82:1068–1075.
3. Girard JP, Sommacal-Schopf D, Bigliardi P, et al. Double-blind comparison of astemizole, terfenadine and placebo in hay fever with special regard to onset of action. J Int Med Res 1985;13:102–108.
4. Gastpar H, Aurich R, Petzold U, et al. Intranasal treatment of perennial allergic rhinitis. Comparison of azelastine nasal spray and budesonide nasal aerosol. Arzneimittelforschung 1993;43:475–479.
5. International Rhinitis Management Working Group. International Consensus Report on the diagnosis and management of rhinitis. Allergy 1994;49(19 suppl): 1–34.

SECTION 12
Dermatologic Disorders
L. Michael Posey, RPh, Section Editor

86 ACNE VULGARIS

▶ **The Graduate** (Level II)

Rebecca M. Law, PharmD
Wayne P. Gulliver, MD, FRCPC

An 18-year-old female with polycystic ovarian syndrome who has been recently treated with two courses of minocycline and topical adapalene for acne presents to her physician because of an acne flare accompanied by some scarring and cyst formation. The patient is a candidate for systemic isotretinoin because she has failed both topical therapies and systemic antimicrobials and has some facial scarring. Systemic hormonal therapy with oral contraceptives containing low doses of estrogen may also be considered because of the influence of elevated testosterone levels associated with polycystic ovarian syndrome. In this situation, the oral contraceptive can help improve acne, regulate her menstrual cycle, reduce excessive facial hair, and prevent pregnancy during treatment with the teratogenic drug isotretinoin. With isotretinoin therapy, some improvement in acne may occur within 4 to 6 weeks, but complete clearing may take up to 3 or 4 months. Isotretinoin has a number of adverse effects that require periodic clinical and laboratory monitoring and comprehensive patient education.

▶ Questions

Problem Identification

1. a. Create a drug-related problem list for this patient.

- Facial acne, inadequately or inappropriately treated with the present regimen.
- Dysmenorrhea due to polycystic ovarian disease, presently untreated.

b. What signs and symptoms consistent with acne does this patient demonstrate?

- The patient has comedones on her forehead, nose, and chin; papules and pustules on her nose and malar area; and a few cysts on her chin.
- She also has scars on the malar area and an increased amount of facial hair. The scarring is of some concern.

c. How does polycystic ovarian disease contribute to this patient's acne and other physical findings?

- Polycystic ovarian disease results in increased free testosterone levels that can result in mild hirsutism and a tendency to acne.

Desired Outcome

2. What are the treatment goals for this patient?

- Induce complete remission of her acne to prevent additional scarring (both physical and psychological)
- Discontinue aggravating factors
- Prevent future flare-ups
- Minimize drug toxicity

Therapeutic Alternatives

3. *What feasible therapeutic alternatives are available for management of this patient's acne?*

- *Topical therapy* is usually used for patients with non-inflammatory comedones or mild to moderate inflammatory acne, with the goal of opening the skin pores and reducing *Propionebacterium acnes* infection.[1] Products include mild and gentle cleansers and the following pharmacologic agents.
  - ✓ *Benzoyl peroxide*
  - ✓ *Azelaic acid*
  - ✓ *Tretinoin* (a retinoid)
  - ✓ *Tazarotene* (a retinoid pro-drug)
  - ✓ *Adapalene* (a naphthoic acid derivative with retinoid-like activity)[2]
  - ✓ *Topical antibiotics* (erythromycin and clindamycin)
  - ✓ *Salicylic acid* and other anti-inflammatory/keratolytic agents.

  These can be used singly but are more effective when used in combination; the best combinations are those that combine a retinoid and a benzoyl peroxide-containing product.

- *Systemic therapy* is used when moderate to severe inflammatory acne does not respond to topical treatments.
  - ✓ *Minocycline, doxycycline, tetracycline,* and *erythromycin* are oral antibiotics that suppress *P. acnes* and decrease the percentage of free fatty acids in surface lipids. At appropriate doses, they are both bactericidal and anti-inflammatory. Doxycycline and especially minocycline are more lipid soluble and are considered more effective than tetracycline or erythromycin.[1]
  - ✓ *Isotretinoin (Accutane)* is an oral agent useful for patients who have failed combination therapy with oral antibiotics and topical tretinoin.[1,3,4] It affects abnormal follicular keratinization and inhibits sebaceous gland function, causing a marked decrease in sebum production within 2 weeks of therapy. It is indicated for patients with nodular and/or inflammatory acne and for recalcitrant acne unresponsive to other therapies. The usual starting dose is 0.5 to 1 mg/kg/day in 1 daily dose or 2 divided daily doses for 4 to 6 weeks, followed by a maintenance dose between 0.1 to 1 mg/kg/day for a total of 12 to 16 weeks. European recommendations use lower daily doses given over a longer period of time; starting at doses < 0.5 mg/kg/day and slowly titrating upward helps to minimize the flare-up of acne that may occur upon initiating therapy. Remission tends to be long lasting even after stopping therapy. Even if clearance is incomplete, patients usually continue to improve for 4 to 5 months after therapy is discontinued. Because this patient has failed topical therapies, has required two courses of oral antibiotics in the past year, and has facial scarring, she is a candidate for isotretinoin therapy.
  - ✓ *Systemic hormonal therapy* (limited to female patients), reduces sebum production by counteracting androgenic effects on the sebaceous gland. This is useful in females where hormonal influences are evident, such as those with polycystic ovary syndrome, which may also be manifested by the presence of hirsutism, menstrual irregularities, elevated free testosterone levels, and hair loss.[5] Hormonal therapy consists of ovarian suppression using oral contraceptives with low-dose estrogens (35 to 50 µg); antiandrogens such as spironolactone, cyproterone acetate, or flutamide; low-dose glucocorticoids using prednisone or dexamethasone to suppress adrenal androgen; or a combination of oral contraceptives and dexamethasone.[5] This patient is a candidate for hormonal therapy because she has menstrual irregularities, hirsutism, and elevated free testosterone levels.

Optimal Plan

4. *What treatment regimen is best suited for this patient?*

- Isotretinoin 40 mg once daily with dinner for 6 weeks then reassess, for a total duration of 4 months.
- A low-dose oral contraceptive such as Tri-Cyclen-28 should also be started immediately and continued after isotretinoin is completed. The oral contraceptive will help reduce facial acne and hirsutism, regulate her menstrual cycle, and minimize the likelihood of conception while taking isotretinoin, a known teratogen.
- Topical therapies are probably inappropriate for this patient. Products containing benzoyl peroxide were found to be too drying for her previously and should not be used in conjunction with isotretinoin, which also commonly causes drying of the mucosa of the mouth, nose, and eyes. Topical therapies do not usually act any faster than systemic therapies; achievement of clinical response using any therapeutic regimen may take 4 to 8 weeks. Occasionally, there is an exacerbation of acne after initiation of topical comedolytic therapy.
- Systemic antibiotics for acne should not be used in conjunction with isotretinoin and oral contraceptives because they may decrease contraceptive effectiveness, but topical antibiotics may be used.[6]
- The patient may benefit from stress reduction exercises and guidance counseling. Her anxiety about graduation is likely a factor in her multiple flare-ups this past year.

Outcome Evaluation

5. *How would you monitor the therapy you recommended for efficacy and adverse effects?*

Efficacy

- Improvement (as indicated by a decrease in lesion count) may take 4 to 6 weeks, and complete clearance often requires 3 to 4 months. However, clearance may occur by 2 months in some cases. The patient should return to clinic in 6 weeks for reassessment.
- If isotretinoin and the oral contraceptive are found to be beneficial (as indicated by a decrease in lesion count), the isotretinoin should be continued for a total of 4 months and the oral contraceptive should be continued indefinitely.
- For patients using isotretinoin alone, it is important to recognize that the patient may continue to improve after the isotretinoin is discontinued.

Adverse Effects

- Isotretinoin may cause hypervitaminosis A-induced mucocutaneous or dermatologic side effects including cheilitis, facial dermatitis, dry or cracked lips, dry mouth, dry nose leading to nosebleeds, and dry eyes causing decreased tolerance to contact lenses. Drying of the skin with scaling, thinning, erythema, and pruritus may also occur. Hair loss may occur but is usually transient.
- Systemic effects of isotretinoin include photosensitivity, skeletal hy-

perostosis, joint pains, headaches, pseudotumor cerebri (rare), ocular opacities, and diminished night vision.
- Isotretinoin may cause increased serum triglycerides and cholesterol, transient increases in liver transaminases, leukopenia, and anemia. A complete blood count and serum chemistries, liver function tests, cholesterol and triglycerides should be obtained before starting treatment and at monthly intervals. If clinically significant increases are seen, isotretinoin may be discontinued or the dose reduced. If triglycerides exceed 800 mg/dL (4 times normal) or if the patient complains of abdominal pain, amylase and lipase levels should be obtained to rule out pancreatitis.[4]
- Isotretinoin may cause depression, psychosis, and (rarely) suicidal ideation, suicide attempts, and suicide. If these effects occur, discontinuation of therapy may be insufficient, and further evaluation may be necessary. However, patients with acne often have poor self-image, are depressed, and have difficulty getting jobs and interacting socially. These problems may be greatly improved with oral isotretinoin, and this fact should be emphasized to patients rather than the possibility that the drug causes depression.
- Isotretinoin is teratogenic, and an effective means of contraception must be used consistently and for at least a month after stopping therapy. The drug should be started on day 2 or 3 of the upcoming menstrual cycle for a sexually active woman to ensure the absence of pregnancy and avoid the risk of teratogenicity. All patients on isotretinoin, including males, should be told to avoid donating blood during therapy and for at least 1 month after stopping isotretinoin.
- Oral contraceptives may occasionally cause nausea and/or vomiting especially during the first cycle. Spotting or light breakthrough bleeding may also occur transiently during the first 3 months.

Patient Counseling

6. *How would you counsel the patient about this treatment regimen to enhance compliance and ensure successful therapy?*

General Information
- It may take 4 to 6 weeks for you to notice improvement in your acne condition. We will see you again in clinic in 6 weeks. Complete clearance may occur by 2 months but often requires 3 to 4 months of treatment.
- To minimize aggravating acne, use oil-free make-up and avoid make-up regimens that require multiple layering. Avoid hair sprays since they may clog pores.
- Wash your face no more than twice daily with a mild, non-alkaline soap or soapless cleanser. Avoid vigorous scrubbing, as this may rupture lesions and cause additional inflammation.
- Your acne condition may have been exacerbated by recent stresses in your life. Stress reduction exercises and guidance counseling may help. We can arrange for you to meet regularly with a counselor.

Isotretinoin
- Start this medication on day 3 of your upcoming normal menstrual cycle. Take 1 capsule (40 mg) daily with dinner.
- This medication can cause serious birth defects in a growing fetus. You MUST use birth control during and for at least 1 month after stopping this drug because you are sexually active. In your case, an oral contraceptive will be started and continued after the isotretinoin course is completed.
- Do not donate blood while taking isotretinoin and for at least 1 month thereafter. If the blood is given to a pregnant mother, there may be enough medication present to cause malformations in her growing baby.
- Avoid excessive use of alcohol while taking this medication. This drug may increase your triglyceride levels, and concurrent alcohol use can make this effect more likely.
- Dryness of your eyes, mouth, and nose (possibly resulting in nosebleeds) may occur. Moisturizing eye drops or eye ointments may be helpful. Use of hard sugarless candies or ice chips may help the dry mouth. If excessive skin dryness occurs, it may help to use a water-based moisturizer.
- You may be more sensitive to sunburn while taking this medication. Avoid prolonged exposure to sunlight and always use a sunscreen with at least SPF 15 protection when you are outdoors.
- Thinning of the hair occurs rarely and is usually a temporary effect. Hair may grow back while treatment is still ongoing. If it does not, it usually regrows once treatment is stopped.
- If you greatly increase your exercise level, you may notice aching and painful muscles that may sometimes be severe. Please let us know if this occurs.
- Contact your doctor or me if you consistently feel more sad or depressed than usual. This drug occasionally causes patients to feel depressed, or even suicidal. Please talk to us immediately if you have any of those feelings. Actually, it is more likely that you are going to feel better and have a more positive self-image as your acne improves.
- You will also need blood tests from time to time while taking this medication, because this drug occasionally causes increases in cholesterol and triglycerides and changes in blood cell counts.

Oral Contraceptive Example: Tri-Cyclen-28
- This medication is an oral contraceptive (birth control pill) that will help to improve your acne, reduce the excess facial hair growth you have experienced, help to regulate your menstrual periods, and prevent you from becoming pregnant while taking the isotretinoin.
- Take 1 tablet each day at approximately the same time of day. There are 28 tablets in a pack; 21 tablets contain medication and 7 contain no medication.
- Start the first tablet of each pack on the first day of your upcoming menstrual cycle. This should also help to regulate your period so that it occurs on the last 7 days of each pack.
- Many women have some spotting or light bleeding or feel sick to their stomach during the first 3 months on the pill. Do not stop taking the pill if this occurs because these effects usually go away with continued treatment. Contact your doctor if you experience excessive menstrual bleeding.
- Missing pills can also cause spotting or light bleeding, even if you make up the missed pills. Follow the instructions in the pack if you do happen to miss 1 or 2 doses.
- Continue taking the oral contraceptive even after your isotretinoin is completed. This medication will help control your acne, regulate your menstrual cycle, and reduce the amount of facial hair.

References

1. Leyden JJ. Therapy for acne vulgaris. N Engl J Med 1997;336:1156–1162.
2. Brogden RN, Goa KE. Adapalene: A review of its pharmacological properties and clinical potential in the management of mild to moderate acne. Drugs 1997;53:511–519.
3. al-Khawajah MM. Isotretinoin for acne vulgaris. Int J Dermatol 1996;35:212–215.
4. James M. Isotretinoin for severe acne. Lancet 1996;347:1749–1750.
5. Cheung AP, Chang RJ. Polycystic ovary syndrome. Clin Obstet Gynecol 1990;33:655–667.
6. Berson DS, Shalita AR. The treatment of acne: The role of combination therapies. J Am Acad Dermatol 1995;32(5 Pt 3):S31–S41.

87 PSORIASIS

▶ The Harried School Teacher   (Level II)

Rebecca M. Law, PharmD

A 55-year-old woman with a 30-year history of psoriasis is admitted with an extensive flare-up of plaque psoriasis. She had been taking methotrexate 25 mg once weekly, and periodic flare-ups had been treated with SCAT (short contact anthralin therapy). Because the patient has failed topical therapies and is receiving the maximum recommended methotrexate dose, the optimal treatment plan should involve replacing methotrexate with other systemic therapies such as acitretin or cyclosporine used alone or on a rotating basis (to minimize toxicities and increase efficacy). Azathioprine, tacrolimus, or hydroxyurea would be acceptable options if she fails acitretin and cyclosporine. Topical therapies such as salicylic acid in bath oil applied to the scalp and continuation of SCAT to heavily crusted lesions would be beneficial. Careful clinical and laboratory monitoring is required because of the potential toxicities of cyclosporine and acitretin.

▶ Questions

Problem Identification

1. a. Create a list of this patient's drug-related problems.

- Psoriasis inadequately controlled or inappropriately treated with current treatments (methotrexate and SCAT).
- Work-related stress that may require evaluation and drug or other treatments.
- Postmenopausal state and receiving HRT, which may require assessment.

b. What signs and symptoms consistent with psoriasis does this patient demonstrate?

- The patient has confluent plaques with extensive lesions on her abdomen, arms, legs, back, and scalp. She also has thick crusted lesions on her elbows, knees, palms, and soles. These areas of involvement are consistent with a severe flare-up of psoriasis.
- The color and description of the lesions (red to violet in color with sharply demarcated borders except where confluent, and loosely covered with silvery-white scales) are consistent with plaque psoriasis.
- There are no pustules or vesicles to indicate this is pustular psoriasis. There are no indications of psoriatic arthritis.

c. What risk factors for a flare-up of psoriasis are present in this patient?

- She complains of feeling jumpy and appears to be under some stress in her work with the school board. The increasing stress could explain the frequent flare-ups of her psoriasis in the past 4 months.

d. Could the signs and symptoms be caused by any drug therapy she is receiving?

- She is not receiving any drugs known to precipitate psoriasis (e.g., lithium, β-blockers, indomethacin, antimalarials, fluoxetine).
- Withdrawal of corticosteroids after prolonged use and hypocalcemia may also exacerbate psoriasis; neither of these is a cause in this patient.
- Neither progesterone nor conjugated estrogens have been reported to precipitate psoriasis.

Desired Outcome

2. What are the goals of pharmacotherapy for psoriasis in this patient?

- Eliminate plaque-like skin lesions and achieve remission if possible
- Prevent future flare-ups (relapses) of the psoriasis
- Relieve her work-related stress through non-pharmacologic and/or pharmacologic means
- Minimize drug-related toxicity and ensure no significant drug interactions with current medications

Therapeutic Alternatives

3. a. What non-pharmacologic alternatives are available for managing the patient's psoriasis?

- Stress reduction (e.g., psychotherapy that includes stress management, guided imagery, and relaxation techniques) has been shown to improve the extent and severity of psoriasis.

b. *What feasible pharmacotherapeutic alternatives are available for controlling the patient's disease at this point?*

- Pharmacotherapy for plaque psoriasis consists of topical treatments, phototherapy, and systemic therapies.
- *Topical therapies* include *crude coal tar, corticosteroids, calcipotriol, anthralin including SCAT* with high anthralin concentrations [2% to 4%] for 20 minutes to 2 hours, and tazarotene 0.05% or 0.1% gel. These treatments constitute first-line therapy.
- *Phototherapy* includes UVB alone, or photochemotherapy using UVB with topical crude coal tar, UVB with topical anthralin, or UVA with oral psoralens (PUVA).
- *Systemic therapies* are second- to third-line and are used for moderate to severe psoriasis insufficiently managed by topical treatments. Systemic therapies are used in a rotating fashion to minimize drug toxicities (e.g., methotrexate, acitretin, cyclosporine or methotrexate, PUVA, acitretin).
  - ✓ *Sulfasalazine* has variable efficacy and is of limited potency. However, its side-effects profile is better than other systemic therapies.
  - ✓ *Methotrexate* (variable dosage range of 2.5 to 25 mg once/week) is more effective than sulfasalazine but carries a risk of hepatotoxicity. A liver biopsy should be performed prior to use and repeated when a cumulative dose of about 1.5 g is reached. Periodic CBCs, renal function tests, and pulmonary toxicity tests should also be conducted.
  - ✓ *Acitretin* is the free-acid metabolite of etretinate and is more potent when used with PUVA. It may produce a more rapid initial response than methotrexate for patients with severe inflammatory forms of psoriasis, and it has antineoplastic properties. Although not a problem in this case, it is teratogenic and relatively contraindicated in women of childbearing potential. Other side effects include ophthalmologic, neuromuscular, and hyperlipidemic changes (see "outcome evaluation: Adverse effects").
  - ✓ *Cyclosporine* is generally reserved for treatment failures. The risk of nephrotoxicity is higher in psoriatic patients than renal transplant recipients; drug-induced hypertension and possible carcinogenesis are also of concern. Intermittent cyclosporine used in < 6-month cycles with other systemic agents such as a retinoid is useful in prolonging the disease-free period and in minimizing drug toxicities. The recommended starting dose of cyclosporine is 2.5 mg/kg/day given orally in 2 divided doses. If an inadequate response is observed by 3 months, the dose may be gradually increased to a maximum of 5 mg/kg/day. Cyclosporine should be discontinued if there is insufficient response after 3 months at the maximum dose.[1,2]
  - ✓ *Azathioprine* has been used in doses of 50 mg twice daily. However, the response time is slower than methotrexate or cyclosporine.
  - ✓ *Tacrolimus (FK506)* is an immunosuppressive agent used to prevent organ transplant rejection that has shown dramatic effectiveness for patients with psoriasis. However, similar to cyclosporine, side effects include nephrotoxicity and hypertension.[3]
  - ✓ *Hydroxyurea* (500 mg twice daily) is an option in patients who have contraindications to methotrexate due to liver disease.
  - ✓ *Oral corticosteroids* are reserved for severe or life-threatening conditions such as severe psoriatic arthritis or exfoliative psoriasis; prolonged steroid use should be avoided.
- *Intralesional corticosteroid injections* (triamcinolone acetonide 5 to 10 mg/mL or triamcinolone hexacetonide 5 mg/mL) may be useful for small, localized, recalcitrant plaques.

Optimal Plan

4. *What drug regimen is best suited for treating this flare of the patient's psoriasis?*

- The patient has failed topical and photochemotherapies with the exception of SCAT for defined limited lesions, and her current regimen of weekly oral methotrexate appears to be inadequate. Increasing the methotrexate dose is not an appropriate option, since a recent dosage increase has not been beneficial. Also, she has already received a cumulative lifetime dose of 2.2 g, although a recent liver biopsy showed no hepatocellular changes as yet.
- The most appropriate options are other systemic therapies such as acitretin or cyclosporine used alone, or preferably *both* agents used on a rotating basis to minimize toxicities and increase efficacy. Retinoids such as acitretin may be effective for her since they have not been used previously; and she is now postmenopausal so teratogenicity is no longer a concern. Retinoids and cyclosporine have differing toxicities and different target sites and may have a synergistic therapeutic effect. Therefore, it is preferable to use them in alternating sequence rather than either agent alone, even though single-drug use is acceptable and often done in practice.
- Sulfasalazine is not appropriate for her since it is less effective than methotrexate.
- Azathioprine, tacrolimus, or hydroxyurea would be acceptable options if she fails acitretin and cyclosporine. Azathioprine has a slower onset of effect, and there is less experience with tacrolimus for psoriasis.
- In addition to systemic therapy, topical therapies such as salicylic acid in bath oil applied to the scalp and continuation of SCAT to heavily crusted lesions would be beneficial.
- The methotrexate should be discontinued, and a trial of low-dose cyclosporine every 3 to 4 months alternating with acitretin should be started, together with SCAT to the heavily crusted lesions. Intermittent low-dose cyclosporine should be started at 2.5 mg/kg/day given in 2 divided doses for 3 months. Although cyclosporine has been suggested to be gradually withdrawn (decrease dose by 0.5 to 1 mg/kg/day every 1 to 2 weeks until discontinued) to theoretically avoid rebound psoriasis, current research indicates that this is not necessary. Cyclosporine can be discontinued abruptly when acitretin is started. The specific drug regimen is as follows: cyclosporine microemulsion (Neoral) 75 mg twice daily for 3 months, followed by acitretin (Soriatane) 25 mg once daily with dinner for 3 months, and repeat. There is a potential for HRT to interact with cyclosporine but the clinical significance would be minor.
- For the scalp, an appropriate regimen is salicylic acid 10% in bath oil applied nightly to the scalp and covered with a shower cap overnight

plus a tar shampoo used 3 times weekly until the scalp lesions clear. An alternative therapy is betamethasone 0.1% lotion for the scalp applied twice daily.
- SCAT (4% anthralin paste applied twice daily for 2 hours then wiped off) should be continued on thickly crusted lesions until improvement is seen.

Outcome Evaluation

5. How should you monitor the therapy you recommended for efficacy and adverse effects?

Efficacy

- Psoriatic lesions do not improve overnight. However, some improvement should be apparent within 1 week for topical therapies and within 2 to 4 weeks for systemic therapies. Scalp lesions should have less scaling and erythema (due to salicylic acid and shampoo treatments) and the thickly crusted lesions on her body should be reduced (due to SCAT treatment) within 1 week.
- She should see an overall improvement within a month (due to cyclosporine). Improvement after 1 month on cyclosporine may be modest, but it may be appropriate to continue at the same dose for up to 3 months before concluding that a higher dose is warranted.[2]

Adverse Effects of Cyclosporine[2]

- Prior to starting therapy, a serum creatinine should be measured after a 12-hour fast on at least 2 separate occasions. If these values vary by more than 10 μmol/L (0.11 mg/dL), additional measurements are recommended. The mean value of these measurements is used as her baseline creatinine during subsequent monitoring.
- Serum creatinine and BP should be measured every 2 weeks for the first 6 weeks of therapy and monthly thereafter. More frequent monitoring is recommended if the cyclosporine dose is increased or if a rise in creatinine or BP is noted.
- Serum cyclosporine concentrations are not routinely measured in patients receiving the drug for psoriasis.
- If hypertension develops (mean diastolic BP > 95 mm Hg on 2 consecutive occasions), the cyclosporine dose may be decreased or nifedipine may be added. If the creatinine rises to > 30% above her baseline value, it should be repeated within 2 weeks. If the rise in creatinine is sustained, the cyclosporine dose should be decreased by at least 1 mg/kg/day for at least 1 month. The cyclosporine should be continued only if the creatinine drops back to < 30% above baseline value. Otherwise, cyclosporine should be withheld and resumed only when the creatinine is within 10% of her baseline value. If the repeated creatinine rises > 30% upon reintroduction of cyclosporine, alternate therapy is recommended, or a nephrologist should be consulted concerning continued cyclosporine use.
- Baseline measurements of liver enzymes, serum potassium, and screening for proteinuria are also recommended. Bilirubin, uric acid, fasting lipids, and serum magnesium measurements may also be useful but are not obligatory. Hepatotoxicity or hyperlipidemia during cyclosporine treatment may require a dosage reduction. Bilirubin, liver enzymes, fasting lipids, and serum potassium measurements should be followed periodically during therapy (e.g., every 2 months).
- Advise the patient to comply with screening procedures for malignancy.
- Other possible adverse effects include tremor, hypertrichosis, gingival hyperplasia, and headache.

Acitretin Adverse Effects

- Hypervitaminosis A induced mucocutaneous side effects include dry or cracked lips, dry mouth, dry nose leading to nosebleeds, and dry eyes causing conjunctivitis. Drying of the skin with scaling, thinning, erythema, and pruritus may also occur. Hair thinning and frank alopecia may occur within the first 3 months of use but is usually transient.
- Systemic effects include hyperostosis (hypertrophy of bone), aching muscles, increased serum triglycerides and cholesterol, transient increases in liver transaminase levels, hepatitis, leukopenia, and posterior subcapsular cataracts. Liver function tests should be performed every 1 to 2 weeks for the first 1 to 2 months of therapy, then every 1 to 3 months thereafter depending on the changes seen.
- Although teratogenicity is not a concern for this patient, she should be told not to be a blood donor during therapy and for 2 years after stopping acitretin use.

Patient Counseling

6. What information should be provided to the patient to enhance compliance and ensure successful therapy?

General Information

- There should be less scaling and redness for your scalp lesions and a reduction in the thickly crusted areas within 1 week. You should notice general improvement in your condition within a month. Your palms, soles, elbows, and knee areas may take longer to clear.
- It is important to keep all follow-up appointments with your physician.

Cyclosporine

- Take a 25-mg capsule and a 50-mg capsule (total dose 75 mg) twice daily with breakfast and dinner. Do not drink grapefruit juice with it. Do not use salt substitutes (containing potassium) while on this medication.
- This medication sometimes causes high blood pressure and kidney damage. Periodic blood pressure checks and blood tests are needed to detect and treat these changes early.
- Headaches and tremors can also occur; contact your doctor if these become troublesome or persistent.
- Rarely, this medication causes cancers to develop. Make sure you keep all your clinic appointments, including screening procedures for malignancy.

Acitretin

- Take 1 capsule daily with dinner.
- Do not donate blood while taking this medication and for 2 years after you stop taking it. If the blood is given to a pregnant mother, there may be enough medication present to cause malformations in her growing baby.
- Dryness of your eyes, mouth, and nose (possibly resulting in nosebleeds) may occur. Moisturizing eye drops may be helpful. Use of hard sugarless candies or ice chips may help the dry mouth.
- You may notice some hair thinning, which infrequently leads to baldness. This is a temporary effect that is often seen within the first 3 months of use. The hair may grow back again while treatment is

still ongoing. If it does not, it usually regrows once treatment is stopped.
- If you greatly increase your exercise level, you may notice aching and painful muscles that sometimes can be severe. Please let us know if this occurs.
- You will also need blood tests periodically while taking this medication.

SCAT
- While wearing gloves, apply the anthralin paste *only* on the thickly crusted areas. Leave the paste on for 2 hours and then wipe it off. Contact us if you notice severe burning.

Salicylic Acid in Bath Oil
- Apply the oil to the roots of your hairs (that is, your scalp) every night before sleeping. Cover with a shower cap overnight. The next morning shampoo it off.
- Use the tar shampoo 3 times a week.

References

1. Finzi AF. Individualized short-course cyclosporin therapy in psoriasis. Br J Dermatol 1996;135(suppl 48):31–34.
2. Berth-Jones J, Voorhees JJ. Consensus conference on cyclosporin A microemulsion for psoriasis, June 1996. Br J Dermatol 1996;135:775–777.
3. Jegasothy BV, Ackerman CD, Todo S, et al. Tacrolimus (FK506): a new therapeutic agent for severe recalcitrant psoriasis. Arch Dermatol 1992;128:781–785.

SECTION 13

Hematologic Disorders
Gary C. Yee, PharmD, FCCP, Section Editor

88 IRON DEFICIENCY ANEMIA

▶ **Bertha's Belly Pain** (Level I)

William E. Wade, PharmD, FASHP, FCCP
William J. Spruill, PharmD

A 40-year-old woman with a history of heavy menses and nonprescription NSAID (naproxen) use presents to the pharmacy complaining of abdominal pain and fatigue. Referral to a physician for evaluation reveals laboratory findings of iron deficiency anemia. An esophagogastroduodenoscopy (EGD) reveals the presence of extensive gastritis, presumably secondary to NSAID use. Treatment of iron deficiency anemia is directed toward removing underlying causes, relieving the patient's symptoms, and correcting abnormal laboratory values. In addition to a diet high in iron content, the usually recommended pharmacotherapy consists of treatment for 3 to 6 months with an oral ferrous salt (sulfate, fumarate, or gluconate) given in 2 to 3 divided doses sufficient to provide about 200 mg of elemental iron per day. The reticulocyte count may be used as an initial indicator of response to iron therapy. Hemoglobin values will increase by 1 to 2 g/dL per week until normalization occurs. Therapy must be continued until iron stores are repleted, which may take as long as 3 to 6 months. The serum ferritin is the best indicator of repletion of iron stores.

▶ **Questions**

Problem Identification

1. a. *What potential drug-related problems does this patient have?*

    - Iron deficiency anemia requiring treatment.
    - Gastritis secondary to non-prescription naproxen use in this patient with a history of ranitidine treatment for PUD/gastritis and no information on length of treatment, healing, or recurrence.
    - No current GI cytoprotective therapy for NSAID-induced gastritis.
    - Higher than recommended dose of non-prescription naproxen.

   b. *What signs, symptoms, and laboratory findings are consistent with the finding of iron deficiency anemia secondary to blood loss?*

Signs
- Spooning of nails (koilonychia)
- Pale conjunctivae
- Guaiac (+) stool
- Endoscopy indicated severe gastritis with multiple bleeding gastric erosions
- The patient does *not* have the signs of angular stomatitis and glossitis that are sometimes seen

Symptoms
- Mild fatigue and tiring easily
- History of heavy menses
- History of routine naproxen use in a patient with a history of gastritis/PUD may increase GI blood loss

Laboratory Values
- Low hemoglobin, hematocrit, and RBC count

- Elevated RDW
- RBC indices indicate a low MCV (microcytosis) and a low MCH and MCHC (hypochromia)
- Decreased serum iron and an elevated TIBC result in a low transferrin saturation
- Low serum ferritin level is most diagnostic of iron deficiency anemia
- Normal vitamin B_{12} and folic acid levels rule out the presence of a megaloblastic anemia

c. *Could any of the patient's symptoms or laboratory abnormalities be drug-related?*

- NSAID-induced gastropathy can in result in "belly pain."
- NSAID-induced gastropathy can in result in bleeding that contributes to iron deficiency anemia (and fatigue).

Desired Outcome

2. *What are the goals of pharmacotherapy for this patient's anemia?*

- Remove underlying causes of iron loss if possible (e.g., eliminate use of NSAIDs for osteoarthritis)
- Correct the anemia and relieve the patient's fatigue with appropriate iron replacement therapy
- Assess arthritis symptoms to determine the most appropriate therapy
- Counsel the patient about NSAID-related gastropathy and recommend periodic reassessment

Therapeutic Alternatives

3. a. *What non-drug therapy may be effective in managing this anemia?*

- Ingestion of food substances high in iron (e.g., meat, fish, poultry, and orange juice)
- Intake of foods high in ascorbic acid
- Avoidance of foods that reduce dietary iron absorption (e.g., tea, milk, and dairy products)

b. *What alternative drug therapy could be used to treat this patient's anemia?*

- In most cases, the recommended treatment is oral iron therapy with a soluble ferrous iron salt that delivers approximately 200 mg of elemental iron per day in 2 to 3 divided doses. The ferrous salt forms are all absorbed equally well but contain different amounts of elemental iron, as shown in Table 88–1. For this reason, the dose required to administer the required daily dose varies depending upon which salt is used. Ferric salts are not recommended because they are not as well absorbed as ferrous salts.

TABLE 88–1. Ferrous Salt Forms

Salt	Mg/Tablet	Iron Content (mg)	Elemental Iron (%)
Ferrous sulfate	325	65	20
Ferrous sulfate, dried	159	50	30
Ferrous fumarate	300	99	33
Ferrous gluconate	325	38	11.6

- The ferrous salts are available generically as non-enteric coated products. They are also available as various brand name sustained-release products of ferrous sulfate (e.g., slow-FE, Ferro-Gradumet, Ferospace, Ferra-TD), ferrous fumarate (e.g., Ferrosequels, Span-FF), and ferrous gluconate (e.g., Ferralet). These sustained-release forms generally offer little therapeutic advantage. Claims of less GI side effects or better bioavailability have not been proven to be clinically significant. In addition, sustained-release forms may transport iron past the major absorption sites of the small intestine, thereby attenuating the hematinic response.[1]
- Some iron products contain extra ingredients such as ascorbic acid (e.g., Ferro-Grad 500, Ferancee) to enhance iron absorption, or a stool softener (e.g., Ferro-DSS, Hemaspan) to decrease iron-related constipation. Products containing ascorbic acid have been shown to only slightly increase iron absorption and should not be routinely recommended.[2] Some products contain a only small dose of the stool softener docusate, which is not enough to be effective. If needed, docusate should be recommended in optimal doses of 50 to 100 mg per day.
- Parenteral iron (iron dextran) may be required for patients who are truly intolerant of oral iron therapy or who have a significant compliance problem with oral iron.[3] The dose may be administered as either weekly IM injections or as a larger IV infusion of parenteral iron (total dose infusion). IM iron dextran is quite painful upon injection, whereas IV iron dextran may cause a hypersensitivity reaction during infusion.
- Packed red blood cell transfusions can be used for patients who are severely anemic.

Optimal Plan

4. *Outline an optimal pharmacotherapy plan for this patient.*

- One of the most common regimens is ferrous sulfate 300 to 325 mg po TID, preferably given on an empty stomach, for 3 to 6 months. Therapy may be initiated at a reduced dosage to decrease initial GI side effects and may be taken with food if GI upset is a problem. Anemic patients need approximately 200 mg of elemental iron per day.
- Other acceptable therapies include ferrous gluconate 325 mg or ferrous fumarate 200 mg po TID on an empty stomach for at least 3 to 6 months. Both of these alternative therapies provide less elemental iron per day, but may also decrease GI intolerance. However, it will take proportionately longer to correct the anemia with these reduced doses.

Outcome Evaluation

5. *What clinical and laboratory parameters are necessary to evaluate the therapy for achievement of the desired therapeutic outcome and to detect and prevent adverse effects?*

Efficacy

- Symptomatic improvement may be documented by resolution of complaints verbalized by the patient (e.g., fatigue, lethargy).
- An increased reticulocyte count 7 to 10 days after beginning iron therapy (reticulocytosis) can be used to confirm that the patient is responding to oral iron therapy. This initial reticulocytosis is only seen for the first 2 weeks of treatment and should not be used as a monitoring parameter after this time.

- Normalization of the hemoglobin, hematocrit, RBC count, MCV, MCH, MCHC, RDW, serum iron, TIBC, transferrin saturation, and serum ferritin occur at different time intervals. Serum hemoglobin values should increase by 1 to 2 g/dL per week until normalization occurs. After correction of the hemoglobin and hematocrit, serum ferritin may be performed at 6 months and 1 year.

Adverse Effects

- Potential GI effects include nausea, constipation, diarrhea, abdominal pain, and dark stools. Administration of iron with meals may be necessary if GI adverse effects are experienced.

Patient Counseling

6. *What information should be provided to the patient to enhance compliance, ensure successful therapy, and minimize adverse effects?*

- Take this medication 3 times a day on an empty stomach (1 hour before or 2 hours after meals).
- Take each dose with a full glass of water or fruit juice.
- Possible side effects include nausea, abdominal pain, and constipation or diarrhea. These effects usually resolve with continued therapy. If stomach or abdominal side effects continue, take this medication with meals, but less iron is absorbed into your system when it is taken with food. This medicine will cause your stools to turn dark or black.
- Avoid milk and dairy products at the time iron tablets are taken; these foods can greatly reduce the amount of iron that is absorbed into your system.
- Do not take antacids or calcium supplements with the iron supplement, as they can also reduce its absorption. If an antacid is needed, take the iron product 1 hour before or 3 hours after the antacid.
- If you forget to take a dose, take it as soon as you remember. However, if it is almost time to take the next scheduled dose, omit the missed dose and go back to your regular schedule.
- Follow the suggested diet carefully, as it is also important in providing necessary iron.
- Keep this medicine out of the reach of children because an iron overdose is extremely poisonous to children.
- Keep all follow-up appointments with your physician.

References

1. Middleton E, et al. Studies on the absorption of orally administered iron from sustained release preparations. N Engl J Med 1966;274:136.
2. Bairiel I. Absorption of sustained release iron and the effects of ascorbic acid in normal subjects and after partial gastrectomy. BMJ 1974;4:505–508.
3. Swain RA, Kaplan B, Montgomery E. Iron-deficiency anemia—when is parenteral therapy warranted? Postgrad Med 1996;100:181–185.

89 VITAMIN B_{12} Deficiency

▶ **Treatment for Life** (Level I)

Barbara J. Mason, PharmD
Beata Saletnik, PharmD

After a year of feeling weak and "terrible," a 74-year-old man with multiple medical problems seeks attention at a Veterans Affairs Medical Center. Laboratory tests reveal a low hemoglobin, hematocrit, and vitamin B_{12} level. A Schilling test to differentiate between malabsorption and intrinsic factor deficiency (pernicious anemia) was not performed. Several options for replacement of vitamin B_{12} are available. A tapering regimen of intramuscular (IM) cyanocobalamin injections is the most common method of replacing the vitamin, but oral and intranasal preparations are also available. In cases of pernicious anemia, IM injections are generally given monthly for life.

▶ **Questions**

Problem Identification

1. a. *Create a drug-related problem list for this patient.*

   - Drug use without indication: pseudoephedrine, famotidine.
   - Inadequately controlled diabetes: HbA_{1c} 8.4% (target level is < 7%, if feasible).
   - Inadequately controlled hyperlipidemia: LDL goal is ≤ 100 mg/dL in this patient with a history of stroke.
   - Untreated condition: cobalamin deficiency (normal B_{12} level is 200 to 900 pg/mL).

   b. *What information indicates the presence or severity of the B_{12} deficiency?*

   - Diminished vibratory sensation in the lower extremities
   - Decreased hemoglobin, hematocrit, and RBC count
   - Decreased cobalamin level
   - Low reticulocyte count in the face of anemia
   - Complaint of weakness
   - Tissue levels of B_{12} decrease before the MCV, which may explain why the MCV value is still normal (rather than increased in B_{12} deficiency, which is a megaloblastic anemia). Patients with underlying cobalamin deficiency frequently have unusual or atypical clinical and laboratory features.[1] There is evidence that macrocytosis is becoming less common as a presenting feature of B_{12} deficiency.[2] With minimal clinical evidence of cobalamin deficiency, the distinction between low-end normal and true early biochemical cobalamin deficiency may be blurred.[3]

   c. *Could the B_{12} deficiency have been caused by drug therapy?*

   - The patient does not have any apparent drug-induced causes of B_{12} deficiency. He does not drink alcohol and has not had cancer chemotherapy, zidovudine, colchicine, metformin, para-aminosalicylic acid, neomycin, or nitrous oxide.

- He has also not recently received antibiotics, anticonvulsants, oral contraceptives, or high dose vitamin C.

d. *What additional information is needed to assess this patient's B_{12} deficiency?*

- Dietary history is needed to determine if intake of vitamin B_{12} is sufficient to replace daily B_{12} losses. Because humans are not able to synthesize vitamin B_{12}, it must be provided nutritionally. Animal protein is the primary dietary source of vitamin B_{12}.
- A peripheral blood smear should be performed to determine red blood cell shape. Oval red blood cells are predominant in patients with megaloblastosis (defective DNA synthesis), and round in shape in patients with liver disease, hemolysis, or bleeding. Hyposegmented neutrophils would suggest myelodysplasia while hypersegmented neutrophils would suggest B_{12} or folate deficiency.
- A Schilling test evaluates cobalamin absorption and can be used to distinguish dietary B_{12} deficiency from pernicious anemia (i.e., lack of intrinsic factor). This test is performed to assess the absorption of orally ingested radiolabeled cyanocobalamin with and without intrinsic factor. A patient with pernicious anemia would always have an abnormal test without intrinsic factor, and a normal test result with intrinsic factor would confirm the diagnosis of pernicious anemia. (*Note to instructors:* Although results of this test may have indicated that oral therapy would be acceptable, a decision to use intramuscular B_{12} therapy made this test unnecessary in this patient and it was not performed.)
- Elevated serum levels of methylmalonic acid and homocysteine may be present in patients with cobalamin deficiency. These tests may help distinguish between folate and vitamin B_{12} deficiency, but this information is not necessary in this particular case.

Desired Outcome

2. *What are the goals of pharmacotherapy in this case?*

- Eliminate symptoms related to B_{12} deficiency anemia
- Replenish vitamin B_{12} stores
- Prevent complications of B_{12} deficiency
- Correct abnormal laboratory values associated with vitamin B_{12} deficiency anemia
- Correct the underlying cause of the anemia
- Prevent future anemia with prophylactic pharmacotherapy or diet
- Ensure that folic acid deficiency does not concurrently exist

Therapeutic Alternatives

3. a. *What non-drug therapies might be useful for this patient?*

- Dietary management to increase nutritional intake of vitamin B_{12} is indicated if that is deemed to be the source of the deficiency.
- Patients with hemoglobin values below 5 g/dL may require transfusion therapy with packed red blood cells. Packed cells may also be indicated if patients with chronic anemia have dyspnea, anginal pain, or evidence of cerebral hypoxia.

b. *What feasible pharmacotherapeutic alternatives are available for treatment of the B_{12} deficiency?*

- *Cyanocobalamin* and *hydroxocobalamin* are the two agents used to replace vitamin B_{12}. Treatment recommendations vary because of differences between these two agents. Hydroxocobalamin is excreted slower, provides higher and more sustained blood levels, and may allow for use of smaller doses. However, it is not more effective in stabilizing hematocrit levels and is not available in the United States. It is also associated with a higher incidence of antibodies to the transcobalamin–hydroxocobalamin complex.
- Vitamin B_{12} is customarily administered IM with a dose schedule ranging from 100 μg to 1000 μg per day for the first 7 to 14 days to saturate B_{12} stores in the body. This may be followed with weekly IM doses of 100 to 1000 μg for 1 month, or until normalization of the hemoglobin and hematocrit occurs. Monthly injections may then be given monthly for life.
- The most common cyanocobalamin dosing regimen is 1000 μg/week IM for 4 weeks followed by 1000 μg/month for lifetime. Lack of patient acceptance of daily injections or inability to self-administer daily injections and the inconvenience of frequent physician office trips may explain why this regimen is commonly used. With longstanding vitamin B_{12} deficiency, symptoms may take months to resolve, which also may explain the widespread use of this dosage regimen.
- Although 100 μg/month IM may be adequate in some patients, there is no generic dosage form available in this strength. Because there are no reports of toxicity due to vitamin B_{12}, the higher dose is frequently used to ensure adequate replacement. Parenteral replacement administered in the medical office is more expensive than self-administration but will ensure compliance.
- The role of oral B_{12} is controversial.[3,4] Cobalamin can be absorbed by both intrinsic factor dependent and independent routes. The independent route is less effective, and larger doses of B_{12} are needed to provide adequate absorption. Only 1% to 3% of vitamin B_{12} is absorbed by the intestine without intrinsic factor, which necessitates individualized dosing to ensure optimal replacement. Oral preparations containing animal intrinsic factor have been associated with antibody formation, although preparations without intrinsic factor are available. The main role of oral therapy is for those patients who are deficient due to nutritional causes. Daily oral treatment is less expensive than monthly IM injections.
- A nasal gel dosage form is also available. The nasal absorption of water-soluble vitamin B_{12} depends on contact time with the nasal mucosa and molecular size. This dosage form may be an option for patients intolerant of or unwilling to receive injections, those who are unable to self-administer injections, or those with difficult access to health care facilities where periodic injections could be obtained.

Optimal Plan

4. *What drug, dosage form, dose, schedule, and duration of therapy are best for this patient?*

- As stated in the social history, the patient has frequent medical appointments at the VAMC and lives nearby. For this reason, it is feasi-

ble to give cyanocobalamin 1000 µg IM daily for 2 weeks, followed by 1000 µg once weekly until the hemoglobin and hematocrit normalize. Monthly injections of 1000 µg should be given for life thereafter.
- Oral cyanocobalamin doses of 500 to 1000 µg daily may be used if the patient does not tolerate parenteral therapy.
- If the nasal dosage form is used, the dose is 500 µg once weekly. Given this patient's close proximity and frequent visits to the VA, this option is not optimal. It may also be a non-formulary item and may be more expensive than injections.

Outcome Evaluation

5. *What clinical and laboratory parameters are necessary to evaluate the therapy for achievement of the desired therapeutic outcome and to detect or prevent adverse effects?*

Efficacy Parameters
- Patients subjectively improve within hours after initiation of cyanocobalamin therapy. Given this patient's other serious medical problems (e.g., prostate cancer), the patient's complaints of feeling "weak and terrible" may not be solely related to B_{12} deficiency and symptom relief may not be a reliable monitoring parameter.
- Morphologic changes of megaloblastic maturation in the marrow revert to normal within 24 to 48 hours. This is monitored only if the accuracy of the diagnosis is in question.
- Reticulocytosis occurs by day 3 and peaks by the end of the first week if there is no concomitant deficiency of iron. A reticulocyte count may be checked around day 5 of therapy if the accuracy of the diagnosis is in question.
- The hemoglobin and hematocrit should begin to rise after about the first week. Hematologic abnormalities should revert to a target hemoglobin level of 16 to 18 g/dL within 2 months. In this patient, a hematocrit should be obtained in 1 month and repeated at 2 months.
- Neurologic symptoms such as paresthesias or ataxia have been reported to worsen after cobalamin therapy was initiated. Most patients respond neurologically completely or partially depending on pretreatment severity and duration of symptoms. Most improvements should occur during the first 6 months of therapy. Baseline assessment of symptoms in individual patients should be measured to document drug therapy effects.
- In cases of true pernicious anemia, the Schilling test will remain abnormal for a lifetime. This is important to note, because clinicians frequently encounter patients who have been receiving B_{12} injections for years with an undocumented past medical history and who therefore require reevaluation of need for B_{12} therapy.
- Patients with B_{12} deficiency will respond hematologically to treatment with either folic acid or vitamin B_{12}, but bone marrow conversion to normoblastic morphology would not occur with folic acid treatment alone in B_{12} deficiency.

Adverse Effect Parameters
- Adverse effects possibly associated with reticulocytosis include hyperuricemia, hypokalemia, and sodium retention.
- Adverse effects of vitamin B_{12} may include urticaria and anaphylaxis. A sensitivity history should be obtained from the patient prior to administration of vitamin B_{12}.

Patient Counseling

6. *What information should be provided to the patient to enhance compliance, ensure successful therapy, and minimize adverse effects?*

Cyanocobalamin
- This medication is called vitamin B_{12} or cyanocobalamin. It is a water-soluble vitamin that can be stored by the body and is needed for normal growth and building of red blood cells, muscle, and nerve tissue. Vitamin B_{12} deficiency may occur because of inadequate amounts in the diet, pernicious anemia (inability to absorb the vitamin after dietary intake), stomach disorders, infections, or surgery.
- The medication comes in an oral form, nasal gel, and injection. The frequency of dosage administration depends on the dosage form used. Initially, vitamin B_{12} may be given daily or weekly as an injection into the muscle, and then monthly. In most cases, it is needed for the rest of your life to prevent return of the deficiency and to prevent damage to the central nervous system. If the oral route is used, the medication must be taken daily.
- If you forget to take an oral dose of vitamin B_{12}, do not take double doses the next dose; skip the missed dose and continue to take one dose each day. It is important to receive the vitamin B_{12} for as long as your prescriber indicates (which may be lifelong).
- If you are self-administering injections, you will need appropriate size needles and syringes and a needle disposer. Injections should be given into the muscle or deep subcutaneously.
- Possible side effects include skin rash, itching or bruising, mild diarrhea, and visual difficulties. If the injectable product is used, discomfort may occur at the site of injection.
- Vitamin B_{12} injection should be protected from light.
- If the nasal gel is used, it should be applied using a finger cot into the mucous membranes of the nose after gently blowing the nose. The medication will be absorbed and may cause slight stinging. Wash your hands after administration.
- During treatment with vitamin B_{12}, it will be necessary to have laboratory tests performed to monitor how well your body is responding to therapy.

▶ Follow-up Question

1. *If this patient had been taking the H_2-receptor antagonist (famotidine) for a documented history of gastritis, how might that have related to vitamin B_{12} deficiency?*

- Long-standing gastritis leads to atrophy of secretory cellular components of the stomach. This causes malabsorption of ingested cyanocobalamin and may lead to megaloblastic anemia. Vitamin B_{12} deficiency has many causes. Pernicious anemia is the most common cause, and the term applies to the condition associated with chronic atrophic gastritis.

References

1. Carmel R. Pernicious anemia: The expected findings of very low serum cobalamin levels, anemia, and macrocytosis are often lacking. Arch Intern Med 1988;148:1712–1714.
2. Metz J, Bell A, Flicker L, Bottligliera T, et al. The significance of subnormal serum vitamin B_{12} concentration in older people: A case control study. J Am Geriatr Soc 1996;44:1355–1361.
3. Reisner E Jr, Weiner L, Schittone M, et al. Oral treatment of pernicious anemia with Vitamin B_{12} without intrinsic factor. N Engl J Med 1955;253:502–506.
4. Thompson R, Ashby D, Armstrong E. Long-term trial of oral vitamin B_{12} in pernicious anemia. Lancet 1962;2:577–579.

90 FOLIC ACID DEFICIENCY

▶ The Piano Man (Level I)

Beata Saletnik, PharmD
Barbara J. Mason, PharmD

A 90-year-old man with a history of bipolar disorder and other medical problems complains of increasing irritability and restlessness. Physical examination reveals some muscle weakness, and laboratory evaluation indicates an anemia with low RBC folate levels. The patient does not have laboratory evidence of macrocytosis, which is a common finding in folic acid deficiency anemia. Correction of folic acid deficiency is usually accomplished by oral administration of exogenous folic acid for approximately 4 months. The patient should also be counseled on the types of foods that are high in folate content. Patient symptoms should begin to improve early in the course of therapy, but it may take several months to normalize the hematocrit and clear all folate-deficient red blood cells. The importance of adherence to the regimen for the full course of therapy should be emphasized to the patient.

▶ Questions

Problem Identification

1. a. *What drug-related problems exist in this patient?*

    - Untreated folic acid deficiency.
    - History of non-adherence to medications.
    - Potential subtherapeutic dosing of Divalproex.
    - No medical indication for ascorbic acid.
    - Chronic stable problems that apparently require no intervention at this time include: 1) osteoarthritis treated with acetaminophen; and 2) benign prostatic hyperplasia (BPH) treated with prazosin.

    b. *What signs, symptoms, and laboratory values indicate this patient has anemia secondary to folate deficiency?*

    - *Signs.* Muscle weakness in left upper extremity.
    - *Symptoms.* Irritability and restlessness. Severe folate deficiency is often associated with depression and sometimes with dementia.
    - *Laboratory values.* Low RBC count, decreased hemoglobin and hematocrit. This patient does not exhibit megaloblastosis (i.e., the MCV is within the normal range), which indicates the production of normocytic erythrocytes. The MCH can be increased in the presence of folate deficiency, but this is not seen in this patient. The MCHC is usually in the normal range in folate deficiency; the only situation in which it is routinely low is in patients with iron deficiency anemia.

    c. *Could the patient's folate deficiency have been caused by drug therapy?*

    - It is unlikely that the folate deficiency is attributable to drug therapy. He is not receiving any concurrent medications that impair folate absorption or inactivate folate (e.g., phenytoin, phenobarbital, primidone, sulfasalazine) or inhibit dihydrofolate reductase (e.g., methotrexate, trimethoprim, triamterene).[1]

    d. *What additional information is needed to satisfactorily assess this patient?*

    - A peripheral blood smear to demonstrate macrocytosis and hypersegmented polymorphonuclear leukocytes.
    - Reticulocyte count to evaluate recent red blood cell production.
    - Lactate dehydrogenase and indirect bilirubin values would be elevated in the presence of hemolysis. However, the total bilirubin (0.4 mg/dL) is well within the normal reference range (0.1 to 1.2 mg/dL), so it would be unlikely that obtaining these tests would provide any additional useful information.
    - A complete medication history should always be obtained to identify use of medications that may cause anemia or folate deficiency (e.g., anticonvulsants, alcohol, sulfasalazine, methotrexate, trimethoprim, triamterene, long-term metformin therapy).
    - It is also important to know whether the patient has multiple prescribers, the amount of alcohol intake (liver disease can result in anemia), history of travel (i.e., tropical sprue), and the function of the GI tract.
    - The presence of disease states wherein hyperutilization of folic acid may cause deficiency should be ruled out. These conditions

include hemolytic anemia, myelofibrosis, malignancy, chronic inflammatory disorders such as Crohn's disease or rheumatoid arthritis, exfoliative skin disease, or long-term dialysis.

e. *Why is it important to differentiate folate deficiency from vitamin B_{12} deficiency, and how is this accomplished?*

- It is necessary to ensure that vitamin B_{12} deficiency does not concurrently exist with folate deficiency because folate supplementation does not prevent or alleviate the neurologic manifestations of vitamin B_{12} deficiency. These neurologic manifestations may become irreversible if left untreated. Therefore, a vitamin B_{12} level should be measured during the evaluation of folate deficiency.
- Also, it has been postulated that large amounts of folate may precipitate neurologic symptoms in some patients with coexisting vitamin B_{12} deficiency by decreasing myelin methylation.[2] Routine folate supplementation in the general population past the point of deficiency resolution is controversial due to potential safety issues.[3]
- As a general rule, the major difference in symptoms between folate deficiency and vitamin B_{12} deficiency is the scarcity of neurologic manifestations with folate deficiency megaloblastic anemia. Laboratory changes are similar except for a decrease in folate for folic acid deficiency and a decrease in vitamin B_{12} for vitamin B_{12} deficiency.[4]

Desired Outcome

2. *What are the goals of pharmacotherapy for this patient's anemia?*

- Correct the underlying cause of the anemia if it is identifiable
- Attempt to resolve symptoms such as irritability and muscle weakness
- Reverse the laboratory abnormalities (i.e., RBC folate, hemoglobin, hematocrit, RBC count)
- Correct the deficiency of folic acid with appropriate pharmacotherapy and duration of treatment
- Discourage the development of future episodes of folic acid deficiency with proper counseling about a diet high in folic acid

Therapeutic Alternatives

3. a. *What non-drug therapies may be used to correct this patient's folic acid deficiency?*

- Counsel the patient about ingesting a diet high in folate. This diet includes items such as liver, kidneys, foods prepared from dried yeasts, fruit (e.g., bananas, oranges), dried beans, peas, lentils, and fresh leafy green vegetables (e.g., asparagus, broccoli, spinach, brussels sprouts). Educate the patient that lengthy cooking can destroy up to 90% of the folate content of food.
- Administration of packed red blood cells will also correct folate deficiency, but this should be reserved for patients with severe cardiovascular compromise.

b. *What pharmacotherapeutic alternatives are available for the treatment of this patient's anemia?*

- *Folic acid* is the only pharmacotherapeutic agent available for the treatment of folic acid deficiency. It is available in oral and parenteral formulations.
  ✓ The drug is usually given orally and may be initiated at 50 μg/day for 2 days, followed by 2 mg orally twice a week or 0.5 to 1 mg daily. Doses >1 mg do not enhance correction of folate deficiency, and most of the excess is excreted unchanged in the urine. Therapy should generally be continued for about 4 months to ensure that all red blood cells deficient in folate have been cleared from the circulation. Long-term folate replacement may be necessary in chronic hemolytic states, refractory malabsorption, and myelofibrosis.
  ✓ Parenteral administration of folic acid is not recommended except in severe cases of intestinal malabsorption, including patients receiving parenteral or enteral alimentation. The parenteral formulation may be administered IM, IV, or SC if the disease is very severe.
  ✓ Low-dose chronic folate therapy (0.5 mg/d) may be necessary if an anticonvulsant drug (e.g., phenytoin) produces the megaloblastic anemia due to impairment of folate absorption. Controversy exists as to whether routine supplementation of folic acid should be initiated with the start of phenytoin therapy or if folic acid would decrease phenytoin's anticonvulsant activity by increasing phenytoin's metabolism.[1]

c. *What economic or psychosocial issues are applicable to this patient and may contribute to the development of folic acid deficiency?*

- Potential problems in this patient include his age and lack of steady income. Although no information on his financial status was given in the case, a low or fixed income may preclude him from purchasing foods high in folate, such as fruits and green leafy vegetables, due to the expense of these products.
- Poor eating habits are often seen in elderly patients. The patient's bipolar disorder may undermine his ability to think about his welfare and the ability to properly care for himself. The patient may be exhibiting signs of dementia (e.g., memory loss), which may be a barrier to proper self-care and nutrition.

Optimal Plan

4. *What is the most appropriate drug, dosage form, dose, schedule, and duration of therapy for the resolution of this patient's anemia?*

- This patient's anemia should be treated with the exogenous administration of folic acid. As stated above, oral folic acid may be initiated at 50 μg/day for 2 days, followed by 2 mg orally twice a week or 0.5 to 1 mg daily. The duration of therapy should be approximately 4 months. This patient is not a candidate for parenteral therapy because there is no evidence of intestinal malabsorption.

Outcome Evaluation

5. *What parameters should be used to evaluate the efficacy and adverse effects of folic acid replacement therapy in this patient?*

Efficacy

- The patient should be monitored for symptomatic improvement in irritability, restlessness, weakness, appetite, and depression. Improvement in these symptoms should be noted shortly after initiation of replacement therapy.

- Unlike macrocytic anemia due to vitamin B_{12} deficiency, folic acid deficiency rarely, if ever, exhibits neurologic symptoms. If the patient is found to have abnormalities in vibratory and position sense or in motor and sensory pathways, this rules against an isolated decrease in folic acid.
- Reticulocytosis occurs within 2 to 3 days after replacement therapy is initiated and peaks in 5 to 8 days due to the proliferative state of the marrow.
- Hematocrit begins to increase within 2 weeks of replacement therapy and should be within the normal range in approximately 2 months.
- In order to monitor the clearance of all folate-deficient red blood cells, the erythrocyte folate level should be measured. This test is not sensitive to short-term changes in folate intake because these levels are established during the erythrocyte formation and endure the life span of the cell. The erythrocyte level is a better indicator of true tissue folate stores since serum folate levels are very sensitive to short-term changes in folate.
- Last, the MCV will initially rise due to an increase in reticulocytes and therefore an increase in the average volume of red blood cells. The reticulocytes will then slowly decrease to normal limits.
- If iron levels are elevated initially, the concentration of iron in the plasma may decrease to normal or below normal as effective erythropoiesis begins.
- Other corrections that may be seen in certain patients include normalization of leukocytes and platelets (may be mildly depressed) and normalization of lactate dehydrogenase and bilirubin levels (which may be elevated due to hemolysis or ineffective erythropoiesis).

Adverse Effects
- Rare side effects of folate therapy include skin rash, itching, redness, and difficulty breathing.

Patient Counseling

6. What information would you provide to this patient about his folic acid replacement therapy?

- This is a B complex vitamin needed by the body to produce red blood cells. An anemia develops when you are deficient in this compound.
- Take this medication once a day as directed.
- You will probably feel better quickly after you start taking this medication, but do not stop taking it until you have been instructed by your doctor to do so.
- Keep all of the appointments with your doctor and the laboratory so that your response to the medication can be monitored.
- Follow the suggested diet carefully. Good sources of folic acid include liver, kidneys, foods prepared from dried yeasts, fruit, and fresh leafy green vegetables.
- If you forget to take a dose, take it as soon as you remember; if it is close to your next scheduled dose, eliminate the missed dose and continue your regular schedule.
- Adverse effects are not common with this medication. Rare side effects include skin rash, itching, redness, and difficulty breathing.
- Tell your doctor and pharmacist what prescription and non-prescription drugs you are taking.
- Do not allow anyone else to take your medication.
- Keep this medication out of reach of children.
- Store the medication at room temperature and away from direct sunlight.

References

1. Lewis DP, Van Dyke DC, Willhite LA, et al. Phenytoin–folic acid interaction. Ann Pharmacother 1995;29:726–735.
2. Tucker KL, Mahnken B, Wilson PW, et al. Folic acid fortification of the food supply: Potential benefits and risks for the elderly population. JAMA 1996;276:1879–1885.
3. Campbell NR. How safe are folic acid supplements? Arch Intern Med 1996;156:1638–1644.
4. Swain RA, St. Clair L. The role of folic acid in deficiency states and prevention of disease. J Fam Pract 1997;44:138–144.

91 SICKLE CELL ANEMIA

▶ **One Crisis After Another** (Level I)

R. Donald Harvey III, PharmD, BCPS
Celeste C. Lindley, PharmD, MS, FASHP, FCCP, BCPS

A 23-year-old pregnant woman with a history of sickle cell anemia presents with a 2-day history of pain in her arms, legs, and back that is unrelieved with oxycodone/acetaminophen. Based on her history, physical examination, and laboratory findings, the patient is considered to be in sickle cell crisis. Relief of the patient's pain is the most immediate goal, and consideration must be given to the fact that the patient is in the first trimester of pregnancy. Hydration and red cell transfusions are also indicated in this patient. The case is unusual in that the patient had a low erythropoietin concentration on a single determination, and epoetin alfa therapy was initiated. Most patients with sickle cell disease have increased endogenous erythropoietin production secondary to chronic anemia and do not benefit from epoetin therapy. After completion of pregnancy, hydroxyurea therapy should be considered to prevent future crises in this patient who has a history of 5 to 10 episodes per year.

▶ **Questions**

Problem Identification

1. a. Create a list of the patient's drug-related problems.

- Painful sickle cell crisis during first trimester pregnancy unresolved by present analgesic regimen.
- Possible multifactorial anemia currently treated with iron, folic acid, and erythropoietin.

b. *What signs, symptoms, and laboratory values are consistent with an acute sickle cell crisis in this patient?*

- *Signs.* None
- *Symptoms.* Acute onset of pain unrelieved by Percocet (oxycodone/acetaminophen). Pain is the only presenting feature in patients experiencing vaso-occlusive crises.
- *Laboratory values.* None; the hematocrit falls acutely only during splenic sequestration crises and hemolytic crises. The moderately elevated LDH in this patient reflects chronic hemolysis seen in sickle cell disease. Although her reticulocyte count is elevated, it is not appropriate for her degree of anemia. Patients who are responding to anemia should be producing a reticulocytosis that is sufficient to not only maintain the current hematocrit (i.e., 1% of red cells replaced daily), but also to respond to the deficiency in red cell number. A corrected reticulocyte count reflects a true response to anemia and can be calculated by:

$$\text{Corrected reticulocyte count} = \text{measured reticulocyte count} \times \frac{\text{current Hct}}{\text{goal HCT}}$$

$$= 4.1\% \times \frac{11.5\%}{30\%}$$

$$= 1.57\%$$

A reticulocyte count in patients with a normal hematocrit is 0.5 to 1.5%. Therefore, her response to an anemia of this degree is blunted. The bone marrow is capable of increasing red cell production by at least ten-fold if there is a physiologic demand (i.e., anemia) and all elements required to make new cells are present. It is not unusual for patients with sickle cell disease to have chronic reticulocyte counts of 10% to 20%. Erythropoietin is required to stimulate a reticulocytosis, and patients with sickle cell disease typically have elevated endogenous erythropoietin concentrations in response to their anemia. Reduced production in this patient, although atypical, is the etiology of her decreased reticulocyte response to this degree of anemia.

c. *What additional information is needed to satisfactorily assess this patient?*

- Medical record and clinic notes for history and assessment of baseline hemoglobin and hematocrit to determine the severity and time course of prior crises.
- Current erythropoietin concentration to assess compliance with therapy.
- Folate concentration along with iron and iron binding studies to assess compliance.
- Vaccination status including pneumococcal and *Haemophilus B* vaccines.

Desired Outcome

2. *What are the goals of pharmacotherapy in this case?*

- Relief of pain secondary to sickle cell crisis
- Appropriate drug selection in the first trimester of pregnancy
- Resolution of anemia and adequate fetal oxygen delivery
- Reduction in frequency of crises

Therapeutic Alternatives

3. a. *What non-drug therapies might be useful for this patient?*

- *Hydration.* Patients in crises may have diminished urine concentrating ability due to renal infarcts and/or hemodynamic changes associated with chronic anemia. Hydration using intravenous fluids to provide 3 to 5 liters/day during crises aids in rehydration and mobilizing sickled cells. Fluid therapy should include 5% dextrose in water (D_5W) because it allows free water to enter red cells, decreasing the relative intracellular hemoglobin concentration. This reduces the tendency of hemoglobin to polymerize and sickle. The addition of 0.45% or 0.9% sodium chloride to fluid therapy increases intravascular volume to a greater extent than D_5W or water alone, thereby aiding in the mobilization of sickled cells in capillaries. Caution should be used in patients with underlying renal or cardiac dysfunction to avoid fluid overload.
- *Red cell transfusions.* This patient's presentation was unusual for her degree of anemia. Patients with hemoglobin values < 7.5 g/dL typically are symptomatic at rest (e.g., fatigue, palpitations) and compensate for hypoxemia through cardiac mechanisms such as tachycardia and increased stroke volume. The presence of a mild systolic ejection murmur in this patient reflects a hyperdynamic cardiac state; and mild mitral and tricuspid regurgitation suggest early valvular disease secondary to chronic anemia. In acute sickle cell crises, the hematocrit does not fall below precrisis values, except during splenic sequestration or aplastic crises. Red cell transfusions are not routinely administered during sickle cell crises. However, in cases of cerebrovascular accidents (CVAs), priapism, severe anemia, and aplastic crises, administering normal red cells to aid in oxygen delivery is indicated.[1] Transfusions decrease the relative number of sickled cells in circulation by providing normal cells for oxygen delivery. Transfusion support is indicated in pregnancy to maintain fetal oxygenation if hemoglobin values fall below 6 g/dL.[2] This patient was not transfused because of a lack of symptoms and because of fear of the further development of antibodies. Sickle cell patients are predisposed to developing anti-E, anti-C, Kell's, and Duffy's red cell antibodies. Blood banks have the capability to screen red cells for these antibodies to avoid immune-mediated hemolysis. Therefore, given her low hemoglobin, transfusion support may have been indicated. For prevention of crises, the role of prophylactic transfusions in decreasing the number of events during pregnancy is controversial.
- *Oxygen.* The use of oxygen during crises improves patient comfort but has no demonstrable effect on oxygen saturation or on the course of sickle cell crises. However, patients often perceive it to be useful and therefore, it may relieve anxiety. Oxygen is typically provided at lower rates (e.g., 2 L/min) via nasal cannula.

b. *What feasible pharmacotherapeutic alternatives are available for treatment of the patient's pain and chronic anemia?*

- *Fentanyl, hydromorphone, meperidine,* and *morphine* are opioids that have been used safely and effectively for pain control in sickle cell crises and during pregnancy.[3] Caution should be employed with the use of prolonged, higher dose meperidine in sickle cell disease patients with renal dysfunction due to accumulation of the neurotoxic metabolite normeperidine. Accumulation of this metabolite predisposes patients to seizures.[4] Pain control is best achieved initially through the parenteral route, but the oral route may be employed provided that the agents used have a rapid onset and adequate doses are given for relief. Patient-controlled analgesia (PCA) is an option that allows patients to dictate their own regimens. Continuous infusions with patient-controlled doses as needed provide around-the-clock pain control with an "on demand" dose for breakthrough needs. Consideration of prior opioid therapy should be used in determining a patient's tolerance to therapy and the need for dosage increases.

- *Erythropoietin* therapy is indicated for chronic anemia *only* in patients with adequately documented low endogenous erythropoietin production. The majority of patients with sickle cell disease have increased endogenous erythropoietin production secondary to chronic anemia and therefore do not benefit from erythropoietin therapy.[2] It is very unusual to see erythropoietin benefit patients with sickle cell disease, and the moderate degree of renal insufficiency in this patient is inconsistent with decreased erythropoietin production. The patient in this case had only one measured low erythropoietin concentration, which led to the use of erythropoietin. A second concentration prior to initiation of therapy should have been obtained to confirm low endogenous production. Erythropoietin use in sickle cell patients during pregnancy has been shown to be safe.[5] Titration of erythropoietin doses should occur every 6 to 8 weeks.

Optimal Plan

4. *Outline a detailed therapeutic plan to treat all facets of this patient's acute sickle cell crisis. For all drug therapies, include the dosage form, dose, schedule, and duration of therapy.*

- *Pain.* Hydromorphone 0.5 to 1 mg bolus, followed by 0.15 to 0.3 mg/hr continuous infusion, along with a PCA pump that delivers 0.25 mg bolus up to every 10 to 20 minutes. The PCA should be adjusted and continued until her pain begins to resolve, when it may be possible to convert her back to her home oxycodone/acetaminophen regimen. Hydromorphone was selected because the patient had an adverse reaction to morphine in the past and the use of meperidine doses adequate for pain control may lead to accumulation of normeperidine with underlying renal dysfunction.
- *Hydration.* Dextrose 5% with 0.45% sodium chloride at 125 mL/hr. Although the patient has renal insufficiency, rehydration is necessary to expand intravascular volume and mobilize sickled cells. Sodium chloride 0.9% could also be used. Fluids such as lactated Ringer's and 0.9% sodium chloride alone are not optimal for rehydration because of a lack of free water. Continued hydration should be governed by clinical signs of fluid overload (peripheral/pulmonary edema, decreased urine output).
- *Oxygen.* Oxygen at a rate of 1 to 2 L/min via nasal cannula may be initiated if the patient feels it to be helpful.
- *Anemia.* Continue folate, iron, and erythropoietin doses as per her home regimen.

Outcome Evaluation

5. a. *What clinical and laboratory parameters are necessary to evaluate therapy for achievement of the desired therapeutic outcome and to detect or prevent adverse effects?*

- *Pain.* Monitor for subjective relief of pain and the ability to tolerate conversion to oral therapy. Monitor PCA adverse effects through monitoring vital signs every 8 hours (O_2 saturation, pulse, respiratory rate). As pain resolves, the patient should return to her oral home regimen.
- *Hydration.* Monitor for resolution of crisis through daily assessments of pain control, hematocrit, and presence of sickled cells on peripheral smear. Fluid accumulation could produce pulmonary edema (wheezes, crackles on lung exam) and/or peripheral edema. Daily physical exams should be performed to assess hydration status.
- *Anemia.* A follow-up erythropoietin concentration would help to determine compliance and response to therapy but was not obtained during the patient's admission. Erythropoietin therapy should be assessed through improvements in hematocrit. A goal hematocrit of 25% to 30% should be established prior to therapy. The risk of increased sickling rates with increased abnormal red cell production should be weighed against the risks associated with transfusions. Adverse effects of erythropoietin include headache and hypertension. However, these adverse effects are very rare in patients who do not have end-stage renal disease.

Adequate iron, folate, and B_{12} must be provided for erythropoiesis. During pregnancy, patients also have increased folate and iron requirements regardless of the presence or absence of anemia. Most patients with sickle cell disease do not require iron therapy because it is highly conserved by the body. This patient probably has low stores because she is a menstruating female. She also has an increased demand due to pregnancy, necessitating iron therapy. A baseline documentation of iron stores is necessary to determine the degree of supplementation needed. Iron studies prior to the initiation of therapy including ferritin, serum iron, and total iron binding capacity (TIBC) would have been helpful in determining the contribution of iron deficiency to her anemia. Low serum ferritin in combination with a high TIBC would indicate a component of iron deficiency anemia. Possible gastrointestinal and menstrual losses should be investigated. In addition, iron requirements double during pregnancy. Dietary intake of iron should be reviewed and increased if necessary.

b. *Considering this information, what changes (if any) in the pharmacotherapeutic plan are warranted?*

- *Chronic anemia.* After 6 weeks of therapy (assuming compliance), the end point of a goal hematocrit of 25% to 30% on erythropoietin has not been achieved. If the erythropoietin concentration remains inappropriately low for her degree of anemia, the dose should be increased to 100 to 150 U/kg rounded to the nearest vial size (2000; 3000; 4000; 10,000; 20,000 Units) 3 times weekly. The importance of folate and iron therapy in conjunction with erythropoietin should be emphasized.
- *Pain.* The continuous infusion of her PCA pump should be discontinued while keeping a bolus dose for breakthrough pain. Her

home oral regimen should be reinstituted as her opioid needs decrease and her pain resolves.
- *Hydration.* Fluids should be discontinued if hydration is adequate and her pain is resolving.

Patient Counseling

6. *What information should be provided to the patient to enhance compliance, ensure successful therapy, and minimize adverse effects?*

Erythropoietin

- Erythropoietin stimulates the production of new red blood cells. It is given as an injection under the skin every Monday, Wednesday, and Friday to raise your blood counts. Erythropoietin is very well tolerated in most patients. It should be stored in the refrigerator prior to use.

Folic Acid

- This vitamin is needed for the production of red blood cells, and it improves the effectiveness of erythropoietin. It will also help to prevent birth defects.

Ferrous Sulfate

- Iron is also necessary for producing red blood cells and helping maximize the effectiveness of erythropoietin.
- It should be taken on an empty stomach if possible but may be taken with food if it causes stomach cramping.
- Iron may also cause constipation or diarrhea, and/or a burning sensation in your throat (called reflux) if you take it shortly after eating. It will also cause your stools to turn a darker color. Stool softeners can be used to prevent constipation.
- If you experience reflux, you may need to reduce your dose to 1 tablet in the morning with a small amount of food. It may be necessary to avoid lying down for 3 or more hours after you take a dose to prevent reflux from occurring.

▶ Follow-up Question

1. *What therapies may be effective in reducing the frequency of crises in this patient who presently has up to 10 episodes per year?*

- Increasing fetal hemoglobin concentration in sickle cell patients has proven to be effective in inhibiting red cell sickling and leads to a reduction in the frequency of painful crises. Hydroxyurea (Droxia) is approved for use in sickle cell patients who experience recurrent severe crises, with the greatest benefit seen in patients with 6 or more crises in the previous 12 months. Patients should be started on 15 mg/kg/day and increased by 2.5 mg/kg/day increments until myelosuppression, the dose limiting toxicity, is reached. Therapy should be withheld if myelosuppression occurs (defined as an absolute neutrophil count $< 2.0 \times 10^3/mm^3$, a platelet count $< 80 \times 10^3/mm^3$, or hemoglobin < 4.5 g/dL). It is recommended that complete blood counts be monitored every 2 weeks. Hydroxyurea also has carcinogenic and teratogenic potential. Patients should be informed of these risks prior to therapy initiation and counseled to use effective birth control measures during treatment.
- Hydroxyurea would be indicated in this patient after completion of her pregnancy because she experiences 5 to 10 crises per year necessitating hospitalization.
- Other therapies including bone marrow transplantation, azacytidine, and pentoxifylline have produced varying results in the reduction of crises. Allogeneic marrow transplantation treats sickle cell anemia by providing stem cells capable of producing normal red cells. However, toxicities including graft-versus-host disease and those associated with prolonged immunosuppression are concerning. Azacytidine also increases fetal hemoglobin concentrations, but its effects are transient. Pentoxifylline has been shown to reduce the frequency of crises in some studies, but results have been inconsistent.

References

1. King KE, Ness PM. Treating anemia. Hematol Oncol Clin North Am 1996; 10:1305–1320.
2. El-Shafei AM, Dhaliwal JK, Sandhu AK, et al. Indications for blood transfusion in pregnancy with sickle cell disease. Aust NZ J Obstet Gynecol 1995;35:405–408.
3. Howard RJ. Management of sickling conditions in pregnancy. Br J Hosp Med 1996;56:7–10.
4. Tang R, Shimomura SK, Rotblatt M. Meperidine-induced seizures in sickle cell patients. Hosp Formul 1980;15:764–772.
5. Bourantas K, Makrydimas G, Georgiou J, et al. Preliminary results with administration of recombinant human erythropoietin in sickle cell/β-thalassemia patients during pregnancy. Eur J Haematol 1996;56:326–328.

PART THREE

Diseases of Infectious Origin

Joseph T. DePiro, PharmD, FCCP, Section Editor

92 USING LABORATORY TESTS IN INFECTIOUS DISEASES

▶ No More Vanco for Me (Level I)

Steven J. Martin, PharmD, BCPS

A 59-year-old woman with a history of an epidural abscess and septicemia caused by methicillin-resistant *Staphylococcus aureus* (MRSA) presents with worsening back pain, tenderness over the lumbar spine, low-grade fever, and leukocytosis with a left shift. Blood cultures are subsequently reported as positive for MRSA. During her previous infectious episode, the patient developed toxic epidermal necrolysis from vancomycin therapy, and she refuses retreatment with this agent. In the case questions that follow, students are asked to interpret minimum inhibitory concentration (MIC) data and discuss the value of also obtaining minimum bactericidal concentrations (MBCs). Case questions also discuss additional testing that may be performed to help select an appropriate antimicrobial regimen. When the patient is started on combination therapy with quinupristin/dalfopristin and rifampin, questions are directed toward use of serum bactericidal titers (SBTs) to predict the efficacy of the regimen *in vivo* and to use SBT testing to optimize drug dosing.

▶ Questions

Problem Identification

1. a. *Create a list of this patient's drug-related problems.*

    - Skin/soft tissue infection with possible osteomyelitis requiring appropriate anti-infective therapy and possible debridement in the future if an abscess develops.
    - Pain inadequately controlled with acetaminophen/codeine and naproxen.
    - Penicillin, cephalosporin, sulfa, and vancomycin allergies that may complicate selection of appropriate antimicrobial therapy.
    - Chronic stable problems not requiring intervention at this time include: 1) hypertension, adequately controlled on propranolol; 2) coronary artery disease, controlled with nitroglycerin; and 3) postmenopausal status receiving estrogen replacement.

    b. *What subjective and objective data indicate the presence of infection?*

    Subjective Data
    - Pain at the suspected infection site
    - History of previous infection in the area

    Objective Data
    - Elevated body temperature
    - Chills witnessed during the physical exam
    - Elevated systemic WBC count with an increase in PMNs and bands
    - Elevated erythrocyte sedimentation rate

Desired Outcome

2. *What are the desired treatment goals for this patient's current medical problems?*

- Eradicate her spinal infection
- Relieve her pain
- Restore temperature to normal and prevent further episodes of chilling and fever
- Normalize WBC count
- Restore sedimentation rate to normal

Therapeutic Alternatives

3. a. *The microbiology laboratory provided both a minimum inhibitory concentration (MIC) and an interpretation of that MIC for each antimicrobial agent tested. How are the MIC and the interpretation correlated?*

- The interpretation correlates the MIC with the expected clinical outcome. Breakpoint concentrations are determined using several criteria:
    - ✓ The pharmacokinetic properties of the drugs in humans, which determine the serum and tissue concentrations of the agent and the duration of organism exposure to the antimicrobial agent.
    - ✓ The natural distribution of MICs for that organism–drug combination.
    - ✓ The clinical efficacy of the agent against bacteria with a given MIC value.
- The definitions of the interpretations are:[1]
    - ✓ *Susceptible.* Infection due to the strain may be appropriately treated with the dosages of antimicrobial agent recommended for that type of infection and infecting species (i.e., the organism is likely to be eradicated during therapy with usual drug doses). Susceptible organisms are inhibited *in vitro* by concentrations of antibiotics achievable in serum.
    - ✓ *Intermediate susceptibility.* Response rates may be lower than for susceptible isolates, but antibiotic concentrations that inhibit bacterial growth *in vitro* are usually attainable clinically in blood and tissue. Clinical efficacy is likely in body sites where the drugs are physiologically concentrated.
    - ✓ *Resistant.* The organisms are not inhibited *in vitro* by usually attainable serum antibiotic concentrations, and clinical efficacy is not reliable when normal dosage schedules are used. This category also includes organisms that may have MICs that fall within the range where specific microbial resistance mechanisms are likely (e.g., β-lactamase production) and clinical efficacy has not been reliable in treatment studies.

b. *Should the laboratory be asked to provide minimum bactericidal concentration (MBC) data for these antibiotics? If so, how would those data be of value in selecting antimicrobial therapy?*

- The MBC describes the ability of an antimicrobial agent to exert bactericidal effect at clinically achievable drug concentrations. Bactericidal activity is important in treating osteomyelitis, because penetration of most antimicrobial agents into the bone tissue is poor, and infection in this area is not readily cleared by the host's immunologic defenses.
- MBCs are time-consuming for the laboratory and are most efficiently performed when the MICs are performed. MBCs should not be ordered indiscriminately, and the value of the data to be obtained must be weighed against the time and effort necessary to obtain them.
- MBCs could be ordered in cases of bacterial endocarditis, meningitis, sepsis in the immunocompromised patient, infections in those unable to mount an immune response, osteomyelitis, chronically infected implants, and other types of chronic infection. The clinical goal of this testing is to attain a drug concentration at the site of infection during all or part of the dosing interval that exceeds the MBC of the infecting pathogen.
- The MICs for this organism against rifampin, quinupristin/dalfopristin, trimethoprim-sulfamethoxazole, and vancomycin were at the breakpoint for susceptibility. The MIC for tetracycline was in the intermediate-susceptibility range. The MBCs for these agents are likely one or more two-fold dilutions higher than the MICs and may be difficult to achieve clinically at the site of infection. If any of these antibiotics is to be used to treat this infection, MBC data would be helpful in tailoring the dosing regimen to achieve adequate serum (and tissue) concentrations.

c. *What additional testing should be performed in the microbiology laboratory to provide information that might be helpful in choosing antimicrobial therapy for this patient? How should this information be interpreted?*

- *Perform additional susceptibility testing.* Most clinical labs use a predetermined panel of antibiotics for routine testing (disk diffusion or broth dilution). These panels are different for gram-positive and gram-negative organisms. The panels typically mimic the institution's antimicrobial formulary. However, often newer, older, or limited-use antimicrobial agents are not included in routine testing.
- *Test other antimicrobial agents for activity against this organism.* Potential drugs include levofloxacin, sparfloxacin, grepafloxacin, trovafloxacin, and teicoplanin (investigational). Disk diffusion testing is rapid (overnight) and easy to perform, and most clinical labs have these commercially prepared antibiotic-containing disks. This information could potentially expand the choice of drugs for use in treating her infection. It is important for the clinician to recognize situations that fall outside of routine or normal and request additional information from the microbiologist when it is necessary.
- *Perform combination testing.* This can be used to determine a synergistic interaction of two or more antibiotics against the organism cultured. Experimental animal data suggest that rifampin combined with another anti-staphylococcal drug such as nafcillin or vancomycin provides better results than does single-drug therapy for chronic staphylococcal osteomyelitis.[2] *Checkerboard testing* using either broth media or agar media is the simplest, most versatile, and most frequently used method for testing antimicrobial combinations. Specifically, checkerboard tests could be performed with:
    - ✓ Rifampin + quinupristin/dalfopristin

- ✓ Rifampin + tetracycline
- ✓ Quinupristin/dalfopristin + tetracycline
- ✓ An aminoglycoside + quinupristin/dalfopristin
- ✓ An aminoglycoside + oxacillin

Antibiotic combinations that demonstrate an additive or synergistic potential (as described by the *FIC index* or by an *isobologram plot*) may be chosen for this patient's therapy.

- *Time-kill methodology* could also be used to determine the extent of bactericidal activity of these combinations of antimicrobial agents if laboratories have the necessary resources. These data may help predict efficacy, particularly in osteomyelitis. However, time-kill curves are generally reserved for research purposes and are seldom used in clinical practice.

Optimal Plan

4. *The patient was started on quinupristin/dalfopristin 850 mg IV Q 8 H after meeting criteria for compassionate use from the drug's manufacturer. In addition, she was started on rifampin 300 mg po Q 12 H.*

Outcome Evaluation

5. a. *Determination of serum concentrations for either of these antibiotics is not readily available. What other laboratory testing could be used to determine more precisely the efficacy of this regimen in vivo? How is it interpreted? What is the pharmacist's role in performing this test?*

- *Serum bactericidal titers (SBTs)* are commonly used in the setting where bactericidal activity is required for complete eradication of the pathogen. This test integrates both pharmacokinetic and pharmacodynamic properties in determining the highest dilution of the patient's serum that provides ≥ 99% eradication of the pathogen. The largest volume of literature regarding the clinical effectiveness of SBT determination is in the treatment of osteomyelitis. Most studies suggest that dosage regimens that achieve a peak bactericidal titer of 1:8 or greater predict successful outcome.
- The clinician must be certain the patient has reached a steady state level in his/her therapeutic regimen and that serum samples are obtained at the correct times. Generally, both a peak and a trough serum concentration are obtained with the SBT.[3] The peak concentration is obtained:
  - ✓ 60 minutes after completion of a 30-minute IV infusion
  - ✓ 60 minutes after an intramuscular dose
  - ✓ 90 minutes after an oral dose

The trough concentration is obtained just prior to administering a dose. If more than one antimicrobial agent is being used, the peak sample should be obtained 1 hour after administration of the second agent. If one of the agents is administered infrequently (e.g., Q 12 H) and the other one is administered frequently (e.g., Q 4 H), peak concentrations should be obtained 1 hour after the completion of the infusion of the second antimicrobial agent at a time when the administration of both agents coincides. Trough concentrations may be obtained based on the timing of the less frequently administered agent. The assumption is made that the agent administered every 4 hours will have a more constant level.

b. *Outline a follow-up plan for monitoring the efficacy of this therapeutic regimen.*

- Three to 5 days after initiation of the regimen, the patient's serum should be collected for SBT testing at peak and trough concentrations. Dosing of the antibiotics should be increased if necessary to achieve optimal SBT ratios. SBTs should be repeated as necessary to assure adequate dosing.
- The CBC and ESR should be followed weekly, and blood cultures should be obtained after therapy has been initiated and repeated until sterile.
- Repeat MRI or other radiologic evidence of infection remission will be necessary at the conclusion of therapy.

References

1. National Committee for Clinical Laboratory Standards. Performance Standards for Antimicrobial Disk Susceptibility Tests, 6th ed. Approved Standard. NCCLS, 940 West Valley Road, Suite 1400, Wayne, PA 19087-1898, 1997.
2. Dworkin R, Modin G, Kunz S, et al. Comparative efficacies of ciprofloxacin, pefloxacin, and vancomycin in combination with rifampin in a rat model of methicillin-resistant *Staphylococcus aureus* chronic osteomyelitis. Antimicrob Agents Chemother 1990;34:1014–1016.
3. National Committee for Clinical Laboratory Standards. Methodology for the Serum Bactericidal Test: Tentative Guideline. NCCLS document M21-T (ISBN 1-56238-143-1) NCLS, 771 East Lancaster Avenue, Villanova, PA 19085, 1992.

93 BACTERIAL MENINGITIS

▶ **Trouble on Day One** (Level II)

Sherry Luedtke, PharmD

A full-term neonate develops tachypnea, grunting, intercostal retractions, leukopenia, hypotension, and metabolic acidosis shortly after birth. Empiric antibiotics are initiated; urine and CSF serology are subsequently positive for Group B streptococcus. Urine and blood cultures are also positive for this organism, which is shown to be sensitive to ampicillin. Gentamicin should be added to ampicillin because of a synergistic effect against Group B streptococcus. The usual duration of therapy for neonatal meningitis is 14 to 21 days. In some cases that respond favorably to combination therapy, it may be appropriate to discontinue the aminoglycoside after the first 5 to 7 days or after the CSF has cleared. Careful clinical and laboratory monitoring is required to ensure eradication of the infection and to prevent neurologic sequelae such as abscess formation.

Questions

Problem Identification

1. a. *What drug-related problems does this infant have?*

   - Group B streptococcus meningitis and sepsis in this patient are indicated by his deteriorating clinical status with metabolic acidosis, respiratory distress despite oxygen supplementation, poor peripheral perfusion unresponsive to fluid resuscitation, and hypotonia.
   - Severe leukopenia with an elevated immature-to-total ratio of neutrophils and the positive CSF latex agglutination for group B streptococcus point to group B streptococcus meningitis as the pathogen.
   - Metabolic acidosis is apparent in this patient by the capillary blood gas pH of 7.26 with respiratory compensation as indicated by the pco_2 of 29.6 mm Hg, tachypnea (normal respiratory rate in an infant is 30 to 50/min), grunting, and intercostal retractions.
   - Hypoperfusion is evidenced by low blood pressure and poor peripheral perfusion with capillary refill time > 4 seconds. Hypoperfusion is the cause of the metabolic acidosis.
   - Neutropenia is apparent in this infant with a total WBC of 3.2×10^3 (8% neutrophils, 13% bands) with a resulting absolute neutrophil count of only $0.672 \times 10^3/mm^3$.

   b. *What risk factors does this patient have for bacterial meningitis?*

   - Newborns account for the highest age-specific attack rate of bacterial meningitis compared to other age groups. This is believed to be due in part to immaturity of the immune system during the first 2 months of life.
   - Risk factors for bacterial meningitis in newborns include:[1,2]
     - ✓ Prematurity < 35 weeks' gestation
     - ✓ Low birth weight
     - ✓ Rupture of amniotic membranes (especially if prolonged > 72 hours)
     - ✓ Maternal group B strep positive
     - ✓ Signs of maternal infection (fever, elevated WBC)
   - The only risk factor in this infant is the premature rupture of amniotic membranes for 41 hours prior to delivery.

   c. *What clinical findings indicate the presence of meningitis and its severity?*

   - Infants typically present with subtle signs of meningitis, including fever (~50%), lethargy, irritability, respiratory distress, jaundice, feeding intolerance, vomiting/diarrhea, hypotonia, and hepatosplenomegaly.[1,2]
   - Seizures and bulging fontanel occur in < 50% of infants who present with meningitis.
   - This infant presents with respiratory distress, slight hypotonia, and hypoperfusion as indicated by a capillary refill of > 4 seconds.
   - Indicators of severity include neutropenia (< $1.5 \times 10^3/mm^3$) and elevated immature-to-total (I:T) neutrophil ratio. An I:T > 0.2 is highly indicative of overwhelming infection in the neonate.[3] This patient is severely neutropenic with an ANC of $0.672 \times 10^3/mm^3$ and has an elevated I:T ratio of 0.62, indicating a systemic infection. Although an elevated WBC/neutrophil count may be present in some infants, it is usually not as indicative of systemic infection as is neutropenia.
   - Hypoperfusion with secondary severe metabolic acidosis and tachypnea are other indicators of the severity of the infection. Respiratory distress and tachypnea occur in the neonate as the body attempts to compensate for the acidosis by blowing off CO_2.
   - The latex agglutination test is positive. Latex agglutination tests take only minutes to perform and are designed to detect bacterial antigens in an otherwise sterile fluid. The tests involve mixing beads that have been coated with antibody against the specific antigens one is wishing to detect in the sample fluid. If antigen is present, it binds with the antibody causing the beads to clump. This is a good early indicator of infection. False positives may occur, particularly in the urine, due to rectal/perineal contamination. Therefore, positive tests in such circumstances should also take the clinical picture into consideration. Common organisms for latex agglutination tests include pneumococcus, group B streptococcus, meningococcus, and *Haemophilus influenzae*.
   - A CSF glucose < 50% of serum glucose and a CSF protein > 150 mg/dL in the neonate is indicative of infection. CSF protein concentrations in newborns are often difficult to evaluate because the normal CSF protein is elevated in premature infants relative to the amount found in adults. The presence of blood in CSF due to intraventricular hemorrhages may also complicate evaluation of CSF protein. The CSF studies here indicate meningitis; the glucose is only 40 mg/dL (serum glucose 103 mg/dL); the protein is elevated (281 mg/dL) despite the presence of relatively few red blood cells.
   - An elevated CSF WBC count is indicative of infection, but healthy term infants often have normal WBC counts of up to $0.032 \times 10^3/mm^3$ in the absence of infection. The classical picture of > 95% PMNs is also often complicated in neonates. The CSF of healthy term neonates may contain up to 60% PMNs (which is high relative to adult values) and antibiotics are often administered prior to transport to the appropriate neonatal intensive care facilities. In this case, the WBC count is elevated (0.306) with only 33% PMNs. The mild elevation in PMNs in this case may be the result of antibiotic administration prior to obtaining the lumbar puncture or the patient's severe leukopenia.

   d. *Is there any drug-related therapy that may have prevented the infection?*

   - Prophylaxis for early group B streptococcal infections may be accomplished by intrapartum administration of penicillin. Intrapartum prophylaxis is indicated if one or more of the following is present: gestation < 37 weeks, intrapartum fever > 38°C, rupture of membranes >18 hours, group B streptococcal bacteriuria during pregnancy, or a previous infant with invasive group B streptococcal infection.[2] Prophylaxis in this patient's mother may have been beneficial since she had rupture of the amniotic membranes for >18 hours. However, prophylaxis was not indicated in light of a negative GBS culture.

Desired Outcome

2. *What are the goals of drug therapy in this situation?*

- The primary goal of pharmacotherapy in this patient is to eliminate the infection.
- Secondary outcomes are aimed at preventing complications such as subdural effusions, hearing impairment, SIADH, and cerebral infarctions.

Therapeutic Alternatives

3. a. What non-drug therapies might be useful in this patient?

- Supplemental oxygen is useful in this situation to improve oxygenation, but elimination of the cause of respiratory distress (metabolic acidosis secondary to infection) is essential.
- In light of the severe neutropenia, granulocyte transfusions may be considered to boost the systemic immunity. Currently, intravenous immunoglobulin (IVIG) is generally preferred over the use of granulocyte transfusions.

b. Describe the antimicrobial alternatives available for the management of meningitis in this patient.

- Common pathogens in newborns differ from those in young children. The common organisms causing sepsis and meningitis in newborns include group B streptococcus, *Escherichia coli*, and *Listeria* species, whereas in older children pneumococcus, *Neisseria meningitidis*, and *H. influenzae* are most common. Empiric coverage of these organisms should be initiated in all neonates with suspected meningitis and continued pending culture results 48 to 72 hours later. Early discontinuation of therapy may lead to inappropriate antibiotic coverage and potentially devastating neurologic morbidity.
- A penicillin *plus* an aminoglycoside or a penicillin *plus* a third-generation cephalosporin should be chosen for empiric antimicrobial treatment of meningitis in newborns. Examples include:
  ✓ Ampicillin or penicillin G *plus* gentamicin or amikacin
  ✓ Ampicillin or penicillin G *plus* cefotaxime or ceftriaxone or ceftazidime
- Ampicillin is generally preferred over penicillin G because it offers increased gram-negative coverage and is active against *Listeria*.
- Gentamicin is the preferred aminoglycoside because of concerns about ototoxicity with amikacin, although resistance patterns might necessitate the use of amikacin in some institutions.
- Cefotaxime is the preferred third-generation cephalosporin because of the extensive experience with its use in neonates. Ceftriaxone is generally avoided in neonates due to concerns of biliary sludging as an adverse effect, whereas ceftazidime use is limited to avoid the development of pseudomonal resistance.
- Ampicillin *plus* cefotaxime is the preferred empiric regimen when gram-negative infection is highly suspected (e.g., maternal *E. coli* sepsis). Cefotaxime has excellent CNS penetration and greater bactericidal activity than the aminoglycosides.
- Ampicillin *plus* gentamicin is the preferred regimen when group B streptococcal infection is suspected (because of maternal risk factors) because of gentamicin's synergism with ampicillin against group B streptococcus. Ampicillin *plus* cefotaxime may be employed when the patient has renal dysfunction to avoid the use of an aminoglycoside.

- IVIG may be considered as adjunctive treatment to antimicrobial therapy to increase serum immunoglobulin concentrations. However, pooled IVIG has not been shown to increase survival.
- Granulocyte colony-stimulating factors could also be considered in this case. However routine use of these agents is not currently recommended in neonates due to limited information regarding potential toxicity.
- Dexamethasone in combination with antimicrobial therapy has been shown to decrease the incidence of neurologic and hearing impairments in children with *H. influenzae* meningitis and may be beneficial in pneumococcal meningitis.[1] Studies have not been performed in children < 2 months of age or in cases of meningitis due to other pathogens. Therefore use of adjuvant dexamethasone in neonates is not recommended.

Optimal Plan

4. Given this new information, what therapy would you recommend for the management of this infant?

- Ampicillin (150 to 200 mg/kg/day divided every 8 hours)[4] = 175 to 235 mg IV Q 8 H

  plus

  gentamicin (2.5 mg/kg/every 8 to 12 hours)[4] = 8.8 mg IV Q 12 H
- Since group B streptococcus has been isolated, the infant should be changed to a combination of ampicillin and gentamicin. Ampicillin must be dosed at "meningitic" doses to ensure adequate penetration into the CNS.
- Ampicillin monotherapy may be employed at the same doses, but the benefit of synergy with gentamicin is preferred during the initial days of treatment for meningitis.
- The use of cefotaxime (150 mg/kg/day divided Q 8 H)[4] and ampicillin may have been appropriate as initial empiric therapy, but once the organism has been identified as group B streptococcus, cefotaxime should be discontinued because it provides no greater coverage than ampicillin monotherapy.
- The duration of therapy ranges from 14 to 21 days. Most practitioners recommend treatment for 14 days after the CSF has been cleared.[1] Although the gentamicin may be continued with ampicillin for the entire duration of the course of treatment, some practitioners continue it only for the first 5 to 7 days, or until the CSF is cleared. There is no data to support one treatment regimen over the other, but short courses of gentamicin reduce the need for serum concentration monitoring, may reduce toxicity, and often make it easier to complete the antibiotic course at home.
- (*Note to Instructors:* This patient was actually treated with ampicillin 235 mg IV Q 8 H and gentamicin 8.8 mg IV Q 12 H. The patient responded well (see "Clinical Course"), and after 5 days of combination therapy, gentamicin was discontinued and the treatment course was completed with ampicillin monotherapy. The patient was discharged after completing 7 days of therapy and completed an additional 7 days of ampicillin monotherapy as an outpatient.)

Outcome Evaluation

5. *Describe the monitoring parameters necessary to evaluate the efficacy and safety of the therapy.*

- Repeat CSF culture and cell counts are recommended after 48 to 72 hours of antimicrobial therapy to ensure sterilization of CSF. If the CSF is not sterilized, this may indicate inadequate treatment or further complications such as abscess formation. The goals are CSF glucose > 50% of serum glucose, protein <150 mg/dL, WBC < 32, and < 60% PMNs. The CSF should contain no organisms. Some specialists argue against follow-up lumbar punctures in infants who have clinically improved, since the clinical improvement itself is indicative of clearing and because those who develop complications (abscess) will generally not improve clinically.
- Evaluate the patient for signs of improvement in metabolic acidosis and tissue perfusion. The goal is to achieve a RR of 30 to 50/min. Continuous respiratory measurements and oxygen saturation measurements (goal sat > 93%) should be performed until the acidosis and respiratory compromise have improved. Capillary blood gas measurements should be performed every 4 to 6 hours until the acidosis has resolved (goals are pH 7.35 to 7.45, po_2 60 to 80 mm Hg, pco_2 35 to 45 mm Hg, HCO_3 19 to 22 mEq/L, BE −5 to +5 mEq/L). Once the acidosis resolves, CBGs can be reduced to every 12- to 24-hours until the infant can be weaned to room air.
- Measurements of mean arterial pressure (MAP) should be performed continuously during the acute stages of sepsis to maintain MAP > 45 mm Hg. Dopamine may need to be increased to maintain appropriate perfusion or other inotropic agents added (e.g., dobutamine). Reduced capillary refill times (goal < 2 sec) and skin color changes (i.e., absence of dusky or cyanotic appearance) may also be used as indicators of improved perfusion. Improvements in perfusion and acidosis should occur within the first 24 to 48 hours of appropriate antibiotic therapy.
- Urinary output should be monitored continuously during the acute stages of infection to maintain urine output > 1 mL/kg/hr at all times.
- Daily serum electrolyte monitoring is indicated to assess fluid status during the first 2 to 3 days of treatment to monitor for signs of reduced renal perfusion (secondary to hypoperfusion) that may signify the need to adjust gentamicin dosing.
- Electrolyte and serum creatinine monitoring is also essential to monitor for signs of SIADH, a common complication of meningitis in infants. Suggestive signs include a serum sodium < 135 mEq/L and serum potassium K > 6 mEq/L.
- Neurologic testing should be performed to monitor the infant for improvements in muscle tone and reduction in lethargy. The patient should be observed for clinical evidence of seizures and an EEG should be performed if necessary.
- Audiometry testing is indicated after completion of the antibiotic course in patients with meningitis to evaluate for auditory or vestibular disturbances. Auditory brainstem response (ABR) and vestibular brainstem response measurements are performed in infants to assess auditory and vestibular responses in young infants unable to cooperate with standard testing.
- Gentamicin levels are indicated if therapy is to be continued throughout the treatment course (> 3 to 5 days) primarily to avoid accumulation. Low serum gentamicin levels are needed for synergy with ampicillin (peak 3 to 4 μg/ml; trough < 1 μg/ml).
- Repeat CBC with differential should be performed within 24 to 48 hours to evaluate for improvement in neutropenia and elevated bands. Goals are an ANC >$1.5 \times 10^3/mm^3$ and an I:T ratio < 0.2.
- Head circumference measurements should be performed to observe for complications such as hydrocephalus. Increases in head circumference > 0.5 to 1 cm within a 1- to 2-day period indicate a need for further diagnostic evaluation.
- Further radiographic imaging (e.g., CT scan or neurosonogram) is indicated to evaluate for abscess formation or infarction if the patient develops a complicated course or requires a prolonged time to sterilization of CSF.

References

1. Feigin RD, McCracken GH Jr, Klein JO. Diagnosis and management of meningitis. Pediatr Infect Dis J 1992;11:785–814.
2. American Academy of Pediatrics Committee on Infectious Diseases and Committee on Fetus and Newborn. Revised guidelines for prevention of early-onset group B streptococcal (GBS) infection. Pediatrics 1997;99:489–496.
3. Gerdes JS, Polin RA. Sepsis screen in neonates with evaluation of plasma fibronectin. Pediatr Infect Dis J 1987;6:443–446.
4. Taketomo CK, Hodding JH, Kraus DM. Pediatric Dosage Handbook, 3rd ed. Hudsen, OH, Lexi-Comp, 1996.

94 COMMUNITY-ACQUIRED PNEUMONIA

▶ **Vern's Visit to the Hospital** (Level I)

Patrick P. Gleason, PharmD, BCPS

A 28-year-old man with a history of asthma presents with pleuritic chest pain, dyspnea, orthopnea, fever, chills, and a cough productive of brown sputum. Chest x-ray reveals consolidation of the left lower lobe, and a sputum Gram stain contains many WBC and moderate gram-positive cocci in chains and pairs. Students are asked to recommend initial empiric therapy for this case of community-acquired pneumonia. Therapy is directed toward the most likely organism, *Streptococcus pneumoniae*, and other common etiologies. Reasonable therapeutic alternatives include second- or third-generation cephalosporins, β-lactam/β-lactamase inhibitors, carbapenems, fluoroquinolones, and macrolides. When this patient fails to respond to the single agent chosen initially, students must recommend appropriate changes in the antimicrobial therapy.

Diseases of Infectious Origin 309

influenzae by latex agglutination, and/or urine antigen testing for *Legionella pneumophila* may be helpful in establishing the diagnosis.

► Questions

Problem Identification

1. a. *Create a list of the patient's drug-related problems.*

    - Untreated indication: newly diagnosed episode of community-acquired pneumonia.
    - Failure to receive the drug prescribed: patient ran out of albuterol MDI for control of mild asthma.

   b. *What information (signs, symptoms, laboratory and other diagnostic tests) indicate the presence of community-acquired pneumonia?*

    - *Signs.* Tachycardia, tachypnea, and E-to-A changes in the LLL and across the middle of the right lung field.
    - *Symptoms.* Patient reported 2-day history of left-sided pleuritic chest pain, dyspnea, orthopnea, intermittent fever and chills, intermittent headaches, decreased appetite, and cough productive of yellow and then brown sputum; one episode of emesis. He currently reports mild headache and left-sided pleuritic chest pain radiating to the proximal LUE during coughing.
    - *Laboratory and other diagnostic tests.* Leukocytosis with left shift (13% bands); sputum Gram stain with many WBC and moderate gram-positive cocci in chains and pairs; chest x-ray showing consolidation of the inferior segments of the LLL and the superior segment of the LLL.

   c. *What signs and symptoms indicate the severity of community-acquired pneumonia in this patient?*

    - Patients at low risk for mortality (i.e., 30-day mortality risk of < 0.5%) from community-acquired pneumonia can be identified at presentation by assessing 11 key variables.[1] Low-risk patients are defined as patients < 50 years of age and having none of the following comorbidities: neoplastic disease, CHF, cerebrovascular disease, and renal or liver disease; and none of the following physical exam findings: altered mental status, pulse >125 bpm, RR > 30/minute, systolic BP < 90 mm Hg, or temperature < 35°C or > 40°C.
    - This patient is < 50 years of age, and had none of the comorbidities or physical finding abnormalities listed. Therefore, his likely risk of mortality is low and he could be treated as an outpatient.[1]

   d. *What additional information is needed to satisfactorily assess this patient?*

    - Sexual history and risk factor assessment for HIV with potential HIV testing in this young, otherwise healthy man with pneumonia, increased CPK, dysuria, and proteinuria.
    - Pulse oximetry to assess oxygenation status.
    - Results of sputum and blood cultures to help identify the organism and guide proper antimicrobial selection; however, results generally take 48 to 72 hours.
    - Serologic testing is usually not helpful because the results may require up to 1 week to reach diagnostic titers.
    - Specific antigen testing for *Streptococcus* species or *Haemophilus*

Desired Outcome

2. *What are the goals of pharmacotherapy in this case?*

    - The primary goal is cure of the community-acquired pneumonia and avoidance of mortality.
    - Secondary goals include:
      ✓ Relief of the symptoms of pleuritic chest pain, cough, and shortness of breath.
      ✓ Return to work and usual activities.
      ✓ Avoidance of adverse drug reactions.
      ✓ Conversion of IV to oral antimicrobial therapy when the patient becomes stable.
      ✓ Discharge of the patient once the patient is taking oral therapy successfully and is stable.
      ✓ Potential prevention of further episodes by influenza vaccination. Secondary pneumococcal infections are common after influenza in patients with asthma. The pneumococcal vaccine is not presently recommended for young, otherwise healthy patients with asthma.

Therapeutic Alternatives

3. *What feasible pharmacotherapeutic alternatives are available for treatment of community-acquired pneumonia?*

    - The causative agent of community-acquired pneumonia is usually unknown, and antimicrobial therapy is empiric. Antimicrobial selection is based upon the most likely pathogens and on the patient's specific test results (i.e., Gram stain, sputum culture, blood culture, urine antigen test for *Legionella pneumophila,* and latex agglutination tests). The leading etiologic agent in virtually all studies of community-acquired pneumonia is *Streptococcus pneumoniae*. Other pathogens implicated less frequently in likely order of frequency among hospitalized patients are atypical organisms (*Legionella* species, *Mycoplasma pneumoniae, Chlamydia pneumoniae*), *Haemophilus influenzae,* respiratory viruses, *Staphylococcus aureus,* and gram-negative bacilli (e.g., *Klebsiella pneumoniae, Moraxella catarrhalis*).
    - Therapeutic antimicrobial alternatives for this patient should be directed initially toward *Streptococcus pneumoniae* because the Gram stain indicated gram-positive cocci in chains and pairs.
    - *Penicillin* historically has been the antimicrobial of choice for treatment of *S. pneumoniae,* but increasing resistance due to altered penicillin binding proteins has resulted in decreased organism sensitivity to penicillin. In addition, penicillin generally lacks activity against other potential pathogens such as *H. influenzae* due to penicillinase production. For these reasons, most clinicians would select an alternative antimicrobial agent.
    - *First-generation cephalosporins* (e.g., cefazolin) are not a good first-line empiric choice in this patient due to poor activity against penicillin-resistant *S. pneumoniae.*
    - *Second-generation cephalosporins* (cefuroxime, cefoxitin, cefote-

tan) would be a reasonable choice. Cefotetan and cefoxitin have less activity against gram-positive organisms and are less likely to be effective than cefuroxime. The usual dose of cefuroxime is 750 mg to 1.5 g IV Q 8 H.

- *Third-generation cephalosporins* could also be used. Usual dosage regimens are:
  ✓ *Ceftriaxone* 1 to 2 g IV Q 24 H; doses ≥ 2 g/day have not been shown to result in improved outcomes in patients with community-acquired pneumonia.
  ✓ *Cefotaxime* 1 to 2 g IV Q 8 H
  ✓ *Ceftizoxime* 1 to 2 g IV Q 8 to 12 H
  ✓ *Ceftazidime* (0.5 to 1 g IV Q 8 H); this drug has less activity against gram-positive organisms and is less likely to be effective than other third-generation cephalosporins.
  ✓ *Cefepime* 1 g IV Q 12 H; this drug has a very broad spectrum and there is concern for development of resistance if it is not used judiciously; it is also an expensive agent.
- *Beta-lactam/β-lactamase inhibitors* have less activity against penicillin resistant *S. pneumoniae* than other therapeutic alternatives and are more expensive. Usual doses are:
  ✓ *Ticarcillin/clavulanic* acid 3.1 g IV Q 6 to 8 H.
  ✓ *Piperacillin/tazobactam* 2 to 4 g IV Q 4 to 8 H.
  ✓ *Ampicillin/sulbactam* (1.5 to 3 g IV Q 6 H); this product has less activity against penicillin-resistant *S. pneumoniae* and gram-negative organisms than other alternatives. Therefore, it would not be a good first-line empiric antimicrobial in this patient.
- *Carbapenems* have a very broad spectrum and there is concern for the development of resistance if they are not used judiciously. They are also expensive agents. Usual doses are:
  ✓ *Imipenem/cilastatin* 500 mg IV Q 6 H.
  ✓ *Meropenem* 1 to 2 g IV Q 8 H.
- *Fluoroquinolones* have good activity against atypical organisms, but some have relatively poor gram-positive activity. Ciprofloxacin and ofloxacin have less activity against gram-positive organisms than the other fluoroquinolones listed in this section and are not recommended as first-line therapy.
  ✓ *Levofloxacin* 500 mg IV or po Q 24 H.
  ✓ *Alatrovafloxacin* 200 mg IV Q 24 H or *trovafloxacin* 200 mg po Q 24 H.
  ✓ *Ciprofloxacin* 400 mg IV Q 12 H; not recommended.
  ✓ *Ofloxacin* 400 mg IV Q 12 H; not recommended.
- *Macrolides* are bacteriostatic agents that possess good activity against atypical organisms. They are generally considered for use in combination with a cephalosporin or β-lactam antimicrobial when atypical organisms are suspected (*Mycoplasma* spp., *Legionella* spp., or *Chlamydia* spp.). Azithromycin has been FDA approved for single-agent treatment of moderately ill patients with community-acquired pneumonia. These agents and dosage regimens include:
  ✓ *Erythromycin* 500 mg to 1 g IV or po Q 6 H.
  ✓ *Azithromycin* 500 mg IV or po Q 24 H.
  ✓ *Clarithromycin* 250 to 500 mg po Q 12 H.
- *Vancomycin* does not provide activity against likely pathogens other than *S. pneumoniae* and *S. aureus*. Its use could contribute to vancomycin-resistant pathogens. Therefore, it should not be considered a first-line agent. The usual dose is 1000 mg IV Q 12 H initially, with subsequent doses adjusted based on pharmacokinetic monitoring.

Optimal Plan

4. a. *What drug, dosage form, dose, schedule, and duration of therapy are best for this patient?*

- The Infectious Disease Society of America (IDSA) guidelines for treatment of community-acquired pneumonia[2] for a patient not severely ill (i.e., not admitted to an ICU) suggest initial use of IV antimicrobial therapy with one of the following regimens.
  ✓ A second- or third-generation cephalosporin with good gram-positive coverage (i.e., cefuroxime, cefotaxime, ceftriaxone, or ceftizoxime).
  ✓ The cephalosporin selected may be used with or without an IV or po macrolide (erythromycin or azithromycin).
  ✓ Alternatively, an IV fluoroquinolone with extended gram-positive activity (levofloxacin or alatrovafloxacin) or the macrolide azithromycin may be used.
- Any of these regimens is appropriate. Due to the generic availability of cefuroxime, at our institution it would be most clinically effective and economical to treat this patient initially with cefuroxime 750 mg IV Q 8 H.
- Within the IDSA guidelines, a table of recommended first-line empiric therapies for patients admitted to the hospital includes β-lactam/β-lactamase inhibitors (e.g., ampicillin/sulbactam). However, in the text of the guidelines, β-lactam/β-lactamase inhibitors are not listed as a recommended empiric therapy.[2] Due to concern for the development of penicillin-resistant *S. pneumoniae*, it is this author's recommendation to avoid β-lactam/β-lactamase inhibitors whenever possible.

b. *What changes in the antimicrobial therapy would you recommend, since the initial treatment is apparently failing?*

Possible Alternatives

- Add an IV macrolide (erythromycin or azithromycin) and continue the initial therapy.
- Discontinue the initial therapy and start an IV fluoroquinolone with gram-positive activity (levofloxacin or alatrovafloxacin).
- If a second-generation cephalosporin was used initially, discontinue it and start a third-generation cephalosporin (ceftriaxone, cefotaxime, or ceftizoxime).
- If cefuroxime 750 mg IV Q 8 H was used initially, increase the dose to 1.5 g IV Q 8 H. This option may not be optimal, because increasing the serum drug concentration is not likely to overcome the resistance of *S. pneumoniae*, the most likely organism.
- (*Note to instructors:* At the conclusion of your discussion, you may wish to disclose to students that this patient was actually started on cefuroxime 750 mg IV Q 8 H initially. Erythromycin 500 mg IV Q 6 H was added when the patient continued spiking fevers. When substantial improvement was still not apparent after several days, erythromycin was replaced with ofloxacin 400 mg IV Q 12 H. The patient gradually began to improve on the combination of cefuroxime and ofloxacin. His asthma was controlled with respiratory therapy and MDI albuterol therapy. His very mild rhabdomyolysis ceased.)

Outcome Evaluation

5. a. *What clinical and laboratory parameters are necessary to eval-*

uate the therapy for achievement of the desired therapeutic outcome and to detect or prevent adverse events?

Clinical Parameters for Efficacy

- Take the patient's temperature every 8 hours until it decreases to ≤ 38.0°C for 24 hours, then daily.
- Check heart rate (goal < 100 bpm) every 8 hours for 24 hours, then daily.
- Measure BP (goal systolic >100 mm Hg) every 8 hours for 24 hours, then daily.
- Count spontaneous respiratory rate (goal < 24 breaths/min) every 8 hours, then daily.
- Assess the patient's ability to tolerate oral foods and medications.
- Ask the patient daily about the presence of pleuritic chest pain, severity of cough, and dyspnea. Fifty percent of patients will have resolution of pleuritic chest pain by 7 days and 75% by 30 days.[3]

Laboratory Parameters for Efficacy

- Check WBC count daily until < $10.0 \times 10^3/mm^3$, then every 2 to 3 days.
- Check for results of sputum and blood cultures and antigen testing, then tailor the therapy appropriately if positive.
- Chest x-ray, cough, and shortness of breath take 30 days to resolve; therefore, they should not be considered important clinical outcomes in the initial 7 days.[3]
- Obtain a chest x-ray if the patient does not improve in the first 48 to 72 hours or begins to worsen.

Monitoring for Adverse Reactions

- Ask the patient to report any rash, pruritus, or worsening shortness of breath.
- Ask the patient about pain at the IV access site.
- Ask the patient to report any hearing loss (ototoxicity can occur with erythromycin).
- Ask the patient to report abdominal discomfort or nausea (nausea can occur with any antimicrobial, but it is more likely with erythromycin).
- Record bowel movement frequency and consistency (diarrhea can occur with any antimicrobial).
- Ventricular dysrhythmias can occur with erythromycin. However, in this patient with no history of cardiovascular disease and young age, cardiovascular monitoring is not required.
- For patients taking penicillin, aminopenicillins, and extended spectrum penicillins, have the patient report any unusual bleeding due to the potential for coagulation abnormalities.

b. At what point is it suitable to change from IV to oral therapy?

- Consider switching from IV to oral therapy when the patient has:[4]
   ✓ Stable vital signs for > 24 hours (temperature < 38.0°C, heart rate < 100 bpm, spontaneous respiratory rate < 24 breaths/min, systolic BP > 90 mm Hg without vasopressor support).
   ✓ Tolerated liquids and is able to take oral tablets or capsules.
   ✓ Negative blood cultures.
   ✓ Not been infected with a high-risk pneumonia (e.g., *Staphylococcus aureus*).
   ✓ A WBC count trending downward toward normal.

Patient Counseling

6. What information should be provided to the patient about azithromycin to enhance compliance, ensure successful therapy, and minimize adverse events?

Azithromycin (Zithromax)

- Take this medication exactly as prescribed.
- Azithromycin capsules and suspension should be taken on an empty stomach (1 hour before or 2 hours after meals). Azithromycin tablets may be taken with or without food, but they may be tolerated better if taken with food.
- Take this medication 2 hours before or 4 hours after taking any antacid or iron preparations.
- If you miss a dose, take it as soon as you remember; then resume your regular schedule.
- The most common side effects of azithromycin are diarrhea/loose stools, nausea, and abdominal pain.
- Antibiotics in this class (fluoroquinolones) may make your skin sensitive to the sun. Avoid prolonged exposure to the sun and sun tanning booths. Use a sunscreen if you will be outdoors in the sun for prolonged periods.
- Contact your physician if any of these effects become troublesome or severe.
- Keep all follow-up appointments with your physician.

References

1. Fine MJ, Auble TE, Yealy DM, et al. A prediction rule to identify low-risk patients with community-acquired pneumonia. N Engl J Med 1997;336:243–250.
2. Bartlett JG, Breiman RF, Mandell LA, et al. Community-acquired pneumonia in adults: Guidelines for management. The Infectious Diseases Society of America. Clin Infect Dis 1998;26:811–838.
3. Metlay JP, Fine MJ, Schulz R, et al. Measuring symptomatic and functional recovery in patients with community-acquired pneumonia. J Gen Intern Med 1997;12:423–430.
4. Ramirez JA, Srinath L, Ahkee S, et al. Early switch from intravenous to oral cephalosporins in the treatment of hospitalized patients with community-acquired pneumonia. Arch Intern Med 1995;155:1273–1276.
5. Meehan TP, Fine MJ, Krumholz HM, et al. Quality of care, process, and outcomes in elderly patients with pneumonia. JAMA 1997;278:2080–2084.

95 OTITIS MEDIA

▶ **Ears and Tears** (Level II)

Carla Wallace, PharmD, BCPS

A 15-month-old boy with a history of asthma is brought to his pediatrician because of fever, decreased appetite, and coughing. He has had 7 episodes of acute otitis media (AOM) in the past year; the most recent episode began 14 days ago and was treated with amoxicillin/clavulanic acid. On physical examination, the right and left tympanic membranes are erythematous, bulging, and non-mobile. In this patient with recurrent AOM within 1 month of the previous episode, the causative organism should be presumed to be the same for both infections. However, a different antibiotic effective against β-lactamase-producing organisms should be selected because of the possible development of resistance. Antibiotic selection should be based on the likely causative organisms, antibiotic efficacy against resistant organisms, and patient factors such as prior antibiotic tolerance and likely patient adherence to the complete regimen. After treatment of the AOM, this patient should be considered for prophylactic therapy because he has experienced more than 5 episodes in a 12-month period.

▶ Questions

Problem Identification

1. a. *Create a drug-related problem list for this patient.*

    - Recurrent AOM in need of acute treatment and potentially prophylactic therapy.
    - Asthma exacerbation despite maintenance therapy with albuterol, cromolyn, and beclomethasone.
    - Report of fever, which has apparently been adequately treated with acetaminophen.

    b. *What subjective and objective data support the diagnosis of AOM?*

    - *Subjective.* Irritability and crying; history of anorexia.
    - *Objective.* History of fever (101°F as per mother); tympanic membranes erythematous, bulging, and non-mobile.

    c. *What information indicates the type and severity of otitis media?*

    - The patient's last episode of AOM was 14 days ago. If signs and symptoms of AOM occur within 1 month of the previous episode, it should be assumed that the same organism caused both infections. Resistance may have occurred; therefore, this is a recurrent infection. A different antibiotic should be selected to treat this infection.
    - Prophylactic antibiotics for AOM may be attempted because the patient has experienced 7 episodes over the past year. Prophylaxis may be tried if 4 episodes occur in a 6-month period or if 6 episodes occur in a 12-month period.

    d. *What risk factors for OM are present in this child?*

    - *Age at first episode.* He had his first episode of AOM at 4 months. Infants with a first episode before the age of 6 months have a relative risk of 1.5 of acquiring AOM in the next 24 months compared with children who have a first episode at an age older than 6 months.
    - *Environmental factors.* He attends day care. The incidence of AOM, recurrent episodes, and otitis media with effusion is greater for children who attend day care.
    - *Season.* It is currently January. Otitis media increases in the winter months. This goes along with viral infections of the respiratory tract.
    - *Gender.* Joseph is male and is therefore more at risk for AOM and recurrent disease.
    - *Race.* Compared to African Americans, Caucasians have an increased incidence of AOM. One factor that may explain this increased incidence is the anatomic differences of the eustachian tube.

Desired Outcome

2. *What are the goals of pharmacotherapy for OM in this child?*

    - Eliminate his symptoms
    - Cure the otitis media
    - Prevent recurrence
    - Prevent complications of untreated otitis media
    - Prevent adverse effects of drug treatment

Therapeutic Alternatives

3. a. *What bacterial organisms typically cause OM?*

    - *Streptococcus pneumoniae* (30%)
    - *Haemophilus influenzae* (21%)
    - *Moxarella catarrhalis* (12%)
    - *Streptococcus pyogenes* (3%) and *Staphylococcus aureus* (2%) are uncommon causes

    b. *What pharmacotherapeutic alternatives are available for treatment of AOM in this patient?*

    - *Amoxicillin* would not be an appropriate choice for this child because it does not have activity against β-lactamase producing bacteria.
    - *Amoxicillin/clavulanic acid* cannot be used due to resistance in this patient (infection within the prior month). A different agent must be used.
    - *Trimethoprim-sulfamethoxazole* (TMP-SMX) could be used because it covers β-lactamase producing strains of *H. influenzae* and *M. catarrhalis,* but it is considered to be in the same category as amoxicillin/clavulanate and would not be the first choice because amoxicillin/clavulanate failed. If antibiotic cost is an issue, however, TMP-SMX is less expensive.
    - *Erythromycin/sulfisoxazole* is similar to TMP-SMX but has the disadvantage of requiring multiple administrations per day.
    - *Cefaclor* does not cover all strains of *H. influenzae* and *M. catarrhalis* and is inferior to amoxicillin/clavulanate, cefixime, and cefuroxime axetil in terms of efficacy.
    - *Cefixime* has excellent β-lactamase coverage but reduced activity against pneumococcus. Because of increasing pneumococcal resistance and failure to rule out the organism, cefixime should not be a first choice cephalosporin in this patient's case.
    - *Cefpodoxime proxetil* and *cefuroxime axetil* are ester suspensions that taste bitter and are generally not well tolerated by infants and children. They do have excellent β-lactamase coverage.
    - *Cefprozil* has excellent β-lactamase coverage and requires only twice-daily dosing.

- *Ceftriaxone* is available only parenterally and has been shown to be equally effective to TMP-SMX and cefaclor.[1,2] Results regarding comparison to amoxicillin/clavulanic acid are not as clear.[3] It would not be indicated for a patient such as this who has good follow-up care and can tolerate oral medication. Another consideration is that the 50 mg/kg dosage may require 2 injections in some toddlers.
- *Clarithromycin* and *azithromycin* are newer macrolides used in otitis media. They both have good activity against β-lactamase producing strains of *H. influenzae* and *M. catarrhalis*. Azithromycin has the advantage of administration for only 5 days versus the traditional 10 days for AOM.
- *Loracarbef* has excellent β-lactamase coverage and twice daily dosing.
- *Cefdinir* is a cephalosporin indicated for once-daily treatment of otitis media. Oral capsules and an oral suspension are both available. In a randomized study, patients receiving cefdinir were found to have similar response rates to those receiving amoxicillin/clavulanate. However, the incidence of side effects was lower in patients receiving cefdinir.[4]

c. Other than antibiotics, what other drug or non-drug therapies may be beneficial to this patient?

- Analgesics and antipyretics may comfort the infant or child with OM.
- Local heat to the ear may comfort the infant.
- Decongestants and antihistamines have not been shown to be of benefit.

Optimal Plan

4. Which of the above alternatives would you recommend to treat this child's AOM? Include the dose, duration of therapy, and rationale.

- Because his AOM occurred within 1 month of a previous episode, it was most likely caused by the same pathogen. Therefore, the emergence of resistance has to be assumed. Since amoxicillin/clavulanate was used to treat the previous episode, a different agent needs to be selected to treat the current episode.
- Another agent with β-lactamase coverage should be selected.[5] Cefixime, cefpodoxime proxetil, cefuroxime axetil, cefprozil, azithromycin, clarithromycin, and loracarbef are effective second-line agents in the treatment of AOM caused by resistant stains of *H. influenzae* and *M. catarrhalis*, which are probably the cause in this situation.
- Patient factors should be considered when choosing the optimal therapy. This child has tolerated cephalosporins and macrolides in the past. Compliance should be considered, especially because he attends day care. An antibiotic requiring dosing 3 or 4 times a day may not be given completely. An appropriate antibiotic that requires the fewest daily doses should be selected. Although cost varies with geographic location, in general, all cephalosporins and the newer macrolides are high in price/kilogram, but the differences among them are usually not significant. All of the therapies discussed above are available in oral liquid formulations, with the exception of ceftriaxone.
- Based on these considerations, the "best" drugs and regimens for this child are:
  - ✓ Cefprozil suspension 200 mg (4 mL) po Q 12 H × 10 days
  - ✓ Azithromycin suspension 120 mg (3 mL) po QD on day 1, then 60 mg (1.5 mL) QD on days 2 through 5
  - ✓ Clarithromycin suspension 100 mg (4 mL) po Q 12 H × 10 days
  - ✓ Loracarbef suspension 200 mg (5 mL) po Q 12 H × 10 days
- Cefpodoxime proxetil 70 mg (3.5 mL) po Q 12 H and cefuroxime axetil 200 mg (8 mL) po Q 12 H have appropriate coverage and would be reasonable choices, but bad taste might compromise patient compliance.

Outcome Evaluation

5. How should the therapy you recommended be monitored for efficacy and adverse effects?

Efficacy

- Improvement of irritability and return of appetite within 48 to 72 hours.
- Resolution of eardrum bulging and return of eardrum mobility; a follow-up ear exam would be appropriate after completion of therapy.
- Normalization of temperature within 48 hours.

Adverse Effects

- Ask the patient's mother about the frequency of stools to monitor for diarrhea.
- Tell the parent to monitor the skin for rashes.
- Cefprozil has been associated with serum sickness, so ask about fever, skin eruptions, and arthralgias.
- The newer macrolides may still cause GI distress, although less frequently than erythromycin.

Patient Counseling

6. How would you provide important information about this therapy to the child's mother?

General Information

- It is very important that Joseph finish all of this medication so that his infection will be treated completely. The duration of treatment will be 10 days (5 days if azithromycin is used).
- Joseph's symptoms should start to improve within 48 hrs; notify your physician or me if he does not improve by this time.
- You may continue to give Joseph acetaminophen (Tylenol) for his fever. However, antihistamines and decongestants have not been shown to be effective for treatment of ear infections.

Cefprozil (Example)

- Cefprozil is a suspension, so it should be shaken well before using. It also requires refrigeration.
- Joseph's dose of cefprozil is 4 milliliters given every 12 hours. Do you have a measuring spoon or syringe you can use for his dose? Can you show me how you use it? A special measuring syringe or spoon should be used instead of a regular tablespoon.
- If Joseph develops a rash, it could be caused by the antibiotic. If this occurs, stop giving Joseph the medicine and notify your physician or me right away.

- This medication could also cause diarrhea; notify your physician or me if it occurs and is severe.

▶ Follow-up Questions

1. *Will this child benefit from further antibiotic treatment after this course of therapy for AOM? Include the rationale for your response and suggest appropriate drug regimens.*

   - He has had 7 episodes of OM in the past 12 months, so prophylaxis should be considered.
   - Reasonable therapeutic alternatives include:
     ✓ Amoxicillin 20 to 30 mg/kg/day in 1 to 2 divided doses.
     ✓ Sulfisoxazole 80 to 100 mg/kg/day in 1 daily dose.
     ✓ TMP-SMZ 4 mg/kg/day (TMP component) in 1 daily dose.
   - Treat an acute recurrence with a different antibiotic if amoxicillin was used for prophylaxis. Resume prophylaxis after a full course of antibiotic therapy.

2. *How should Joseph's acute exacerbation of asthma be addressed? Provide specific recommendations for therapy.*

   - Increase the frequency of albuterol (but not cromolyn) to Q 6 H.
   - A burst of oral prednisolone (1 to 2 mg/kg/day = 15 mg po QD) for 3 to 5 days may be considered.

References

1. Barnett ED, Teele DW, Klein JO, et al. Comparison of ceftriaxone and trimethoprim-sulfamethoxazole for acute otitis media. Pediatrics 1997;99:23–28.
2. Chamberlain JM, Boenning DA, Waisman Y, et al. Single-dose ceftriaxone versus 10 days of cefaclor for otitis media. Clin Pediatr (Phila) 1994;33:642–646.
3. Varsano I, Volovitz B, Horev Z, et al. Intramuscular ceftriaxone compared with oral amoxicillin-clavulanate for treatment of acute otitis media in children. Eur J Pediatr 1997;156:858–863.
4. Adler M, McDonald PJ, Trostmann U, et al. Cefdinir versus amoxicillin/clavulanic acid in the treatment of suppurative acute otitis media in children. Eur J Clin Microbiol Infect Dis 1997;16:214–219.
5. Rosenfeld RM. An evidence-based approach to treating otitis media. Pediatr Clin North Am 1996;43:1165–1181.

96 STREPTOCOCCAL PHARYNGITIS

▶ It's Not Just a Sore Throat   (Level I)

Denise L. Howrie, PharmD
Elaine McGhee, MD

A 5-year-old girl is brought to the pediatrician because of a sore throat, fever, decreased appetite, and headache. Physical examination reveals pharyngeal erythema, and a rapid streptococcal antigen test is positive. Oral penicillin VK for 10 days remains the treatment of choice for Group A β-hemolytic streptococcal (GABHS) pharyngitis. A single dose of IM benzathine penicillin G with or without procaine penicillin may obviate the need for adherence to an oral regimen. Oral amoxicillin may be more palatable than penicillin VK, but its use should be discouraged to prevent development of antimicrobial resistance. Oral erythromycin may be used for penicillin-allergic patients; other macrolides such as clarithromycin and azithromycin should be limited to patients unable to tolerate erythromycin. Selected first-generation cephalosporins (e.g., cephalexin, cefadroxil) may be used in penicillin-allergic patients, but the broader-spectrum second- and third-generation agents should not be routinely used. Symptoms of GABHS pharyngitis generally resolve within several days of initiating therapy, but patients or their caregivers should be advised to continue the antimicrobial regimen for the entire duration prescribed.

▶ Questions

Problem Identification

1. a. *Create a list of the patient's drug-related problem(s).*

   - GABHS pharyngitis requiring antimicrobial therapy.
   - Fever requiring an antipyretic for symptomatic relief.

   b. *What information indicates the presence or severity of pharyngitis?*

   - Relevant patient-specific history includes sore throat for 2 days, temperature 100.8°F, headache, and nausea.
   - Objective evidence includes tonsillar hypertrophy and erythema without exudate, erythema of the soft palate and tongue, cervical lymphadenopathy, and a positive rapid strep antigen test.
   - Findings that may be present in other patients with GABHS include pain with swallowing, emesis, abdominal pain without coryza, cough, conjunctivitis or diarrhea. These episodes generally occur in winter and spring seasons in children ages 5 to 15 years. When symptoms are accompanied by a fine, diffuse erythematous rash, a diagnosis of "scarlet fever" is made.[1]

   c. *How can the diagnosis of streptococcal pharyngitis best be made in a timely manner?*

   - No findings in the patient history or physical examination will conclusively identify GABHS as the cause of infectious pharyngitis. When findings suggest streptococcal infection as a cause of pharyngitis, a rapid antigen detection test using a well-collected throat swab sample may, within minutes, confirm the presence of GABHS and strongly suggest a diagnosis of GABHS pharyngitis. False-positive test results are unusual. However, because rapid antigen detection tests have a 10% to 20% incidence of false-negative results, a confirmatory throat culture may be useful in cases where rapid strep screen results are negative in the presence of active symptoms.[1,2]

- Empiric antibacterial therapy may be initiated pending results of throat cultures in patients with symptoms strongly suggestive of GABHS. Antibiotics should be discontinued if subsequent cultures are negative for GABHS or other pathogenic bacteria.[2]

Desired Outcome

2. *State the goals of treatment of GABHS pharyngitis in this case.*

   - Rapidly resolve symptoms with return of the patient to normal activities as soon as possible.
   - Reduce contagiousness.
   - Prevent the development of rheumatic fever.
   - Prevent complications such as peritonsillar abscess, fasciitis, and toxic shock syndrome.
   - Antimicrobial treatment should be cost-effective, associated with minimal and tolerable adverse effects, have a high compliance rate, and have a low likelihood of acquired drug resistance. No treatment regimen will eradicate GABHS from the pharynx in all patients, nor is this required for symptom resolution or prevention of post-streptococcal complications.[3]

Therapeutic Alternatives

3. a. *What non-drug therapies may be helpful in this child?*

   - Comfort measures for pharyngitis may include the use of a humidifier to reduce environmental dryness, avoidance of smoke and other irritants, and oral lozenges to provide topical lubrication.

   b. *What therapeutic alternatives are available for treatment of pharyngitis?*

   - Most episodes of infectious pharyngitis are the result of respiratory viruses. However, when GABHS is identified in patients with clinical symptoms of pharyngitis, many antibacterial agents may be selected for treatment. Characteristics of an "ideal" antibacterial agent include:
     ✓ Narrow antibacterial spectrum directed against streptococcal species
     ✓ Documented reliability in organism eradication and prevention of rheumatic fever
     ✓ Tolerable adverse effects including no significant drug–drug or drug–food interactions
     ✓ High rates of regimen compliance
     ✓ Low cost
   - *Oral penicillin V* has been the regimen of choice since the 1950s, with estimated bacteriologic failure rates of 10% to 25%.[4] Despite the availability of more extended-spectrum antibacterial agents, oral penicillin VK for 10 days in age-adjusted doses as low as 250 to 500 mg TID in children and adults remains the most cost-effective regimen for initial episodes of streptococcal pharyngitis in patients who do not demonstrate penicillin allergy. Its narrow antibacterial spectrum, low cost, documented efficacy over decades of use, and rare serious adverse effects contribute to the continued recommendation of oral penicillin as the drug of choice.[1–3] However, the bitter taste of penicillin in tablet or liquid formulations may discourage compliance, especially in children.
   - *IM benzathine penicillin G* in a single dose of 600,000 units (if < 27 kg) or 1.2 million units (if > 27 kg) may be administered alone or in combination with *procaine penicillin* to reduce pain; this improves compliance and may be especially useful for patients with a history of rheumatic fever.[1,3]
   - *Oral amoxicillin* in suspension or chewable tablet formulations may be better tolerated by children due to its more pleasant flavor[1,2] and is routinely prescribed by pediatricians. However, it is not recommended for routine use due to its broader antibacterial spectrum and the potential development of drug resistance.
   - *Oral erythromycin* for 10 days is a recommended alternative in penicillin-allergic patients.[1–3] Erythromycin estolate 20 to 40 mg/kg/day or erythromycin ethyl succinate 40 mg/kg/day (1 g/day total dose) may be given in 2 to 4 divided doses. Although BID dosing may improve compliance, GI toxicity generally necessitates more frequent dosing. Also, the efficacy of BID dosing in adults has not been studied.
   - *Clarithromycin* suspension or tablets (about 15 mg/kg/day in 2 divided doses for 10 days) and azithromycin suspension (12 mg/kg/day in a single daily dose for 5 days) are more expensive alternatives that may reduce GI toxicity. However, their increased cost and extended antibacterial activity should limit routine use of these agents to patients intolerant of other agents.
   - *Cephalexin, cefadroxil (first-generation cephalosporins), or other cephalosporins* could be used for 10 days in selected penicillin-allergic patients.[1,3] The increased cost and extended spectrum are counter-balanced with the convenience of cefadroxil QD dosing or the improved taste of liquid cephalexin products. Second- and third-generation cephalosporins should be reserved for other indications due to their increased cost, unnecessarily broad antibacterial spectrum, and often increased adverse effect profiles. Although these antibiotics may successfully treat GABHS pharyngitis, efficacy in preventing rheumatic fever has not been determined. Pediatric cephalosporin doses are provided as follows.
     ✓ *Cephalexin* 25 to 50 mg/kg/day in 2 divided doses
     ✓ *Cefadroxil* 30 mg/kg/day in 1 or 2 divided doses
     ✓ *Cefaclor* 20 mg/kg/day in 2 divided doses
     ✓ *Cefixime* 8 mg/kg/day in 2 divided doses
     ✓ *Cefprozil* 15 mg/kg/day in 2 divided doses
     ✓ *Cefuroxime* axetil 20 mg/kg/day in 2 divided doses
     ✓ *Loracarbef* 15 mg/kg/day in 2 divided doses
     ✓ *Ceftibuten* 9 mg/kg/day in a single daily dose
     ✓ *Cefpodoxime proxetil* 10 mg/kg/day in 2 divided doses
   - *Clindamycin* is not usually used for initial therapy but may be considered in doses of 20 to 30 mg/kg/day in 2 to 4 divided doses for 10 days in patients with multidrug allergies to penicillins, cephalosporins, and macrolides. Clindamycin may be used in symptomatic patients with repeated episodes of GABHS pharyngitis.
   - A small number of studies have investigated the use of shorter antibiotic courses with drugs such as amoxicillin and selected cephalosporins for GABHS; however, none of these shorter regimens is presently FDA approved.[4]
   - Tetracyclines, sulfonamides, trimethoprim-sulfamethoxazole, and quinolone antibacterial agents should not be used for streptococcal pharyngitis infections due to inadequate spectrum against GABHS.[1,3]

Optimal Plan

4. a. *What drug, dosage form, dose, schedule, and duration of therapy are best for this patient?*

   - The preferred regimen for this child is penicillin VK 250 mg/5 mL suspension in a dose of 250 mg (1 teaspoonful) by mouth 3 times a day for 10 days. As previously stated, this is the most cost-effective regimen for this patient who does not have a history of drug allergy to penicillins. The suspension would be most convenient for this child, given the difficulty most young children have with swallowing solid dosage forms that cannot be chewed.
   - Acetaminophen may be used every 4 hours as needed for patient comfort and to reduce fever in a dose of 240 mg (about 10 mg/kg/dose) using either 1½ 160-mg chewable tablets or 1½ teaspoonful of the 160 mg/5 mL elixir. Families should be cautioned about the various acetaminophen concentrations available in tablets and liquid forms to ensure accurate and safe dosing in infants and young children.

   b. *What alternatives would be appropriate if the initial therapy cannot be used?*

   - In this child who may not be compliant with penicillin due to its bitter taste in both tablet and liquid forms, amoxicillin 250 mg by mouth TID in either chewable tablet or liquid suspension form could be used to complete a 10-day course. However, this practice should be reserved for children who are non-compliant with penicillin products to reduce potential drug resistance.
   - If signs of penicillin allergy develop during treatment, erythromycin estolate for 10 days may be substituted. If the allergic reaction is limited to a mild urticaria or other rash reaction, cefadroxil or cephalexin could also be considered.

   c. *If the child's symptoms recur after completion of the prescribed regimen, what options are then available?*

   - Recurrence of symptoms after completion of a 10-day course of penicillin may be the result of poor compliance; the presence of β-lactamase-producing flora, which impedes penicillin effects; reacquisition of the same or a new strain of GABHS; or development of pharyngitis unrelated to streptococcal disease.[1]
   - Poor compliance is a frequent cause of treatment failure with a 10-day course of penicillin. Reasons for variable compliance include symptomatic improvement within 1 to 3 days of initiation of treatment, with reduced incentive to complete the prescribed course; reported bitter penicillin taste or gastrointestinal toxicity; and use of penicillin QID instead of a more convenient TID or BID schedule. Unfortunately, the use of 5- to 7-day courses of oral penicillin less effectively eradicates infecting organisms.
   - Although streptococcus organisms have remained exquisitely sensitive to penicillin through decades of use, β-lactamase-producing bacteria in the pharyngeal area may "protect" GABHS, resulting in failure to eradicate an infecting strain. Patients may reacquire streptococcal organisms from contacts, so symptom recurrence may actually represent a new infectious episode. Also, patients may be asymptomatic carriers of streptococcus species with incidental symptoms of pharyngitis unrelated to the colonizing streptococcal organisms harbored in the nasopharynx.
   - In patients who do not experience symptom resolution with treatment or who complain of recurrent pharyngitis within several days of appropriate treatment, a first-generation cephalosporin for 10 days or azithromycin for 5 days may be used. Alternatively, oral clindamycin or IM benzathine penicillin G may be considered.
   - A patient with multiple episodes of apparent GABHS pharyngitis within several months presents a management dilemma. Close contacts such as family members may be screened using throat cultures to determine the presence of asymptomatic carriers who may benefit from treatment with clindamycin, sometimes in combination with rifampin, to eradicate the carrier state and prevent reinfection.

Outcome Evaluation

5. *What clinical and laboratory parameters are necessary to evaluate the therapy for achievement of the desired outcome and to detect or prevent adverse effects?*

   Efficacy
   - Patients with streptococcal pharyngitis frequently experience symptom resolution within several days, regardless of whether antibiotics are used. Therefore, the clinician should evaluate patients who have persistent and/or increasingly severe fever, pharyngitis, or other constitutional symptoms. In most patients, no further diagnostic tests are necessary to document organism eradication.

   Adverse Effects
   - In general, regardless of the antibacterial agent chosen, patients should be evaluated for the development of moderate or severe GI symptoms, especially nausea, emesis, pain, or diarrhea, which may prevent completion of the prescribed regimen.
   - Evidence of drug allergy, such as shortness of breath, urticaria, throat or tongue swelling, or fever should be monitored.
   - Oral or vaginal superinfections with yeast and *Clostridium difficile* colitis should be considered when extended-spectrum agents such as cephalosporins are used.

Patient Counseling

6. *What information should be provided to the patient's parents to enhance compliance, ensure success of therapy, and minimize adverse effects?*

   Penicillin VK
   - The antibiotic penicillin has been prescribed because your daughter has strep throat. Although she may feel better in a day or two, she will have the best cure if she takes every dose for 10 days.
   - After she has taken the drug for a full day, she may return to day care, pre-school, or kindergarten if she feels well.
   - I suggest that you give a dose when she wakes up (at least 1 hour before breakfast) and a second dose at bedtime (at least 2 hours after dinner or snacks).
   - Shake the bottle for about a minute and measure the dose using this mouth syringe that I have marked at "1 teaspoon."
   - Taking the liquid with a glass of water will help reduce or prevent upset stomach.
   - If you forget to give a dose or two, don't give a "double-dose" but just add the dose(s) to the total 10-day course.

- If there is any medication left after 10 days and she has taken all her doses, discard the remaining medicine.
- Call your pediatrician if she still has a sore throat or fever in 2 days or if her sore throat comes back after the 10-day treatment course.
- Please call me or your pediatrician if your daughter develops a skin rash, itching, hives, shortness of breath, joint pain, or any other new problem. About 2% of people are allergic to penicillin.

References

1. Gerber MA. Strep pharyngitis: Update on management. Contemporary Pediatr 1997;14:156–165.
2. Schwartz B, Marcy SM, Phillips WR, et al. Pharyngitis—principles of judicious use of antimicrobial agents. Pediatrics 1998;101S:171–174.
3. Dajani AS. Current therapy of Group A streptococcal pharyngitis. Pediatr Ann 1998;27:277–280.
4. Pichichero ME, Cohen R. Shortened course of antibiotic therapy for acute otitis media, sinusitis and tonsillopharyngitis. Pediatr Infect Dis J 1997;16:680–695.

97 RHINOSINUSITIS

▶ Head Case (Level II)

Aaron D. Killian, PharmD, BCPS

A 25-year-old man with head pressure, fever, and leukocytosis is ultimately diagnosed with chronic infectious rhinosinusitis. Appropriate empiric antimicrobial therapy directed toward the most common infecting organisms includes β-lactams, fluoroquinolones, and macrolides/azalides for 3 to 6 weeks. Inhaled corticosteroids may also be beneficial for this patient. Several other adjunctive therapies may also be considered to relieve symptoms and improve mucociliary clearance. When the patient returns after 4 months of appropriate therapy with improved but persistent symptoms, students are asked to recommend appropriate changes in therapy.

▶ Questions

Problem Identification

1. a. Identify all of the drug-related problems of this patient.

- Multiple clinical findings of malaise, arthralgias, fevers, head pressure/tenderness, abdominal cramping, diarrhea, and neutrophilia/eosinophilia. All require further diagnostic evaluation and possible drug therapy if found to be unrelated to a solitary treatable problem.
- Use of PRN medications; the clinician must determine their frequency of use, whether he would benefit from regular use or discontinuation of these agents, or if they could be exacerbating any of the patient's symptoms.
- Naproxen use for an unknown indication (possibly arthralgias). NSAIDs should be used with caution, as they may induce nasal polyps with prolonged use in patients with significant nasal/systemic allergy.
- Continued use of levocabastine; evaluate whether or not GPC has resolved.
- Antihistamines may be a cause of drowsiness/lethargy and/or undesirable anticholinergic side effects. Antihistamines are best avoided in sinusitis as they impair mucociliary clearance and elimination of bacteria from sinus passages. The second-generation, non-sedating antihistamines have the least effect on mucociliary clearance. Consequently, this patient might benefit from a switch to loratadine, cetirizine, fexofenadine, or astemizole.

b. What clinical and laboratory features are consistent with a diagnosis of infectious rhinosinusitis rather than nasal allergy (inflammatory rhinosinusitis) in this patient? (Note: Rhinosinusitis is used instead of the term sinusitis since the nose and sinuses are both generally involved in the inflammatory process.)

- *Rhinosinusitis.* Temporal/frontal pressure, ocular/maxillary hyperaesthesia (i.e., facial pain) involving cranial nerve V, maxillary gum discomfort, nasal crusting/mucosal hypertrophy, post-nasal discharge, difficulty concentrating ("swimming" feeling), malaise, fever of 100.3°F, and a previous CT showing sinus opacification are all consistent with rhinosinusitis. With the exception of headache, this patient has a history and symptoms suggestive of multiple sinus involvement.
  - ✓ Ethmoid sinus: retro-orbital pain
  - ✓ Frontal sinus: supra-orbital pain; frontal pressure in a "mask-like" pattern
  - ✓ Maxillary sinus: maxillary tooth/gum discomfort; cheek and ipsilateral temple involvement
  - ✓ Sphenoid sinus: headaches, optic nerve involvement; meningitis
- *Allergy.* Use of a topical mast cell stabilizer (levocabastine) for conjunctivitis and an oral antihistamine (clemastine fumarate) for itchy eyes and paroxysmal sneezing suggest oculonasal allergy. Signs and symptoms such as malaise, "shiners," migratory arthralgias, sleep disturbance, mild GI disturbances, and eosinophilia suggest that this patient may also have significant systemic allergy as well.
- *Differentiating between infectious and inflammatory disease.*[1] The presence of an infectious process is suggested by the classical appearance of a viscous, often purulent, post-nasal discharge (as opposed to thin, watery secretions in allergic disease), persistent facial/sinus pressure (often aggravated by bending down), and hypertrophied nasal mucosa. A simple Gram stain of nasal mucus could also be used to determine the underlying cause; neutrophils predominate in acute bacterial and early viral infections whereas eosinophils are most numerous in allergic rhinitis. An erythematous nasal mucosa may also indicate infection but is less specific in regions of high humidity where a more pale appearance may resemble nasal allergy.

c. *Are this patient's signs and symptoms consistent with acute, recurrent acute, or chronic rhinosinusitis?*

Patients with rhinosinusitis may be classified as follows.[2]
- *Acute rhinosinusitis.* The patient frequently has symptoms such as facial pain, headache, fever, fatigue, nasal congestion, purulent thick nasal discharge for longer than 1 week, and/or evidence of ostial obstruction. Symptoms rarely persist beyond 1 month, and the patient usually has no more than 4 episodes a year. These episodes generally resolve by 1 month requiring no additional therapy.
- *Recurrent acute rhinosinusitis.* While not receiving medical therapy, the patient has recurrent acute episodes, each separated by 2 weeks or more.
- *Chronic rhinosinusitis.* The patient has persistent disease not controlled by medical therapy and mucosal hypertrophy documented by endoscopic exam or radiography/diagnostic imaging. This category also applies to adults with: 1) 2 or more months of persistent symptoms; 2) ≥ 4 episodes a year, each longer than 10 days duration; and/or 3) continued CT abnormalities 2 months after medical therapy (without intercurrent infection).
- The presence of mucosal hypertrophy and 6 months of persistent symptoms in a patient with documented sinus aberrations imply that this patient has developed chronic rhinosinusitis as a result of multiple recurrent acute infections. In addition, he has facial/sinus pressure with viscous post-nasal discharge, yet lacks significant nasal congestion. These features (sometimes accompanied by chronic cough and diminished olfactory sensation) are hallmarks of chronic rhinosinusitis.

d. *What factors predispose this patient to the development of rhinosinusitis?*

- Allergic rhinitis
- Previous dental extraction
- Mucosal hypertrophy
- First-generation antihistamine use (cause reduced mucociliary clearance in patients with nasal allergy)

Desired Outcome

2. *What are the goals of pharmacotherapy in this patient?*

- Treatment with aggressive antibiotic therapy directed toward elimination of infection, prevention of recurrences, and avoidance of surgical intervention.
- Implementation of an adjunctive maintenance regimen that will alleviate facial/sinus pressure and pain, diminish allergic symptomatology, suppress mucosal inflammation, and improve mucociliary clearance/sinus ventilation to reduce bacterial colonization.
- Avoidance of serious sequelae such as brain abscess, frontal bone osteomyelitis, meningitis, and adjacent ocular infection (e.g., orbital cellulitis/abscess).

Therapeutic Alternatives

3. a. *What are the most likely causative pathogens in this patient?*

- *Bacteria.*[3] Acute rhinosinusitis is most often caused by *Streptococcus pneumoniae* (41%), *Haemophilus influenzae* (35%), other streptococci and anaerobes (7%), *Moraxella catarrhalis* (4%), and *Staphylococcus aureus* (3%). *M. catarrhalis* is about 5-fold more prevalent in children where otitis media is a coexisting illness in 50% of the patients.

  In this patient, chronic rhinosinusitis is more likely to be caused by *S. aureus* and also gram-negative bacilli (e.g., *H. influenzae, Klebsiella pneumoniae,* or *Pseudomonas* spp.), α-hemolytic streptococci, and anaerobes (often anaerobic cocci such as *Peptostreptococcus,* or bacilli such as *Porphyromonas, Prevotella, Bacteroides,* and *Fusobacterium* spp.), in addition to those listed.[4] The recent discovery of this microbiologic shift to anaerobes in chronic disease may be related to use of the newer technique of middle meatus endoscopy rather than the historical gold standard maxillary puncture. Interestingly, endoscopic cultures report a higher incidence of anaerobes and staphylococci/aerobes in maxillary and ethmoid disease, respectively. Some theorize that anaerobes may be indirectly pathogenic in that they protect susceptible pathogens via β-lactamase production.[5]

  Chlamydia pneumoniae and *Mycoplasma pneumoniae* have recently been suggested as pathogens in patients with concurrent respiratory illness, atypical pneumonia, and bronchitis. Although serologic evidence exists for the former, the latter has yet to be confirmed from sinus culture, and the precise role of these organisms in rhinosinusitis is unknown.
- *Viruses.* Sinus cultures have revealed influenzae, parainfluenzae, and the rhinovirus in some patients. Viral infections may lead to mucosal thickening, nasal congestion, and increased nasal discharge. Furthermore, sinus drainage/ventilation may be disrupted, allowing for transient bacterial colonization of the ostiomeatal complex.
- *Fungi.* These organisms are uncommonly involved in immunocompetent patients. Fungal infection may occur as allergic fungal sinusitis (AFS), a benign, non-invasive disease caused by allergy to fungal antigens. It usually occurs in patients with chronic disease who exhibit persistent nasal congestion, discharge for months to years, atopy, nasal polyps, and/or peripheral eosinophilia. Most cases are due to phaeohyphomycoses (*Alternaria, Bipolaris,* and *Curvularia*) and *Aspergillus* spp.

b. *What antibiotics are available for the acute empiric therapy of rhinosinusitis?*

- β-*lactams* (e.g., amoxicillin/clavulanic acid,[b,c] cefpodoxime proxetil,[b] cefuroxime axetil,[b,e] cefprozil,[b,c,e,f] and loracarbef[c,e,f]).
- *Fluoroquinolones* (e.g., levofloxacin,[a] sparfloxacin,[a] and trovafloxacin[a]).
- *Macrolides/azalides* (e.g., clarithromycin,[c] azithromycin[c,d]).

  [a] Most active against aerobic rhinosinusitis pathogens (including resistant *S. pneumoniae*).
  [b] Effective against intermediately-resistant *S. pneumoniae*.
  [c] Least desirable agents for the treatment of *highly resistant S. pneumoniae*.
  [d] Least desirable agents for *S. aureus*.
  [e] Increasing resistance to β-lactamase producing *M. catarrhalis*.
  [f] Increasing resistance to β-lactamase producing *H. influenzae*.
- The overall resistance of *S. pneumoniae* to specific antibiotics

used to treat sinusitis is amoxicillin/clavulanic acid 24%, cefuroxime 12%, clarithromycin 10%, and levofloxacin 0%. Cefprozil and loracarbef are both less active than cefuroxime.[6] Due to trends toward antimicrobial resistance, amoxicillin, erythromycin, and trimethoprim-sulfamethoxazole should no longer be considered as first-line agents for empiric therapy in most centers.

Optimal Plan

4. a. Based on the patient's presentation, what would you recommend as initial antibiotic and anti-inflammatory therapy? Include drug(s), dosage form(s), schedule(s), and duration(s) of therapy.

Antibiotics

- Because this patient has chronic rhinosinusitis, the best initial therapy should cover *S. aureus* and gram-negative bacilli in addition to the usual acute rhinosinusitis pathogens. The aforementioned β-lactams and fluoroquinolones cover most of these organisms.
- Antipseudomonal coverage with a fluoroquinolone may not be necessary in this patient but should be used in severe cases or in patients who fail to improve after sinus surgery. This patient is less likely to have atypical or fungal rhinosinusitis (see Question 3.a).
- Since a mixed anaerobic infection is certainly a possibility, amoxicillin/clavulanic acid is preferred, but trovafloxacin or clindamycin plus ciprofloxacin/ofloxacin are rational alternatives. Levofloxacin and sparfloxacin have only moderate activity against anaerobes, especially *Prevotella* and non-*fragilis Bacteroides*. Considering spectrum of activity and side-effect profiles, the most appropriate choices would likely be monotherapy with one of the following for a minimum of 3 to 6 weeks.[7]
  - ✓ Amoxicillin/clavulanic acid 500 mg po TID (875 mg po BID if compliance is an issue)
  - ✓ Cefpodoxime proxetil 200 mg po BID[a]
  - ✓ Cefuroxime axetil 250 to 500 mg po BID[a,b]
  - ✓ Levofloxacin 500 mg po QD[c]
    - [a] No anaerobic activity.
    - [b] May exhibit better activity against resistant *S. aureus* than cefpodoxime.
    - [c] Consider ciprofloxacin/ofloxacin plus clindamycin or monotherapy with trovafloxacin to cover anaerobes in chronic sinusitis.
- The other antibiotics listed in the answer to question 3.b. are acceptable alternatives as long as the clinician recognizes their inherent limitations and monitors closely for resolution of infection.

Intranasal Corticosteroids

- These medications are especially helpful for allergic rhinosinusitis, eosinophilia, and vasomotor (non-allergic) rhinosinusitis.
- A variety of products may be used, including, triamcinolone acetonide (Nasacort 2 sprays QD), flunisolide (Nasalide 2 sprays BID), beclomethasone (Beconase AQ 1 to 2 sprays BID, Vancenase AQ 1 to 2 sprays QD), budesonide (Rhinocort 2 sprays BID or 4 sprays QD), or fluticasone (Flonase 1 to 2 sprays QD). Corticosteroids are more effective than cromolyn sodium for chronic sinusitis with an allergic component.

b. What adjunctive measures can be employed to optimize this patient's medical therapy?

- Decongestants restrict nasal blood flow, widen ostia, and promote sinus drainage/ventilation. Topical products should be used no longer than 3 to 5 days to avoid rhinitis medicamentosa. Systemic products (e.g., phenylpropanolamine 75 mg po BID, pseudoephedrine 120 mg po BID) are the best choice in patients with chronic rhinosinusitis. They should be avoided in patients with prostatic hyperplasia, diabetes, glaucoma, and hypertension.
- Analgesics may be used for relief of sinus pain. Acetaminophen is preferred over NSAIDs to avoid the risk of nasal polyp formation.
- A high-efficiency particulate air (HEPA)/electrostatic filter may be used in the home to reduce allergic symptoms.
- Nasal saline irrigation (using commercial buffered products and bulb syringing) improves mucociliary clearance and provides a mild decongestant effect. Rarely, preservatives in commercial products may be irritating, especially to those with allergy. Use only sterile saline, because non-sterile fluids can introduce gram-negative bacteria into sinuses.
- Steam inhalation also enhances mucociliary clearance; membrane warming can be achieved with saunas, whirlpools, or by boiling water on the stove or in a cup.
- Humidification is especially helpful during winter/cold months. It reduces the viscosity of nasal mucus and prevents drying, irritation, swelling, and secondary infection. Ultrasonic humidification is better than steam humidification, but both may increase molds and dust mites; they should be used with caution in this patient with allergic rhinosinusitis.
- Vigorous exercise may be helpful in improving mucociliary clearance.
- Expectorants (e.g., guaifenesin LA 1.2 g BID) may help to thin tenacious secretions and reduce the adhesiveness of mucus. The guaifenesin component of combination decongestant/expectorant products (e.g., Entex LA) may alleviate the drying effect of the decongestant.
- Eating spicy foods or chicken soup appear to be helpful, but well-controlled studies are lacking.
- Ipratropium bromide (Atrovent) nasal spray is *not* recommended for this patient. It is excellent for perennial allergic and non-allergic (e.g., vasomotor) rhinorrhea. It should be avoided in patients with thick, tenacious secretions and those lacking rhinorrhea.

Outcome Evaluation

5. How should these new medications be monitored for efficacy and adverse effects?

Efficacy

- Patients should be encouraged to report any significant worsening of disease before the next follow-up. If the patient appears to have resolution of symptoms, repeat laboratory testing is not necessary.
- If symptoms persist but the rhinosinusitis has not worsened significantly, the patient may benefit from a second or longer course of an-

tibiotic therapy (e.g., 4 to 6 weeks) without further laboratory work-up.
- If no improvement is observed after 2 to 3 courses of therapy, the patient should have further laboratory/diagnostic testing (i.e., repeat CT scan, endoscopy with culture/sensitivity) and functional endoscopic sinus surgery may need to be considered.

Adverse Effects

- *Antibiotics.* Question the patient about nausea, vomiting, diarrhea (*C. difficile* induced disease is a concern with prolonged β-lactam therapy), dysgeusia (clarithromycin, cefuroxime), and rash and other hypersensitivity reactions. Caution the patient about photosensitivity, especially if taking sparfloxacin. Avoid potential CYP 450 3A4 drug interactions involving clarithromycin and sparfloxacin with antihistamines such as astemizole, as the combination may induce QT prolongation.
- *Intranasal corticosteroids.* Observe for nasal crusting/bleeding at the first follow-up visit. If present, the dose may have to be reduced. With long-term use (i.e., > 6 months), patients should be evaluated at least annually for less common toxicities such as nasal atrophy/mucosal ulceration and septal perforation. It is also important to monitor for both non-adherence and excessive use (which may result in systemic absorption and an increased incidence of adverse effects).

Patient Counseling

6. *How would you counsel the patient about his new therapeutic regimen?*

Antibiotic

- This medication must be taken each day to prevent recurrence of your infection. Take all of the medication even if you begin to feel better before it is finished.
- This medication may be taken with food (β-lactams, clarithromycin, and fluoroquinolones) to minimize stomach upset and increase the amount of drug that enters your body (cefuroxime). If you are taking azithromycin capsules, they should be taken on an empty stomach (at least 1 hour before or 2 hours after a meal). Azithromycin tablets may be taken with or without food.
- If you are taking a fluoroquinolone, do not take any iron, calcium, zinc, or aluminum containing products for at least 4 to 6 hours after taking the antibiotic.
- Some patients experience mild stomach discomfort such as cramping or diarrhea. This usually passes after a few days, but, if it continues, causes a fever, or becomes intolerable, contact your physician or pharmacist.
- If you miss a dose, take it as soon as you remember. If it is almost time for your next dose, skip the missed dose and go back to your regular schedule.
- For cefuroxime/clarithromycin: if you experience a bothersome "metallic" taste, you may find it helpful to suck hard, sugarless candies or ice chips, brush your teeth frequently, or drink flavored beverages.
- For sparfloxacin: avoid exposure to direct sunlight; apply sunblock if you must be out in the sun for prolonged periods. Also avoid ultraviolet lamps during therapy and for 5 days after the antibiotic is finished.

Intranasal Corticosteroids

- This medication should be taken regularly to reduce the inflammation in your nose and lessen the allergic symptoms that you are experiencing. It may take 4 to 7 days before you experience any benefit.
- It should be shaken gently before use. Insert the device fully into your nose (to avoid mist in your eyes) and deliver each spray upward and outward within each nostril.
- This medication may produce a slight burning or irritation initially. It may also cause your nose to feel dry and, occasionally, cause nasal crusting or bleeding. Contact your doctor or pharmacist if the bleeding continues or increases in severity because temporary discontinuation or further evaluation may be necessary.
- Other adverse effects include headaches and sore throat. These effects tend to be mild and transient.

▶ Follow-up Question

1. *If the current regimen cannot be continued, what would you recommend and why?*

- Although the patient may simply be experiencing diarrhea as a result of altered bowel flora, a history of chills, significant cramping, and diarrhea suggest the possibility of antibiotic associated colitis (AAC). The patient should initially be evaluated for evidence of significant fever/leukocytosis and monitored carefully for worsening of the present condition. If fever and leukocytosis are present, a further work-up for AAC is necessary (e.g., fecal leukocytes, *C. difficile* toxin) and amoxicillin/clavulanic acid should be discontinued. Therapy with oral metronidazole may be necessary.
- If there is no evidence of AAC but the patient feels he cannot continue therapy, antibiotic therapy may be changed. Since there was some improvement with the initial therapy chosen, a longer course with that agent would be acceptable. However, levofloxacin would be a rational alternative. The incidence of GI upset/diarrhea is likely to be lower than with amoxicillin/clavulanic acid, and it is less likely to exacerbate AAC (compared with amoxicillin and cephalosporins). The disadvantage of levofloxacin is that if anaerobes are causing the rhinosinusitis, it will likely exhibit only moderate activity against such pathogens.

References

1. Spector SL. The allergy-sinusitis link: Treatment of sinusitis with an allergic component. Hosp Med 1997;33(suppl):28–34.
2. Leopold DA. Management of rhinosinusitis. Hosp Med 1997;33(suppl):40–44.
3. Gwaltney JM Jr. Sinusitis: Pathogenesis and antimicrobial resistance. Hosp Med 1997;33(suppl):35–44.
4. Ramadan HH. What is the bacteriology of chronic sinusitis in adults? Am J Otolaryngol 1995;16:303–306.
5. Nord CE. The role of anaerobic bacteria in recurrent episodes of sinusitis and tonsillitis. Clin Infect Dis 1995;20:1512–1524.
6. Doern GV, Brueggemann A, Holley HP Jr, et al. Antimicrobial resistance of Streptococcus pneumoniae recovered from outpatients in the United States during the winter months of 1994 to 1995: Results of a 30-center national surveillance study. Antimicrob Agents Chemother 1996;40:1208–1213.
7. Sydnor TA Jr. Antibiotic therapy in bacterial sinusitis: New options. Hosp Med 1997;33(suppl):45–49.

98 PRESSURE SORES

▶ When Life Gets You Down   (Level III)

Richard S. Rhodes, PharmD
Catherine A. Heyneman, PharmD, MS

An 82-year-old man who has been bedridden because of multiple medical problems develops several stage I and II pressure (decubitus) ulcers on his buttocks and lower back. Treatment of pressure ulcers involves a comprehensive plan of skin care, proper body positioning, debridement, and perhaps granulation and epithelialization therapies. A variety of wound dressings are available, and each possesses unique advantages and disadvantages. Selection of the most appropriate product for an individual patient depends on the size and depth of wound, presence of infection, frequency of dressing changes required, cost, and other factors. Improvement in the therapy for the patient's osteoarthritis, chronic lung disease, depression, and incontinence is needed to reduce risk factors for the development of recurrent pressure ulcers.

▶ Questions

Problem Identification

1. a. *Create a list of the patient's drug-related problems.*

   - Pressure sores requiring treatment (2 stage II ulcers on the buttocks, 1 stage I ulcer on the coccyx).
   - Overflow incontinence, poorly controlled. Adequate control would help keep the skin free from moisture, decrease friction forces and tissue maceration, inhibit bacterial growth, and prevent chemical irritants from coming into contact with the skin. Increasing the dose of baclofen to 10 mg po TID may be beneficial.
   - Anticholinergic side effects of nortriptyline may contribute to the patient's risk of developing pressure sores. Sedation contributes to immobility, and urinary retention is counterproductive in overflow incontinence. The therapeutic goal in treating overflow incontinence is complete bladder emptying. Anticholinergics strengthen the external sphincter causing outflow resistance. A selective serotonin-reuptake inhibitor (SSRI) may be a better antidepressant choice for this patient.
   - Depression unsatisfactorily controlled with insufficient antidepressant doses. Controlling the patient's depression may help increase his physical activity, decrease insomnia, decrease anxiety, and increase his overall quality of life.
   - COPD inadequately treated as evidenced by difficulty breathing, SOB, compensated ABGs. Addition of a β_2-agonist metered-dose inhaler (e.g., albuterol) may be beneficial.
   - Osteoarthritis inadequately treated with low doses of PRN acetaminophen, which has no anti-inflammatory activity. Better control of both osteoarthritis and COPD would improve ambulation, increase circulation, and decrease pressure on areas susceptible to pressure sore formation. Providing regularly scheduled, adequate doses of acetaminophen (e.g., 1 g po Q 6 H) may be attempted.
   - Difficulty sleeping; treating insomnia will improve energy and strength, facilitating ambulation and decreasing the amount of immobility.
   - Routine benzodiazepine use with no clear diagnosis of anxiety. However, the patient has voiced apprehension about his new surroundings and physical condition.
   - Nicotine dependence, and the patient continues to smoke (as indicated in the SH and by the fact that the patient's CO-Hgb (carboxy-hemoglobin) is > 3%).
   - H/O excessive EtOH abuse × 50+ years.

   b. *Which of the patient's medical problems contributes to the development of pressure sores?*

   - *Immobility.* Confinement to a bed or chair, or a body part immobilized in a cast, causes unrelieved pressure making immobility a major risk factor for development of pressure sores. This patient has several factors that contribute to immobility, including COPD, osteoarthritis, and medications (nortriptyline, lorazepam, and baclofen; the elderly are especially sensitive to the effects of drugs that affect the CNS).
   - *Incontinence.* Urine and feces contain irritants such as urea, bacteria, enzymes, and yeast, which contribute to skin breakdown. Tissue maceration, increasing friction forces, chemical irritation, enhanced bacterial growth, and weakened skin integrity from moisture also increase the risk of pressure sores.
   - *Depression.* This contributes to immobility and predisposes patients to self-neglect and lack of self-care, which enhances susceptibility to pressure sore development and hinders wound healing.
   - *Advanced age.* Structural, physiologic, and immunologic changes in aging skin all contribute to reduced healing, increased skin fragility, a decrease in dermal thickness and subcutaneous mass, and increased susceptibility to shearing forces. A diminished blood supply resulting from the aging process inhibits oxygen transport necessary for the healing of tissue.[1]
   - *Smoking.* This has a negative effect on wound healing by causing vasoconstriction and interfering with blood flow. Carbon monoxide from cigarette smoke has a high binding affinity for hemoglobin, which decreases the amount of oxygen reaching injured tissue.

   c. *List other risk factors (whether or not they are present in this patient) that predispose individuals to the development of pressure sores.*

   - *Malnutrition.* Inadequately nourished tissues break down more easily and inhibit wound healing. Adequate protein, calorie, and fluid intake are essential to prevent negative nitrogen balance, which inhibits wound healing.

- *Dehydration.* This also contributes to ulcer development by decreasing blood volume and interfering with peripheral circulation, resulting in decreased nutrient and oxygen supply.
- *Poor sensory perception.* This can dull patients' response to pain or discomfort and compromise their ability to adjust their bodies for pressure relief. Dementia, stroke, spinal cord injury, psychiatric illness, paralysis, neurologic disorders, and medications that affect the central nervous system can all decrease sensory perception.
- *Medications.* Any pharmacologic agent that inhibits mobility, decreases sensory perception, promotes dehydration, causes incontinence, or inhibits wound healing should be considered a risk factor for the development of decubitus ulcers.

Desired Outcome

2. What are the goals of treatment for this patient's pressure sores?

- Prompt relief of pain and discomfort
- Elimination of risk factors that predispose him to the development and recurrence of decubitus ulcers (e.g., better treatment of overflow incontinence)
- Complete healing of lesions
- Improve mobility and ambulation by optimizing therapy for the patient's other medical conditions (e.g., depression, COPD, osteoarthritis)

Therapeutic Alternatives

3. a. What therapeutic interventions are available for treatment of the patient's pressure sores?

Appropriate therapeutic intervention includes a specific treatment plan and prevention protocol that includes a number of specific measures.

Skin Care
- Examine and assess skin on a regular basis.
- Keep skin clean when soiled with mild cleansing agent and dry thoroughly.
- Avoid using topical products that dry skin, especially in the elderly.
- Prevent contact with moisture and irritants that soil the skin (e.g., perspiration, urine, feces).
- Minimize pressure, friction, and shearing forces by using proper positioning, regular turning and repositioning, and support surfaces (e.g., pillows, wedges, mattress overlays, specialty beds).
- Keep skin lubricated (moisturizers, lubricants, etc.) with cautious application over susceptible bony prominences to prevent skin softening and subsequent breakdown.
- Provide frequent evaluation of nutrition status.

Body Positioning[1]
- Proper body positioning is important to relieve pressure on tissue over vulnerable bony prominences. Gently alternating patients from sides to back every 2 hours is usually recommended. Schedules for repositioning high-risk patients should be more frequent.
- Patients positioned on their side should not be placed directly on the trochanters, and the back should be situated, with wedges or pillows, at a 30-degree angle to the support surface.
- The head of patients lying on their backs should be at the lowest possible angle to prevent sliding downward and increased friction and shearing forces.
- Avoid sliding patients when repositioning to prevent shearing forces and mechanical injury.
- Pressure-relieving devices (pillows, wedges) should be used to completely suspend the heels.
- Gravity increases pressure over vulnerable tissues while sitting. Stress good posture to distribute weight and prevent the body from sliding downward. Thighs should be horizontal. Repositioning patients while sitting in chairs or wheelchairs should be done more frequently.

Disinfecting Agents
- All stage II, III, and IV decubitus ulcers are colonized with bacteria to some extent. However, thorough cleansing and debridement will prevent the ulcer from being clinically infected.
- Routine cultures of wounds are not necessary unless signs of infection are present. The classic signs of infection are erythema, fever (heat), foul odor, and pain.
- Much debate exists as to whether disinfecting agents help or inhibit wound healing, since they may cause tissue damage in existing wounds. Most studies show that disinfectants, like topical antibiotics, exhibit inadequate penetration into the wound and results are inconsistent and inconclusive. (Refer to textbook Chapter 100.)

Debridement
- Debridement of devitalized tissue is the most important aspect of wound healing. There are various methods of debridement.[2-4]
  - ✓ *Chemical debridement* involves the use of enzymatic agents (fibrinolysin and desoxyribonuclease, collagenase, trypsin or papain) that attack specific tissues (protein, fibrin, collagen) in the wound. Their main advantage is ease of application. Disadvantages include injury to adjacent healthy tissue, increased cost, the need for several treatments, and the time required. Also, certain topical antibiotic agents can alter the wound bed pH and inactivate the enzymes.
  - ✓ *Autolytic debridement* allows the body's own endogenous enzymes, under occlusive dressings, to break down necrotic tissue. This method causes no pain and is an alternative for patients who cannot tolerate other forms of debridement. However, the procedure is slow and usually requires surgical debridement before application of the occlusive dressing.
  - ✓ *Surgical debridement* is removal of devitalized tissue, usually by scissors or scalpel. It is the fastest, most efficient, and cost-effective method of debridement. However, it is nonselective and may accidentally result in removal of healthy tissue. It is also painful and may result in possible expansion of the ulcer borders and bleeding complications.
  - ✓ *Mechanical debridement* is usually performed by applying saline-soaked gauze to the wound and removing dead tissue when the gauze dries and the dressing is changed. This method has low cost and ease of application. However, it may be associated with pain and the unintentional removal of healthy tissue.
  - ✓ *Hydrodebridement,* another type of mechanical debridement, uses a whirlpool or pulsed water to remove necrotic

tissue. This method is an effective adjunct to other types of debridement but requires more staff time and may non-selectively remove healthy tissue along with the non-viable tissue.

Granulation and Epithelialization Therapies[2–5]

- *Pharmacologic agents* (karaya, sugar, insulin, benzoyl peroxide, phenytoin, ketanserin) all have shown efficacy in treatment of pressure ulcers. However, poor study design and small sample sizes limit the conclusions that can be drawn from these studies. Consequently, their use is limited to patients refractory to other treatments.
- *Polyurethane film dressings* (e.g., Acu-Derm, Bioclusive, Opraflex, Op-Site, Tegaderm, Uniflex) are transparent and semipermeable, allowing evaporation and exchange of gases and promoting autolysis. These products maintain a moist wound environment, allow water vapors and oxygen to escape to the outside (preventing maceration of surrounding skin), are impermeable to contaminants (urine, feces), decrease pain, are easy to apply, and require only weekly changing. However, they may stick to intact and new tissue and may macerate surrounding skin if the skin is not protected. Some products are hard to apply and may need secondary dressings. These products are most appropriately used on non-infected stage I and stage II decubitus ulcers.
- *Hydrocolloid or occlusive dressings* (e.g., DuoDerm, Tegasorb, Comfeel, Intact, Restore, Exuderm, Cutinova-hydro) are impermeable wafers that retain a moist environment and interact with wound fluids to form a gelatinous mass over the wound and promote autolysis. They are waterproof and moisture retentive; prevent penetration of water, oxygen, and contaminants; and have a changing frequency of up to 1 week. However, premature removal damages tissue, there is odor on removal, they are non-transparent and the wound cannot be seen (obviating their use on infected wounds or wounds with severe dermatitis), and the dressings may be displaced if the wound produces heavy exudate (except for Cutinova-hydro). These products may be used on stage II or shallow stage III pressure ulcers with no signs of infection.
- *Hydrogels* (e.g., Vigilon, Geliperm, Clear-site, Elasto-gel, Nu-gel) are amorphous dressings with a high moisture content that promotes cell migration, hydration of necrotic tissue, and autolysis. They are associated with patient comfort, decreased pain, moisture retention, enhanced topical antibiotic penetration, and they support debridement. On the other hand, they require secondary dressings, are expensive, dehydrate if not correctly covered, may promote *Pseudomonas* and yeast infections, and require changing several times daily. They may be useful for stage II, III, or IV pressure sores with minimal to moderate exudate.
- *Exudate absorbers* (e.g., Bard Absorption dressings, Debrisan, Hydron, Comfeel Powder, Envisan, Duoderm granules, Hollister Exudate) absorb large amounts of fluid and exudate and fill up the wound space as debris is removed by irrigation. They are inexpensive, support autolytic debridement, fill dead space to facilitate expansion, absorb up to 20 times their weight in wound debris, and have no odor. Disadvantages include dehydration of the wound, slight pain, leakage of dressing material, and the need for a secondary dressing and dressing changes every 24 hours. They may be used in stage III or IV deep wounds with large space and heavy exudate.
- *Alginate dressings* (e.g., Kaltostat, Sorbsan, Curasorb) are natural polysaccharides derived from brown seaweed that form a soft gel and absorb wound fluid and exudate. They are good for deep stage III and IV wounds with moderate to heavy exudate, are easy to apply, can be easily flushed or irrigated, cause minimal pain, are soft and comfortable, and cause no odor. However, they can lead to dehydration of the wound, require additional dressing, and may dry without a proper covering. They are used in stage III or IV wounds with heavy exudate or infected wounds.
- *Gauze dressings* comprise wet-to-dry and wet-to-damp sterile moistened gauze that acts as a type of mechanical debridement. When dressings are changed, necrotic tissue attaches to the gauze and is removed. They are cost effective, readily available, soothing, can be used on infected wounds, are compatible with other topicals, and offer good mechanical debridement. Disadvantages include little moisture retention, pain if the dressing dries before removal, need for changing several times a day, increased nursing time, and need for a secondary dressing. They are used on small and large pressure sores, wounds that require "filling," infected wounds, grafts, abrasions, and burns.

b. *What economic issues should be considered when making plans to prevent or treat pressure sores?*

- Prevention, early intervention, and prompt healing of pressure sores can reduce morbidity, mortality, expense, extended hospital stays, labor, and human suffering. The treatment of pressure sores each year in the United States is estimated at $5 billion.[6]

Optimal Plan

4. a. *What drug dosage form, dose, schedule, and duration of therapy are best for this patient?*

- Treatment of this patient's pressure ulcers should include cleansing of the wound and choosing the most appropriate method of debridement and type of wound dressing. Although there are no definitive studies on the most effective method of debridement or which dressing is best suited for all ulcers, there are guidelines (discussed previously) that are helpful in making these selections.
- Surgical debridement is appropriate for this patient because: 1) it is the most rapid and effective method; 2) it is cost effective; 3) it can be done at the bedside for small pressure sores (stage II); and 4) the chance of enlarging the borders of small pressure ulcers is remote.
- There were no signs or symptoms of infection in this patient. However, since acute wounds are more susceptible to bacterial invasion, the presence of infection should be assessed with each dressing change (refer to the textbook section "Pressure Sores" in Chapter 100).
- A polyurethane film wound dressing (e.g., Op-Site) would be a good choice for this patient for several reasons: 1) it is indicated for small non-infected pressure wounds; 2) it is a semipermeable dressing that allows moisture and oxygen to escape to the outside, which prevents skin maceration and promotes healing; 3) it pro-

duces a moist wound environment and promotes autolysis; 4) it is impermeable to bacteria; 5) it is transparent; and 6) weekly dressing changes save nursing time.

b. *What alternatives would be appropriate if the initial therapy fails or cannot be used?*

- The process of wound healing is greatly influenced by many factors (e.g., the patient's health, nutrition status, type and severity of wound), and since there is no single treatment method that is optimum for all wounds, it is imperative to continually assess the patient.
- As a general rule, consider reevaluation of treatment modalities if the wound shows no signs of healing within two weeks. Lack of healing could be due to a number of factors other than the treatment method. At that point, the patient's overall medical condition should be reevaluated, not just the pressure sore. Nutrition status, infection, incontinence care, positioning, pressure relief, and physical functioning could all contribute to a non-healing wound.
- A trial-and-error approach coupled with sound clinical judgment and a knowledge of the advantages and disadvantages of each treatment modality is the best course of action.
- A pressure ulcer may also respond better to a different treatment as the wound heals. Wet-to-dry saline dressings may be switched to an occlusive dressing as the wound improves and healing stops. An occlusive dressing may be changed to a continuously moist saline gauze dressing that maintains a moist environment to allow proliferation of new tissue and when repeated inspection is necessary. Moist saline gauze dressings are used on wounds that are almost healed with little necrotic tissue. If changed often and continually remoistened, they are soothing and the wound bed remains moist to facilitate epithelial migration and prevent damage to tissues on removal.

Outcome Evaluation

5. *What clinical and laboratory parameters are necessary to evaluate the therapy for achievement of the desired therapeutic outcome and to detect or prevent adverse effects?*

- For evaluation of healing, a baseline assessment of the pressure sore should be documented at the beginning of treatment, and a systematic evaluation of the lesions should be recorded with each dressing change. Healing assessment parameters include:
  ✓ Presence or absence of wound discharge. Infection is identified by local inflammation, purulent drainage, and fever. Routine culturing of non-purulent wounds is not warranted.
  ✓ Appearance of healthy granulation tissue, which provides evidence of newly generated tissue.
  ✓ Reduction in ulcer volume. Determination of ulcer size can be performed by one of the commercially available measuring tools (i.e., MediRule). Colored photographs with metric squares superimposed on the film are useful in determining the outer edges and discoloration of the wound and avoid physical contact with the wound to decrease the chance of contamination.
  ✓ Depth of the wound. There is a correlation between the depth of a wound and time to healing.
  ✓ Local pain; its presence may indicate infection.

- Nutrition status should be assessed. Malnutrition is a major risk factor for the development of pressure sores, and adequate nutrition is needed for tissue integrity and wound healing. Serum albumin, total protein, and transferrin levels should be monitored in susceptible individuals.
- Wound cultures should be obtained if there is a foul odor, purulent exudate, fever, edema, or wound pain. Osteomyelitis and sepsis are the most serious possible complications of pressure ulcers.

Patient Counseling

6. *What information should be provided to the patient to enhance compliance, ensure successful therapy, and minimize adverse effects?*

- Education of caregivers
- Pressure sore prevention and risk factors (pressure, shearing forces, friction, moisture)
- Signs and symptoms of infection
- Pressure relief, body positioning and repositioning
- Pressure relief devices (foams, pads, mattress, pillows, wedges)
- Management of incontinence
- Nutrition support
- Skin care and inspection and sterile techniques
- Dressing change procedures
- Knowledge of when to seek medical advice

References

1. Maklebust J, Sieggreen MY. Pressure ulcer treatment. In: Pressure Ulcers: Guidelines for Prevention and Nursing Management, 2nd ed. Springhouse, PA, Springhouse Corporation, 1996:77–94.
2. Yarkony GM. Pressure ulcers: A review. Arch Phys Med Rehabil 1994;75:908–917.
3. Evans JM, Andrews KL, Chutka DS, et al. Pressure ulcers: Prevention and management. Mayo Clin Proc 1995;70:789–799.
4. Maklebust J, Sieggreen MY. Pressure ulcer treatment. In: Pressure Ulcers: Guidelines for Prevention and Nursing Management, 2nd ed. Springhouse, PA, Springhouse Corporation, 1996:104–121.
5. Leigh IH, Bennett G. Pressure ulcers: Prevalence, etiology, and treatment modalities: a review. Am J Surg 1994;167(1A):25S–30S.
6. Kertesz D, Chow AW. Infected pressure and diabetic ulcers. Clin Geriatr Med 1992; 8:835–852.

99 DIABETIC FOOT INFECTION

▶ **Watch Your Step** (Level II)

Renee-Claude Mercier, PharmD

Accidentally stepping on a piece of metal results in erythema and swelling of the right foot in a 39-year-old homeless woman with poorly controlled type 2 diabetes mellitus. Laboratory evaluation reveals leukocytosis with a left shift. The patient underwent incision and drainage of the lesion with removal of a 2-cm metallic foreign body from the foot. Empiric antimicrobial treatment must be initiated before results of wound culture and sensitivity testing are known. Because of this particular patient's condition, parenteral monotherapy with ampicillin/sulbactam, cefotetan, or cefoxitin would constitute appropriate therapy. Other alternatives include ticarcillin/clavulanate, piperacillin/tazobactam, imipenem/cilastatin, or the combination of clindamycin plus cefazolin. When tissue cultures are reported as positive for methicillin-sensitive *Staphylococcus aureus*, students are asked to change to more specific therapy, which might include parenteral penicillinase-resistant penicillins or first-generation cephalosporins. Although parenteral therapy may be completed as an outpatient, attention must be given to the patient's social situation. Better glycemic control and education on techniques for proper foot care are important components of a comprehensive treatment plan for this patient.

▶ Questions

Problem Identification

1. a. Create a list of the patient's drug-related problems.

- Cellulitis and infection of the right foot in a patient with diabetes.
- Poorly controlled type 2 diabetes mellitus, as evidenced by a HbA_{1c} of 11.8% (goal < 7%).
- Non-compliance with medication administration and home glucose monitoring.
- History of depression, which may be inadequately treated (the patient is described as having a "flat affect").
- Poor social conditions; lives in a shelter with minimal family support. This situation may make it difficult for her to afford medications and glucose monitoring supplies and may contribute to non-adherence with therapy.
- Fungal infection of toenails requiring treatment.

b. What signs, symptoms, or laboratory values indicate the presence of an infection?

- Swollen, sore, and red foot.
- 2+ edema of the foot increasing in amplitude.
- WBC elevated (20.45 × 10^3/mm^3) with increased PMNs and bands.
- X-ray showing the presence of a foreign body in the right foot.

c. What risk factors for infection does the patient have?

- Patient stepped on a foreign object
- She is a poorly controlled diabetic patient.
- Vascular calcifications are present in the foot, indicating a decreased blood supply.
- Poor foot care (presence of fungus and overgrown toenails).

d. What organisms are most likely involved in this infection?

- Aerobic isolates: *Proteus mirabilis*, group D streptococci, *Escherichia coli*, *Staphylococcus aureus*.[1]
- Anaerobic isolates: *Bacteroides fragilis*, *Peptococcus*, *Peptostreptococcus*.

Desired Outcome

2. What are the therapeutic goals for this patient?

- Eradicate the bacteria
- Prevent the development of osteomyelitis and the need for amputation
- Improve control of the diabetes mellitus
- Prevent further recurrence of foot infection
- Improve social conditions and depression by providing her with a secure place to live

Therapeutic Alternatives

3. a. What non-drug therapies might be useful for this patient?

- Deep culture of the wound for both anaerobes and aerobes.
- Appropriate wound care by experienced podiatrists (I & D, debridement of the wound, toenail clipping), nurses (wound care, dressing changes of wound, foot care teaching), and physical therapists (whirlpool treatments, wound debridement, teaching about minimal weight bearing with a walker or crutches).
- Bed rest, minimal weight bearing, leg elevation, and control of edema.
- Proper counseling about wound care and the importance of good diabetes control, glucometer use, and adherence with the medication regimens.

b. What feasible pharmacotherapeutic alternatives are available for the empiric treatment of the foot infection?

- Diabetic foot infections are classified into two categories:
    - ✓ *Non-limb-threatening infections.* Superficial, no systemic toxicity, minimal cellulitis extending less than 2 cm from portal of entry, ulceration not extending fully through skin, no significant ischemia.
    - ✓ *Limb-threatening infections.* More extensive cellulitis, lymphangitis, and ulcers penetrating through skin into subcutaneous tissues, prominent ischemia.
- *An aminoglycoside plus ampicillin IV* has been suggested for limb-threatening infections, but this regimen should not be considered a first empiric choice because it does not have good coverage against the most common anaerobes involved in diabetic foot infection. Use of *IV clindamycin* instead of ampicillin would be more appropriate in this case because it has broader anaerobic coverage. Regimens including an aminoglycoside (which have been associated with the development of nephrotoxicity) should probably be avoided in this patient population because they have an increased risk of developing diabetic nephropathy and renal failure.
- *Cefoxitin* or *cefotetan* (second-generation parenteral cephalo-

sporins) monotherapy is attractive because their spectrum of activity covers the most likely causative organisms. Single-drug therapy is also attractive because of the potential advantages of convenience, cost, and avoidance of toxicities.

- *Ampicillin/sulbactam, piperacillin/tazobactam,* and *ticarcillin/clavulanate* are also appropriate as IV monotherapy but are more costly than second-generation cephalosporins.
- *Imipenem/cilastatin* IV could also be considered, but few studies are available to support its use in this situation. It is also an expensive choice and is a very potent β-lactamase inducer.
- *Clindamycin IV plus either gentamicin or an IV fluoroquinolone* could be used in patients allergic to penicillin.
- *Oral clindamycin* plus an *oral fluoroquinolone* (e.g., ciprofloxacin, ofloxacin) or *cephalexin* could be used in patients in whom osteomyelitis has been ruled out and in those with non-limb-threatening infections.[2] Oral fluoroquinolones have poor activity against *Bacteroides* species and should be used in combination if anaerobes are suspected, such as infections with a foul odor.
- An *oral fluoroquinolone, cloxacillin,* or *clindamycin* alone could be used in patients with non-limb-threatening infection who have not previously received antibiotic therapy because they usually have infections caused by only 1 or 2 species of aerobic organisms, staphylococci and/or streptococci.[3]
- *Becaplermin 0.01% Gel (Regranex)* is FDA approved for the treatment of diabetic ulcers on the lower limbs and feet. Becaplermin is a genetically engineered form of platelet-derived growth factor, a naturally occurring protein in the body that stimulates diabetic ulcer healing. In one clinical trial, becaplermin applied once daily in combination with good wound care significantly increased the incidence of complete healing when compared to placebo gel (50% for becaplermin gel versus 35% for placebo gel). Becaplermin gel also significantly decreased the time to complete healing of diabetic ulcers by 32% (about 6 weeks faster). The incidence of adverse events including infection and cellulitis was similar in patients treated with becaplermin gel, placebo gel, or good diabetic wound care alone. Because becaplermin is a new drug with limited clinical experience, further studies are needed to assess which patients might best benefit from its use.

c. *What economic and social considerations are applicable to this patient?*

- Simplified drug regimen (less frequent dosing) should be selected due to her history of poor medication adherence.
- In light of the patient's social status, she probably does not have access to health care insurance, which may become an important consideration in selecting her future therapeutic plan.
- In order for this patient to receive appropriate wound care and home IV therapy if judged necessary, she needs to establish secure and comfortable living arrangements for the time of therapy.

Optimal Plan

4. *Outline a drug regimen that would provide optimal initial empiric therapy for the infection.*

- This diabetic foot infection has significant involvement of the skin and skin structures with deep tissue involvement. Moreover, the area of cellulitis and induration exceeded 2 cm (4 × 5 cm). Even though this is her first foot infection and is more likely to be caused by a single organism, one cannot rule out the presence of a polymicrobial infection because of the extensive skin and skin structure involvement. Initial empiric IV therapy is appropriate in serious cases of diabetic foot infection such as this one.[2-3]
- As discussed, a number of treatment options are appropriate for empiric therapy of diabetic foot infections. The antimicrobial therapy selection may be based on institutional cost and drug availability through the formulary system. Any one of the following regimens is appropriate as monotherapy because each has good coverage of the most commonly involved organisms (including both aerobic and anaerobic bacteria) and a good safety profile.
  ✓ Ampicillin/sulbactam 1.5 to 3 g IV Q 6 H; the higher dosage should be reserved for serious infections in patients with poor peripheral circulation
  ✓ Cefotetan 2 g IV Q 12 H
  ✓ Cefoxitin 1 to 2 g IV Q 8 H
- Other acceptable IV alternatives given as monotherapy include ticarcillin/clavulanate 3.1 g IV Q 6 H, piperacillin/tazobactam 3.375 g IV Q 6 H, or imipenem/cilastatin 500 mg IV Q 6 H. These agents should not be considered first-choice therapy because they are often restricted for more severe/life-threatening nosocomial infections due to their broader spectrum of activity, to prevent the development of resistance, and to reduce treatment costs.
- Clindamycin 900 mg IV Q 8 H in combination with cefazolin 1 to 2 g IV Q 8 H is also appropriate in this case. However, this two-drug regimen is less convenient than monotherapy and is more often associated with *Clostridium difficile* colitis because of clindamycin.

Outcome Evaluation

5. a. *What clinical and laboratory parameters are necessary to evaluate your therapy for achievement of the desired therapeutic outcomes and monitoring for adverse effects?*

- Regardless of the drug chosen, improvement in the signs and symptoms of infection and healing of the wound with prevention of limb amputation are the primary end points.
- Decreased swelling, induration, and erythema should be observed after 72 to 96 hours of appropriate antimicrobial therapy and surgical debridement. The response to therapy is often patient dependent, and in some cases, improvement may not be seen for up to 7 to 10 days of treatment.
- A decrease in cloudy drainage and formation of new scar tissue are signs of positive response to therapy that may take up to 7 to 14 days to be seen.
- A WBC count and differential should be performed every 48 to 72 hours for the first week or until normalization if less than 1 week, and weekly thereafter until the end of therapy. Monitoring should continue until therapy is completed because neutropenia has been associated with many antibiotics (e.g., ampicillin/sulbactam, cefotetan, cefoxitin).
- BUN and serum creatinine should be monitored weekly while on therapy to detect the development of renal toxicity from certain antibiotics such as nafcillin (acute interstitial nephritis) and aminoglycosides.

- Question the patient to detect any unusual side effects related to the drug or infusion (e.g., rash, nausea, vomiting, diarrhea) daily for the first 3 to 5 days and then weekly thereafter.

▶ Follow-up Questions

b. *What therapeutic alternatives are available for treating this patient once results of cultures are known to contain MSSA?*

- Once the culture results are available and the involved organism(s) is (are) considered pathogenic and responsible for the infectious process, therapy should be targeted at the specific organism(s). Penicillinase-resistant penicillins such as nafcillin, oxacillin, or methicillin are the first-line choices for skin and soft tissue infections caused by MSSA. Methicillin may be more nephrotoxic than the other two agents.
- Other IV therapies that could also be considered include the first-generation cephalosporins (e.g., cefazolin) or ampicillin/sulbactam. Ampicillin/sulbactam is a restricted antibiotic in many institutions and is more expensive than the other alternatives.
- Clindamycin and vancomycin are effective alternatives in penicillin-allergic patients. The use of vancomycin should be limited to patients with severe penicillin allergy in whom the use of cephalosporins or other alternatives should be avoided in order to prevent the development of vancomycin-resistance.

c. *Design an optimal drug treatment plan for treating her MSSA infection while she remains hospitalized.*

- Because the patient does not have a penicillin allergy, she should be started on either nafcillin 2 g IV Q 4 H or cefazolin 2 g IV Q 8 H. Due to the severity of the infection (i.e., limb-threatening), the possible decrease in blood supply to the area, and the good renal function of the patient, high doses of the antibiotic (>1 g) should be used to assure appropriate drug concentrations at the site of infection.
- The duration of therapy is controversial and based on the patient's personal situation. Therapy should be continued until all signs and symptoms disappear and for at least 2 to 4 weeks total. Some patients require longer therapy, and wound healing in diabetic patients is often very slow.
- Patients should remain hospitalized until they are afebrile for 24 to 48 hours, have signs of improvement and positive response to therapy (decreased swelling, redness, purulent drainage; normalization of the WBC), and outpatient wound care has been established, either by proper teaching to the patient or through home health care services. This patient will not be able to be discharged until a proper living situation has been found.

d. *Design an optimal pharmacotherapeutic plan for completion of her treatment once she has been discharged from the hospital.*

- The decision about completion of therapy with IV versus oral therapy is often based on clinical experience, because few clinical trials have been performed on long-term treatment of diabetic foot infections.
- Treatment with oral antibiotics should be considered if the wound is healing well with disappearance of signs and symptoms of infection, there is formation of new scar tissue, and the infection is no longer limb-threatening. Available options are dicloxacillin, cloxacillin, cephalexin, or cephradine, each given in doses of 500 mg po Q 6 H. No studies have demonstrated the superiority of one agent over the others, and the choice is often based on experience, availability, and cost.
- Home IV therapy may be more appropriate in this patient because of the severity of the infection and the very slow improvement observed. Home IV drug therapies suitable for MSSA include nafcillin 2 g IV Q 4 H given via a peristaltic pump, cefazolin 2 g IV Q 8 H, or ceftriaxone 2 g IV Q 24 H. No prospective studies have been performed comparing these 3 agents in this patient population against MSSA. Ampicillin/sulbactam 1.5 to 3 g IV Q 6 H is generally not recommended, because the drug is unstable for the period required with a peristaltic pump and is inconvenient because of the dosing frequency. If the patient was started on nafcillin 2 IV Q 4 H in the hospital, it is more appropriate to continue the same regimen as an outpatient.

Patient Counseling

6. *What information should be provided to the patient to enhance compliance, ensure successful therapy, and minimize adverse effects with IV nafcillin?*

- Nafcillin, like most antibiotics, may cause diarrhea that could be caused by bacteria known as *Clostridium difficile*. Contact your health care provider immediately if it occurs and before taking any antidiarrheal medicine.
- Contact your doctor or me if any unusual side effects such as rash, shortness of breath, or decreased urine production occur while taking this medicine.
- Contact your home health care provider if pain, redness, or swelling is observed at the IV site.
- The peristaltic pump will deliver the antibiotic every 4 hours for 24 hours, then the bag will need to be changed. Contact your home health care provider if you have any questions or if you notice abnormalities with the pump, such as noise, clogging of the tubing, or air bubbles.

Note: The patient needs to be made aware that osteomyclitis and limb amputation are possible consequences of these infections in diabetic patients. She also needs to be provided with personnel resources (telephone numbers, addresses) to contact if unusual reactions occur while on therapy, if infection worsens, or if she has questions or concerns. Compliance with outpatient clinic follow-up visits is of prime importance for success in this case.

References

1. Lipsky BA, Pecoraro RE, Wheat LJ. The diabetic foot: Soft tissue and bone infection. Infect Dis Clin North Am 1990;4:409–432.
2. Lipsky BA, Pecoraro RE, Larson SA, et al. Outpatient management of uncomplicated lower-extremity infections in diabetic patients. Arch Intern Med 1990;150: 790–797.
3. Lipsky BA, Baker PD, Landon GC, et al. Antibiotic therapy for diabetic foot infections: Comparison of two parenteral-to-oral regimens. Clin Infect Dis 1997;24: 643–648.

100 INFECTIVE ENDOCARDITIS

▶ If the Heart Could Tell (Level II)

Renata Smith, PharmD
Keith A. Rodvold, PharmD, FCCP, BCPS

A 39-year-old man with a history of IV drug abuse and penicillin allergy develops right-sided infective endocarditis. The organism was identified as *Staphylococcus aureus* sensitive to oxacillin, vancomycin, gentamicin, trimethoprim-sulfamethoxazole, ofloxacin, and cefazolin. Satisfactory resolution of this case involves initiation of an appropriate inpatient regimen taking into consideration the patient's penicillin allergy, determination of appropriate parameters to assess efficacy and toxicity, changing therapy when the patient does not respond to initial recommendations, and developing a penicillin desensitization protocol. Students are also asked to assess the appropriateness of home IV therapy in this patient and to develop an outpatient oral regimen when the patient decides to leave the hospital prior to completion of the IV therapy.

▶ **Questions**

Problem Identification

1. a. *Identify all of the drug-related problems of this patient.*

    - *S. aureus* bacteremia and endocarditis requiring antibiotic therapy.
    - Seizures due to heroin withdrawal requiring anticonvulsant therapy.
    - Heroin withdrawal requiring treatment.
    - Possible tobacco withdrawal during hospitalization that may require treatment.
    - The patient's SLE appears to be a chronic, stable problem presently controlled by daily prednisone.

   b. *What signs, symptoms, and other information indicates the presence of endocarditis in this patient?*

    - *Signs.* Cardiac murmur, clubbing.
    - *Symptoms.* Diarrhea, vomiting, anorexia, 30-pound weight loss.
    - *Other information.* Elevated WBC count with left shift, elevated ESR, mild anemia, positive blood cultures for *S. aureus*; tricuspid vegetation documented by echocardiogram.

   c. *What risk factors does this patient have for developing endocarditis?*

    - Intravenous drug use
    - Previous history of endocarditis

   d. *Based on this patient's risk factors and location of the vegetation, does this patient have right-sided or left-sided endocarditis?*

    - Endocarditis occurs more frequently on the mitral and aortic valves, which is left-sided endocarditis. In patients such as this who are IV drug users with *S. aureus* infection, the vegetation is located on the tricuspid valve 80% to 100% of the time. Therefore, he has right-sided endocarditis.[1]

   e. *What additional information (laboratory tests or patient information) is needed to satisfactorily assess this patient?*

    - *Laboratory tests.* Antibiotic susceptibilities for *S. aureus*.
    - *Patient information.* Duration of cardiac murmur (i.e., is it new or has he had it for some time?); the type of reaction to penicillin; the therapy he received for his last episode of endocarditis.

Desired Outcome

2. *What are the goals of pharmacotherapy for infective endocarditis?*

    - Resolve the patient's symptoms (achieve clinical cure)
    - Eradicate the organism from the body (achieve bacteriologic cure)
    - Use the most effective drug therapy (i.e., bactericidal drugs)
    - Avoid drug toxicity with appropriate monitoring
    - Avoid recurrence by educating the patient about the role of prophylaxis prior to major dental and surgical procedures

Therapeutic Alternatives

3. a. *Identify the therapeutic alternatives for the treatment of* S. aureus *endocarditis based on the organism's susceptibilities. Include the drug name, dose, dosage form, schedule, and duration of therapy in your answer.*

    - Antibiotics used for treating endocarditis should be bactericidal and given for a prolonged period of time in order to clear the blood and sterilize the valve vegetation.
    - *Nafcillin* or *oxacillin* 2 g IV every 4 hours for 4 to 6 weeks with the option to add *gentamicin* 1 mg/kg every 8 hours for the first 3 to 5 days is recommended for patients who have methicillin-susceptible *S. aureus*, no prosthetic (mechanical) heart valves, and no history of immediate-type (anaphylactic) hypersensitivity to β-lactam antimicrobials.[2] The use of aminoglycosides is limited to aminoglycoside-susceptible strains of *S. aureus* in all of the listed regimens. The addition of gentamicin does not improve cure rates, but it clears the bacteremia more rapidly, perhaps minimizing damage to the heart valve and the formation of extracardiac abscesses.
    - *Cefazolin* 2 g IV every 8 hours for 4 to 6 weeks with the option to add gentamicin 1 mg/kg IV every 8 hours for the first 3 to 5 days is recommended for patients with non-immediate type (rash) β-lactam hypersensitivity.[2]
    - *Vancomycin* 15 mg/kg IV every 12 hours for 4 to 6 weeks is the recommended regimen for patients with methicillin-resistant *S. aureus* or immediate-type β-lactam hypersensitivity.[2] The dosage

interval should be lengthened appropriately based on the degree of renal impairment.
- *Nafcillin* or *oxacillin* 2 g IV every 4 hours plus *rifampin* 300 mg po every 8 hours for ≥ 6 weeks and gentamicin 1 mg/kg IV every 8 hours for the first 2 weeks is recommended for patients with prosthetic heart valves, no immediate-type β-lactam hypersensitivity, and methicillin-susceptible *S. aureus*.[2]
- *Vancomycin* 15 mg/kg every 12 hours plus *rifampin* 300 mg po every 8 hours for ≥ 6 weeks and gentamicin 1 mg/kg IV every 8 hours for the first 2 weeks (if the organism is susceptible to gentamicin) is recommended for patients with prosthetic valves *and* either methicillin-resistant *S. aureus* or immediate-type β-lactam hypersensitivity.[2]
- *Nafcillin* 2 g IV every 4 hours plus *gentamicin* 1 mg/kg every 8 hours for 2 weeks has been reported to result in cure rates of at least 85% in IV drug users with uncomplicated *S. aureus* endocarditis localized on the tricuspid valve. The same results were not obtained with a 2-week course of vancomycin plus an aminoglycoside.[3,4] In patients who are candidates for this regimen, a 2-week course of therapy may be used to decrease hospital stay and increase patient adherence. This patient is not a candidate for this regimen because he has a penicillin allergy.

b. *What non-drug therapies might be used to treat this patient's endocarditis?*

- Replacement of the affected valve may be warranted in this patient. Reasons for valve replacement are fungal endocarditis, persistent positive blood cultures while on therapy, relapse after appropriate therapy, uncontrolled sepsis, or hemodynamic instability.[1]

Optimal Plan

4. a. *What is the most appropriate treatment plan for this patient (give drug name, dose, dosage form, schedule, and duration of therapy)?*

- Due to the patient's immediate-type hypersensitivity to β-lactams, vancomycin 15 mg/kg IV every 12 hours for 4 to 6 weeks is the appropriate choice for patients with normal renal function.[2] The dosing interval in this patient should be adjusted because of his decreased renal function. Based on his age (39 years), body weight (54 kg), gender (male), and serum creatinine (2.0 mg/dL), his estimated creatinine clearance (CL_{cr}) by the Cockcroft and Gault equation is 38 mL/min. Several dosing methods for vancomycin therapy in patients with renal impairment are available.[5] A dose of 800 mg Q 24 H is an appropriate initial starting regimen for this patient based on his total body weight (15 mg/kg × 54 kg) and CL_{cr}. The monitoring of serum vancomycin concentrations remains controversial. However, in this patient with renal impairment, a trough concentration once weekly may be necessary to make appropriate dose adjustments. An appropriate target trough level is 5 to 10 μg/mL.

b. *What is an appropriate, non-surgical, therapeutic alternative for this patient?*

- Blood cultures should become negative within 3 to 7 days after starting appropriate antimicrobial therapy.[1] Therefore, this patient is not responding to his present regimen. Vancomycin has been shown to be less effective against *S. aureus* than nafcillin or oxacillin. Changing the patient to nafcillin may be more effective in eradicating the cardiac valve vegetation.[2] However, the patient must undergo penicillin desensitization before this treatment can be initiated because of his history of penicillin hypersensitivity.

c. *Explain how you would desensitize this patient to penicillin, and provide your new treatment recommendations assuming that desensitization is successful.*

- Please refer to Table 81–6 in textbook Chapter 81 for a complete parenteral penicillin desensitization protocol. Desensitization should be done in an ICU setting with a crash cart available and a staff capable of managing anaphylaxis, should it occur.
- Nafcillin 2 g IV every 4 hours for 4 to 6 weeks plus gentamicin 1 mg/kg every 8 hours for the first 3 to 5 days should be initiated if desensitization is successful in this patient. Vancomycin should be discontinued when nafcillin and gentamicin are started.

Outcome Evaluation

5. a. *What clinical and laboratory parameters should be monitored to evaluate the efficacy of therapy and to prevent adverse reactions?*

Clinical Outcome Parameters
- Check temperature at every shift change (patient should be afebrile within 3 to 7 days).
- Monitor for pulmonary emboli (shortness of breath, rales, tachycardia).
- Monitor for congestive heart failure (shortness of breath, rales, pulmonary edema by chest x-ray, and extremity edema).
- Obtain vital signs at every shift change (BP and HR should remain stable unless the patient develops a PE, heart failure, or other complications).

Laboratory Outcome Parameters
- Blood cultures should be obtained prior to starting therapy and then periodically (e.g., every other day) while on therapy and until cultures become negative. Blood cultures should also be obtained if fever recurs.
- Monitor serum gentamicin concentrations with the third dose and every 3 to 4 days thereafter if the patient continues to receive gentamicin. Monitor levels more often if renal function changes rapidly. The target peak should be 3 to 4 μg/mL and the trough < 2 μg/mL.
- Measure serum creatinine every 2 to 3 days if the patient's renal function remains stable or daily if it is rapidly changing.

Gentamicin Adverse Effects
- Nephrotoxicity (monitor serum creatinine as above)
- Ototoxicity (assess the patient for ringing in the ears, muffled voices, or ear fullness)
- Neuromuscular changes (evaluate gait)
- Neurotoxicity (check for vertigo)

Vancomycin Adverse Events
- Drug fever, hypotension, red man syndrome (administer over 1 hour to prevent this)
- Ototoxicity (when high doses are given or with pre-existing kidney dysfunction)
- Nephrotoxicity (when given with other nephrotoxic drugs)
- Skin rash

Nafcillin Adverse Events
- Skin rash and other hypersensitivity reactions (e.g., fever, eosinophilia, pruritus, anaphylaxis).
- Neutropenia (obtain WBC with differential 1 to 3 times weekly during therapy).
- Phlebitis or thrombophlebitis at the injection site; ulceration and necrosis can result if extravasation occurs.

b. *Based on your assessment of this patient's response and his past history, what alternatives are available for completing his course of therapy?*

- Several options are available for this patient including: 1) keeping the patient in the hospital and finishing 4 weeks of nafcillin therapy; 2) transferring the patient to a long-term care facility to finish his therapy; 3) arranging for home IV therapy; and 4) sending the patient home on oral antibiotics.
- Factors that preclude home IV therapy in patients with endocarditis include IV drug use, hemodynamic instability, need for valve replacement, prosthetic valve disease, non-compliance, abnormal mental status, multiple comorbidities, high risk of embolic complications, and large vegetations.[6] This patient is not a candidate for home IV therapy due to his IV drug use.
- Alternatively, he could be discharged on dicloxacillin 1 g po Q 6 H for 4 weeks or minocycline 100 mg po Q 12 H for 4 weeks to finish a 6-week course of therapy.[4,7,8] In addition, right-sided endocarditis in IV drug users may be treated with an oral regimen of ciprofloxacin 750 mg Q 12 H plus rifampin 300 mg Q 12 H.[4,7] However, development of resistance to fluoroquinolones and rifampin may limit the use of this regimen.
- Oral therapy may not be the most effective option because of this patient's recurrent endocarditis and the difficulty in clearing the bacteremia with IV vancomycin. The ideal situation would be for the patient to remain hospitalized and finish 6 weeks of IV nafcillin. Longer therapy (i.e., 6 weeks rather than 4 weeks) may be more appropriate in this patient because he had a delayed clinical response.

Patient Counseling

6. *If this patient is discharged home to complete his regimen on oral antibiotics, what information should be provided to him to enhance adherence and ensure successful therapy?*

General Information
- Infective endocarditis is a very serious infection that can cause heart failure, blood clots in the lungs, or abscesses in other parts of the body if it is not treated with the appropriate antibiotics for 4 to 6 weeks.
- It is important to take the antibiotics at the correct times every day to have high enough blood concentrations of the drug to kill the bacteria.
- Contact your physician or go to the emergency room if you begin to have fever, develop heart palpitations, have difficulty breathing, or feel dizzy.

Dicloxacillin
- This medication is best absorbed when taken on an empty stomach, preferably 1 hour before or 2 hours after meals.
- If you forget to take a dose of this medicine, take it as soon as you remember. However, if it is almost time for your next dose, skip the missed dose and go back to your regular schedule.
- This medicine sometimes causes diarrhea; contact your doctor or me if this becomes troublesome or severe.

Minocycline
- This medication may be taken without regard to meals. You may take it with food if it causes upset stomach or nausea.
- Take each dose with a full glass of water to avoid irritation of the esophagus and stomach.
- If you forget to take a dose of this medicine, take it as soon as you remember. However, if it is almost time for your next dose, skip the missed dose and go back to your regular schedule.
- Minocycline may cause dizziness, lightheadedness, or unsteadiness. Make sure you know how you react to this medicine before you perform activities that may be dangerous, such as driving.
- This medicine rarely causes the skin to become more sensitive to sunlight. Avoid prolonged exposure to sunlight while taking this medicine and for several weeks afterward. Use a sunscreen with SPF of 15 or higher and wear protective clothing (e.g., a long-sleeved shirt and a hat) if you must be exposed to direct sunlight for extended periods.

References

1. Cunha B, Gill V, Lazar JM. Acute infective endocarditis: Diagnostic and therapeutic approach. Infect Dis Clin North Am 1996;10;811–834.
2. Wilson WR, Karchmer AW, Dajani AS, et al. Antibiotic treatment of adults with infective endocarditis due to streptococci, enterococci, staphylococci, and HACEK microorganisms. JAMA 1995;274:1706–1713.
3. DiNuble MJ. Short-course antibiotic therapy for right-sided endocarditis caused by *Staphylococcus aureus* in injection drug users. Ann Intern Med 1994;121: 873–876.
4. Chambers HF. Short-course combination and oral therapies of *Staphylococcus aureus* endocarditis. Infect Dis Clin North Am 1993;7:69–80.
5. Pryka RD, Rodvold KA, Erdman SM. An updated comparison of drug dosing methods. Part IV: Vancomycin. Clin Pharmacokinet 1991;20:463–476.
6. Rehm SJ. Outpatient intravenous antibiotic therapy for endocarditis. Infect Dis Clin North Am 1998;12:879–901.
7. Heldman AW, Hartert TV, Ray SC, et al. Oral antibiotic treatment of right-sided staphylococcal endocarditis in injection drug users: Prospective randomized comparison with parenteral therapy. Am J Med 1996;101:68–76.
8. Lawlor MT, Sullivan MC, Levitz RE, et al. Treatment of prosthetic valve endocarditis due to methicillin-resistant *Staphylococcus aureus* with minocycline. J Infect Dis 1990;161:812–814.

101 PULMONARY TUBERCULOSIS

Someone to Watch Over Me   (Level I)

Susan Shaffer, PharmD
Dennis M. Williams, PharmD, FASHP, FCCP, BCPS

A 50-year-old resident of a homeless shelter presents with a 2-month history of persistent cough, malaise, fever, night sweats, and a 20-pound weight loss. The patient has diffuse rhonchi on physical exam, a chest x-ray reveals bilateral upper lobe infiltrates, and a CT scan of the chest shows a 3 × 4 cm cavity in the left lung. A PPD test is positive, and sputum Gram stains are positive for acid-fast bacilli. Treatment of active tuberculosis (TB) requires multiple drug therapy to quickly sterilize the sputum, eradicate the organisms, and prevent the development of resistance. Isoniazid and rifampin should be a part of the regimen; pyrazinamide and ethambutol (or streptomycin) are usually added. The minimum duration of treatment for adults with culture-positive TB is 6 months. Directly observed therapy (DOT) should be considered as an option to ensure that the patient adheres with the long-term therapy. Students are asked to consider alternative regimens when culture reports later indicate the presence of isoniazid-resistant organisms.

► Questions

Problem Identification

1. a. Create a list of the patient's drug-related problems.

- Active pulmonary TB requiring appropriate antimicrobial therapy.
- Borderline macrocytic anemia, which may be associated with phenytoin-induced folate deficiency and/or malnutrition.
- Chronic, stable problems not requiring attention at this time include: 1) unspecified seizure disorder apparently controlled with phenytoin; and 2) hypertension controlled with hydrochlorothiazide.

b. What signs, symptoms, and other findings are consistent with active TB infection?

- *Signs.* Diffuse rhonchi in upper lung lobes, decreased breath sounds; infiltrate on chest x-ray with possible cavitary lesion.
- *Symptoms.* Productive cough, fever, fatigue, night sweats, and weight loss.
- *Other findings.* Positive PPD skin test (induration of >10 mm in a patient at risk for TB is considered a positive test); presence of AFB in sputum.[1]

c. What factors place this patient at increased risk for acquiring TB?

- Race (the highest incidence of TB is in non-Hispanic blacks)
- Homeless shelter resident (individuals living in closed environments are at a higher risk)

Desired Outcome

2. What are the goals of therapy for this patient with active TB?

- Eliminate the patient's symptoms (cough, fever, fatigue, night sweats, weight loss).
- Institute drug therapy to make the patient non-infectious as soon as possible. Most patients with drug-susceptible organisms become non-infectious within several days to a few weeks after drug therapy is started. Symptom improvement and reduction in AFB on sputum smear are indicators that the patient is less infectious. Three separate-day negative sputum smears or negative culture results virtually assures that the patient is no longer infectious.[2]
- Prevent the transmission of TB to patient contacts.
- Prevent the development of drug resistance (a major factor is patient compliance).
- Minimize costs of drug therapy and drug related toxicities.
- Prevent the relapse of TB.

Therapeutic Alternatives

3. a. What non-drug therapies might be useful in this patient?

- *HIV test counseling.* There is a strong association between HIV infection and TB. For a patient who is infected with TB, the risk of progressing to active disease is 100 times higher. The risk for TB infection with resistant organisms has been reported to be higher in HIV-infected patients.
- *Nutrition consult.* This will be helpful for this homeless patient who has a recent history of weight loss associated with his infection. Assessments of his caloric intake can be made and goals can be set to help him gain and maintain weight. Supplemental calories can be provided during his hospital stay. Attention can also be given to his anemia, which may be due to poor nutrition as well as to phenytoin use.
- *Social work consult.* This patient should undergo an assessment to determine his eligibility for medical coverage as an indigent/homeless person. Resources can be sought for his nutrition needs, medical needs, and for treatment of his active TB.

b. What drug therapies are available for the treatment of active TB?

- Effective treatment of active TB requires use of a multiple-drug regimen to which the organisms are susceptible. At least two medications to which the organism is susceptible are required. Multiple agents must be given for an adequate period of time to ensure that various populations of TB organisms are eradicated. Multiple drugs also help to sterilize the sputum as quickly as possible.
- Mycobacteria can reside as extracellular, rapidly dividing bacteria, as intracellular organisms in macrophages, or as dormant organisms in granulomas. The current minimal acceptable treatment period is 6 months. The drugs must be taken regularly and

for the entire course of therapy to reduce the likelihood of developing drug resistance.
- *Isoniazid* and *rifampin* represent the two most important therapies for active TB and should be part of the regimen unless either is contraindicated or not tolerated. Isoniazid is effective, with a relatively low frequency of side effects and low cost. Rifampin has had the greatest impact on shortening the duration of treatment and in minimizing treatment failures.
- *Pyrazinamide, ethambutol,* and *streptomycin* are other first-line agents that may be selected based on their effectiveness against certain populations of organisms, relative safety, and clinical experience.

c. *What economic and social considerations are applicable to this patient?*

- Since the patient is homeless, the cost of medications is probably an issue. Attempts should be made to minimize costs while maximizing drug compliance. Medications can generally be provided through the local health department.
- Non-adherence is the major factor contributing to drug resistance. An assessment should be made to determine if this patient is a candidate for directly observed therapy (DOT) to ensure compliance with his drug therapy.

Optimal Plan

4. a. *What drug, dosage form, dose, schedule, and duration of therapy are best for this patient?*

- Generally, 3 options exist as initial, empiric therapy for the patient with active TB. All regimens utilize 4 of the 5 first-line agents. Second-line medications should only be employed when these agents fail, are not tolerated, or resistance is known.
- The preferred treatment for this patient involves an initial treatment phase (2 months) consisting of isoniazid, rifampin, and pyrazinamide. Ethambutol (or streptomycin) should be used in the initial phase of treatment until susceptibility results are known, since the potential for drug resistance exists.[2] This 4-drug regimen is effective in treating active TB and in preventing the development of resistance. The minimum duration of treatment for adults with culture-positive TB is 6 months. Using 4 drugs initially is effective even when isoniazid resistance is present, since multiple drugs are still being used that have activity against the organism. The following doses should be given.
  - ✓ Rifampin 600 mg po QD (10 mg/kg/day); maximum 600 mg/day
  - ✓ Isoniazid 300 mg po QD (5 mg/kg/day); maximum 300 mg/day
  - ✓ Pyrazinamide 1500 mg po QD (15 to 30 mg/kg/day); maximum 2000 mg/day
  - ✓ Ethambutol 2 g po QD (15 to 25 mg/kg/day); maximum 2.5 g/day; *or* streptomycin 1 g IM/IV QD (15 mg/kg/day); maximum 1 g/day
  - ✓ Pyridoxine 25 mg po daily

After the initial 2-month treatment phase, therapy should continue for an additional 4 months with isoniazid and rifampin; the total treatment period should be 6 months. The isoniazid and rifampin can be given either daily or 2 to 3 times weekly as DOT.

- Another option is to use daily rifampin, isoniazid, pyrazinamide, and ethambutol (or streptomycin) for 2 weeks followed by twice-weekly doses of the same drugs for 6 weeks as DOT. Then isoniazid and rifampin can be given 2 times weekly as DOT for an additional 16 weeks.
- The last option is continuous DOT with 3 times weekly isoniazid, rifampin, pyrazinamide, and ethambutol (or streptomycin) for a total of 6 months.
- The latter two regimens are less well studied and may result in a higher incidence of side effects due to intermittent therapy. Therefore, the first regimen is recommended for this patient.

b. *What alternatives to daily administration of medicines exist?*

- All patients with active TB should be evaluated for the need for DOT. Since non-compliance is the primary reason for treatment failures and resistance, close monitoring of compliance is imperative.
- In certain circumstances, drug therapy can be administered twice or three times weekly rather than daily. This minimizes costs to patients but often increases the risk for side effects.
- There is evidence that switching to intermittent therapy after 2 weeks of daily administration produces results equal to those of daily administration.[2]
- Rifapentine (Priftin) could be used as an alternative DOT therapy. It is a rifamycin derivative in the same class as rifampin and rifabutin. In the initial treatment of pulmonary tuberculosis, it can be administered twice a week for two months, along with 1 to 3 other daily antitubercular agents. After 2 months of therapy, rifapentine can be continued for 4 months on a once-weekly basis with at least 1 other antitubercular agent. It is likely that future recommendations for treatment of pulmonary tuberculosis will include rifapentine-containing regimens.

Outcome Evaluation

5. *What clinical and laboratory parameters are necessary to evaluate the therapy for achievement of the desired therapeutic outcome and to detect or prevent adverse effects?*

Efficacy

- The patient should be monitored for improvement of his symptoms (e.g., cough, fatigue, fever, night sweats).
- The best indication of response to therapy is a conversion to negative sputum smears and culture; however, many patients will note an improvement in their symptoms within 1 to 2 weeks.
- Sputum should be evaluated at least monthly until sputum conversion is seen (weekly sputum smears with quantification are encouraged).[2] More than 85% of patients will have negative sputums after 2 months of therapy.

Adverse Effects

- Baseline laboratory tests that should be obtained include hepatic enzymes, total bilirubin, serum creatinine, CBC, platelet count, serum uric acid (in patients receiving pyrazinamide), and examination of visual acuity and red-green color perception. If baseline values are normal, follow-up testing is needed only if symptoms of drug toxicity arise.[2] Patients who have abnormalities at baseline should have follow-up testing of these findings.[2]

- Isoniazid
  - ✓ Elevations in hepatic aminotransferase enzymes.
  - ✓ Hepatitis (risk increases with advancing age; 2.3% risk for patients 50 to 64 years of age[2]).
  - ✓ Peripheral neuropathy is rare at doses of 5 mg/kg. Pyridoxine should be given to patients at high risk for pyridoxine deficiency or in whom neuropathies may occur, including those with diabetes, uremia, alcoholism, malnutrition, pregnancy, or a seizure disorder.
  - ✓ Mild CNS side effects may occur (e.g., ataxia, tinnitus, euphoria, dizziness). Seizures and encephalopathy are rare.
- Rifampin
  - ✓ Elevations in hepatic aminotransferase enzymes; overt hepatitis
  - ✓ GI distress (the most common side effect)
  - ✓ Red or orange discoloration of body secretions (e.g., saliva, tears, urine, sweat)
  - ✓ Skin eruptions
  - ✓ Thrombocytopenia (rare)
  - ✓ Cholestatic jaundice (rare)
  - ✓ Intermittent administration of doses >10 mg/kg may be associated with thrombocytopenia, an influenza-like syndrome, hemolytic anemia, and acute renal failure
- Pyrazinamide
  - ✓ Hepatotoxicity
  - ✓ Hyperuricemia (acute gout is uncommon)
  - ✓ Arthralgias (treatment with salicylates generally provides symptomatic relief)
  - ✓ Skin rash
  - ✓ GI distress
- Ethambutol
  - ✓ Retrobulbar neuritis: blurred vision, central scotomata, red-green color blindness, change in visual acuity (dose related). Use of this drug should be avoided in children because they may be too young to assess visual acuity or red-green color discrimination.
- Streptomycin
  - ✓ Ototoxicity (commonly results in vertigo but may lead to hearing loss)
  - ✓ Nephrotoxicity (rare, but may occur in patients with renal dysfunction or who are taking other nephrotoxic drugs)
  - ✓ Pain on injection

Patient Counseling

6. What information should be provided to the patient to enhance compliance, ensure successful therapy, and minimize adverse effects?

General Instructions
- Take these medicines once each day for the full course of treatment, even if you begin to feel better.
- It is important not to miss any doses. If you miss a dose, take it as soon as you remember; if it is almost time for your next dose, skip the missed dose and return to your regular schedule. Do not take double doses.
- Medications may cause stomach upset; taking them with food can decrease this; nausea or vomiting should be reported to your physician.
- Some of these drugs can affect the liver; for this reason, periodic laboratory testing may be performed.
- Liver problems are more likely to occur if alcohol is regularly consumed while taking these medicines.
- It is important to keep all scheduled follow-up appointments with your doctor.

Isoniazid
- Notify your doctor if you develop numbness, burning, tingling, or pain in the hands or feet; unusual tiredness or weakness; clumsiness or unsteadiness; dark urine; or yellowing of the eyes.
- Pyridoxine (vitamin B_6) is given once a day to prevent or lessen the side effects of this medication.

Rifampin or Rifapentine
- This medicine will cause a red or orange discoloration of body fluids, such as sweat, urine, saliva, and tears. Do not wear soft contact lenses while taking this medication because they may become permanently discolored.
- This medication interacts with many other medicines; consult your doctor or me before taking any new medications.

Ethambutol
- Report any changes in vision, such as blurred vision, eye pain, red-green color blindness, or loss of vision to your doctor immediately. Baseline eye exams are recommended before starting this medicine and then periodically during therapy.

Pyrazinamide
- This medicine may precipitate a gout attack in patients with a history of gout. Inform your doctor of pain or swelling in any joints while taking this medication.

▶ Follow-up Questions

1. How should the presence of INH resistance influence the drug therapy?

- Patients who have organisms resistant to 1 or more drugs should be treated with at least 2 drugs to which the organisms are susceptible. The value of the 4-drug regimen initially is that it is effective even if INH resistance is present.
- If INH resistance is noted during the 6-month treatment regimen, INH should be discontinued and therapy should be continued with pyrazinamide for the entire 6 months in place of INH.
- Alternatively, some clinicians continue the remaining 3 drugs for the entire 6 months or use rifampin and ethambutol for 12 months.

2. After 3 months of therapy, an increase in the patient's AST and ALT are noted (AST 160 IU/L; ALT 190 IU/L). Other liver enzymes and total bilirubin are normal. The patient reports no new complaints. What changes would you make to the current therapy and monitoring plan?

- Isoniazid, rifampin, and pyrazinamide are each potentially hepatotoxic. Increases in LFTs, particularly transaminases, commonly occur. Small increases may not warrant changes in drug therapy, especially in asymptomatic patients. Increases in transaminases of 3 to 5 times normal may be well tolerated. If greater increases occur, or if the patient develops symptoms (e.g., nausea, vomiting, malaise, abdominal pain, or jaundice), one or more agents should be discontinued and alternative therapy used.

3. *What potential drug interactions should be evaluated? How should they be managed?*

- In patients taking phenytoin and isoniazid, the serum concentrations of both drugs may be increased. Because isoniazid can increase phenytoin concentrations and rifampin (a potent inducer of CYP2C and CYP3A isoenzymes) can reduce phenytoin concentrations, serum phenytoin levels should be measured frequently and patients should be monitored for signs of phenytoin toxicity (ataxia, drowsiness, nystagmus) or subtherapeutic concentrations (to prevent seizure activity). Serum phenytoin concentrations should be obtained monthly during concomitant therapy for at least the initial 2 or 3 months of therapy. Subsequent monthly monitoring is at the discretion of the clinician in patients who are compliant with therapy.
- The patient also has a borderline macrocytic anemia. This is most likely due to chronic phenytoin therapy in which folic acid is used to metabolize phenytoin. In the absence of significant symptoms, no further intervention is needed.

4. *How should close contacts of the patient be treated (considering that he has INH-resistant organisms)?*

- PPD skin testing should be performed on close contacts. If the results are positive, chemoprophylaxis should be administered once active TB has been ruled out. Isoniazid 300 mg daily should be used initially unless the index case has INH-resistant organisms. In this case, treat positive contacts with rifampin 600 mg daily (or 10 to 20 mg/kg in children). Adults should receive chemoprophylaxis for 6 months, children for 9 months. Some clinicians add a second drug for chemoprophylaxis in this setting (ethambutol 15 mg/kg or pyrazinamide 15 to 30 mg/kg daily), but data on the efficacy of these regimens are lacking. Shorter courses are also being evaluated, such as rifampin for 4 months or rifampin plus pyrazinamide for 2 months.

References

1. Bass JB Jr, Farer LS, Hopewell PC, et al. Treatment of tuberculosis and tuberculosis infection in adults and children. American Thoracic Society and the Centers for Disease Control and Prevention. Am J Respir Crit Care Med 1994;149:1359–1374.
2. American Thoracic Society. Control of tuberculosis in the United States. Am Rev Respir Dis 1992;146:1623–1633.

Note: A document entitled "Core Curriculum on Tuberculosis: What the Clinician Should Know," (3rd ed, 1994) is available from the Centers for Disease Control and Prevention on the Internet at http://www.cdc.gov/nchstp/tb/pubs/corecurr.htm

102 CLOSTRIDIUM DIFFICILE–ASSOCIATED DIARRHEA

▶ When One Antibiotic Requires Another (Level I)

Margaret B. Zak, PharmD

A 70-year-old man with type 2 diabetes mellitus and other medical problems is brought to the emergency department by his sister because of confusion and lethargy. Upon evaluation, the patient is found to have dehydration, hypoglycemia, and hypokalemia. Laboratory results reveal leukocytosis with a left shift, the presence of fecal leukocytes, and a stool culture positive for *Clostridium difficile*. Dextrose, IV fluids, and potassium must be administered to correct the metabolic imbalances. Primary options for treatment of *C. difficile* diarrhea include oral metronidazole or vancomycin. Metronidazole is preferred because of increasing enterococcal resistance to vancomycin. When this patient fails to respond adequately to the initial therapy chosen, students are asked to consider the possible reasons for treatment failure and to recommend alternative treatments.

▶ Questions

Problem Identification

1. a. *Create a complete list of the patient's drug-related problems at the time of admission.*

- Hypoglycemia secondary to continued usage of the oral hypoglycemic glipizide (Glucotrol XL) in a fasting patient.
- Hypertension, diabetic nephropathy, and CHF, which would all likely benefit from addition of an ACE inhibitor.
- Hismanal (astemizole) therapy for unknown indication.
- Hypokalemia requiring supplementation.
- Dehydration requiring fluid replacement.
- Diarrhea secondary to Augmentin usage (amoxicillin/clavulanic acid). Augmentin can cause *C. difficile* associated diarrhea or may cause drug-induced diarrhea not associated with *C. difficile*.
- Magnesium use may also have contributed to diarrhea in this patient.

b. *What signs, symptoms, and laboratory values are consistent with* C. difficile *diarrhea in this patient?*

- *Signs*. Abdominal guarding demonstrating tenderness, hyperactive bowel sounds, and diarrhea. Lack of fever may be secondary to the advanced age of patient; fever may be absent in the elderly.
- *Symptoms*. Reports of abdominal tenderness and cramping; greenish, watery diarrhea during and after antibiotic therapy.
- *Laboratory values*. WBC differential showing a left shift or bandemia (30% bands); fecal leukocytes present and stool culture positive for *C. difficile*. Several other methods for detection of *C. difficile* diarrhea may be used, including tissue culture for the presence of toxin B, enzyme immunoassay for toxin A and/or B,

latex agglutination, or endoscopy that is positive for pseudomembranes characteristic of *C. difficile* pseudomembranous colitis.

c. *Which antibiotics have been shown to cause* C. difficile *diarrhea?*

- Virtually all antibiotics have been associated with *C. difficile* diarrhea. However, the antibiotics most frequently associated include amoxicillin and ampicillin (amoxicillin/clavulanate included), and cephalosporins (most frequently the third-generation cephalosporins), and clindamycin.

Desired Outcome

2. *What are the goals of pharmacotherapy in this case?*

- Relief of symptoms including abdominal tenderness and diarrhea
- Eradicate *C. difficile* from GI tract and permit restoration of normal GI flora
- Correct and prevent hypovolemia, dehydration, and electrolyte disturbances
- Administer effective treatment while minimizing the cost of therapy
- Prevent recurrence
- Ensure compliance with therapy

Therapeutic Alternatives

3. a. *What non-drug therapies may be useful for the treatment of* C. difficile *in this patient?*

- Discontinuation of the inciting antibiotic would be beneficial. Clinical trials have reported that discontinuance of antibiotics alone may be sufficient to cure approximately 23% of patients with mild disease.[1] However, this patient requires antibiotics to manage his wound infection. If possible, alternative agents with less potential for inducing *C. difficile* could be substituted.
- Fluid support and electrolyte supplementation (potassium low). This patient must be managed cautiously, as aggressive management of hypoglycemia with dextrose is occurring concomitantly with potassium supplementation. A further decrease in serum potassium levels will likely be seen while correcting glucose concentrations.

b. *What feasible pharmacotherapeutic alternatives are available for treatment of* C. difficile *diarrhea?*

- *Metronidazole* is recommended by the Centers for Disease Control (CDC) for all cases of *C. difficile* diarrhea with the exception of those that are severe and potentially life-threatening or in patients who have failed to respond to metronidazole.[2] Metronidazole and vancomycin have very similar rates of response to therapy and relapse.[3] Metronidazole is preferred over vancomycin because of the increased rate of vancomycin resistance in *Enterococcus* species. Metronidazole is recommended to be given orally in doses of either 250 mg QID or 500 mg TID for 7 to 10 days. The drug may be administered IV if necessary.
- *Vancomycin* may be given for the treatment of *C. difficile* when the patient has failed metronidazole, is allergic to or intolerant of metronidazole, is pregnant, is a child under the age of 10, is taking other medications that contain ethanol, has severe life-threatening *C. difficile* infection, or has been diagnosed with diarrhea secondary to *Staphylococcus aureus*.[4] Vancomycin must be given by the oral route. The recommended oral dosage is 125 mg QID. Doses larger than 125 mg have not been shown to be more effective and should not be used unless the patient has life-threatening disease.[5]
- *Bacitracin* 25,000 U po QID has also been shown to be effective for the treatment of *C. difficile*. However, the cost of bacitracin is quite high and clinical response with bacitracin is lower than with either metronidazole or vancomycin. Also, the relapse rate is higher.
- *Cholestyramine* and *colestipol* are non-absorbable anion binding agents that may also be effective in the treatment of mild disease. However, these agents are not as effective as either vancomycin or metronidazole and have a slower response time.

Optimal Plan

4. a. *What drug, dosage form, schedule, and duration of therapy are best suited for this patient?*

- This patient may be given metronidazole either 250 mg po QID or 500 mg po TID for 7 to 10 days. Once 50% dextrose has been given and the patient is placed on maintenance fluids, the patient's mentation should improve, permitting reliable administration of oral metronidazole. He is not known to be allergic to metronidazole and has been shown to have *C. difficile* present upon stool culture. The diarrhea should resolve within 5 days of initiation of therapy.

b. *The patient was placed on the regimen you recommended. However, after 7 days his diarrhea is still present (5 to 7 watery stools per day) and a repeat* C. difficile *stool culture is reported as positive. What possible explanations do you have for his treatment failure?*

- *C. difficile* resistant to metronidazole.
- Diarrhea secondary to *Staphylococcus aureus*; this organism may also cause infectious diarrhea. Metronidazole will not cure *S. aureus* diarrhea because its spectrum of activity does not include this organism.
- Failure to attain adequate concentration of metronidazole in the gastrointestinal lumen. Metronidazole is 100% absorbed and then secreted into the GI tract. However, the amount secreted is quite variable and is diminished in healthy volunteers and as the diarrhea subsides.
- Metronidazole has occasionally been implicated as a cause of *C. difficile* diarrhea.
- Non-compliance could be the cause, but this occurs much less frequently in the inpatient setting.

c. *What changes, if any, should be made in the pharmacotherapeutic plan for the patient at this time?*

- The metronidazole should be discontinued and vancomycin 125 mg po QID should be initiated.
- If the lower-dose metronidazole regimen (250 mg po QID) had been selected initially, one might be tempted to simply increase the dose. Clinical trials that directly compare the response to different dosages of metronidazole for the treatment of *C. difficile* have not been performed. Current opinion is that once failure to

metronidazole has been established, alterations in dosage regimen probably have minimal effect, and therapy should be changed to an alternative agent such as vancomycin.
- Therapy with vancomycin or metronidazole could be continued for an additional month after the diarrhea subsides with either intermittent dosing or using a gradual taper.
- Anion-binding regimens may be added to therapy during the intermittent or taper phase or after the metronidazole or vancomycin therapy is discontinued. It should be noted that cholestyramine has been shown to bind vancomycin and reduce its absorption when given concomitantly.
- Oral rifampin can be added to oral vancomycin.
- Oral *Lactobacillus* preparations or *Saccharomyces boulardii* can be given at the end of therapy with vancomycin or metronidazole for several weeks to restore the GI tract flora.

Outcome Evaluation

5. *What clinical and laboratory parameters are necessary to evaluate the therapy for achievement of the desired therapeutic outcome and to detect or prevent adverse effects?*

Efficacy

- The diarrhea should subside, which can be measured by monitoring the patient's number, volume, and consistency of stools on a daily basis.
- Symptoms such as abdominal cramping and tenderness should resolve as the diarrhea subsides and can be measured by asking the patient daily how he feels.
- The WBC count and differential should return to normal. A WBC count with a differential can be obtained every 1 to 2 days until they begin to normalize.
- If the temperature was elevated (not in this case), the patient's temperature curve should be recorded and evaluated on a daily basis.
- A repeat culture for *C. difficile* or assay for toxins A or B should not be repeated unless the patient does not respond after approximately 5 days of therapy.

Adverse Effects

- Monitor patients taking metronidazole for nausea, vomiting, diarrhea, and loss of appetite, as these occur in >10% of patients. These adverse reactions can be monitored daily by asking the patient how he feels and how his appetite is. The nurse or caregiver should also be asked how much he is eating at meals. This is especially important for this patient, as his hypoglycemia was due to poor appetite while he continued to take an oral hypoglycemic.
- Daily monitoring of his diarrhea is also important to detect the onset of drug-induced diarrhea.
- Rare adverse reactions of metronidazole include seizures, peripheral neuropathy, metallic taste, black hairy tongue, leukopenia, ataxia, dark urine, and a disulfiram reaction with alcohol. These adverse reactions do not need to be monitored routinely.
- Patients taking oral vancomycin should be monitored for nausea, vomiting, and bitter taste in their mouths, as these reactions occur in >10% of patients. Chills, drug fever, ototoxicity, and renal impairment are rare adverse reactions that do not need to be monitored in this patient. Serum vancomycin levels should not be obtained, because oral vancomycin is poorly absorbed from the GI tract.

Patient Counseling

6. *What information should be provided to the patient to enhance compliance, ensure successful therapy, and minimize adverse effects?*

General Information

- You are being treated with metronidazole (Flagyl) 250 mg by mouth 4 times a day for 10 days for the treatment of your diarrhea. (He is later treated with vancomycin 125 mg orally every 6 hours for 1 month.)
- Spread the doses out evenly during the day (try to take the drug about every 6 hours).
- Take all of the metronidazole (vancomycin) until the prescription is gone to prevent recurrence of the infection or antibiotic resistance to the drug.
- Your diarrhea should go away in 5 days or sooner. Call your doctor if it does not go away or gets worse after this time.
- If you miss a dose of your metronidazole (vancomycin), take the dose as soon as you remember. However, if it is almost time to take the next dose, skip the missed dose and just take your next dose at the scheduled time.
- Store this medicine in a dry, cool place.

Metronidazole

- You may take this medicine with food to minimize stomach upset.
- Avoid alcohol-containing beverages and medicines while taking this medicine and for at least 1 day after you finish taking it.
- This medicine sometimes causes nausea, diarrhea, vomiting, loss of appetite, and a metallic taste.
- Notify your doctor if you experience numbness or tingling in your hands or feet while on this medicine.
- This medicine may darken the color of your urine.

Vancomycin

- This medicine may be taken either with food or between meals.
- This medicine may cause nausea or vomiting.

(*Note to instructors:* You may convey to students that the patient's metronidazole was replaced with vancomycin 125 mg po QID, and he was noted within 4 days to have diminished frequency of stools and increased stool consistency (no longer watery). He was discharged 2 days later with a prescription for vancomycin for an additional 22 days (total course of 4 weeks). A CBC with a differential at the time of discharge revealed a WBC of $7.4 \times 10^3/mm^3$ with 60% neutrophils and 2% bands. The patient has not had any subsequent recurrences of *C. difficile*.

References

1. Teasley DG, Gerding DN, Olson MM, et al. Prospective randomised trial of metronidazole versus vancomycin for *Clostridium difficile*-associated diarrhea and colitis. Lancet 1983;2:1043–1046.
2. Centers for Disease Control and Prevention. Preventing the spread of vancomycin resistance—a report from the hospital infection control practices advisory committee. Fed Reg 1994;59:25758–25763.
3. Kelly CP, Pothoulakis C, LaMont JT. *Clostridium difficile* colitis. N Engl J Med 1994:330:257–262.
4. Fekety R. Guidelines for the diagnosis and management of *Clostridium-difficile*-associated diarrhea and colitis. Am J Gastroenterol 1997;92:739–750.
5. Fekety R, Silva J, Kauffman C, et al. Treatment of antibiotic-associated *Clostridium difficile* colitis with oral vancomycin: Comparison of two dosage regimens. Am J Med 1989;86:15–19.

103 INTRA-ABDOMINAL INFECTION

▶ Like Mother, Like Son   (Level II)

Renee-Claude Mercier, PharmD

A 67-year-old man with a history of alcoholic cirrhosis and encephalopathy is brought to the ED because of nausea, vomiting, severe abdominal pain, and altered mental status. Physical examination reveals fever, tachypnea, and a distended abdomen with positive guarding. A CBC indicates leukocytosis with a left shift, and a paracentesis is positive for numerous white cells but no organisms. Because the Gram stain is often negative in primary bacterial peritonitis, initial antimicrobial therapy is frequently empiric. Third-generation cephalosporins (e.g., cefotaxime) cover the most likely organisms when used as monotherapy in many cases. They also avoid the risk of nephrotoxicity associated with aminoglycoside use. Other potential alternatives include broad-spectrum penicillins (mezlocillin, ticarcillin, piperacillin), carbapenems (e.g., imipenem), and β-lactam/β-lactamase inhibitor combinations (e.g., ticarcillin/clavulanate, piperacillin/tazobactam, ampicillin/sulbactam). When this patient's blood cultures are reported positive for *Escherichia coli* sensitive to ampicillin, the antibiotic regimen may be simplified to ampicillin alone for a total therapy duration of 10 days. Provision of appropriate hemodynamic and nutrition support should also be considered in this case.

▶ Questions

Problem Identification

1. a. *Create a list of the patient's drug-related problems.*

   - Primary bacterial peritonitis, requiring treatment.
   - Cirrhosis with ascites and hepatic encephalopathy, requiring treatment.
   - Alcohol abuse/possible withdrawal symptoms that may require treatment.
   - Hypertension, inadequately controlled (elevated systolic BP).
   - Potential problem: if an aminoglycoside is used, close monitoring of the dosing is required to prevent nephrotoxicity and ototoxicity. Patients with severe primary bacterial peritonitis tend to be volume depleted, and multiple organ failure could be an important complication.
   - Potential problem: antacids and H_2-antagonists increase the risk of developing bacterial peritonitis in patients with cirrhosis and ascites.

   b. *What signs, symptoms, and laboratory values indicate the presence of primary bacterial peritonitis?*

   - *Signs.* Fever; distended abdomen with ascites and decreased bowel sounds; tachycardia; shallow, frequent breathing.
   - *Symptoms.* Severe abdominal pain, nausea, vomiting.
   - *Laboratory values.* Elevated WBC count with left shift; ascitic fluid with elevated leukocyte count.

   c. *What risk factors for infection are present in this patient?*

   - Cirrhosis with ascites is associated with portal hypertension, which poses an increased risk for bacteria to be transported from the bloodstream to the peritoneal cavity where the inflammatory process begins.
   - Alcohol abuse results in decreased phagocytic activity and impaired intracellular killing activity.
   - Antacids/H_2-antagonists increase gastric pH, which may promote bacterial growth. Due to the high risk of aspiration in an alcoholic patient with altered mental status, the antacids and/or H_2-antagonist may increase the likelihood of aspiration pneumonia.

   d. *What organisms are the most likely cause of this infection?*

   - *Escherichia coli, Klebsiella pneumoniae, Streptococcus pneumoniae,* and enterococci.[1]
   - *Staphylococcus aureus* and anaerobes are infrequent causes of primary bacterial peritonitis.

Desired Outcome

2. *What are the therapeutic goals for this patient?*

   - Cure of the infectious process should be seen if the following antimicrobial therapeutic goals are achieved.
     - ✓ Control bacteremia if present and prevent establishment of metastatic foci of infection
     - ✓ Reduce suppurative complications
     - ✓ Prevent local spread of existing infection
   - Physiologic/hemodynamic support of the patient; maintain BP, HR, and RR within normal limits; maintain good urinary output without compromising intravascular volume; decrease the amount of ascites.
   - Improve hepatic encephalopathy.
   - Prevent alcohol withdrawal symptoms.

Therapeutic Alternatives

3. a. *What non-drug therapies might be useful for this patient?*

   - This infectious process requires antibiotics for treatment. However, concomitant conditions may require non-drug therapies such as proper ventilation/oxygen support, hemodynamic support with fluids, and counseling for the alcohol abuse and hepatitis C positivity.
   - Drainage of the abdomen is not required for the treatment of primary peritonitis.

   b. *What feasible pharmacotherapeutic alternatives are available for the treatment of the primary bacterial peritonitis?*

   - Because the Gram stain is often negative in primary bacterial peritonitis, the initial antimicrobial therapy is frequently empiric, based on the most likely pathogens. The regimen can be modified once the results of the culture and susceptibility testing are available.

- *Ampicillin plus an aminoglycoside* has been used effectively in primary bacterial peritonitis.
- Some *third-generation cephalosporins (e.g., cefotaxime, ceftizoxime)* have been demonstrated to be as effective as ampicillin/aminoglycoside.[2] They also avoid the risk of nephrotoxicity, which is sufficiently frequent in this group of patients to warrant the avoidance of aminoglycosides if an equally effective alternative can be used. Ceftazidime is not considered a first-line agent because of its lack of activity against gram-positive bacteria such as *S. pneumoniae*. It would also be preferable to avoid ceftriaxone in this patient because it is primarily metabolized in the liver and this patient has significant liver impairment.
- *Broad-spectrum penicillins (e.g., mezlocillin, ticarcillin, piperacillin), carbapenems (e.g., imipenem/cilastatin), and β-lactam/β-lactamase inhibitor combinations (e.g., ticarcillin/clavulanate, piperacillin/tazobactam, ampicillin/sulbactam)* are potential alternatives.[3]
- *Clindamycin* or *metronidazole* should be added if anaerobes cannot be ruled out.
- *Aztreonam* would be an appropriate alternative for gram-negative bacteria but has no activity against enterococci and anaerobes.
- *Ofloxacin* 400 mg IV or po Q 12 H could be used in patients allergic to penicillin and/or cephalosporins.
- Refer to Table 104–6 in textbook Chapter 104 for a complete listing of recommended initial antimicrobial therapy for intra-abdominal infections.

Optimal Plan

4. a. *Given this patient's condition, which drug regimens would provide optimal therapy for the infection?*

- Cefotaxime 2 g IV Q 8 H covers the most common pathogens, including resistant strains of *S. pneumoniae*, with a simplified and well tolerated single-drug regimen. The patient will not require an aminoglycoside, which will decrease the likelihood of developing nephrotoxicity. The interval should be increased to Q 4 H if the infection becomes life threatening. The duration of therapy for bacterial peritonitis is controversial, but this patient should be treated for at least 10 to 14 days to prevent recurrence.
- If enterococci are highly suspected (e.g., because of immunosuppression due to chronic alcohol intake), an aminoglycoside in combination with penicillin or ampicillin should be considered.
- Other alternatives include ticarcillin/clavulanate 3.1 g IV Q 4 to 6 H, piperacillin/tazobactam 3.375 g IV Q 6 H, or ampicillin/sulbactam 1.5 to 3 g IV Q 6 H. These agents would provide good gram-negative and anaerobic coverage. They are also effective against penicillin-sensitive *S. pneumoniae* but lack activity against the resistant strains.

b. *In addition to antimicrobial therapy, what other drug-related interventions are required for this patient?*

- Lactulose 30 ml po QID should be started for treatment of hepatic encephalopathy.
- An IV multivitamin (10 mL/day), thiamine 100 mg/day, and folic acid 1 mg/day should be started to prevent alcohol withdrawal symptoms.
- Diuretic use is controversial in the treatment of ascites because they may decrease intravascular volume and cause hypovolemia since mobilization of fluid from the third space is a relatively slow process.
- Blood pressure should also be controlled by continuing Procardia XL 60 mg QD and adjusting the dose if required.
- Appropriate nutrition support should also be provided.

Outcome Evaluation

5. *What clinical and laboratory parameters are necessary to evaluate the therapy for achievement of the desired therapeutic outcome and to detect or prevent adverse effects?*

- If proper antimicrobial treatment is selected, the patient's condition should improve within 24 to 48 hours.[2–3]
- Check for resolution of abnormal laboratory findings, urine output, renal function (BUN/SCr), and electrolytes daily while in the ICU, then 3 to 4 times/week if the patient's status is stable.
- Monitor for improvement in signs and symptoms of infection daily. The patient's temperature should be taken 3 to 4 times/day while febrile, then daily. If further ascitic fluid needs to be removed while the patient is on antimicrobial therapy, a portion of the fluid should be sent for fluid analysis and culture to assess the response to antibiotics.
- Improvement in mental status should be assessed daily.
- Be observant for the onset of unusual diarrhea. Lactulose may cause loose stools, and diarrhea should not be assumed to be due to *C. difficile* without testing for it in the stool.

Patient Counseling

6. *What information should be provided to the patient to enhance compliance, ensure successful therapy, and minimize adverse effects?*

- The patient should receive at least 10 to 14 days of inpatient IV therapy. Before discharge, he should receive counseling about his alcohol abuse and be given the names and addresses of organizations that can help him with his drinking problem.
- He should also be aware that his long-term prognosis from liver failure is poor if he does not stop drinking.
- He should also be told about his hepatitis C status and his increased risk of liver failure.

References

1. Conn HO, Fessel JM. Spontaneous bacterial peritonitis in cirrhosis: Variations on a theme. Medicine (Baltimore) 1971;50:161–197.
2. Felisart J, Rimola A, Arroyo V, et al. Cefotaxime is more effective than is ampicillin-tobramycin in cirrhotics with severe infections. Hepatology 1985;5: 457–462.
3. Bohnen JM, Solomkin JS, Dellinger EP, et al. Guidelines for clinical care: Anti-infective agents for intra-abdominal infection. A Surgical Infection Society policy statement. Arch Surg 1992;127:83–89.

104 PELVIC INFLAMMATORY DISEASE AND OTHER SEXUALLY TRANSMITTED DISEASES

▶ Frankie and Jenny Were Lovers   (Level II)

Denise L. Howrie, PharmD
Pamela J. Murray, MD, MPH

A 28-year-old man and a 22-year-old woman who are involved in an intimate relationship present to a health clinic with a variety of complaints suggesting multiple sexually transmitted diseases (STDs). The man is ultimately found to require treatment for gonococcal urethritis, *Chlamydia*, trichomoniasis, and herpes simplex. The woman has evidence of pelvic inflammatory disease (PID). Students are asked to consider the appropriate therapeutic alternatives for each STD and recommend an appropriate comprehensive treatment strategy for each patient. The current treatment guidelines from the Centers for Disease Control and Prevention should be consulted for recommended STD treatment alternatives.

▶ Questions

Problem Identification

1. a. For each patient, create a list of drug-related problems.

- Frankie's current problems include 1) gonococcal urethritis; 2) recurrent genital herpes; 3) trichomoniasis; and 4) lack of appropriate contraceptive use.
- Jenny's current problems include 1) pan-genital tract infection including pelvic inflammatory disease (PID), cervicitis, vaginitis, and urethritis; and 2) lack of appropriate contraceptive use.

b. What information indicates the presence or severity of each STD in each patient?

- Frankie, who is sexually active with multiple partners and does not use a barrier contraceptive method reliably, has dysuria and a urethral discharge for 5 days. These are common symptoms of urethritis, which is the most common presentation of an STD in males. The presence of 15 WBC/hpf in the urethral discharge and a positive Gram stain for gram-negative intracellular diplococci provides a presumptive diagnosis of gonococcal infection that may be confirmed through bacterial culture.[1] Because a coexisting *Chlamydia* infection may be present in up to 50% of patients in some geographic areas,[1] a *Chlamydia* PCR test would be helpful to confirm this but would generally not be available for several days. Flagellated organisms visualized by microscopy indicate the presence of trichomoniasis, which may cause urethritis or asymptomatic infection in males. Frankie also reports a history of genital herpes two years ago and has 4 vesicles ("blisters") in the genital area, suggesting recurrent genital herpes.
- Jenny is sexually active without use of a barrier method and has had recent intercourse with a partner with STDs. She has evidence of cervicitis including purulent discharge and erythema, commonly associated with *Chlamydia trachomatis* and gonococcus.[1] Symptoms of vaginal discharge, erythema and excoriation suggest vaginitis, most often due to candida or trichomonas infection.[1] Trichomonal infections may also present with vulvar, vaginal, urethral, and cervical symptoms. Constitutional symptoms of nausea, vomiting, fever, lower abdominal pain, elevated body temperature, tachycardia, abdominal guarding, and leukocytosis with a left shift suggest the presence of gonococcal-related PID. Her pelvic examination reveals cervical motion tenderness, adnexal tenderness, and discharge from the cervical os, consistent with a diagnosis of PID.[1] She has no evidence of herpes genitalis and therefore does not require evaluation or treatment at this time.
- The diagnosis of PID is suspected in women with lower abdominal, cervical, and adnexal tenderness; rebound tenderness and guarding of the abdomen.[1,2] Abnormal cervical or vaginal discharge or bleeding, dysuria, fever, vomiting, and diarrhea increase the specificity of the diagnosis. Evaluation of the cervical or vaginal discharge by Gram stain for gonococcus in women is not helpful because this test has a higher rate of false-negative results in women than men and may also reveal organisms that are normal vaginal flora. Bacterial culture of secretions should therefore be performed. When available, more sensitive tests for the presence of *Chlamydia trachomatis* such as a polymerase chain reaction (PCR) test may be helpful in confirming the presence of this commonly infecting organism in women with PID.
- Vaginal redness with excoriations suggesting pruritus and a colored vaginal discharge are consistent with a diagnosis of vaginitis, which may be due to candidiasis, herpes, or trichomoniasis. Examination of the discharge was not consistent with a diagnosis of candidiasis, which is usually caused by *Candida albicans*. Bacterial vaginosis is also unlikely, given the low pH of vaginal secretions, lack of clue cells, and a negative whiff test after addition of 10% KOH. The presence of flagellated organisms confirms the diagnosis of trichomoniasis, which is commonly associated with pruritus, dysuria, abdominal pain, and a yellow-green malodorous discharge.

c. Should any additional tests be performed in these patients?

- Because of the history of unprotected sexual intercourse and Frankie's multiple sexual partners, more complete screening for other STDs such as HIV, syphilis, and hepatitis B should be performed in each patient, as these may be coexisting asymptomatic infections. Although viral cultures may be performed in Frankie to confirm a diagnosis of herpes simplex infection, a clinical diagnosis of recurrence is usually sufficient to begin empiric therapy, given the high frequency of recurrence of this infection and the delay in laboratory confirmation.

- Jenny should undergo a beta human chorionic gonadotropin (β-HCG) test[1] to detect pregnancy, although her last menses ended 10 days ago by history. Also, patients with PID may receive further diagnostic procedures including pelvic ultrasound and laparoscopy to better evaluate the extent of disease. The cervical secretions should be cultured to determine the presence of *Neisseria gonorrheae* or other infecting organisms. Blood cultures are not routinely obtained but may be helpful in severe episodes with high fever when bacteremia is suspected.

d. *What complications of infection can be reduced or avoided with appropriate therapy?*

- For Frankie, treatment of gonococcus, *Chlamydia,* and *Trichomonas* should reduce infectivity and prevent acute complications including epididymitis. Treatment directed against herpes simplex will not result in eradication of the virus but will shorten the duration and severity of the viral disease, shorten the duration of viral shedding, and reduce infectivity.
- For Jenny, treatment may prevent acute complications of bacteremia and sepsis. Treatment may also reduce the frequency of later complications, which occur in 25% of cases, including infertility (20%, with increased risk with other episodes of PID), chronic abdominal pain syndromes (5% to 20%), and ectopic pregnancy (6- to 10-fold increased risk) due to damage of the fallopian tubes.[2] Early treatment is imperative, as delay will increase the risk of infertility and other complications.[2]

Desired Outcome

2. *State the goals of treatment for each patient.*

- For Frankie, goals include: 1) resolution of infection and relief of symptoms using a cost-effective treatment plan; 2) improved education about the risks of sexual intercourse with regard to infection and possible pregnancy; and 3) identification of all sexual partners for evaluation and treatment. It is important to consider the public health risks of untreated and/or asymptomatic carriers of *Chlamydia trachomatis,* gonococcus, *Trichomonas,* and *Treponema pallidum.*[1]
- For Jenny, goals include: 1) eradication of infecting organisms for symptomatic relief; 2) initiation of treatment as soon as possible to reduce complications; 3) use of a cost-effective regimen with minimal toxicity; 4) education about the risks of sexual intercourse with regard to pregnancy and infection; and 5) provision of women's health support including yearly screening tests and contraceptive methods appropriate for her. Psychosocial support should be provided in this time of stress with her relationship with Frankie.

Therapeutic Alternatives

3. *What therapeutic options are available for treatment of each patient?*

- For Frankie, gonococcal urethritis requires concurrent therapy for *Chlamydia trachomatis* urethritis, because *Chlamydia* is a frequent co-infecting organism. In addition, he requires treatment for trichomoniasis and may benefit from treatment of recurrent genital herpes.
  ✓ Single doses of oral *ciprofloxacin* 500 mg, *ofloxacin* 400 mg or *cefixime* 400 mg, or intramuscular *ceftriaxone* 125 mg (in combination with lidocaine to reduce local injection pain) are the treatments of choice for *Neisseria gonorrheae* because of the high frequency of penicillin-resistant strains.[3] Oral therapy, although more convenient and less expensive than parenteral therapy, may eventually result in the development of drug-resistant strains, as has been demonstrated in some geographic areas where ciprofloxacin has been extensively used. Compliance with oral single-dose therapy should be assured by observation of dose ingestion and careful monitoring for drug-related nausea or vomiting, which may require retreatment.
  ✓ *Doxycycline* 100 mg po BID × 7 days or *azithromycin* 1 g po as a single dose (using the 1-g single-dose packet for oral suspension) are two treatments of choice for chlamydial urethritis or cervicitis.[3]
  ✓ *Metronidazole* 2 g in a single dose or 500 mg po BID × 7 days may be prescribed for treatment of trichomoniasis. Metronidazole 375 mg capsules po BID × 7 days may also be used.
  ✓ *Acyclovir, famciclovir,* or *valacyclovir* may be used for 5 days to treat episodic recurrent genital herpes infections.[3] When considering issues of compliance and dosing frequency, acyclovir 800 mg po BID compares favorably with famciclovir 125 mg po BID or valacyclovir 500 mg po BID. Acyclovir may also be prescribed in doses of 400 mg po TID or 200 mg po 5 times a day. Treatment must be begun during the prodromal stage of illness or within 1 day of development of lesions to have a clinically significant effect on the duration of the episode.
- For Jenny, PID poses the risk of serious infectious complications. PID is a polymicrobial infection in which *Neisseria gonorrheae, Chlamydia trachomatis,* aerobes such as *Escherichia coli,* and anaerobes such as *Bacteroides* and *Peptostreptococcus* may be present.[1,2] Empiric, broad-spectrum antibacterial agents should be prescribed in combinations that provide optimal coverage of these organisms. Studies are ongoing to determine the need for routine hospitalization in PID management. At this time, many patients may be successfully treated in the ambulatory setting when symptoms are mild, compliance with oral medications is likely, and compliance with follow-up visits is assured to monitor the efficacy of treatment. It should be emphasized that lack of compliance can greatly increase the risk of disease sequelae. Hospitalization may be indicated for treatment of patients with tubo-ovarian abscess, bacteremia or sepsis, pregnancy, or those who cannot retain oral medications or comply with the medical follow-up needed to assess treatment outcome.
  ✓ *Cefoxitin* 2 g IV Q 6 H or cefotetan 2 g IV Q 12 H *plus doxycycline* 100 mg IV or po Q 12 H × 14 days are the recommended regimens for inpatient management of PID.[3]
  ✓ *Gentamicin* 2 mg/kg (ideal weight) IV/IM loading dose followed by 4.5 mg/kg/day given Q 8 H *plus clindamycin* 900 mg IV Q 8 H followed by *doxycycline* 100 mg po BID × 14 days total is an alternative regimen. Parenteral regimens should be con-

tinued for a minimum of 24 to 48 hours after significant clinical improvement.
- ✓ *Azithromycin* 500 mg IV for 2 days (or for 24 to 48 hours after significant clinical improvement), followed by 500 mg po once daily for a total of 10 days is FDA approved for PID, but this regimen lacks anaerobic coverage, which may be needed in more serious infections.
- ✓ *Ofloxacin* 400 mg po BID with *metronidazole* 500 mg po BID × 14 days or *ceftriaxone* 250 mg IM plus *doxycycline* 100 mg BID for 14 days may be used for ambulatory treatment of PID.[3] Other parenteral second- or third-generation cephalosporins may be substituted for ceftriaxone if needed. At this time, oral azithromycin is not recommended in place of oral doxycycline for chlamydial infection in PID.

Optimal Plan

4. a. *What treatment regimen (drug, dosage form, dose, schedule, and duration) is appropriate for these patients?*

- Frankie should be treated with a multidrug combination such as: 1) cefixime 400 mg po × 1 dose; 2) metronidazole 2 g po × 1 dose; 3) azithromycin 1 g po × 1 dose; and 4) acyclovir 800 mg po BID × 5 days. Single-dose regimens were chosen for gonococcal, trichomonal, and chlamydial infection due to concerns of non-adherence with longer antibiotic courses such as doxycycline × 7 days for *Chlamydia* or metronidazole × 7 days for trichomoniasis. Ibuprofen 400 to 600 mg or acetaminophen 650 to 1000 mg po QID may be given as needed for patient comfort. Acetaminophen with codeine 30 mg may be required for the intense discomfort of genital herpes in some patients. Appropriate attention to cleanliness, with sitz baths for genital herpes, should be encouraged.
- Jenny should be hospitalized for treatment because she has nausea and vomiting precluding oral therapy and has evidence of moderate-to-severe infection. The combination of parenteral cefotetan and doxycycline in the dosage regimens described above provides appropriate antibacterial activity against *Neisseria gonorrheae, Chlamydia trachomatis,* anaerobes, and *E. coli.* She should also begin metronidazole 500 mg po BID × 7 days for trichomoniasis, because single-dose therapy may provoke emesis in her case. Acetaminophen 650 mg po Q 4 H for fever and pain may be administered; more severe pain episodes may require other analgesic strategies such as parenteral ketorolac or opioids.

b. *What alternatives would be appropriate if the initial therapy cannot be used?*

- For Frankie, oral ofloxacin in a single 400 mg dose could be used for gonococcal urethritis if he had a cephalosporin or serious penicillin allergy. Although doxycycline can be used in place of azithromycin, the multiday treatment course required may result in poor compliance and treatment failure in this particular patient.
- For a hospitalized patient such as Jenny, gentamicin 110 mg IV loading dose and 75 mg Q 8 H plus clindamycin 900 mg Q 6 H is an appropriate alternative, to be followed by oral doxycycline for a total of 14 days. Other antibiotic regimens have been included as alternatives in the 1998 CDC guidelines.[3] Agents such as ofloxacin or ciprofloxacin possess broader antibacterial spectrum, higher cost, and a need for a greater total number of drugs for treatment without obvious advantages, except in patients with drug allergies or renal dysfunction. If Jenny had been pregnant, alternative regimens to avoid potentially teratogenic medications could have been recommended.

Outcome Evaluation

5. a. *What clinical and laboratory parameters are necessary to evaluate the therapy for achievement of the desired outcome and to detect or prevent adverse effects?*

- Frankie should have improvement and eventual resolution of the urethral discharge and dysuria within several days of treatment. Single-dose therapy was chosen to ensure compliance in this patient; careful observation for severe nausea and emesis is appropriate, as repeated doses or changes in therapy may be required. Signs of drug hypersensitivity, including drug rashes and anaphylaxis, sun sensitivity, or diarrhea may occur but should be self-limiting due to single-dose use. Metronidazole may produce dizziness and acute disulfiram-like reactions with concurrent ethanol use or within a day of treatment. As acyclovir reduces the severity and duration of recurrent herpes episodes, the blisters may increase in number or progress to ulcers before slowly improving over days to weeks. Oral acyclovir is generally well tolerated, with mild nausea the most likely toxicity in this patient.
- Jenny should be monitored for improvement in symptoms during the first 2 to 3 days of treatment by evaluating temperature, heart rate, blood pressure, abdominal pain, and vaginal discharge. Repeat pelvic examination is indicated if there is minimal or no improvement in pain. Because systemic symptoms may resolve quickly, improvement in pelvic symptoms and findings are important parameters of treatment effects. Adverse effects may include diarrhea, nausea, drug hypersensitivity reactions, and phlebitis.

b. *What changes, if any, in antibacterial therapy are required?*

- No changes are required for either patient, as each received appropriate presumptive therapy for both gonococcal and chlamydial infections. The expected delay in receiving definitive results illustrates the need for broad spectrum antibacterial agents, particularly for Frankie who may be unwilling or unavailable to return for treatment.

Patient Counseling

6. *What information should be provided to Frankie to enhance compliance, ensure success of therapy, and minimize adverse effects?*

- You have several infections that are spread through sexual intercourse, which could have been spread to your partners. It is important that you contact anyone that you had sex with in the last 4 weeks and have them come to our clinic or their doctor to be checked and treated, whether they have any problems or symptoms or not, since some infections are silent. The only reliable way to avoid getting some of these infections is to use condoms whenever you have sex, no matter when or with whom.

- It is possible to spread one infection called trichomoniasis (or "trich") even with use of a condom, so it is important to avoid sex and sexual contact if you or a partner may have this infection.
- Also, you can spread herpes infections to your partners without a condom, because this infection is never cured. Avoid having sex for at least a week after all the blisters have healed so you do not infect anyone else. Herpes infections can come back and drugs can help shorten the illness if taken within the first day of symptoms. Call us or come in to be seen as soon as possible if you notice any tingling or blisters.
- Do not drink beer, wine, or any alcohol within 2 days of taking the medicine Flagyl, or you may have headaches, an upset stomach, or vomiting. If you notice a skin rash, fever, difficulty breathing, or any other problems, call the clinic or me as soon as possible, since any of these medications can rarely cause an allergy.
- Return to the clinic if you notice any pain with urinating, if the discharge does not stop, or if it comes back after initially going away.

References

1. Lappa S, Moscicki A. The pediatrician and the sexually active adolescent: A primer for sexually transmitted diseases. Pediatr Clin North Am 1997;44:1405–1445.
2. Carson DS, Wild SW. Pelvic inflammatory disease. US Pharmacist 1997;22:187–196.
3. Centers for Disease Control and Prevention. 1998 Guidelines for Treatment of Sexually Transmitted Diseases. MMWR 1998;47(No. RR-1):1–116. http://www.cdc.gov/diseases/diseases.html

105 LOWER URINARY TRACT INFECTION

▶ **Yearning and Burning** (Level I)

Christine A. Lesch, PharmD
Keith A. Rodvold, PharmD, FCCP, BCPS

A 21-year-old woman presents to an outpatient clinic with complaints of urgency, frequency, and dysuria for 24 hours. She had one bladder infection 6 months ago. She denies fever, vomiting, back pain, or being sexually active. Urinalysis reveals the presence of bacteriuria and pyuria. A presumptive diagnosis of lower urinary tract infection (UTI) is made. A urine culture is not necessary in this patient. Factors to be considered in choosing an antimicrobial regimen include activity against the most likely infecting organisms, dosing frequency and duration, urinary antibiotic concentrations achieved, effect on fecal and vaginal flora, clinical response rates, adverse-effect profile, patient allergies, presence or absence of pregnancy, compliance rates, and cost. Short-course (3-day) therapy with trimethoprim-sulfamethoxazole (TMP-SMX) double-strength tablets is one of the regimens that possesses favorable characteristics for the treatment of uncomplicated lower UTIs. However, because she has an allergy to TMP-SMX, a 3-day regimen of a fluoroquinolone is a reasonable alternative.

▶ **Questions**

Problem Identification

1. a. *What clinical and laboratory features are consistent with the diagnosis of an acute uncomplicated lower UTI (cystitis) in this patient?*

   - *Clinical features.* Dysuria, frequency, and urgency.
   - *Laboratory features.* Pyuria, bacteriuria.
   - The absence of fever, flank pain, and hematuria suggests the presence of a lower UTI (i.e., cystitis) rather than an upper UTI (pyelonephritis).
   - The patient had a UTI 6 months ago. This is probably a reinfection rather than a relapse of the same infection, since the prior infection was 6 months earlier.

   b. *How does one differentiate cystitis from urethritis (caused by* Chlamydia trachomatis, Neisseria gonorrhoeae, *or herpes simplex virus) or vaginitis (due to* Candida *or* Trichomonas *species)?*

   - Urethritis is more common in women who have had a new sex partner in the previous few weeks, her sex partner complained of urethral symptoms, there is a past history of an STD, symptoms developed gradually over the prior few weeks, and she has had other vaginal symptoms such as discharge or odor.
   - Symptoms of vaginitis include vaginal discharge or odor, pruritus, dyspareunia (painful coitus), and external dysuria, with no increased frequency or urgency.[1]

   c. *Should a urine culture be obtained in this patient experiencing her second episode of cystitis?*

   - The presence of pyuria, bacteriuria, and clinical symptoms confirm the diagnosis of an uncomplicated UTI, and empiric anti-infective therapy can be selected based on this information alone. A culture and sensitivity test should be ordered if the patient remains symptomatic after 72 hours of empiric therapy.
   - A urine culture is necessary in a patient with symptoms suggestive of pyelonephritis, such as fever, flank pain, nausea, and vomiting, or if this episode is a relapse (a reinfection within 2 weeks of completing an appropriate regimen).
   - A urine culture is most useful before therapy is started in cases where the medical history, physical examination, and urinalysis cannot differentiate among cystitis, urethritis, and vaginitis. A standard urinalysis or a leukocyte esterase test (for detecting pyuria) are rapid, reliable, and inexpensive methods for determining infection in a symptomatic patient.[2]

   d. *What are the most likely pathogens and frequency of occurrence causing this patient's infection?*

   - *Escherichia coli* (85%)
   - *Staphylococcus saprophyticus* (5% to 15%)
   - Other Enterobacteriaceae (e.g., *Proteus mirabilis, Klebsiella* species, *Pseudomonas aeruginosa*) (5% to 10%)

e. *What factors can increase the risk of developing a UTI?*

- Structural abnormalities of the urinary tract (e.g., obstruction due to prostatic hyperplasia, urethral strictures, calculi, and tumors).
- Neurologic malfunction causing incomplete bladder emptying (e.g., stroke, diabetes, spinal cord injuries).
- Urinary catheterization or mechanical instrumentation.
- Pregnancy.
- Female gender.
- Increased sexual activity.
- Diaphragm and/or spermicide use.

f. *Create a list of this patient's drug-related problems.*

- Acute cystitis requiring antimicrobial therapy.
- Allergy to trimethoprim-sulfamethoxazole, which will impact on the treatment regimen selected.
- Bulimia, which may require drug therapy in the future.

g. *Since this is her second episode of an uncomplicated UTI, should she receive prophylactic antibiotics to prevent further episodes?*

- If she had a history of recurrent episodes of uncomplicated UTIs > 2 times/year, then she may benefit from patient-administered self-treatment. Single-dose therapy was demonstrated to be effective in a crossover study of 38 women for 12 months.[3] Patients with > 3 infections/year should be considered for continuous, low-dose antimicrobial prophylaxis or postcoital prophylaxis. Since this is only the second episode she has ever had, giving prophylaxis or self-administered treatment is premature.[2]

Desired Outcome

2. *What are the goals of pharmacotherapy in this case?*

- Achieving clinical resolution of symptoms, rather than microbiologic response, is the most important outcome measure, since a urine culture is not necessary in this patient.
- Using the most effective and least expensive anti-infective therapy.
- Minimizing the incidence of adverse events.
- Avoiding relapse by educating the patient about the importance of adherence to the therapy.
- Avoiding reinfection by educating the patient about the role of risk factors.

Therapeutic Alternatives

3. a. *What are the desirable characteristics of an anti-infective agent selected for the treatment of this uncomplicated UTI?*

- A spectrum of antimicrobial activity that will cover the most common uropathogens.
- Minimal resistance to the anti-infective by the common uropathogens.
- A prolonged duration of adequate urinary levels.
- QD or Q 12 H dosing frequency.
- Minimal adverse drug reactions.
- Activity against *E. coli* without disturbing normal vaginal or fecal flora such as *Lactobacillus*.
- Low cost.
- Oral route of administration.

b. *What feasible pharmacotherapeutic alternatives are available for empiric first-line and second-line treatment of an uncomplicated UTI?*

Three-day Regimens

- *Trimethoprim-sulfamethoxazole* (TMP-SMX) double-strength, 1 tablet po Q 12 H, is frequently a regimen of choice due to effectiveness against common UTI pathogens, a low adverse-event rate, and low cost. It results in eradication rates of 78% to 83%, which is equivalent to > five-day regimens with fewer adverse effects.[4]
- *Fluoroquinolones* are not used as first-line agents due to high cost and concern for resistance. However, development of resistance may be of negligible concern with 3-day regimens. Eradication rates range between 81% to 94%. Three-day regimens that have been used include:
  - ✓ *Ciprofloxacin* 250 mg po Q 12 H
  - ✓ *Enoxacin* 400 mg po Q 12 H
  - ✓ *Levofloxacin* 250 mg po QD
  - ✓ *Lomefloxacin* 400 mg po QD
  - ✓ *Norfloxacin* 400 mg po Q 12 H
  - ✓ *Ofloxacin* 200 mg po Q 12 H
  - ✓ *Trovafloxacin* 100 mg po QD
  - ✓ *Sparfloxacin* 400 mg × 1 day, then 200 mg po QD × 2 days
- *Trimethoprim* 100 mg po Q 12 H is inexpensive, but there is increasing resistance among outpatient strains (range 5% to 60%).
- *Nitrofurantoin macrocrystals* 100 mg po Q 12 H is also inexpensive, but some studies have shown that 3-day regimens are not as effective as 7-day regimens.
- *Amoxicillin* 500 mg po Q 8 H is inexpensive but produces cure rates lower than with TMP-SMX. Eradication rates are in the range of 50% to 85%. Beta-lactam antimicrobials have a shorter duration of high concentrations in urine. In addition, they are ineffective in eradicating *E. coli* in the vaginal and fecal reservoirs.
- *Amoxicillin/clavulanate* 500 mg po Q 8 H or 875 mg po Q 12 H is an expensive agent that has the same limitations noted for amoxicillin. It also has a higher incidence of GI adverse effects (e.g., diarrhea).
- *Cefixime* 400 mg po QD is moderately expensive and has poor *in vitro* activity against staphylococci, which raises concerns for its use against *S. saprophyticus*. Overall eradication rates are about 77%.

Seven-day Regimens

- Seven-day regimens are recommended for male patients, patients with diabetes mellitus, patients with symptoms for > 7 days, childhood urinary tract infections, cases involving recent antimicrobial use, and patients more than 65 years of age.
- *TMP-SMX DS* 1 tablet po Q 12 H provides eradication rates of 87% to 96%. It is associated with more frequent adverse effects than the 3-day regimen.
- *Nitrofurantoin macrocrystals* 100 mg po Q 12 H may not be effective against *Proteus* species. Some studies show that 3-day regimens are not as effective as 7-day regimens.
- *Cefpodoxime proxetil* 100 mg po Q 12 H has been shown to be as

effective as 7-day regimens of amoxicillin and cefaclor. There are no studies comparing it to TMP-SMX or fluoroquinolones.
- *Sulfisoxazole* 1 g po Q 6 H is inexpensive, but sulfonamides alone have generally been replaced by more active agents because of resistance formation.
- *Cephalosporins (cephalexin, cephradine, cefaclor, cefadroxil, cefuroxime axetil, and cefixime)* offer no advantages over other classes and are more expensive. They may be useful in cases resistant to amoxicillin or TMP-SMX.
- Other agents included under the three-day regimens have also been used in 7-day regimens (refer to Table 106-3 in textbook Chapter 106 for complete information).

One-day Regimens
- *TMP-SMX DS* 1 or 2 tablets has been shown to produce eradication rates of 55% to 100% but is generally considered to be inferior to the 3-day regimen.
- *Amoxicillin* 3 g po has demonstrated eradication rates of 50% to 91%, but it has higher relapse rates than TMP-SMX.
- *Sulfisoxazole* 2 g po has shown early eradication rates of 94%, but no data exist regarding relapse rates.
- *Fosfomycin tromethamine* 3 g (as granules dissolved in 4 ounces of water) is indicated for single-dose treatment of acute cystitis due to susceptible strains of *E. coli* and *Enterococcus faecalis*.

c. *Which non-pharmacologic therapies may be useful in treating uncomplicated UTIs?*

Conflicting evidence exists that certain behaviors may decrease the risk of UTI:[2]
- Increasing fluid intake causes more frequent micturition and may cause a "flushing out" of bacteria from the bladder and urethra.
- Do not ignore the urge to void; retaining urine may increase the risk of UTI.
- Postcoital urination may "flush out" transient bacteria because sexual activity may promote movement of vaginal and fecal flora into the urethra.
- Drinking cranberry juice may cause inhibition of bacterial adherence because of a substance in the juice.
- Avoiding use of a diaphragm with spermicide for contraception may decrease colonization of the vagina with uropathogens.

Optimal Plan

4. *What drug, dosage form, dose, schedule, and duration of therapy are best for this patient?*

- As shown in Table 106-3 in textbook Chapter 106, and in question 3.b., a variety of regimens would provide effective therapy for this patient. Patient compliance, adverse effects, and cost should also be considered.
- Effective 3-day regimens include TMP-SMX and fluoroquinolones such as norfloxacin, ciprofloxacin, and ofloxacin. However, current literature favors TMP-SMX because of its relative efficacy, safety, and cost.[5]
- Although it is highly effective, TMP-SMX is not a feasible choice for this patient due to her history of rash. Therefore, a 3-day regimen of a fluoroquinolone, cefpodoxime, or cefixime would be reasonable alternatives.[1] Although there are no clinical studies using cefpodoxime in a 3-day regimen, it may be considered because of its longer half-life compared to other β-lactams and its broad spectrum of activity.[1]
- Three-day regimens of ampicillin, amoxicillin, and first-generation cephalosporins are not recommended first-line empiric agents because higher cure rates have been seen with TMP-SMX and trimethoprim alone.
- Nitrofurantoin is another alternative, but the duration of therapy should be for a minimum of 7 days because contradictory evidence exists with a 3-day regimen.
- One-day regimens have been shown to be less efficacious than 3-day regimens. It appears that TMP-SMX is the most efficacious single-dose therapy.[4] These regimens may be a feasible option for initial therapy of acute uncomplicated cystitis in non-compliant women.

Outcome Evaluation

5. *What clinical and laboratory parameters are necessary to evaluate the therapy for achievement of the desired therapeutic outcome and to detect or prevent adverse effects?*

Outcome Parameters
- Resolution of clinical symptoms by 72 hours is a reasonable goal. The patient should be counseled to contact the clinic if symptoms continue or recur. A follow-up call after completion of therapy is advised to ensure that symptoms have not recurred.
- A follow-up urine culture is not necessary unless a relapse has occurred.

Adverse Effect Parameters
- Side effects commonly associated with fluoroquinolones include rash, vomiting, nausea, diarrhea, and headache.

Patient Counseling

6. *What information should be provided to the patient to enhance compliance, ensure successful therapy, and minimize adverse effects?*

Fluoroquinolones
- Take this medication for the full duration of therapy to ensure eradication of the bacteria.
- Take each dose with a full 8-ounce glass of water, and continue to drink at least 8 × 8-ounce glasses of water for the duration of therapy.
- The most common side effects of this medicine include rash, headache, nausea, vomiting, and diarrhea.
- Take this medication on an empty stomach, 1 hour before or 2 hours after meals.
- Avoid taking this medicine with antacids, calcium, iron, zinc, or multivitamins. If you take these medicines, take them either 4 hours before or 2 hours after the antibiotic.

References

1. Hooton TM, Stamm WE. Diagnosis and treatment of uncomplicated urinary tract infections. Infect Dis Clin North Am 1997;11:551–581.
2. Stapleton A, Stamm WE. Prevention of urinary tract infection. Infect Dis Clin North Am 1997;11:719–733.
3. Wong ES, McKevitt M, Running K, et al. Management of recurrent urinary tract infections with patient-administered single-dose therapy. Ann Intern Med 1985; 102:302–307.

4. Norrby SR. Short-term treatment of uncomplicated lower urinary tract infections in women. Rev Infect Dis 1990;12:458–467.
5. Hooton TM, Winter C, Tiu F, et al. Randomized comparative trial and cost analysis of 3-day antimicrobial regimens for treatment of acute cystitis in women. JAMA 1995;273:41–45.

106 ACUTE PYELONEPHRITIS

▶ The Stone Glazer (Level III)

Margaret E. McGuinness, PharmD

A 75-year-old man with small cell cancer of the prostate develops fatigue, vomiting, back pain, and chills 2 weeks after receiving combination antineoplastic therapy. Clinical and laboratory evaluation reveals that the patient has a urinary tract infection, with systemic signs and symptoms suggesting pyelonephritis and perhaps bacteremia. Students are asked to design an appropriate empiric antimicrobial regimen that takes into consideration the patient's weakened immune system. In this case, monotherapy with a third-generation cephalosporin, extended-spectrum penicillin, or aminoglycoside would provide effective initial therapy. When urine and blood cultures are subsequently reported as positive, students are asked how they would modify the original regimen and to create a plan for completing therapy on an outpatient basis. This patient has a number of other diseases and drug-related problems that must be addressed for complete management of the patient.

▶ Questions

Problem Identification

1. a. *Create a list of the patient's drug-related problems.*

   - *Untreated indication.* The patient has a UTI, with systemic signs and symptoms suggesting that he has pyelonephritis and is also bacteremic or septic.
   - *Untreated indication.* Volume depletion; the patient has been vomiting, has not eaten in > 24 hours, and appears dry on PE and by laboratory result (increased BUN, serum creatinine, and BUN-to-creatinine ratio 19:1).
   - *Untreated indication.* The patient had an MI 3 years ago but is not on recommended β-blocker therapy, which has been shown to reduce mortality and reinfarction after MI.
   - *Untreated indication.* Patient is stated to be receiving dietary management of type 2 DM. However, on admission, he has hyperglycemia and glycosuria. These may be elevated because of infection and vomiting with no intake in the last 24 hours. Uncontrolled diabetes is a risk factor for developing UTIs. He should be screened with an HbA_{1c} to evaluate long-term diabetes control, provided with dietary consultation, and drug therapy considered if the HbA_{1c} is elevated.
   - *Untreated indication.* Hypokalemia; this may have resulted from low intake and/or wasting in the urine. Check the serum magnesium, as he may be wasting this also, which will exacerbate potassium loss.
   - *Drug therapy without indication.* Patient is receiving quinine sulfate, presumably for nocturnal cramps, but this condition is not included in the PMH. Furthermore, there are no convincing clinical data that support quinine use as effective treatment or prophylaxis for nocturnal leg cramps.
   - *Possible adverse effects.*
     - ✓ The patient has osteoarthritis for which he takes salsalate and Tylenol #3 (acetaminophen/codeine). He is complaining of nausea, vomiting, anorexia, and back pain. It is possible that he may have consumed Tylenol #3 for relief of the fever and pain associated with his current condition. Obtain a history of the use of Tylenol #3 and other acetaminophen-containing preparations. Acetaminophen toxicity can present with anorexia, vomiting, nausea, and abdominal pain. The total daily dose of acetaminophen should not exceed 4 g.
     - ✓ Reconsider the continued use of codeine. Although the patient states he has no constipation, he does take Metamucil and Senokot S. If codeine is not necessary to control pain, acetaminophen alone is a preferred therapy.
     - ✓ There is no evidence that salsalate or other NSAIDs are superior to acetaminophen for the treatment of osteoarthritis pain. If salsalate exacerbates his GERD symptoms, it should be discontinued and the osteoarthritis managed with acetaminophen alone. Because carboplatin causes significant thrombocytopenia, it is advisable to avoid use of NSAIDs during chemotherapy. However, salsalate has less effect on platelet aggregation than other NSAIDs.

   b. *What information (signs, symptoms, laboratory tests) indicates the presence and severity of pyelonephritis in this patient?*

   Signs
   - Fever; reported to appear ill during the physical examination; abdominal tenderness on deep inspiration with mild rebound tenderness; costovertebral angle (CVA) tenderness; and seems confused at times. The patient does not have tachycardia and has adequate blood pressure. However, he has a pacemaker and may not be able to mount a significant increase in heart rate. The normalcy of vital signs does not exclude the possibility of pyelonephritis or bacteremia.

   Symptoms
   - Chills, dysuria, back pain, anorexia, nausea, vomiting, and weakness.

Laboratory Tests

- The urine is cloudy, bloody, and contains a significant number of white cells and bacteria. The urine is also very concentrated (high specific gravity) and is foul-smelling. The positive nitrite and leukoesterase tests indicate the presence of gram-negative organisms. Pyelonephritis and lower UTI are the two most common causes of hematuria.
- The abdominal CT scan demonstrated concentration of the contrast material within the kidney in a patchy manner, which suggests areas of inflammation with decreased dye clearance. This is a common finding in pyelonephritis.

c. *List any potential contributing factors, including drug therapy, that may have predisposed this patient to developing pyelonephritis.*

- Although he has an appropriate increase in WBC count for an infection, his overall immune status is compromised after chemotherapy, and he is susceptible to infection.
- Potential urinary retention from obstruction of the urethra by the cancer could also increase likelihood of infection.
- Kidney stone formation can occur with high-dose salicylates, and stones are a risk factor for UTI. The patient takes salsalate and has had back pain and pain on urination, so salsalate could be a contributing factor. This is not likely, given the length of treatment with salsalate and the fact that this is his first UTI.
- Volume depletion may increase the likelihood of stone formation, and he is volume depleted.

d. *What additional information is needed to fully assess the patient?*

- The urine and blood should be cultured prior to starting empiric antimicrobial therapy. The patient should be recultured for fever > 38.0°C or BP < 80/50 mm Hg. The culture results will help to elucidate the organism(s) involved and determine if the patient is systemically infected (i.e., bacteremic). If the organisms in the blood and urine are not the same, a source of infection other than the kidney should be investigated.
- The antimicrobial sensitivities of any organisms cultured from the patient should be obtained.[1] If the patient is indeed bacteremic, minimum bactericidal concentrations (MBCs) may be helpful to ensure that adequate therapy is being used. MBCs are not usually required to treat pyelonephritis because most antimicrobials are excreted renally in an active form, providing adequate bactericidal concentrations.

Desired Outcome

2. *What are the goals of pharmacotherapy in this patient?*

- Treat the infection to ensure elimination of organism(s).
- Resolve the patient's symptoms related to infection and other causes.
- Provide nutritional, fluid volume, and electrolyte support until the patient is able to maintain these on his own with a normal diet.
- Improve and maintain blood glucose concentrations within the target range for diabetic patients.
- Assess the patient for the presence of complications of diabetes such as nephropathy, retinopathy, and neuropathy. Pharmacotherapy should be considered if the patient has signs of microalbuminuria.

Therapeutic Alternatives

3. a. *What non-drug therapies might be useful for this patient?*

- A *nutritious diet* aimed at preventing weight loss is appropriate for this patient who is immunocompromised and at risk for poor nutrition. Dietary therapy is also an important component of the management of diabetes mellitus.
- *Fluid intake* may help resolve the painful urination by promoting frequent urination, decreasing urine concentration, and reducing residence time of infected urine in the bladder.
- An *exercise program* to maintain mobility should be considered for the patient's osteoarthritis.

b. *What organisms are commonly associated with pyelonephritis?*

- Most cases of pyelonephritis are caused by gram-negative bacilli, such as *Escherichia coli*, *Klebsiella* spp., and *Proteus* spp. These organisms represent more than 95% of all UTIs, whether hospital or community acquired.
- Patients with risk factors such as nephrostomy tubes, urinary catheters, and ureteral stents are susceptible to infections with gram-positive organisms.
- Immuncompromised patients are susceptible to infection by opportunistic organisms such as *Pseudomonas aeruginosa*.

c. *What feasible pharmacotherapeutic alternatives are available for the empiric treatment of pyelonephritis?*

- The goal of antimicrobial therapy of pyelonephritis is to eliminate the organism by using drugs that are active against the organism (*in vitro*) and that obtain adequate bactericidal concentrations within the kidney. Bactericidal agents are preferred over bacteriostatic agents to ensure elimination of all microorganisms. Beta-lactams (penicillins and cephalosporins) and aminoglycosides achieve excellent concentrations within the kidney and cover most of the likely organisms.
- *Third-generation cephalosporins* are commonly used for empiric therapy of pyelonephritis.[2] Potential drugs and regimens include:
  - ✓ *Ceftriaxone* 1 g IV Q 24 H
  - ✓ *Cefotaxime* 1 g IV Q 8 H
  - ✓ *Ceftazidime* 1 g IV Q 8 H

  In addition to the advantage of once-daily dosing, ceftriaxone is cleared by glomerular filtration and tubular secretion, and very high concentrations are obtained throughout the kidney. It is not necessary to reduce the dose in renal impairment until the estimated creatinine clearance (CL_{cr}) is < 50 mL/min.
- *Second-generation cephalosporins* (e.g., *cefuroxime*) may also be used in some situations.
- *First-generation cephalosporins* (e.g., *cefazolin*) may be chosen in geographic locations where the sensitivity of common organisms to these agents is known to be high (> 90%).
- *Extended-spectrum penicillins* (e.g., *piperacillin* 3 to 4 g IV Q 6 to 8 hours) are commonly used for empiric therapy for pyelonephritis. Ampicillin is no longer recommended for empiric therapy due to the high resistance rates of *E. coli* (about 60%).
- *Aminoglycoside monotherapy* (e.g., *gentamicin* 3 to 5 mg/kg Q 24 H) might also be considered, especially since once-daily dosing is appropriate in many patients. It may be prudent to avoid

aminoglycosides in patients with impaired renal function. Some patients require contrast studies that may further compromise renal function.
- Monotherapy is appropriate for empiric therapy unless there is a high suspicion for *Pseudomonas* spp. or *Enterococcus faecalis*. In cases of *Pseudomonas,* monotherapy may in fact be adequate with ceftazidime or ciprofloxacin because these drugs achieve excellent concentrations within the kidney and urinary tract.
- Double-drug coverage (e.g., vancomycin plus an aminoglycoside) is required for pyelonephritis due to enterococci.
- Drugs with β-lactamase protection should be considered if staphylococcal organisms are suspected or found.
- Drugs suitable for single-daily dosing are cost effective in pyelonephritis, so agents such as aminoglycosides (in immunocompetent patients) or ceftriaxone are frequently used. Such therapy reduces nursing and pharmacy costs and provides the patient with a greater degree of freedom. Selection of agent(s) frequently depends on formulary issues and local antibiotic susceptibility patterns.
- Intravenous therapy has traditionally been used as initial therapy in pyelonephritis because patients are frequently nauseated and/or vomiting. However if patients are not vomiting, certain drugs can be considered for oral therapy (e.g., fluoroquinolones such as ciprofloxacin).[3]
- Patients with uncomplicated pyelonephritis usually begin to respond to drug therapy within 24 hours of the first dose. It is not uncommon for patients to continue to spike temperatures and experience flank pain, chills, and rigors for 24 hours. Thus, it is important not to switch antimicrobial therapy within the first 24 hours. It is preferable to await culture results prior to adjusting therapy. If urine cultures are taken prior to initiating antimicrobial therapy, the yield of positive cultures is high and one is able to adjust therapy once these results are known.
- Doses of all antibiotics should be adjusted appropriately according to the degree of renal impairment.

Optimal Plan

4. Outline an antimicrobial regimen that will provide appropriate empiric therapy for pyelonephritis in this patient.

- The patient is 2 weeks past his last chemotherapy cycle, and the WBC count indicates that he is not neutropenic, so it is unlikely that *Pseudomonas* is a pathogen. Broad-spectrum empiric antimicrobial therapy is appropriate to cover the likely organisms (e.g., *E. coli, Klebsiella, Proteus*). Gram-positive organisms are unlikely to be a concern.
- In this elderly man with slight impairment of renal function who is potentially immunocompromised, a third-generation cephalosporin such as ceftriaxone 1 g IV Q 24 hours could be selected. Unless an institution is known to have problems of organism resistance, ceftriaxone is an excellent choice for empiric therapy for the reasons discussed above.
- Other potential choices in this patient include another third-generation cephalosporin or a broad-spectrum penicillin. The primary disadvantage of such therapy over ceftriaxone is the need for multiple daily doses.
- Single daily dosing of an aminoglycoside could also be considered. In this patient, a 12-hour post-dose level is imperative to assess the patient's clearance. With an estimated CL_{cr} of about 40 mL/min, the gentamicin clearance would be about 0.03 L/kg/hour with a half-life of 6 to 8 hours. Based on population pharmacokinetic parameters with standard once daily dosing of gentamicin or tobramycin at 3 to 5 mg/kg every 24 hours, the peak level would be 15 mg/L, the expected level at 12 hours would be about 3 to 4 mg/L, and the level at 24 hours would be about 1 mg/L. If the patient demonstrates low clearance, a change to a Q 36 H or Q 48 H regimen may be necessary.
- Trimethoprim-sulfamethoxazole is not a suitable alternative, even though it has good penetration into the kidney. It is a bacteriostatic combination, and the cost of IV therapy is much greater than oral therapy. Depending on culture results, this might be an acceptable oral alternative for definitive therapy. Trimethoprim-sulfamethoxazole is best avoided in patients with impaired renal function.
- The initial empiric therapy should be given until culture results are known, at which time more organism-specific therapy may be implemented. IV therapy should be continued for at least 24 hours after the patient is afebrile. If the patient is also found to be bacteremic, the current recommendation is 7 to 10 days of IV therapy followed by oral therapy for a total antibiotic course of 10 to 14 days.

Outcome Evaluation

5. a. What clinical and laboratory parameters are necessary to evaluate the antibiotic therapy for achievement of the desired therapeutic outcomes and to detect or prevent adverse effects?

Microbiologic Monitoring of Efficacy
- Empiric therapy should be adjusted on the basis of urine and blood culture results that are usually available within 72 hours. Ideally, adjustments are made based on both the organism and its sensitivity patterns. Formulary medications, dose adjustments for renal insufficiency, and total treatment costs (e.g., drug cost, administration frequency) should also be considered. If the patient is responding to therapy, it may be possible to switch to oral therapy at that time.
- Some clinicians recommend follow-up blood cultures every 24 to 48 hours until negative if the patient is found to be bacteremic. Repeat culturing aids in judging how long to continue therapy as well as patient response. If the patient continues to be bacteremic, an additional source of infection should be sought, and the possibility of endocarditis or an abscess that continues to seed the blood should be considered. If the organism in the blood and urine are different, an alternative source of bacteremia also must be sought. Follow-up urine cultures may be taken during therapy and several days after completion of the antibiotic course to ensure eradication of organisms.

Laboratory Monitoring
- Serum chemistries and hematologic parameters should be monitored at least every other day. This is of particular importance in this patient who had hyperglycemia, hypokalemia, and elevated BUN and creatinine levels. He also had an elevated WBC count with a significant left shift. The WBC count should drop as antibiotic therapy is commenced; a rising count suggests a secondary infection, inappropriate antibiotic selection, or an adverse drug reaction.
- If an aminoglycoside is chosen, it is important to check renal function tests for nephrotoxicity and to ensure that dose adjustments are made if necessary.

- A repeat urinalysis should be performed within 24 to 48 hours to assess resolution of microscopic hematuria and bacteriuria. Observation of the patient's voided urine can be used to identify the presence of gross hematuria.

Adverse Reaction Monitoring

- Daily observance of dermatologic reactions to antibiotics and every-other-day assessment of the WBC count is recommended. The presence of fevers and/or chills could indicate allergy and are part of daily monitoring of antibiotic therapy.
- Because of the patient's penicillin allergy, monitor for cross-sensitivity reactions if a cephalosporin is chosen to treat the patient. If a cross-reaction occurs, it will manifest early in the course of therapy, probably during or shortly after the first dose.

b. *What recommendations, if any, do you have for changes in the initial drug regimen?*

- *E. coli* grew from both blood and urine and have the same sensitivities, suggesting that the organism is the same one. The clinician should switch to a bactericidal drug with the narrowest spectrum that achieves good renal and urinary concentrations of active drug.
- Ampicillin is not a good choice because of the patient's penicillin allergy. Because the reaction was manifested as a rash, an IV first-generation cephalosporin (e.g., cefazolin) is a reasonable choice. It can be dosed 2 to 3 times a day depending on renal function and can subsequently be switched to an oral first-generation cephalosporin (e.g., cephradine, cephalexin). Because the patient is progressing well after more than 3 days of IV therapy, changing to an oral agent could be considered at this time. Urinalysis indicates that the urine is now sterile, and the patient's WBC count and other laboratory indices have improved considerably (see Casebook Table 106–1).
- Because he was bacteremic, the patient should complete a 10- to 14-day course of antibiotics. The presence of bacteremia may warrant continued IV therapy until subsequent blood cultures are negative.
- In summary, it would be appropriate to switch to cefazolin 1 g IV Q 12 H based on his calculated CL_{cr} of 47 mL/min. For a CL_{cr} between 35 and 54 mL/min, the recommended dose for severe infections is 0.5 to 1 g Q 8 to 12 H. Cefazolin therapy could be continued until day 6 or 7 when, if blood cultures from day 2 are negative, oral therapy with cephradine or cephalexin 500 mg Q 6 H could be initiated for a total antibiotic course of 10 to 14 days.

Patient Counseling

6. *What information should be provided to the patient upon discharge to enhance adherence, ensure successful therapy, and minimize adverse effects?*

Cephradine or Cephalexin

- This medicine is effective against the bacteria found in your blood and urine and can be taken by mouth until you finish a total of 14 days of antibiotic treatment. The course will last for another 7 days because you have already been on antibiotics for 7 days in the hospital.
- Take 500 mg (1 capsule) 4 times a day about 6 hours apart until the full course has been taken.
- This medicine can be taken either with food or between meals. Take each dose with a full 8-ounce glass of water.
- Possible side effects include upset stomach and diarrhea. Contact your physician if these become severe. Also contact your doctor if a rash occurs while taking this medication or for 1 to 2 weeks afterward.
- Because you have recently had chemotherapy and your immune system is weakened, antibiotics may increase your risk of developing a fungal infection ("thrush") in the mouth or throat. Contact your doctor if you notice white patches in your mouth and/or a sore throat. Brush your teeth thoroughly, taking particular care around the gum lines, on the top of your mouth, and under your tongue.
- Some signs of a recurring infection include back pain, abdominal pain, problems with urination, fever, and chills. We will check your blood counts and obtain another urine culture after you finish taking the medication.
- It is important for you to control your blood sugar by checking your capillary blood glucose levels 4 times a day over the next 2 weeks. This will help to clear the infection and reduce the chance of subsequent infections.
- If you miss a dose of the medicine, take it as soon as you remember. If you miss more than 1 dose, take the missed doses at equal intervals until the next dose, then continue with the rest of the regimen.

References

1. Jinnah F, Islam MS, Rumi MA, et al. Drug sensitivity pattern of *E. coli* causing urinary tract infection in diabetic and non-diabetic patients. J Int Med Res 1996;24:296–301.
2. Sandberg T, Alesig K, Eilard T, et al. Aminoglycosides do not improve the efficacy of cephalosporins for treatment of acute pyelonephritis in women. Scand J Infect Dis 1997;29:175–179.
3. Bailey RR, Begg EJ, Smith AH, et al. Prospective, randomized controlled study comparing two dosing regimens of gentamicin/oral ciprofloxacin switch therapy for acute pyelonephritis. Clin Nephrol 1996;46:183–186.

107 SYPHILIS

▶ **Hitting Below the Belt** (Level I)

Alex K. McDonald, PharmD
Dennis M. Williams, PharmD, FASHP, FCCP, BCPS

A 28-year-old woman who is 14 weeks pregnant is found to have an RPR titer of 1:16 and a positive FTA-ABS test. She has no clinical signs or symptoms of syphilis. Because the duration of infection is unknown, it should be considered to be more than 1 year. The treatment of choice for this case of late latent syphilis is benzathine penicillin G 2.4 million units IM once weekly for three injections. This regimen effectively prevents disease transmission to the fetus and eradicates fetal infection, if present. There are no satisfactory alternatives to penicillin G for the treatment of syphilis in pregnant patients. Pregnant women who are allergic to penicillin should undergo a desensitization procedure followed by standard treatment with penicillin G using a preparation, dosage, and treatment duration that are appropriate for the patient's stage of disease.

Questions

Problem Identification

1. *What information (signs, symptoms, laboratory values) indicates the presence or stage of syphilis?*

   - The patient has no signs or symptoms of syphilis.
   - Positive serology tests indicating syphilis include the positive RPR titer (1:16) followed by a reactive FTA-ABS test. The RPR (Rapid Plasma Reagin) test is a non-treponemal test used to screen patients and follow therapy. In general, patients with a true-positive non-treponemal test will have a titer >1:8. Another non-treponemal test used during screening is the VDRL (Venereal Disease Research Laboratory). False-positives can occur due to other acute and chronic diseases, and false negatives can occur in early and late syphilis with these non-specific tests. For this reason, patients with clinical symptoms who have a negative nontreponemal test should be retested using a treponemal test.
   - Patients who have reactive RPR or VDRL serology should be tested with a treponemal test to confirm an infection using the FTA-ABS (Fluorescent Treponemal Antibody-Absorption Test) or the MHA-TP (Microhemagglutination-Treponema Pallidum); the latter test is less costly and simpler to perform.
   - The non-treponemal tests are quantitated, and if the infection is treated adequately, the titer will fall. Conversely, the treponemal tests remain positive for life and are therefore of no benefit in monitoring therapy.
   - Seroreactivity with no clinical evidence of disease is definitive for latent syphilis. This patient meets the criteria for latent syphilis of unknown duration. She denies any history of symptoms, so it is not known when she was initially infected.

Desired Outcome

2. *What are the goals of pharmacotherapy in this case?*

   - Eradicate the organism, halt disease progression, and prevent late complications of the disease
   - Eliminate infectivity of the patient
   - Prevent infection of the fetus/offspring

Therapeutic Alternatives

3. a. *What non-drug recommendations should be given to this patient?*

   - The patient should be educated about the transmission of STDs, with suggestions to avoid sexual contact or to use latex condoms during intercourse or intimate contacts.
   - Sexual partners should be evaluated and treated.
   - Very importantly, patients diagnosed with syphilis should be tested for the human immunodeficiency virus (HIV). Risk factors for HIV infection and syphilis are similar. Also, the compromised defense barrier caused by genital lesions increases the potential for HIV transmission. Patients with HIV who are anergic may produce false-negative reactivity to RPR and VDRL tests when infected with *Treponema pallidum*.

   b. *What pharmacotherapeutic alternatives are available for this patient?*

   - *Parenteral penicillin G* is preferred for all stages of syphilis. The preparation(s) used (i.e., benzathine, aqueous procaine, or aqueous crystalline), the dosage, and the duration of treatment depend on the stage and clinical manifestations of the disease.[1]
   - *Parenteral penicillin G* is the only therapy with documented efficacy for syphilis during pregnancy.[1] It is effective for preventing disease transmission to the fetus and for treating established fetal infection. The penicillin regimen given during pregnancy should be dictated by the patient's stage of syphilis.
   - *Benzathine penicillin G* 2.4 million units IM at 1-week intervals for 3 doses is recommended for adults with late latent syphilis or latent syphilis of unknown duration. Because this patient has syphilis of unknown duration, it is assumed to be greater than 1 year; therefore, treatment for late latent syphilis is indicated.
   - *Non-pregnant*, penicillin-allergic patients with latent syphilis may be treated with either:
     - ✓ *Doxycycline* 100 mg po BID or
     - ✓ *Tetracycline* 500 mg po QID

     Treatment should be given for 2 weeks if the duration of infection is known to have been < 1 year; it should be given for 4 weeks if the duration of infection is unknown.
   - *Erythromycin* 500 mg po QID for 14 days is an alternative only in those penicillin-allergic patients with syphilis of < *1 year's duration*.
   - The treatment regimen for HIV-infected patients with syphilis is similar to that of HIV-negative patients.

Optimal Plan

4. a. *What is the recommended treatment (drug, dose, and duration) for this patient?*

   - Benzathine penicillin G 2.4 million units IM at 1-week intervals for 3 doses is the optimal treatment for the reasons described.

   b. *What alternatives would you recommend if this patient were allergic to your first suggestion?*

   - There are no proven alternatives to penicillin for treating pregnant women with syphilis. If a penicillin allergy is present, the CDC recommends a desensitization protocol followed by treatment with penicillin G. The process of desensitization involves serial administration of increasing doses of the drug and takes place in the hospital where resuscitation is readily available (refer to textbook Chapter 81, for a specific desensitization protocol). Doxycycline and tetracycline are generally avoided during pregnancy. Erythromycin should not be used in pregnancy because it does not reliably cure an infected fetus.
   - There is insufficient data to support the use of other drugs including azithromycin and ceftriaxone in this population.

Outcome Evaluation

5. *What clinical and laboratory parameters are necessary to evaluate the therapy for achievement of the desired therapeutic outcome and to detect or prevent adverse effects?*

   - Non-treponemal antibody titers usually correlate with disease activity.

A four-fold change in titer (equivalent to a change of two dilutions, e.g., 1:16 to 1:4) suggests a clinically significant response. RPR titers should be repeated during the third trimester and at delivery.
- Repeat serologic testing in the third trimester and at delivery to determine the adequacy of therapy and the risk to the fetus. The newborn should also undergo serologic testing.

Patient Counseling

6. a. *What information should be provided to the patient to enhance compliance, ensure successful therapy, and minimize adverse effects?*

- It is important for you to receive each of the 3 weekly injections of penicillin to avoid future complications of syphilis.
- Abstain from sexual activity during treatment.
- The intramuscular penicillin injection may cause pain and swelling at the injection site.
- Some patients experience a fever (which may be accompanied by headache, muscle pain, and other symptoms) within 24 hours after receiving therapy for syphilis. Contact your obstetrician if you experience severe symptoms. (*Note to instructors:* In pregnant patients, this reaction may cause fetal distress or induce early labor; therefore, the supervision of an obstetrician may be warranted. However, treatment for syphilis should not be postponed or delayed because of this reaction.)

b. *What information should be provided to the patient to prevent a future sexually transmitted disease?*

- It is important for you to know about prevention measures to prevent sexual transmission of HIV and other sexually transmitted diseases. These strategies include avoiding sexual intercourse with an infected partner, being testing for these diseases (including HIV) before sexual intercourse, and using a new condom for each act of intercourse.
- It is recommended that you receive testing for HIV infection; you are at risk for this infection because you have a sexually transmitted disease.

▶ Follow-up Questions

1. *What are potential explanations for this finding?*

- The mother had an adequate response to treatment for syphilis. Her non-treponemal titer decreased by four-fold. The infant's test was negative. Testing the infant's blood is preferred over testing the cord blood, which may be contaminated with the mother's blood.

2. *What further assessment and treatment should be considered for the patient?*

- No additional tests are required for the mother. If the titer had not decreased by four-fold, central nervous system disease would have to be ruled out by a lumbar puncture because the regimen used to treat the patient may not have been adequate for neurosyphilis.

3. *What assessment and treatment should be considered for the infant?*

- Despite the negative serologic test, the infant should be examined for signs of congenital syphilis (i.e., jaundice, hepatosplenomegaly, rhinitis, skin rash, or paralysis of an extremity). In light of a nonreactive RPR, a treponemal test (MHA-TP) is not warranted.

Reference

1. Centers for Disease Control and Prevention. Syphilis. 1998 guidelines for treatment of sexually transmitted diseases. MMWR 1998;47(RR-01):28–49. www.cdc.gov

108 GENITAL HERPES AND CHLAMYDIAL INFECTIONS

▶ Double Trouble (Level II)

Suellyn J. Sorensen, PharmD, BCPS

The development of genital lesions and a vaginal discharge causes a 20-year-old woman to seek treatment at a county STD clinic. Viral cultures reveal the presence of herpes simplex type 2 (HSV2) and rectal and cervical cultures are positive for *Chlamydia trachomatis*. The HSV-2 infection may be treated with acyclovir (400 mg po TID or 200 mg 5 times/day for 7 to 10 days), valacyclovir (1 gram po BID for 7 to 10 days), or famciclovir (250 mg po TID for 7 to 10 days). The recommended treatment for *Chlamydia* is either azithromycin 1 gram po in a single dose or doxycycline 100 mg po BID for 7 days. The case also addresses the issues of treatment for recurrent episodes and use of suppressive therapy.

▶ Questions

Problem Identification

1. a. *Create a list of the patient's drug-related problems.*

- Untreated primary genital HSV2 infection
- Untreated *C. trachomatis* infection
- Untreated vaginal candidiasis
- Possible failure of oral contraceptive (LMP 6 weeks ago)
- Potential drug-interaction between ciprofloxacin and Loestrin
- Potential drug-interaction between multivitamin with iron and ciprofloxacin
- Inappropriate antimicrobial for prophylaxis of recurrent urinary tract infections
- Untreated sexual partners

b. *What subjective and objective clinical data are consistent with a primary genital herpes infection?*

- *Symptoms.* Headache, muscle aches.
- *Signs.* Extensive shallow, small, painful vesicular lesions over her vulva and labia; inguinal adenopathy; fever.
- Other data associated with either primary, first-episode non-primary, or recurrent herpes genitalis infection are painful vesicular lesions; history of recent sexual activity (anal and vaginal intercourse); and HSV2 isolated on viral culture and DFA monoclonal stain.

c. *Could any of the patient's problems have been caused by drug therapy?*

- Oral contraceptives predispose women to vaginal candidiasis, especially high-dose estrogen products. However, Loestrin is a low-dose estrogen contraceptive.
- Women taking broad-spectrum antimicrobials are at increased risk of *C. albicans* overgrowth because of suppression of the normal vaginal flora, including lactobacillus, which are protective against *C. albicans*.
- Oral contraceptive failure may be caused by the administration of antibiotics. Ciprofloxacin may reduce the population of intestinal bacteria, interrupting the enterohepatic circulation of the estrogen, which results in a decreased concentration of circulating estrogen. This drug interaction is most commonly associated with penicillins and tetracyclines, but contraceptive failures have been reported with other antibiotics. Use of low-dose estrogen contraceptives such as Loestrin increases the possibility of failure when administered with antibiotics.

Desired Outcome

2. *What are the goals of pharmacotherapy in this case?*

- The goals for herpes simplex infection are to control the signs and symptoms, decrease viral shedding, prevent recurrences, prevent transmission to sexual partners, prevent complications associated with the spread to extragenital sites, prevent transmission during pregnancy, minimize adverse effects from drug therapy, and promote adherence with the drug regimen selected.
- The goals of therapy for *Chlamydia* are to eradicate the infection; prevent sequelae such as PID, ectopic pregnancy, and infertility; identify and treat sexual partners; prevent spread to other sexual partners; minimize adverse effects and drug interactions from drug therapy; and promote adherence with the drug regimen selected.
- The goals for vaginal candidiasis are to eradicate the infection, eliminate or reduce the predisposing factors, and decrease signs and symptoms of infection.

Therapeutic Alternatives

3. a. *What non-drug therapies might be useful for this patient?*

- Condoms may act as an effective barrier to viral transmission, although this method does not offer complete protection for the transmission of HSV2. When used properly, condoms provide a high degree of protection against the acquisition and/or transmission of *Chlamydia*. Furthermore, if prophylaxis of recurrent UTIs is indicated, an alternative form of birth control may be necessary.
- Counseling about the natural history of genital herpes, sexual and perinatal transmission, and methods to reduce transmission is an essential component of HSV2 management.

b. *What feasible pharmacotherapeutic alternatives are available for treatment of genital herpes and* Chlamydia?

Genital Herpes Infection

- *Acyclovir* is FDA approved for the treatment of initial genital HSV2 infections. The 1998 CDC guidelines recommend a dosage of 400 mg po TID for 7 to 10 days or 200 mg 5 times/day for 7 to 10 days.[1] Oral acyclovir has demonstrated efficacy in reducing viral shedding, duration of symptoms, and time to healing of first episode genital herpes infections. It is FDA approved for use in immunocompromised patients.
- *Valacyclovir* is FDA approved for the treatment of initial genital HSV2 infections. Valacyclovir is an acyclovir prodrug with enhanced bioavailability compared to acyclovir. This enhanced bioavailability allows for less frequent dosing, which should improve adherence to therapy. The recommended dosage is 1 g po BID for 7 to 10 days.[1] This 10-day regimen for initial infections has equivalent efficacy to acyclovir 200 mg po 5 times/day for 10 days. Valacyclovir is more expensive than acyclovir but comparable in cost to famciclovir for the treatment of initial episode genital herpes.[2] Valacyclovir is not FDA approved for use in immunocompromised patients. Thrombotic thrombocytopenia purpura/hemolytic uremic syndrome (TTP/HUS) was reported in clinical trials in immunocompromised patients receiving 8 g per day and in some cases resulted in death.[3] This syndrome has not been reported in otherwise healthy patients treated with lower doses.
- *Famciclovir* is a pro-drug of penciclovir with enhanced bioavailability compared to acyclovir, allowing for less frequent dosing, which should improve adherence to therapy. Famciclovir is not FDA approved for the treatment of initial genital HSV2 infections. However, it has been studied at various dosing regimens for initial infections and demonstrated equivalent efficacy to acyclovir. The 1998 CDC guidelines recommend a dosage of 250 mg po TID for 7 to 10 days.[1] Famciclovir is not FDA approved for use in immunocompromised patients.
- Topical formulations of acyclovir and penciclovir provide little to no benefit in most patients with initial episode genital herpes. Topical therapy used along with oral therapy does not appear to offer any additional advantage over oral therapy alone.

Chlamydial Infection

- *Azithromycin* 1 g po in a single dose or *doxycycline* 100 mg po BID for 7 days is recommended in the CDC guidelines.[1] The results of clinical trials indicate that these drugs are equally efficacious. These investigations were conducted primarily in populations in which follow-up was encouraged and adherence to a 7-day regimen was good. Doxycycline costs less than azithromycin and has been used extensively for a longer period of time. In populations with poor compliance or minimal follow-up, azithromycin may be more cost-effective because it provides single-dose, directly observed therapy.

- *Erythromycin* base 500 mg po QID for 7 days or *ofloxacin* 300 mg po BID for 7 days are alternative regimens. Erythromycin is less efficacious than either azithromycin or doxycycline, and GI side effects frequently discourage patients from adhering to this regimen. Ofloxacin is similar in efficacy to doxycycline and azithromycin but is more expensive and offers no advantages.
- *Ciprofloxacin* is not reliably effective against chlamydial infections, and this patient became infected despite chronic UTI prophylaxis with this agent.

Optimal Plan

4. *What drug, dosage form, dose, schedule, and duration of therapy are best for treating this patient's genital herpes and chlamydial infections?*

Genital Herpes

- Any of the 4 treatment regimens discussed previously would provide acceptable treatment for most patients. It is important to assess adherence to therapy prior to selecting either acyclovir or valacyclovir.
- Acyclovir 200 mg po 5 times/day for 7 to 10 days is the dosing regimen that is FDA approved for the treatment of genital herpes. However, 400 mg po TID should improve adherence and is recommended in the 1998 CDC STD treatment guidelines based on results from ongoing studies and expert opinions.
- If it appears that a 5 times/day or TID regimen will be difficult for this patient to adhere to, then valacyclovir 1 g po BID for 7 to 10 days may be the most appropriate regimen, even though it is more expensive.
- If the patient indicates that she can adhere to a TID regimen, then acyclovir 400 mg po TID for 7 to 10 days would be the most appropriate treatment regimen because it is the least expensive agent and equally efficacious compared to valacyclovir and famciclovir.
- It is important to determine the results of her pregnancy test prior to treatment because the safety of these drugs during pregnancy has not been established. Although current registry findings do not indicate an increased risk for major birth defects after acyclovir treatment, these case histories represent an insufficient sample to reach a definitive conclusion. Prenatal exposure to valacyclovir and famciclovir is too limited to provide useful information on pregnancy outcomes. Acyclovir and famciclovir are pregnancy category B, and valacyclovir is category C. The 1998 CDC treatment guidelines indicate that the first episode of genital herpes during pregnancy may be treated with oral acyclovir. The benefits of treatment must clearly outweigh the risks to the fetus. If it were at or near term, acyclovir therapy would probably be appropriate. The optimal treatment during early pregnancy (as would be the case in this situation) is less clear.
- If the patient is found to be HIV positive, then acyclovir is probably the most appropriate drug therapy because it is FDA approved for and has been used extensively in this patient population.

Chlamydia

- Appropriate treatment may be given with either azithromycin 1 g po single-dose therapy directly observed in the clinic or doxycycline 100 mg po BID for 7 days.
- If she is found to be pregnant, doxycycline and ofloxacin are contraindicated. The safety and efficacy of azithromycin has not been established in pregnancy, but it is considered an alternative to erythromycin or amoxicillin. If she is treated with erythromycin or amoxicillin she needs a repeat culture 3 weeks after the completion of therapy because neither regimen is highly efficacious and the frequency of side effects with erythromycin might discourage compliance.

Outcome Evaluation

5. *What clinical and laboratory parameters are necessary to evaluate the therapy for achievement of the desired therapeutic outcome and to detect or prevent adverse effects?*

Efficacy of Herpes Treatment

- Resolution of the signs and symptoms of primary herpes simplex infection (crusting of the lesions; disappearance of pain, headache, muscle aches, and fever) should occur within 2 to 3 weeks.
- The patient should return to the clinic in 1 week for a follow-up appointment and to provide her with the results of laboratory tests that are pending.

Efficacy of *Chlamydia* Treatment

- The majority of women with chlamydial infections are asymptomatic.
- Post-treatment cultures are not necessary unless reinfection is suspected. A test to see if the patient is cured may be considered 3 weeks after treatment with erythromycin.

Adverse Effects of Herpes Treatment

- In general, side effects from all three drugs are mild and infrequent and include headache, nausea, vomiting, fatigue, and diarrhea.
- Elevated liver function tests have been reported with all three drugs. Baseline AST and ALT studies are not needed for short-term treatment. Baseline and periodic (every 4 months) AST and ALT studies may be advisable for long-term suppressive therapy regimens, especially if the patient is taking other hepatotoxic agents.
- Acyclovir and valacyclovir have been rarely associated with increases in serum creatinine concentrations. This transient increase in serum creatinine is most commonly seen with IV acyclovir and is a result of drug crystallizing in the renal tubules.
- Valacyclovir has caused TTP/HUS in immunocompromised patients as described previously.

Adverse Effects of *Chlamydia* Treatment

- Azithromycin may cause nausea, vomiting, diarrhea, and abdominal pain.
- Doxycycline may cause rash, photosensitivity, anorexia, nausea, vomiting, and diarrhea.

Patient Counseling

6. *What information should be provided to the patient to enhance compliance, ensure successful therapy, and minimize adverse effects?*

Herpes Simplex

- The patient should be told about the natural history of the disease, with an emphasis on the potential recurrent episodes, asymptomatic viral shedding, and sexual transmission.
- Do not have sex when lesions or early symptoms are present, and inform your sex partners that you have herpes. Condoms should be used with all new and uninfected partners.

- Herpes can be passed to others when you do not have active lesions or symptoms.
- If you are pregnant, tell your OB/GYN doctor that you have herpes, because it can be passed to your unborn child.
- Antiherpes drugs given within 48 hours of future outbreaks may shorten the duration of lesions, so call your doctor as soon as you have symptoms.
- Acyclovir is a drug used to treat herpes infections. Take one tablet (400 mg) by mouth 3 times a day for 10 days. Acyclovir can be taken with or without food. This medication may cause nausea, vomiting, diarrhea, and tiredness. Call your doctor if these side effects become severe. If you miss a dose of your medication, you may take the dose as soon as you remember; however, if it is almost time for your next dose don't double your dose. Skip the missed dose and take your regularly scheduled dose.

Chlamydia

- Your sex partners should be seen by a doctor for evaluation, testing, treatment, and counseling. You should avoid sexual intercourse until 7 days after your first dose of *Chlamydia* medication.
- Azithromycin is a drug used to treat chlamydial infections. Take all 4 of these 250 mg tablets at once to receive the desired single-dose treatment of 1000 mg. This drug is long acting, so you only need to take 1 dose of the medication. The tablets may be taken with or without food. This medication may cause nausea, vomiting, diarrhea, and abdominal pain. Call your doctor if these side effects persist or if you notice any other unusual side effects.

▶ Follow-up Questions

1. *Six months later Lisa calls the STD clinic complaining of genital lesions that look and feel the same as the lesions she had 6 months earlier when seen and treated in the clinic. Should this episode of recurrent genital herpes be treated? If so, what therapies would be appropriate?*

   - When treatment is started during the prodrome or within 1 day after the onset of lesions, many patients who have recurrent disease benefit from episodic therapy. If it is decided to provide episodic treatment, the patient should be provided with a prescription for antiviral therapy so that treatment can be initiated at the first sign of prodrome or genital lesions. Any of the following episodic treatment regimens listed below may be prescribed.
     - ✓ Acyclovir 400 mg po TID × 5 days
     - ✓ Acyclovir 200 mg po 5 times/day × 5 days
     - ✓ Acyclovir 800 mg po BID × 5 days
     - ✓ Famciclovir 125 mg po BID × 5 days
     - ✓ Valacyclovir 500 mg po BID × 5 days

2. *Is daily suppressive therapy indicated because she had a recurrent episode?*

   - No, daily suppressive therapy is not indicated since she has only had one recurrent episode. It is indicated after 6 or more recurrences per year. Daily suppressive therapy reduces the frequency of genital herpes recurrences by ≥ 75% among patients who have frequent recurrences. Any of the following episodic treatment regimens listed below may be prescribed.
     - ✓ Acyclovir 400 mg po BID
     - ✓ Famciclovir 250 mg po BID
     - ✓ Valacyclovir 250 mg po BID
     - ✓ Valacyclovir 500 mg po QD (this regimen appears less effective than other valacyclovir dosing regimens in patients who have very frequent recurrences [i.e., ≥10 episodes per year])
     - ✓ Valacyclovir 1000 mg po QD

3. *When is Chlamydia treatment indicated for sex partners?*

   - Sex partners should be evaluated, tested, and treated if they had sexual contact with the patient during the 60 days preceding the onset of symptoms in the patient or the diagnosis of *Chlamydia*.
   - The most recent sexual partner should be treated even if the time of the last sexual contact was > 60 days before symptom onset or diagnosis.

4. *What additional pharmacotherapeutic interventions should be made to address the problems that were identified in question 1.a.?*

   - The vaginal candidiasis should be treated with an imidazole or triazole vaginal cream, tablet, or suppository inserted vaginally at bedtime for 1, 3, or 7 days depending on the product selected. Examples of such products include:
     - ✓ Clotrimazole 500 mg vaginal tablet, inserted vaginally at bedtime for one dose only
     - ✓ Butoconazole 2% cream, one full applicator inserted vaginally at bedtime for 3 consecutive days
     - ✓ Terconazole 80 mg vaginal suppositories, inserted vaginally at bedtime for 3 consecutive days
     - ✓ Terconazole 0.4% vaginal cream, one full applicator inserted vaginally at bedtime for 7 consecutive days

   The single dose therapy regimens are appropriate for uncomplicated mild-to-moderate vulvovaginal candidiasis, especially in situations where compliance may be a problem.

   - A 150 mg po single dose of fluconazole would also be an appropriate treatment regimen in non-pregnant patients that may be more favorably accepted by women and would improve patient adherence.
   - An adequate history should be taken to determine if chronic prophylaxis for recurrent UTIs is indicated. If therapy is indicated, then a more cost-effective antimicrobial should be selected such as TMP-SMX 80/400 mg (single strength) 0.5 to 1 tablet po QD or 1 tablet 3 times/week. Fluoroquinolones should be reserved for patients with antimicrobial resistance or when the patient is intolerant to other recommended antimicrobials. Multivitamins containing iron should be given 2 to 4 hours before or after the ciprofloxacin to avoid decreased absorption of ciprofloxacin.
   - If the decision is made to continue chronic prophylaxis of her recurrent urinary tract infections, then an alternative form of birth control (in addition to the condoms) should be prescribed because of the drug interaction between antibiotics and oral contraceptives. Depo-Provera 150 mg IM Q 3 months would be a reasonable alternative.

References

1. Centers for Disease Control and Prevention. Genital herpes simplex (HSV) infection; Chlamydial infection. 1998 guidelines for treatment of sexually transmitted diseases. MMWR 1998;47(RR-01):20–26, 53–59. Also see http://www.cdc.gov/
2. Anon. Drugs for non-HIV viral infections. Med Lett 1997;39:69–76.
3. Valtrex Caplets Package Insert. Research Triangle Park, NC, Glaxo Wellcome, 1997.

109 OSTEOMYELITIS

▶ My Brother's Kicker (Level I)

Edward P. Armstrong, PharmD, BCPS, FASHP
Victor A. Elsberry, PharmD, BCNSP
Leslie L. Barton, MD

An 8-year-old boy develops osteomyelitis of the right distal femur after being kicked by his brother while playing soccer. The patient's symptoms persist for 1 month and adjacent septic arthritis of the right knee ensues due to inadequate treatment with subtherapeutic doses of cefazolin. Because *Staphylococcus aureus* is the most common causative organism in pediatric osteomyelitis, initial empiric therapy should consist of parenteral therapy with a penicillinase-resistant penicillin (e.g., nafcillin or oxacillin) or a first-generation cephalosporin (e.g., cefazolin or cephalothin). Therapy may be changed to an equivalent oral regimen after a good response to parenteral treatment has been demonstrated. Clindamycin may be used in children allergic to penicillins or cephalosporins. Prolonged therapy (a total of 4 to 6 weeks) is required for successful treatment of osteomyelitis.

▶ Questions

Problem Identification

1. a. Create a list of the patient's drug-related problems.

- Inadequately treated osteomyelitis with an initial dose of cefazolin of 75 mg/kg/day in 4 divided doses, rather than 100 mg/kg/day in 3 divided doses. The initial dosing regimen resulted in subtherapeutic bone concentrations, which probably explains the patient's inadequate response.

b. What information (signs, symptoms, laboratory values) indicates the presence or severity of acute osteomyelitis?

- *Signs.* Local tenderness and swelling; findings on x-ray of involved bones.
- *Symptoms.* Bone pain.
- *Laboratory values.* Elevated ESR.
- In this patient, concurrent septic arthritis is indicated by adjacent knee joint pain, tenderness, swelling, and markedly decreased range of motion.

Desired Outcome

2. What are the goals of pharmacotherapy in this case?

- Arrest the acute infection and eradicate the infecting organism
- Prevent further tissue damage and progression to chronic osteomyelitis

Therapeutic Alternatives

3. a. What non-drug therapies might be useful for this patient?

- Initially, surgical drainage is needed to relieve the pressure of pus, which in itself may cause articular damage. Surgical drainage of the area of infection also decreases both the burden of organisms and mediators of inflammation in the infected tissue.
- Physical therapy will be beneficial as pain resolves to restore mobility and strength and to decrease the risk of further damage due to nonuse of the involved joint.

b. What feasible pharmacotherapeutic alternatives are available for the empiric treatment of acute osteomyelitis?

- Empiric antimicrobial therapy should be directed against *Staphylococcus aureus,* the most common organism in children with osteomyelitis. Intravenous therapy is recommended for initial treatment of acute osteomyelitis. After demonstration of a good clinical response, therapy may then be switched to an equivalent oral regimen.
- A parenteral *penicillinase-resistant penicillin* (e.g., *nafcillin* or *oxacillin*) is appropriate initial therapy. The regimen may be subsequently changed to oral therapy (e.g., *dicloxacillin* or *cloxacillin*).
- A parenteral *first-generation cephalosporin* (e.g., *cefazolin* or *cephalothin*) is also appropriate initial therapy. Therapy may later be changed to oral *cephalexin.*
- *Clindamycin* IV may be used if the patient is allergic to penicillins or cephalosporins. Therapy may later be changed to oral clindamycin.
- A *third-generation cephalosporin (cefotaxime or ceftriaxone)* should also be used in patients with sickle cell anemia because *Salmonella* is the most common infecting organism.[1]
- *Ampicillin* should be included in the therapy of young infants because group B streptococcal osteomyelitis is a serious consideration.
- *Fluoroquinolones* such as ciprofloxacin should *not* be used in children due to the risk of cartilage damage.

Optimal Plan

4. What drug, dosage form, dose, schedule, and duration of therapy are best for this patient?

- A penicillinase-resistant penicillin is generally considered the treatment of choice for all serious *Staphylococcus aureus* infections.
- In the outpatient setting, the longer dosing interval for first-generation cephalosporins makes them the agents of choice. Because this young boy was treated at home, the first-generation cephalosporin cefazolin offers the advantage of every-8-hour dosing compared to every 4 to 6 hours for nafcillin.

- An acceptable regimen for this patient is cefazolin 100 mg/kg/day in 3 divided doses for a total of 4 to 6 weeks (including conversion to equivalent oral therapy).[2]

Outcome Evaluation

5. *What clinical and laboratory parameters are necessary to evaluate the therapy for achievement of the desired therapeutic outcome and to detect or prevent adverse effects?*

- Culture and sensitivity testing of bacterial isolates at initiation of treatment.
- White blood cell count initially and repeated if clinically indicated.
- Erythrocyte sedimentation rate weekly.
- Observation for clinical signs of inflammation (redness, pain, swelling, tenderness, fever) daily during the initial phase of therapy.
- Confirm adherence to outpatient therapy. Reinforce the importance of compliance before starting oral therapy and with each health care visit.
- Documentation of resolution of major radiographic abnormalities after conclusion of therapy.
- Asking the patient's mother about the presence of adverse effects of oral cephalosporins, such as GI intolerance, diarrhea, and rash with each health care visit.

Patient Counseling

6. *What information should be provided to the patient's caregiver to enhance compliance, ensure successful therapy, and minimize adverse effects?*

General Information[3,4]

- Acute osteomyelitis is a serious infection of the bone. If inadequately treated, it can lead to chronic disability; therefore, it is important for your child to take every dose for the entire duration of therapy; this may be 4 to 6 weeks.

Cephalexin

- Give your child each dose about 8 hours apart, 3 times a day, and at the same time each day.
- This medication can be taken without regard to meals.
- It may upset your child's stomach or cause diarrhea or rash. Contact your doctor immediately if your son has trouble taking the medication. Also contact your physician if your child develops another illness resulting in nausea, vomiting, or diarrhea.
- Have all laboratory and x-ray tests performed when requested. Keep all follow-up appointments with your doctor. Contact your doctor immediately if your son's condition does not improve or worsens.

Dicloxacillin

- This medication should be taken 1 hour before or 2 hours after meals.
- If you forget to take a dose of this medicine, take it as soon as you remember. However, if it is almost time for your next dose, skip the missed dose and go back to your regular schedule.
- This medicine sometimes causes diarrhea; contact your doctor or me if this becomes troublesome or severe.

References

1. Burnett MW, Bass JW, Cook BA. Etiology of osteomyelitis complicating sickle cell disease. Pediatrics. 1998;101:296–297.
2. Nelson JD. Skeletal infections in children. Adv Pediatr Infect Dis 1991;6:59–78.
3. Dagan R. Management of acute hematogenous osteomyelitis and septic arthritis in the pediatric patient. Pediatr Infect Dis J 1993;12:88–92.
4. Lew DP, Waldvogel FA. Osteomyelitis. N Engl J Med 1997;336:999–1007.

110 GRAM-NEGATIVE SEPSIS

▶ Bottomed Out (Level II)

Mary M. Hess, PharmD

A 77-year-old man with a history of alcoholic cirrhosis is brought to the emergency department with weakness, dyspnea on exertion, and altered mental status. Treatment for hypotension and hyperkalemia were instituted, the patient was intubated, and cultures were obtained from urine, blood, and sputum. Readers are asked to consider treatment alternatives for sepsis-induced hypotension and to design an appropriate initial empiric antibiotic regimen for presumed sepsis. The case follows the patient's course throughout his stay in the intensive care unit, where periodic changes in the patient's status require adjustments in the regimens for hypotension and infection. The patient is ultimately discharged to complete an oral antimicrobial regimen on an outpatient basis; proper patient counseling on the medication must be provided.

▶ Questions

Problem Identification

1. a. *Devise a drug-related problem list for this patient.*

- Possible sepsis [primary source abdomen (ascites) or lung (pneumonia)], requiring antimicrobial treatment.
- Metabolic acidosis (secondary to hyperkalemia and hypotension), requiring treatment.
- Acute renal failure (hyperkalemia, increased SCr), requiring treatment.
- Liver dysfunction secondary to alcoholic cirrhosis that may affect subsequent drug dosing.
- Potential for alcohol withdrawal that would require pharmacologic treatment.
- Stress ulcer prophylaxis required.
- Deep vein thrombosis prophylaxis needed.
- Nutrition support required (patient is unable to eat with ventilator tube in place).

b. *What clinical signs does this patient exhibit that are consistent with infection? What elements must be present to confirm the presence of sepsis?*

Criteria for Sepsis[1]	Patient Values
Temperature > 38° or < 36°C	35.6°C
SBP < 90 mm Hg or 40 mm Hg decrease from baseline	76/palp
Heart rate > 90 bpm	74, paced
Respiratory rate > 20/min or $PaCO_2$ < 32 mm Hg	20
WBC > 12.0 or < 4.0 × 10³/mm³ or ≥ 10% bands	WBC 11.0 × 10³/mm³, 15% bands

- Prolonged hypotension states will lead to perfusion abnormalities resulting in lactic acidosis, oliguria, and altered mental status. In general, two or more of the criteria in the table above are required to make the diagnosis of sepsis. There must also be clinical suspicion of infection or the presence of a documented infection.

Desired Outcome

2. *What are the short-term and long-term goals of therapy when managing a patient with sepsis?*

- *Short-term goals.* Stabilization of cardiac output is the key initially. This may be accomplished through stabilization of the blood pressure, which will help maintain an adequate urine output and maintain oxygenation and perfusion to vital organs.
- *Long-term goals.* Once the hemodynamic parameters are stabilized, begin to work up the proposed source that caused the destabilization. In this case, a thorough evaluation for potential infectious sources should be considered. Prevent development or further progression of organ failure by maintaining short-term goals and adjusting drug therapy as necessary to decrease the risk of adverse effects (e.g., development of acute tubular necrosis from aminoglycoside therapy,[2] pulmonary edema from overhydration).

Therapeutic Alternatives

3. a. *What are the treatment alternatives for sepsis-induced hypotension?*

- Aggressive fluid resuscitation is the first intervention for sepsis-induced hypotension. Reversal of the hypotension may require several liters of fluid. Crystalloid solutions are the preferred initial therapy (i.e., normal saline or lactated Ringer's solution) unless the patient has a serum albumin < 2 g/dL. Patients with heart failure may receive smaller volumes of crystalloid therapy. The total volume is dependent upon clinical parameters and the severity of the patient's heart failure. Patients with volume restrictions (e.g., heart failure) should receive albumin plus crystalloid in order to keep the volume provided in the intravascular space. Once crystalloid therapy has been maximized (2 L within 2 hours), colloid therapy may be used. Hetastarch is the initial agent of choice except in patients who have albumin levels < 2 g/dL or a coagulopathy.[3,4] In those settings, one may move directly to albumin.

b. *What colloids are commercially available?*

- *Dextran* is available but rarely used because of adverse events.
- *Hetastarch* 6% is the preferred agent in all patients except those with documented coagulopathy or a serum albumin < 2 g/dL. The recommended dose range is 500 to 1500 mL per day.
- *Albumin* 5% becomes the agent of choice once crystalloid or hetastarch criteria have been met except in those patients with a serum sodium ≥ 145 mEq/L. Dosing may be initiated in 12.5-g increments.
- *Albumin* 25% is the agent of choice in patients with fluid restrictions or in patients with serum sodium concentrations > 145 mEq/L. Dosing is the same as for albumin 5% (i.e., in 12.5-g increments).
- *Plasma protein fraction* (PPF) may be therapeutically interchanged with albumin. The albumin factor recommendations may be followed with the exception of the serum sodium cutoffs. Because there is only one concentration of PPF, the sodium concentration is irrelevant. A pre-determined volume is given in 250- or 500-mL increments.

c. *Outline a reasonable alternative antibiotic regimen for empiric treatment of this patient (include dosing and duration of therapy). In formulating your answer, consider the potential sources of infection and the most common infecting organisms for those sources.*

- Potential sources of infection in this patient include:
  - ✓ Urinary tract: older persons may have some urinary retention.
  - ✓ Device: the patient may have a skin or internal source because of recent device placement (pacemaker).
  - ✓ Pulmonary: he may have a community-acquired pneumonia.
  - ✓ GI tract: the presence of ascites is a risk factor.
- The most common organisms for the suspected sources are:
  - ✓ Urinary tract: *Escherichia coli*, *Staphylococcus* spp., and *Proteus* spp.
  - ✓ Device (pacemaker): *Staphylococcus* spp.; if the infection is internal the most likely organisms are gram-negative (e.g., *Pseudomonas* and *Klebsiella* spp.).
  - ✓ Pulmonary (community-acquired pneumonia): *Streptococcus* spp., *Staphylococcus* spp., *Haemophilus influenzae*, and atypical organisms (e.g., *Legionella* and *Chlamydia* spp.).
  - ✓ GI tract (ascites): *E. coli*, *Klebsiella*, *Enterobacter*, and *Enterococcus*.
- Initial empiric antimicrobial therapy should cover organisms that are typically found in community-acquired pneumonia and GI tract infections.
- Empiric antimicrobial coverage should be broad initially and narrowed as cultured organisms are identified and sensitivities determined. Empirically, an antibiogram may be used to help select the most appropriate agent. Antibiograms are institution-specific, providing information about the prevalence of an organism and its corresponding sensitivity profile. Antibiograms may also report the source of the culture and the frequency of organism identification at each source. The information may be sorted by medical service or institutional unit and should have separate inpatient and outpatient data. Antibiograms are useful tools that assist in empiric selection but are of minimal value once specific information is available.

- Penicillins, cephalosporins, fluoroquinolones (second-, third-, or fourth-generation of any of these three classes) with or without an aminoglycoside (e.g., gentamicin, tobramycin) may be used as initial empiric antimicrobial coverage. Aminoglycoside dosing may follow either traditional dosing for ICU patients (3 mg/kg loading dose followed by a maintenance regimen) or the alternative once-daily dosing regimen (7 mg/kg loading dose with the maintenance dose to be determined by random concentration monitoring).[5]

Optimal Plan

4. a. *Based on this information, what do you recommend as the next therapeutic intervention?*

   - Ideally, the goal is to achieve and maintain a systolic BP > 90 mm Hg. There is room to increase the dopamine drip rate. Dopamine is generally titrated upward in increments of 2 to 3 µg/kg/min if the patient is close to achieving the goal BP, and in increments of 5 µg/kg/min if the desired BP cannot be achieved quickly. A sustained low BP increases the risk of ischemia and multiple organ failure. The maximum rate for dopamine is 20 µg/kg/min.

   b. *One hour after your recommendation was implemented, his BP was 85/45 and pulse was 74. What is the next therapeutic option to achieve your BP goal?*

   - Once dopamine has been maximized, the addition of an α-agonist may be indicated (i.e., norepinephrine or phenylephrine). Initial infusion rates are norepinephrine 0.05 µg/kg/min and phenylephrine 0.03 µg/kg/min.

   c. *What adjustments in therapy do you recommend for the patient at this point?*

   - *Blood pressure.* Begin to wean the α-agonist vasopressor agent to off. One could also begin to wean both dopamine and the vasopressor. As you are able to decrease the α-agonist, you may begin tapering dopamine prior to turning off the α-agonist. For example, a recommendation could be given to wean norepinephrine to off while maintaining SBP > 90 mm Hg with dopamine. This will help reduce the risk of decreased organ function secondary to vasoconstriction and subsequent decreased peripheral perfusion.
   - *Antimicrobial therapy.* No change should be made until the specific organism and its sensitivities are known.

   d. *What is your plan at this point?*

   - *Blood pressure.* Continue to wean the vasopressors. If not already done, discontinue the α-agonist and continue weaning the dopamine to off (if not already done) while maintaining the BP parameter written for yesterday.
   - *Antimicrobial therapy.* Review the antimicrobial agents you are utilizing and assess whether you need to continue all of them or whether you can narrow the spectrum to what has been identified. You have potentially identified a source for the infection and identified the organism. The patient's clinical picture has improved, based on his WBC count and temperature (afebrile) for the past 24 hours. If the agent you previously selected does not cover *Klebsiella* spp., change to an agent that does. Examples include cephalosporins, penicillins, fluoroquinolones (second-, third-, or fourth-generations of any of these three classes), carbapenems, and aztreonam. If an aminoglycoside is used, it should be combined with one of the other agents.

   e. *What adjustments, if any, do you want to make now that all of the information is available?*

   - Confirm that the previous agents selected are appropriate based upon the organism's sensitivities. In addition, if therapy can be narrowed, now is the time to do so.
   - All agents that are sensitive to the organism could be considered for treatment. Agents that may be used as monotherapy include all drugs that the organism is sensitive to with the exception of the aminoglycosides. Aminoglycosides are almost always used as a part of a combination regimen. They may occasionally be used as monotherapy in the treatment of urinary tract infections.
   - The primary advantage of using cefepime instead of ceftazidime (or trovafloxacin instead of ampicillin/sulbactam) is related to β-lactamase production. Ceftazidime is a potent inducer of β-lactamase whereas cefepime is a low inducer. The sulbactam component of ampicillin/sulbactam is also a β-lactamase producer; trovafloxacin is not an inducer.

   f. *What are your final recommendations regarding the antimicrobial therapy?*

   - Determine an appropriate duration of treatment (e.g., 7, 10, or 14 days). Although there is no single correct answer, the author's recommendation is to continue treatment for a full 14 days.
   - Consider when therapy can be switched from the IV to the oral route. This decision should be based upon his ability to absorb oral medications, defervescence of the infection (e.g., normalization of the WBC count and temperature, decrease in sputum production), and the overall bioavailability of the drug.

Outcome Evaluation

5. *What parameters should be monitored to evaluate the efficacy and toxicity of your interventions?*

   - *Adequate oxygenation.* Pao_2 may be evaluated 1 to 2 times per day depending upon the mode of ventilation. The O_2 saturation is monitored continuously. The Pao_2/Fio_2 ratio monitoring is performed continuously.
   - *Hemodynamic parameters.* Monitor BP, CVP, and if a Swan–Ganz catheter is placed monitor PCWP, CO/CI, and SVR/SVRI. The frequency of monitoring is variable based upon patient stability and clinician preference. In most ICU patients, BP is documented every 2 hours, and CVPs are obtained at least 1 to 2 times per day.
   - *Adequate perfusion.* Assess skin color, temperature of extremities, urine output, and mental status (e.g., ability to respond appropriately to questions every shift).
   - *Antibiotic efficacy.* Obtain WBC with differential and temperature daily. Time points for monitoring serum aminoglycoside concentrations depend upon the regimen selected. The frequency of serum level monitoring is dependent upon the dynamic status of the patient (e.g., changes in organ function or hemodynamics).
   - *Antibiotic toxicity.* Measure serum creatinine, urine output, serum aminoglycoside concentrations, and watch for neutropenia and thrombocytopenia. Assess the patient for skin rash and diarrhea. These parameters are monitored daily in the ICU.

Patient Counseling

6. *What information should be provided to the patient about his antimicrobial regimen upon discharge?*

- This patient could be converted to an oral cephalosporin or fluoroquinolone. Counseling information that should be provided for each agent is included below.

Cephalosporin

- Take this medication exactly as prescribed by your doctor.
- Take the doses at the intervals prescribed; this medication may be taken with food.
- Continue to take this until all doses have been taken, even though you may begin to feel better.
- If you miss a dose, take it as soon as you remember. If it is nearly time for the next dose, skip the missed dose and continue your regular schedule; do not take 2 doses at once.
- Possible side effects of this medication may include nausea, vomiting, and mild diarrhea.
- Allergic reactions sometimes occur. Stop taking the medicine and contact your doctor immediately if you develop a rash, hives, or shortness of breath.

Fluoroquinolone

- Take this medication exactly as prescribed by your doctor.
- Take each dose on an empty stomach (about 1 to 2 hours after meals).
- Do not take iron, antacids containing aluminum, or calcium- or magnesium-containing products within 2 hours of taking a fluoroquinolone dose.
- (Dosing instructions regarding full duration and missed doses are the same as for cephalosporins.)
- Possible side effects include nausea, vomiting, loss of appetite, dizziness, headache, nervousness, or trouble sleeping. Contact your doctor as soon as possible if you develop tendon pain, joint pain, trouble breathing, or severe diarrhea.

References

1. Bone RC, Balk RA, Cerra FB, et al. Definitions for sepsis and organ failure and guidelines for the use of innovative therapies in sepsis. The ACCP/SCCM Consensus Conference Committee. Chest 1992;101:1644–1655.
2. Boucher BA, Coffey BC, Kuhl DA, et al. Algorithm for assessing renal dysfunction risk in critically ill trauma patients receiving aminoglycosides. Am J Surg 1990;160:473–480.
3. Yim JM, Vermeulen LC Jr, Erstad BL, et al. Albumin and nonprotein colloid solution use in U.S. academic health centers. Arch Intern Med 1995;155:2450–2455.
4. Vermeulen LC Jr, Ratko TA, Erstad BL, et al. A paradigm for consensus. The University Hospital Consortium guidelines for the use of albumin, nonprotein colloid, and crystalloid solutions. Arch Intern Med 1995;155:373–379.
5. Nicolau DP, Freeman CD, Belliveau PP, et al. Experience with a once-daily aminoglycoside program administered to 2,184 adult patients. Antimicrob Agents Chemother 1995;39:650–655.

111 SYSTEMIC FUNGAL INFECTION

▶ Solving a Budding Problem   (Level III)

Aaron D. Killian, PharmD, BCPS

A 57-year-old woman admitted for a COPD exacerbation develops nosocomial pneumonia and a perforated cecum requiring treatment with broad-spectrum antimicrobials and a right hemicolectomy. Five days post-operatively, the patient develops leukocytosis, hypotension, and positive cultures for *Candida* in the urine and blood. Because the patient has three sites previously colonized with *Candida*, she is thought to have disseminated fungal disease. The patient fails to respond initially to fluconazole 400 mg IV daily, and amphotericin B therapy is initiated. The case requires students to develop an appropriate dosage regimen and monitoring parameters for amphotericin B in this complex patient situation.

▶ Questions

Problem Identification

1. a. *Identify the patient's initial drug-related problems and provide recommendations for managing each of them.*

    - Administration of prophylactic subcutaneous heparin in a patient with a recent GI hemorrhage (guaiac positive reddish-black NG aspirate). Discontinue the heparin and, if possible, use pneumatic compression devices instead.
    - No pharmacologic prophylaxis for stress ulceration. Prophylaxis with an H_2-antagonist should be instituted because this patient is at high risk for stress ulcers. This may also help reduce transfusion requirements in the event of continued GI bleeding.
    - Metoclopramide is not controlling the gastric residuals (i.e., the residuals are > twice the hourly feeding rate). The patient's delirium may be at least partially attributable to this agent. Consider discontinuing metoclopramide.
    - Nasogastric administration of potassium chloride in a patient with borderline hypokalemia and no bowel sounds (reduced intestinal peristalsis). Recommend IV administration until peristalsis improves; if the serum level is still low, increase the dose to 40 mEq daily and monitor renal function carefully to avoid potassium accumulation.
    - Administration of high-dose corticosteroids in a COPD patient without an asthmatic component. Re-evaluate this situation and consider tapering methylprednisolone to a maximum dose of 30 mg IV Q 8 H.
    - Theophylline may be contributing to tachycardia (HR 122 bpm). Assess the need for theophylline in COPD and consider discontinuing it during this acute illness.
    - Terazosin may contribute to hypotension during this acute illness. Recommend holding the drug at present. Once the acute ill-

ness is over, evaluate the patient for low-dose thiazide therapy, which is preferred by JNC-VI and, according to the SHEP study, should not affect lipid control significantly.
- Morphine may be contributing to absent bowel sounds. Temporarily hold the drug until bowel sounds return and RUQ abdominal tenderness resolves.
- Hypermagnesemia and hyperphosphatemia are present. Monitor electrolytes carefully.
- Frequent administration of a potent loop diuretic (furosemide). Evaluate the need for continued diuresis (i.e., pulmonary edema, JVD, central venous or pulmonary artery pressures, hemodynamics, weight, edema in extremities, urine output, BUN/SCr, fractional excretion of sodium, and/or urine electrolytes).
- Presence of hyperglycemia during an acute illness. Add insulin to improve glucose control and maintain blood glucose < 200 mg/dL while the patient has an active infection.
- Untreated fungal skin infection. Recommend a topical antifungal cream to be applied to the affected area.

b. *What risk factors for disseminated fungal infection are present in this patient?*

- Acute renal failure.
- Age > 40 years.
- Antibiotics for ≥ 7 days.[1]
- Parenteral nutrition.
- Multiple organ system dysfunction/trauma.
- Serum glucose persistently > 200 mg/dL.
- Corticosteroid administration.
- A recent study found an APACHE II score >10, ventilator dependence > 48 hours, and multiple antibiotic use to be associated with an increased risk of fungal infection.[2] However, severity of underlying illness and use of multiple antibiotics have been the only factors consistently proven to result in an increased risk of fungal colonization/invasion. It is likely that many ICU patients, including those who are not severely ill, are at risk for the development of fungal infections.

c. *Does this patient meet the criteria for colonization or invasive/disseminated fungal infection?*

- *Definitive invasive infection.* Burn wound invasion; culture of fungus from peritoneal fluid or tissue (e.g., kidney, liver, lung); endophthalmitis (present in 30% of patients).[3]
- *Likely invasive infection.* Two sets of positive blood cultures at least 24 hours apart, without a central line; 2 sets of positive blood cultures with the second obtained >24 hours after removal of a central line; 3 or more colonized sites.
- Although this patient does not have positive blood cultures, she has 3 previously colonized sites (tracheal aspirate, urine cultures, skin folds). Given this information, it is likely that this patient has invasive/disseminated disease.

Desired Outcome

2. *What are the goals of pharmacotherapy in this patient?*

- Prompt clinical and microbiologic eradication of the infecting pathogen to avoid definite dissemination, prolonged antimicrobial therapy, and/or the systemic inflammatory response syndrome (SIRS).
- Short-course IV therapy with conversion to oral therapy as soon as possible following the disappearance of all signs and symptoms of infection.
- Therapy should be directed towards decreasing mortality and preventing relapse while maintaining quality of life.

Therapeutic Alternatives

3. a. *What non-drug measures would you recommend for treatment of this fungal infection?*

- In the event that the urinary catheter is the source, both symptomatic patients and asymptomatic patients who are likely to have disseminated candidiasis should have their catheters changed or removed.[4]
- It is important to have a physician perform a funduscopic examination of the eyes to check for endophthalmitis and evaluate the patient for the presence of any GI tract obstruction or genitourinary tract abnormality that may be predisposing the patient to hematogenous spread of fungi.
- Two sets of blood cultures should be taken, and consideration should be given to replacement and culture of the central line.
- The patient's antibiotic regimen needs to be evaluated to determine if she has received sufficient treatment for her nosocomial pneumonia/sinusitis. Disseminated fungal infections can be difficult to treat in the face of continued broad-spectrum antimicrobial use.
- The importance of tight glucose control cannot be overemphasized.
- The lowest possible dose of corticosteroids should be encouraged to limit the degree of immunosuppression.

b. *What are the most likely causative pathogens in this patient?*

- In this patient, it is unknown whether the *Candida* in the urine represents the source or the spread of candidemia. However, candidemia in patients with preceding surgical procedures is most frequently caused (in descending order) by: *Candida albicans, Candida tropicalis,* and *Torulopsis glabrata*. More specifically, the presence of "germ tubes" indicates infection due to *Candida albicans*.
- The *S. epidermidis* is most likely a contaminant, but any further cultures should increase the index of suspicion and may warrant empiric antibiotic therapy. *S. epidermidis* is now the most common cause of catheter-related infections and is a common blood-borne pathogen in ICU patients.

c. *What pharmacotherapeutic agents are available for the acute therapy of this infection?*

Polyene Antifungals
- *Amphotericin B* IV is the drug of choice for serious deep seated fungal infections.
- *Nystatin* IV remains in clinical trials; the oral form is not suitable due to its poor absorption profile.

Azoles
- *Ketoconazole* given orally has multiple adverse effects and drug interactions that make it least desirable.
- *Miconazole* IV has significant adverse effects that relegate its use primarily for resistant pathogens.

- *Fluconazole* IV followed by po therapy has the most literature support.
- *Itraconazole* orally lacks documentation of efficacy in clinical trials, but it has shown promise in candiduria.

Antimetabolites
- *5-fluorocytosine* (5-FC) given orally has demonstrated synergy with amphotericin B and fluconazole.

d. *What is the significance of the catheter tip cultures and the continued positive blood and urine cultures?*

- A CFU count < 15 is likely representative of catheter contamination from the blood rather than a true catheter-related infection (CRI). Of interest, *S. epidermidis* is a common finding in patients prior to and during fungemia.[1]
- A probable CRI occurs when a common skin organism (coagulase-negative staphylococci, micrococci, *Bacillus, Corynebacterium, Propionibacterium*), *S. aureus*, or *Candida* is isolated from a single blood culture in a patient with clinical signs of sepsis and no other identifiable source of infection except the catheter (unlike this patient). Coagulase-negative staphylococci, the predominant aerobes on human skin, are now the most common cause of CRIs (43%). *S. aureus* (18%), enterococci (13%), and *Candida* spp. (9% to 11%) are also frequently isolated. Approximately 75% of *Candida* spp. are due to *C. albicans*, with many of the remaining cases due to *C. parapsilosis*. *Corynebacterium* (esp. JK strains) and *Bacillus* spp. are skin contaminants, whereas gram-negative bacilli (e.g., *Pseudomonas, Acinetobacter, Xanthomonas*) are usually acquired from nosocomial settings.
- Definite CRIs occur when there is/are: 1) pus at the insertion site; 2) resolution of sepsis after catheter removal; 3) positive cultures of the same organism from the catheter or pus compared to blood; and 4) 10-fold higher CFU from blood drawn through the catheter compared with a peripheral vein.
- The persistent candidemia/candiduria and hypotension are of concern. Non-catheter associated candidemia is associated with a higher mortality rate than is catheter-associated disease. In fact, the absence of amphotericin B has been shown to be a negative factor related to outcome in patients who have died as a result of candidemia. High-grade candidemia (> 25 CFU/mL or > 2 days of candidemia while on antifungal therapy) may necessitate a funduscopic exam, transesophageal echocardiography (TEE), or venography to rule out retinitis, endocarditis, and septic thrombosis of a central vein, respectively. Central venous catheters should be removed if candidemia persists longer than 48 hours or if patients still have signs and symptoms after 96 hours of therapy.[5]

Optimal Plan

4. *What drug therapy (including dose and route of administration) would you recommend for this patient?*

- Amphotericin B IV is the treatment of choice since this patient has hemodynamic instability. Although it is controversial, some clinicians prefer to initiate combination amphotericin B plus 5-FC therapy in any patient with hemodynamic instability.
- Most clinicians would initiate amphotericin B IV 0.7 mg/kg/day and consider increasing the dose to 1 mg/kg/day and/or adding oral 5-FC if there is inadequate response within 48 hours (i.e., reduction in temperature and WBC, improved hemodynamics).
- Although one could argue that the dose of fluconazole may have been inadequate (i.e., a dose < 800 mg QD was utilized), the patient has presumably failed to respond to initial therapy with fluconazole as well.
- The first few milligrams of the initially scheduled amphotericin B dose may be administered at a slower rate over 20 to 30 minutes. If the patient shows signs of toxicity, then premedication may be necessary (see question below). Amphotericin B has traditionally been administered over 4 to 6 hours, but more recently, 1- to 2-hour infusions have been successful. Shorter infusions do NOT increase nephrotoxicity, fever spikes, phlebitis, or nausea (phlebitis and nausea may actually be reduced), but they may increase the severity/duration of chills. Shorter infusions must *not* be given if the dose is >1 mg/kg or if patients have significant electrolyte disorders (e.g., hypokalemia, hyperkalemia, hypomagnesemia) or renal disease (CL_{cr} < 25 mL/min), because they are more predisposed to cardiotoxicity (e.g., hypotension and dysrhythmias).

Outcome Evaluation

5. *How should the antifungal regimen be monitored for efficacy and adverse effects?*

Efficacy
- Resolution of fever, hypotension, and leukocytosis with left shift. Temperature and blood pressure should be monitored hourly until the patient is hemodynamically stable, then every 4 to 6 hours until the parameters normalize (usually 48 to 72 hours). They can then be monitored once each shift thereafter during therapy. A CBC with differential should be monitored daily until it normalizes and then every 2 to 3 days thereafter during therapy.
- Amelioration of positive fungal cultures from urine and blood (cultures should be re-evaluated after 48 to 72 hours of amphotericin B therapy and repeated every 3 to 4 days until negative).
- Given the immunosuppressed status of the patient, treatment should continue for 2 weeks after negative cultures are documented.

Adverse Effects
- Infusion-related reactions (> 50%) may be related to tumor necrosis factor or prostaglandin E production from macrophages. Fever, chills, and rigors are most common. These symptoms may be reduced by administration of acetaminophen, aspirin, or NSAIDs (e.g., ibuprofen 10 mg/kg up to 600 mg) 30 minutes prior to the infusion. Caution should be exercised with NSAIDs during acute renal failure. Meperidine (25 to 50 mg) and hydrocortisone (25 mg) have also been employed. The latter is *not* very effective whereas the former, although useful for chills and rigors, cannot be used in this case due to the patient's allergy. Generally, routine premedication before the first dose is *not* recommended. If the patient shows signs of any reaction, then premedication for subsequent doses may be necessary. Similarly, patients who develop significant electrolyte or cardiac abnormalities should have the drug infused over a longer period of time (see question 4).
- Thrombophlebitis (10% to 50%) is common with prolonged infusions. It may be reduced by using a central IV line or by adding heparin (1000 units) to each infusion bag.

- Nephrotoxicity (80%) is thought to be due, in part, to an alteration of the tubuloglomerular feedback mechanism in the proximal or distal tubule. This leads to loss of electrolytes (especially sodium and potassium) and, possibly, a reduction in blood flow due to vasoconstriction of the afferent arterioles of individual nephrons in an attempt to reduce solute loss. This most likely explains the increased serum creatinine and azotemia. This is fairly predictable and persistent in those requiring prolonged therapy. It is potentiated by sodium depletion and diuretic use. Concomitant nephrotoxic agents should be avoided if possible. Possible dehydration and azotemia necessitate daily BUN and serum creatinine monitoring, and electrolytes should be checked frequently for abnormalities in potassium, magnesium, and/or bicarbonate. The incidence is significantly reduced with a minimum of 90 mEq of sodium/day (1 L of normal saline contains 154 mEq sodium).
- A normochromic, normocytic anemia (60% to 90%) is a frequent complication after 2 or more weeks of therapy and is probably related to suppression of erythropoietin production.
- Miscellaneous effects (10% to 50%) include anorexia, nausea, vomiting, and headache.

▶ **Follow-up Questions**

1. Would liposomal amphotericin B be an appropriate alternative to consider at this time?

- Since the renal toxicity occurred after several days of therapy with amphotericin B, it would be more appropriate to continue therapy with this agent. Moreover, the rise in serum creatinine, although significant, is lower than that generally recommended for substitution with liposomal amphotericin B.
- If the renal function declined early in therapy and the serum creatinine was > 2.5 mg/dL, then one might conceivably consider switching to liposomal amphotericin B (especially if the patient is likely to require 14 or more days of therapy).
- In this situation, if the serum creatinine continues to rise, one might consider alternate-day therapy (i.e., doubling the daily dose and giving it every other day) to complete the course of therapy.

2. How much longer should therapy be continued?

- In the absence of complications (e.g., endocarditis, thrombophlebitis, retinitis, or other organ involvement), this patient should be treated for hematogenous candidiasis. Since she is at high risk for morbidity and mortality due to fungemia because of the severity of the illness, she should be treated for 10 to 14 days after the disappearance of all signs and symptoms of infection.[6]

References

1. Burchard KW, Minor LB, Slotman GJ, et al. Fungal sepsis in surgical patients. Arch Surg 1983;118:217–221.
2. Dean DA, Burchard KW. Fungal infection in surgical patients. Am J Surg 1996;171:374–382.
3. Slotman GJ, Shapiro E, Moffa SM. Fungal sepsis: Multisite colonization versus fungemia. Am Surg 1994;60:107–113.
4. Fisher JF, Newman CL, Sobel JD. Yeast in the urine: Solutions for a budding problem. Clin Infect Dis 1995;20:183–189.
5. Maki DG. Infections caused by intravascular devices used for infusion therapy: Pathogenesis, prevention, and management. In: Infections Associated With Indwelling Devices, 2nd ed. American Society for Microbiology, 1994:155–211.
6. Uzun O, Anaissie EJ. Problems and controversies in the management of hematogenous candidiasis. Clin Infect Dis 1996;22(suppl 2):S95–S101.
7. Edwards JE Jr, Bodey GP, Bowden RA, et al. International conference for the development of a consensus on the management and prevention of severe candidal infections. Clin Infect Dis 1997;25:43–59.

112 DERMATOPHYTOSIS

▶ **Skin and Nails** (Level II)

Winnie M. Yu, PharmD, BCPS

A 46-year-old man presents with clinical findings of tinea pedis (athlete's foot) and tinea unguium (onychomycosis) involving both feet. Tinea pedis may be effectively treated with one of a number of topical antifungal preparations for two weeks. Onychomycosis requires oral therapy, preferably with terbinafine or itraconazole for 12 weeks. Griseofulvin and ketoconazole could also be used, but these agents require treatment for 6 months. Recurrence rates are high with both conditions. For this reason, predisposing factors should also be addressed, which include wearing nonocclusive footwear, employing good foot hygiene, and drying the feet thoroughly after showering.

▶ **Questions**

Problem Identification

1. a. Create a list of the patient's drug-related problems.

- Athlete's foot (tinea pedis) requiring topical antifungal therapy.
- Onychomycosis (tinea unguium) requiring systemic antifungal therapy.
- Hypercholesterolemia, presently inadequately treated with pravastatin (goal LDL < 160 mg/dL).
- Recurrent peptic ulcer disease, presently treated with omeprazole (unknown *Helicobacter pylori* status).
- Use of topical hydrocortisone without medical indication and which may promote fungal growth.
- Use of echinacea without medical indication or knowledge of its effect on concurrent drug therapy.

b. What are the subjective and objective signs and symptoms of tinea pedis and onychomycosis in this patient?

Tinea Pedis

Subjective. Itchy feet; white flakes on the feet.
Objective. Mild erythematous skin on the feet; fine silvery white

flakes on the plantar surfaces of both feet; dry scales and hyperkeratotic skin covering the soles.

Onychomycosis

Subjective. Yellow and brittle toenails.

Objective. Yellow-brown discoloration and thickening of the first, second, and third toenails of both feet; microscopy of toenail debris revealed branching and filamentous hyphae consistent with dermatophyte infection.

c. *What are the common pathogens associated with tinea pedis and onychomycosis?*

- Tinea pedis, also known as athlete's foot, is the most common form of dermatophyte infection that involves the plantar surface and the sole of the foot. Onychomycosis, also known as tinea unguium, is a dermatophytic infection that involves the nail plate such as fingernails and toenails.
- Both infections are caused by dermatophytes such as *Trichophyton rubrum, Trichophyton mentagrophytes,* and *Epidermophyton floccosum* in > 80% of cases. Yeasts such as *Candida albicans* account for 5% to 17% of infections. Approximately 5% of the cases are caused by non-dermatophytic molds such as *Scopulariopsis, Scytalidium,* and *Fusarium* species, which may develop secondary to dermatophytic infection and trauma.[1]

d. *What are the risk factors for tinea pedis and onychomycosis in this patient?*

- In general, the incidence of tinea pedis increases with increasing age.
- Poor foot hygiene and prolonged exposure of the feet to moisture and heat (e.g., hot and humid weather, occlusive footwear, or excessive sweating) also favor the growth of fungus. Risk factors in this patient include possible poor foot hygiene because of frequent traveling, occlusive footwear (old tennis shoes), and constant exposure to moisture because of jogging in rainy weather for the past 2 weeks.
- Pre-existing tinea pedis has been shown to be a risk factor for onychomycosis.
- Trauma that weakens the seal between the nail plate and nail bed also creates a portal of entry for fungal invasion of the nail plate.
- Patients who are immunosuppressed due to HIV infection or immunosuppressive agents such as prednisone, cyclosporine, and tacrolimus are also at higher risk for tinea pedis and onychomycosis.[2] This patient's use of hydrocortisone cream promotes further growth of fungal pathogens.

Desired Outcome

2. *What are the goals of treatment for tinea pedis and onychomycosis in this patient?*

- Relieve symptoms (itching)
- Prevent further progression of the fungal infection on his feet and toenails
- Restore activities of daily living (e.g., jogging and traveling)
- Minimize side effects of antifungal therapy

Therapeutic Alternatives

3. a. *What non-drug therapies might be useful for this patient?*

- Non-occlusive footwear (e.g., thick cotton socks) with frequent changes
- Good foot hygiene
- Dry the feet thoroughly after showering
- Wear leather rather than vinyl shoes

b. *What feasible pharmacotherapeutic alternatives are available for treatment of the tinea pedis and onychomycosis?*

Tinea Pedis

- Azoles, allylamines, and miscellaneous products are topical agents that can effectively treat tinea pedis (see Table 112–1 below). However, relapse is common after treatment of the initial episode. The agents available differ by mechanism of action, efficacy, and prescription status. Cure rates with the azoles, allylamines, and ciclopirox are similar. Efficacy rates are lower with tolnaftate and undecylenic acid. These antifungal agents are usually applied twice daily until clearance of the infection, which may take 2 weeks or longer.
- Resistant cases may respond to systemic oral antifungal agents such as griseofulvin, fluconazole, itraconazole, and terbinafine. Amphotericin B and nystatin ointment are not effective for dermatophytes.

Onychomycosis

- Systemic oral antifungal agents achieve high drug concentrations in the nail plate and have been proven to be valuable in the management of onychomycosis.[3] Possible options include:
  - ✓ *Griseofulvin* 500 mg po BID × 6 months
  - ✓ *Ketoconazole* 200 mg po QD with meals × 6 months
  - ✓ *Itraconazole* 200 mg po QD with meals × 12 weeks
  - ✓ *Terbinafine* 250 mg po QD × 12 weeks

TABLE 112–1. Topical Antifungal Preparations

Drug	Formulations	Prescription (Rx) or OTC
Azoles		
Clotrimazole	Cream, lotion, solution	Rx or OTC
Econazole	Cream	Rx
Ketoconazole	Cream, shampoo	Rx
Miconazole	Cream, powder, spray	OTC
Oxiconazole	Cream, lotion	Rx
Sulconazole	Cream, solution	Rx
Allylamines		
Butenafine	Cream	Rx
Naftifine	Cream, gel	Rx
Terbinafine	Cream	Rx
Miscellaneous		
Ciclopirox	Cream, lotion	Rx
Tolnaftate	Cream, gel, powder, solution, spray liquid, spray powder	OTC
Clioquinol	Cream, ointment	OTC
Triacetin	Cream, spray, solution	Rx
Undecylenic acid	Cream, ointment, powder, foam, soap	OTC

- Griseofulvin and ketoconazole were the drugs of choice before the availability of itraconazole and terbinafine. However, a prolonged treatment duration of 6 months is necessary, and cure rates are low and associated with high rates of relapse. Griseofulvin also has a high incidence of GI side effects such as nausea and abdominal pain. The side effects of ketoconazole (e.g., hepatotoxicity and endocrine effects) are also troublesome.
- The newer agents itraconazole and terbinafine have high activities against dermatophytes with low MIC values. Both agents are highly lipophilic and achieve high-drug concentrations in the infected nails, and therapeutic concentrations persist for months after treatment.
- Itraconazole is more active than terbinafine against infections caused by *Candida* species, and terbinafine is at least as effective as itraconazole in dermatophyte infections.
- Itraconazole requires an acidic gastric pH and food for optimal absorption, and steady-state concentrations are usually reached within 3 weeks after initiation of therapy. Because itraconazole is metabolized by cytochrome P450 3A4, enzyme inducers such as phenytoin and rifampin decrease itraconazole levels. Itraconazole inhibits CYP 450 3A4 enzymes, and concurrent administration with terfenadine (no longer marketed) or cisapride is contraindicated.[4]
- Terbinafine is a squalene epoxidase inhibitor. It is well absorbed, and food or gastric pH does not influence its absorption. It has a long elimination half-life of 22 days, and plasma concentrations are detectable for up to 3 months after treatment. It has a more favorable drug-interaction profile than itraconazole since it is a substrate of cytochrome P450 but does not induce or inhibit CYP 450 enzymes. Common side effects of terbinafine include GI upset, skin reactions, and loss of taste.[5]
- Few pharmacoeconomic analyses have been performed to compare the cost-effectiveness of itraconazole and terbinafine in the management of onychomycosis. Recent data suggest that terbinafine is probably more cost-effective than itraconazole due to its low cost and similar efficacy rates.
- If oral systemic therapy is unsuccessful or shorter duration of therapy is desired, avulsion of the nail plate may be useful as an adjunctive therapy. After removal of the nail plate, the course of antifungal therapy may be shortened with increased duration of remission.
- Topical therapy may be helpful in fungal infections of the nail. However, efficacy rates are low due to poor penetration of the medication into keratinous tissue.

Optimal Plan

4. What drug, dosage form, dose, schedule, and duration of therapy are best for this patient?

- Because this patient has both tinea pedis and onychomycosis unrelieved by tolnaftate and hydrocortisone cream, a different topical agent and an oral antifungal agent are warranted.
- Topical agents that are superior to tolnaftate include the azoles and allylamines. Since the patient is going to be started on terbinafine, one may want to use a topical azole cream such as clotrimazole cream 1% to cover for possible *Candida* species. The cream should be applied to affected areas twice daily for at least 2 weeks.
- As discussed, itraconazole or terbinafine is preferred over griseofulvin or ketoconazole due to the shorter duration of treatment and higher efficacy rates. Terbinafine is probably the best choice for this individual because he is taking omeprazole, which may decrease the absorption of itraconazole, and administration of itraconazole with acid juices is also prohibited because he cannot tolerate citrus juices. As stated above, the dose of terbinafine is 250 mg once daily for 12 weeks.
- Topical hydrocortisone cream should be discontinued because he has been using it for more than a month, and it has no antifungal activity.

Outcome Evaluation

5. What clinical and laboratory parameters are necessary to evaluate the therapy for achievement of the desired therapeutic outcome and to detect or prevent adverse effects?

Efficacy

- Itching should resolve within 1 to 2 weeks.
- Color and appearance of toenails should improve within 3 months.
- The degree of scaling on the plantar surfaces of the feet should improve within 1 month.

Adverse Effects

- Ask the patient about the presence of GI upset and loss of taste; the latter effect usually resolves on its own after 6 weeks of therapy.
- Hypersensitivity reactions such as skin rash, skin eruptions, and Stevens–Johnson syndrome may occur.
- Obtain baseline liver function tests (AST, ALT, alkaline phosphatase) and monitor for signs and symptoms of liver toxicity such as abdominal pain, dark urine, and jaundice. Drug discontinuation may be required if symptoms of hepatotoxicity develop when other etiologies are ruled out or if liver function tests rise 3 to 5 times higher than baseline values.

Patient Counseling

6. What information should be provided to the patient to enhance compliance, ensure successful therapy, and minimize adverse effects?

- Treatment of toenail infections requires at least 3 months of oral antifungal therapy. Cure rates are fairly high with the newer therapies such as terbinafine, but relapse is common.
- The onset of therapy is slow, and improvement in symptoms and appearance of toenails is usually not seen until 1 month after initiation of therapy.
- Take one 250-mg terbinafine tablet once daily with or without food.
- Common side effects of terbinafine include stomach upset and taste disturbance. These symptoms usually resolve a few weeks after initiation of therapy. Contact your physician immediately if you experience any rash, skin eruptions, or signs of liver toxicity such as abdominal pain, dark urine, and jaundice.
- Apply the clotrimazole topical cream twice daily (morning and evening) to the affected areas. Clean and dry the areas before each application. You will need to use this cream for at least 2 weeks.

- Non-drug therapies are essential to treatment success and prevention of relapse. Wear thick cotton socks and non-occlusive footwear such as leather shoes rather than vinyl shoes. Frequent changes are also necessary to maintain good foot hygiene. Because fungal infection of the feet is a contagious infection spread by infectious particles, avoid using communal bathing places, swimming pools, and saunas. A warm and humid environment favors the growth of fungus, so clean and dry your feet thoroughly after jogging. Air-dry your shoes and socks before re-wearing them.

References

1. Elewski BE, Hay RJ. Update on the management of onychomycosis: Highlights of the Third Annual International Summit on Cutaneous Antifungal Therapy. Clin Infect Dis 1996;23:305–313.
2. Odom R. Pathophysiology of dermatophyte infections. J Am Acad Dermatol 1993;28(5 Pt 1):S2–S7.
3. Gupta AK, Scher RK, De Doncker P. Current management of onychomycosis. Dermatol Clin 1997;15:121–135.
4. Como JA, Dismukes WE. Oral azole drugs as systemic antifungal therapy. N Engl J Med 1994;330:263–272.
5. Abdel-Rahman SM, Nahata MC. Oral terbinafine: A new antifungal agent. Ann Pharmacother 1997;31:445–456.

▶ Follow-up Questions

1. *What are the cardiovascular risk factors in this patient?*

   - Male and age > 45 years
   - Hypertension
   - Family history of premature cardiac disease

2. *How does his risk factor status affect your management of his hypercholesterolemia?*

   - Because his LDL is 175 mg/dL and he has multiple risk factors, he is at risk for heart disease. Since he has no established CAD and has ≥ 2 risk factors, his goal LDL for primary prevention therapy is <160 mg/dL.
   - According to the West of Scotland study on primary prevention of heart disease, pravastatin 40 mg/day reduced cardiovascular disease morbidity and mortality in patients with average LDL of 180 mg/dL. Therefore, pravastatin use is appropriate; since he has been on the 20 mg dose for more than 1 year, increasing the dose to 40 mg/day is warranted to maximize the benefits of pravastatin therapy.
   - An appropriate diet should also be encouraged, but adherence may be difficult because of his frequent traveling.

113 BACTERIAL VAGINOSIS

▶ Competition Among Bacteria (Level I)

Charles D. Ponte, PharmD, BCPS, CDE, FAPhA, FASHP, FCCP

A 20-year-old woman presents with clinical and laboratory findings consistent with bacterial vaginosis. In this disorder, the normal vaginal flora of *Lactobacilli* is replaced by a variety of aerobic and anaerobic bacterial species including *Gardnerella vaginalis*; the anaerobic gram-negative rods *Prevotella* spp., *Porphyromonas* spp., and *Bacteroides* spp.; *Peptostreptococcus* spp.; *Mycoplasma hominis*; *Ureaplasma urealyticum* and *Mobiluncus* spp. Appropriate treatment consists of oral metronidazole 500 mg twice daily for 7 days; a 2-gram single dose is an effective alternative regimen, but recurrence rates are higher. Oral clindamycin 300 mg twice daily for 7 days is as effective as oral metronidazole. Intravaginal preparations of both metronidazole and clindamycin are also available and may be preferred in certain circumstances.

▶ Questions

Problem Identification

1. a. *Create a list of the patient's drug-related problems.*

   - Asymptomatic, untreated bacterial vaginosis

   b. *What clinical or laboratory information indicates the presence of bacterial vaginosis (see Table 113–1)?*

   - Thin white discharge; the typical discharge is malodorous, thin, white or gray, adherent, and may be copious.
   - Positive whiff test (a fishy odor when vaginal secretions are mixed with 10% KOH; the test has an 80% positive detection rate).
   - Vaginal pH > 4.5 (normal pH is 3.8 to 4.2).
   - Absence of *Lactobacilli* (the normal predominance of *Lactobacilli* has been replaced by other bacteria).
   - Presence of clue cells (vaginal epithelial cells studded with coccobacilli).
   - The diagnosis of bacterial vaginosis cannot be made on the basis of patient symptoms alone. Microscopic examination of vaginal secretions typically reveals a lack of *Lactobacilli* and no mycelia, trichomonads, or leukocytes. At least 3 of the following findings must be present for the diagnosis: 1) a homogenous discharge; 2) a vaginal pH > 4.5; 3) a positive whiff test; and 4) the presence of clue cells.[1]

   c. *What is the pathophysiologic basis for the development of bacterial vaginosis?*

   - Normal vaginal flora is primarily composed of facultative hydrogen peroxide-producing *Lactobacilli*. In bacterial vaginosis, this normal vaginal ecosystem is disrupted. *Lactobacilli* are replaced with a variety of aerobic and anaerobic bacterial species including *Gardnerella vaginalis*; the anaerobic gram-negative rods

TABLE 113–1. Characteristics of Different Types of Vaginitis

Characteristic	Candida	Bacterial	Trichomonas	Chemical
Pruritus	++	+/–	+/–	++
Erythema	+	+/–	+/–	+
Abnormal discharge	+	+	+/–	–
Viscosity	Thick	Thin	Thick/thin	–
Color	White	Gray	White, yellow, green-gray	–
Odor	None	Foul, "fishy"	Malodorous	–
Description	Curd-like	Homogeneous	Frothy	–
pH	3.8–5.0	> 4.5	5.0–7.5	–
Diagnostic tests	KOH prep. shows long, thread-like fibers of mycelia microscopically	+ "whiff test," "clue cells"	Pear-shaped protozoa, cervical "strawberry" spots	–

Prevotella spp., *Porphyromonas* spp., and *Bacteroides* spp.; *Peptostreptococcus* spp.; *Mycoplasma hominis*; *Ureaplasma urealyticum* and *Mobiluncus* spp.[1–3]

d. *Could the patient's problem have been caused by drug therapy?*

- No. The use of birth control pills and antibiotics (e.g., doxycycline) has not been associated with the development of bacterial vaginosis.

Desired Outcome

2. *What are the goals of pharmacotherapy in this case?*

- Eradicate the causative organisms responsible for bacterial vaginosis
- Ameliorate the patient's symptoms or complaints
- Minimize adverse effects and drug interactions from the recommended drug therapy
- Prevent the subsequent development of pelvic inflammatory disease and other gynecologic illnesses (e.g., plasma-cell endometritis and cervical intra-epithelial neoplasia)
- Prevent recurrence of bacterial vaginosis

Therapeutic Alternatives

3. a. *What feasible pharmacotherapeutic alternatives are available for the treatment of bacterial vaginosis?*

- Although it is typically not life threatening, bacterial vaginosis is amenable to either topic or systemic drug therapy.
- *Oral metronidazole (Flagyl, generics)* is considered the drug of choice for bacterial vaginosis, even though it is not FDA approved for this indication.[4] The drug is active against most pathogens associated with bacterial vaginosis (including *Mobiluncus* spp. and gram-negative anaerobes). The usual dosage is 500 mg po BID for 7 days. Cure rates are typically > 90%. A 2-gram single dose is an alternative regimen and is nearly as effective, but recurrence rates are higher. The FDA has recently approved an extended-release formulation of the drug (Flagyl ER 750 mg) for the treatment of bacterial vaginosis. A single 750-mg daily oral dose is administered on an empty stomach for 7 days.
- *Metronidazole 0.75% vaginal gel (MetroGel-Vaginal)* was approved by the FDA in 1992 for the treatment of bacterial vaginosis. It exhibits comparable efficacy to oral metronidazole. The usual dose is one full applicator intravaginally twice daily for 5 days. Although the drug is well tolerated, *Candida* cervicitis (6% incidence) has been associated with its use. The drug should be used with caution in pregnancy and in those who consume alcohol.
- *Oral clindamycin (Cleocin, generics)* is an equally effective alternative to oral metronidazole, but it also does not carry an FDA-approved indication for this use. It may be preferred over metronidazole in pregnancy and in patients refusing to abstain from alcohol. The usual dose is 300 mg BID for 7 days.
- *Clindamycin 2% vaginal cream (Cleocin Vaginal Cream)* was approved by the FDA in 1992 for the treatment of bacterial vaginosis. It produces cure rates comparable to oral metronidazole regimens. The usual dose is one full applicator (100 mg clindamycin/5 g cream) intravaginally at bedtime for 7 days. A recent study suggested that an abbreviated 3-day regimen may also be effective. Although the drug is well tolerated, *Candida* cervicitis (11% incidence) has been associated with its use. Importantly, the preparation contains a mineral oil vehicle that can adversely affect the strength of latex condoms. Despite minimal systemic absorption, intravaginal clindamycin is not considered a suitable alternative for the treatment of bacterial vaginosis in pregnancy because pre-term deliveries have been reported.
- Triple-sulfa vaginal cream, oral antibiotics (e.g., tetracycline, erythromycin, ampicillin, amoxicillin), acetic acid gel, and povidone-iodine douches are not recommended because they have been shown to exhibit poor efficacy in the treatment of bacterial vaginosis.
- Intravaginal boric acid suppositories, which require extemporaneous compounding by a pharmacist, are not recommended because efficacy has not been established in bacterial vaginosis.

b. *What economic, psychosocial, and ethical considerations are applicable to this patient?*

- Because bacterial vaginosis has not been definitively linked to sexual activity, there is no requirement to treat the sexual partners of this patient.
- Because she is a college student, the cost of therapy becomes an important consideration. The cheapest therapy is generic oral

metronidazole (multiple or single doses). Also, if she continues to drink alcohol, the use of either oral or topical metronidazole may be contraindicated.

Optimal Plan

4. a. *What drug, dosage form, dose, schedule, and duration of therapy are best for this patient?*

- Oral metronidazole 500 mg po BID for 7 days may be the treatment of choice. The drug is active against the mixed microbial flora associated with bacterial vaginosis, and the cure rate exceeds 90%. Because it is available generically, the cost of treatment is compatible with the financial status of a college student. A 2-gram single dose of metronidazole would be an acceptable alternative if the patient expresses adherence concerns about a 7-day regimen or wishes to continue drinking alcohol. Importantly, pregnancy should be ruled-out before initiating metronidazole.

b. *What alternatives would be appropriate if the initial therapy fails or cannot be used?*

- Metronidazole 0.75% vaginal gel in a dose of one full applicator intravaginally BID for 5 days is an acceptable alternative. The preparation has also been shown to be effective in a single daily dose for 5 days. Intravaginal metronidazole is equally effective to oral metronidazole and may be preferred to the oral drug if the patient is pregnant, continues to drink alcohol, or experiences gastrointestinal distress with the oral tablets. However, the gel may be unacceptable to some patients due to the application technique required or the perceived messiness of the preparation.
- Oral clindamycin 300 mg po BID for 7 days or topical clindamycin 2% cream 100 mg intravaginally once daily for 7 days are also acceptable alternatives. A 3-day course of topical clindamycin is also effective. The drug has equal efficacy to metronidazole and may be preferred in patients who refuse to abstain from alcohol or where pregnancy cannot be ruled out.

Outcome Evaluation

5. *What clinical and laboratory parameters are necessary to evaluate the therapy for achievement of the desired therapeutic outcome and to detect or prevent adverse effects?*

Efficacy

- *Clinical parameters.* Resolution of malodorous discharge, especially after intercourse; resolution of mild, irritative vaginal or vulvar complaints (if present). Clinical improvement should be noted during therapy and uniformly at the conclusion of the treatment course. Further clinic follow-up is unwarranted if signs and symptoms resolve.
- *Laboratory parameters.* Although not used to routinely guide follow-up, microscopic examination of vaginal secretions should reveal the presence of *Lactobacilli* and a lack of clue cells; vaginal pH should be < 4.5.

Adverse Effects

- *Oral metronidazole:* GI distress, metallic taste, discoloration of urine (brown), vaginal candidiasis, lightheadedness, dizziness, and disulfiram-like reaction with alcohol.

- *Vaginal metronidazole:* vaginal itching or irritation, vaginal candidiasis, abdominal pain, irritation of the penis of the male partner, and painful intercourse.
- *Oral clindamycin:* GI distress, diarrhea, rectal or vaginal itching, skin rash, sore throat or fever, and unexplained bruising or bleeding.
- *Vaginal clindamycin:* vaginal itching or irritation, vaginal candidiasis, abdominal pain, skin irritation or rash, and painful intercourse.

Patient Counseling

6. *What information should be provided to the patient to enhance compliance, ensure successful therapy, and minimize adverse effects?*

Metronidazole

- This medication eliminates bacteria and other organisms that are responsible for your vaginal infection.
- It should be taken by mouth twice a day for 7 days. Follow the prescription label directions carefully. Take this with food to minimize upset stomach.
- If you have intercourse while taking this medication, your partner should consider wearing a condom to avoid possible reinfection. However, the sexual transmission of bacterial vaginosis is unlikely.
- Wear clean cotton underclothing and/or pantyhose with cotton crotches.
- Take all of the medication, even though you may feel fine or have no symptoms. Contact your doctor if your symptoms do not get better or if they worsen.
- Do not drink alcohol while taking this medication and for 2 days after your last dose.
- If you forget a dose, take it as soon as you remember and evenly space out the remaining doses. Do not take a double dose.
- Common side effects include nausea, metallic taste, urine discoloration (dark or reddish-brown), rash, or vaginal irritation or discharge. Consult your physician or me if these become troublesome or severe.
- Do not let anyone else use this medication.
- Keep the medication in the original container and out of the reach of children.

▶ Follow-up Questions

1. *What is the most likely cause of this patient's vaginal candidiasis?*

- The use of oral metronidazole has been associated with the development of *Candida* superinfection. The temporal relationship between the initiation of metronidazole and the development of symptoms strongly suggests the drug as the cause. However, it is important to rule out other reasons, including inadequately treated bacterial vaginosis, recent use of broad-spectrum antibiotics, high estrogen content oral contraceptives, HIV infection, diabetes, and orogenital sex.

2. *What other issues should be addressed with the patient during this follow-up visit?*

- Prevention strategies: consistent use of condoms (despite use of oral contraceptives) and avoidance of multiple sexual partners if possible.
- Treatment issues: the routine treatment of sexual partners is not

presently recommended for women experiencing bacterial vaginosis or vulvovaginal candidiasis.

3. What is the role of the pharmacist in the management of patients with infectious vaginitis?

- Consultation and triage: the community pharmacist should thoroughly question the patient who presents with vaginal complaints; referral can be made to a physician for further diagnostic evaluation, or an appropriate non-prescription product may be recommended. Patient misunderstandings and confusion can be remedied.
- Information source: provision of information about women's health care concerns can be provided to the public and patients using a variety of media tools (e.g., pamphlets and videotapes).
- Patient education: discuss proper use of medication and prevention strategies and ensure adherence to medication regimen.
- Resource to health care professionals: sharing unique knowledge about women's health care product selection, therapeutic alternatives, and monitoring parameters.

References

1. Joesoef MR, Schmid GP. Bacterial vaginosis: Review of treatment options and potential clinical indications for therapy. Clin Infect Dis 1995;20(suppl 1): S72–S79.
2. Sobel JD. Vaginitis. N Engl J Med 1997;337:1896–1903.
3. Ries AJ. Treatment of vaginal infections: Candidiasis, bacterial vaginosis, and trichomoniasis. J Am Pharm Assoc 1997;NS37:563–569.
4. Centers for Disease Control and Prevention. Diseases characterized by vaginal discharge. 1998 guidelines for treatment of sexually transmitted diseases. MMWR 1998;47(RR-01):70–79. www.cdc.gov

114 ANTIMICROBIAL PROPHYLAXIS FOR SURGERY

▶ To Be Able to Walk Down the Aisle
(Level II)

Susan J. Skledar, RPh, MPH
Paige Robbins Gross, RPh

A 68-year-old woman with severe osteoarthritis of the left knee is scheduled to undergo a total knee replacement. Pre- and post-operative antimicrobial prophylaxis and post-operative pain management are the two drug-related problems addressed in this case. First-generation cephalosporins (e.g., cefazolin) are the recommended agents for "clean" orthopedic procedures, but this patient is allergic to both penicillins and cephalosporins. In this situation, clindamycin is preferred over vancomycin due to concerns of antimicrobial resistance, adverse effects, and cost. Prophylaxis is given within 2 hours prior to the procedure and for 24 to 48 hours post-operatively. Initial pain management should consist of IV opioid analgesics, which can be changed to oral opioids and then peripherally acting analgesics as the patient recovers.

▶ Questions

Problem Identification

1. a. Prepare a complete drug-related problem list for the patient.

- Impending left TKR from degenerative osteoarthritis that will require surgical antimicrobial prophylaxis.
- Post-surgical analgesia for control of pain will be required.
- Chronic, stable problems not requiring intervention at this time include: 1) asthma, controlled with Serevent (salmeterol) and Aerobid (flunisolide); and 2) postmenopausal state treated with Premarin (conjugated estrogens).

b. What are the risk factors for surgical wound infection (SWI) in patients undergoing surgical procedures?

- Surgical wound infections depend on patient-related and procedure-related factors.[1-3] (See textbook Chapter 112.)
- Patient-related factors that can contribute to SWI include diabetes mellitus, chronic immunosuppression, advanced age, cancer, recent corticosteroid use, prolonged hospitalization, preoperative hospitalization, pre-existing unresolved infection prior to surgery, and malnutrition.
- Procedure-related factors that may contribute to SWI include type/length of surgery, operative technique, surgeon skill, National Research Council (NRC) surgical procedure risk classification, pre-operative preparation of surgical site, and pre-operative antimicrobials given > 2 hours before surgical incision.

c. What organisms are the most likely causes of infection in orthopedic surgery patients?

- Orthopedic surgery is typically considered a "clean" surgery (the term "clean" suggests that antimicrobial prophylaxis may not be necessary), but when prosthetic devices are implanted, prophylaxis has been shown to be beneficial.
- The five most common organisms seen in SWI include *Staphylococcus aureus*, *Enterococcus* spp., coagulase-negative *Staphylococci*, *Escherichia coli*, and *Pseudomonas* spp.
- When determining adequate prophylaxis for orthopedic surgery in particular, commonly encountered skin flora organisms that may cause SWI include *S. aureus* and *S. epidermidis*. Infrequently, gram-negative anaerobes may also cause infection.

d. What recent event in this patient's PMH should be a caution for close monitoring of this patient for postoperative SWI?

- The patient had a previous SWI 6 months ago, an infected left knee after arthroscopy, which was treated with IV vancomycin for 6 weeks.

Desired Outcome

2. What are the therapeutic goals for this patient?

- The overall goal is optimal management to prevent SWI and postoperative complications
- Prevention of pain and discomfort
- Improving patient mobility and quality of life with osteoarthritis after surgery
- Continued control of her asthma is also an important goal

Therapeutic Alternatives

3. a. What non-pharmacologic interventions should be considered in this patient pre- and post-surgery?

- Prior to surgery, the patient should be informed of the risks of the procedure and expectations for the post-operative course (including expected recovery time, how to watch for signs and symptoms of infection, and the importance of postoperative rehabilitation).
- Non-pharmacologic interventions essential to minimizing SWI risk include maintaining sterile technique, proper preparation of surgical site (antisepsis, hair removal by clipping), use of closed drains, and confirmation of lack of infection prior to operation.

b. What pharmacotherapeutic alternatives are available to minimize post-operative wound infection in this type of surgery?

- Prophylactic parenteral antimicrobials have been shown to be protective against SWI.[1–5] The antimicrobial should be administered as close to the incision time as possible and no more than 2 hours before the surgical incision to have the greatest effect on reducing the risk of SWI.[1–4] An often used dose timing recommendation is at induction of anesthesia.
- If there is excessive blood loss or if the procedure is prolonged, repeat dosing is indicated.
- *Cephalosporins* are widely chosen for prophylaxis due to coverage against commonly encountered organisms, favorable pharmacokinetics, and relative safety. First-generation cephalosporins (e.g., cefazolin) are preferred over second-generation (e.g., cefuroxime, cefoxitin, cefotetan) and third-generation agents (e.g., cefotaxime, ceftazidime, ceftriaxone) due to similar efficacy, narrower spectrum, and lower cost.
- *Vancomycin* and *clindamycin* are two additional options for prophylaxis in penicillin-allergic patients (see Question 4 for additional discussion).

c. What pharmacotherapeutic alternatives are available to manage post-operative pain for this patient?

- Post-operative pain is at its peak immediately after surgery and lessens with time. Systemic opioids are generally used in the immediate post-operative period, and then patients are gradually transitioned to peripherally acting analgesics until they have recovered and their pain is relieved.
- IV administration is the parenteral route of choice after major surgical procedures. The oral route, being both inexpensive and convenient, is indicated as soon as the patient can tolerate oral intake. Oral analgesia is the cornerstone of pain management in the ambulatory surgical patient population.
- Around-the-clock pain relief is essential in the immediate post-operative period. This can be changed to a PRN schedule late in the post-operative course.
- Options for immediate post-operative pain management in this patient include patient-controlled analgesia (PCA) or continuous epidural analgesia. The choice of technique may vary depending on practice standards at individual institutions. Opioids commonly administered via the PCA or epidural route include morphine and fentanyl. Morphine is traditionally the standard of therapy for opioid analgesia for moderate to severe pain. When converting to oral intake, care must be taken to use equianalgesic doses to estimate the new oral dose. In addition, modifications to the initial estimate will be needed based on the specific drugs involved and the patient's response.

Optimal Plan

4. What antimicrobial drugs, dosage form, schedule, and duration of therapy are best for this patient?

- Antimicrobial prophylaxis is recommended for a 24 or 48 hour duration for total joint replacement. Either duration is appropriate, and the decision is generally institution specific.
- Regarding agent selection, prophylaxis should be designed to cover for the most likely organisms that cause post-surgical wound infection. Severity of patient allergies and institution sensitivity patterns also are key considerations in agent selection.
- This patient has penicillin and cephalexin allergies with a reaction of severe hives. As mentioned previously, vancomycin and clindamycin are viable options for penicillin-allergic patients. Routine use of vancomycin for prophylaxis is not recommended due to resistance development, adverse effects, and cost.[4] Vancomycin may be considered if an institution has a high incidence of MRSA or methicillin-resistant, coagulase-negative Staphylococci.
- Thus, clindamycin is the most appropriate antimicrobial prophylaxis for this patient. It has similar gram-positive coverage to cefazolin, and for certain surgical procedures, clindamycin may be preferred over cefazolin due to better biliary penetration and better gram-positive and anaerobic coverage. The recommended regimen is clindamycin 600 mg IV at induction of anesthesia and then 600 mg IV Q 8 H × 24 or 48 hours postoperatively.
- In patients without penicillin-allergy, cefazolin 1 g IV within 2 hours before the incision is the recommended pre-surgical antimicrobial regimen for orthopedic procedures.[3,4] Cefazolin 1 g IV Q 8 H × 24 hours is a standard post-operative regimen.
- Third-generation cephalosporins, although they have a longer half-life and broader gram-negative coverage, are not recommended for prophylaxis due to emergence of resistance, higher cost, and less activity against gram-positive and anaerobic organisms.
- If an indwelling drain is placed, this should be viewed as not only a route for infective fluids to exit the knee area, but also as a potential route for infection to originate. The literature is controversial as to whether to continue antibiotics until the drain is removed. Consensus has not yet been reached on this issue. It is important to remember that post-operative infections can surface up to a full year after insertion of a prosthetic device.

Outcome Evaluation

5. What clinical and laboratory parameters are necessary to evaluate therapy for achievement of desired outcomes and to detect and prevent adverse drug reactions?

Efficacy

- SWI is the second most common nosocomial infection among hospitalized patients.[2] Immediate concerns post-operatively are stabilization of the patient and adequate pain control enabling the move to a general post-surgical unit. The focus of monitoring then shifts to signs of post-surgical infection, continued pain control, and rehabilitation.
- Clear liquids will be encouraged immediately post-operatively, and a regular diet will be advanced as tolerated beginning on the day after surgery.
- Monitoring parameters for volume status and the need for transfusion or additional fluids include hemoglobin, hematocrit, and vital signs (temperature, pulse, respiratory rate). A CBC is obtained daily and BUN, creatinine, and electrolytes can be checked at least on postoperative day 1. Intake and output should be monitored regularly (e.g., each shift, or until the patient is tolerating oral liquids well and bladder function returns to normal).
- Once the patient is stabilized, she will be moved to a general patient care unit. Vital signs are measured frequently, initially Q 4 H and then progressing to Q 12 H. Temperatures > 38.5°C should be reported immediately to the doctor, as this can be the first indication of an SWI.
- Hydration will continue until the patient is tolerating oral liquids, which will be slowly encouraged upon arrival to the general unit. Drainage will be collected, and the need for re-infusion as well as drain removal will be determined by the surgeon.
- Pain service consultation may be obtained for patient management for the first post-operative day.
- An x-ray of the knee joint will also be performed in the recovery room to assure proper alignment and placement of the new joint and once again on discharge day to assure proper alignment.
- The Foley catheter is normally discontinued in 24 hours.
- The surgical dressing will be monitored very closely on the day of surgery and on post-operative days on a Q 2 H to Q 4 H basis. The incision and dressing will be changed daily for the first several postoperative days, and then as needed. When the dressing is changed, it should be checked for signs of heavy bleeding or pus drainage, and the incision should be checked for redness, swelling, and excessive tenderness to light touch.
- The patient will be required to wear elastic stockings at all times post-operatively to prevent deep venous thrombosis until he or she becomes ambulatory.
- Pain control should be monitored by having the patient use a verbal pain rating scale (e.g., 0–10, where 0 is no pain and 10 is the worst possible pain). A patient report of post-operative pain should be believed, while the possibility of excessive sedation with liberal opioid use should be cautioned. By post-operative day 2 or 3, an oral pain regimen is usually initiated using a medication such as oxycodone/acetaminophen, and allowing for a range of doses (1 to 2 tablets) in a range of time (Q 4 to 6 H), so that the patient may increase or decrease requests for medication based on the severity of pain.
- Physical therapy will usually be initiated on postoperative day 1, whereby the patient and therapist begin to develop a treatment plan and strategy for rehabilitation and review exercises at the bedside in the morning, and begin ambulation of the patient by evening.
- Occupational therapy will also begin on postoperative day 2 or 3 to address activities of daily living.

Adverse Effects

- Gastrointestinal distress, specifically nausea, vomiting, and constipation, caused by the antimicrobials or the pain medications should be monitored by observation and questioning of the patient and can be treated with the use of antiemetics, stool softeners, and a laxative if needed.

Patient Counseling

6. *What information should be provided to the patient to enhance compliance, ensure successful therapy, and minimize adverse events?*

General Information

- It is extremely important for you to watch for any signs of infection. These signs include fever (an increased temperature), not feeling like you are getting well (malaise), or any redness, swelling, or discharge from where your knee was cut. A home health care nurse will be checking on your incision, but contact your physician immediately if you notice any of these signs.
- As a precaution, please notify your physician before undergoing any dental procedures, including a simple cleaning. Your doctor may want you to take a dose of antibiotics prior to your dental appointment as a precaution against infection.
- Since you are not at high risk for developing blood clots, your doctor has chosen not to put you on any oral medication to thin your blood. By doing all of the necessary physical therapy and exercises discussed with you, you can help decrease the chance of developing any complications from blood clots.

Opioid Analgesic (Vicodin)

- Your doctor has prescribed a pain medication called Vicodin. You are to take 1 or 2 tablets every 4 to 6 hours as you need it. If your pain is more intense in the morning, you may want to take 2 tablets then, or if your pain is most intense before and after your therapy sessions, this may be where you would take 2 tablets for several doses and then go back to 1 tablet.
- This medication can make you drowsy, so use caution when performing your everyday tasks. Do not drive while you are taking this medication.
- Take this medicine with food or milk to minimize any stomach upset.
- Other possible side effects include dry mouth and constipation. Contact your doctor or me if any of these become intolerable.
- This medicine contains acetaminophen, so do not take any extra acetaminophen unless checking with your doctor or me first.

References

1. Classen DC, Evans RS, Pestotnik SL, et al. The timing of prophylactic administration of antibiotics and the risk of surgical-wound infection. N Engl J Med 1992;326:281–286.
2. Lizan-Garcia M, Garcia-Caballero J, Asensio-Vegas A. Risk factors for surgical-

wound infection in general surgery: A prospective study. Infect Control Hosp Epidemiol 1997;18:310–315.
3. Page CP, Bohnen JM, Fletcher JR, et al. Antimicrobial prophylaxis for surgical wounds. Guidelines for clinical care. Arch Surg 1993;128:79–88.
4. Antimicrobial prophylaxis in surgery. Med Lett 1997;39:97–102.
5. Silver A, Eichorn A, Kral J, et al. Timeliness and use of antibiotic prophylaxis in selected inpatient surgical procedures. The Antibiotic Prophylaxis Study Group. Am J Surg 1996;171:548–552.
6. Deacon JM, Pagliaro AJ, Zelicof SB, et al. Prophylactic use of antibiotics for procedures after total joint replacement. J Bone Joint Surg 1996;78:1755–1770.

115 PEDIATRIC IMMUNIZATION

▶ Ensuring a Healthy Start   (Level II)

Daniel T. Casto, PharmD, FCCP

A 6.5-month-old infant is seen for a follow-up evaluation 3 weeks after experiencing a generalized tonic-clonic seizure thought to be due to high fever associated with otitis media. The patient has received no immunizations other than hepatitis B vaccine, given at birth. The focus of the case is directed toward beginning necessary immunization and ensuring that all series are completed. Several commercial alternatives are available for some of the vaccines, and knowledge of the differences among them is important in ensuring optimal therapy for this child. Counseling of the child's mother on the adverse effects that may be expected and ways to minimize them is required. The case highlights the psychosocial factors that may serve as barriers to the successful completion of a full vaccination schedule.

▶ Questions

Problem Identification

1. Create a list of the patient's drug-related problems.

- Patient is in need of immunization. As long as immunizations are incomplete, the child remains susceptible to potentially life-threatening illnesses. Completion of recommended series of vaccination will drastically reduce the risk of serious illness.
- The patient's small size and low weight, although not grossly abnormal, may be the result of poor nutrition, considering the financial problems this family faces.

Desired Outcome

2. What immediate and long-term goals are reasonable in this case?

- Begin immunization series in this child today; continue regular follow-up to completion.
- Refer to social services for possible enrollment in WIC, which will provide nutrition supplementation. WIC is a federally funded program that provides dairy products (including infant formula) to needy women and young children. The WIC program also provides nutrition education and has assumed a greater role in matters such as screening for needed vaccines and administering them when patients come in for their nutrition products.
- Educate the family about available medical resources and the importance of health maintenance visits.
- Complete needed immunization in all family members.

Therapeutic Alternatives

3. What vaccines should be administered to this child today? (Helpful

hint: The following Web sites may be useful in answering this and other questions: www.cdc.gov/nip and www.aap.org)

- *Diphtheria toxoid/tetanus toxoid/acellular pertussis vaccine (DTaP).* Historically, a combination that included "whole-cell" pertussis vaccine (DTwP) was used. However, DTaP has been shown to cause fewer adverse effects than DTwP. However, DTwP is an acceptable alternative if DTaP is not available. Several DTaP vaccines are commercially available (Acel-Immune; Infanrix; Tripedia), but they differ in their FDA-approved uses. At the time of this writing, not all DTaP vaccines have been approved for use in the entire series.[1]
- *Haemophilus influenzae, type b conjugate vaccine (Hib-conjugate).* Four different Hib conjugate products are available in the United States. They each contain the outer polysaccharide capsule of Hib (polyribosylribitol phosphate, or "PRP"), but they differ in the protein carrier to which it is covalently linked.
  ✓ PRP-OMP (PedvaxHIB): the carrier is an outer membrane protein from *Neisseria meningitidis.*
  ✓ PRP-D (ProHIBit): the carrier is diphtheria toxoid.
  ✓ PRP-T (Omni-HIB): the carrier is tetanus toxoid.
  ✓ HbOC (HibTITER): the PRP has been modified to an oligosaccharide, and the carrier is a non-toxic mutant diphtheria toxin.
  In this child there is only a choice of three products, because PRP-D is not immunogenic enough to be used below 12 months of age. This product is being phased out and replaced by the other alternatives but may still be in some inventories. The use of PRP-D or PRP-T does not change the need for giving diphtheria or tetanus toxoids; DTaP or DTwP is still indicated.[1]
- *Oral poliovirus vaccine (OPV; Orimmune) or inactivated poliovirus vaccine (IPV; IPOL).* For years, OPV was the preferred polio vaccine in the United States because it confers intestinal as well as systemic immunity. However, it is a live vaccine and has the potential

to cause paralytic polio in the vaccine recipient (although the risk is very low). IPV, which is an inactivated vaccine, is the polio vaccine of choice for individuals who are immunocompromised or are receiving immunosuppressive medications. The risk of vaccine-associated paralytic polio (VAPP) is greatest after the first dose of OPV; therefore, in immunocompetent children, the preferred regimen uses IPV for the first two doses of the polio series. However, an all-IPV or all-OPV schedule is also acceptable.[1]

- *Hepatitis B vaccine (HepB; Recombivax HB and Engerix-B).* This represents a continuation of the HepB series that was started in the hospital at the time of the child's birth. The two different brands of HepB differ in their strengths and recommended doses, and care must be exercised to ensure that the appropriate dose is being administered.[1]

Optimal Plan

4. a. What immunization schedule should be followed for this patient?

- This child's immunization status cannot be brought up-to-date at a single clinic visit; multiple visits will be necessary. Assuming compliance with scheduled clinic visits, the schedule in Table 115–1 below is recommended.
- The number of Hib-conjugate doses required depends upon the commercial product used. PRP-OMP requires a 2-dose primary series with a booster at age 12 to 15 months. PRP-T and HbOC require a 3-dose primary series, with a booster at age 12 to 15 months. This patient does not get the entire regimen, due to the age at which the series is started.[1]
- Comvax (PRP-OMP + HepB), Tetramune (DTwP + HbOC), and ActHib (DTaP + PRP-T) are multi-antigen products that can be used to minimize the number of injections necessary at any one visit. The introduction of combination products reduces the number of injections required and should help increase parents' compliance with recommended immunization schedules.
- The exact timing of HepB vaccine administration is less important than assuring that all 3 doses are given.
- In this patient with a history of febrile convulsions, every effort should be made to use DTaP rather than DTwP. DTaP causes fewer local side effects as well as less frequent and less severe fever. Using DTaP should be associated with a lower risk of post-vaccination seizures, since fewer patients have significant fever after this vaccine, and since most DTP-associated seizures are febrile convulsions.[1]
- In many cases DTaP, MMR, Hep B, and VAR will all be administered at the same clinic visit. However, this case is slightly different than the routine schedule. The fourth dose of DTaP can be given as early as 12 months of age, *provided* that there has been an interval of at least 6 months since the third dose. In this child's case, the necessary 6-month interval will not have occurred by age 15 months; therefore, the fourth DTaP is not scheduled for the visit at 12 to 15 months of age.[1]
- Post-vaccination febrile reactions can be reduced by administering prophylactic acetaminophen at the time of DTP vaccination and for 24 hours after the dose. Lowering the risk of fever in this patient should reduce the risk of febrile convulsions.

b. In addition to vaccination, what additional therapy is warranted in this case, considering the patient's dietary history and laboratory values?

- The patient's diet does not contain sufficient iron to prevent development of iron deficiency anemia. This can be corrected through the use of iron-fortified infant formula (Enfamil with Iron; Similac with Iron) or ferrous sulfate (ferrous sulfate drops; FeoSol). Elemental iron 1 mg/kg/day should be given for the first year of life.

Outcome Evaluation

5. How should the response to the pharmacotherapeutic plan be assessed?

Documentation of Vaccination

- The immunization status of every child should be determined each time he or she is seen by a health care provider. Parents' recollection of what vaccinations a child has had is often inaccurate. Therefore, the history should be confirmed by reviewing the patient's personal immunization card, the medical record, or an up-to-date immunization registry in which the patient's records are listed. In the clinic setting, an immunization record should be a prominent part of each patient's record.
- Reminder systems (e.g., post cards) are used by some clinics and physician offices to encourage compliance with return visits for vaccinations.

Assessment of the Response to Therapy

- Serologic response to vaccination does not have to be confirmed because the vaccines in use today are highly immunogenic. However, confirmation of administration of each of the required doses is important. The mother should be taught to bring the child's immunization record to every doctor visit, even if she does not think that any shots are due.

TABLE 115–1. Immunization Schedule

Visit Number	DTaP	Hib-conj	Polio	HepB	MMR	Varicella
1 (today)	Dose 1	Dose 1	Dose 1	Dose 2		
2 (2 mo from visit 1)	Dose 2	Dose 2	Dose 2			
3 (2 mo from visit 2)	Dose 3	Dose 3	Dose 3			
4 (age 12 to 15 months)				Dose 3	Dose 1	Dose 1
5 (6 mo from visit 3)	Dose 4					
6 (age 4 to 6 years)	Dose 5		Dose 4		Dose 2	

- The response to any nutrition intervention can be assessed at periodic clinic visits by plotting growth parameters (height, weight, FOC) and hematologic screening tests (hemoglobin, hematocrit).

Assessment of Adverse Events

- The mother should be asked about any side effects to previous doses of vaccine, because serious reactions to previous doses may indicate a need to avoid subsequent use.
- Federal law requires that parents have the potential benefits and risks explained to them prior to vaccination of their children. To assist with the explanation of risks, the Centers for Disease Control and Prevention (CDC) has developed Vaccine Information Pamphlets (VIPs) that explain the risk of adverse events at about an eighth-grade reading level. After the risks have been explained, signed informed parental consent must be obtained prior to administration of any federally purchased vaccine. Even if the vaccine was not purchased with federal funds, it is highly recommended that informed consent be obtained.
- No vaccine is totally free from side effects. The most common adverse events associated with the vaccines that this infant needs are as follows.
    - ✓ DTP: redness, swelling, soreness at the injection site, fever, fussiness, seizures (related to fever), inconsolable crying for more than 3 hours. These adverse effects can occur with either DTwP or DtaP but are less common with the acellular products.
    - ✓ Hib: local reactions at the injection site.
    - ✓ OPV: none that are common; rare symptoms of polio (which can lead to permanent paralysis).
    - ✓ IPV: local reactions at the injection site.
    - ✓ HepB: redness, soreness at the injection site.
    - ✓ MMR: stinging on injection; redness, soreness at the injection site, fever, rash (seen 1 to 2 weeks after vaccination), joint stiffness (more common in susceptible post-pubertal females).
- Any serious side effects are to be reported to the Vaccine Adverse Event Reporting System (VAERS), a program run by the U.S. Department of Health and Human Services. The VAERS toll-free telephone number to obtain reporting forms and information is 1-(800)-822-7967.
- This child's history of seizures is not a contraindication to DTwP or DTaP administration. The family history of seizures is also not a contraindication.

Patient Counseling

6. *What important information about vaccination needs to be explained to this infant's mother?*

- Vaccination is one of the most important things for keeping your children well. Without the shots they need, they could get very sick. Although it seems like a lot of shots, they are all important, and you should see that all of your children get every shot that they need. It is also important that they get their shots on time.
- Bring your baby's shot card with you every time you go to see the doctor or nurse, even if you don't think they will need it.
- Some of the shots may cause your baby to have a fever. You can help prevent the fever by giving her this acetaminophen (fever medicine) every 6 hours for the first day after her shots.
- The shots may also cause some redness and swelling where the needle goes in. This usually lasts only a couple of days.
- If your baby starts acting differently (being a lot more fussy, being very sleepy, or having seizures) for several days after the vaccination, call you doctor, pharmacist, or nurse.
- Adults also need to have some shots to keep them healthy. If you would like, we can see what shots you and your husband may need, as well as taking care of your children's needs.

Reference

1. American Academy of Pediatrics. Active and passive immunization. In: Red Book—Report of the Committee on Infectious Diseases, 24th ed. Elk Grove Village, IL, American Academy of Pediatrics, 1997:1–71.

116 CYTOMEGALOVIRUS (CMV) RETINITIS

▶ **The Case for Compliance** (Level II)

Winnie M. Yu, PharmD, BCPS

A 27-year-old man with a 2-year history of HIV infection presents with blurred vision and "floaters" in his right eye. He has missed follow-up clinic visits and has been non-adherent with his antiretroviral therapy regimen. Funduscopic examination reveals retinal changes only in the right eye that are consistent with CMV retinitis. He has no signs or symptoms of systemic CMV disease. Therapeutic alternatives include ganciclovir (IV or ocular implant), IV foscarnet, and IV cidofovir. Oral ganciclovir should be used only in patients with early stage disease who do not have IV access. Because the patient has unilateral localized CMV retinitis without systemic involvement, the ganciclovir ocular implant may be the optimal choice for this patient. The patient should be followed clinically for progression of retinitis, and monthly ophthalmologic examinations should be performed. The patient should also be evaluated for signs of systemic CMV disease. Strict adherence to the antiretroviral regimen is critical in maintaining immune function and preventing future episodes of CMV and other HIV-related opportunistic infections.

▶ **Questions**

Problem Identification

1. a. *Create a list of this patient's drug-related problems.*

- CMV retinitis requiring antiviral therapy.
- Advanced AIDS disease with a low CD4 count and high viral load.
- Non-adherence to antiretroviral therapy, contributing to the high viral load.
- Oral thrush while receiving systemic antifungal therapy without an initial trial of topical therapy.

- Depression treated with sertraline, which may contribute to his poor appetite.
- Poor appetite/weight loss, requiring nutritional intervention.

b. *What are the signs and symptoms of CMV retinitis in this patient?*

- *Signs.* Testing by the Snellen chart indicates decreased visual acuity in the right eye. The funduscopic exam reveals unilateral disease of the right eye. The presence of white, fluffy lesions with focal hemorrhages on the retina is a classic presentation of CMV retinitis. A positive CMV antibody usually means that the host has been exposed previously to the virus, but it does not necessarily indicate the presence of active disease.
- *Symptoms.* Blurred vision, floaters.
- CMV retinitis can be manifested as unilateral or bilateral disease. For patients with unilateral disease, the frequencies of CMV retinitis in the contralateral eye and other organs are 50% and 30% at 6 months, respectively.
- Other common symptoms of CMV retinitis not noted in this patient include loss of visual fields, scotomata (blind spots), and photopsia (flashing lights). Other funduscopic presentations include retinal detachment or atrophy of the retina.

c. *What are the risk factors for CMV retinitis in this patient?*

- CD4 counts of 15 cells/mm^3. The disease usually occurs in patients who have CD4 counts < 50 cells/mm^3.
- Advanced HIV infection secondary to non-adherence to medication or to failure of antiretroviral therapy.
- CMV end-organ disease is a common opportunistic infection in advanced HIV-infected patients, with the incidence ranging from 20% to 40% in patients diagnosed with AIDS. CMV disease can manifest as retinitis, esophagitis, colitis, pneumonia, and encephalitis. Retinitis is the most common presentation, accounting for 85% of the total cases of CMV infection.[1]

Desired Outcome

2. *What are the goals of therapy for CMV retinitis in this patient?*

- Prevent progressive retinal destruction that may lead to additional partial or complete vision loss (if left untreated)
- Improve vision
- Provide effective therapy with few adverse effects
- Improve the patient's quality of life

Therapeutic Alternatives

3. *What feasible pharmacotherapeutic alternatives are available for treatment of CMV retinitis in this patient?*

- *Ganciclovir* is an acyclic nucleoside analogue that is active against CMV, HSV, EBV, and hepatitis B virus and is commonly used for induction and maintenance treatment of CMV disease. Intracellular activation to an active triphosphate form is necessary for its antiviral activity.
  - ✓ *IV ganciclovir (Cytovene IV)* has similar efficacy as IV foscarnet as maintenance therapy of CMV retinitis, and it delays first progression of retinitis by approximately 60 days.[2] It is renally eliminated and the dose-limiting toxicities are neutropenia, anemia, and thrombocytopenia. Due to the need for lifelong daily IV infusions, indwelling catheter infections are also common. Despite numerous therapy-related morbidities, IV ganciclovir remains one of the first-line agents for patients who have disseminated CMV disease or have sight-threatening CMV retinitis.
  - ✓ *Oral ganciclovir (Cytovene)* was developed in an effort to eliminate the need for lifelong IV therapy as maintenance treatment of CMV retinitis. It has a maximum bioavailability of 9% when given with meals at doses of 1000 mg po TID. The efficacy of oral ganciclovir as maintenance treatment has been compared to IV ganciclovir in several studies. Overall, the results have been disappointing, with significantly shorter mean times to disease progression in patients who received oral therapy.[3] Currently, monotherapy using oral ganciclovir is considered a suboptimal therapy for patients who have sight-threatening CMV retinitis. It may be considered in patients who do not have IV access and are in an early stage of disease. However, frequent ophthalmologic examinations are necessary to detect disease progression, and the risks of oral therapy must be discussed with patients before initiation of therapy. Adherence to oral therapy can also be difficult due to the large number of capsules (12 per day) that must be taken.
  - ✓ *Ganciclovir ocular implant (Vitrasert)* is a sustained-release drug delivery device that is surgically placed in the posterior segment of the eye. Each implant consists of 4.5 mg of ganciclovir and is designed to deliver therapeutic levels of ganciclovir in the eye over 5 to 8 months. The efficacy of the ganciclovir implant has been compared to IV ganciclovir in a randomized, controlled, multicenter trial.[4] The study showed that the ganciclovir implant is more effective than IV ganciclovir in the prevention of disease progression; however, the risks of extraocular CMV disease and CMV infection in the untreated eye are much higher in the ganciclovir implant treatment group due to low systemic drug levels. Common adverse effects of the implant include vitreous hemorrhage (14.9%) and retinal detachment (11.8%) of the implanted eye. The advantages of the implant over systemic IV therapy are its low systemic toxicity and the high levels of drug achieved in the diseased eye. Moreover, it eliminates the need for a long term IV catheter, which can potentially improve quality of life.
- *IV foscarnet (Foscavir)* is a pyrophosphate analogue that selectively inhibits CMV DNA polymerase. In contrast to ganciclovir, foscarnet does not require intracellular activation, and it also possesses anti-HIV activity by inhibiting HIV reverse transcriptase. Foscarnet and IV ganciclovir have similar efficacy rates in induction and maintenance treatment of CMV retinitis. One study demonstrated longer median length of survival in foscarnet-treated patients, which may have been due to the anti-HIV activity of the drug. However, with the availability of the highly active antiretroviral therapies such as protease inhibitors, the potential benefit from the antiretroviral activity of foscarnet is probably insignificant. The dose-limiting toxicities of foscarnet are nephrotoxicity and electrolyte imbalances (e.g., hypocalcemia, hypomagnesemia, and hypophosphatemia). Severe hypocalcemia has been reported in patients receiving concomitant foscarnet and parenteral pentamidine therapy. Foscarnet therapy should be discontinued in patients with creatinine clearances < 4 mL/min/kg. In general, IV ganciclovir is better tolerated than foscarnet and is preferred over foscarnet in patients who have no con-

traindications to ganciclovir therapy (e.g., thrombocytopenia or neutropenia). Foscarnet may be considered in patients who have good renal function and have pre-existing bone marrow suppression or in patients who have ganciclovir-resistant CMV strains.

- *IV cidofovir (Vistide)* is a cytidine nucleoside analogue that is active against CMV, VZV, acyclovir-resistant HSV, and ganciclovir-resistant CMV. The efficacy of cidofovir has been evaluated in randomized clinical trials in patients with newly diagnosed CMV retinitis or with refractory CMV retinitis who have failed ganciclovir and/or foscarnet. Both studies demonstrated that cidofovir is efficacious in the treatment of CMV retinitis with median time to retinitis progression of approximately 100 days.[5] The long half-life of the active intracellular metabolite of cidofovir allows for more convenient weekly dosing and avoids the cost and complications of an IV indwelling catheter. However, nephrotoxicity limits the widespread use of this agent. In order to reduce the incidence of nephrotoxicity, probenecid must be given 3 hours prior to and at 2 and 8 hours post-infusion. Prehydration with 1 L normal saline is also essential. Cidofovir is contraindicated in patients who have pre-existing renal impairment (serum creatinine ≥ 1.5 mg/dL, creatinine clearance ≤ 55 mL/min, urine protein ≥ 100 mg/dL or 2+ proteinuria) or who are receiving nephrotoxic drugs (e.g., aminoglycosides, amphotericin B). Intolerance to probenecid is also common. Adverse reactions such as fever, rash, and nausea are usually responsive to antihistamine, antiemetic, and analgesic therapies. Owing to the dose-limiting toxicity of cidofovir, its role in the management of CMV disease has been limited to patients with refractory disease or in patients who require systemic IV therapy and have no long-term IV access.
- *Fomivirsen (Vitravene)* is an antisense compound intended for intravitreal injection in AIDS patients with CMV retinitis. The drug is indicated as second-line therapy for patients who are intolerant of or have contraindications to other treatments for CMV retinitis, or who did not respond sufficiently to previous treatments. The most common adverse effects are transient increase in intraocular pressure, cataracts, anterior chamber inflammation, vitritis, and uveitis. The drug is not recommended in patients who have recently (within 2 to 4 weeks) been treated with cidofovir because of the risk of exaggerated ocular inflammation.
- Recommended regimens for the management of CMV retinitis are summarized in Table 116–1 below. With IV regimens, induction therapy is necessary for treatment of active disease, and lifelong maintenance therapy is indicated for chronic suppression of recurrent disease. Median time to progression of retinitis differs among these agents, as shown in the table.

Optimal Plan

4. *Which agent and regimen would you recommend for management of this patient's CMV retinitis?*

- Because he has localized CMV retinitis in the right eye without systemic involvement, the ganciclovir ocular implant is probably the best choice for this patient. It avoids the cost and complications associated with IV therapy of ganciclovir and foscarnet. It can also potentially improve the quality of life of CMV-infected patients.
- Oral ganciclovir should not be used since it is only FDA approved for maintenance (suppressive) therapy. Moreover, since the patient has a history of non-adherence with oral medications, the "pill burden" of oral ganciclovir makes it a suboptimal choice for him.
- Cidofovir is not preferred due to its nephrotoxicity and the need to give probenecid with it, as discussed previously.
- Fomivirsen should be reserved for second-line therapy, as discussed.
- Therefore, the patient needs to be scheduled for outpatient surgery for placement of the ganciclovir ocular implant. The surgery usually lasts about an hour, and possible complications include vitreous hemorrhage and retinal detachment, which usually occur within the first 2 months after surgery.

Outcome Evaluation

5. *What clinical and laboratory parameters are necessary to evaluate the therapy for achievement of the desired therapeutic outcome and to detect adverse effects?*

Efficacy

- Evaluate the patient for signs and symptoms of retinitis progression, such as the sudden onset of multiple floaters, flashing lights, loss of visual fields, and decreased vision. Monthly ophthalmologic examination of both eyes should be performed, and a new implant should be placed in 5 to 8 months as evidenced by progression of retinitis.
- Monitor for signs of extraocular CMV disease such as fever, myalgias, leukopenia, mental status changes, generalized wasting, shortness of breath, diarrhea, and GI symptoms.

TABLE 116–1. Comparative Efficacy of Agents Used as Maintenance Therapy for CMV Retinitis

Drug	Induction Dose	Maintenance Dose	Median Time to Retinitis Progression (days)
Ganciclovir			
Ocular implant	None	4.5 mg SR implant	221
IV	5 mg/kg IV Q 12 H × 14 days	5 mg/kg IV QD	56
Oral	Not indicated	1000 mg TID with meals	57[a]
Foscarnet IV	60 mg/kg IV Q 8 H × 14 days	90 mg/kg IV Q 12 H	60
Cidofovir IV	5 mg/kg IV Q week × 2 weeks	5 mg/kg IV Q 2 weeks	115
Fomivirsen intravitreal injection	330 μg intravitreal injection every 2 weeks for 2 doses	330 μg intravitreal injection every 4 weeks	80

[a] Number denotes mean time to first progression of retinitis with oral ganciclovir; mean time to first progression for IV ganciclovir was 71 days in the study.

Adverse Effects

- Monitor carefully for signs of eye bleeding and acute loss of vision after surgery. Vitreous hemorrhage, retinal detachment, and visual acuity loss of 3 lines or more occur in 10% to 20% of individuals within 2 months after implantation.
- Monitor for signs of rash and other hypersensitivity reactions to ganciclovir.

Patient Counseling

6. *What information should be provided to the patient to ensure successful therapy?*

- The ganciclovir ocular implant is not a cure for CMV retinitis. Disease progression can occur after 5 to 8 months of implantation. Periodic ophthalmologic examination of both eyes is necessary to monitor for disease progression.
- Because the amount of drug in the implant only lasts for 5 to 8 months, replacement of the old implant will eventually be necessary.
- The ganciclovir implant only protects against disease progression in your right eye, and you are still at risk for CMV infection in the left eye and in other organs such as the lung, brain, and gastrointestinal tract. Contact your physician immediately if you develop fever, sore throat, diarrhea, stomach pain, headaches, or mental status changes.
- During the first 2 to 4 weeks after surgery, almost all patients experience immediate and temporary decrease in the sharpness of vision. However, your vision should improve over several weeks. Notify your physician if you experience any acute change in vision or worsening of vision after surgery.
- Finally, you should be aware that CMV infection is a complication of your HIV infection. Strict compliance to the antiretroviral therapy is probably the best way to prevent you from getting other complications of AIDS and progression of CMV disease. Missing doses of your medicine can result in low drug levels in the body and promote the development of resistant HIV strains that can lead to treatment failure.

▶ Follow-up Questions

1. *Do you agree with the changes that were made in his HIV therapy 2 months ago? Provide a rationale for your answer.*

- Since he had a high viral load (128,860 copies/mL) and low CD4 count (15 cells/mm^3) at his last clinic visit, he is at high risk for further disease progression and development of other opportunistic infections of AIDS.
- Since he failed indinavir, zidovudine, and lamivudine therapy 2 months ago, a change in antiretroviral therapy is warranted; at least 2 agents should be changed at the same time to prevent the emergence of resistance. The choice of ritonavir, saquinavir, stavudine, and lamivudine as salvage therapy is appropriate, since it involved the introduction of at least 2 new agents to the regimen.
- The use of ritonavir together with saquinavir results in at least a 10-fold increase in saquinavir levels, which constitutes a potent regimen for patients who have failed 3-drug regimens that contain one protease inhibitor.

- Since the patient has not been able to be compliant with his medication schedule due to his depression and poor appetite, he should be given the option to withhold antiretroviral medications until he is emotionally stable enough to cope with the medication schedule. Once therapy is restarted, strict adherence to the schedule should be encouraged because subtherapeutic drug levels can lead to emergence of resistant HIV strains.

2. *If the patient received the ganciclovir ocular insert as treatment for his CMV retinitis, how would you manage the disease if he developed extraocular CMV disease 6 months after the implantation?*

- Development of extraocular disease in the future necessitates systemic IV therapy consisting of 2 weeks of induction therapy and lifelong maintenance therapy.
- IV ganciclovir should be considered the first-line agent unless he has pre-existing bone marrow suppression (i.e., neutropenia, thrombocytopenia, or anemia) that predicts a tolerability problem. In that case, foscarnet may be considered, but his renal function and electrolytes should be carefully monitored to prevent the development of overt renal failure.
- Cidofovir should be reserved as a third-line agent after ganciclovir and foscarnet therapy due to the limited clinical experience with this new agent and its potential for nephrotoxicity.

References

1. Jacobson MA. Treatment of cytomegalovirus retinitis in patients with the acquired immunodeficiency syndrome. N Engl J Med 1997;337:105–114.
2. Mortality in patients with the acquired immunodeficiency syndrome treated with either foscarnet or ganciclovir for cytomegalovirus retinitis. Studies of Ocular Complications of AIDS Research Group, in collaboration with the AIDS Clinical Trials Group. N Engl J Med 1992;326:213–220.
3. Drew WL, Ives D, Lalezari JP, et al. Oral ganciclovir as maintenance treatment for cytomegalovirus retinitis in patients with AIDS. N Engl J Med 1995;333:615–620.
4. Musch DC, Martin DF, Gordon JF, et al. Treatment of cytomegalovirus retinitis with a sustained-release ganciclovir implant. N Engl J Med 1997;337:83–90.
5. Parenteral cidofovir for cytomegalovirus retinitis in patients with AIDS: The HPMPC peripheral cytomegalovirus retinitis trial. A randomized, controlled trial. Studies of Ocular Complications of AIDS Research Group in Collaboration With the AIDS Clinical Trials Group. Ann Intern Med 1997;126:264–274.

117 TREATMENT OF HIV INFECTION

▶ The Antiretroviral-naive Patient (Level II)

Susan Chuck, PharmD
Keith Rodvold, PharmD, FCCP, BCPS

A 41-year-old man with a 2-year history of HIV infection presents to clinic requesting antiretroviral therapy after a long discussion on this topic during the last clinic visit. The patient's CD4 lymphocyte count from his last visit 2 weeks ago is 234 cells/mm^3 and his viral load (HIV RNA) is 33,995 copies/mL. Antiretroviral therapy is indicated in this man to delay further disease progression, prevent opportunistic infections, and improve survival. Prophylaxis against *Pneumocystis carinii* is not indicated with a

CD4 lymphocyte count of 234 cells/mm³, no history of a CD4 lymphocyte count less than 200 cells/mm³, and no prior episodes of *Pneumocystis carinii* pneumonia. After initiation of therapy, the surrogate markers indicate that the regimen is effective with improvements in the immune system and a decline in viral load. These findings are confirmed at the 4-month follow-up visit. Although the viral load is detectable at the 4-month follow-up visit, no change in therapy is indicated because the increase is < 0.5 log.

► Questions

Problem Identification

1. a. *What information (signs, symptoms, laboratory values) indicates the severity of HIV disease? Provide an assessment of this patient's HIV disease at this visit and his risk of progression to AIDS.*

   - *Signs.* None; the physical examination reveals no abnormalities. He has no current or previous history of opportunistic infections.
   - *Symptoms.* He has no symptoms associated with the HIV infection.
   - *Laboratory values.* HIV RNA is detectable; the CD4 lymphocyte count is between 200 to 499 cells/mm³.
   - The duration of HIV infection is 2 years. According to the 1993 AIDS surveillance case definition for adolescents and adults, he is clinical category A2.
   - His risk of progression to AIDS is 40% in 3 years, 73% in 6 years, and 86% in 9 years (based on the Multicenter AIDS Cohort Study [MACS] data using last visit's CD4 lymphocyte count and HIV RNA).

   b. *Is it rational to begin antiretroviral therapy in this patient?*

   - According to current guidelines, treatment is indicated in all persons with: 1) HIV-related symptoms; 2) a CD4 lymphocyte count < 200 cells/mm³; or 3) an HIV RNA >10,000 copies/mL (bDNA) or >20,000 copies/mL (RT-PCR) regardless of the CD4 lymphocyte count.
   - Clinical categories not requiring therapy are A1 and A2 (asymptomatic with CD4 lymphocyte count ≥ 200 cells/mm³) with HIV RNA < 10,000 copies/mL (bDNA) or < 20,000 copies/mL (RT-PCR). Some clinicians recommend only close observation for patients with HIV RNA < 10,000 copies/mL (bDNA) or < 20,000 copies/mL (RT-PCR) with CD4 lymphocyte count between 350 to 500 cells/mm³.
   - Because this patient has an HIV RNA > 20,000 copies/mL by RT-PCR, he is a candidate for antiretroviral therapy, even though his CD4 count is > 200 cells/mm³. If the test were performed by bDNA, the requirement would be >10,000 copies/mL.

   c. *Is prophylactic therapy for any HIV-associated opportunistic pathogen indicated in this patient?*

   - *Pneumocystis carinii* prophylaxis is indicated in the following groups: 1) present CD4 count < 200 cells/mm³; 2) history of a CD4 count < 200 cells/mm³; 3) prior episodes of *Pneumocystis carinii* pneumonia; 4) HIV-associated thrush; or 5) unexplained fever (>100°F) for > 2 weeks.
   - Other significant CD4 levels for starting prophylaxis are ≤ 50 cells/mm³ for *Mycobacterium avium* complex and ≤ 100 cells/mm³ for toxoplasmosis when serology is positive.
   - Therefore, prophylaxis against *Pneumocystis carinii*, *Mycobacterium avium*, or toxoplasmosis is not presently indicated in this patient.

Desired Outcome

2. *What are the goals of pharmacotherapy in this case?*

   - Prevent further immune system destruction
   - Delay further disease progression
   - Improve survival
   - Prevent opportunistic infections
   - Avoid adverse drug effects

Therapeutic Alternatives

3. a. *What therapeutic options are available for the treatment of this antiretroviral-naive man?*

   - Table 117–1 contains a list of the agents categorized by mechanism of action that were commercially available at the time of this writing.
   - The preferred regimen includes three drugs: one protease inhibitor (PI) and two nucleoside analog reverse transcriptase inhibitors (NRTIs).
     ✓ The preferred PIs are indinavir, ritonavir, nelfinavir, or saquinavir (soft gel capsule or SGC). The hard gel capsule (HGC) of saquinavir is not considered a preferred PI due to its poor bioavailability.
     ✓ The combination of ritonavir with saquinavir is also a preferred PI choice. Low-dose ritonavir serves to increase saquinavir serum concentrations. This 4-drug regimen is often reserved for salvaging failed initial regimens.
     ✓ The preferred combinations of NRTIs are: 1) zidovudine plus didanosine; 2) zidovudine plus zalcitabine; and 3) zidovudine plus lamivudine. These combinations have at least one randomized trial with clinical end points (i.e., reduced opportunistic infections, AIDS defining events, or deaths). The combinations of: 4) stavudine plus didanosine; and 5) stavudine plus lamivudine are also in the preferred category of NRTI combinations. However, these two combinations have only laboratory end points available to judge efficacy (beneficial surrogate marker effects) and have been studied only very recently.
   - Alternative regimens that are less likely to provide sustained virus suppression include: 1) a non-nucleoside analog reverse transcriptase inhibitor (NNRTI) in combination with two NRTIs; or

TABLE 117–1. Antiretroviral Agents Categorized by Mechanism of Action

Generic Name	Brand Name	Other Names	Usual Oral Dose (> 60 kg)
Nucleoside Analog Reverse Transcriptase Inhibitor (NRTI)			
Zidovudine	Retrovir	ZDV (avoid AZT)	200 mg TID or 300 mg BID
Lamivudine	Epivir	3TC	150 mg BID
Zalcitabine	Hivid	ddC	0.75 mg TID
Didanosine	Videx	ddI	200 mg BID
Stavudine	Zerit	D4T	40 mg BID
Lamivudine and Zidovudine [a]	Combivir		One BID
Non-nucleoside Analog Reverse Transcriptase Inhibitor (NNRTI)			
Nevirapine	Viramune		200 mg BID
Delavirdine	Rescriptor		400 mg TID
Efavirenz	Sustiva		600 mg QD
Protease Inhibitor (PI)			
Saquinavir	Invirase	Hard gel capsule (HGC)	600 mg TID
	Fortovase	Soft gel capsule (SGC)	1200 mg TID
Indinavir	Crixivan		800 mg TID
Ritonavir	Norvir		600 mg BID
Nelfinavir	Viracept		750 mg TID

[a] A combination of zidovudine and lamivudine in a single tablet.

2) the hard gel capsule (HGC) of saquinavir in combination with one of the preferred combinations of NRTIs above.
- Using only a 2-drug regimen consisting of one of the preferred combinations of NRTIs is not generally recommended due to incomplete and transient virus suppression.
- The following NRTI combinations are *not* recommended due to antagonism or overlapping toxicities: 1) stavudine plus zidovudine; 2) zalcitabine plus didanosine; 3) zalcitabine plus stavudine; and 4) zalcitabine plus lamivudine.

b. *What economic, psychosocial, racial, and ethical considerations are applicable to this patient?*

- Check medication coverage (e.g., private insurance, AIDS Drug Assistance Program or ADAP, indigent programs, clinical drug trials, expanded access programs) to ensure an uninterrupted supply of medications.
- Aspects of lower socioeconomic class associated with non-adherence include unstable or poor housing, low income, low level of education, and lack of medical insurance.
- African Americans may be less likely to accept pharmacotherapy (especially enrollment in a clinical drug trial) due to the Tuskegee incident.
- Pharmacotherapy should not be denied to IVDU or illegal substance users; these patients should be educated about the benefits, options, and importance of adherence so they can make an informed decision about starting therapy or deferring therapy until a time when they can commit to therapy and be adherent.

Optimal Plan

4. a. *Design an individualized antiretroviral regimen for this man. State the drug name, dosage form, dose, schedule, and duration of therapy for the regimen you choose.*

- Any of the preferred regimens described above would be acceptable initial antiretroviral therapy in a treatment-naive patient. Therapy duration is life-long. Factors other than treatment efficacy that should be considered include the following issues.
  ✓ Many patients may not remember to take the middle dose of a Q 8 H schedule or may not be able to ingest the fluid intake required with indinavir.
  ✓ Consider avoiding Q 8 H agents (i.e., indinavir, saquinavir, nelfinavir, zalcitabine, delavirdine) and choose agents that allow for Q 12 H dosing (i.e., ritonavir, ritonavir plus saquinavir, zidovudine, didanosine, lamivudine, stavudine, nevirapine).
  ✓ Ritonavir 600 mg po Q 12 H with any of the following combinations is an excellent Q 12 H regimen: 1) zidovudine 300 mg plus lamivudine 150 mg Q 12 H; or 2) stavudine 40 mg plus lamivudine 150 mg Q 12 H.
  ✓ These regimens require 16 tablets/capsules per day; but zidovudine plus lamivudine is available in a single-tablet formulation (Combivir). Combivir 1 tablet Q 12 H plus ritonavir 6 × 100 mg Q 12 H minimizes the number of tablets/capsules in the regimen (14/day).
  ✓ Less frequent dosing is currently being investigated for di-

danosine (QD), lamivudine (QD), nevirapine (QD), and nelfinavir (Q 12 H). Indinavir Q 12 H has proven to be suboptimal.
- ✓ Because diarrhea is not well tolerated (especially if restrooms are not readily available), offer an antidiarrheal medication (e.g., diphenoxylate/atropine or loperamide) to the patient to be taken as needed.

b. *Design an antiretroviral regimen that would be appropriate if the patient informs you that he has difficulty swallowing large pills.*

- All of the PIs (indinavir, ritonavir, saquinavir, nelfinavir) are large tablets or capsules. Consider ritonavir liquid as an alternative, but patient adherence may be a problem. Opening indinavir capsules is not recommended due to the bitter taste of indinavir powder. Saquinavir gel capsules should not be opened. Nelfinavir tablets can be split in two to decrease their size.
- All of the RTIs are small tablets/capsules or chewable tablets (didanosine). Combivir 1 tablet Q 12 H plus ritonavir 600 mg liquid Q 12 H is a good regimen in this situation.

c. *Design an antiretroviral regimen that would be appropriate if the patient states that medicines often upset his bowels, and he prefers to avoid anything that may cause him trouble.*

- All of the PIs are associated with diarrhea or GI upset (nausea, vomiting).
- The buffer in didanosine formulations provides the optimal pH for maximal absorption, but it is associated with diarrhea and GI upset.
- Two options exist for this situation.
  - ✓ Use a PI and offer an antidiarrheal; reassure him that tolerance to the side effects develops over time and that using an antidiarrheal will minimize diarrhea.
  - ✓ Also, gradual dosage escalation of ritonavir and taking nelfinavir with food will minimize diarrhea.
  - ✓ Use ritonavir 400 mg Q 12 H plus saquinavir 400 mg Q 12 H, because this combination of protease inhibitors allows for lower doses of each agent and is associated with a lower frequency of diarrhea.

Outcome Evaluation

5. *What parameters should you select to monitor the clinical efficacy and toxicity of the pharmacotherapeutic regimen? Specify the frequency with which you would monitor these parameters. For laboratory parameters, state the range of values or significant change in values (i.e., log change, x-fold change, and specific HIV RNA values) that would indicate that the desired therapeutic outcome has been achieved.*

Efficacy Parameters

- Monitor the CD4 lymphocyte count and HIV RNA at baseline (start of therapy), in 4 to 8 weeks, and then every 3 to 4 months. The desired end point in CD4 count is an increase from baseline or no decrease. The optimal end point for HIV RNA is for it to become non-detectable or at least > 0.5 log or a 3-fold decrease from baseline.
- To detect the occurrence of new opportunistic infections, question the patient at each clinic visit about potential signs and symptoms (i.e., fever, chills, night sweats, diarrhea, shortness of breath).

Adverse Effect Parameters

- For diarrhea, ask the patient at each clinic visit about the consistency, frequency, odor, and color of his stool. The goal is to have normal bowel movements.
- To detect peripheral neuropathy, question the patient at each clinic visit about the presence of numbness, tingling, and its distribution and severity if present.
- The patient should also be asked at each visit whether he has noticed any taste perversion, circumoral paresthesia, nausea, vomiting, headache, insomnia, fatigue, or weakness.
- Hepatic transaminases, serum triglycerides, creatine kinase, and uric acid should be obtained every 2 to 3 months to detect abnormal elevations.
- A CBC with differential should be checked every 2 to 3 months to detect anemia (hemoglobin, hematocrit), and neutropenia. The WBC and neutrophil counts should be used to calculate the absolute neutrophil count (ANC) to assess the patient's risk of infection.

Patient Counseling

6. a. *What important information would you provide to this patient about his therapy?*

- It is important to take the exact number of capsules, tablets, or liquid doses prescribed each day. We have devised a schedule so that you only have to take medicine once every 12 hours. You must take the doses within 2 hours of their scheduled time.
- Your adherence to this schedule is crucial to prevent the virus from developing resistance to the treatment.
- If you do happen to miss a dose, take it as soon as possible; however, if it is almost time for your next dose; skip the missed dose and return to your regular schedule; do not take double doses.
- With regard to dosing and meals, ritonavir should be taken with meals; zidovudine and lamivudine can be taken without regard to meals.
- Store the ritonavir capsules in the refrigerator and the liquid at room temperature.
- The most common side effects of these medicines include:
  - ✓ Ritonavir: diarrhea and tingling or numbness around the mouth.
  - ✓ Zidovudine: low red and white blood cell counts and weakness.
  - ✓ Lamivudine is generally well tolerated.
- Loperamide is a common non-prescription antidiarrheal medication that can be used as needed to minimize diarrhea. Also, the diarrhea tends to become more tolerable with time.
- Contact your physician or me if you become concerned about any possible side effects. Do not discontinue therapy or reduce doses if they occur.
- It is important for you to return to clinic periodically to assess your tolerance of the medicines and to monitor for benefit and side effects. A small blood sample will be required every 2 to 3 months to check necessary laboratory tests.
- Check with your physician or pharmacist before starting other prescription medications, herbal products, vitamins, or over-the-

counter medications to be sure that they are compatible with your HIV medications.

b. *Explain in non-technical terms the surrogate markers and their use in monitoring HIV disease.*

- The CD4 T-cell count measures the immune system responsible for fighting off bacteria and other infections. An uninfected person has 800 to 1200 cells in a certain amount of blood. Counts below 700 cells occur when something is destroying the immune system, such as an HIV infection. AIDS (acquired immunodeficiency syndrome) is the term used to describe a severely damaged immune system with < 200 CD4 cells.
- The viral load measures the number of HIV viruses in your blood. A test is used to count how much HIV is in your body. This number can be as high as hundreds of thousands. A high viral load means that there is a lot of HIV present, which is capable of damaging your immune system. The test we use for viral load only counts down to 400 or 500. When the viral load is less than 400 to 500, it is called an "undetectable viral load." Even if your load is undetectable, you can still infect someone else through sharing needles or sex because there is still HIV present in your brain, blood, and genitals.
- We obtain blood samples from you at baseline before treatment (now) and in 4 to 8 weeks when you return to clinic to determine whether the immune system is improving/healing and the viral load is decreasing (i.e., the HIV virus is being destroyed). If there is improvement in your viral load and CD4 count, we continue the medications and check every 3 months to make sure they continue to work. If no improvement is seen, this indicates that the medications are not working and the HIV may be resistant to the medications.
- There are 12 HIV drugs available, so we can switch to other medications to see if they work. We are not experimenting or using trial-and-error; the viral load and CD4 tests let us know early if the medications are working or not.

c. *If this man changed his mind about starting antiretrovirals, what questions would you ask him? Explain in non-technical terms when therapy is indicated and what the potential benefits are.*

- The following questions should be asked. Why did you change your mind about starting? What are your concerns? (Identify problems/issues.) Are you aware of the benefits of HIV therapy? (Check knowledge base.) Is the HIV treatment too complex for you? (Identify problems/issues.)
- HIV therapy is started to stop or slow down the destruction of the immune system by HIV. HIV-infected patients have symptoms when infections occur due to a poor immune system. These infections can be life threatening and reduce the quality of life. Therapy is started when the immune system has started to be destroyed (CD4 count about 500 cells) and if the viral load is detectable.
- Benefits of HIV therapy include prolonged survival and reduced numbers of infections. HIV should be considered a chronic disease, similar to high blood pressure or diabetes, in that you may not feel sick but life-long therapy is needed. Untreated disease causes many serious problems and is deadly in the long run. Treatment can prevent many of these problems and prolong life. Close follow-up is needed with your doctor, and medications are required for the rest of your life.

▶ **Follow-up Question**

1. *Considering this new information, provide an assessment of the patient's HIV disease status at each of the two visits.*

1 Month Later

- This patient's HIV disease is stable with no current or new opportunistic infections and no decline in CD4 count.
- Improvements in surrogate markers were noted with an 80-cell increase in CD4 count and a drop in viral load to non-detectable levels after 1 month of antiretroviral therapy.
- An exact estimate of the risk of progression to AIDS is not available, but it is expected to be < 4% in 3 years.

4 Months Later

- This patient's HIV disease remains stable with no current or new opportunistic infections and no decline in CD4 count.
- Improvement in CD4 count (40 cell increase) was noted with a slight increase in viral load to detectable levels after 4 months of antiretroviral therapy. The risk of progression to AIDS is slightly increased with a now detectable viral load. The risk is 4.4% in 3 years, 22% in 6 years, and 47% in 9 years.

2. *Provide an assessment of the antiretroviral regimen efficacy at each follow-up visit.*

1 Month Later

- There was at least a 1.87 log drop in viral load, from 36,873 copies/mL to < 500 copies/mL, and an 80-cell increase in CD4 count compared to baseline.
- Antiretroviral regimens that achieve at least a 0.5-log decline in viral loads 4 to 6 weeks post-initiation are thought to be effective. Less than a 0.5-log change may simply represent diurnal or test variation. The optimal target for viral load is to non-detectable levels, which was accomplished in this patient.

4 Months Later

- There was a 0.03-log increase in viral load, from < 500 copies/mL to 538 copies/mL, and a 40-cell increase in CD4 count compared to the 1-month post-initiation surrogate marker values.
- Although the viral load is now detectable, this regimen continues to be effective. The increase in viral load was not greater than 0.5 log, which is consistent with diurnal or test variability.

References

1. Report of the NIH panel to define principles of therapy of HIV infection and guidelines for the use of antiretroviral agents in HIV-infected adults and adolescents. MMWR 1998;47(RR-05):1–82.
2. Drugs for HIV infection. Med Lett 1997;39:111–116.
3. Carpenter CC, Fischl MA, Hammer SM, et al. Antiretroviral therapy for HIV infection in 1997. Updated recommendations of the International AIDS Society—USA Panel. JAMA 1997;277:1962–1969.
4. 1993 AIDS surveillance case definition for adolescents and adults. MMWR 1992;41(RR-17):1–9.

5. CDC 1997 USPHS/IDSA guidelines for the prevention of opportunistic infections in persons infected with HIV. MMWR 1997;46(RR-12):1–46.
6. Carpenter CC, Fischl MA, Hammer SM, et al. Antiretroviral therapy for HIV infection in 1998: Updated recommendations of the International AIDS Society—USA Panel. JAMA 1998;280:78–86.

118 HIV INFECTION AND PCP PNEUMONIA

▶ A Treatment-experienced Patient

(Level III)

Linda M. Page, PharmD
Peter L. Anderson, PharmD
Courtney V. Fletcher, PharmD

A 31-year-old man with HIV infection who has been receiving didanosine, stavudine, and indinavir for the past year presents with shortness of breath and fever. Over the past 6 months, he has had 2 episodes of oral thrush, his CD4 count has declined, and his HIV RNA levels have increased. A chest x-ray reveals bilateral infiltrates, and bronchoscopy with BAL is positive for *Pneumocystis carinii*. The two issues that must be addressed in this case are treatment of *Pneumocystis carinii* pneumonia (PCP) and reversal of HIV treatment failure. Although trimethoprim-sulfamethoxazole (TMP-SMX) is the treatment of choice for PCP, it cannot be used in this case because the patient is allergic to sulfas (skin rash). Second-line therapy is pentamidine isethionate 4 mg/kg/day by IV infusion for 21 days, or use of one of several other alternatives. Prednisone is added early to reduce the risk of respiratory failure and improve survival. The HIV therapy should be changed to at least two new antiretroviral drugs that are not cross-resistant with agents the patient has received previously. Potential treatment alternatives are discussed in the case questions and answers. Students are also asked to establish monitoring parameters for PCP and HIV therapy and to provide appropriate patient education about the treatment for both diseases.

▶ Questions

Problem Identification

1. a. *Create a list of the patient's drug-related problems.*

   - HIV treatment failure evidenced by: 1) CD4 cell return to baseline; 2) rebound in plasma HIV RNA; and 3) HIV-associated opportunistic infections (recent oral thrush, PCP while on prophylaxis).
   - Potential drug–drug interactions: didanosine has been shown to decrease the absorption of indinavir when administered at the same time. Therefore, treatment failure could be a result of inadequate systemic indinavir.
   - Increased liver function tests can occur with all of the patient's current medications.
   - Incomplete history of immunizations, which may increase the risk of future infections.

   b. *What information (signs, symptoms, laboratory values) indicates the presence or severity of the PCP and HIV disease progression?*

   - *PCP.* 1) presenting symptoms of SOB, nonproductive cough, fever, fatigue; 2) positive BAL for PCP; 3) increased serum LDH; 4) chest x-ray with bilateral subtle infiltrates; and 5) CD4 count < 200 cells/mm^3 is associated with increased risk for PCP.
   - *HIV disease.* 1) CD4 count < 200 cells/mm^3 meets the CDC definition of AIDS; 2) CD4 cell decline; 3) increasing HIV RNA (viral load); and 4) presence of opportunistic infections (PCP, recent oral thrush).

   c. *Could any of the patient's problems have been caused by drug therapy?*

   - Yes; assess overall compliance with assigned drug regimens because poor adherence is one contributing factor to HIV treatment failure.
   - Query the patient about how he takes his medications because of the interaction between didanosine and indinavir when administered at the same time. In addition, indinavir should be taken on an empty stomach (or with a small, low-fat meal) for optimal absorption.

   d. *Are any of the patient's problems amenable to pharmacotherapy?*

   - HIV therapy should suppress plasma HIV RNA to low or undetectable levels. This patient may need a new regimen (options covered later).
   - PCP is susceptible to drugs (listed later) with a 25% to 80% cure rate depending on severity. This patient has a moderate case with a 70% to 80% chance of recovery with appropriate treatment.
   - A complete history of immunizations should be obtained and treatment arranged, if needed.
   - Patient education will enhance understanding of HIV disease and the role of medications, and ensure that the patient knows how and when to take medications.

   e. *What additional information is needed to satisfactorily assess this patient?*

   - *Arterial blood gases.* 80% of patients with PCP have Pao$_2$ < 80 mm Hg; a Pao$_2$ < 70 mm Hg correlates with fatal outcomes.
   - *History/nature of drug allergy.* TMP-SMX is the drug of choice for PCP. Desensitization of sulfa allergies can be attempted depending on severity.
   - *Compliance history.* History of how and when the patient takes his medications (to clarify the drug interaction described above).

Verify that the patient takes the correct doses at the correct intervals and with the correct relation to meals.
- *Past antiretroviral therapy.* Previous antiviral therapy can cause HIV to be resistant to both the drugs used, and in some cases, to other drugs in the same class.[1]

Desired Outcome

2. *What are the desired goals of pharmacotherapy in this case?*

- Resolve PCP infection
- Prevent further immune system destruction
- Delay further HIV disease progression
- Improve survival
- Prevent further opportunistic infections

Therapeutic Alternatives

3. a. *What non-drug therapies might be useful for this patient?*

- Support groups may be helpful. HIV infection still carries a social stigma. Groups may help with this and provide education about the disease.

b. *What feasible pharmacotherapeutic alternatives are available for treatment of PCP and HIV infection in this patient?*

Pneumocystis Carinii Pneumonia[2]

- *TMP-SMX 15 to 20 mg/kg/day IV* (based on the TMP component) given in 3 to 4 divided doses for 21 days is the therapy of first choice and is associated with a 60% to 80% response rate. Oral therapy may suffice in mildly ill and reliable patients. Adverse reactions include fever, rash, neutropenia, thrombocytopenia, and hepatitis. This patient has a reported history of sulfa allergy, which may preclude its use.
- *Pentamidine isethionate 4 mg/kg/day IV* infused over 1 to 2 hours × 21 days is also associated with a 60% to 80% response rate. Adverse reactions include hypotension, cardiac arrhythmias, azotemia, pancreatitis, hypoglycemia followed by hyperglycemia, irreversible diabetes mellitus, nephrotoxicity, hypocalcemia, hypomagnesemia, and neutropenia. Some reactions appear infusion-rate related (hypotension, tachycardia) and can be minimized by infusing the drug over 1 hour or longer. Pentamidine given via aerosol has been used in the past for treatment of PCP; it is associated with slower clinical response and higher rates of therapeutic failure and PCP relapse. Therefore, its use is no longer recommended.
- *Dapsone 100 mg po QD plus trimethoprim 20 mg/kg/day po* in 4 divided doses has also been used. In controlled trials, the response rate was > 90%. Dapsone should not be used alone in the treatment of PCP because the response rate is less than TMP-SMX and dapsone plus trimethoprim. Adverse reactions to dapsone are methemoglobinemia, rash, fever, nausea, and vomiting; hemolysis can occur in patients who have glucose-6-phosphate dehydrogenase (G6PD) deficiency.
- *Clindamycin 600 mg po TID plus primaquine 30 mg po QD* has been used in a number of uncontrolled trials to successfully treat mild and moderate PCP. It may be associated with serious adverse reactions, including rash, neutropenia, anemia, and methemoglobinemia.
- *Atovaquone suspension 750 mg po BID with meals* is less effective than TMP-SMX in the treatment of mild to moderate PCP but is better tolerated. Side effects are usually mild and include skin rash, abnormal liver function tests, and GI complaints.
- *Trimetrexate 45 mg/m² per day IV* is useful for salvage therapy. Its major adverse reaction is myelosuppression; *leucovorin (20 mg/m² po Q 6 H)* must be administered concurrently during treatment and for 48 to 72 hours after the last dose of trimetrexate. This regimen is used in patients who do not respond to or cannot tolerate standard PCP therapies.
- *Corticosteroids* added early as adjunctive therapy to anti-PCP regimens have been shown to decrease the risk of respiratory failure and improve survival in patients with AIDS and moderate to severe PCP. The regimen currently recommended is prednisone 40 mg po BID days 1 to 5; 40 mg po QD days 6 to 10; and 20 mg po QD days 11 to 21, or for the duration of therapy. Data supporting the use of corticosteroids are based on initiation within the first 24 to 72 hours of the start of anti-PCP therapy.

HIV Infection[1,3]

- Combinations of three primary groups of agents are used for therapy of HIV infection.
  - ✓ *Nucleoside reverse transcriptase inhibitors (NRTIs)*: didanosine (ddI), lamivudine (3TC), stavudine (d4T), zalcitabine (ddC), and zidovudine (ZDV).
  - ✓ *Non-nucleoside reverse transcriptase inhibitors (NNRTIs)*: delavirdine (DLV), nevirapine (NVP), and efavirenz (EFV).
  - ✓ *Protease inhibitors (PIs)*: indinavir (IDV), nelfinavir (NFV), ritonavir (RTV), and saquinavir (SQV).
- As a general guide, any of the following events should prompt serious consideration for changing therapy.[3]
  - ✓ Less than one-log reduction in HIV-RNA 4 weeks after the initiation of therapy, or failure to achieve maximal suppression of HIV replication within 4 to 6 months.
  - ✓ Persistent decline in the CD4 cell count or a return to pretreatment value.
  - ✓ Clinical disease progression, usually the development of a new opportunistic infection.
- In patients deemed to be failing HIV therapy, the guiding principles of treatment are to change to at least 2 new antiretroviral drugs that are not cross-resistant with agents the patient has received previously.[3]
- Given that the patient's prior regimen included didanosine (NRTI), stavudine (NRTI), and indinavir (PI), the patient should be changed to two different NRTIs, such as zidovudine and lamivudine *and* either one of the two following combinations.
  - ✓ A combination of PIs: saquinavir (soft gelatin capsule) plus ritonavir; *or* saquinavir (soft gelatin capsule) plus nelfinavir.
  - ✓ A PI plus an NNRTI: nelfinavir (PI) plus either nevirapine, delavirdine, or efavirenz (NNRTIs); clinical trials support use of nevirapine or efavirenz over delavirdine.
- There is no single best alternative regimen nor has the clinical efficacy of any alternative regimen in patients failing therapy been established.

Optimal Plan

4. *What drug, dosage form, schedule, and duration of therapy are best for treating this patient's PCP and HIV infections?*

PCP Infection and Prophylaxis[2]

- Infuse pentamidine 4 mg/kg/day IV over 1 to 2 hours for 21 days. The patient has a documented allergy to sulfa, and therefore TMP-SMX (the drug of first choice) should not be used.
- Start adjunctive corticosteroid therapy immediately to decrease the risk of respiratory failure and improve survival. Give prednisone 40 mg po BID days 1 to 5; 40 mg po QD days 6 to 10; and 20 mg po QD days 11 to 21, or for the duration of pentamidine therapy.
- Increase the dapsone dose to 100 mg po QD after resolution of the acute episode of PCP. The patient is currently receiving 50 mg po QD for PCP prophylaxis. Controlled studies have indicated that dapsone failure rates are higher with 50 mg/day than with 100 mg/day. An alternative to increasing the dapsone dose could be a desensitization regimen and then a trial of TMP-SMX at the usual dose (one double-strength tablet daily) for PCP prophylaxis.

HIV Infection[1,3]

- Change the antiretroviral regimen to one of those suggested above. At the time of this writing, the NIH Guidelines for Antiretroviral Therapy (April, 1998) suggest changing to two new NRTIs and a new two-drug PI combination. Given these guidelines and current knowledge and experience, the following alternative regimen would be considered "best."
- ✓ Two new NRTIs: zidovudine 300 mg po BID *plus* lamivudine 150 mg po BID (given as Combivir) *plus*
- ✓ Two new PIs: saquinavir (soft gelatin capsule) 400 mg po BID *plus* ritonavir 400 mg po BID.
- There is no requirement to immediately change the antiretroviral regimen. The acute episode of PCP can be treated and then the antiretroviral regimen changed.

Outcome Evaluation

5. *What clinical and laboratory parameters are necessary to evaluate the PCP and HIV therapy for achievement of the desired therapeutic outcome and to detect or prevent adverse effects?*

Monitoring PCP Resolution

- Measure serum LDH at baseline and then every 3 to 5 days; a declining LDH suggests a response to therapy. It may take 3 to 8 days for improvement to be seen, which should be followed by continued improvement during therapy.
- Obtain a chest radiograph at baseline, if therapeutic failure is suspected, and at the end of treatment. Expected time to improvement is 3 to 8 days, but total resolution may take 20 to 30 days or more.
- Measure Pao_2 initially, then O_2 saturation until improved. Improvement may take 3 to 8 days, and a transient worsening may occur 3 to 5 days into therapy despite successful drug treatment.
- Assess the patient for fever, dyspnea, and chest tightness every 4 to 6 hours. Improvement in the patient's symptoms should be seen within 3 to 8 days.

Monitoring Pentamidine Toxicity[4,5]

- Monitor BP for hypotension at baseline, during the infusion, and every 4 hours thereafter. The patient should be supine for the infusion. Administer IV fluid boluses if there is a ≥ 30% drop in pressure.
- Monitor serum creatinine and BUN at baseline and daily to detect nephrotoxicity. Ensure good hydration to minimize its occurrence. Pentamidine dosage reduction may be necessary if nephrotoxicity occurs.
- Obtain serum electrolytes at baseline and every 3 to 4 days to detect hypocalcemia and hypomagnesemia. Replace these electrolytes if necessary.
- Monitor the ECG at regular intervals during therapy (i.e., by telemetry) to detect cardiac arrhythmias, including *torsades de pointes*. Rapid infusion of magnesium sulfate or lidocaine may be required for treatment.
- Monitor serum glucose at least daily for hypoglycemia followed by hyperglycemia (due to pancreatic islet cell necrosis). Glucose infusions may be needed for hypoglycemia; conversely, hyperglycemia may require insulin therapy.
- Monitor liver function tests (total bilirubin, AST, ALT, and alkaline phosphatase) at baseline and then every 3 to 4 days to detect liver toxicity. Treatment with an alternative agent may be needed if severe abnormalities occur.
- Obtain a complete blood count at baseline and every 3 to 4 days to detect leukopenia, thrombocytopenia, and anemia. A change to an alternative agent may be necessary if abnormalities are severe.

Monitoring HIV Disease[1]

- Question the patient at each follow-up visit about the presence of AIDS symptoms (e.g., unexplained fever, oral thrush). Treatment and expected time to improvement are dependent upon the type of opportunistic infection present.
- Obtain a CD4 count at baseline and then every 3 to 4 months. It may take several months for improvement to be seen after initiation of the new regimen. Trends over time are more important than single values.
- Measure HIV RNA at baseline, 2 to 4 weeks later, then every 3 months. A decline should be observed within 2 to 4 weeks of starting the new regimen. The levels should fall by 1 to 2 logs within the first 4 weeks.

Patient Counseling

6. *What information should be provided to the patient to enhance compliance, ensure successful therapy, and minimize adverse effects?*

- Because this patient is hospitalized, the information is provided to help the patient understand the purpose of the therapy and what to expect during treatment.

Pentamidine[4]

- This drug is used to treat *Pneumocystis carinii* pneumonia (PCP), a very serious kind of pneumonia. To help clear up your infection completely, you will remain in the hospital, and pentamidine must be given for the full time of treatment, even after you start to feel better.
- The dose or the amount of drug given to you will be determined by

how much you weigh. This will be given by injection slowly into a vein over a 1- to 2-hour period every day for 21 days.
- The most common side effects are heart rhythm problems, low blood pressure, and low or high blood sugar; you will be followed in the hospital for these and treated as necessary.

Prednisone
- This medicine is being used to help reduce inflammation in your lungs so that you can breathe easier. You will gradually reduce the amount you are taking before stopping it completely.
- The most common side effects are increased thirst, increased appetite, and restlessness. Most of these go away as your body adjusts to the medicine. You will only take this drug while in the hospital, and we will follow laboratory tests to check for side effects.

Dapsone
- This drug is used to prevent PCP infection in the future. It needs to be taken every day to be effective.
- The most common side effects of dapsone are itchy skin and rash. If you become short-of-breath easily, have pale skin, or fatigue easily, this could indicate anemia, and you should call your doctor immediately.

Zidovudine[4]
- Zidovudine is used for HIV infection. It works by stopping the virus from reproducing. It is common to combine this drug with other anti-HIV drugs to obtain the best response possible.
- The most common side effects from this medication are nausea (this drug can be taken with food), malaise (a "crummy" feeling), headache, and insomnia. These side effects tend to get better over time. If you notice that you are very weak or get short-of-breath easily, this may indicate anemia and you should contact your doctor.

Lamivudine
- Lamivudine works similarly to zidovudine by blocking virus from reproducing.
- This drug has few side effects. It may cause some nausea (this drug can also be taken with food), headache, or insomnia. Again, these effects tend to improve with time. Some people on both zidovudine and lamivudine experience neuropathy (tingling, pin-prick feelings, or burning) in the arms, feet, legs, or hands. Report this to your doctor if it occurs.

Ritonavir
- Ritonavir works in a different way than zidovudine and lamivudine. It ruins the "machinery" of assembling new viruses. The result is that the viruses do not work.
- Ritonavir works best if taken with food.
- It is important to store the capsules in the refrigerator; if you are taking the solution, it should be stored at room temperature.
- The most common side effects of this drug are nausea, diarrhea, a different taste of food, and malaise (a "crummy" feeling). These side effects may get better with time. Some people experience tingling or altered sensation in the arms, legs, or around the mouth. Report very dark urine or a yellowing of the skin or eyes to your doctor.
- Your doctor may take small blood samples periodically to monitor how your body is responding to the medicine.
- This drug can cause very serious drug interactions if taken with certain medications. It is very important that your doctor and pharmacist know all of the medications that you currently take.

Saquinavir
- Saquinavir works similarly to ritonavir. These drugs work well together because ritonavir may increase the amount of saquinavir in your body.
- It is important to take this drug with a meal.
- Possible side effects include nausea, diarrhea, and headache. These effects tend to get better over time. Report dark urine or yellowing of your eyes or skin to your doctor.
- Your doctor may take small blood samples periodically to monitor how your body is responding to this drug.

▶ **Follow-up Questions**

1. How would you assess the patient's cardiac event? What is the most likely cause?

- *Torsades de pointes* may be due to corticosteroids and/or pentamidine, most likely pentamidine.
- Hypokalemia and hypomagnesemia may occur from a variety of causes and may independently predispose to such arrhythmias in patients being treated with pentamidine.
- Corticosteroids can result in electrolyte abnormalities and may increase the potential for arrhythmias in patients receiving pentamidine.
- Pentamidine has structural similarities to procainamide.
- Pentamidine has a high tissue binding affinity and a long serum elimination half-life of 6.5 hours. It is still detectable in tissues after 8 weeks and therefore may have a delayed effect.

2. Considering this new information, what pharmacotherapeutic recommendation would you make?

- Electrolyte replacement as needed, particularly magnesium and potassium. It should be noted that serum magnesium levels correlate poorly with intracellular magnesium, so the goal serum level is the high end of the normal range.
- Consider stopping the pentamidine therapy and switching to an alternative drug.
- Evaluate for potential drug interactions: are any other cardiotoxic drugs being used? Are any nephrotoxic drugs being used that might cause accumulation of pentamidine?

References

1. NIH Panel to Define Principles of Therapy of HIV Infection. Report of the NIH panel to define principles of therapy of HIV infection. MMWR 1998;47(RR-5):1–42.
2. Santamauro JT, Stover DE. Pneumocystis carinii pneumonia. Med Clin North Am 1997;81:299–318.
3. Panel on Clinical Practices for Treatment of HIV Infection. Guidelines for the use of antiretroviral agents in HIV-infected adults and adolescents. MMWR 1998;47(RR-5):43–83.
4. Drug Information for the Health Care Professional. USP-DI, 18th ed. Taunton, MA, 1998.
5. Eisenhauer MD, Eliasson AH, Taylor AJ, et al. Incidence of cardiac arrhythmias during intravenous pentamidine therapy in HIV-infected patients. Chest 1994;105:389–395.

PART FOUR

Oncologic Disorders

Gary C. Yee, PharmD, FCCP, Section Editor

119 BREAST CANCER

▶ The Role of Neoadjuvant
 Chemotherapy   (Level II)

Laura Boehnke Michaud, PharmD

Development of a painful breast mass causes a 69-year-old woman to seek medical evaluation. A complete diagnostic work-up leads to the diagnosis of intraductal carcinoma with skin, pectoral muscle, and axillary lymph node involvement (Stage IIIB). Neoadjuvant (or primary) chemotherapy is indicated in this patient to provide systemic disease control and reduce tumor size, thereby permitting less extensive surgical resection later. Local radiotherapy will also be required due to skin and muscle involvement. The addition of hormonal therapy with tamoxifen after completion of chemotherapy may prolong survival in women with estrogen-receptor positive tumors. This patient developed bone and lung metastases 9 months after initial treatment, requiring additional systemic chemotherapy with 6 cycles of docetaxel. Eighteen months after completing docetaxel, the patient returned with new hip and rib metastases. Therapy with anastrozole was initiated for progressive metastatic breast cancer. The case questions require students to develop monitoring and patient counseling plans for each portion of the patient's disease course.

▶ Questions

Problem Identification

1. a. *Identify all of the patient's drug-related problems.*

   - *Untreated indication.* Newly diagnosed breast cancer requiring treatment.
   - *Drug use without indication.* Use of Paxil (paroxetine) without a defined indication.
   - *Improper drug selection (possible).* Back pain of unknown origin for which she takes Tylenol #3 (codeine/acetaminophen).
   - Hypertension is a chronic, stable drug-related problem not requiring intervention at this time as it is well controlled on Procardia (nifedipine) and Zestril (lisinopril).
   - The etiology of the eosinophilia was not pursued.

   b. *Given the above clinical information, what is this patient's current clinical stage of cancer?*

   - $T_4 N_1 M_0 \rightarrow$ Stage IIIB.

Desired Outcome

2. a. *What is the goal of therapy for this patient?*

   - The goal of therapy is to cure the patient of breast cancer.

   b. *What is the prognosis for this patient based on tumor size and nodal status?*

   - The rate of relapse is 70% to 80% at 5 years.

   c. *In addition to stage of disease, what other factors may be helpful in determining the prognosis for breast cancer?*

   - Prognostic factors include ER/PR status, S-phase fraction, angiogenic growth factors, cathepsin D, EGF receptor, Her-2/neu oncogene, nuclear grade, p53 gene, and DNA content.

Therapeutic Alternatives

3. List the general types of treatment options that are available for the patient at this time, and briefly discuss their advantages and limitations.

- *Surgery* would be difficult at this time. Due to the extent of skin involvement, primary closure of the wound may not be possible. If the patient has a good response to chemotherapy, surgery would be an option in the future.
- *Radiation* will only address the local disease but will not address the systemic spread of the cancer. The cancer has at least spread to the lymph node basin (based on ultrasound evidence), so radiation therapy is not optimal at this time. If she eventually undergoes surgery, radiation therapy afterward would be required because of the initial skin involvement.
- *Chemotherapy* is recommended at this time because of the need for systemic therapy. Chemotherapy works faster than hormonal therapy and is therefore the systemic treatment of choice for primary pharmacotherapy.
- *Hormonal therapy* works slower than chemotherapy and would not achieve the results needed quickly enough. In rare selected patients (e.g., elderly patients with comorbid conditions limiting the use of chemotherapy) hormone therapy may be used as primary systemic therapy, but this is not routine.

Optimal Plan

4. Outline the optimal treatment plan for this patient that includes both pharmacologic and non-pharmacologic measures. If antineoplastic chemotherapy is part of your plan, identify the specific regimen you would use and provide your rationale.

- *Primary (neoadjuvant) chemotherapy* should be administered initially. Surgery would be very difficult now due to the size of the tumor, skin and pectoral muscle involvement, and location of tumor in the breast and axilla. She is at very high risk for metastases (she is stage IIIB, with involvement of skin and possibly the pectoralis muscle). Despite her advanced age, she has an aggressive tumor requiring the faster response of chemotherapy over hormonal therapy. The specific advantages of neoadjuvant chemotherapy in this setting include: 1) the ability to demonstrate tumor sensitivity to chemotherapy; 2) downstaging the tumor to permit less extensive surgery and potentially breast-conserving surgery; and 3) the systemic control provided from chemotherapy allows for subsequent local control through surgery and/or radiation in advanced tumors that are initially inoperable.[1]
- The neoadjuvant regimen used should contain doxorubicin. It is the most active agent against breast cancer, and regimens containing it offer the best chance for a favorable response. Example regimens include:
    ✓ FAC (5-fluorouracil, cyclophosphamide, doxorubicin)
    ✓ AC (doxorubicin, cyclophosphamide)
    ✓ CAF (cyclophosphamide, doxorubicin, 5-fluorouracil)
- If the patient responds to chemotherapy and is then considered operable, she should subsequently undergo surgery. Current surgical techniques include modified radical mastectomy or lumpectomy plus radiation therapy.
- Additional adjuvant chemotherapy usually follows surgery. The choice of regimen is determined by the findings at surgery. If residual tumor is present, a different regimen may be chosen. However, if there was a good response to the initial chemotherapy despite the presence of residual tumor, a similar regimen may be used after surgery.
- Radiotherapy is required regardless of the type of surgery performed due to skin involvement and possible pectoralis muscle involvement. Radiation therapy usually follows chemotherapy and can be given concomitantly with hormone therapy.
- Hormonal therapy (e.g., tamoxifen) added after chemotherapy is completed has been shown to prolong disease-free survival and overall survival in women with estrogen-receptor positive tumors.[2]

Outcome Evaluation

5. a. What adverse effects can be anticipated with this regimen?

- Docetaxel can cause total body alopecia, leukopenia, fluid retention, nail ridging/onycholysis, mucositis, hand/foot syndrome, mild nausea, peripheral neuropathy, skin hyperpigmentation/rash, hypersensitivity reactions, diarrhea, and myalgias.[3]

b. What information is needed before calculating an appropriate dose of docetaxel for this patient? What dose would you recommend for this patient?

- Because docetaxel is primarily eliminated through biliary excretion, liver function tests (LFTs) should be performed before determining the docetaxel dose. Although the patient's AST, alkaline phosphatase, and total bilirubin were normal at disease presentation 9 months ago, they should be repeated now because of the length of time that has elapsed and because of the treatments that she has received since that time.
- The drug's manufacturer recommends the following dose reduction for patients with elevated LFTs:
    ✓ Total bilirubin > 1.5 times the upper limit of normal (ULN): Docetaxel dose reduction cannot be recommended, and the drug should not be used unless strictly indicated.
    ✓ Normal total bilirubin but alkaline phosphatase > 2.5 × ULN *and* AST/ALT > 1.5 × ULN: Docetaxel should be given at doses of 75 mg/m^2.
- The dose range for docetaxel is 60 to 100 mg/m^2. Most patients are started at full dose (100 mg/m^2) unless they have undergone extensive prior therapy or have some other reason for suspecting they will not tolerate full doses. The drug is given IV over 1 hour every 3 weeks. Dexamethasone (e.g., 8 mg po BID) is given for 3 days beginning 24 hours before the infusion to prevent or delay fluid retention and hypersensitivity reactions. Two or three cycles are given, and the response is then determined. If the patient is responding, the chemotherapy is continued. If the tumor is growing, treatment will be changed.

Patient Counseling

6. What information should the patient be given about the general effects she should expect to experience after this treatment?

- This therapy will cause a lowering of your white blood cell counts, which increases your risk of getting infections. Contact your doctor or go to the closest emergency room if you develop a fever of 101°F or higher, chills, or a sore throat.
- This therapy may cause mild nausea, but the medication you are taking before and after the chemotherapy will prevent you from having nausea. You will also be given medication to take at home in case you have nausea at home.
- This therapy may cause mouth sores, which may be painful and may become infected if the mouth is not kept clean. It is important to rinse with salt water and/or baking soda solution in the morning, after each meal, and at bedtime. This will keep the mouth clean and prevent infections. When you brush your teeth, use a soft toothbrush and avoid toothpaste with mint flavoring, which may burn your mouth. If these sores become painful, contact your doctor for other medications to reduce the pain.
- You may have some diarrhea with this chemotherapy. It is usually mild and lasts only a few days. You may take any over-the-counter medications as long as you do not have a fever. Call your doctor if you have diarrhea with a fever. The diarrhea may be a mechanism for your body to get rid of infection in the intestines, so you do not want to stop this. Be sure to drink a lot of fluid so you do not become dehydrated.
- This therapy may cause some fluid retention. It is very important to take your dexamethasone tablets for all 6 doses. This will help to prevent or lessen the fluid retention. The first sign of fluid retention is weight gain. We will monitor your weight very closely at each visit; however, keeping track of your weight at home also is a good idea. Call your doctor or nurse if you notice any swelling in your feet, ankles, hands, or arms. If you notice any shortness of breath or trouble breathing, go to the closest emergency room to be evaluated.
- This therapy may cause changes in your skin, nails, palms, and soles. The skin may become darker and dry or you may have a rash. Your nails may become ridged and lift up from the nail bed. If this happens, let the clinic know, and be very careful of infections under the nails. You may also notice some redness of the palms of the hands and soles of the feet that may be painful. Let your doctor know if this occurs, and he or she can give you medication that may help this.
- This therapy may cause numbness and tingling in your fingers or toes. This is usually mild but may worsen with every course of chemotherapy. If this becomes a problem, let us know and we may be able to help with medications.
- Some patients may have an allergic reaction to this chemotherapy. We will give you premedication that will help to prevent allergic reactions. If you notice any rashes, shortness of breath, difficulty breathing, or wheezing during the infusion, let your nurse know immediately. These reactions are rare with this chemotherapy.
- This chemotherapy causes total body hair loss. Your hair will start to fall out in about 10 to 14 days after the first chemotherapy. It usually falls out quickly, so you may want to plan ahead for this. Most of our patients prefer to shave off their hair before chemotherapy starts to avoid the trauma of having hair fall out unexpectedly. This also allows for matching a wig to your original hair color if that is your preference.

▶ Follow-up Questions

1. What are the patient's drug-related problems at this time?

- Rib and hip pain, uncontrolled with acetaminophen; the patient may be exceeding the maximum recommended daily dose of 4 g.
- Microcytic anemia (from iron deficiency, potentially resulting from lack of dietary iron intake or occult blood loss).
- Progressive metastatic breast cancer.

2. What are the treatment goals at this time?

- Cure is not a reasonable goal at this point. Once the cancer has spread to distant organs, the likelihood of 10-year survival is less than 5%.
- Appropriate goals are palliation of symptoms and prolongation of life.

3. What pharmacotherapeutic alternatives are available for each of the patient's current problems?

Rib and Hip Pain
- Stronger pain meds (e.g., opioid analgesics)
- Bisphosphonates (see "Self-study Assignments")
- Steroids and NSAIDs
- Systemic therapy of the cancer

Microcytic Anemia/Iron Deficiency (Not Related to Chemotherapy)
- Iron supplementation
- The role for erythropoietin in this setting has not established (see "Self-study Assignments").

Progressive Metastatic Breast Cancer
- Local treatment will only control the symptoms as stated above.
- Hormonal therapy would probably be used first due to the time between therapy and progression of disease and because of the fact that she has disease in only bone at this time. Bone metastases respond very well to hormonal therapy, and there is no oncologic emergency that requires immediate results. Refer to textbook Chapter 116 for more information regarding choice of agent.
- Chemotherapy is generally not very effective as third-line treatment in this setting. However, chemotherapy would be chosen if there were an oncologic emergency or other situation that required a rapid response.

▶ Follow-up Question

4. What important information would you provide to the patient about her new therapy for breast cancer?

- This medication may cause mild nausea; take it with food or milk or at bedtime to prevent this side effect.[4]
- It may cause headaches; these are usually mild and can be controlled with over-the-counter pain medications. Tell your doctor if these are not adequate for the pain, and stronger medications can be prescribed.
- This medicine may cause mild diarrhea; you can take over-the-counter medications such as loperamide for relief. Tell your doctor if these are not effective, and he or she may prescribe stronger medication.

- Many people experience hot flashes with this medication. There are medications that can help decrease their severity. Beware of herbal remedies, as some of these preparations contain hidden estrogens or may promote the production of estrogens in the body.
- This medicine may cause unwanted blood clots in the arms, legs, and elsewhere. This is not common but can be severe. Signs to look for are painful, red, hot areas in the legs or arms; sudden onset of shortness of breath; dizziness; or visual changes. Contact your doctor immediately if any of these effects occur.
- You may experience a feeling of overall weakness or decreased energy. This is uncommon, usually mild, and disappears after taking the medication for a while.

References

1. Bonadonna G, Valagussa P. Primary chemotherapy in operable breast cancer. Semin Oncol 1996;23:464–474.
2. Fisher B, Dignam J, Wolmark N, et al. Tamoxifen and chemotherapy for lymph node-negative, estrogen receptor-positive breast cancer. J Natl Cancer Inst 1997;89:1673–1682.
3. Fulton B, Spencer CM. Docetaxel: A review of its pharmacodynamic and pharmacokinetic properties and therapeutic efficacy in the management of metastatic breast cancer. Drugs 1996;51:1075–1092.
4. Buzdar A, Jonat W, Howell A, et al. Anastrozole, a potent and selective aromatase inhibitor, versus megestrol acetate in postmenopausal women with advanced breast cancer: Results of overview analysis of two phase III trials. Arimidex Study Group. J Clin Oncol 1996;14:2000–2011.

120 NON–SMALL CELL LUNG CANCER

▶ Remember the Surgeon General's Warning (Level II)

Kimberly Heying, PharmD
Jane M. Pruemer, PharmD, FASHP

A 58-year-old woman presents with hemoptysis, a non-productive cough, and dyspnea on exertion. After extensive evaluation, she is found to have surgically unresectable Stage IIIB non–small cell lung cancer (NSCLC). Long-term survival rates are low in this situation, and platinum-based combination chemotherapy regimens are commonly given with radiation therapy. There is no single standard chemotherapy regimen for NSCLC, and any one of several regimens may be chosen. A number of laboratory and other tests must be performed at specified intervals to detect adverse effects of therapy. Readers are also asked to devise prophylactic antiemetic regimens, calculate the patient's body surface area, calculate a serum calcium level corrected for hypoalbuminemia, and recommend appropriate treatment for hypercalcemia.

▶ Questions

Problem Identification

1. a. Identify the patient's drug-related problems.

- *Untreated indication.* Unresectable NSCLC requiring antineoplastic chemotherapy.
- *Adverse drug reaction.* Hypokalemia from HCTZ, requiring potassium supplementation.
- *Drug use without indication.* Patient is receiving Axid (nizatidine), an H_2-receptor antagonist, with no history of peptic ulcer disease, GERD, or other reason for its use.
- Other chronic drug-related problems include: 1) anemia of unknown etiology treated with ferrous sulfate and folic acid; 2) postmenopausal state receiving estrogen replacement; 3) dyslipidemia, treated with Zocor (simvastatin); disease control cannot be assessed with the information provided; and 4) hypertension, apparently controlled on HCTZ and Cardizem CD (sustained-release diltiazem).

b. What signs, symptoms, and other information indicate the presence of NSCLC in this patient?

- This woman presented with hemoptysis, which is the initial presenting symptom in about 30% of patients.
- In addition, she presented with coughing and dyspnea, which are other symptoms of lung cancer (refer to textbook Chapter 117 for additional symptoms).
- Her chest x-ray and CT scan revealed a right upper lobe mass.
- The bronchoscopy revealed squamous cell carcinoma, and the mediastinoscopy showed NSCLC with metastases to the contralateral mediastinal nodes.

Desired Outcome

2. What is the desired goal for this patient, and what is the likelihood of it being achieved?

- This patient has Stage IIIB NSCLC that is not surgically resectable. The ultimate goal is to cure the patient using chemotherapy and radiation.
- Unfortunately, patients who present with Stage IIIB NSCLC have a 10-month overall median survival rate and a 5-year survival rate of less than 5%. The patient would be considered cured of NSCLC if she achieved 5-year disease-free survival.

Therapeutic Alternatives

3. a. What chemotherapeutic regimens may be considered for NSCLC?

- There is no standard regimen for NSCLC. It is recommended that combination platinum-based (cisplatin or carboplatin) regimens be used because they are associated with increased survival.[1] A recent meta-analysis of 14 randomized clinical trials of chemotherapy plus radiation therapy versus radiation therapy alone in patients with Stage III unresectable NSCLC showed an advantage for the combination therapy group.[2] Most of the trials used a cisplatin-based regimen. The combination of cisplatin-based chemotherapy plus radiation reduced the relative risk of death by 12% at 1 year, 13% at 2 years, and 17% at 3 years. Adverse effects of cisplatin include significant nausea/vomiting, risk of neurotoxicity, and nephrotoxicity. Carboplatin-based regimens are associated with less neurotoxicity and nephrotoxicity than those containing cisplatin. However, carboplatin causes thrombocytopenia. Inclusion of paclitaxel has resulted in increased survival. Adverse effects of paclitaxel include alopecia, neurotoxicities, myalgias, hypersensitivity reactions, and bradycardia.

Examples of Chemotherapy Regimens

- *CE.* Cisplatin 60 to 100 mg/m^2 IV day 1 and etoposide 80 to 120 mg/m^2 IV × 3 days; the course is repeated every 3 to 4 weeks.
- Carboplatin AUC of 6 mg/mL·min IV on day 1 and paclitaxel 175 mg/m^2 IV on day 1; the course is repeated every 21 to 28 days.
- *MVP.* Mitomycin 8 mg/m^2 IV days 1 and 29; vindesine 3 mg/m^2 IV days 1, 8, 29, and 36; and cisplatin 80 mg/m^2 IV days 1 and 29; the cycle is repeated every 6 weeks.
- Vinorelbine 30 mg/m^2 IV once weekly with or without cisplatin 100 mg/m^2 IV on days 1 and 29; the regimen is repeated every 6 weeks until toxicity.

Information Regarding Chemotherapy

- The regimens given as examples are now being used instead of some of the other regimens because of similar or better response rates with better toxicity profiles. Platinum-based regimens (such as cisplatin/paclitaxel) and vinorelbine with or without cisplatin have been shown to produce improved survival in controlled clinical trials.
- The duration of chemotherapy should be 2 to 8 cycles depending on response.
- Refer to textbook Tables 117–4 and 117–6 for a more complete listing of combination regimens used.
- Investigational regimens may include topotecan, gemcitabine, taxotere, and ifosfamide.
- Single-agent chemotherapy generally has no significant overall effect on survival.
- The issue of two-drug versus three-drug combinations is still controversial, given the newer agents used to treat NSCLC.

b. What non-drug therapies may be used for NSCLC?

- Combined modality therapy that includes radiation and chemotherapy has been shown to prolong survival for patients with unresectable Stage III disease. This is preferred over radiation alone for patients with good performance status.[1]
- Radiation can also palliate symptoms such as hemoptysis, coughing, bone pain, and post-obstructive pneumonia.
- Radiation to the lung should not exceed a total of 7000 cGy. Radiation may be given concurrently, subsequently, or "sandwiched" between chemotherapy cycles.
- Surgery is of little benefit in patients with Stage IIIB disease but has been used with patients in Stage IIIA. Patients with Stage IIIB disease who have a significant response to chemotherapy may be rendered surgically resectable, resulting in improved survival.

Optimal Plan

4. a. Design a specific chemotherapeutic regimen to treat this patient, and explain why you chose this regimen.

- As discussed, there is no standard regimen for NSCLC, and many different combination regimens have been used. A platinum-based combination regimen should be used because survival is prolonged with platinum-based chemotherapy.
- This patient began combined modality treatment consisting of combination chemotherapy with concomitant radiation. The chemotherapy regimen given was cisplatin 100 mg/m^2 IV on day 1 and etoposide 100 mg/m^2 IV on days 1, 2, and 3. The course was repeated every 28 days. She received 3000 cGy of chest radiation.
- This regimen was chosen because of the good response rates associated with platinum-based regimens and because it was believed that she could tolerate this regimen, given that she did not have heart failure and had a good performance status.

b. What additional measures should be taken to ensure the tolerability of the regimen and to prevent adverse effects?

- To decrease the risk of nephrotoxicity, hyperhydration before, during, and after the administration of cisplatin using normal saline at 150 to 200 mL/hr is recommended to maintain a urine output of ≥ 100 mL/hr.
- Antiemetics are also indicated in this highly emetogenic regimen and should consist of a 5HT$_3$ antagonist (e.g., ondansetron, granisetron, or dolasetron) with dexamethasone. Example antiemetic regimens include ondansetron 16 mg IVPB plus dexamethasone 20 mg IV or ondansetron 24 mg po plus dexamethasone 20 mg po given for 1 dose prior to the cisplatin.
- Because cisplatin is also known to cause delayed nausea and vomiting (occurring more than 24 hours after administration), additional oral prophylactic antiemetics should be prescribed for the patient to take on a scheduled basis at home, such as: metoclopramide 10 to 20 mg every 6 hours; dexamethasone 8 mg BID × 2 days, then 4 mg BID × 2 days; ondansetron 8 mg TID; or a phenothiazine such as prochlorperazine 10 mg every 6 hours.
- The patient may also require potassium and magnesium supplementation due to cisplatin-induced renal wasting of these electrolytes.
- Etoposide should be infused over at least 1 hour to prevent hypotension associated with rapid infusion.
- After the first cycle of chemotherapy, nadir neutrophil counts should be monitored. If the patient develops a neutropenic fever after any cycle of chemotherapy, a colony-stimulating factor such as filgrastim (G-CSF) should be administered prophylactically after the next cycle.
- In addition, epoetin alfa may be administered to patients who have anemia due to cisplatin therapy.

c. What additional laboratory and clinical information is needed prior to administration of the chemotherapy?

- The patient's body surface area (BSA) needs to be calculated (based on height and weight) to calculate drug dosages.
- Laboratory tests should be obtained to assess the patient's renal

function (BUN/SCr), hepatic function (AST, ALT, bilirubin), and hematologic status (CBC with differential).
- Baseline neurologic testing (such as sensory system tests or gait tests) and hearing tests (audiogram) should also be performed.

d. *Calculate the patient's BSA and the amount of each drug to be administered based on the regimen chosen.*

- BSA = Square root of [{height (in.) × wt (lb.)} ÷ 3131]
  = Square root of [{63 × 154} × 3131]
  = 1.76 m²
- Regimen: cisplatin 100 mg/m² IV on day 1 = 176 mg IV on day 1
  etoposide 100 mg/m² on days 1, 2, and 3 = 176 mg IV on days 1, 2, and 3

Outcome Evaluation

5. *What clinical and laboratory parameters are necessary to evaluate the therapy for achievement of the desired therapeutic outcome and the occurrence of adverse effects?*

Efficacy Parameters
- A repeat chest x-ray or chest CT scan is used to evaluate any reduction in tumor mass. The unofficial standard is to evaluate the response to therapy after 2 cycles to determine if there is decrease in tumor size or stable disease.

Adverse Effect Parameters
- Cisplatin can cause nausea and vomiting both acutely (within the first 24 hours) and delayed (24 hours after cisplatin and can last up to 7 days). The number of emesis episodes and their severity should be monitored either by nurses' notes as an inpatient or by a patient self-diary as an outpatient.
- Because cisplatin can cause nephrotoxicity, the BUN and SCr should be monitored within 3 days after cisplatin. The BUN and SCr are not routinely monitored on an outpatient basis.
- Fluid balance (intake and output, body weight) should be monitored during the administration of cisplatin and for the first 24 hours afterward. Because urine output should be ≥ 100 mL/hour prior to the start and for 24 hours after cisplatin, fluid intake should be at least 100 mL/hour. Body weight should not change.
- Serum electrolytes (especially magnesium and potassium) should be monitored for imbalances 5 to 7 days after treatment. If low, electrolytes should be replaced appropriately and reevaluated prior to the next treatment.
- The occurrence of peripheral neuropathy and ototoxicity should be determined prior to each cycle. These would be assessed based upon patient signs and symptoms, using repeated sensory neurologic testing and repeat audiograms.
- The hemoglobin and hematocrit should be monitored prior to each cycle because cisplatin can cause anemia.
- Etoposide is associated with neutropenia (the nadir occurs 7 to 14 days after treatment), thrombocytopenia (the nadir occurs 9 to 16 days after treatment), and anemia. Consequently, monitoring the CBC with differential 7 to 10 days after chemotherapy is warranted.
- Etoposide is associated with hypotension during the infusion (monitor BP), mucositis, mild nausea, alopecia, and peripheral neuropathy.

- Radiation can cause irritated skin in the treatment area, fatigue, nausea and vomiting, esophagitis, and mucositis.

Patient Counseling

6. *What information should be provided to the patient to optimize therapy and minimize adverse effects?*

- Maintain proper hydration by drinking 8 to 10 8-ounce glasses of water or other fluids per day.
- This treatment will lower your white blood cell count, increasing your risk of infection. Notify your doctor or nurse of any fever over 100°F, chills, cough with sputum production, a change in sputum color, or a burning feeling with urination.
- Take the antinausea medications exactly as directed to prevent nausea and vomiting. Contact your doctor if you have vomiting that is not relieved by your antinausea medicine.
- Report any bleeding episodes or easy bruising, changes in your hearing, or numbness or tingling in your hands or feet.

▶ Follow-up Questions

1. *Calculate the patient's corrected calcium level and provide an interpretation of that value.*

   Corrected calcium = (4.0 − serum albumin level) × (0.8) + measured serum calcium value
   = 1.6 + 11.5 = 13.1 mg/dL

- Because calcium is bound to albumin in the bloodstream, hypoalbuminemia results in more unbound (free) calcium that is available to interact at tissue receptor sites. Therefore, the measured serum calcium level in this situation underestimates the degree of hypercalcemia. The equation is used to correct the serum calcium level for the degree of hypoalbuminemia, thereby providing a more accurate estimate of the severity of hypercalcemia.

2. *What treatment modalities may be used to correct hypercalcemia?*

- Patients with hypercalcemia are dehydrated. Consequently, the first step involves hydration with normal saline.
- Loop diuretics (e.g., furosemide, bumetanide, torsemide) promote calciuresis, but they should be reserved until the patient is well hydrated, because overdiuresis may cause dehydration.
- Specific agents used to lower serum calcium levels include the bisphosphonates (e.g., pamidronate), calcitonin, plicamycin, gallium nitrate, and corticosteroids. Typically a bisphosphonate is used, such as pamidronate 90 mg IV in 500 mL of normal saline infused over 3 hours × 1. Calcium levels should begin to decrease within 24 to 48 hours and nadir in about 7 days.

References

1. Clinical practice guidelines for the treatment of unresectable non-small cell lung cancer. Adopted on May 16, 1997 by the American Society of Clinical Oncology. J Clin Oncol 1997;15:2996–3018.
2. Pritchard RS, Anthony SP. Chemotherapy plus radiotherapy compared with radiotherapy alone in the treatment of locally advanced, unresectable, non-small-cell lung cancer. A meta-analysis. Ann Intern Med 1996;125:723–729.

121 COLON CANCER

▶ The Editor (Level I)

Daniel Sageser, PharmD

Recurrence of colon cancer occurs in a 54-year-old man who had the primary tumor resected 10 months ago and subsequently underwent 9 months of chemotherapy with a regimen containing 5-fluorouracil (5-FU) and levamisole. The recurrent masses were surgically resected, and he now presents to begin a second regimen of cancer chemotherapy. Potential regimens include either weekly or monthly 5-FU plus leucovorin or weekly irinotecan. Irinotecan may be preferred in this patient because of the possible development of tumor resistance to 5-FU. Case questions relate to designing regimens to assess both regimen efficacy and adverse effects and patient counseling on recognition and treatment of irinotecan adverse effects.

▶ Questions

Problem Identification

1. Create a list of the patient's drug-related problems.

- *Untreated indication.* Recurrent colon carcinoma, requiring aggressive chemotherapy.
- *Possible inadequate dosage.* Type 2 diabetes mellitus, which may be inadequately controlled on present dose of metformin (the goal fasting blood glucose is <120 mg/dL, but it is unknown whether the present glucose value of 187 mg/dL was taken in the fasted state).
- *Improper drug selection.* Patient takes diphenhydramine as often as twice daily for unknown reasons; because of its anticholinergic effects, diphenhydramine has been used as a sleep aid, but its other anticholinergic properties (e.g., dry mouth, urinary retention) make it undesirable as a hypnotic agent.
- Insufficient information is available to assess the appropriate use of and current need for temazepam (hypnotic), prochlorperazine (antiemetic), and loperamide (antidiarrheal). The patient should be questioned about his current use of these medications.

Desired Outcome

2. What is the desired outcome for chemotherapy in this patient?

- Metastatic colorectal cancer is presently incurable. Because this patient is relatively young and tolerated his previous regimen well, treatment will be given with intent to palliate, or decrease colon cancer symptoms.
- Important outcome measures include the effects of treatment on patient symptoms, daily activities and performance status, and other quality of life indicators.
- Positive prognostic indicators in this patient include his young age and prior ability to tolerate chemotherapy. Negative prognostic indicators include: 1) metastatic recurrence after surgery and adjuvant chemotherapy; 2) relatively short time to recurrence; 3) male gender; and 4) symptomatic initial presentation.

Therapeutic Alternatives

3. What chemotherapeutic options are available for this patient?

- *5-fluorouracil (5-FU) plus levamisole* is not a viable option because the patient's malignancy progressed on this therapy.
- *5-FU plus leucovorin* is an option, which can be given in one of two regimens.
  - ✓ Weekly 5-FU (500 mg/m^2) + leucovorin (500 mg/m^2) IV once weekly for 6 weeks with 2 weeks off between cycles
  - ✓ Monthly 5-FU (425 mg/m^2) + leucovorin (20 mg/m^2) IV given on days 1 through 5 of a 28-day cycle.

  One of these two regimens may be advantageous because the patient has tolerated 5-FU-based therapy well in the past with a good quality of life. However, this regimen would employ the same mechanism of antineoplastic activity as his previous regimen. One difference is that it adds the biochemical modulating effects of leucovorin. Nevertheless, if the patient's neoplastic cells have developed resistance to 5-FU, he may relapse quickly.
- *Irinotecan* is indicated as second-line therapy for colon cancer in patients who experience recurrence while on 5-FU-based regimens. It has a different mechanism of action than 5-FU, inhibiting DNA synthesis of rapidly dividing cells by decreasing the ability to unwind DNA for replication by inhibiting the enzyme topoisomerase I.[1] In contrast, 5-FU inhibits pyrimidine synthesis by inhibiting the enzyme thymidylate synthetase. However, irinotecan can cause more severe diarrhea and bone marrow suppression than 5-FU-based regimens. It is also much more expensive. One cycle consists of irinotecan 125 mg/m^2 IV given over 90 minutes once weekly for 4 weeks followed by a 2-week rest period. If the patient has minimal toxicity, the dose can be increased to 150 mg/m^2 in subsequent cycles. The regimen is continued until there is evidence of progression on imaging scan or a rise in the CEA level, patient intolerance, or if the patient's oncologist feels that further treatment would not benefit the patient. Irinotecan may cause moderate nausea/vomiting, so adjuvant pharmacotherapy should include a 5HT$_3$ antagonist (e.g., ondansetron 16 mg IV or granisetron 1 mg po) and dexamethasone 10 mg IV 30 minutes prior to irinotecan. Dexamethasone should be used with caution in this diabetic patient because it may contribute to glucose intolerance. The patient should also be instructed to take the prochlorperazine as prescribed if he experiences nausea or vomiting at home.

Optimal Plan

4. Design a chemotherapy regimen for treating this patient's recurrent colon carcinoma.

- The irinotecan regimen is preferred because it has a different mechanism of action and has been shown to be effective in patients who re-

ceived prior treatment with 5-FU-based regimens.[2] This is the most aggressive line of therapy.
- A case can also be made for 5-FU + leucovorin therapy because the patient's previous regimen did not have the biochemical modulating effect of leucovorin. Adding leucovorin may result in increased activity against the patient's colon cancer cells.

Outcome Evaluation

5. *What parameters should be monitored to evaluate the efficacy and adverse effects of the regimen you recommended?*

Efficacy
- Repeat serum CEA levels at the beginning of each cycle.
- Perform imaging studies (CT or MRI scan) after the first or second cycle. The patient should be restaged after 2 cycles of chemotherapy.
- Question the patient about the presence of disease symptoms such as a change in bowel habits, changes in stool caliber, or nonspecific GI distress, pain, or cramping.
- Check stools for occult blood every 3 to 4 months for the first 3 years.

Adverse Effects of Irinotecan
- The diarrhea from irinotecan has an acute onset (< 24 hours post-dose) and is considered to be a cholinergic reaction. It may be treated with atropine sulfate 0.25 to 1.0 mg SC × 1 dose.[3] Diarrhea is usually accompanied by diaphoresis and or abdominal cramping.
- Diarrhea with a delayed onset (> 24 hours post-dose) can be serious or even life threatening and must be treated immediately.[4] First-line therapy is loperamide 4 mg initially, then 2 mg po every 2 hours until 12 hours after the last loose stool.
- Neutropenia (ANC < $1.0 \times 10^3/mm^3$) may occur starting after week 2 of each cycle. If severe, dosage reduction may be warranted or cytokine therapy initiated (e.g., filgrastim).
- Nausea, vomiting, and dehydration are most likely to occur for 1 to 2 days after the infusion of irinotecan. Rescue therapy can be initiated with a phenothiazine (e.g., prochlorperazine, promethazine, or thiethylperazine) or a moderate dose of metoclopramide (e.g., 20 mg po or IV Q 6 H). Observe for signs of extrapyramidal symptoms with these medications because the patient is at moderate risk for these side effects because he is a male and is still relatively young. Dehydration can be detected by a careful history of fluid intake and urine output. It can be detected clinically by examining the oral mucosa and skin turgor. A BUN-to-SCr ratio of greater than 20:1 may also indicate dehydration.
- Stomatitis and mucositis can begin any time after day 5 of a cycle and can be minimized by proper oral hygiene during therapy. It is commonly palliated with compounded mouthwashes containing diphenhydramine, lidocaine, and antacid.

Patient Counseling

6. *What information should be provided to the patient to ensure the safety and efficacy of your regimen?*

- Both irinotecan and 5-FU can cause diarrhea. It is imperative that the patient receive verbal teaching and written material on the treatment of delayed diarrhea due to either medication, and be instructed to call his physician if he develops this side effect.
- This treatment can lower the number of your white blood cells, increasing your risk of developing an infection. Notify your doctor immediately if you get a fever.
- This medication may cause nausea and vomiting. You will be given some antinausea medications to take home and use as your doctor prescribed them. Call your doctor or the cancer center if the nausea or vomiting is not controlled by the medication.
- This medicine may cause ulcers inside your mouth. Report any white patches or sore spots in your mouth to your physician, even if they do not hurt. If they become irritated, mouthwashes can be prescribed that will decrease the pain until they heal.

References

1. Kawato Y, Aonuma M, Hirota Y, et al. Intracellular roles of SN-38, a metabolite of the camptothecin derivative CPT-11, in the antitumor effect of CPT-11. Cancer Res 1991;51:4187–4191.
2. Rothenberg ML, Eckardt JR, Kuhn JG, et al. Phase II trial of irinotecan in patients with progressive or rapidly recurrent colorectal cancer. J Clin Oncol 1996;14:1128–1135.
3. Camptosar package insert. Kalamazoo, MI, Pharmacia & Upjohn, 1997.
4. Abigerges D, Armand JP, Chabot GG, et al: Irinotecan (CPT-11) high-dose escalation using intensive high-dose loperamide to control diarrhea. J Natl Cancer Inst 1994;86:446–449.

122 PROSTATE CANCER

▶ **For Men Only** (Level II)

Judith A. Smith, PharmD
Barry R. Goldspiel, PharmD, FASHP

A 69-year-old man with stage D_2 prostate cancer seeks additional treatment options after experiencing disease progression on combined androgen blockade with goserelin acetate and bicalutamide. Antiandrogen withdrawal is recommended as the first manipulation because objective responses lasting 3 to 14 months have been observed after drug discontinuation. Combination chemotherapy with estramustine plus vinblastine or mitoxantrone plus corticosteroids has also been shown to palliate hormone-refractory prostate cancer. Androgen ablation is usually continued when chemotherapy is initiated. This patient desired treatment with chemotherapy but failed to respond, and his disease progressed during his second cycle. Chemotherapy was discontinued at that time, and further efforts were focused on pain control and other comfort measures.

▶ Questions

Problem Identification

1. a. Create a list of this patient's drug-related problems.

- Metastatic prostate cancer that has progressed despite combined androgen blockade.
- Pain from bone metastases, inadequately treated with present medications.
- Type 2 diabetes with blood glucose concentrations currently uncontrolled.
- Anemia of chronic disease, which is not responsive to treatment with iron, folate, or vitamin B_{12}.

b. What signs, symptoms, and other information are consistent with progressive prostate cancer in this case?

- *Symptoms.* The most common complaints in patients with advanced disease arise from ureteral dysfunction or impingement including urinary frequency, hesitancy, and dribbling. Bone-related pain is common in patients with bone metastases, the most common metastatic site for prostate cancer. Patients with progressive advanced prostate cancer while receiving androgen-deprivation therapy (such as this patient received with goserelin plus bicalutamide) present with increasing pain at prior known metastatic sites or new onset pain at new metastatic sites.
- *Signs.* An enlarged prostate containing a firm nodule that is biopsy-positive along with increasing urinary symptoms suggests either local recurrence or increased tumor size.
- *Other information.* In this patient's case, the bone scan revealing new sites in the ribs, left shoulder, and pelvis along with new onset pain in the affected shoulder gives the initial suspicion of progressive disease. The marked PSA increase, well out of the normal range even corrected for age, confirms the presence of progressive disease.[1] The elevated alkaline phosphatase is also consistent with bony metastases.

c. What is your assessment of the appropriateness of the initial therapy (goserelin plus bicalutamide) that this patient received for Stage D_2 prostate cancer?

- Because prostate gland and prostate cancer growth are dependent on androgens, the major initial treatment modality for advanced prostate cancer (stage D_2) is androgen-ablative therapy.[2,3] (Refer to textbook Table 119–2.) Approximately 85% of patients have an initial objective response to hormonal manipulation, usually manifested as symptom relief and PSA reductions. Local radiation therapy is also commonly used to palliate painful skeletal metastases in patients where bone fracture is imminent, whose pain cannot be controlled by analgesics, or who have relapsed after endocrine therapy.
- The initial hormonal manipulation should be based on physician assessment, patient preference, cost, and adverse effects. Despite their relatively high-cost, LHRH agonists (leuprolide or goserelin) have become the usual initial treatment for advanced prostate cancer. However, LHRH agonists should not be used, or should be used very cautiously (with concomitant radiation or antiandrogens), as initial therapy in patients with impending urinary obstruction or spinal cord compression. The sustained-action formulations that can be given every 3 or 4 months have almost completely replaced those that must be given daily. There are no direct comparative studies of these two agents, but equivalent response rates and adverse effects are observed for each preparation.
- Some investigators consider combined androgen ablation [i.e., adding an antiandrogen (flutamide, bicalutamide, or nilutamide) to LHRH agonist therapy or orchiectomy] to be the initial hormonal therapy of choice for newly diagnosed stage D_2 patients; the costs of combined therapy must be weighed against potential benefits because of conflicting results from randomized trials.[2] For those trials that did show an advantage for combined androgen blockade, whether these effects are testosterone deprivation method-specific (i.e., orchiectomy versus LHRH agonist), antiandrogen-specific (flutamide versus bicalutamide versus nilutamide), or patient selection-specific, is not clear. Some studies have demonstrated a major benefit in patients with minimal disease. Consequently, this may be the ideal population for combined androgen ablation.
- Although specific information that would exclude any of the initial therapies mentioned was not given, this patient's initial combination therapy with LHRH agonist and an antiandrogen can be considered appropriate. One could question whether adding the antiandrogen was essential, but justification can be strengthened if information was provided that the patient had minimal disease at initial presentation.

d. Would you consider this patient an appropriate candidate for a clinical research trial?

- According to the NCCN Prostate Cancer Practice Guidelines[3] (see textbook Figure 119–3), suggested treatment for patients with progressive disease depends on the initial treatment, the patient's medical status, and patient preference. When patients have become hormone-refractory, consideration for a clinical trial is an ethical option because there is no standard hormonal or chemotherapy regimen that prolongs survival.
- In patients initially treated with combined androgen deprivation (goserelin plus bicalutamide in this case), the NCCN guidelines suggest that antiandrogen withdrawal should be the first manipulation. Objective and subjective responses have been noted following the discontinuation of flutamide, bicalutamide, or nilutamide in patients receiving these agents as part of combined androgen ablation with an LHRH agonist.[4] Mutations in the androgen receptor have been demonstrated that allow antiandrogens such as flutamide, bicalutamide, or nilutamide (or their metabolites) to become agonists and activate the androgen receptor. Patient responses to androgen withdrawal manifest as significant PSA reductions and improved clinical symptoms that may start to manifest 3 to 6 weeks after androgen discontinuation. Androgen withdrawal responses lasting 3 to 14 months have been noted in about 35% of patients, and predicting response seems to be most closely related to longer antiandrogen exposure times. Incomplete cross-resistance has been noted in some patients who received bicalutamide after they had progressed while receiving flutamide.
- Although a clinical trial would be an ethical option for this pa-

tient and he might meet other general clinical trial entry criteria such as having good performance status and adequate laboratory values, he would not be eligible at this time because the bicalutamide was discontinued only 1 week ago. Because of the potential for response after antiandrogen withdrawal, a sufficient observation and assessment period (usually 4 to 6 weeks) combined with clear objective evidence for disease progression, is usually required before a patient can be enrolled on a clinical trial evaluating a new agent or therapy for advanced prostate cancer.

Desired Outcome

2. *Considering this patient's disease stage and treatment history, what are the reasonable therapeutic goals?*

- Advanced (Stage D) prostate cancer is not currently curable, but patients can experience symptom palliation for an average of 2 to 3 years after starting androgen ablative therapy. The prognosis for patients with progressive prostate cancer after receiving androgen ablative therapy is poor, with a median survival of 6 to 9 months. In these patients, symptom palliation and maintaining quality of life should be the main goals.
- In this patient's case, symptom palliation and quality of life maintenance are the most appropriate goals; these efforts should focus on pain control and urinary symptom relief.

Therapeutic Alternatives

3. *What pharmacotherapeutic options are available for the treatment of this patient?*

- Secondary or salvage therapies for patients who progress after their initial therapy depend on what was used for initial management (see textbook Figure 119–4).[3]
- *Androgen withdrawal* should be the first salvage manipulation considered if the patient initially received combined androgen blockade with an LHRH agonist with an antiandrogen. Adding an agent that blocks adrenal androgen synthesis, such as aminoglutethimide, at the time androgens are withdrawn may produce a better response than androgen withdrawal alone.[5]
- *Chemotherapy* with approved agent(s) or combinations that have demonstrated palliative activity is another option. However, despite extensive testing of single agents, combination regimens, and combination chemotherapy/hormonal regimens, significant response rates are rare and no currently approved antineoplastic agent or combination prolongs survival in patients with advanced prostate cancer. Recently, PSA reductions and/or clinical improvements (such as quality of life, improved pain, and reduced analgesic requirements) have been adopted as accepted end points for trials evaluating chemotherapy agents in prostate cancer patients.[1] Androgen ablation is usually continued when chemotherapy is initiated.
    - ✓ *Estramustine plus vinblastine* has been evaluated in several trials.[6] Response is manifested as objective tumor regression (partial response rate up to 50%), PSA declines, pain relief, and delay in bone scan progression. The toxicities of estramustine combined with vinblastine are nausea, gynecomastia, fatigue, and fluid retention.
    - ✓ *Mitoxantrone plus corticosteroids* is another combination regimen that can palliate hormone-refractory prostate cancer.[7] In a 160-patient trial, palliative responses were noted in 29% of patients in the mitoxantrone plus prednisone group and 12% of patients in the prednisone alone group ($p = 0.01$). The duration of palliative response was greater and quality of life scores for pain, physical activity, constipation, and mood were better in patients who received mitoxantrone plus prednisone. Patients treated with mitoxantrone plus prednisone experienced tolerable adverse effects, but 5 patients did develop some cardiac-related adverse effects. More than 30% of patients developed hyperglycemia while receiving mitoxantrone combined with hydrocortisone. Mitoxantrone plus corticosteroids is an FDA-approved therapy for hormone-refractory prostate cancer.
    - ✓ *Ketoconazole plus doxorubicin, estramustine plus etoposide,* and *estramustine plus paclitaxel* are other possible chemotherapeutic regimens suggested by the NCCN guidelines and investigated in clinical trials.[3]
- Strong consideration should be given to entering eligible patients into clinical trials investigating new therapies for advanced prostate cancer because better therapy that prolongs life or cures patients is needed.
- If the patient is not eligible for a clinical trial, supportive care, chemotherapy, or local radiotherapy can be used in patients who have failed all forms of androgen ablation manipulations, because these patients are considered to have androgen-independent disease.

Optimal Plan

4. *Design an optimal pharmacotherapeutic plan for this patient, considering that he is not eligible for a clinical research study at this time and wants to receive some chemotherapy in addition to adjusting his pain control medications.*

- After explaining to the patient that chemotherapy may improve his symptoms but will probably not prolong his life, the two most tested regimens to consider are estramustine plus vinblastine or mitoxantrone plus corticosteroids.
- Because the patient is a poorly controlled diabetic on many antidiabetic medications, it would probably be best to avoid corticosteroids, which may worsen his glucose control.
- In this case, the physician chose to start the patient on estramustine 600 mg/m^2 po daily on days 1 through 42 plus vinblastine 4 mg/m^2 IV once weekly for 6 weeks starting on day 1, with courses to be repeated every 8 weeks.[8] Goserelin was continued in the hope that continued androgen ablation would provide some benefit.

Outcome Evaluation

5. *How should the therapy you recommended be monitored for efficacy and adverse effects?*

Efficacy Parameters

- In a patient with symptomatic progressive prostate cancer treated with palliative intention, invasive tests and procedures should be minimized and performed only as patient symptoms dictate.
- Clinical responses are documented by assessing the patient's performance status, pain intensity, analgesic requirements, and weight changes.
- If pain is the patient's main symptom, assessment should be done at each clinic visit, and the patient should be instructed to maintain

communication with his health care providers about his pain levels between clinic visits.
- Bone scans and other scans (x-rays, CT, MRI) can be repeated when symptoms worsen to help establish the presence of new metastatic sites.
- The PSA can be monitored if the patient gets worse, but there is no need to routinely monitor PSA in an asymptomatic or stable patient. Most clinicians agree that, outside of a clinical trial, there is no obligation to treat an asymptomatic or stable patient with a rising PSA as the sole possible manifestation of progressive disease.

Adverse Effect Parameters
- The main adverse effects associated with the estramustine plus vinblastine regimen are leukopenia, anemia, nausea, edema, fatigue, and breast tenderness. To monitor for adverse effects, hematologic indices should be monitored at least weekly during chemotherapy prior to the vinblastine infusion. Weight measurement, edema assessment, and nausea and vomiting assessment should be performed with each chemotherapy cycle.

Patient Counseling

6. *What information should be provided to the patient about his new therapy?*

Goserelin
- Goserelin is given by injection under the skin every 3 months.
- If you miss a dose of this medicine, get it as soon as possible.
- Goserelin may decrease your desire and ability to have sexual relations. You may also notice sudden feelings of warmth and a sudden onset of sweating ("hot flashes"). These adverse effects usually go away with continued treatment. Rarely, some patients experience anxiety or depression, constipation, dizziness, headache, loss of appetite, nausea, breast enlargement, swelling in the feet or lower legs, trouble sleeping, and weight gain.
- Inform your doctor immediately if you develop pain in your groin or legs (especially calves) or shortness of breath, because goserelin can, rarely, cause blood clots.

Estramustine
- Estramustine is a capsule that should be taken exactly as directed by your physician. Your total daily dose is divided into 3 doses that should be taken at evenly spaced intervals throughout the day.
- You will take this medicine each day for 42 days (6 weeks) and then have 2 weeks off before starting it again. It may be helpful to speak with your pharmacist about designing a schedule to take all your medications.
- If you miss a dose, skip the missed dose and resume your regular dosing schedule. Do not double doses.
- Take this medication on an empty stomach (1 hour before or 2 hours after a meal) and spaced at least 2 hours from the time any milk, milk formulas, or dairy products are consumed.
- If significant nausea or vomiting occurs, it may be taken with a light meal or antacid to decrease these problems. Your doctor may also prescribe antiemetics to reduce or eliminate the nausea and vomiting.
- Inform your doctor of any drug allergies and the names of prescription and non-prescription medications that you take regularly, or if you start a new medication.

- Do not have any immunizations (vaccinations) while taking estramustine without your physician's approval.
- Tell your doctor about any history of blood clots, chicken pox (including a recent exposure), herpes zoster (including shingles), stomach ulcer, stroke, or if you smoke.
- Estramustine may cause some swelling in your feet or lower legs. It may decrease your desire and ability to have sexual relations. Also, you may experience some breast tenderness or enlargement and diarrhea while taking estramustine. Rarely, a skin rash and unusual tiredness or fatigue may occur.
- Notify your doctor if you develop black, tarry stools; blood in your urine or stools; severe or sudden headaches; new cough or hoarseness; lower back pain; and painful or difficult urination. Because estramustine increases the risk of blood clots, notify your doctor if you develop pain in the chest, groin, or leg (especially calf), or shortness of breath.

Vinblastine
- Vinblastine is given into one of your veins once weekly for 6 weeks. You will then have 2 weeks off before receiving the next cycle.
- Vinblastine temporarily lowers your white blood cell count and increases your risk for infection. Because fever is an important sign of an infection while your white blood cell count is low, your physician or other health care provider will instruct you how and when to take your temperature and what to do if it is elevated.
- Vinblastine may also lower the number of platelets in your blood that are needed for proper clotting.
- To prevent complications while your blood counts are low, try to avoid contact with others who have active infections (such as a cold), use good hygiene practices (e.g., do not touch your eyes or inside of your nose unless you have just washed your hands, and try not to cut, bruise, or injure yourself).
- Vinblastine may cause a temporary loss of hair, constipation, mouth sores, jaw pain, dizziness, or fatigue. Less often, it may cause joint pain, cough, fever, chills, lower back pain, or nausea and vomiting.
- Immediately report to your doctor any changes in urination, changes in hearing, a sensation of "pins and needles," or new rashes (i.e., pinpoint red spots on skin). Also report any signs of bleeding such as black, tarry stools, blood in your urine or stool, or unusual bleeding or bruising.

▶ Follow-up Question

1. *Given the patient's wish to not receive any chemotherapy agents and his probable ineligibility for clinical trials (based on his poor performance status), what therapeutic options are available for him at this time?*

- Because chemotherapy does not prolong survival in patients with progressive advanced prostate cancer, it is appropriate to provide only supportive care to patients who do not want to receive chemotherapy, who are poor candidates for chemotherapy, or who are ineligible for clinical trials.
- The patient's wishes should be honored and if available, a pain management team should be consulted to review the options for pain control. Alternatives include analgesics, corticosteroids, local radiotherapy, and radioisotope therapy for bone pain. Because this pa-

tient's diabetes-related symptoms may worsen with corticosteroids and it is desirable to avoid compromising his quality of life further, corticosteroid administration may not be a suitable option.
- Efforts should focus on optimizing his pain control, making him comfortable, and preparing both the patient and his family for his eventual death.

References

1. Roach M, Small EJ. Using the serum prostate specific antigen (PSA) to screen for and manage prostate cancer. Princ Pract Oncol Updates 1997;11:1–14.
2. Garnick MB. Hormonal therapy in the management of prostate cancer: From Huggins to the present. Urology 1997;49(3A suppl):5–15.
3. Millikan R, Logothetis C. Update of the NCCN guidelines for treatment of prostate cancer. Oncology (Huntingt) 1997;11(11A):180–193.
4. Kelly WK, Slovin S, Scher HI. Steroid hormone withdrawal syndromes. Pathophysiology and clinical significance. Urol Clin North Am 1997;24:421–431.
5. Sartor O, Cooper M, Weinberger M, et al. Surprising activity of flutamide withdrawal, when combined with aminoglutethimide, in treatment of "hormone-refractory" prostate cancer. J Natl Cancer Inst 1994;86:222–227.
6. Hudes G. Estramustine-based chemotherapy. Semin Urol Oncol 1997;15:13–19.
7. Tannock IF, Osoba D, Stockler MR, et al. Chemotherapy with mitoxantrone plus prednisone or prednisone alone for symptomatic hormone-resistant prostate cancer: A Canadian randomized trial with palliative end points. J Clin Oncol 1996;14:1756–1764.
8. Hudes GR, Greenberg R, Krigel RL, et al. Phase II study of estramustine and vinblastine, two microtubule inhibitors, in hormone-refractory prostate cancer. J Clin Oncol 1992;10:1754–1761.

123 MALIGNANT LYMPHOMA

▶ The French Chef   (Level I)

Krista M. King, PharmD, BCOP

A 68-year-old man presents for recommendations regarding treatment of a newly diagnosed gastric large cell lymphoma, stage IEB. His PMH is significant for hypertension, type 2 diabetes, and chronic renal insufficiency. The standard treatment recommendation for this aggressive primary gastric lymphoma is CHOP (cyclophosphamide, doxorubicin, vincristine, and prednisone) for 6 to 8 cycles, followed by consolidative radiotherapy. Although several second- and third-generation regimens have been introduced, CHOP has been shown to be as effective as these regimens with fewer fatal toxicities. The acute and delayed toxicities of the chemotherapy regimen must be monitored. Appropriate treatment measures must be initiated to prevent and treat nausea and vomiting, mucositis, and tumor lysis syndrome. Antineoplastic treatment must be administered while maintaining control of the patient's concomitant diabetes, chronic renal insufficiency, and hypertension.

▶ Questions

Problem Identification

1. a. *Identify all of the drug-related problems of this patient.*

   - Large cell lymphoma, requiring chemotherapy.
   - Hypertension that may be inadequately controlled with low doses of captopril.
   - Chronic renal insufficiency likely, secondary to diabetes, which may benefit from ACE inhibitors to prevent further progression. However, the patient has hyperkalemia that may necessitate use of other agents to slow progression of renal disease.
   - Type 2 diabetes treated with low doses of glipizide; long-term control is difficult to assess with the information provided.

   b. *What clinical and other information is consistent with the diagnosis of non-Hodgkin's lymphoma?*

   - *Signs.* Epigastric mass 10 to 12 cm in diameter, guaiac (+) stools.
   - *Symptoms.* Epigastric pain, fatigue, early satiety, and B symptoms (fever, night sweats, and weight loss).
   - *Laboratory values.* Increased LDH, β-2 microglobulin, and uric acid.
   - *Pathology.* Diffuse large cell lymphoma, B-cell type. The diagnosis of non-Hodgkin's lymphoma must be established by an appropriate biopsy to provide tissue for pathologic review.
   - *Scans.* Positive gallium scan and CT scan of the abdomen.

   c. *Explain what system of staging was used and how his stage of disease was determined.*

   - The staging system used is the Ann Arbor Staging System, which is the same staging system originally developed for Hodgkin's Disease. Refer to the section "Diagnosis and Staging" in textbook Chapter 120 for more detailed information.
   - The following staging procedures were performed to determine the extent of disease: complete H & P; laboratory values; detailed history of lymphadenopathy; CXR; endoscopy; CT scans of chest, abdomen, and pelvis; gallium scan; and bilateral bone marrow biopsies.
   - Stage I was determined because the patient has involvement of a single lymph node region or structure (the stomach) with associated perigastric lymphadenopathy.
   - Subset "E" describes involvement of a single extranodal site, in this case the stomach.
   - Subset "B" indicates the presence of B symptoms (fever, night sweats, and weight loss), which are seen in approximately 20% of NHL patients.

d. *What laboratory and clinical features does this patient have that may affect his prognosis?*

- The prognosis and treatment of non-Hodgkin's lymphoma is dependent on the histologic type and the presence of certain adverse clinical features.
- The International Prognostic Index was developed from pooled data on previously untreated patients with aggressive lymphoma. The patients were evaluated for clinical features predictive of overall survival and relapse-free survival. Features determined to adversely affect prognosis are: age > 60, Ann Arbor Stage III–IV, >1 extranodal site, poor performance status, and elevated LDH.[1]
- Tumor Score is yet another proposal for prognostic features for intermediate grade lymphomas and immunoblastic lymphomas. Poor prognostic features include: Ann Arbor Stage III–IV, presence of bulky mass, elevated β-2 microglobulin, elevated LDH, and B symptoms.[2]
- In summary, the laboratory and clinical features that this patient exhibits that indicate a poor prognosis include: age > 60, elevated LDH, elevated β-2 microglobulin, B symptoms, and presence of a bulky mass.

Desired Outcome

2. *What are the goals of therapy in this case?*

- The main goal of therapy is to cure the lymphoma. Diffuse large cell lymphoma, an aggressive neoplasm once considered uniformly fatal, is now among the most successfully treated non-Hodgkin's lymphomas. Chemotherapy with involved-field radiation has yielded 80% to 90% 5-year disease-free survival rates for stage I disease.
- Minimize acute treatment toxicities.
- Prevent long-term treatment toxicities.
- Promote gastric ulcer healing to prevent chronic blood loss and anemia.
- Improve hypertension control and avoid ACE inhibitors because of hyperkalemia.
- Avoid progression of chronic renal insufficiency.
- Control diabetes mellitus during corticosteroid treatment.

Therapeutic Alternatives

3. *What alternative drug therapies are available for the treatment of this non-Hodgkin's lymphoma?*

- CHOP (cyclophosphamide, doxorubicin, vincristine, and prednisone) is considered the standard chemotherapy regimen for the treatment of non-Hodgkin's lymphoma. In the 1980s, increasingly complex chemotherapy regimens were introduced (second- and third-generation regimens) with reports of improved remission and cure rates. When compared with these second- and third-generation regimens in a prospective randomized trial, CHOP was found to be as effective as m-BACOD, ProMACE-CytaBOM, and MACOP-B, and caused less fatal toxicity.[3]

Optimal Plan

4. a. *What drug, dosage form, schedule, and duration of therapy are best for treating this patient's non-Hodgkin's lymphoma?*

- The standard treatment recommendation for this aggressive primary gastric lymphoma is CHOP for 6 to 8 cycles, followed by consolidative radiotherapy to the stomach and lymphatic beds.
- Drug regimen:
  ✓ Cyclophosphamide 750 mg/m² IVPB on day 1
  ✓ Doxorubicin 25 mg/m²/day by IV continuous infusion over 24 hours QD on days 1 and 2
  ✓ Vincristine 1.4 mg/m² (maximum 2 mg) IVPB on day 1
  ✓ Prednisone 100 mg po QD on days 1 through 5
  ✓ The regimen is repeated every 21 days
- Due to the bulk of his tumor and other concurrent medical problems, it is recommended that the first chemotherapy treatment be administered in the hospital with very close follow-up in the outpatient setting upon discharge.
- Doxorubicin should be used with caution in this patient because he has an LVEF of 48%. The risk of cardiac toxicity from doxorubicin is related to peak drug levels. Therefore, it should be administered by continuous infusion rather than IV bolus. Shifting from bolus drug administration to weekly dosing or prolonged infusions has resulted in a significant reduction in the incidence of cardiac toxicity.[4–7] However, in community practice, the bolus administration of doxorubicin may sometimes still be used.

b. *What other interventions should be made to maintain control of the patient's other concurrent diseases?*

- Continue treatment with omeprazole 20 mg po QD to treat gastric ulcers.
- Continue glipizide 2.5 mg po QD and cover with sliding scale insulin during prednisone therapy. Obtain an HbA_{1c} level to evaluate the long-term control of diabetes.
- The patient is anemic from chronic blood loss. Start iron supplementation to replace lost iron stores.
- The patient's blood pressure is inadequately controlled. Signs of long-term uncontrolled hypertension include: cotton wool exudates on the funduscopic exam, reduced LVEF, chronic renal insufficiency, and an S_4 heart sound. Although captopril and other ACE inhibitors may slow progression of renal disease in patients with diabetes mellitus, they may also cause hyperkalemia (the patient's serum potassium is already elevated at 5.9 mEq/L). Consideration should be given to changing to another class of antihypertensive agent. Non-dihydropyridine calcium channel blockers (e.g., diltiazem) may have some efficacy in slowing progression of renal disease.

c. *What non-drug therapies might be useful for this patient?*

- Diabetic teaching for proper dietary management.
- Blood transfusions when necessary for severe anemia.

Outcome Evaluation

5. a. *How is the response to the treatment regimen for the non-Hodgkin's lymphoma assessed?*

- Response is determined by follow-up radiologic studies that initially showed positive findings, gallium scanning, and endoscopy evaluation. These tests should be performed every 2 to 4 cycles. The exact timing depends on physician preference, institutional guidelines, and sometimes, insurance coverage.

- The treatment response should also be assessed by monitoring the following signs and symptoms: epigastric mass and associated stomach pain; presence of B symptoms; and elevated LDH, uric acid, and β-2 microglobulin. These can be monitored every cycle.

b. *What acute adverse effects are associated with the chemotherapy regimen, and what parameters should be monitored?*

- Myelosuppression (doxorubicin, cyclophosphamide): obtain CBC, differential, and platelets twice weekly for 3 weeks after each course of chemotherapy. The patient should monitor himself for signs of infection or bleeding.
- Nausea/vomiting (moderate with doxorubicin and cyclophosphamide, mild with vincristine): record the number and severity of nausea and vomiting episodes. Monitor electrolytes twice weekly for 3 weeks after each course of chemotherapy.
- Stomatitis/mucositis (doxorubicin): mucous membranes should be examined for erythema, ulcers, or breakdown daily by the patient and by a clinician during each physical exam.
- Cardiotoxicity (doxorubicin): acute cardiotoxicities of the anthracyclines are usually self-limiting and rarely life-threatening. During and shortly after administration, transient nonspecific ECG abnormalities, arrhythmias, and vasospasm may occur. Transient CHF, pericarditis/myocarditis syndrome, and myocardial infarction have also been described as acute toxicities.
- Other adverse effects of the regimen include: alopecia (doxorubicin, cyclophosphamide, vincristine); darkening of the skin or fingernails (cyclophosphamide); hemorrhagic cystitis (cyclophosphamide); constipation (vincristine); and increased appetite, indigestion, nervousness/restlessness, insomnia, and hyperglycemia (prednisone). Doxorubicin and vincristine are vesicants.
- Gastric perforation is also a potential complication in this patient.
- Tumor lysis syndrome (TLS) is a potential complication of rapid tumor breakdown that occurs most commonly in diseases characterized by large tumor burdens and rapid growth rates that are extremely sensitive to cytotoxic treatment. TLS results in the rapid release of intracellular contents into the bloodstream. These contents can increase to life-threatening concentrations. Hyperuricemia, hyperkalemia, hyperphosphatemia, and hypocalcemia characterize TLS and can result in cardiac arrhythmias, acute renal failure, tetany, and muscle cramps. TLS is often an avoidable complication of treatment that is most commonly observed in the treatment of high-grade lymphomas or aggressive lymphomas that are growing rapidly.

c. *What pharmacologic measures should be instituted to treat or prevent the acute toxicities associated with the chemotherapy regimen?*

- *Myelosuppression.* If infectious complications occur after chemotherapy cycles, or if prolonged myelosuppression prevents the timely administration of subsequent cycles, growth-factor support with filgrastim (G-CSF) or sargramostim (GM-CSF) may be considered.
- *Nausea/vomiting.* A $5HT_3$-receptor antagonist should be given prior to each treatment because doxorubicin and cyclophosphamide are moderately emetogenic. Medication for breakthrough nausea and vomiting should also be prescribed.
- *Stomatitis/mucositis.* Good oral hygiene should be encouraged. Oral rinses with salt and soda solutions or chlorhexidine can help maintain a clean mouth. Topical management of mucositis may also include the use of viscous lidocaine, sucralfate suspension, or extemporaneously prepared suspensions containing combinations of viscous lidocaine, diphenhydramine, and magnesium/aluminum hydroxide.
- *Tumor lysis syndrome.* Recognizing the risk and instituting measures of prevention are essential to the management of TLS. Intravenous hydration including sodium bicarbonate or sodium acetate should be initiated 24 to 48 hours before the administration of the chemotherapy if possible, along with allopurinol to minimize hyperuricemia. Serum electrolytes, phosphorus, calcium, creatinine, and uric acid should be checked routinely after starting chemotherapy. Hyperkalemia should be treated with sodium polystyrene sulfonate (an oral sodium-potassium exchange resin) or combined IV glucose and insulin therapy. If renal function acutely worsens, dialysis should be considered to gain rapid control of serum concentrations of potassium, phosphorus, and uric acid.

d. *What are potential late complications of the chemotherapy regimen, and how can they be detected and prevented?*

- *Cardiotoxicity (doxorubicin).* Chronic anthracycline associated cardiotoxicity is characterized by cardiomyopathy and is frequently life threatening. Patients present with typical symptoms of ventricular failure. The frequency and severity of this chronic toxicity is related to the cumulative dose. Doxorubicin associated cardiac injury is unusual at cumulative doses < 450 mg/m^2 but increases at doses > 450 to 550 mg/m^2. Several risk factors that increase the frequency and severity of anthracycline induced cardiotoxicity include hypertension, pre-existing cardiac disease, prior thoracic radiation, and very young or very old age. A MUGA scan should be obtained at baseline prior to starting therapy to evaluate the ejection fraction. Follow-up exams at appropriate intervals are important especially in patients with risk factors for cardiotoxicity or for those who require > 450 mg/m^2 of doxorubicin. Few clinicians would continue therapy with doxorubicin if the LVEF is < 45% without a cardiology evaluation, as additional therapy could result in irreversible heart failure. Doxorubicin is contraindicated in patients with LVEF < 30%.[8]
- *Peripheral neuropathy (vincristine).* The dose-limiting adverse effect of vincristine is neurotoxicity. The most frequent neurotoxic manifestation is peripheral neuropathy. Patients with underlying neurologic disease and geriatric patients may be more susceptible to the neurotoxic effects. This is typically a cumulative effect occurring after several treatments. Neurologic examinations should be performed at baseline and prior to each treatment. If this patient exhibited peripheral neuropathy from long-standing diabetes mellitus, vincristine could compound this effect.
- *Carcinogenicity (cyclophosphamide).* Cyclophosphamide-treated patients can develop secondary malignancies that include malignancy of the urinary bladder and myeloproliferative and lymphoproliferative malignancies.

- *Sterility (cyclophosphamide).* Cyclophosphamide interferes with oogenesis and spermatogenesis. Amenorrhea, azoospermia, or oligospermia has been reported in 10% to 30% of patients. Sterility usually occurs only after prolonged use.

Patient Counseling

6. *What information would you provide to the patient about the chemotherapy agents?*

Doxorubicin

a. This drug interferes with the growth of cancer cells. Since the growth of normal cells may also be affected, side effects will occur. The drug is administered intravenously (injected into a vein).

b. The most common side effects include nausea and vomiting, temporary loss of hair (normal hair growth should return after treatment has ended), sores in the mouth and on the lips, red urine, and possible sterility.

c. Contact your doctor immediately if any of these less common side effects occur: fast or irregular heartbeat, cough or hoarseness, shortness of breath, or swelling of the lower legs or feet.

d. This drug can lower the number of platelets in your blood, which are needed for proper blood clotting. This may increase your risk of bleeding. Contact your doctor immediately if you notice any unusual bleeding or bruising, blood in the urine or stools, black-tarry stools, or pinpoint red spots on your skin.

e. This drug temporarily lowers the number of white cells in your blood, increasing your chance of getting an infection. Try to avoid coming into contact with people who have infections. Contact your doctor immediately if you experience any of the following symptoms: fever or chills, lower back or side pain, painful or difficult urination, or cough or hoarseness.

f. If this drug accidentally seeps out of the vein into which it is injected, it may damage the adjacent tissue and cause scarring. Contact your doctor immediately if you notice redness, pain, or swelling at the site of injection.

g. There is a chance that this drug may cause birth defects if it is taken during pregnancy, or if either the male or female is receiving it at the time of conception. A reliable form of birth control should be used while receiving the drug.

Cyclophosphamide

- Side effects a, d, e, and g as with doxorubicin.
- The most common side effects of this drug include nausea or vomiting, loss of appetite, darkening of the skin or fingernails, dizziness, temporary hair loss, and possible sterility.
- If too much of this drug appears in the urine or if the urine stays in the bladder too long, it can cause dangerous bladder irritation. Contact your doctor immediately if you notice blood in the urine or painful urination. It is important to drink extra fluids so that you will pass more urine. Also, empty your bladder frequently, including at least once during the night.
- Contact your doctor immediately if any of these less common side effects occur: fast heartbeat, joint pain, shortness of breath, or swelling of the lower legs or feet.

Vincristine

- Side effects a, f, and g as with doxorubicin.
- The most common side effects of this drug include blurred or double vision, constipation, numbness or tingling in fingers and toes, difficulty walking, and temporary hair loss.
- Contact your doctor immediately if any of these less common side effects occur: confusion, convulsions, agitation, dizziness, hallucinations, or problems with urination.

Prednisone

- This drug may lower your resistance to infection.
- The most common side effects of this drug include increased appetite, indigestion, nervousness/restlessness, trouble sleeping, and increased blood sugars in patients with diabetes mellitus.
- Contact your doctor immediately if any of these less common side effects occur: decreased or blurred vision, frequent urination, or increased thirst, which are all symptoms of an elevated blood sugar.

▶ Follow-up Question

1. *What could be the possible causes of the epigastric pain experienced by the patient?*

- Necrosis of tumor
- Worsening gastric ulcers
- Perforation of the gastric wall
- Blood loss into the peritoneum

References

1. The International Non-Hodgkin's Lymphoma Prognostic Factors Project. A predictive model for aggressive non-Hodgkin's lymphoma. N Engl J Med 1993;329: 987–994.
2. Rodriguez J, Cabanillas F, McLaughlin P, et al. A proposal for a simple staging system for intermediate grade lymphoma and immunoblastic lymphoma based on the "tumor score." Ann Oncol 1992;3:711–717.
3. Fisher RI, Gaynor ER, Dahlberg S, et al. Comparison of a standard regimen (CHOP) with three intensive chemotherapy regimens for advanced non-Hodgkin's lymphoma. N Engl J Med 1993;328:1002–1006.
4. Doroshow JH. Anthracyclines and anthracenediones. In: Chabner BA, Longo DL, eds. Cancer Chemotherapy and Biotherapy, 2nd ed. Philadelphia, Lippincott-Raven, 1996:409–429.
5. Steinherz LJ, Yahalom J. Cardiac complications of cancer therapy. In: DeVita VT Jr, Hellman S, Rosenberg ST, eds. Cancer: Principles & Practice of Oncology, 4th ed. Philadelphia, JB Lippincott, 1993:2370–2385.
6. Carlson RW. Reducing the cardiotoxicity of the anthracyclines. Oncology (Huntingt) 1992;6:95-100, 104, 107-108.
7. Basser RL, Green MD. Strategies for prevention of anthracycline cardiotoxicity. Cancer Treat Rev 1993;19:57–77.
8. Ganz WI, Sridhar KS, Ganz SS, et al. Review of tests for monitoring doxorubicin-induced cardiomyopathy. Oncology 1996;53:461–470.

124 OVARIAN CANCER

▶ **Dorothy Walker's Ordeal** (Level II)

William C. Zamboni, PharmD
James A. Trovato, PharmD

A 46-year-old woman with stage IV epithelial ovarian cancer presents for her first cycle of consolidative chemotherapy after undergoing primary cytoreductive therapy (total abdominal hysterectomy and left oophorectomy). The combination of paclitaxel plus either cisplatin or carboplatin has replaced cyclophosphamide plus a platinum analog as first-line consolidative treatment in women with stage III or IV disease. When this patient experiences nephrotoxicity and neurotoxicity after 3 cycles of paclitaxel plus cisplatin, readers are asked to recommend an alternative chemotherapeutic regimen. This involves replacing cisplatin with carboplatin, the dose of which must be calculated by an equation to achieve a target AUC. Although the patient achieved a clinical complete response after 6 total cycles of chemotherapy, she relapsed 8 months after the last cycle. Readers are then asked to recommend a regimen for relapsed epithelial ovarian cancer.

▶ **Questions**

Problem Identification

1. a. *What are the patient's drug-related problems?*

    - *Untreated indication.* Ovarian cancer requires systemic chemotherapy to prolong survival and/or cure disease.
    - *Subtherapeutic dosage.* Hypertension currently uncontrolled on present dose of Procardia XL (nifedipine); goal BP in a patient with diabetes is < 130/85 mm Hg.
    - *Untreated indication (possible).* Peripheral neuropathy possibly secondary to diabetes, which may benefit from pharmacotherapy.
    - *Drug use without indication.* The patient does not require the progestin agent medroxyprogesterone contained in Prempro because she has had a hysterectomy. A progestin is used in postmenopausal women with an intact uterus to reduce the risk of endometrial cancer from unopposed estrogen therapy.
    - Chronic, stable problems not requiring intervention at this time include: 1) type 2 diabetes mellitus presently well controlled on glipizide; and 2) post-menopausal state currently without symptoms.

   b. *What clinical and other information indicates the presence and severity of ovarian cancer?*

    - *Symptoms.* Abdominal pain, bloated feeling, and weight gain at the time of presentation.
    - *Signs.* 20 cm × 10 cm left adnexal mass at the time of presentation.
    - *Laboratory values.* Elevated CA-125, which is a tumor marker found in more than 80% of ovarian tumors. Rising or falling titers correlate with the extent of disease.
    - *Other information.* Soft-tissue pelvic mass on CT scan; tumor mass on laparotomy with microscopic disease and positive lymph nodes; ovarian and liver tumor biopsies positive for epithelial ovarian cancer.

   c. *What stage of ovarian cancer does this patient have, and how does the stage of disease affect the choice of therapy?*

    - The cancer has metastasized outside of the peritoneal cavity to the presacral spine and para-aortic region. This is defined as stage IV epithelial ovarian cancer, thus requiring primary cytoreductive surgery and consolidative chemotherapy.

   d. *What is the significance of the size of residual tumor after primary cytoreductive surgery?*

    - The amount of residual tumor burden affecting chemotherapeutic response is theoretically due to improved tumor perfusion and increased growth fraction in smaller sized residual tumors. Stage III patients with optimal debulking (less than 1 to 2 cm of residual disease tumor) have a 4-year survival rate of 30%. Stage III or IV patients with suboptimally debulked disease (> 2 cm of residual tumor) have a 5-year survival rate of < 10%.[1]

Desired Outcome

2. *What are the goals of therapy for this patient?*

    - Cure of disease, defined as pathologically negative at second-look laparotomy. Unfortunately, cure of disease occurs in only 10% to 20% of patients with stage III or IV disease.
    - Prolong life: from the time of diagnosis, the median survival in patients with stage III or IV disease is approximately 25 to 37 months, with a 5-year survival rate of 10% to 20%.
    - Increase the quality of the patient's life.
    - Minimize treatment-related toxicities.

Therapeutic Alternatives

3. *What consolidative chemotherapy options are available for this patient?*

    - *Cyclophosphamide plus cisplatin or carboplatin.* The combination of cyclophosphamide and a platinum analog was until recently the adjuvant therapy of choice in women with advanced-stage ovarian cancer. Carboplatin has equal efficacy to cisplatin when combined with cyclophosphamide and may have more acceptable toxicity (i.e., less nephrotoxicity, neurotoxicity, nausea, and vomiting).[2] Carboplatin does have a higher incidence of neutropenia and thrombocytopenia than cisplatin. Consequently, cisplatin may be more appropriate in patients at increased risk of severe myelosuppression. Carboplatin may be more appropriate in patients with sufficient marrow reserve.
    - *Paclitaxel plus cisplatin or carboplatin.* The combination of paclitaxel plus cisplatin achieved better response rates and survival outcomes than cyclophosphamide plus cisplatin in patients with newly

diagnosed, suboptimally debulked stage III or IV ovarian cancer.[3] The complete response rates were 51% and 31% after treatment with paclitaxel–cisplatin and cyclophosphamide–cisplatin, respectively. The median progression-free survival was 18 months with the paclitaxel-containing regimen and 13 months with the cyclophosphamide-containing regimen. The National Comprehensive Cancer Network (NCCN) Ovarian Cancer Practice Guidelines recommend paclitaxel in combination with cisplatin or carboplatin as first-line consolidative treatment in women with stage III or IV disease.[4]

- The dose-limiting toxicity (DLT) associated with high-dose paclitaxel (250 mg/m^2 over 24 hours repeated every 21 days) is peripheral neuropathy. A complicating factor in this patient is that she already has peripheral neuropathy. However, lower doses of paclitaxel (135 mg/m^2 IV over 3 hours) with carboplatin or lower paclitaxel doses (135 mg/m^2 IV over 24 hours) with cisplatin have a DLT of myelosuppression. In addition, due to the poor prognosis of patients with stage III or IV disease, the combination of paclitaxel with a platinum analog may be the most appropriate first-line therapy regardless of the peripheral neuropathy.

Optimal Plan

4. *Which consolidative chemotherapy regimen and ancillary treatment measures would you recommend for this patient?*

- For the reasons described, the optimal consolidative chemotherapy regimen is:
  ✓ Paclitaxel 135 mg/m^2 IV (24 hour infusion) on day 1
  ✓ Cisplatin 75 mg/m^2 IV on day 1
  ✓ Repeat the regimen every 21 days for 6 cycles
  Carboplatin could be used in place of cisplatin because the patient is newly diagnosed and therefore may not be at increased risk of severe myelosuppression (i.e., neutropenia, thrombocytopenia) from the drug. However, cisplatin may be more appropriate to reduce the duration of severe myelosuppression and its associated risks.
- Prophylaxis of chemotherapy-associated nausea and vomiting should be initiated with a regimen such as the following.
  ✓ Granisetron 2 mg po single dose 30 minutes prior to chemotherapy
  ✓ Dexamethasone 4 mg po 30 minutes prior to chemotherapy, and Q 6 H × 3 days
  ✓ Prochlorperazine 10 mg po Q 4 H PRN for breakthrough nausea and vomiting
- Prophylaxis for paclitaxel hypersensitivity reactions should be initiated with a regimen such as the following.
  ✓ Diphenhydramine 50 mg po 30 minutes prior to paclitaxel
  ✓ Ranitidine 150 mg po 30 minutes prior to paclitaxel

Outcome Evaluation

5. *How would you monitor the therapy for efficacy and adverse effects?*

Efficacy Monitoring

- CA-125 is a cell surface glycoprotein common to most nonmucinous epithelial ovarian cancer cells. CA-125 levels > 35 IU/mL are found in 82% of ovarian cancer patients, in 25% of patients with non-gynecological malignancies, and in 1% of healthy women. The CA-125 should be evaluated at the time of diagnosis, and every 3 to 4 months as part of the patient's follow-up.

- Repeat abdominal imaging studies are usually performed after 6 to 7 cycles of chemotherapy. Once a complete remission has been achieved, repeat abdominal MRI scans are not usually performed unless signs and/or symptoms suggest a local recurrence.
- Local signs of progression and/or relapse (e.g., pain, ascites) are monitored at each follow-up visit by physical examination and by questioning the patient.
- Second-look laparotomy has been used in clinical trials and is usually used clinically to determine pathologic response after 6 to 7 cycles of chemotherapy. However, its clinical utility is controversial. A study of stage I or II ovarian carcinoma suggests that second-look laparotomy may not be warranted in asymptomatic patients with early-stage disease. In addition, the NCI consensus conference recommends that second-look operations should only be performed when the results will change management or as part of a clinical trial.[4]

Adverse Effect Monitoring

- Paclitaxel
  ✓ Neutropenia (dose-limiting toxicity) results in an increased risk of infection when the ANC is < 0.5 to 1.0 × 10^3/mm^3. The nadir occurs 7 to 10 days after administration. Obtain a WBC count with differential every 2 to 3 days until the ANC has risen above 0.5 to 1.0 × 10^3/mm^3. Also, observe the patient for signs of infection, such as fever and redness at IV access sites.
  ✓ Thrombocytopenia results in an increased risk of bleeding when the platelet count is < 20 × 10^3/mm^3. The nadir occurs 7 to 10 days after administration. Obtain a platelet count every 2 to 3 days until it rises above > 50 × 10^3/mm^3. Also observe the patient for signs of bleeding (e.g., easy bruising, bleeding from the nose, mouth, or GI tract).
  ✓ Assess for hypersensitivity reactions such as anaphylaxis and rash by monitoring for difficulty breathing, shortness of breath, skin rash or hives, hypotension, and tachycardia. Hypersensitivity reactions occur within the first 24 hours.
  ✓ Neurotoxicity may be manifested as numbness, tingling, and/or burning pain in the extremities. Monitor for loss of touch sensation of the hands and feet and decreased ability to ambulate. Neurotoxicity occurs after repeated treatments.
  ✓ Cardiac dysrhythmias such as transient bradycardia and ventricular dysrhythmias may occur when paclitaxel is used in combination with platinum analogs. Dysrhythmias occur within the first 24 hours after administration. Monitor heart rate, blood pressure, and ECG in the first 24 hours after administration.
  ✓ Mucositis (necrotic inflammation of the mucous membranes associated with agranulocytosis) may be very painful and is associated with an increased risk of infection. It is primarily associated with continuous infusions of paclitaxel, high drug exposures, and hepatic impairment. The development of mucositis coincides with the fall in ANC, occurring 7 to 10 days after drug administration. Regrowth of the mucous membranes follows recovery of neutrophil counts. Monitor for red, inflamed areas of the oral mucous membranes, diarrhea, pain, and the ability to eat and drink.
- Cisplatin
  ✓ Nephrotoxicity (dose-limiting toxicity) is manifested as a decreased creatinine clearance and electrolyte abnormalities (hypomagnesemia, hypokalemia). Monitor serum creatinine, potas-

sium, and magnesium once weekly. If problems develop, then monitor more frequently as indicated. Nephrotoxicity may occur within the first 24 hours and may persist for several days after administration.
- ✓ The frequency and severity of nausea and vomiting should be assessed by recording the number of vomiting or retching episodes. Nausea can be evaluated using a visual analog scale or daily life scale. Nausea and vomiting occurs within the first 8 to 24 hours after administration and may persist for several days.
- ✓ Hypersensitivity reactions (e.g., anaphylaxis) may occur; monitor as for paclitaxel. Reactions occur within the first 24 hours after administration.
- ✓ Ototoxicity (at high doses) may manifest as loss of hearing. High-tone audiometry can be used, but this is not routinely performed. This effect is related to total dose administered and peak concentrations. It occurs within the first 24 to 48 hours after administration and may persist for several days to weeks.
- ✓ Neurotoxicity may occur and should be monitored as for paclitaxel. It occurs with repeated administration and may persist for several days to weeks.
- Carboplatin
  - ✓ Thrombocytopenia is the dose-limiting toxicity; monitor as for paclitaxel.
  - ✓ Neutropenia should be monitored as for paclitaxel.
  - ✓ Nausea and vomiting are much less common and severe than with cisplatin; monitor as for cisplatin.
  - ✓ Nephrotoxicity is much less common and severe than with cisplatin; monitor as for cisplatin.
  - ✓ Neurotoxicity is much less common than with cisplatin and rarely produces disabling symptoms; monitor as for cisplatin.
- Cyclophosphamide
  - ✓ Neutropenia is the dose-limiting toxicity; monitor as for paclitaxel.
  - ✓ Thrombocytopenia primarily occurs at high doses; monitor as for paclitaxel.
  - ✓ Hemorrhagic cystitis (bleeding from the bladder due to accumulation of toxic metabolites) may occur. Monitor for hematuria continuously for the first 48 hours, as it usually occurs within the first 24 to 48 hours after administration. Inform patients to report any blood in the urine immediately.
  - ✓ The acute period of nausea and vomiting occurs within the first 24 hours after administration. The delayed period occurs more than 24 hours after administration; monitor as for cisplatin.

Patient Counseling

6. *What information would you provide to the patient about this therapy?*

Paclitaxel
- The major toxicity associated with paclitaxel is a reduction in the number of your bone marrow cells. In particular, a low white blood cell count may increase your risk for infection. Monitor your temperature closely and report any fevers (a single temperature higher than 101.3°F or three temperatures higher than 100.4°F over a 24-hour period) to your doctor immediately.
- You may also have a reduction in platelets that increases your risk of bleeding. Notify your doctor immediately of any abnormal bruising or bleeding.
- Allergic reactions sometimes occur. These may be prevented by administrating steroids and antihistamines prior to your chemotherapy.
- Numbness, tingling, and pain in your hands and feet may occur, but this is usually reversible with discontinuation of the chemotherapy.

Cisplatin
- The nausea and vomiting associated with cisplatin usually starts within the first hour after chemotherapy and may persist for 1 to 5 days. This effect may be prevented by administering additional medication, called antiemetics, before and after the chemotherapy.

Carboplatin
- Like paclitaxel, the major toxicity associated with carboplatin is a reduction in your bone marrow cells. With this drug, the primary effect is a reduction in platelets, which will increase your risk of bleeding. A lowering of white blood cells may also occur.
- Carboplatin may also cause nausea and vomiting that is much less severe than with cisplatin; it rarely lasts beyond 24 hours.

Cyclophosphamide
- The major toxicity of this drug is a reduction in the number of your bone marrow cells. In particular, a low white blood cell count may increase your risk for infection. Monitor your temperature closely as described for paclitaxel.
- You may also have a reduction in platelets that increases your risk of bleeding. Notify your doctor immediately of any abnormal bruising or bleeding.
- Cyclophosphamide may also cause bleeding from your bladder. Call your doctor immediately if you have blood in your urine. This may be prevented by giving you a large volume of fluids, causing you to urinate frequently. Another medication called mesna may also be given to help prevent this side effect.

▶ Follow-up Questions

1. *What chemotherapeutic regimen would you recommend for this patient for her next cycle? Provide the rationale for your answer.*

- It is appropriate to change the next cycle to the following regimen.
  - ✓ Paclitaxel 135 mg/m² IV (3-hour infusion) on day 1
  - ✓ Carboplatin dose to AUC 7.5 mg/mL • min IV on day 1
  - ✓ Repeat the regimen every 21 days for 3 additional cycles
- The decline in renal function and development of numb toes (peripheral neuropathy) may be related to cisplatin therapy. A possible facilitating factor in this patient could be uncontrolled diabetes. Carboplatin has less frequent and severe nephrotoxicity and neurotoxicity than cisplatin.

2. *Describe how you would calculate a carboplatin dose for this patient based on a target AUC.*

- *Calvert equation.*
  Carboplatin dose (mg) = target AUC (mg/mL·min) × (GFR + 25)
  GFR (mL/min) can be estimated by creatinine clearance determined

from a 24-hour urine collection, ethylenediamine tetra-acetic acid (^{51}Cr-EDTA) clearance, ^{99m}Tc-diethylene triaminepentaacetic acid (^{99m}Tc-DTPA) clearance, or creatinine clearance calculated by the Cockcroft–Gault equation.
- *Chatelut equation.*

    carboplatin dose (mg) = target AUC (mg/mL • min) × carboplatin CL (mL/min)

    carboplatin clearance (CL) = 0.134 × weight + [218 × weight × (1 − 0.00457 × age) × (1 − 0.0314 × sex)] / serum creatinine

    with weight in kg, age in years, serum creatinine in micromolar, and sex = 0 if male and sex = 1 if female.

▶ Follow-up Questions

1. *What chemotherapeutic options are available for this patient's relapsed ovarian cancer?*

    - Refer to textbook Table 121–3. Examples of systemic chemotherapeutic regimens include:
        - ✓ Paclitaxel plus cisplatin or carboplatin
        - ✓ Cyclophosphamide plus cisplatin or carboplatin
        - ✓ Cisplatin (high dose)
        - ✓ Paclitaxel (high dose)
        - ✓ Paclitaxel plus cisplatin plus cyclophosphamide
        - ✓ Topotecan
    - Intraperitoneal (IP) chemotherapeutic regimens include:
        - ✓ Cisplatin IP plus carboplatin IV
        - ✓ Single agents: cisplatin, carboplatin, paclitaxel, mitoxantrone

3. *Which of the chemotherapeutic regimens would you suggest for the patient's locally relapsed ovarian cancer and why?*

    - One appropriate regimen would consist of the following agents.
        - ✓ Paclitaxel 135 mg/m^2 IV (3-hour infusion) on day 1
        - ✓ Carboplatin dose to AUC 7.5 mg/mL • min IV on day 1
        - ✓ Repeat the regimen every 21 days for 6 cycles
    - The NCCN guidelines for refractory disease that recurs more than 6 months after initial chemotherapy recommend paclitaxel alone or in combination with a platinum analog.[4] The decision to add a platinum analog depends on the time frame in which the disease recurs. If the disease recurs more than 6 months after initial treatment with a platinum analog, a significant response rate can be achieved with subsequent platinum-containing regimens.
    - In patients with disease that recurs less than 6 months after initial treatment with a platinum analog, high-dose cisplatin (150 to 200 mg/m^2) is a viable option due to the dose response curve associated with the platinum analogs. In addition, the use of dose-intensive paclitaxel (250 mg/m^2/day) is an alternative.
    - A useful guideline when treating a patient with refractory or relapsed disease is to administer the salvage regimen for 2 courses and then evaluate for response. If no response is observed, then an alternative salvage regimen may be selected.
    - In the case of topotecan, current evidence suggests continuation of treatment for 4 cycles before evaluating for response.
    - Patients who do not respond to salvage therapy should receive supportive care or be referred to a clinical trial.

- Significant advances have occurred in our understanding of the advantages and limitations of IP administration of chemotherapeutic agents for the treatment of ovarian cancer. A trial of previously untreated women with stage III disease (residual tumors < 2 cm) reported increased survival and decreased toxicity in patients treated with IP cisplatin and IV cyclophosphamide compared to IV cisplatin and IV cyclophosphamide.[5] However, further studies are needed to confirm the advantage of IP compared to IV administration of cisplatin.

References

1. Cannistra SA. Cancer of the ovary. N Engl J Med 1993;329:1550–1559.
2. Alberts DS, Green S, Hannigan EV, et al. Improved therapeutic index of carboplatin plus cyclophosphamide versus cisplatin plus cyclophosphamide: final report by the Southwest Oncology Group of a phase III randomized trial in stages III and IV ovarian cancer. J Clin Oncol 1992;10:706–717.
3. McGuire WP, Hoskins WJ, Brady MF, et al. Cyclophosphamide and cisplatin compared with paclitaxel and cisplatin in patients with stage III and stage IV ovarian cancer. N Engl J Med 1996;334:1–6.
4. Morgan RJ Jr, Copeland L, Gershenson D, et al. NCCN Ovarian cancer practice guidelines. The National Comprehensive Cancer Network. Oncology (Huntingt) 1996;10 (11 suppl):293–310.
5. Alberts DS, Liu PY, Hannigan EV, et al. Intraperitoneal cisplatin plus intravenous cyclophosphamide versus intravenous cisplatin plus intravenous cyclophosphamide for stage III ovarian cancer. N Engl J Med 1996;335:1950–1955.

125 ACUTE LYMPHOCYTIC LEUKEMIA

▶ Jenny's Long Battle (Level II)

Mark T. Holdsworth, PharmD, BCPS

A 3-year-old girl presenting with fatigue, low-grade temperature, and easy bruising is ultimately found to have acute lymphocytic leukemia and pancytopenia. She is admitted to receive supportive transfusion of blood products and induction chemotherapy with vincristine, prednisone, and asparaginase, plus intrathecal medications. Readers are asked to develop pharmacotherapeutic plans for febrile neutropenia, constipation, nausea, and vomiting that occurred during induction. The patient achieves a complete remission by the completion of the 4-week therapy and then enters a consolidation phase with intermediate-dose methotrexate that lasts from weeks 5 through 24. Case questions ask readers to develop plans for supportive measures during this phase and to assess the methotrexate therapy based on serum concentrations. A maintenance regimen with oral, parenteral, and intrathecal medications is then given for 2.5 years to ensure a successful outcome.

▶ Questions

Problem Identification

1. a. *Identify the patient's drug- and disease-related problems upon initial presentation to the hospital.*

    - Acute lymphocytic leukemia requiring combination drug therapy.
    - Pancytopenia requiring support with blood products.

   b. *What drug-related problems developed during her initial hospitalization, and which of these could have been prevented by pharmacotherapy?*

    - *Fever on day 1 while neutropenic.* Fever in the presence of an ANC < 0.5×10^3/mm^3 is known as febrile neutropenia. Due to a high rate of morbidity and occasional mortality if untreated, this condition warrants the immediate institution of broad-spectrum antibiotic therapy, and thus represents the most urgent of her three main problems during induction therapy.
    - *Nausea, vomiting, abdominal pain, and constipation.* These are common drug-induced diseases in this patient population. Recently, it has been demonstrated that the majority of children who receive a TIT treatment without antiemetic protection develop moderate nausea/vomiting. This trial also demonstrated the value of reduced-dose ondansetron in alleviating nausea/vomiting secondary to TIT treatment.[1] This patient should receive prophylactic ondansetron prior to future TIT courses. Most patients who receive vincristine for successive weeks become constipated. This patient should therefore be receiving at least a stool softener (e.g., docusate) to decrease the risk of severe constipation. The nausea from TIT is short-lived and will resolve spontaneously. However, the constipation may become quite severe and should be effectively treated at this juncture.

   c. *If vincristine and the TIT are to be administered on the same day, what precautions must be observed to avoid severe drug toxicity?*

    - If vincristine and TIT are scheduled for the same day, it is important to be extremely careful when both preparing and administering these agents. Inadvertent intrathecal administration of vincristine almost always results in death. If scheduled for the same day, the vincristine and the TIT should be prepared in strict isolation from each other and should not be delivered to the patient care area at the same time.

Desired Outcome

2. a. *What are the initial goals of pharmacotherapy in this patient, and were they achieved?*

    - The initial goal is complete remission (CR), or the absence of any measurable disease. This does not indicate a cure but merely that the patient successfully responded to induction therapy. The vast majority of pediatric ALL patients treated with 3- or 4-drug induction regimens achieve a CR by the end of induction therapy.
    - The low level of blasts (2%) in her peripheral blood on day 7 of induction therapy indicates a greater likelihood of achieving long-term disease-free survival. Data from children with leukemia have shown that a peripheral blast count < 1.0×10^3/mm^3 by day 7 will significantly improve chances for long-term survival.[2]
    - Based upon a normal bone marrow aspirate at the end of induction therapy, this patient has achieved a CR.

   b. *What are the long-term treatment goals, and what indicators of achieving these goals exist in this patient?*

    - The long-term goal of therapy in this patient is prolonged survival and eventual cure. To be truly considered a cure, the patient would need to return to the same average life expectancy of a female born in the 1990s. Thus, definite cure in pediatric ALL is still unknown at the present time. Given this patient's good risk features, her chances for long-term survival are about 80% to 85%.[2]

Therapeutic Alternatives

3. *List the therapeutic alternatives for this patient's drug- and disease-related problems that developed during induction therapy (see question 1.b.) and discuss the risks and benefits of these therapies.*

   Febrile Neutropenia
   - Reasonable therapeutic regimens include:
     - ✓ Ceftazidime or cefepime monotherapy 150 mg/kg/day IV (divided Q 8 H)
     - ✓ Ceftazidime as above + vancomycin 40 mg/kg/day IV (divided Q 8 to 12 H)
     - ✓ Ceftazidime as above + gentamicin or tobramycin 5 to 7.5 mg/kg/day (divided Q 6 to 8 H)
     - ✓ Ceftazidime as above + aminoglycoside as above + vancomycin as above
     - ✓ Imipenem 50 mg/kg/day (divided Q 6 H)
   - These regimens result in similar outcomes in febrile neutropenia. It is important to initiate therapy with an agent that has adequate coverage against serious gram-negative pathogens, because these organisms can quickly lead to the patient's demise.
   - Because ceftazidime monotherapy is much simpler to administer and has a lower rate of adverse reactions than the other regimens, this choice may be optimal.
   - Although cefepime may be administered every 12 hours, it has only been used in this manner for the treatment of febrile neutropenia when it is combined with an aminoglycoside.[3] In addition, there is no published experience with cefepime for treating febrile neutropenia in children.
   - Monotherapy for febrile neutropenia is not ideal in patients with unstable vital signs or at institutions with a significant prevalence of highly resistant organisms such as *Enterobacter, Citrobacter,* or *Serratia* spp.[4]
   - Although cultures in febrile neutropenic patients have revealed more gram-positive than gram-negative infections in the past decade, this has not led to decreased efficacy of ceftazidime, suggesting an adequate gram-positive spectrum for this agent.
   - In multiple studies examining the value of using vancomycin at the initiation of therapy, no differences in outcome were noted. Thus, it

appears that this agent can be withheld until needed for an infectious etiology unresponsive to the initial therapy.[5]
- The use of filgrastim in this setting is still controversial, and studies to date have not demonstrated a consistent benefit.[6,7]

Constipation
- No well-controlled studies have been performed on vincristine-induced constipation.
- Docusate sodium with or without small doses of a stimulant laxative such as senna benefits most patients.
- Lactulose is another useful alternative.
- Suppositories or enemas should not be used in patients with significant myelosuppression because they may increase the risk for perirectal abscess formation.

Nausea and Vomiting
- TIT chemotherapy commonly causes nausea and vomiting in this patient population, and chemotherapy-induced nausea/vomiting is much easier to prevent than to treat.
- Adequate hydration should be ensured, as it was in this patient.
- Lorazepam or promethazine may be given IV in PRN doses if nausea is particularly problematic.
- There are no data regarding the value of 5-HT$_3$ antagonists as rescue therapy, and these agents are not recommended for use in this manner. However, for the patient's next TIT treatment, ondansetron 0.15 mg/kg IV × 2 doses (pre- and post-TIT) or 0.3 mg/kg pre-TIT will provide protection from nausea/vomiting in the majority of patients.[1]

Optimal Plan

4. Outline the optimal treatment schedule and duration for each of the drug-related problems described in the previous answer. What therapeutic alternatives should be considered if initial therapy fails?

Febrile Neutropenia
- The author's choice is ceftazidime 50 mg/kg IV Q 8 H until the patient has been afebrile for 48 hours and has recovered from neutropenia. If there are positive blood cultures, treatment should be continued for a minimum of 7 days.
- If the patient remains febrile after 5 days, consider adding amphotericin 0.5 mg/kg IV QD.
- If signs of sepsis develop (e.g., hypotension despite fluid resuscitation, tachycardia, tachypnea, respiratory failure), add an aminoglycoside.

Constipation
- For prevention and treatment of constipation, initiate docusate sodium 50 mg po BID either alone or with a stimulant laxative such as Senokot ½ to 1 tablet po QD. If this is ineffective, consider adding lactulose.

Nausea and Vomiting
- Prevent nausea/vomiting from TIT by giving ondansetron 0.3 mg/kg IV pre-TIT.
- Lorazepam or chlorpromazine may be used to treat acute episodes of nausea/vomiting, but there is no objective evidence that these or other agents are successful as rescue agents in the acute treatment of this complication.

Outcome Evaluation

5. Which key laboratory parameters are indicative of an adequate response at the end of induction therapy?

- The primary laboratory parameter that is relied upon to document adequate initial response to chemotherapy is the bone marrow aspirate at the completion of induction therapy. If this aspirate demonstrates < 5% leukemic lymphoblasts, the patient has achieved complete remission. This does not indicate cure, but merely represents that the patient's leukemic cell burden is now below the limit of detection. Interestingly, this patient's day 15 bone marrow also indicated complete remission. This is a favorable prognostic finding and has been shown to be predictive of an increased chance for long-term survival.[2]

Patient Counseling

6. What information should be provided to the patient's parents about the potential beneficial and adverse effects from the chemotherapy agents used during induction therapy?

- Jenny will have decreased immune function from these medications and from her disease, and she may develop a serious infection at any time. Therefore, monitor her for fevers, which may be the only sign of infection when her blood counts are low. If she develops a fever, immediately contact the pediatric oncologist on call so that appropriate antibiotic therapy may be initiated.
- Each of her chemotherapy medications has certain adverse effects, only some of which may be prevented.
  - ✓ Vincristine may result in constipation, which can often be reduced by using the stool softener docusate. Vincristine can also cause muscle weakness (especially in the wrists or ankles) or painful tingling sensations (especially in the jaw area after the first dose). The painful sensations can be treated with pain medications. If she develops significant muscle weakness, the vincristine will be postponed until recovery, since further doses will only worsen this effect and extend the time necessary for recovery.
  - ✓ The most troublesome adverse effects from prednisone when given for 1 month are behavioral disturbances such as mood swings and difficult behaviors. There is no treatment known to prevent this complication, but your awareness of this possibility may help in successfully coping with difficult behavior. Another common side effect is a marked increase in Jenny's appetite. These side effects will resolve once prednisone is discontinued.
  - ✓ The adverse effects of asparaginase include allergic reactions (usually seen as a rash with intramuscular injections), and a rare possibility of bleeding or clotting abnormalities, and/or pancreatitis (inflammation of the pancreas). Report any rashes, abdominal pain, or continued nausea/vomiting to your doctor.
- It is very important to continue the chemotherapy for a total of 3 years. Even though the initial bone marrow aspirate indicates complete remission, the majority of ALL patients will relapse and subsequently die from their leukemia without an extended duration of treatment.
- The successful treatment of ALL depends on the ability to avoid the development of resistance by the leukemia cells to the chemotherapy

medications. The two key factors that are thought to be most important for decreasing this risk of relapse are the use of different rotations of combination chemotherapy regimens with different agents and the use of maximally tolerated doses of each agent.

- In addition, it is imperative that Jenny undergo periodic intrathecal injection treatments since the central nervous system (CNS) is an important site for leukemia relapse. Most drugs used to treat leukemia do not achieve adequate penetration into the CNS. Before intrathecal injections or other methods of CNS prophylaxis became routine practice, most children relapsed in the CNS and then subsequently relapsed in the bone marrow. Once relapse occurs, the child's chances for long-term survival are markedly diminished.
- To decrease the risk of relapse, all chemotherapy doses should be taken when they are scheduled, and clinic appointments for IV chemotherapy should be closely followed. Report any missed doses of oral chemotherapy medications immediately to the pediatric oncologist.

▶ Follow-up Questions

1. *During week 7 of consolidation, Jenny is scheduled to receive her first course of intermediate dose methotrexate (1 g/m^2). Which additional medications and supportive measures will be necessary for administration of this dose of methotrexate?*

- When this dose of methotrexate is administered, it is essential that an adequate urine output be maintained by providing sufficient IV hydration. The hydration should be initiated at a rate of at least 1500 mL/m^2/24 hr.
- The hydration should include sodium bicarbonate because methotrexate is hydroxylated to a metabolite that is likely to precipitate in the renal tubules at a neutral or acidic pH.
- This dose of methotrexate is moderately emetogenic, so ondansetron 0.3 mg/kg IV should be administered prior to the methotrexate infusion.

2. *What laboratory tests and examinations must be performed prior to the methotrexate administration?*

- A urine pH of 6.5 to 7.0 should be achieved prior to starting the methotrexate infusion.
- Adequate renal function should be ensured prior to initiation of the methotrexate. Patients with a $CL_{cr} < 60$ mL/min are not candidates for this dose of methotrexate.
- The patient should be closely examined for the presence of a pleural effusion, which can delay methotrexate elimination and place the patient at risk for toxicity.

3. *After the methotrexate administration, the 24-hour peak concentration is 8.7 µmol. The 48-hour concentration is undetectable (< 0.1 µmol). What is the significance of these findings, and what additional changes in therapy should be made based on these concentrations?*

- At approximately hours 36 to 42, IV leucovorin rescue should be initiated at a dose of 10 mg/m^2 IV every 6 hours for 5 doses. If methotrexate concentrations drawn at 42 to 48 hours are considered to be above the toxicity threshold, increased doses of leucovorin and an increase in the hydration and alkalinization schedule will be initiated and continued until methotrexate concentrations drop below this toxic threshold.
- The methotrexate peak concentration at the end of the infusion is not predictive of toxicity. It was initially thought that this peak concentration was predictive of long-term survival, but further analysis of more mature survival data did not demonstrate this.[8]
- However, methotrexate concentrations at 42 to 48 hours are very predictive of the risk for toxicity and form the basis for adjusting the dose of leucovorin and the hydration schedule. This patient's 48-hour concentration is below the toxic threshold, and does not necessitate any changes in the hydration/alkalinization and leucovorin rescue protocol.

4. *It is now week 63, and Jenny is receiving the maintenance phase of her chemotherapy protocol. Which laboratory test is closely monitored to gauge the adequacy of her chemotherapy doses?*

- During maintenance treatment, the WBC differential is relied upon as a surrogate marker for the adequacy of dose intensity. It is believed that failure to achieve adequate myelosuppression will increase the risk of relapse, since leukemic lymphoblasts are less likely to be killed by doses of chemotherapy that are insufficient to result in myelosuppression.

5. *What is the target value for this laboratory measurement, and how will the chemotherapy doses be changed if the laboratory test(s) is above the target range?*

- The target range for the ANC is generally between 0.750 and 1.5 × 10^3/mm^3. If the ANC is continually above this target range, the dose of either mercaptopurine or methotrexate is increased by 25%, and if an adequate level of myelosuppression is not achieved within 2 to 3 weeks, the other agent is also increased by 25%.[8]

References

1. Holdsworth MT, Raisch DW, Winter SS, et al. Assessment of the emetogenic potential of intrathecal chemotherapy and response to prophylactic treatment with ondansetron. Support Care Cancer 1998;6:132–138.
2. Reiter A, Schrappe M, Ludwig WD, et al. Chemotherapy in 998 unselected childhood acute lymphoblastic leukemia patients. Results and conclusions of the multicenter trial ALL-BFM 86. Blood 1994;84:3122–3133.
3. Cordonnier C, Herbrecht R, Pico JL, et al. Cefepime/amikacin versus ceftazidime/amikacin as empirical therapy for febrile episodes in neutropenic patients: A comparative study. Clin Infect Dis 1997;24:41–51.
4. Pizzo PA. Management of fever in patients with cancer and treatment-induced neutropenia. N Engl J Med 1993;328:1323–1332.
5. Rubenstein EB, Rolston K. Outpatient management of febrile episodes in neutropenic cancer patients. Support Care Cancer 1994;2:369–373.
6. Mitchell PL, Morland B, Stevens MC, et al. Granulocyte colony-stimulating factor in established febrile neutropenia: A randomized study of pediatric patients. J Clin Oncol 1997;15:1163–1170.
7. Pui CH, Boyett JM, Hughes WT, et al. Human granulocyte colony-stimulating factor after induction chemotherapy in children with acute lymphoblastic leukemia. N Engl J Med 1997;336:1781–1787.
8. Pearson AD, Amineddine HA, Yule M, et al. The influence of serum methotrexate concentrations and drug dosage on outcome in childhood acute lymphoblastic leukaemia. Br J Cancer 1991;64:169–173.
9. Shurtleff SA, Buijs A, Behm FG, et al. TEL/AML1 fusion resulting from a cryptic t(12;21) is the most common genetic lesion in pediatric ALL and defines a subgroup of patients with an excellent prognosis. Leukemia 1995;9:1985–1989.

126 CHRONIC MYELOGENOUS LEUKEMIA

▶ A Long Arm Translocation   (Level II)

Terri G. Davidson, PharmD
Catherine A. Smith, PharmD

A 4-month history of shortness of breath, weight loss, early satiety, and fatigue causes a 51-year-old man to seek medical attention. The clinical, laboratory, and bone marrow biopsy results are consistent with chronic myelogenous leukemia in chronic phase (CML-CP). Interferon alfa is the treatment of choice for CML-CP with the goal of achieving a hematologic and cytologic remission. Interferon alfa requires careful monitoring because of potential adverse effects. Hydroxyurea is added when the patient's white blood cell count remains elevated after 4 weeks of interferon alfa treatment. When this patient fails to achieve a cytogenetic response after 6 months of treatment, an allogeneic marrow transplant from an HLA-matched sibling donor is undertaken.

▶ Questions

Problem Identification

1. a. What information in the patient's history is consistent with a diagnosis of CML-CP (see Casebook Figure 126–1)?

- *Symptoms.* Tiredness, fatigue, weight loss, left upper quadrant fullness, and early satiety.
- *Signs.* Splenomegaly on physical exam, palpable inguinal lymph node.
- *Laboratory values.* Thrombocytosis, leukocytosis, anemia, and increased LDH; myeloblasts seen only on examination of the bone marrow biopsy; Philadelphia chromosome (Ph$^+$) or a t(9q;22q) chromosomal aberration. Hypoalbuminemia and hyperbilirubinemia may be indicative of cancer but are not specific for CML.

b. Describe the natural progression of CML.

- CML usually begins with a chronic stable phase (CML-CP), progressing to an accelerated phase (CML-AP), then progressing to an acute or blastic phase termed "blast crisis" (CML-BC). The chronic phase may last 3 to 5 years. Presenting signs and symptoms may include malaise, fatigue, heat intolerance, splenic enlargement, dyspnea, pallor, and weight loss. Patients in the chronic phase typically have 20% or fewer myeloid cells in the peripheral blood and 30% or fewer in the marrow. The mean WBC is $225 \times 10^3/mm^3$ (range 20 to $600 \times 10^3/mm^3$); fewer than 5% are myeloblasts. The platelet count is $> 450 \times 10^3/mm^3$ in 50% of the cases and $> 1000 \times 10^3/mm^3$ in 25% of cases. Leukocyte alkaline phosphatase (LAP) is absent or low.
- In patients with Philadelphia chromosome negative (Ph$^-$) CML, splenomegaly is less prominent. The WBC count is 50 to $75 \times 10^3/mm^3$, and the median platelet count is $170 \times 10^3/mm^3$. LAP is normal to increased and survival ranges from 10 to 19 months compared to 40 to 45 months in Ph$^+$ disease.
- The transition from CML-CP to CML-AP is usually gradual and is characterized by progressive splenomegaly, anemia, basophilia, quantitative platelet abnormalities, increased myelopoiesis, and circulating myeloblasts (with or without additional cytogenetic abnormalities). Bone marrow may have increased reticulin and fibrosis. CML-AP typically lasts from a few weeks to 6 months.
- The blastic phase is associated with the appearance of an aggressive and often resistant form of acute leukemia. The presence of circulating or marrow myeloblasts ($\geq 20\%$), myeloblasts or progranulocytes ($\geq 30\%$ in the peripheral blood or $\geq 50\%$ in the marrow), or extramedullary blastic infiltrates are required for the diagnosis of CML-BC. Patients present with fever, night sweats, weight loss, splenic pain, bone pain, weakness, fatigue, easy bruisability, and hepatosplenomegaly. The hemoglobin is usually less than 10 g/dL; the WBC is more than $50 \times 10^3/mm^3$; the platelet count is $< 100 \times 10^3/mm^3$. LAP is normal or increased. About one-third of the CML-BC leukemias are lymphoid in nature with the remaining two-thirds being of myeloid origin. BC usually lasts only 2 to 6 months (Refer to the sections "Clinical Presentation" and "Clinical Course" in textbook Chapter 123 for more information.)

c. List factors that signal a poor prognosis for CML patients in chronic phase.

- *Clinical features.* Older age (≥ 60 years), presence of symptoms at diagnosis, significant weight loss ($> 10\%$ of dry weight), hepatomegaly, splenomegaly (≥ 10 cm below costal margin), poor performance status, black race.
- *Laboratory features.* Increased number of blasts or blasts plus promyelocytes in the blood ($\geq 3\%$) or marrow ($\geq 3\%$), increased basophils in blood ($\geq 7\%$) or marrow ($\geq 3\%$), thrombocytosis (platelets $\geq 700 \times 10^3/mm^3$), thrombocytopenia (in blast crisis phase), anemia, collagen or reticulin fibrosis of the marrow, cytogenetic clonal evolution.
- *Treatment-associated features.* Longer time to achieve hematologic remission, short remission duration, failure to suppress the Ph$^+$ metaphases.

Desired Outcome

2. What are long-term therapy goals for this patient?

- Delay the onset of blastic crisis
- Control the signs and symptoms associated with the disease
- Eradicate the malignant clone

Therapeutic Alternatives

3. *What pharmacologic and/or non-pharmacologic alternatives should be considered for this patient?*

   - *Splenectomy or splenic irradiation* is reserved for patients with symptomatic splenomegaly that is unresponsive to chemotherapy (busulfan, hydroxyurea, interferon alfa) or patients with anemia and/or thrombocytopenia related to hypersplenism. Randomized studies comparing splenectomy with no splenectomy in early chronic-phase CML patients or before allogeneic BMT have not shown a survival advantage for splenectomy. The surgical procedure may increase the patient's risk of infections, thereby increasing morbidity and mortality.
   - *Leukapheresis* is used for emergent complications of leukostasis (WBC >150 to 200 × 10^3/mm^3) including visual disturbances, mental status changes, respiratory distress, and/or priapism; or in pregnant females, to avoid teratogenic drugs.
   - *Chemotherapy agents (e.g., busulfan, hydroxyurea)* may be used to achieve hematologic remission. Until recently, hydroxyurea (1 to 3 g/d) was the treatment of choice for CML-CP.[1] Although hematologic remissions are obtained in 70% to 80% of patients with CML-CP, the Ph$^+$ cells persist in over 90% of the marrow metaphases, indicating that the malignant clone has not been eliminated. However, hydroxyurea is more effective in increasing survival than other agents including busulfan, melphalan, 6-mercaptopurine, and chlorambucil, as well as radiotherapy. In addition, it has the advantage of oral administration and low cost. Median survival is 30 to 55 months with hydroxyurea compared to 19 months in untreated patients. Its adverse effects are relatively infrequent but are not innocuous. This agent is most often used in patients who are not candidates for BMT or who cannot tolerate the subcutaneous injections and adverse-effect profile of interferon alfa.
   - *Allogeneic bone marrow transplantation (BMT)* using matched (or one-antigen mismatched) related or unrelated donors offers CML-CP patients the only chance for cure. Transplantation in the chronic phase produces significantly better disease-free survival than transplantation in the accelerated or blastic phases. Early allogeneic BMT may be justified in patients with an average or poor prognosis, but a conservative approach is advisable for patients with good prognostic factors. With the median survival after interferon alfa therapy or interferon-based therapies averaging between 40 to 65 months, BMT may be reserved for CML patients not achieving a cytogenetic remission with interferon.

     Long-term results with allogeneic human leukocyte antigen (HLA)-identical sibling donor BMT have demonstrated event-free survival rates of 39% to 75% at 3 years.[2] The relapse rate is 20%, and treatment-related deaths occur in 15% of patients. Younger patients (< 30 years old) are better candidates because they have a lower risk of graft-versus-host disease (GVHD). The results appear to be better if the BMT is performed within 1 year of diagnosis.

     Matched-unrelated donor (MUD) transplants are associated with an overall survival of 37% at 2 years and 35% at 5 years.[3] Treatment-related mortality is 61%, which is higher than HLA-identical sibling transplants. However, in younger patients transplanted in the first chronic phase from an HLA-matched donor without T-cell depletion, the 2-year leukemia-free survival, treatment-related mortality, and relapse incidence rates are 51%, 47%, and 2%, respectively. Thus, in selected patients, MUD transplants are an attractive option.
   - *Interferon alfa* is a biologic response modifier that has been shown to produce hematologic response rates of 55% to 75%. Importantly, complete or partial cytogenetic response (disappearance of Ph$^+$ metaphases) occurs in 20% to 40% of cases. A higher cytogenetic response rate occurs when therapy is started within 1 year of diagnosis. The duration of complete hematologic response may be up to 41 months. Remission duration is longer (62 to 66 months) in patients who achieve a cytogenetic response. When compared to hydroxyurea, interferon alfa demonstrates an increased response, increased time to progression, and a survival advantage, suggesting that it should be the preferred treatment for CML-CP.[4] In addition, hydroxyurea produces only minor and transient cytogenetic responses, whereas interferon alfa has shown durable cytogenetic responses. Its mechanism of action remains unclear, but its effect on the leukemic clone is thought to be related to its antiproliferative, antiviral, and/or immune-modulating properties.
   - *Interferon gamma* is also active in CML but acts by a different mechanism than interferon alfa. Several trials have examined the use of single-agent interferon gamma or alternating interferon alfa and interferon gamma. However, the use of interferon gamma alone or in combination with interferon alfa has not yielded superior results to interferon alfa alone.[5]

Optimal Plan

4. *Considering all patient factors, describe the optimal initial treatment plan for this patient.*

   - The treatment of choice is interferon alfa in a dosage of 9 × 10^6 units/m^2/day by SC or IM injection; the median time to achieve a complete hematologic response is 5 months. Based on clinical experience, short-term tolerance may be improved by gradually increasing the dose of interferon over the first week of administration from 3 million units/day × 3 days, to 6 million units/day × 3 days, and then to 9 million units/day for the duration of the treatment period.
   - Because of the potential for cytogenetic remission, it is reasonable to give all patients with CML a trial of interferon alfa early in the course of disease. The minority of patients who achieve cytogenetic remission should continue receiving this agent. The majority of patients who do not obtain cytogenetic remission could then be treated with hydroxyurea or intensive chemotherapy followed by BMT. This strategy allows younger patients being considered for BMT to avoid the potential risks of the procedure.

Outcome Evaluation

5. *Describe parameters for monitoring disease response and toxicity for the treatment option you recommended.*

   Interferon Alfa
   - Early toxicities include flu-like symptoms (fever, chills, malaise, myalgias, fatigue, and headache). Monitor by physical examination and questioning the patient daily or 2 to 3 times weekly until symptoms resolve, which is usually within 1 to 2 weeks.
   - Late toxicities:
     - ✓ Increased hepatic transaminases: measure AST and ALT at baseline and every 3 to 6 weeks.

- ✓ Nausea/vomiting: monitor fluid status using body weight, fluid intake and output, and serum electrolytes at baseline and every 3 to 6 weeks. It is rare that nausea and vomiting require a dosage change or antiemetic treatment.
- ✓ Diarrhea: monitor number/volume of loose stools, fluid status, and serum electrolytes at baseline and every 3 to 6 weeks. If diarrhea exceeds 6 large stools per day, treat with nonspecific antidiarrheal medications. Reduce interferon alfa dosage if antidiarrheal medications are ineffective.
- ✓ CNS symptoms (frontal-lobe syndrome of apathy, memory or concentration problems, a parkinsonism-like syndrome, depression, and psychosis): monitor physical examination and question the patient or caregiver(s) every 3 to 6 weeks; discontinue therapy if symptoms persist.
- ✓ Hair thinning (reversible): monitor by physical examination.
- ✓ Skin rash: monitor by physical examination; treat symptomatically unless symptoms are severe.
- ✓ Neutropenia and thrombocytopenia: monitor complete blood counts with differential (to calculate ANC) and platelet count weekly until nadir is obtained, then every 3 to 6 weeks; neutropenia and thrombocytopenia are rare with standard doses. Low blood counts and signs and symptoms of infection or bleeding should be addressed and treated.
- ✓ Proteinuria: monitor urinalysis at baseline and every 2 to 3 months or with symptoms; if symptoms are accompanied by evidence of kidney damage, discontinue interferon therapy.
- ✓ Hypothyroidism: measure serum TSH and T_4 at baseline and every 2 to 6 months, or with symptoms; treat hypothyroidism until therapy is discontinued.
- ✓ Immune hemolysis: perform Coombs' test (direct and indirect) at baseline, weekly for 2 to 4 weeks, and then as needed. Discontinue interferon only if all other causes have been ruled out.

Patient Counseling

6. *What information should be given to the patient prior to treatment?*

- Interferon alfa is a substance normally found in the white blood cells and other cells of the human body. When prepared and given by injection, it affects several different cellular functions. Although the exact mechanisms by which it treats CML are not fully understood, it is believed to decrease the rate at which the leukemic cells grow by interfering with the cell growth process.
- Your physician will determine the precise dose and frequency of administration, but it can be given from 3 to 5 times per week as a subcutaneous (under the skin) injection (similar to how a diabetic patient injects insulin).
- Call your doctor immediately if you experience irregular heartbeat, chest pain that lasts longer than 15 minutes, unexplained fever, numbness or tingling in the hands or feet, or mental status changes.
- If the following side effects become problematic, seek advice from a health care professional about how best to alleviate or prevent the symptoms.
  - ✓ Flu-like symptoms (fever, chills, malaise, muscle pain, fatigue, and headache); acetaminophen may be taken before each injection to prevent or decrease the severity of these symptoms if they become a problem.
  - ✓ Tiredness, drowsiness; be careful when driving or performing other activities that require you to be alert.
  - ✓ Loss of appetite, nausea, vomiting, or weight loss.
  - ✓ Dry mouth, nose, and throat.
  - ✓ Changes in your sense of taste.
- Store interferon vials in the refrigerator; the refrigerated solution is good for 1 month after it has been mixed as instructed. Do not shake or freeze the solution.
- Dispose of needles and syringes in the special container provided.
- Talk to your doctor before getting flu shots or other vaccines because the vaccines may not work as well while you are taking this medication.

▶ **Follow-up Questions**

1. *What is the rationale for adding hydroxyurea, cytarabine, or hydroxyurea plus cytarabine in this patient at the 4-week follow-up visit? What outcomes would be expected from using this combination therapy?*

- Hydroxyurea, busulfan, initial or cyclic intensive chemotherapy, and low-dose cytarabine have been combined with interferon alfa in an effort to improve its effect on prognosis. Combinations with busulfan and intensive chemotherapy have been unsuccessful. Busulfan and interferon alfa result in cumulative myelotoxic effects, and intensive chemotherapy given over 2 to 3 months may be insufficient time to allow adequate exposure of the cytotoxic agents to the malignant clone.
- The combination of hydroxyurea and interferon alfa has demonstrated several advantages including ease of administration, rapid disease control, better complete hematologic response rates, a lower incidence of leukocytosis-associated adverse effects, and longer disease control. However, when compared to interferon alfa alone, no improvement in cytogenetic response rates have been documented.
- Complete hematologic response rates are significantly higher and survival is significantly longer in CML patients in the late chronic phase who received combination therapy with interferon alfa and cytarabine when compared with interferon alfa alone.[6] The combination also shows a trend toward better cytogenetic responses in these patients. More recently, a trial comparing interferon alfa plus hydroxyurea combined with cytarabine versus interferon alfa and hydroxyurea was conducted.[7] Complete hematologic responses were seen in 66% and 55%, respectively, and complete and major cytogenetic responses were seen in 41% and 24%, respectively. A significant improvement in survival was seen in the interferon alfa/hydroxyurea/cytarabine group (85.7% versus 79.1% at 3 years).
- Thus, it is reasonable to add hydroxyurea and/or cytarabine to single-agent interferon alfa in this patient, with the goals being to increase the response rate, prolong the hematologic and/or cytogenetic remission, and to more rapidly decrease the malignant clone as represented by the high WBC count.

2. *What is the goal of therapy for allogeneic BMT in the management of CML-CP?*

- The goal of therapy for allogeneic BMT is long-term disease-free survival and cure. The best outcome occurs in patients transplanted in the first chronic phase as opposed to the accelerated, second chronic, or blastic phases. Results of allogeneic BMT in CML show a 50% to 60% disease-free survival for patients transplanted in first chronic phase, 30% for those transplanted in accelerated phase, and 10% to 20% for those transplanted in blastic phase. The incidence of relapse increases with disease progression. The optimal timing of BMT in chronic phase is controversial. MUD and allogeneic BMT with mismatch at one locus have also been performed, but these procedures have an increased risk of infection, graft failure, and GVHD.

3. *Is this CML patient an optimal candidate for a BMT? Why or why not?*

- Characteristics of the optimal CML patient for BMT are those who: 1) are less than 55 years of age; 2) have an HLA-matched sibling donor; 3) are in chronic phase within 1 year of diagnosis; and 4) have never received busulfan.
- This patient is a good candidate for BMT because he is less than 55 years old, enjoyed excellent health prior to his diagnosis, has a matched sibling donor, is in the first chronic phase of his disease, and has never received busulfan. Additionally, he did not respond well to initial therapy. BMT represents his only chance for cure or long-term disease-free survival.

4. *List common complications of allogeneic BMT and this preparative regimen.*

- GVHD: rash, diarrhea, LFT abnormalities
- Febrile neutropenia: infections (bacterial, fungal, and viral)
- Hemorrhagic cystitis
- Pulmonary fibrosis
- Veno-occlusive disease
- Mucositis

5. *Identify important laboratory/clinical values to monitor during the BMT course.*

- GVHD: obtain serum electrolytes at baseline and every 3 to 6 weeks unless symptoms are present; check immunosuppressive serum drug concentrations (i.e., cyclosporine, tacrolimus) twice weekly until levels are stable and within the therapeutic range; obtain bilirubin and alkaline phosphatase at baseline and every 3 to 6 weeks unless symptoms are present.
  - ✓ Acute GVHD (< 100 days post BMT): maculopapular rash, diarrhea, abdominal pain.
  - ✓ Chronic GVHD (> 100 days post BMT): early effects include raised papules or diffuse skin erythema. Late findings include sclerodermatous lesions, dry eyes, photophobia, or ocular pain; oral dryness, erythema, or sensitivity to acidic or spicy foods; dysphagia; and weight loss.
- Graft-versus-leukemia effect (associated with the presence of acute and chronic GVHD).
- Neutropenia: check CBC with differential, ANC, and platelets until counts nadir, then every 3 to 6 weeks unless symptoms are present. Obtain blood cultures if temperature rises above 100.5°F.
- Lung and airway complications (i.e., interstitial pneumonitis, infection, restrictive lung disease, bronchiolitis obliterans): assess by chest x-rays, physical examination (cough), sputum cultures, and pulmonary function tests, if necessary.
- Veno-occlusive disease: assess weight gain, left upper quadrant pain, total bilirubin.
- Renal toxicity: measure BUN, serum creatinine, and fluid intake and output.
- Hemorrhagic cystitis: assess fluid status, perform urinalysis if symptoms develop.
- Other: check liver function tests, examine for mucositis, obtain cytomegalovirus surveillance cultures.

6. *When the patient is discharged after BMT, what important information should be relayed to him?*

- Information about the immunosuppressive agent(s) used to prevent GVHD.
- Information related to other drug therapies the patient will be taking at home (i.e., potassium supplements, magnesium supplements, hypnotics).
- Contact your physician if you notice unusual bruising or bleeding, shaking chills, or fever > 100.5°F, persistent diarrhea or vomiting.
- Have your blood counts checked regularly.

7. *If relapse occurs after allogeneic BMT, what treatment alternatives remain for this patient?*

- Continue interferon alfa therapy alone or in combination with hydroxyurea (higher doses)/cytarabine.
- Investigational agents (e.g., interleukin-1, other interferons): interferon gamma has been used as a single agent or alternating with interferon alfa. Preliminary studies examining interferon gamma alone have shown definite but modest hematologic activity with a response rate between 20% to 30%.[5]
- Donor leukocyte (buffy-coat) infusions are widely used in this setting to reinduce hematologic and cytogenetic remission, perhaps by enhancing the graft-versus-leukemia effect.

8. *If the patient progresses to CML-blast crisis despite BMT, what is the best treatment option for him?*

- If he progresses to blast crisis of myeloid origin, an acute myeloid leukemia (AML) regimen should be used (e.g., doxorubicin 60 mg/m^2/day × 3 days plus cytarabine 2 to 3 g/m^2/day × 7 days). Twenty to thirty percent of patients receiving this regimen will respond by conversion into a second Ph$^+$ chronic phase. However, responses are of short duration and median survival is 2 to 12 months.
- If the patient progresses to blast crisis of lymphoid origin, an acute lymphocytic leukemia (ALL) regimen should be used (e.g., vincristine 2 mg IV once weekly and prednisone 60 mg/m^2/day with or without an anthracycline and cytarabine. Patients with lymphoid blast crisis have a better outcome than those with a myeloid blast crisis; 40% to 70% respond to therapy. Remission durations range from 6 to 10 months, with a median survival of 9 to 12 months. Overall, the outlook for patients with CML-BC is poor.

References

1. Hehlmann R, Heimpel H, Hasford J, et al. Randomized comparison of busulfan and hydroxyurea in chronic myelogenous leukemia: Prolongation of survival by hydroxyurea. Blood 1993;82:398–407.
2. Kantarjian HM, O'Brien S, Anderlini P, et al. Treatment of myelogenous leukemia: Current status and investigational options. Blood 1996;87:3069–3081.

3. Devergie A, Apperley JF, Labopin M, et al. European results of matched unrelated donor bone marrow transplantation for chronic myeloid leukemia. Impact of HLA class II matching. Bone Marrow Transplant 1997;20:11–19.
4. Chronic Myeloid Leukemia Trialists' Collaboration Group. Interferon alfa versus chemotherapy for chronic myeloid leukemia: A meta-analysis of seven randomized trials. J Natl Cancer Inst 1997;89:1616–1620.
5. Kurzrock R, Talpaz M, Kantarjian H, et al. Therapy of chronic myelogenous leukemia with recombinant interferon-gamma. Blood 1987;70:943–947.
6. Kantarjian HM, Keating MJ, Estey EH, et al. Treatment of advanced stages of Philadelphia chromosome-positive chronic myelogenous leukemia with interferon-alpha and low-dose cytarabine. J Clin Oncol 1992;10:772–778.
7. Guilhot F, Chastang C, Michallet M, et al. Interferon alfa-2b combined with cytarabine versus interferon alone in chronic myelogenous leukemia. N Engl J Med 1997;337:223–229.

127 MELANOMA

▶ **Remember Your ABCDEs** (Level I)

Jennifer A. Torma, PharmD
Rowena N. Schwartz, PharmD

An excisional biopsy of a suspicious-looking mole leads to the diagnosis of superficial spreading melanoma in a 38-year-old man. The patient underwent wide excision of the primary tumor, and regional lymph node dissection revealed metastases to local lymph nodes; no distant metastases were found. Use of adjuvant interferon alfa-2b in this situation is employed to increase relapse-free and overall survival as well as to improve quality of life. The patient is scheduled to receive high-dose IV therapy for 4 weeks followed by low-dose subcutaneous treatment for 48 weeks. Students are asked to develop an interferon treatment plan that includes calculation of the doses required for each phase of therapy and preparation of the dosage form for administration to the patient. Many clinical and laboratory parameters must be assessed regularly to detect and prevent adverse effects from interferon therapy. Providing information to the patient on dosage preparation, self-administration of subcutaneous interferon at home, and monitoring for adverse effects during the low-dose phase is critical to the successful completion of the therapy.

▶ **Questions**

Problem Identification

1. a. Create a list of the patient's drug-related problems.

- Newly diagnosed melanoma s/p wide excision to begin IFNα-2b therapy.
- Seasonal allergic rhinitis is a chronic, stable problem, adequately self-treated with non-prescription antihistamines.

b. What risk factor(s) does this patient have for the development of melanoma?

- He has a history of severe sunburns. As a child, his fair complexion put him at a greater risk for sunburns. One of the greatest risks for melanoma is severe, blistering sunburns during childhood and adolescence.
- As an adult, he has been at an increased risk of sunburns because of his complexion, potentially having summers off of work because of his occupation as a school teacher, and possibly because of the altitude of Colorado offering less protection from the sun.
- The presence of multiple nevi alone is not a risk factor for the development of melanoma without the presence of the familial atypical multiple mole syndrome or hereditary dysplastic nevus syndrome. Given his family history, this was not a risk factor for this patient's development of melanoma.

c. What are the characteristics of Stage III melanoma, in terms of tumor size/thickness, nodal involvement, and metastases?

- Staging of melanoma has been performed by two methods, the Breslow method that measures the thickness of the lesion, and the Clark method that accounts for the depth of the lesion into the underlying tissues. The American Joint Committee on Cancer (AJCC) has developed a uniform staging system for melanoma that incorporates the Clark and Breslow methods and accounts for lymph node involvement and metastatic disease (refer to textbook Chapter 124 for a more complete discussion of the staging of melanoma).
- According to the AJCC criteria, this patient has stage III melanoma, which is characterized by a tumor of any thickness, regional lymph node involvement, and no distant metastases.

Desired Outcome

2. What are the goals of using adjuvant IFNα-2b in this patient?

- Use of adjuvant IFNα-2b in patients with high-risk melanoma has been shown to increase relapse-free and overall survival compared to patients who received only observation after tumor excision.[1] In a randomized trial, patients at high risk for relapse after curative surgery (Stage IIb and IIIa) were randomized to either treatment with IFNα-2b for 52 weeks or to observation only. Patients randomized to the IFNα group received 4 weeks of high-dose IV therapy followed by 48 weeks of lower-dose subcutaneous therapy. Patients who were maintained on IFNα had a prolonged relapse-free survival time compared to patients in the observation arm of the study. Overall median survival time was also increased for patients who received IFNα compared with patients who received no therapy (3.8 versus 2.8 years, respectively).

- Another goal of the adjuvant therapy is to improve or maintain overall quality of life. The improvement in quality of life depends on the individual patient and his or her preferences regarding improved survival versus the treatment toxicities of interferon. A quality-of-life-adjusted survival analysis using Quality-Adjusted Time Without Symptoms and Toxicity (Q-TWiST) found that adjuvant IFNα therapy afforded patients more quality-of-life-adjusted time than patients who were only observed after surgery for melanoma.[2] For patients who are willing to experience toxicity in exchange for increased survival and delayed disease relapse, this was statistically significant. For patients who value avoiding toxicity equally to improved relapse-free survival, the quality-of-life-adjusted time did not reach statistical significance. Therefore, the issue of this patient improving his quality of life with IFNα therapy depends on his preferences regarding toxicity from treatment and relapse-free survival gained from treatment, as well as his ability to tolerate continued therapy.

Therapeutic Alternatives

3. *If IFNα-2b therapy was not chosen for this patient, are other feasible pharmacotherapeutic options available?*

- Chemotherapy has not been shown to increase overall and relapse-free survival in the adjuvant setting. Options include observation only or participation in a clinical trial (e.g., a study of melanoma vaccines).

Optimal Plan

4. a. *As the first step in developing a treatment plan for adjuvant treatment with IFNα-2b for this patient, calculate his body surface area.*

- BSA (m^2) = the square root of [(wt in kg) × (ht in cm)/3600]
- BSA = the square root of [(83.2 kg × 175.3 cm)/3600] = 2.01 m^2

b. *Determine dose of interferon for high-dose intravenous therapy and describe how the dose should be prepared for administration.*

- The recommended dosage of high-dose IFNα-2b is 20 million units (MU) per square meter BSA given once daily 5 days a week for 4 weeks.

  20 MU/m^2 = 20 MU × 2.01 m^2 = 40 MU/day IV Monday through Friday × 4 weeks

- Reconstitute the vial of alfa-interferon powder by adding 1 mL of diluent provided by the manufacturer (bacteriostatic water for injection) to a 50 MU vial of IFNα-2b and gently swirl the vial or roll it between your hands. Do not shake the vial, because that will cause foaming of the solution, which makes it difficult to draw up an accurate dose.
- Withdraw IFNα 40 MU (0.8 mL) from the vial and add it to 100 mL of normal saline; administer the dose IV over 20 minutes into a peripheral vein.
- The multidose vial containing the remaining 0.2 mL may be stored in the refrigerator for future use; it is stable for 30 days under refrigeration.

c. *Determine dose of interferon for the subcutaneous 48-week phase.*

- The low-dose phase of IFNα-2b is 10 MU/m^2 given SC 3 times a week.

  10 MU/m^2 = 10 MU × 2.01 m^2 = 20 MU SC Q Monday, Wednesday, and Friday for 48 weeks

- Mr. Neilson should be counseled on the storage of the product, the handling and disposal of the needle and syringe, and the reconstitution and administration of the interferon as described below.

d. *What supportive measures may be used to minimize adverse effects of the IFNα-2b therapy?*

- Administer acetaminophen 650 mg po prior to interferon and then Q 4 H for the remainder of that day to relieve the constitutional symptoms of fever, malaise, and muscle/joint pain.
- Encourage oral hydration.

Outcome Evaluation

5. a. *What parameters will you monitor to assess interferon efficacy?*

- Local recurrence of melanoma on physical exam when the patient returns for follow-up
- The presence of lymphadenopathy on physical exam

b. *What parameters will you monitor for adverse effects of interferon during the high-dose phase?*

- Vital signs before and after interferon infusion
- CBC for leukopenia, anemia, and thrombocytopenia twice weekly
- LFTs for increases in transaminases twice weekly
- Neuro checks weekly to detect mental status changes
- Daily weight to assess fluid status
- Question the patient about the presence of arthralgias/myalgias

c. *What parameters will you monitor for adverse effects of interferon during the low-dose maintenance phase?*

- CBC for leukopenia, anemia, and thrombocytopenia weekly
- LFTs for increases in transaminases weekly
- Neuro checks weekly to detect mental status changes
- Weekly weight for changes in fluid status

Patient Counseling

6. a. *What information should the patient receive prior to his high-dose phase?*

- Fatigue is the most common complaint of patients who receive interferon. You may start to feel very tired and weak and unable to complete your usual tasks around the house. It will be helpful if you can delegate activities to your friends and family members if you do not feel that you are up to your regular activities. Rest when you feel that you need to and try not to push yourself.
- Chills and fever may occur during the interferon injection. We will give you acetaminophen (Tylenol) before the injection, and

you should continue to take it every 4 hours afterwards if you need it; this will help prevent or reduce fever. If you do develop a high fever, this is sometimes accompanied by shaking chills. If this occurs, we can give you medicine in the clinic to stop the chills.
- You may experience muscle and joint pain after you begin interferon therapy. The acetaminophen may also help prevent this problem. If the aches become severe, tell your oncologist or clinic nurse. Do not take any over-the-counter pain medicine without discussing it with your doctor first.
- When you receive the interferon every day in the clinic, you may notice that the fever and aches become less severe as the week goes by. This is because your body starts to become tolerant to the drug's effects. After having the weekend with no therapy, these problems may seem worse again on Monday.
- You may notice that your appetite is decreased. This could be because you feel nauseated or because food does not taste the same. If you can, try to eat small meals throughout the day. You can also drink dietary supplements if you are not eating a sufficient amount of food. It is very important that you drink plenty of fluid so that you do not become dehydrated.
- We will monitor your blood counts when you come into clinic because your white and red blood cells and platelets will probably decrease while you are receiving the interferon. We follow the numbers closely; if they become too low, we will withhold the interferon therapy until they come back up again.
- We will also check blood tests that tell us how well your liver is functioning. These numbers sometimes become elevated during interferon therapy. We will follow them closely, and if they become too high we may have to modify your regimen by withholding some interferon doses or decreasing the dose.
- Other side effects that some patients report are difficulty concentrating, slower thinking, and trouble with memory. If you experience these or any other unusual effects, be sure to call the clinic or tell your oncologist, nurse, or pharmacist.

b. *What information should the patient receive prior to initiating the low-dose phase of the regimen?*

Drug Storage and Administration
- These are the supplies that you will need at home to administer your interferon: two syringes, the vials of interferon 50 million units, the vials of water, alcohol swabs, and a container in which you can dispose of the syringe and empty vials. When you get home, store all of the interferon vials in your refrigerator in a single container.
- When it is time for your evening dose, take out one vial of interferon powder 50 MU and one vial of water. Wash your hands first and then work in a clean area. Remove the caps of both vials and swab the rubber stops with an alcohol pad. Carefully remove the plastic cover of the syringe, being careful not to touch any part of the needle. Insert the needle into the vial of water, turn it upside down, and pull back on the plunger to the 1 mL mark. Make sure the tip of the needle is in the water so that you withdraw water into the syringe and not air. Turn the vial right-side up and withdraw the needle.
- Insert the needle into the vial of interferon and slowly push on the plunger to add the water to the interferon powder. Aim for the side of the vial so the water doesn't foam when it mixes with the powder. Withdraw the needle and throw the needle and syringe, uncapped, into the "sharps" container.
- Gently swirl the vial or roll it between your hands; do not shake the vial or the solution will foam, making it difficult for you to withdraw an accurate dose. Take the second syringe, carefully remove the plastic cover, and insert the needle into the vial. Turn the vial upside down and pull back on the plunger to 0.4 mL, again ensuring that the tip of the needle is in the solution. Tap out any air bubbles that are in the syringe. Your dose of interferon is 20 MU, which is what will be contained in the 0.4 mL of solution.
- Swab your skin with the alcohol pad and administer the dose into the skin as your nurse has shown you. When you are finished, throw the syringe, uncapped, into the "sharps" container.
- Put the unused remainder of the interferon back into the refrigerator; you will be able to draw two and a half doses out of each vial. The mixed solution of interferon is stable for 1 month when refrigerated, but try to use it as soon as possible. Be sure to swab the top of the rubber stopper each time you use the vial.
- When the syringes in the "sharps" container reach the filled line, start using a new container and bring the full one in to us. Overfilling the container will put you at risk for sticking yourself.
- Store the syringes in a safe place, especially with children in the house who could harm themselves.

Adverse Effects
- Fatigue is usually a problem for patients during the low-dose chronic phase of this regimen. Continue to rest when you need to and ask others to help you with activities you do not feel up to doing.
- Administer the dose of interferon in the evening, but don't schedule the dose too late, because symptoms such as fever and chills may interfere with your sleep. Getting enough sleep at night may prevent some of the fatigue.
- If your appetite has been normal throughout the high-dose phase, it still may decrease during continued therapy. Remember to try to eat small meals throughout the day and drink plenty of fluids. You may also want to try some dietary supplements to keep up your caloric intake.
- We will continue to check your blood counts and liver function tests when you come to the clinic. If your liver numbers become too high, we may have to withhold some of your interferon doses and decrease the dose that you receive.
- You may begin to notice that your mood changes as you continue therapy. Some patients report that they feel depressed, mentally slow, and don't feel like participating in their normal activities. If any of these problems occur, be sure to call the clinic or tell your oncologist, nurse, or pharmacist.

c. *What information would you give to the patient regarding sun exposure?*

- When you will be outdoors in the sun for a significant time, always apply sunscreen with an SPF of at least 15 to sun-exposed areas; wear a broad-brimmed hat and a long-sleeved shirt.

- Avoid exposure during the peak sun-exposure hours; these hours depend on geographic location, but typically occur during midday.
- Use a waterproof sunscreen when swimming outdoors. Reapply the sunscreen once out of the water to replace any that may have washed off. Reapply sunscreen at least every 2 to 3 hours, or more frequently if sweating.
- Even during the winter months, excess exposure to the sun can cause a burn, especially when snow on the ground causes reflection of the ultraviolet rays.
- Make sure that your sons are adequately protected from harmful ultraviolet rays. They are at a crucial age because children and adolescents who have high sun exposure are at greater risk for developing melanoma later in life.

▶ Follow-up Questions

1. *Given this new information, what changes, if any, should be made in the patient's interferon therapy?*

- The patient's SCr is increased from his baseline of 0.8 mg/dL. Renal toxicity from interferon therapy is uncommon and is usually seen as mild proteinuria. Other causes of an elevated SCr, such as dehydration, should be ruled out, and caution should be used in patients receiving concurrent nephrotoxic agents. For example, if the patient were taking an NSAID to prevent or treat myalgias and fevers, this could have an additive nephrotoxic effect, and the NSAID should be discontinued.
- Hepatic toxicity, a dose-related interferon effect, usually manifests as increases in hepatic aminotransferases. These are typically transient and will return to baseline after interferon discontinuation. Interferon should be withheld until the patient's LFTs are less than 5 times normal and then restarted with a 50% dose reduction.
- Weight loss secondary to decreased appetite is a common adverse effect of interferon therapy. When patients lose between 5% to 10% of their baseline weight, the dose of interferon should be reduced by 50%. The effect of appetite stimulants has not been sufficiently evaluated for interferon-induced anorexia. Corticosteroids should be avoided because it is hypothesized that they may interfere with the immunostimulatory effects of the interferon. Cannabinoids could worsen the patient's sedation, and megesterol acetate may have adrenal effects and should, therefore, also be avoided. The patient could also be losing weight from decreased oral intake secondary to fatigue or taste changes. At this point, nutritional education and behavioral therapy are appropriate interventions to decrease his weight loss in addition to the previously mentioned interferon dose reduction.

2. *What information is needed to fully assess the patient's acute mental status changes?*

- A complete physical exam that includes a thorough neurologic examination
- Medication history and current medication list
- Current laboratory data, including serum electrolytes, renal function tests, CBC, and LFTs
- CT or MRI of the brain to evaluate for brain metastasis or hemorrhage

3. *What possible complications resulting from the interferon therapy might account for his acute mental status changes?*

- Dehydration
- Electrolyte abnormalities
- Fatigue
- Anemia

4. *Should any changes be made in the patient's interferon therapy at this point?*

- Neurologic side effects of interferon can manifest as depression, anxiety, lethargy, somnolence, and fatigue, as previously described. They can also be more severe and debilitating such as stupor and confusion. Side effects such as these can prevent patients from performing their normal activities of daily living, leading to a decreased performance status.
- If a patient presents with persistent somnolence, interferon therapy should be withheld until there is improvement; at that time it can be restarted at a dosage reduction of up to 50%.
- However, if a patient is disoriented and confused, as is this patient, and other causes have been ruled out, interferon therapy should be discontinued until the etiology is determined.

5. *If the patient develops metastatic disease, what pharmacotherapeutic options are available?*

- Single agents with the greatest activity in patients with melanoma include dacarbazine and the nitrosoureas, carmustine (BCNU) and lomustine (CCNU), which have response rates of approximately 20% to 25% and 10% to 20%, respectively.
- Dacarbazine has been combined with cisplatin, hormonal agents, and immunotherapy. Although response rates have been greater with combination chemotherapy, there have been no direct comparisons with the single agent dacarbazine. Toxicity is more severe with combination regimens, and improvements in survival have been minimal.
- Dacarbazine and interleukin-2 (IL-2) are the only approved agents for the treatment of metastatic melanoma. Several other therapies, such as monoclonal antibodies and intralesional chemotherapy, are undergoing clinical investigation. Clinical trials are always an option for patients with metastatic melanoma who have failed conventional therapies.

References

1. Kirkwood JM, Strawderman MH, Ernstoff MS, et al. Interferon alfa-2b adjuvant therapy of high-risk resected cutaneous melanoma: The Eastern Cooperative Oncology Group Trial EST 1684. J Clin Oncol 1996;14:7–17.
2. Cole BF, Gelber RD, Kirkwood JM, et al. Quality-of-life-adjusted survival analysis of interferon alfa-2b adjuvant treatment of high-risk resected cutaneous melanoma: An Eastern Cooperative Oncology Group study. J Clin Oncol 1996;14: 2666–2673.
3. Cocconi G, Bella M, Calabresi F, et al. Treatment of metastatic malignant melanoma with dacarbazine plus tamoxifen. N Engl J Med 1992;327:516–523.

128 BONE MARROW TRANSPLANTATION

▶ A Dilemma in Antibiotic Therapy   (Level II)

Simon Cronin, PharmD, MS

This case follows the clinical course of a man with non-Hodgkin's lymphoma who received intensive chemotherapy followed by autologous peripheral stem cell transplantation. While receiving antibiotic therapy during the period of neutropenia, the patient developed vancomycin-resistant *Enterococcus* (VRE) bacteremia. The patient also developed other adverse effects related to the chemotherapy, including mucositis and liver function abnormalities. Minimizing the use of antibiotic therapy is essential in preventing the incidence of VRE infections in transplant patients.

▶ Questions

Problem Identification

1. a. *What risk factors did this patient have for developing VRE sepsis?*

   - Prior to the transplant admission, there had been several admissions for IV antibiotic therapy. *E. faecium* is intrinsically resistant to most antibiotics, including the cephalosporins; therefore, it is possible that VRE had already colonized the GI tract.
   - The chemotherapy regimen causes severe mucositis. Loss of mucosal cell lining is not confined to the oral mucosa and was probably located at several places along the GI tract of this patient, thereby allowing VRE access to the venous system.
   - The problem was further compounded by the fact that ceftazidime (which has no coverage against enterococci) was administered after the first fever spike. This may have preferentially selected the overgrowth of the VRE in the GI tract during the transplant admission.

   b. *What other potential drug-related problems does this patient have?*

   - The major chemotherapy-induced toxicity at the present time is severe oral mucositis.
   - High-dose cyclophosphamide is associated with cardiac necrosis (which manifests as heart failure) and hemorrhagic cystitis. There is no evidence of either of these disorders.

Desired Outcome

2. *What are the therapeutic goals in this patient?*

   - Resolve the patient's fever
   - Eradicate the VRE from the patient
   - Prevent or minimize antibiotic-associated side effects
   - Minimize further chemotherapy-related toxicity
   - Produce a normal functioning bone marrow with a rapid recovery of neutrophil production
   - Achieve complete remission or cure of the NHL (a longer-term goal)

Therapeutic Alternatives

3. *What alternative antibiotic(s) would effectively treat the VRE infection in this patient?*

   - The genus *Enterococcus* is classified as a group D *Streptococcus*, which is a lower bowel inhabitant that can become pathogenic in neutropenic patients, especially when the lining of the GI tract becomes denuded by chemotherapy.[1] The antibiotics that are routinely tested for *Enterococcus* sensitivity include ampicillin, levofloxacin, ciprofloxacin, vancomycin, doxycycline, and gentamicin.
   - It is usual to select two antibiotics with different mechanisms of action for the treatment of *Enterococcus* isolated from blood in order to prevent development of resistance over the course of therapy.
     ✓ *Ampicillin plus low-dose gentamicin* (desired serum peaks of 3 to 4 μg/mL) is a regimen of choice if the organism is sensitive to ampicillin.
     ✓ *Vancomycin plus gentamicin* is usually used if the patient is penicillin-allergic or if the *Enterococcus* is resistant to ampicillin.
   - Bacterial resistance is normally determined by reviewing the MIC of the antibiotic against the organism (the minimum concentration of antibacterial necessary to inhibit the growth of the microorganism). The MIC for gram-positive streptococci that are sensitive to vancomycin is usually ≤ 4 μg/mL. Organisms with vancomycin MICs > 4 μg/mL but < 16 μg/mL are considered to be intermediately sensitive. If the MIC is > 16 μg/mL, the organism is considered to be resistant to vancomycin because too much vancomycin would have to be administered to achieve the necessary MIC *in vivo*. Because the organism in this case is of the genus *Enterococcus* and the vancomycin MIC is >16 μg/mL, it is considered to be a vancomycin-resistant *Enterococcus* or VRE.
   - *Doxycycline* is the only other commercially available antibiotic on the sensitivity panel that shows sensitivity (the MIC is < 4 μg/mL), making doxycycline an obvious treatment choice. The usual dose is 100 mg IV Q 12 H. To prevent emergence of doxycycline resistance over the course of therapy, it is preferable to add a second agent.
   - *Quinupristin/dalfopristin* is a streptogramin antibiotic that was investigational at the time of this writing. However, the drug may be

available from the manufacturer through an emergency use program for patients with vancomycin-resistant gram-positive infections unresponsive to available antibiotic therapy. In early 1998, The FDA's Anti-Infective Drugs Advisory Committee recommended its approval for treatment of infections due to vancomycin-resistant *E. faecium*, among other indications. Its two compounds work synergistically to kill susceptible bacteria by inhibiting protein synthesis. The combination of quinupristin/dalfopristin with doxycycline may provide synergistic activity against VRE, although this has not been conclusively established. The usual dose is 7.5 mg/kg IV Q 8 H. Adverse effects include local reactions (inflammation, pain, and infusion-site reactions), arthralgias, myalgias, nausea, diarrhea, vomiting, rash, and elevated serum bilirubin concentrations.

- *Nitrofurantoin* sometimes has activity against VRE. However, this patient's VRE was cultured from the blood, and nitrofurantoin does not achieve satisfactory blood levels to be effective. Nitrofurantoin is a good option for urinary tract infections caused by VRE because high enough urinary tract concentrations are easily achieved.
- *Imipenem* sometimes shows activity against enterococci. Although it is not routinely tested for sensitivity against gram-positive aerobic bacteria, in this instance the organism was also found to be resistant to imipenem (the MIC is > 16 µg/mL, so concentrations in the blood high enough to reach the MIC cannot safely be achieved without developing toxicity).
- *Erythromycin* shows good activity against streptococci in general, but rarely shows activity against enterococci. In this case, the isolate is clearly insensitive, making erythromycin a poor choice for the patient.
- *Fluoroquinolones (levofloxacin, ciprofloxacin)* are generally weaker in their activity toward gram-positive cocci than toward gram-negative bacilli. Ofloxacin has somewhat better activity than ciprofloxacin against streptococci, but in this instance, the MIC data clearly show resistance of the VRE isolate.

Optimal Plan

4. a. Outline an appropriate antibiotic regimen for treating this patient's VRE infection.

- Start doxycycline 100 mg IV Q 12 H (infused over 1 hour) plus quinupristin/dalfopristin 7.5 mg/kg IV Q 8 H (infused over 1 hour). If quinupristin/dalfopristin is still an investigational agent at the time of your case discussion, discuss with students the need for the patient to read and sign an approved informed consent document prior to initiation of the investigational agent.

b. What other pharmacotherapeutic measures should be implemented to enhance the patient's defense mechanisms against infection and to prevent other types of infection?

- The patient is still neutropenic (WBC count < 0.5×10^3/mm^3), greatly reducing his defenses against infection by endogenous and exogenous organisms. A colony-stimulating factor can be added to assist the patient's WBC recovery. G-CSF (filgrastim) 5 µg/kg/day SC should provide adequate therapy. An alternative is GM-CSF (sargramostim) 5 µg/kg/day.
- Acyclovir can be continued for herpes simplex prophylaxis.
- Vancomycin should not be restarted. There are no other sites of infection, and there is already an organism that is resistant to vancomycin.

Outcome Evaluation

5. What parameters should you monitor to assess the response to therapy and to detect adverse effects?

Efficacy Parameters

- Monitor the patient's temperature at least 3 times a day as long as the patient is febrile (temperature >100.5°F) and/or neutropenic (WBC < 0.5×10^3/mm^3). The WBC may remain low until about 14 days post-transplant.
- Draw daily blood cultures while the patient is febrile and neutropenic (WBC < 0.5×10^3/mm^3) to rule out another micro-organism as the cause of the fever. Once the patient's temperature is < 100°F for 24 hours or longer, daily blood cultures are no longer necessary. Blood cultures should remain negative and should be repeated at the end of therapy (2 weeks).
- If the patient is responding clinically, the temperature should begin to normalize within about 48 hours after initiating therapy.

Adverse Effect Parameters

- Quinupristin/dalfopristin can cause myalgias (muscle aches), arthralgias (joint pains), and infusion-site reactions that sometimes require discontinuation of therapy. The patient should be asked daily about these effects.
- Both doxycycline (< 1% of patients) and quinupristin/dalfopristin can cause elevations in liver function tests. Bilirubin, ALT, AST, and alkaline phosphatase should be monitored 3 times a week during therapy. If they become elevated to > 2 times baseline, discontinuation of antibiotic therapy should be considered until the LFTs return to baseline.
- Monitor for the development of a rash, pruritus, nausea, vomiting, and diarrhea during antibiotic therapy.
- G-CSF (filgrastim) can cause fever and bone pain. An increase in baseline temperature can rarely occur shortly after the injection and then slowly returns to baseline (temporal association). Pain is typically described by the patient to be located deep in the bones and is usually distinct from muscle aches and pains. The patient should be asked about this daily. The G-CSF should be discontinued when the neutrophil count is $\geq 0.5 \times 10^3$/mm^3 for 48 hours. The subcutaneous injection sites should be observed daily for bruising. If bruising is evident, the IV route can be used.

Patient Counseling

6. How will you explain to the patient that he has an antibiotic-resistant infection?

- A certain kind of bacteria in your gastrointestinal tract has found its way into your blood and is the probable cause of your fever. In order to treat this, we have to modify your antibiotic therapy.
- To treat it adequately, we would like to use an investigational antibiotic that is showing promise for the treatment of this type of infection. Because it is not yet approved for general use in this country, we would like for you to read this statement of informed consent. If you understand and agree with its contents, we will ask you to sign the consent form. We will be available to answer any questions you may

have about this antibiotic at any time during the course of your therapy.

▶ Follow-up Questions

1. *Review the clinical and laboratory data on day +11 and suggest a possible reason for the change in liver function tests.*

    - Elevation in LFTs can be associated with drug toxicity. Fluconazole has rarely been associated with a non-infectious hepatitis; however, the AST and ALT were within normal limits in this case.
    - There was a slight increase in alkaline phosphatase and a larger increase in total bilirubin. Because the patient did not receive an allogeneic transplant, graft-versus-host disease is an extremely unlikely explanation for the alteration in the LFTs.
    - There was RUQ abdominal tenderness and a 2-kg weight gain. Mild hepatic veno-occlusive disease (VOD) is a distinct possibility. This patient is within the time frame for development of VOD post-transplant (usually 8 to 20 days) and has had prior exposure to chemotherapy (including high-dose cyclophosphamide). Diagnosis of VOD should be made by liver biopsy, but this procedure is contraindicated in most transplant patients because of thrombocytopenia and the associated risk of bleeding. Therefore, a diagnosis of VOD is often made on clinical grounds, usually based on the following criteria: jaundice plus any 2 of the following 3 signs: hepatomegaly, ascites, or weight gain (≥ 5% of baseline).[2]

2. *Assume that the LFT changes are not related to infection. Outline a therapeutic plan aimed at treating this new problem, should it progress.*

    - The patient probably has mild VOD. Supportive care with sodium and fluid restriction should be attempted, as well as the judicious use of diuretics and a low dose of dopamine (2 to 4 µg/kg/min) to prevent the onset of renal dysfunction.
    - Mild VOD is usually reversible, and patients should make a complete recovery with resolution of all the clinical signs (weight gain, hyperbilirubinemia, abdominal pain). Severe VOD, on the other hand, is associated with a high mortality of 50% to 98%. Options for management of VOD include the use of prostaglandin PGE_1 or tissue-plasminogen activator (rt-PA) with heparin.[3] rt-PA is used in low doses (10 mg/day IV over 4 hours) for 2 days with low-dose heparin (1000-unit loading dose followed by 150 units/kg/day by continuous IV infusion for 10 days.
    - Because of the dismal outcome associated with severe VOD, more emphasis is usually directed at prevention. To that end, pharmacologic maneuvers have been aimed at preventing the venous plugging caused by platelet activation and thrombus formation. Low-dose heparin use is controversial. Other drugs that have been used to prevent VOD include pentoxifylline (aimed at limiting the damage caused by the production of tumor-necrosis factor),[4] and PGE_1 (to oppose the vasoconstriction). In this case, there was no attempt to prevent VOD through use of any of the agents listed. Fortunately, the patient did not progress to severe VOD and recovered.

References

1. Murray BE. Vancomycin-resistant enterococci. Am J Med 1997;102:284–293.
2. Jones RJ, Lee KSK, Beschorner WL, et al. Venoocclusive disease of the liver following bone marrow transplantation. Transplantation 1987;44:778–783.
3. Terra S, Spitzer TR, Tsunoda SM. A review of tissue plasminogen activator in the treatment of veno-occlusive disease after bone marrow transplantation. Pharmacotherapy 1997;17:929–937.
4. Bianco JA, Applebaum FR, Nemunaitis J, et al. Phase I-II trial of pentoxifylline for the prevention of transplantation related toxicities following bone marrow transplantation. Blood 1991;78:1205–1211.

PART FIVE

Nutrition and Nutritional Disorders

Gary R. Matzke, PharmD, FCP, FCCP, Section Editor

129 PARENTERAL NUTRITION

▶ To Diet in Vein   (Level III)

Douglas D. Janson, PharmD, BCNSP

A 28-year-old obese man with acute necrotizing pancreatitis is started on total parenteral nutrition (TPN) to minimize exocrine stimulation of the pancreas during the initial phase of the disease course. Readers are asked to assess the patient's nutrition risk and to calculate the body mass index (BMI) prior to estimating the patient's nutrient requirements. A TPN formulation must then be designed that includes final concentrations of amino acids, dextrose, lipid emulsion, electrolytes, vitamins, trace elements, and the rate of infusion. Measures to control hyperglycemia while on TPN also need to be considered. Numerous monitoring parameters require assessment during TPN therapy; in this case, readers are also asked to interpret the results of a nitrogen balance study. Patient counseling includes information on both TPN and the transition to enteral nutrition as the patient begins recovery.

▶ Questions

Problem Identification

1. a. *Create a list of this patient's problems related to nutrition, fluid, and electrolytes.*

   - He is at high risk for developing protein and calorie malnutrition because of NPO status × 7 days with only IV fluids infusing, a dysfunctional GI tract preventing oral ingestion, and complicated acute pancreatitis.
   - There is the potential for fluid, electrolyte, and acid–base imbalances because of NG tube aspiration, medication side effects, and the necrotizing pancreatitis.
   - Hyperglycemia and hypertriglyceridemia are possible because of the pancreatitis, obesity, and institution of nutrition therapy.
   - Deficiencies of selected micronutrients may be present given his history of chronic ethanol abuse.
   - GI complications such as "gut atrophy" with subsequent alteration of the gut barrier function and cholestasis may occur during NPO status. For more details, refer to the discussion on the rationale for enteral nutrition in textbook Chapter 129.

   b. *What is acute pancreatitis and what are the common causes?*

   - Acute pancreatitis is pancreatic inflammation resulting from premature activation of proteolytic enzymes within the organ and subsequent autodigestion of the gland and peripancreatic tissues.
   - Common causes include obstruction (choledocholithiasis) and toxins (e.g., EtOH). For other causes, refer to Table 37–2, in textbook Chapter 37.

   c. *What are the clinical, laboratory, and radiologic characteristics of acute pancreatitis in this patient?*

   - *Signs/symptoms.* Abdominal pain with radiation to the back, abdominal distension, history of N/V, fever, and jaundice.[1]

- *Laboratory findings.* Elevated serum lipase, hyperglycemia, elevated total bilirubin and ALT, and increased WBC count.
- *Radiologic findings.* Contrast-enhanced CT can delineate the pancreas, and ultrasonography can assess the biliary tract and help determine the cause of pancreatitis.

d. *What clinical, laboratory, and radiologic characteristics indicate that this patient has severe (or complicated) acute pancreatitis?*

- *Signs/symptoms.* Marked abdominal pain and tenderness (rated 7 out of 10); history of fever with symptom onset; distended and hypoactive bowel sounds; large NG tube output/24 hours; systemic effects of elevated pulse, BP, and RR; diaphoresis; and SOB on supplemental oxygen delivery.
- *Laboratory findings.* Persistently elevated WBC and bandemia, suboptimal oxygenation (decreased Pao_2 and Sao_2).
- *Radiologic findings.* CT scan indicates extensive peripancreatic inflammation and evidence of necrosis in the head and body of pancreas; possible small bowel ileus.

e. *Describe why this patient is at nutrition risk and characterize the type of malnutrition he will likely develop.*

- The patient is 7 days into the disease course that is becoming more clinically complicated, and he is receiving only IVF and is NPO with an NG tube in place for decompression (on low continuous suction).
- The dextrose 5% at 125 mL/hour that he is receiving supplies 150 g/day dextrose (or 510 kcal/d), which only meets about 20% of his energy requirements and does not sufficiently retard the rate of his daily nitrogen losses or meet daily micronutrient requirements.
- The systemic effects of acute pancreatitis cause a catabolic state evidenced by an increased resting energy expenditure, gluconeogenesis, protein degradation, and urea generation.[2]
- Despite his obesity, this patient is at high risk for developing protein malnutrition (referred to as kwashiorkor); it can develop quickly in response to protein deprivation in the setting of catabolic stress.

f. *What additional nutritional assessment data should you request and why?*

- Serum albumin is used as an indirect measure of protein nutriture or lean body mass. It can also be used to interpret the serum calcium level and to assess the relative intravascular oncotic pressure.
- Hypocalcemia accompanies acute pancreatitis as a result of hypoalbuminemia and the saponification of calcium by free fatty acids during peripancreatic fat necrosis.[1]

Desired Outcome

2. *What are the goals of specialized nutrition support in this patient?*

- Specialized nutrition support has not been shown to have a primary role in the natural history of acute pancreatitis; it is viewed as adjuvant or supportive care.[2,3]
- Major goals are to: 1) reduce the net rate of daily nitrogen loss (i.e., achieve a less negative or positive nitrogen balance) and maintain micronutrient homeostasis; 2) minimize the potential for therapy-related complications; and 3) reduce the effects of malnutrition as a comorbidity during the disease course.

Therapeutic Alternatives

3. *What are the therapeutic options for specialized nutrition intervention in this patient?*

- Withholding oral food intake in order to minimize exocrine stimulation of the pancreas conservatively manages the initial 4 to 5 days of the disease course. For more information, see the discussion on physiology of exocrine pancreatic secretion and treatment of acute pancreatitis in textbook Chapter 37.
- Currently, enteral nutrition through a feeding tube is not a feasible option based on the signs and symptoms of small bowel ileus and other complications of the acute pancreatitis.
- Parenteral nutrition delivered through a peripheral or central vein is a feasible option. However, during this catabolic illness, the patient requires a parenteral formulation that completely meets his estimated nutritional requirements. Therefore central venous access is required because of the increased solution hyperosmolarity; a peripheral vein would develop thrombophlebitis and infiltrate the subcutaneous tissues if such a hyperosmolar parenteral nutrition formulation were infused. The patient already has a suitable central venous catheter (a subclavian vein triple lumen port) in which a designated port is used for the TPN.

Optimal Plan

4. a. *What method is used to classify this patient as obese?*

- Body mass index (BMI), defined as weight in kg divided by height in square meters (kg/m^2), is an accurate method for assessing body fatness. This patient's calculated BMI is $130/(1.98)^2 = 33.1$ kg/m^2.
- A BMI ≥ 30 kg/m^2 is defined as obesity by an expert panel published in the 1998 NIH Obesity Clinical Guidelines.[4]

b. *What body weight would be used to estimate the nutrient requirements in this obese man?*

- Weight is used to calculate daily nutrient requirements. However, if the actual body weight of an obese patient is used, this will overestimate the actual energy requirement since adipose tissue is less metabolically active than lean body mass.
- Adjustment of body weight for obesity (kg):
adjusted body weight = ({actual weight − ideal weight*} × 0.25) + ideal weight*
= (\{130 − 91.4\} × 0.25) + 91.4
= 101 kg

*ideal weight = 50 kg + {(number of inches over 5′0″) × 2.3}
= 50 kg + {(18) × 2.3}
= 91.4 kg

c. *What are the ranges of estimated daily goals for calories (kcal/kg/day), protein (g/kg/day), and hydration (mL/kg/day) for this patient?*

- Refer to "Assessment of Nutrient Requirements" in textbook Chapter 126 (see Table 129–1).

- The ranges for nutrition requirements are as follows:

Substrate/Hydration	Goals for Maintenance and Preventing Malnutrition	Estimated Daily Requirements
Nonprotein	30 to 35 kcal/kg/d	3030 to 3535 kcal/d
Protein	1.5 to 2.0 g/kg/d	152 to 202 g/d
Hydration	30 mL/kg/d	3030 mL/d[a]

[a] This hydration volume does not take into account the amount of extraordinary fluid lost via gastric decompression.

d. Design a TPN formulation for the first day of treatment that includes the volume and rate (mL/hour), final amino acids (g/L), dextrose (g/L), lipid emulsion (g/L), electrolytes (mEq/day or mmol/day), vitamins, trace elements, and other additives (see Table 129–1).

e. What other order(s) would you suggest at the initiation of the TPN?

- Discontinue the scheduled famotidine, as it will be contained within the TPN.

TABLE 129–1. Recommended TPN Formulation for the First Day of Treatment

TPN Components	Considerations	Formulation[5]
Hydration	Estimated maintenance hydration of 3000 mL selected for TPN with the IVF used to replace extraordinary NG tube outputs; goal is to maintain adequate intravascular volume, given the risk of pancreatic edema (third spacing of fluid) and without complicating respiratory function, given possible pulmonary edema.	3000 mL/d infused over 24 hours at a rate of 125 mL/hour
Protein (amino acid or AA) Generally up to 20% of daily calories	Initially begin with lower range of estimated requirement and adjust according to monitoring parameters.	Final AA = 150 g/d $\frac{150 \text{ g/d}}{3 \text{ L/d}} = 50 \text{ g/L}$
Dextrose (D) Generally 40% to 60% of daily calories with dextrose infusion range of 3 to 5 mg/kg/min	Patient is mildly hyperglycemic on 5% dextrose; at risk for greater hyperglycemia with increasing dextrose delivery because of impaired endocrine function of pancreas, increases in counterregulatory hormones, and stress-induced insulin resistance at peripheral receptor sites.	3–5 mg/kg/min = 436–727 g/d dextrose Select: Final D = 450 g/d $\frac{450 \text{ g/d}}{3 \text{ L/d}} = 150 \text{ g/L}$
Lipid Generally 20% to 40% of daily calories with lipid dosed at 1.0-1.5 g/kg/d	IV lipid emulsion is commonly used as a substrate in pancreatitis, except during complications of significant hypertriglyceridemia, which can exacerbate or cause pancreatitis; lipid can be a desirable source of nonprotein calories during hyperglycemia.	1.0–1.5 g/kg/d = 100–150 g/d of lipid emulsion Select: Final lipid = 100 g/d $\frac{100 \text{ g/d}}{3 \text{ L/d}} = 33.3 \text{ g/L}$
Electrolytes Daily doses depend on serum levels, organ function, acid–base status, concomitant drug therapy, extraordinary fluid loss content, and anabolic feeding goals	Patient has low-normal values for sodium, phosphate, and calcium; ticarcillin supplies 57 mEq/d sodium, and furosemide induces losses of sodium, potassium, magnesium, and calcium; the IVF will continue to replace the extraordinary losses of sodium, chloride, and potassium.	Sodium chloride = 40 mEq/d Sodium acetate = 40 mEq/d Potassium acetate = 15 mEq/d Potassium chloride = 16 mEq/d Potassium Phosphate = 40 mmol/d (phosphate content = 40 mmol/d and potassium content of salt = 59 mEq/d) Calcium gluconate = 15 mEq/d Magnesium sulfate = 18 mEq/d
Vitamins	Multivitamin injection containing the RDA for 12 vitamins is routinely provided for adults receiving TPN; chronic ethanol abuse predisposes this patient to thiamine (vitamin B_1) and folate deficiency.	Multivitamin injection Thiamine 50 mg/d Folic acid 1 mg/d
Trace minerals	Multi-trace minerals are routinely provided for adults receiving TPN.	Multi-trace mineral injection (zinc, copper, manganese, selenium and chromium)
Other additives	Insulin is compatible in TPN; initial starting dosage 0.05 to 0.1 units/g of dextrose/d; famotidine is compatible with TPN and provides convenient delivery.	Humulin insulin 20 units/d and famotidine 40 mg/d delivered through the TPN

- Reduce the rate of the IV fluid to replete the extraordinary losses from the NG tube (decrease to 90 mL/hour) to prevent dehydration and hypochloremic metabolic alkalosis.
- Initiate bedside monitoring of blood glucose QID.
- Order a sliding scale subcutaneous regular insulin coverage, such as shown below.

Blood Glucose (mg/dL)	Regular Insulin SC (units/dose)
< 200	0
200–250	3
251–300	6
301–350	9
351–400	12
> 400	Notify physician

Outcome Evaluation

5. a. *What monitoring parameters and frequency are required for monitoring the TPN regimen?*

- See Figure 128–4 in textbook Chapter 128.
- Obtain daily weight, vital signs, nutrition intake, fluid balance (input/output), and fingerstick glucose as needed (initially QID).
- Measure serum sodium, potassium, chloride, bicarbonate, calcium, magnesium, phosphorous, BUN, and creatinine daily for the first 3 to 4 days, then 2 to 3 times weekly (depending on metabolic stability).
- Assess nitrogen balance, transferrin, triglyceride, alkaline phosphatase, AST, total bilirubin, PT, and INR weekly as necessary.

b. *Within the first week of TPN, a nitrogen balance study was performed with the following results: 19.5 grams of urine urea nitrogen (UUN) measured from a 24-hour urine collection. Why is a nitrogen balance study done during specialized nutrition support?*

- A nitrogen balance study is an indirect measure of preservation or erosion of lean body mass. As the level of physiologic stress increases, there is a concomitant increase in body protein catabolism, resulting in an increase in the urinary nitrogen excretion. UUN accounts for 60% to 90% of the total nitrogen excreted.
- The UUN is affected by renal function and the accuracy of the 24-hour urine collection.
- The study results are useful in evaluating the adequacy of protein and calorie support in critical illness when visceral proteins (albumin and/or transferrin) are affected by non-nutritional factors (see Table 126–3 in textbook Chapter 126).

c. *Interpret the aforementioned data to calculate the nitrogen balance. Hint: refer to the section "Assessment of Nutrient Requirements" in textbook Chapter 126 for this information.*

- The study is performed by collecting 24 hours of urine and assaying it for the amount of UUN (grams/24 hr specimen); therefore, evaluating the volume of urine assayed with the record of the patient's urine output is required.

- N_{out} (g/d) = (UUN [g] × 1.2) + 1
  = (19.5 × 1.2) + 1
  = 24.4
- Nitrogen balance = $N_{in} - N_{out}$
  = (150 g/d × $\frac{1 \text{ g nitrogen}}{5.98 \text{ g amino acid}}$) − 24.4
  = 25.1 − 24.4
  = (+) 0.7 or rounded to (+) 1.0
- This is an acceptable positive balance with the current level of protein and caloric support during acute catabolic illness.

Patient Counseling

6. a. *What information should be provided to the patient and family during his hospitalization regarding the parenteral and enteral nutrition therapy?*

- Total parenteral nutrition (or TPN) is an artificial form of nourishment that is directly infused into a vein (intravenously) through a catheter, such as the triple lumen central venous device that is in the large vessel near your heart.
- TPN completely bypasses your gastrointestinal tract (stomach and intestines). The sterile solution contains all of your required nutrients in a large bag infused through a pump into your vein over 24 hours a day.
- As the person assisting with your nutritional care, I will assist your surgeon in defining your nutrient prescription and monitor your blood chemistries to assure that we are adequately meeting your requirements.
- TPN is required for you because your pancreas is very inflamed and the movement of your stomach and intestines is abnormally slow. Allowing you to eat or putting liquid nutrition solutions into your gastrointestinal tract would cause further pain, nausea, and vomiting. It is your surgeon's goal to rest your pancreas now by using TPN and not feeding through your stomach or intestines. The pancreas is stimulated by food in your stomach and upper small intestine.
- The TPN will probably be needed for at least a week or more, depending on the duration of time it takes to bring your pancreas and gastrointestinal tract to better health and function.

b. *Explain to the patient the transition from parenteral to enteral nutrition through use of the jejunostomy port of the transgastric jejunostomy tube.*

- Now that you have had surgery to remove the diseased and infected portions of your pancreas, it is reasonable to slowly instill a liquid nutrition solution into the small intestine. Your pancreas is not completely healthy yet, so we do not want to feed directly into your stomach by having you eat food.
- Your surgeon has placed a feeding tube device that permits us to infuse nutrition solutions into a portion of your small intestine called the jejunum. This form of artificial nutrition is called enteral nutrition. By feeding into your small intestine beyond the pancreas, we can allow your pancreas more time to heal.
- As we continue to advance the amount of enteral nutrition that is

delivered through the pump, we can eventually discontinue the TPN. The enteral nutrition can completely meet your nutrient requirements. Enteral nutrition requires less intensive monitoring than TPN and is as effective.

c. *Explain the anticipated course for enteral nutrition and the transition back to oral food ingestion.*

- As the surgeon determines that your pancreas is healing and that you are making clinical improvement (no fevers, ambulating), the gastric port of your transgastric jejunostomy will be closed for increasing periods of time. This is done to determine how well your stomach is emptying gastric contents into the intestines.
- Soon, a clear liquid diet will be initiated. Your gastrointestinal function (nausea, vomiting) will be assessed, and soon your diet will be advanced to more solid foods. You will be required to be on a low-fat diet, and a dietitian will provide dietary counseling to you and your caregiver. A low-fat diet has less potential to stimulate your pancreas to work.
- The rate of enteral nutrition will be decreased as your oral caloric intake increases. Eventually, the enteral nutrition will be discontinued completely as you make successful progress in advancing your oral food ingestion. This entire process is dependent on the time it takes to heal your pancreas.

References

1. Steinberg W, Tenner S. Acute pancreatitis. N Engl J Med 1994;330:1198–1210.
2. Kusske AM, Katona DR, Reber HA. Nutritional support in pancreatic disease. In: Rombeau JL, Rolandelli RH, eds. Clinical Nutrition: Enteral and Tube Feeding, 3rd ed. Philadelphia, Saunders, 1997:429–438.
3. Marulendra S, Kirby DF. Nutrition support in pancreatitis. Nutri Clin Pract 1995;10:45–53.
4. National Institutes of Health. Clinical guidelines on the identification, evaluation, and treatment of overweight and obesity in adults—the evidence report. Obes Res 1998(6 suppl 2):51S–209S.
5. National Advisory Group on Standards and Practice Guidelines for Parenteral Nutrition. Safe practices for parenteral nutrition formulations. J Parenter Enteral Nutr 1998;22:49–66.
6. De Beaux AC, Plester C, Fearon KCH. Flexible approach to nutritional support in severe acute pancreatitis. Nutrition 1994;10:246–249.

130 ADULT ENTERAL NUTRITION

▶ **Down the Tube** (Level III)

Carol J. Rollins, MS, RD, PharmD, BCNSP

A 68-year-old man with gastric/esophageal cancer and weight loss after chemotherapy is referred to home health care for initiation of tube feedings. Before implementing the physician's orders, the clinician must obtain the necessary information to properly evaluate the orders and recommend an appropriate feeding plan. Readers are asked to calculate the protein, calorie, and fluid requirements for the patient and select the type of formula and administration rate. Methods for continued administration of the patient's current oral mediations must also be considered. Finally, a plan for clinical and laboratory monitoring must be created to ensure tolerance of the feedings and achievement of the desired nutritional end points.

▶ Questions

Problem Identification

1. a. *What other information is necessary or would be helpful to evaluate the orders and provide recommendations for a feeding plan?*

   - The patient's height will be needed to calculate his nutrition requirements.
   - His usual weight or his weight prior to illness.
   - The amount of weight loss and the time period of the loss.
   - Recent laboratory data to evaluate visceral protein status, glucose tolerance, and electrolyte status are most important.
   - Laboratory data to evaluate renal function, hepatic function, and hematologic status would be helpful, but are not essential at this particular time.
   - Information related to the presence of nausea, vomiting, diarrhea, constipation, and strength or exercise capacity would be helpful.
   - Physical examination information including evidence of nutritional lesions, muscle wasting, loss of subcutaneous fat stores, ascites, and edema would be helpful in assessing nutrition requirements.

   b. *How can you obtain this information for your home health care company, which is located across town from the clinic and hospital?*

   - Contact the clinic where the patient receives chemotherapy; request the necessary information from a nurse, or request permission for a representative from the home health care company to review the patient's chart.
   - You could also contact the patient or his caregiver.
   - Contact the nutrition support professional at the hospital where surgery was performed. A brief operative report and history of parenteral or enteral support during that time may be available.
   - Request permission to review the patient's record yourself at the hospital.

   c. *Is insurance coverage an issue in this situation?*

   - Verification of insurance coverage is one of the first steps for home therapy. The patient is financially responsible for the cost of therapy if criteria for insurance coverage are not met. This patient's Medicare Part B covers home parenteral and enteral therapy when specific criteria listed in the *Medicare Coverage Issues Manual* (HCFA Publication 6 through revision 42) and *Durable Medical Equipment Regional Carrier Suppliers Manual* are met. (*Note to instructors:* It may be difficult for students to obtain these publications or to find this information elsewhere. You may wish to provide them with the following information.) Criteria for Medicare coverage of enteral nutrition include all of the following items.

- ✓ Functional impairment of the GI tract, such as dysphagia due to neurologic disease or CVA; coverage is included under the prosthetic device benefit. The impairment must involve dysfunction of structures that normally allow food to reach the site of digestion and absorption. For example, weight loss in a patient who forgets to eat because of Alzheimer's disease is *not* covered.
- ✓ Permanent impairment, defined as at least 90 days.
- ✓ Tube feeding must be medically necessary to maintain weight and strength commensurate with overall condition; tube feeding must be the primary and essential source of nutrition (not supplemental).
- ✓ Additional documentation is required to justify the following components:
  - —An enteral pump (orders for this patient included feedings "via enteral pump")
  - —More than 35 kcal/kg/day (*note*: this patient's weight is subsequently given as 52.5 kg, so this prescription order calls for 43.8 to 45.7 kcal/kg/day)
  - —Less than 20 kcal/kg/day

d. *Create a drug-related problem list for this patient.*

- *Untreated indication.* Malnutrition, requiring supplementation.
- *Subtherapeutic dosage (potential).* Persistent abdominal and back pain, requiring continued attention to morphine and cyclobenzaprine dosing.
- *Over/underdosing (potential).* Patient is receiving warfarin with no INR value available.
- *Adverse drug reaction.* Constipation from morphine, requiring relief.
- *Drug interaction (potential).* Morphine plus cyclobenzaprine may have an additive effect on decreasing alertness.
- *Improper drug selection (potential).* Megestrol acetate therapy with apparent lack of response; may potentially contribute to DVT.
- *Overdosage.* Serum magnesium level slightly above normal in patient receiving magnesium oxide.
- *Adverse drug reaction.* Macrocytic anemia, possibly associated with 5-fluorouracil (a folate antagonist). There is also a risk of vitamin B_{12} deficiency with a near-total gastrectomy and reduced B_{12} absorption because of decreased gastric acidity from Pepcid (famotidine, an H_2-antagonist).
- It should also be noted that the patient has difficulty swallowing large tablets.

e. *What information indicates the presence or severity of malnutrition?*

- Weight loss of 21.5 kg (29%) over 6 months.
- Weight at about 70% of ideal (75.3 kg) and pre-surgery (74 kg) weights.
- Compromised visceral protein status (hypoalbuminemia).
- Dysphagia secondary to esophageal stricture.
- Poor tolerance to solids for 2 weeks.
- Decreased functional status as indicated by fatigue and weakness.
- Presence of a pressure ulcer on buttocks.
- Potential skin breakdown or infection at site of implanted venous access device and jejunostomy (redness around both areas).
- Recent infection (just completed 10 days of cephalexin).
- Peripheral edema.
- Subcutaneous fat loss: prominence of implanted venous access device.
- Decreased wound healing, skin breakdown, increased risk of infection, and decreased functional capacity are consequences of malnutrition.

f. *What type and degree of malnutrition does this patient exhibit? What evidence supports your assessment?*

- Severe protein-energy malnutrition or marasmic kwashiorkor. Energy malnutrition is indicated by severely depressed weight. Protein malnutrition is indicated by hypoalbuminemia and edema.

Desired Outcome

2. a. *What are the goals of nutrition support in this patient?*

- Repletion of visceral protein stores, manifested by transferrin or prealbumin in the mid-normal range within 2 weeks
- Weight gain of 0.5 to 2 pounds/week to a goal close to ideal weight
- Healing in areas of skin breakdown; prevention of further skin breakdown
- Improvement in functional status (decreased weakness and fatigue)
- Prevention of mechanical, infectious, and metabolic complications
- Avoidance of incompatibilities with feedings and medications
- Design of a feeding regimen that is appropriate for home care
- Documentation of the information required for insurance coverage

b. *What outcomes should be considered for the patient's other medical problems?*

- Correct constipation.
- Maintain appropriate anticoagulation with warfarin by dosage adjustments based on INRs.
- Provide therapy for macrocytic anemia if appropriate.
- Adjust medication doses for renal function. The patient's estimated CL_{cr} is about 50 mL/min. However, his true renal function is probably less because muscle mass (and therefore, creatinine) is decreased in a patient who is at 70% of his ideal weight.

Therapeutic Alternatives

3. a. *What are the potential alternatives for improving nutritional*

status in this patient other than initiating specialized nutrition support?

- *Esophageal dilation.* This procedure was ruled out due to risk of perforation.
- *Appetite stimulant.* Megestrol acetate apparently failed in this patient. The clinician should determine whether medication adherence is an issue and whether the dose is optimized for the severity of this patient's anorexia.
- *Diet modification.* Dietary education for anorexia was provided previously. A modified oral "dysphagia" diet or full liquid diet may be tried, but the friability of esophageal tissue may be considered at least a relative contraindication to foods due to the risk of perforation.

b. *What are the potential routes for specialized nutrition support and the reason(s) why each is or is not appropriate for this patient?*

- *Total parenteral nutrition (TPN).* A central line (implanted venous access device) is in place, but this route should be reserved for situations in which the GI tract cannot be used.
- *Peripheral parenteral nutrition (PPN).* This is indicated for short-term use only. It requires frequent IV access site changes, so it is rarely considered when a central line is in place. Also, serum triglycerides should remain in the range of 200 to 300 mg/dL with 45% to 60% of calories obtained from IV lipids; achieving this is highly unlikely when his baseline triglyceride level is 350 mg/dL. In addition, the significant reaction that the patient has to tofu means that an allergic reaction to soybean oil in IV lipids is a potential issue.
- *Tube feeding into the stomach or small bowel.* The GI tract is functional, except for a near-total gastrectomy and dysphagia due to an esophageal stricture. A surgically placed jejunostomy is present. Refer to Figure 129–2, Table 129–5, and the section "Enteral Access" in textbook Chapter 129 for more information on types of access for enteral tube feeding. Enteral nutrition is the route of choice unless motility or absorptive problems preclude adequate nutrition by this route or feeding tube placement is contraindicated.[1] The textbook chapter provides detailed information on the rationale for initiating enteral nutrition versus parenteral nutrition.

c. *A major economic issue is Medicare coverage for home enteral therapy. Based on the information now available to you, does this patient meet the necessary criteria?*

- Dysphagia due to esophageal stricture meets the requirement that a functional impairment of the GI tract exists.
- The impairment is expected to meet the test of permanence (> 90 days) because the Taxol plus 5-FU regimen and radiotherapy are not yet complete. Tissue friability is unlikely to allow esophageal dilation for several months.
- Weight loss has continued despite appetite stimulants and dietary counseling, supporting the medical necessity of enteral tube feeding.
- See question 4 below for a discussion of caloric requirements > 35 kcal/kg and the need for a feeding pump.

Optimal Plan

4. a. *Estimate the protein, calorie, and fluid requirements for this patient.*

- Protein requirements are about 1 g/kg/day in healthy elderly individuals but increase up to 1.5 to 2 g/kg/day during metabolic stress. This patient needs about 1.5 g protein/kg/day (range 1.4 to 1.6 g/kg/day or 73 to 84 g/day) considering the pressure ulcer, potential areas of skin breakdown or infection around the jejunostomy site and implanted venous access site, and the ongoing need for tissue repair associated with chemotherapy. Protein may be reduced if azotemia develops because of renal insufficiency.
- Caloric requirements for patients over 60 years of age can be estimated using the equation for calculating basal energy expenditure (BEE): BEE (kcal/day) = $8.8W + 1128H - 1071$, where W is actual weight in kg and H is height in meters. For this patient, BEE = 1425 kcal/day. The BEE $\times$ 1.2 to 1.5 meets caloric requirements for active healthy adults. This patient is not very active but has moderate metabolic stress; thus, BEE $\times$ 1.3 to 1.4 (1853 to 1995 kcal/day) is reasonable. Calories for a gradual weight gain of 0.5 to 2 pounds/week must also be added. For each pound of weight gain, an additional 3500 kcal must be added, or 500 kcal/day for a pound/week weight gain. Caloric needs are therefore about 2353 to 2495 kcal/day to achieve a weight gain of 1 pound/week.
- Maintenance fluid requirements are 30 to 35 mL/kg/day for elderly persons. Formulas with 1.0 to 1.2 kcal/mL provide about 82% to 85% free water.

b. *What type of formula (e.g., polymeric, monomeric) is most appropriate for this patient?*

- A polymeric formula can be used because a distal pancreatectomy does not usually alter digestive function. Pancreatic enzymes can be added to the medication regimen if necessary. Polymeric formulas are generally "ready-to-use."
- Monomeric (elemental) formulas often require reconstitution, which is inconvenient and may introduce contamination or mixing error, especially in the home setting. Monomeric formulas are also much more expensive and require documentation of need for Medicare. Textbook Table 129–8 and the sections of the Enteral Nutrition chapter on characteristics of enteral formulas and selecting an enteral formula provide more detailed information.
- A standard caloric density formula (1.0 to 1.2 kcal/mL) with 13% to 14% of calories as protein provides the desired ratio of calories and protein. Isocal, Isosource, and Resource are example products.
- It is best to use a lactose-free formula due to potential lactose intolerance, especially in an adult of non-Northern European descent. See textbook Table 129–8 for more details on formula characteristics.
- An isotonic formula may be better tolerated for jejunal feedings.
- Fiber may decrease constipation but also requires adequate fluid to avoid fecal impaction. Fibersource and Resource with Fiber are formulas with appropriate calories and protein for this patient.

c. What administration regimen should be used for tube feedings?

- Steady infusion at a controlled rate (e.g., via pump) is desired for jejunostomy feedings because no reservoir exists for a "bolus."
- Start with full-strength isotonic formula. Dilution of hypertonic formula to half-strength may be necessary because the jejunum has limited capacity to handle hypertonic loads.
- Initiate feedings as a steady infusion over 18 to 24 hours using an enteral pump. Let the patient help determine the infusion duration to give him some control over the process and to avoid conflicts with his schedule.
- Infuse the feeding at about 30 to 40 mL/hr initially. Advance by 25 to 35 mL/hr at set time intervals until the goal rate is achieved (about 95 mL/hr). Slow advancement (preferably every 2 to 3 days) for home patients at risk of metabolic complications allows time to respond to electrolyte and fluid issues before they become critical.
- The safety of initiating tube feedings in the home for this patient should be discussed with his physician. Fluid overload and electrolyte depletion associated with refeeding syndrome can be life-threatening problems in a severely malnourished patient such as this man.
- A 1.0 to 1.2 kcal/mL formula provides the patient with about 35 mL of free water/kg, which meets maintenance fluid requirements. Extra fluid "flushes" should not be needed to provide free water.

d. Assuming that the patient is to continue his current medications during tube feedings, how should each of these be administered?

- Medications are generally administered through the feeding tube using liquid dosage forms, finely crushed tablets, or contents from an opened capsule. When available, alternate dosage forms such as transdermal patches, topical pastes, ointments, and rectal suppositories may be convenient, cost-effective methods of medication administration. See textbook Tables 129–9, 129–10, and 129–11, and the Enteral Nutrition chapter sections on drug compatibility with enteral formulas and complications of concomitant drug administration for more complete information.
- Morphine sustained release tablets: change to immediate-release solution with more frequent dosing; administer the oral sustained release tablets as long-acting rectal suppositories; change to a fentanyl transdermal patch; or change to the much smaller sustained-release oxycodone tablets, which the patient may be able to swallow.
- Famotidine tablets: change to oral suspension (40 mg/5 mL).
- Megestrol acetate tablets: change to suspension (200 mg/5 mL) if this therapy is to continue, given the questionable response.
- Magnesium oxide: discontinue this therapy because of the high serum level. Reduced losses can now be expected since cisplatin has been replaced by 5-FU in the chemotherapy regimen.
- Warfarin sodium: there is no liquid dosage form. The compatibility of the injectable form with enteral formulas has not been tested. Subcutaneous heparin is an alternative if problems develop with swallowing or crushing the tablets.
- Docusate sodium capsules: change to a syrup that is combined with casanthranol (e.g., Peri-Colace has 10 mg/5 mL) since the patient appears to also need a stimulant laxative to counter the effects of morphine.
- Cyclobenzaprine: this drug is only available in film-coated tablets that are often difficult to crush thoroughly, thereby increasing the risk of tube blockage. There are no therapeutic alternatives in liquid dosage forms. Evaluate the continued need for the drug versus the ability to continue taking it orally.

Outcome Evaluation

5. *What clinical and laboratory parameters are necessary to evaluate the therapy for detection and/or prevention of adverse effects and to evaluate achievement of the desired response?*

- Refer to the textbook section "Complications and Monitoring of Enteral Nutrition" in the Enteral Nutrition chapter for general guidelines.
- Obtain serum potassium, magnesium, and phosphate levels before rate increases and within 48 hours of reaching the goal rate. These tests should also be obtained daily or every other day for 7 to 8 days initially, then 2 to 3 times/week until stable, due to the risk of refeeding syndrome.
- Obtain transferrin or prealbumin (transthyretin) levels weekly for 2 or 3 weeks to assess short-term response to the tube feeding.
- Observe for and ask the patient about GI tolerance (e.g., bloating, pain, diarrhea) daily for several days.
- Evaluate fluid status daily for 7 to 8 days due to the risk of refeeding syndrome. Assess changes in body weight and perform clinical assessment of hydration status (e.g., check for pulmonary and peripheral edema and changes in blood pressure) while a nurse is still seeing the patient for teaching about tube feedings or for laboratory venipunctures.

Patient Counseling

6. *What information should be provided to the patient or his caregiver to enhance compliance, ensure successful therapy, and minimize adverse effects of enteral nutrition therapy?*

- Include the caregiver in counseling, with a Spanish translator if needed.

Isocal (Example)

- Isocal is an enteral liquid formula that can be given into the feeding tube that the doctor placed in your abdomen during your surgery. Between 9 and 10 cans per day will meet your nutritional needs, but you will need to slowly work up to this amount.
- You will start with 3 cans of the formula daily for the first 2 to 3 days. The home care nurse or I will tell you when to increase the number of cans of formula per day.
- Some people have cramping or diarrhea when feedings start or the amount per day increases, and some patients feel very full. You could also feel weaker if certain elements in your blood decrease; that is why it is very important for a nurse to take blood several times during the first week or 2 of the feedings. Please contact the home care nurse, the doctor, or me if you are having any problem tolerating the feedings.

- Sometimes the feeding schedule or formula need to be changed. The nurse who comes to your home will teach you how to give the feedings and review use of the pump and supplies with you. The nurse will see you 2 or 3 times for teaching, or more often if it is necessary.
- I will send a folder home with you that contains phone numbers you may need and some information on the feeding set-up, pump, and supplies. There is also information on safe handling and storage of the formula. This is like a food, so you should keep opened cans covered and in the refrigerator; use opened cans within 24 hours. Fresh formula is added to the feeding container about every 4 to 6 hours during the day, or about every 8 to 9 hours for overnight feedings. The nurse will review this information with you. What questions do you have about the feeding procedure?
- I understand from your primary care physician that you are having problems swallowing some of your medications. I will be reviewing your medications with him so that you can take some of them through the feeding tube. To prevent clogging the feeding tube, it is very important to flush the tube with a small amount of water (10 mL) before and after each medication. You can use tap water for this. The amount of water for flushing is written on the therapy page in your folder and will be reviewed by the home nurse. The doctor or I will let you know which medications will change. Please remember to call if you have any questions or are having problems with the feedings.

References

1. ASPEN Board of Directors. Guidelines for the use of parenteral and enteral nutrition in adult and pediatric patients. JPEN 1993;17(suppl 4):1SA–52SA.

131 OBESITY

▶ **Stomach Staples and a Tummy Tuck?**
(Level II)

Dannielle C. O'Donnell, PharmD, BCPS

A 55-year-old woman weighing 80 kg and with a body mass index (BMI) of 30.5 kg/m^2 seeks surgical treatment for obesity after failing to lose weight on nonprescription anorexiants and water pills, fad diets, and "herbal fen-phen." Her obesity is complicated by dyslipidemia, hyperglycemia, osteoarthritis, depression, and a history of cholelithiasis. The goals of therapy are a modest 10% weight loss over several months, prevention of weight regain, and avoidance of drug-related adverse effects. Non-pharmacologic therapies include an appropriate food plan, exercise program, and behavior modification. Pharmacotherapeutic alternatives include noradrenergic agents (phentermine, diethylpropion, mazindol, benzphetamine), sibutramine, and orlistat. Initial outcome evaluations should include biweekly assessment of weight, waist and hip circumference, diet and exercise logs, and subjective improvement in clothing fit, energy level, and exercise ability. Improvements in the patient's other comorbid conditions may also be expected gradually after the goal weight has been achieved.

▶ Questions

Problem Identification

1. a. *Create a drug-related problem list for this patient.*

    - Obesity, inadequately treated with various diets, nonprescription drugs, and herbal therapies.
    - Osteoarthritis, inadequately treated with PRN acetaminophen.
    - Hyperlipidemia that may be suboptimally treated with the present simvastatin dose (goal LDL-C = 130 mg/dL if she has the two CAD risk factors of age $\geq$ 55 and diabetes mellitus); triglycerides > 200 mg/dL is possibly secondary to hyperglycemia.
    - Depression, currently untreated.
    - Post-menopausal not receiving ERT.
    - Possible type 2 diabetes (one fasting glucose measurement > 126 mg/dL; the test should be repeated on another day).
    - A chronic, stable problem not requiring intervention at this time is hypothyroidism, which is presently controlled on levothyroxine (TSH is within the normal range).

    b. *Calculate the patient's BMI and WHR and contrast with weight the clinical implications of these values on defining obesity and on stratifying mortality risk.*

    - BMI = Wt (kg)/Ht (m)^2
      = 80 kg/(1.62 m)^2
      = 80 kg/2.62 m^2
      = 30.5 kg/m^2
      WHR = 102 cm/112 cm = 0.91

    - Weight is not an accurate indicator of health, whereas the BMI is a more reliable indicator of obesity (peripheral body fat) in the general population that can be calculated without having to actually measure body fat. A BMI between 25 and 30 kg/m^2 is considered overweight (or "mild obesity"); a BMI between 30 to 40 kg/m^2 defines moderate obesity; and > 40 kg/m^2 is severe or morbid obesity. Overall, as body mass increases (primarily above 27 kg/m^2) there is an increase in morbidity and all causes of death.
    - The WHR is also valuable for determining central obesity, and waist girth alone may be adequate. A WHR > 0.9 in women and > 1.0 in men is also associated with greater morbidity and mortality.[1]

    c. *What information (signs, symptoms, laboratory values) indicates the presence or severity of obesity?*

    - *Signs.* BMI > 30 kg/m^2, WHR > 0.9, abdominal striae, lower extremity varicosities, history of gall bladder disease.

- *Symptoms.* Complaints of fatigue, osteoarthritis, depression, and previous weight loss attempts.
- *Laboratory values.* Hyperglycemia, abnormal lipid profile.

d. *Could any of the patient's problems have been caused by drug therapy?*

- No. Although systemic corticosteroids may promote weight gain or increase blood glucose or lipids, a single intra-articular steroid injection is unlikely to result in significant systemic steroid adverse effects. Also, this patient's obesity and hyperlipidemia predate the injection, and the length of time since the injection make even a temporal relationship improbable.

e. *What other medical conditions should be considered to exclude primary causes of her obesity?*

- Untreated or undertreated hypothyroidism
- Polycystic ovary syndrome
- Cushing's syndrome
- Hypothalamic injury or tumor

Desired Outcome

2. *What are the goals of pharmacotherapy for the patient's obesity?*

- The primary outcome is a modest 10% weight loss over several months and prevention/minimization of weight regain while minimizing drug-related adverse effects. The aim of weight reduction is to decrease morbidity, and as little as a 5% to 10% weight loss has been shown to produce clinically beneficial improvements in blood glucose, lipids, physical performance, and patient well-being. Although greater weight loss has been associated with even greater benefit, reasonable short-term goals should be set, and in general obesity medications approved in the United States need only demonstrate weight loss > 5% over placebo.[2,3]
- Secondary outcomes include improvement in obesity-related comorbidities of osteoarthritis (i.e., reduced pain, improved range of motion, physical performance, quality of life), hyperlipidemia (attain LDL-C < 130 mg/dL and triglycerides < 200 mg/dL), hyperglycemia (FBG < 120 mg/dL), and prevention of symptomatic cholelithiasis.[2]

Therapeutic Alternatives

3. a. *What non-drug therapies might be useful for this patient?*

- *Dietary evaluation.* A registered dietician should devise a food plan and review it with the patient. This should also include evaluation of a food diary that includes portion sizes, noting moods/behaviors during eating, food preferences, and shopping habits. Positive reinforcement of low-fat, low-cholesterol choices should be coupled with introduction of diabetic diet instruction, given her hyperglycemia and modest caloric reduction. A very low calorie diet (VLCD, 500 to 800 kcal/day) is probably not indicated at this point as every effort should be given to promoting a good life-long food plan, and the brief diet history provided gives a clear indication of room for significant improvement with less cost than a VLCD.
- *Exercise program.* Although limited by her osteoarthritis, she should be encouraged to find exercises that cause less stress on the knees. Some examples include a stationary bicycle or water aerobics. A regular exercise program is a strong predictor of successful weight maintenance and also has cardiovascular benefits. An exercise physiologist or trainer may be consulted if necessary.
- *Behavior modification/support group.* These techniques are very beneficial for addressing attitudes toward food, internal and external feeding cues, trigger avoidance, and stress minimization, as well as congratulating success and preventing weight regain. Support groups may include commercial programs, church groups, or patient groups.[1]
- *Surgery.* Gastroplasty or gastric bypass, although desired by the patient and proven successful in promoting significant weight loss, is indicated only in the severely obese (BMI > 40 kg/m^2 or BMI > 35 kg/m^2 with comorbidities) who have not responded to the non-drug therapies described above plus pharmacologic interventions.[1]

b. *What pharmacotherapeutic alternatives are available for this patient's obesity?*

- *Noradrenergic agents (phentermine, diethylpropion, mazindol, benzphetamine, phenylpropanolamine)* are anorexiants that primarily enhance norepinephrine (NE) transmission.[3,4] These compounds have been available for years, and some immediate-release preparations may be more economical than sustained-release products. However, the noradrenergic agents are more frequently associated with the development of tolerance to the anorectic effects and have an increased incidence of adverse reactions, including overstimulation, nervousness, restlessness, palpitations, and dry mouth. This class may also have a greater potential for physical and psychological dependence than sibutramine and orlistat. Phenylpropanolamine (PPA) is available over the counter, but because this patient has not had success with it previously, it is probably not the best choice at this time. The entire class of noradrenergic agents is comparable with respect to efficacy and adverse effects, with the exception of diethylpropion, which may be less likely to increase blood pressure. These agents are often associated with tolerance to the stimulating and appetite-suppressing effects within a few weeks at recommended dosages.
- *Sibutramine HCl monohydrate (Meridia)* inhibits central norepinephrine, serotonin, and possibly dopamine reuptake. It is recommended for obese patients with an initial BMI ≥ 30 kg/m^2 or ≥ 27 kg/m^2 in patients with other risk factors (e.g., hypertension, diabetes, dyslipidemia). It enhances weight loss as an adjunct to diet and exercise. Its lack of anticholinergic and potentially less frequent CNS effects may enable sibutramine to have a more favorable side-effect profile than older agents that primarily enhance NE transmission. In placebo-controlled studies, the most common adverse effects were headache, dry mouth, loss of appetite, insomnia, and constipation; patients did not discontinue therapy more often than did patients receiving placebo. Sibutramine has been associated with dose-dependent increases in blood pressure and pulse rate, but clinical studies did not find an increased incidence of heart valve abnormalities. The sibutramine dose is 10 mg po QD, given without regard to meals (usually in the morning). If there is inadequate weight loss (i.e., less than 4

pounds in the first 4 weeks), the dose may be increased to 15 mg QD. Tolerance (significant weight regain while on the drug) does not appear to develop, and patients may be maintained on the same dose for 1 year to aid in weight maintenance.
- *Orlistat (Xenical)* inhibits gastric and pancreatic lipases, decreasing the GI absorption of fat by approximately 30%. This provides additional caloric deficit for weight loss and control. In clinical studies, orlistat produced a mean weight loss of 4% more than placebo, and one-third of patients lost at least 10% of baseline weight. Its local action and association with negative reinforcement of dietary indiscretions (i.e., adverse effects of fecal urgency, fatty or oily stool, fecal incontinence) make this a theoretically attractive choice. In 2-year studies, GI adverse effects decreased significantly in the second year, which may be explained by increased dietary adherence. There is also decreased absorption of vitamins A, D, E, K, and beta carotene. The dose of orlistat is 120 mg po TID, given with main meals. However, since its duration of action is short, patients may choose not to take it prior to high-fat meals because of its predictable GI side effects. Although tolerance appears to develop to adverse effects, tolerance to weight loss and maintenance effects did not appear to develop in 2-year studies.

Optimal Plan

4. a. *What drug(s), dosage form(s), dose(s), schedule(s), and duration are appropriate to treat this patient's obesity and why?*

   - Orlistat 120 mg po TID with main meals, in combination with a diet having less than 30% of calories from fat, may be a preferred option for this patient because orlistat is not systemically absorbed and may enhance dietary compliance. In controlled clinical trials, orlistat has been shown to improve LDL-C levels, normalize oral glucose tolerance tests, and produce small reductions in HbA_{1c} and blood pressure, all of which may be potential benefits for this patient. Also, because her systolic blood pressure is in the "high-normal" range according to JNC-VI guidelines, an anti-obesity agent without the potential for increasing blood pressure may be preferable. Therapy may be continued for up to 2 years to prevent weight regain, which has been a problem for her.
   - Sibutramine 10 mg po QD without regard to meals is also a rational choice if orlistat is not tolerated and if the patient is not taking monoamine oxidase inhibitors (MAOIs) or selective serotonin reuptake inhibitors (SSRIs) for depression. These drugs should be stopped for at least 2 weeks before starting sibutramine. Although initial trials for depression did not prove efficacy, there may be some benefit for this patient, given her history of depression. If there is inadequate weight loss (< 4 lb.) after 4 weeks, the dose may be increased to 15 mg QD. Conversely, 5 mg may be used if she experiences significant adverse effects (i.e., a sustained, significant increase in blood pressure or heart rate, or insomnia). Therapy should generally be continued for at least 1 year to help minimize weight regain.
   - The noradrenergics, while acceptable, are perhaps second-line therapy due to the higher incidence of adverse effects and propensity for tolerance. These drugs are contraindicated if the patient is started on an MAOI. The sustained-release preparations of phentermine and diethylpropion may be preferred over immediate-release formulations to facilitate patient convenience and potentially decrease the occurrence of "peak-dose" adverse effects. Within this class, diethylpropion may have less frequent adverse effects on blood pressure, which may be an advantage in this patient.[4] Acceptable alternative regimens include:
     - ✓ Phentermine HCl 8 mg po TID 30 min AC (or 15 to 37.5 mg sustained-release po Q AM)
     - ✓ Diethylpropion HCl 25 mg po TID 1 hr AC and additional 25 mg PRN midevening (or 75 mg extended-release tablets QD in midmorning)
     - ✓ Mazindol 1 mg po TID 1 hr AC or 2 mg po QD 1 hr before lunch
     - ✓ Benzphetamine HCl 25 to 50 mg po QD in midmorning or midafternoon, increased as needed but not to exceed 50 mg TID

   PPA should probably be avoided, because she has tried this previously and was unsuccessful. Also, there may be enhanced compliance with lifestyle modifications and accountability with a prescription medication. If tolerance develops to the noradrenergic agents and weight gain occurs, the maximum dose should not be exceeded, and the medication should be discontinued.

   b. *What alternatives would be appropriate if initial therapy fails?*

   - In general, primary treatment failure should be evaluated after the first 4 weeks of treatment. This may be defined as those who failed to lose 0.45 kg (1 lb.)/week.[5] If this occurs with orlistat, there is no rationale to support an increased dose, so it should be discontinued and an alternate therapy selected. As stated above, the dose of sibutramine may be increased from 10 to 15 mg. There is no information to suggest that any second choice may be more effective than another. In general, it may be advisable to select an agent from a different class. However, patients with an inadequate response to one noradrenergic agent have demonstrated response to another noradrenergic agent.
   - Some experts have suggested that there may be utility in combination therapy (i.e., using agents from two different classes). While conceptually attractive, there are presently no published studies with currently available agents to support this practice.[5]
   - Some practitioners have advocated combining phentermine with low-dose fluoxetine ("phen-pro") or sertraline; interestingly, paroxetine does not seem to work. Some patients on these combos do receive enhanced results, but there is insufficient evidence that these combinations are safe.[6,7]
   - In the case of initial satisfactory weight loss but an early "plateau," VLCD in combination with continued exercise and behavior modification may be tried for at least 3 months to "jumpstart" weight loss. Although some practitioners use VLCD for an extended period to attain desired or ideal body weight, it is important to remember that significant improvement in morbidity and mortality may be attained with modest weight reduction.
   - Surgery should generally be reserved for the morbidly obese (i.e., BMI > 40 kg/m²) or those with a BMI > 35 kg/m² with comorbidities who are failing conventional therapy.[1]

Outcome Evaluation

5. *What clinical and laboratory parameters are necessary to evaluate the therapy for achievement of the desired therapeutic outcome and to detect or prevent adverse effects?*

Efficacy Parameters

- Initially, body weight should be assessed every 2 weeks using the same office scale. Waist and hip measurements should be taken at the same time.
- The patient should be asked about subjective improvements such as clothing fit, increased energy, and enhanced exercise ability. Diet and exercise logs should be reviewed at each visit.
- Over the longer term, as the goal weight reduction of 10% is attained (6 to 12 months), periodic visits (every 3 to 6 months) should assess for weight regain, decreased osteoarthritic symptoms, prevention of future gallbladder attacks, improvement in blood glucose (FBG < 120 mg/dL, HbA_{1c} < 7.0%), lipid profile (LDL-C < 130 mg/dL, triglycerides < 200 mg/dL), and improvement in depressive symptoms while providing continued encouragement.

Adverse Effect Parameters

- Blood pressure and heart rate should be measured at each clinic visit and the patient queried about symptoms of agitation, insomnia, palpitations, cough, and chest pain.
- An ECG or cardiac ultrasound may be warranted in patients taking noradrenergic agents or sibutramine who have symptoms of heart valve problems.

Patient Counseling

6. *What general and medication-specific information should be provided to the patient to enhance adherence, ensure successful therapy, and minimize adverse effects?*

General Information

- This medication (provide its name) is intended to help you lose weight, but it should be used only in conjunction with a food plan, regular exercise, and behavior modification.
- This will not produce dramatic results overnight; the goal of therapy is to lose approximately 10% of body weight over 6 to 12 months and then to maintain that weight loss over the long term. Modest but sustained weight loss can have definite health benefits, and it is important to set realistic expectations.
- It is not necessary or advisable to weigh yourself each day because these numbers tend to fluctuate. Rather, consider weighing yourself once weekly without clothes the first thing in the morning, after voiding, to monitor your progress. Be sure to take notice of your clothing fit over time as well as your actual weight loss.
- It will be helpful if you begin to view your life-long management of this condition as a long-term investment in your health, just like treatment of high blood pressure or cholesterol: through a combination of both lifestyle changes and medication.

Orlistat

- This medication will not suppress your appetite; it works by decreasing the amount of fat that is absorbed into your system after you eat. It is important to combine taking the medicine with a diet that has less than 30% of total calories from fat.
- Take this medication with each main meal; it is important to minimize snacking, because this medicine will not prevent fat absorption from food taken between the main meals.
- This medicine will probably cause some adverse stomach effects, such as the urge to have a bowel movement, oily stools, and rectal leakage. These effects appear to decrease with time, particularly with improved dietary adherence. You may want to use a sanitary napkin in the beginning as you learn how the drug affects you.
- Orlistat may decrease the absorption of some vitamins, so it may be advisable to take a daily multivitamin. Orlistat is generally a long-term treatment that can also help to prevent weight regain.

Sibutramine

- Take this medicine once daily; it can be taken without regard to meals. If you miss a dose, do not take double doses.
- Some common side effects include headache, dry mouth, insomnia, and constipation. Contact your doctor if these become troublesome or severe.
- Sibutramine may also increase blood pressure, which will be monitored at your return visits.
- Other similar medications for weight loss have been associated with increased blood pressure in the blood vessels of the lungs (primary pulmonary hypertension) and heart valve abnormalities. Although these effects have not been seen with sibutramine, notify your doctor if you develop chest pain or shortness of breath.
- Sibutramine is generally a long-term treatment that will also help maintain weight loss.

Noradrenergics (Phentermine, Diethylpropion, Mazindol, Benzphetamine)

- Take this medication only as directed by your doctor. Do not take it any less than 10 hours before bedtime, because this may produce insomnia.
- If you miss a dose, do not take double doses.
- Notify your doctor if you experience palpitations or episodes of a "racing heart," as well as agitation or insomnia.
- This is generally a long-term treatment with some potential dose increase over time in conjunction with your overall weight loss program.

▶ Follow-up Questions

1. *What changes, if any, should be made in her weight loss regimen?*

- No changes are necessary. She has surpassed her goals of 10% weight loss, LDL-C <130 mg/dL, and improvement in her blood glucose. She should now enter the maintenance phase, focusing on prevention of weight regain. Positive reinforcement and encouragement about goal attainment and appropriateness of goals is critical. This plateau is a common occurrence and should not be confused with tolerance.[5]
- Because she appears to be tolerating the regimen well, she should not discontinue the medication; long-term use appears to prevent weight regain. A revisit with the dietitian may be worthwhile to ensure dietary compliance. If a "jump-start" is desired, this may be effected by modest additional caloric restriction or increase in physical activity. A more aggressive jump-start such as changes in drug ther-

apy or severe dietary restriction are not warranted at this early point in chronic disease management, particularly since progress is still evident.

2. *What, if anything, would you suggest to improve her knee symptoms?*

- Reassure her that acetaminophen is first-line therapy for osteoarthritis and that it may be less irritating to her stomach than other therapies. She should begin to take this on a regular schedule of up to 1000 mg (2 tablets) 4 times a day to better control her symptoms. This change, along with continued exercise and maintenance of a lower weight, will help to decrease arthritic symptoms.

References

1. Rosenbaum M, Leibel RL, Hirsch J. Obesity. N Engl J Med 1997;337:396–407.
2. Pi-Sunyer, FX. A review of long-term studies evaluating the efficacy of weight loss in ameliorating disorders associated with obesity. Clin Ther 1996;18:1006–1035.
3. Popovich NG, Wood OB. Drug therapy for obesity: An update. J Am Pharm Assoc 1997;NS37:31–39, 56.
4. Weiser M, Frishman WH, Michaelson MD, et al. The pharmacologic approach to the treatment of obesity. J Clin Pharmacol 1997;37:453–473.
5. Long-term pharmacotherapy in the management of obesity. National Task Force on the Prevention and Treatment of Obesity. JAMA 1996;276:1907–1915.
6. Anchors JM. Safer than Phen-fen. Rocklin, CA, Prima Publishing, 1997.
7. Bostwick JM, Brown TM. A toxic reaction from combining fluoxetine and phentermine. J Clin Psychopharmacol 1996;168:189–190. Letter.

61